In 2008 Shelf-Life Goes Away

During the first quarter of 2008, the ASCP will begin to extend the real-time value of this and other *ASCP Quick Compendia* with an online update service. Each purchased text in the series entitles you to access (for a 3-year period from date of publication) to a number of features that extend the life and utility of your book:

- updates and postings from the authors to alert you to the working edge of change
- forums connecting you to colleagues and authors
- e-mailing of selected passages to colleagues
- e-notes and bookmarking that will remain attached to your online text service
- full-text search capacity

You need never worry again that the book you buy today will outdate between editions.

The original purchaser of this text is entitled to register for the new ASCP online update service for this text. Watch for an announcement on **www.ascp.org** for the *ASCP Quick Compendia Online* in the first quarter of 2008, then use the unique, one-time-use, registration number printed herein.

5664a05229

ASCP
QUICK COMPENDIUM
OF
SURGICAL PATHOLOGY

Dedication

Gerald D. Abrams, MD

Mentor

Role Model

Colleague

Friend

ASCP

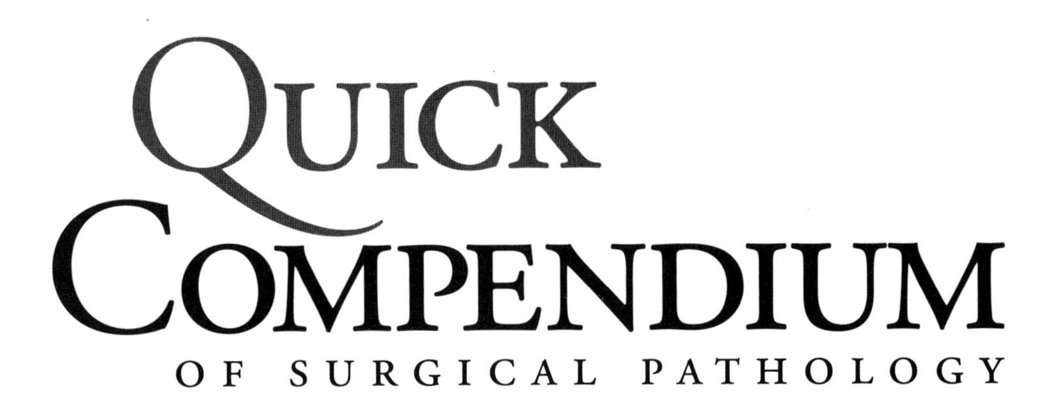

Stephen Ramsburgh, MD

Attending Pathologist
University of Michigan Medical Center
Ann Arbor

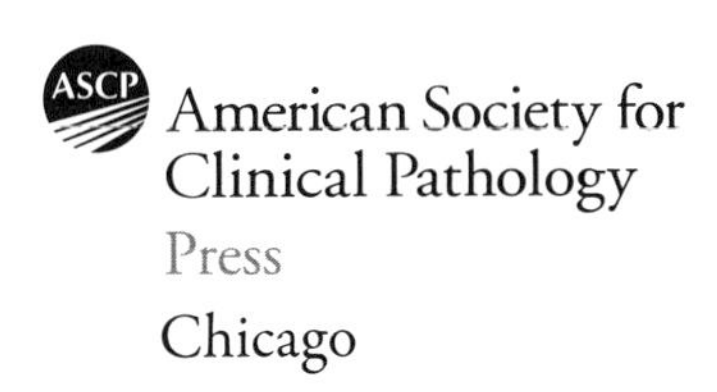

American Society for
Clinical Pathology
Press
Chicago

Publishing Team
Ted Moon and Erik Tanck (design)
Erik Tanck (production)
Joshua Weikersheimer (publishing direction)

Notice
Trade names for equipment and supplies described herein are included as suggestions only. In no way does their inclusion constitute an endorsement or preference by the American Society for Clinical Pathology. The ASCP did not test the equipment, supplies, or procedures and therefore urges all readers to read and follow all manufacturers' instructions and package insert warnings concerning the proper and safe use of products.

12 11 10 09 08 5 4 3 2 1

Printed in the United States of America

Acknowledgments

I am greatly indebted to the faculty, both past and present, of the Department of Pathology of the University of Michigan who used their skill, patience, and compassion to teach me Anatomic Pathology. They are wonderful teachers and incredibly skilled diagnostic pathologists. Their commitment to teaching and enthusiasm for surgical pathology has been, and continues to be, an inspiration to me.

The residents with whom I have worked provided the inspiration for this work; they have taught me far more than I them. They are my friends as well as colleagues, and my relationship with them is the highlight of my professional life.

I am especially grateful to Dr. Gerald Abrams and Dr. Jeffrey Warren for their counsel and support over the time this book has evolved.

Finally, I express special thanks to Dr. Meryem Koker, Dr. Guangming Guo, Dr. Kristen Curlett, Dr. Malti Kshirsagar, Dr. Cohra Mankey, Dr. Matthew, Dr. Christopher Przybcin, and Jason Carvalho my tireless proof-readers and editors. Mrs. Dianna Banka and Ms. Peggy Otto typed the original manuscript and several subsequent editions; their skill and unfailing patience and good humor made the whole endeavor a pleasure.

Joshua Weikersheimer is the only editor of medical textbooks who both understood the premise of the project and had the wherewithal to carry it through. Without his insight and advice this work would still be nothing more than a collection of notes on my shelf.

— S. Ramsburgh, MD

Preface

Readers of this text should understand that it does not represent a compendium of unique, original material. What I have tried to do is assemble in 1 easy-to-use book, the diagnostically relevant information pertaining to many diagnostic entities...information gleaned from diverse sources, most of which are considered "gold standard" books in the field. All of the references used in a given chapter are cited at the end of the chapter. Specific footnotes have not been used in the text, given that each section represents an amalgam of material prepared in conjunction with use of sources listed at the end of the chapter.

Many times I encountered major differences of opinion from one author or editor to another. Some of these differences were on opposite ends of a spectrum. I did my best to resolve as many of these as possible, but often went with the majority opinion. Most of these issues involve differential diagnosis, immunohistochemical stains, or molecular alterations. No text of this type can possibly cover all aspects of all diagnoses, so at times I simply had to stop. Any errors of omission or commission are entirely my responsibility and reflect my own decisions.

I have reviewed the role of both the pathologist and the surgeon concerning both the intraoperative consultation (the frozen section or frozen section diagnosis) and the handling of specimens. Understanding and communication on the part of both surgeon and pathologist is often essential to insure diagnostic accuracy of both frozen and permanent sections. Much of this is a reflection of my observations as both a surgeon and surgical pathologist. I also found *Intraoperative Consultations in Surgical Pathology*, published by the California Society of Pathologists in 1996 under the editorship of Mahendra Ranchod, MB, ChB to be an invaluable resource.

I sincerely hope this text be a helpful reference for those training in anatomic pathology, especially as they prepare for their "Boards." In addition I would like the text to be of use at pathology sign-out, when questions concerning microscopic variants, immunohistochemical stains, molecular alterations, and possible associated conditions come up between faculty and residents. Finally, the book will hopefully serve as a resource for all physicians who come in contact with pathologic specimens and surgical pathology reports. In particular, surgeons in every subspeciality may find this text useful, not only in terms of interpreting the microscopic description provided in most pathology reports, but also as a rapid source of information concerning diagnoses that may be out of his or her realm of expertise.

This is a surgical pathology text without photomicrographs; most unusual to say the least. This is not an atlas to be pulled from the shelf to match slides to images but rather a resource to be used when the diagnosis is either fairly certain or limited to 2 or 3 pathologic entities and additional clinicopathologic information is desired.

— S. Ramsburgh, MD

Table of

Contents

Foreword

Where Worlds Collide: Surgery and Pathology

Chapter 1

Cardiovascular System

Chapter 2

Central Nervous System

Chapter 3

Endocrine

Chapter 4

Breast

Chapter 7
Gastrointestinal Tract

Chapter 8
Liver, Gallbladder, and Extrahepatic Bile Ducts

Chapter 11
Lung

Chapter 12
Pleura and Peritoneum

Chapter 13
Mediastinum

Chapter 14
Lymph Nodes

Chapter 15

Male Reproductive System

Chapter 16

Urinary Tract

Chapter 17

Mandible and Maxilla

Chapter 18
Salivary Glands

Chapter 19
Bones and Joints

Chapter 20
Soft Tissue

Appendix
Syndromes

Index

Foreword

Where Worlds Collide: Surgery and Pathology

The Surgeon and Pathologist

The advanced technology that is so rapidly changing the face of medicine has resulted in an obvious improvement in the quality of care available to patients in every medical discipline. These technological advances, however, have a drawback; the accompanying explosion of knowledge has reached the point that most specialties, even those that work closely together, have become more and more isolated intellectually. Many physicians today not only lack a detailed knowledge of related fields but also an understanding of what their colleagues in those fields can and cannot do. 150 years ago the fields of surgery and pathology were essentially one specialty. Today, there is often limited communication between the two on issues germane to both. As areas of surgical expertise have become more and more specialized, only the pathologist with a particular subspeciality interest has a real understanding of the issues the surgeon faces in a given surgical field. Likewise, as new technologies have come to the aid of pathologists, their diagnostic reports now contain important information not always understood by clinical colleagues.

Interdisciplinary conferences are now common in most academic as well as private institutions and have gone a long way to broadening the knowledge base of both surgeons and pathologists. Unfortunately, many of the most pressing issues facing the pathologist and surgeon, such as intra-operative consultations (frozen section requests), specimen handling, and the wording of diagnostic reports, are still not completely understood by either party. These problems are often compounded by a lack of bilateral communication. Many surgeons no longer routinely discuss with their pathology colleagues the anticipated operative findings, actual intra-operative findings or the concerns the surgeon may have, not only about the diagnosis, but about the adequacy of surgical excision. In a similar vein, because the pathologist does not always understand the surgeon's concerns, he or she may fail to communicate effectively with the surgeon.

In my experience, it is the rare pathologist who does not enjoy the experience of reviewing the pathology of a case with the operating surgeon. This interaction gives the pathologist the opportunity to discuss the nuances of the case in terms of the differential diagnosis and the possible variants of a given diagnosis. It also gives the pathologist the opportunity to explain the meaning of any words in the diagnostic report that may be confusing to the surgeon. There are many areas in pathology that are somewhat "grey," even to pathologists. Words such as "atypia," "dysplastic," "carcinoma-in-situ," "reactive change," "changes indicative of prior injury" can be confusing to a surgeon, especially in terms of their clinical implications. A joint review forces the pathologist to explain to the surgeon his or her criteria for calling a lesion dysplastic and the implications of that diagnosis in terms of patient management. The surgeon, in turn, will begin to appreciate the distinctions between high-grade and low-grade dysplasia, the difficulty of recognizing a focus of microinvasion in what otherwise appears to be a carcinoma in situ, and the difficulties inherent in calling changes dysplastic rather than reactive. Making these types of pathologic diagnoses with precision requires a great deal of training and years of experience; indeed, the pathologist often makes these types of diagnoses only after consultation with other pathologists. It seems obvious when both surgeon and pathologist are making decisions that affect patient care, that at some point the two should get together and discuss the pathological and clinical implications of their actions as they relate to each other. Sitting over the microscope with a pathologist, even for a brief period of time with a single case, can often give the surgeon an appreciation for the pathologist's concerns about a particular diagnosis. This exchange of information, in and of itself, can markedly expand the surgeon's sense of the adequacy of his or her procedure and the need for follow-up.

The Intraoperative Consultation

From the pathologist's perspective there are several valid indications for an intra-operative frozen section diagnosis:

1. ***When the surgeon needs a diagnosis that will determine immediate surgical management.*** This situation arises most frequently during intra-abdominal or intrathoracic procedures when it has not been possible to obtain a diagnosis prior to the laparotomy or thoracotomy. Examples include abdominal explorations for suspected malignancy, such as an ovarian mass or obstructive biliary lesion. A diagnosis of "positive for carcinoma" may lead to a staging proce-

dure in the former and possibly a pancreaticoduodenectomy in the latter.

2. ***When the surgeon needs to know that diagnostic material has been obtained.*** The purpose of this frozen section is not to establish a definitive diagnosis intra-operatively, but rather to ensure that the tissue sample is adequate for eventual diagnosis on permanent section. This situation most frequently arises when a surgeon is attempting to obtain tissue from a site accessible only with difficulty or when tissue is being obtained from a patient who is under general anesthesia. The surgeon must realize that the presence of lesional tissue on a frozen section does not necessarily mean that there is enough tissue for a definitive final diagnosis. This problem may arise in biopsies of large lesions, many of which have a variety of histologic patterns, such as areas of dedifferentiation that can only be accurately assessed after multiple sections from multiple locations have been examined.

3. ***When the surgeon needs information to facilitate a decision as to the scope of a procedure.*** Typical examples include biopsies of liver nodules or mesenteric lymph nodes in cases of suspected metastatic carcinoma. The rendering of a diagnosis, "positive for carcinoma" in this instance will often result in the surgeon abandoning a proposed procedure; while a diagnosis, "negative for carcinoma," may lead the surgeon toward a resection.

4. ***When the surgeon needs to determine the adequacy of resection.*** The surgeon's best chance of obtaining a complete excision is typically at the time of initial surgery. The ideal way to determine the status of surgical margins is for the surgeon to bring the specimen to pathology and discuss the anatomy with a pathologist. If frozen sections are deemed necessary to determine the adequacy of the surgical margins, the appropriate sections can then be taken by the pathologist in conjunction with the operating surgeon. This insures that the operating surgeon knows exactly where the sections were taken that might prove to be positive. Difficulty arises, however, if the neoplasm is not readily visible. The boundaries of well-differentiated soft tissue tumors are notorious for being hard to see within a soft tissue specimen. The risk of a sampling error that can lead to a report of a negative surgical margin, only to be followed by a permanent section report indicating the margin is positive, represents a major error and may have significant consequences for the patient, namely that he or she will likely face a second procedure. The risk of this type of error can be dramatically reduced if the surgeon and pathologist work together to examine the fresh specimen and jointly determine where the most appropriate frozen sections should be taken. Even under the best of circumstances, sampling errors occur; if the surgeon is aware of the types of specimens that generate these types of errors, he or she can modify the operative procedure accordingly.

5. Finally, ***when the presence of lesional tissue must be confirmed.*** Confirmation of lesional tissue is crucial prior to submitting tissue for additional studies (eg, culture, flow cytometry, immunoperoxidase stains on frozen tissue, electron microscopy, gene rearrangement studies or research).

It is important for the pathologist in the rendering of a frozen section report to have some understanding of the actual conduct of the surgical procedure. A case in point is the request for a frozen section of a bronchial margin on a lobectomy or pneumonectomy for malignancy. Another example is a request for a frozen section of pancreatic and biliary margins on a pancreaticoduodenectomy. If the entire specimen is received in pathology with an accompanying frozen section request concerning margins, the pathologist should appreciate that for all practical purposes the surgeon is now in the final phases of the procedure. In the case of the lobectomy or pneumonectomy, the surgeon may well be ready to close the chest. In the case of the pancreaticoduodenectomy, the surgeon has begun the anastomoses to reestablish intestinal continuity. In such cases the pathologist should move immediately to render the frozen section report. This may well mean moving a case to the "front of the line." The surgeon who learns that the bile duct margin is positive on a pancreaticoduodenectomy after the choledochojejunostomy has been performed is now in a position of having to take down the anastomosis, resubmit a new bile duct margin and re-perform the anastomosis, all of which are time consuming, technically challenging, and usually avoidable. By the same token, the thoracic surgeon who has removed a lung may well have to delay closure of the chest if the frozen section on the bronchial margin takes more than 15 to 20 minutes.

Intraoperative Consultation

To the pathologist, certain frozen sections are considered unnecessary or inappropriate. Occasionally a surgeon will submit a frozen section in "the name of patient care." The intra-operative frozen section diagnosis supposedly enables the surgeon to relieve the patient's anxiety or to communicate more effectively with the patient or the patient's family immediately after surgery. This preliminary diagnosis does not, however, truly serve patient care, and in addition, may differ from the final diagnosis. Most patients understand, if they are told, that some time is required to process and examine tissue adequately. It is the rare patient indeed who will balk at waiting 24 to 36 hours for a pathology report that is complete and carries a very small chance (generally thought to be <1%) of being either falsely positive or falsely negative. Frozen section reports may not carry the same degree of accuracy.

Frozen sections are also occasionally submitted because the surgeon is curious about an incidental, intra-operative finding that has no bearing on the course of the procedure or the patient's welfare. This represents the single "most inappropriate" request for a frozen section diagnosis.

Sometimes the rendering of a frozen section can actually compromise the accuracy of the final diagnosis. If limited tissue is available and all or most of it is frozen, the inevitable freezing artifacts in the permanent sections may compromise the final diagnosis. Typical examples involve skin biopsies for melanoma and breast biopsies (especially biopsies done under mammographic direction in which there is no grossly discernible lesion). These types of specimens require complete fixation, careful sectioning, and total submission so that all of the material can be examined under the microscope. Frozen section diagnosis in these settings is associated with unacceptably high false-negative and false-positive rates, and the final, permanent sections may be suboptimal.

The most vexing clinical situation in which a surgeon and pathologist can find themselves is the situation in which a definitive diagnosis cannot be made on frozen section and yet the diagnosis will have a major and immediate effect on the intra-operative management of the patient. A diagnosis, "positive for carcinoma," if incorrect, may lead to an unnecessary major resection or may stop a resection that is indicated. On the other hand, a diagnosis of, "negative for carcinoma," if incorrect, may lead to a futile resection or leave the patient with at least the need for a second procedure. The pathologist feels this dilemma acutely. For their part, surgeons must accept the fact that a frozen section cannot always provide a definitive diagnosis. Consequently, they must be prepared, on occasion, to make intra-operative decisions based largely on gross operative findings and clinical circumstances. When these situations arise, it is of paramount importance that the surgeon and pathologist communicate with each other as openly and honestly as possible. It is never inappropriate for the pathologist to visit the operating room to discuss the problems concerning the frozen section with the surgeon, or for the surgeon, if possible, to leave the operating room and discuss the frozen section findings over the microscope with the pathologist. The pathologist will almost always recommend the least extensive surgical procedure when the frozen section diagnosis is in doubt. The type of consultation outlined above will increase the likelihood that the best course of action will be chosen.

From the surgeon's perspective, the rendering of a frozen section diagnosis from an appropriate request for frozen section diagnosis always seems to take an eternity. 15 to 20 minutes is the usual amount of time it actually takes a pathologist to render a frozen section diagnosis. The surgeon should also keep in mind that frozen sections occasionally arrive in the pathology suite in bunches and there may be some delay in processing as the cryostats are cleared of cases that were received earlier. In addition, a pathologist will frequently consult with a colleague or may request that deeper sections be cut to further evaluate the lesion. These efforts and occasional technical problems may delay the rendering of a frozen section report beyond the usual time. When these delays are imminent it behooves the pathologist to communicate with the surgeon who is anxiously waiting for the results. Communication between the pathologist and surgeon concerning the status of the frozen section, especially if the diagnosis will be delayed, is as important as it is considerate and is an essential part of the pathologist-surgeon relationship.

The appearance of the surgeon in the pathology suite in an effort to "speed up" the performance of the frozen section only adds more stress to an already stressful endeavor. On the other hand, the presence of the surgeon to assist the pathologist in obtaining, with maximum efficiency, the samples absolutely necessary for frozen section examination (such as a particularly close surgical margin) is always appreciated. In addition, pathologists with few exceptions, always welcome the opportunity to examine tissue with the operating surgeon so that a more in-depth analysis of the diagnostic possibilities can be discussed beyond a simple positive or negative for neoplasm. This type of interchange over the microscope can be of benefit to the surgeon in cases where the diagnosis may be in doubt and can help the pathologist understand how the surgeon will proceed based upon the diagnosis rendered.

Most surgeons understand that occasionally a pathologist will confirm that diagnostic tissue is present but will defer a definitive diagnosis until permanent sections are available for examination. Most institutions report a deferral rate of approximately 5%. Most deferrals involve a few particular kinds of specimens. One example of such a problem lesion is the follicular thyroid nodule. Distinguishing a follicular adenoma from a follicular carcinoma from a follicular variant of a papillary carcinoma from a nodule of thyroid hyperplasia is extremely difficult on frozen section. In this instance, the report will simply read, "Follicular lesion, defer to permanents." Another specimen that commonly results in deferral is the lymph node suspected of containing lymphoma. Most institutions do not attempt to make a definitive diagnosis on frozen sections of a lymph node in which there is a possibility of lymphoma. These reports typically read, "Lymphoid tissue present, lymphoma work-up pending."

Occasionally, the diagnosis rendered on a frozen section will not be confirmed when the permanent sections are examined. The discordance rate between frozen section and final diagnosis should be less than 2%. Most reported errors are false-negative diagnoses (a false-negative diagnosis is one in which the frozen section is reported as negative but permanent sections reveal the lesion to be malignant). While this could be the result of an interpretative error, most commonly it is an artifact of sampling. A sampling error occurs when the frozen section is indeed negative but deeper cuts into the specimen (done to create permanent sections) reveal the presence of a neoplasm. False-positive diagnoses (lesions misinterpreted as malignant that are actually benign) are rare. More often a misdiagnosis is the result of incorrect sampling of the specimen, the plane of section of the frozen section, or limitations imposed by the nature of the specimen itself (for example, specimens that are primarily fat, bone or mucoid).

The final consideration for the surgeon in terms of his or her relationship with the pathology department is the importance of providing an accurate clinical history. There is no doubt that the more pertinent clinical history that is provided, the greater the likelihood that the pathologist will not only render an appropriate and accurate frozen section diagnosis but will render an appropriate and accurate permanent section diagnosis. Surgeons need to discard the notion that "too much clinical history" prejudices the pathologist. Such a concept is contrary to the aim of open and honest communication between surgeon and pathologist.

The Resected Surgical Specimen

When appropriate, the processing, sectioning and examination of individual specimens will be discussed in the introduction to each of the following chapters. There are, however, some general considerations that are important to both pathologists and surgeons.

Pathology departments generally have some form of cutting manual that is used as a guideline for processing surgical specimens. These manuals often provide protocols as to how a specimen should be oriented and, more importantly, how it should optimally be sectioned to demonstrate the disease that is present. It is not always necessary for a surgeon to understand the actual intricacies of specimen processing and sectioning, but there are times where the surgeon's input into the sectioning of a specimen and the subsequent understanding that can be gained is of benefit to both parties.

As mentioned under the topic of the frozen section, surgical margins are of paramount importance to both the pathologist and surgeon. Some surgical margins are very straightforward and essentially never present a problem. Classic examples are the resection margins of colon cancer or a bronchial margin of a lobectomy or pneumonectomy for malignancy. Other specimens, however, can cause very real problems to the pathologist in terms of determining the adequacy of a surgical margin. Typically, for instance, the surgical margins of

Resected Surgical Specimen

a specimen containing a soft tissue tumor are inked. Different colors of ink are used for each margin and are recorded in the gross description. The pitfall of this approach, however, is that a large resection specimen will have large margins. If, for instance, the entire lateral margin of a large specimen is inked one color and tumor is seen microscopically at that margin, the issue immediately becomes exactly where along that margin is it positive. In addition, where does the lateral margin become the superior margin, the superior margin become the posterior margin, etc? As mentioned earlier, this problem can be minimized if the surgeon is in attendance when the section is taken. The surgeon can help the pathologist orient the specimen and can point out the areas where the margins are most likely to be closest to the tumor. Margins submitted and labeled under the direction of the surgeon contribute to a more concise and meaningful final report. Other specimens are simply difficult to orient. What may seem to be a very straightforward pancreaticoduodenectomy specimen to the surgeon can be a very complicated and difficult specimen for the pathologist receiving it in a bucket with landmarks distorted. The surgeon who identifies and labels important structures with marking sutures or who spends a few moments with the pathologist to assist in identifying the bile duct margin, the pancreatic margin, and the presence of worrisome peripancreatic lymph nodes, can be of tremendous assistance and can assure that all of the important information will be provided in the final report.

If a surgical margin is violated, either accidentally or intentionally, prior to its arrival in the pathology department, the ability of the pathologist to assess the margins of the specimen is significantly compromised. Intraoperative disruption of a surgical margin may be unavoidable on occasion, but sharing that information with the pathologist who will process the specimen and pointing out the areas that have been violated will help the pathologist ink and orient the specimen so that appropriate sections can be submitted. Obviously, when tissue needs to be harvested for research purposes or if the surgeon desires to see the gross morphology of the excised lesion, this is best done in the pathology suite under the direction of the pathologist. It is easy to appreciate the frustration felt by the pathologist when a surgical specimen resected for neoplasm is received piecemeal, ruptured, partially "harvested" or extensively cauterized, considering that the most important pathologic feature next to the diagnosis is the adequacy of the surgical margins.

The surgeon who has some knowledge of pathology and understands the issues faced by a pathologist in determining a diagnosis, be it on frozen section or permanent section, will be a better surgeon. The converse is also true. The pathologist who understands the issues faced by the surgeon, in terms of preoperative management, the conduct of the procedure and the postoperative management, will be a better pathologist. The road to this mutual understanding is based on open communication and an appreciation for the needs of each.

Chapter 1

Cardiovascular System

board lectures
- Cardiac tumors
- Cardiac path
- Hypersensitivity.

Cardiac Tumors

Cardiac Myxoma

Clinical Manifestations

- Occurs almost exclusively on endocardial surface and typically in left atrium near the fossa ovalis
- Represents 50% of all primary cardiac tumors
- More frequent in women than men
- 90% of patients diagnosed between ages of 30 and 60 years with an average age at presentation of 50 years; rare in children
- Constitutional symptoms include fever, malaise, and weight loss; regardless of the location of the neoplasm, most patients develop anemia and hypergammaglobulinemia during the course of their disease
- Obstruction of the mitral valve results in a clinical picture similar to that of chronic rheumatic mitral valve disease
- Embolic sequelae include ischemia of extremities, viscera, or brain (embolus may represent part of the tumor itself or a thrombus on the tumor)
- Left atrial lesions more commonly present with embolic events (35%) and less commonly with symptoms of mitral stenosis (20%)
- Right atrial lesions less frequently symptomatic; symptoms include syncope, ankle edema, Budd-Chiari syndrome (20%), and pulmonary embolus (15%)
- Lesions that have embolized have the capacity to grow into the arterial wall at the embolic site
- 95% sporadic; remainder have a familial history of both atrial tumors and extracardiac lesions (*Carney syndrome*)
- Familial lesions more frequently multiple, recurrent, and right-sided than sporadic lesions
- Mean age at presentation of patients with familial disease approximately 25 years

Gross Pathology

- 73% occur in the left atrium, 20% in the right atrium, 2% are biatrial, and 2% occur in the left and right ventricles; 3% occur in >1 cardiac chamber
- Tumors typically attached to endocardium by either a broad-base or a narrow pedicle

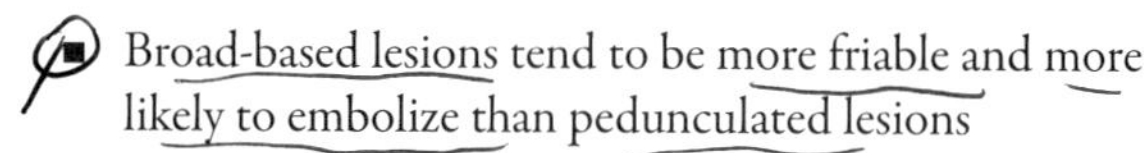

- Broad-based lesions tend to be more friable and more likely to embolize than pedunculated lesions
- Lesions vary from a gelatinous mass with frondlike excrescences to lesions with a smooth firm surface
- Organized thrombi frequently present on surface
- On sectioning, neoplasms have a variegated appearance and may contain areas of calcification and cysts

Microscopic Pathology

- Myxoma cells have abundant eosinophilic cytoplasm, indistinct cell borders, and an oval nucleus with an irregular nuclear membrane, dense chromatin, and an inconspicuous nucleolus
- Many myxoma cells multinucleated
- Myxoma cells typically distributed singly or as complex structures in a myxoid background; most characteristic arrangement that of a ring consisting of 1 or several cell layers surrounding a blood vessel and infiltrated by mononuclear inflammatory cells; in a less common architectural pattern, the myxoma cells form branching cords or tufts that may be quite cellular (often located near the surface of the tumor)
- Rare mitotic figures may be present (particularly near the surface)
- Myxoid matrix rich in proteoglycans and may contain areas of fibrosis, thrombosis, and calcification
- Hemosiderin-laden macrophages almost always present
- Degenerative changes to include ossification (may include bone marrow) and Gamna-Gandy bodies (identical to those seen in the spleen as a result of hemosiderin and calcium deposition in patients with sickle cell disease) may be prominent
- Mononuclear inflammatory infiltrates (aggregates or diffuse) present within myxoid stroma
- Interface between the tumor and intra-atrial septum characterized by presence of lymphoid aggregates with or without germinal centers, bundles of smooth muscle, occasional granulomas, and prominent thick-walled blood vessels
- Foci of extramedullary hematopoiesis present in 5% to 10% (a rare finding in adults)
- Glandular structures lined by mucin-containing cells that resemble goblet cells of the gastrointestinal tract may be present (approximately 1%)
- Embolic fragments have an identical histologic appearance to the parent lesion

Cardiac Tumors>Cardiac Myxoma

Special Stains

- Mucin-containing cells within glandular structures of a myxoma are periodic acid-Schiff (PAS) positive and diastase resistant

Immunohistochemistry

- Myxoma cells typically positive for CD31 and CD34; 80% positive for vimentin and 20% positive for cytokeratin. Cells stain variably for endothelial markers (factor VIII) and *Ulex Europaeus*, muscle markers (desmin and smooth muscle actin), and neural markers (neuron-specific enolase, S-100 protein, and synaptophysin)
- Myxoma cells positive for nonspecific histiocytic markers (lysozyme, α_1-antichymotrypsin, and α_1-antitrypsin), but negative for specific histiocytic marker CD68 (Kp-1)

Electron Microscopy

- Tumor cells are mesenchymal with variable numbers of intermediate filaments
- Cells typically have primitive tight intercellular junctions but lack desmosomes
- Rare tumors that contain mucin-forming glands have true desmosomes, villi, and glandlike structures

Molecular Alterations

- Patients with myxoma syndrome probably have an autosomal dominant transmission

Differential Diagnosis

- Extensively myxoid sarcomas (myxoid fibrosarcoma, myxoid chondrosarcoma, myxoid malignant fibrous histiocytoma)
- Papillary fibroelastoma
- Mural thrombus
- Myxoma embolus may be difficult to differentiate from an organizing thrombus that elaborates myxoid ground substance from proliferating mesenchymal cells
- Embolic sarcoma may resemble embolic myxoma

Treatment

- Simple surgical excision (a biatrial approach with full-thickness excision of the septum and repair of the resulting septal defect)
- Mitral valve involvement may require replacement or repair

Prognosis

- Surgical mortality <1%
- Recurrence approximately 2% and seen almost exclusively in patients with familial disease

Associations

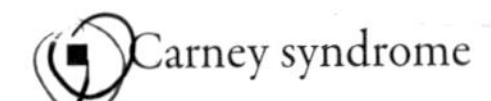

- Carney syndrome
  - □ Autosomal dominant mutation of *PRKAR1A*, type 1x-regulatory subunit of a protein kinase that acts on a tumor suppressor gene on chromosome 17q22-24 in 50%
  - □ Remainder have abnormalities at locus 2p16
  - □ More frequent in whites than blacks
- *Myxomas*
  - □ Cardiac
    - Present in 65%
    - May be multiple
    - Most serious component of disorder
    - Causes death in 20% of patients and responsible for serious embolic sequelae in 20%
  - □ Skin
    - Present in 30%
    - Multiple in 75%
    - Most common site is the head (eyelid, ear canal, scalp, and cheek), followed by trunk (nipples, chest, back and flank); perineum, genitalia, buttocks, and groin; upper limb and lower limb
  - □ Breast
    - Present in 25% of female patients
    - Bilateral in the majority
- *Lentiginosis and blue nevi*
  - □ Distribution, in decreasing order of frequency: Face (periocular and perioral), eyelids, ears, vermilion borders of lips, trunk, neck, conjunctiva or sclera, vulva (especially labia minora), extremities, and backs of hands

- *Endocrine tumors*
    - Adrenal
        - Bilateral pigmented nodular adrenal disease with associated Cushing syndrome in 20%
        - Microscopically, nodules are composed of enlarged, globular, cortical cells with granular, eosinophilic cytoplasm that often contains lipofuscin
    - Testis
        - 30% of male patients
        - Bilateral in 75% and multicentric in each affected testis
        - Median age 14 years (range 5-33 years)
        - Present as sexual precocity
        - Microscopically, lesions are large-cell calcifying Sertoli cell tumor and steroid-type tumor (Leydig cell tumor or adrenocortical rest tumor)
        - No reports of metastasis
    - Pituitary
        - 10% have adenoma associated with gigantism or acromegaly; plasma levels of growth hormone always elevated
- *Schwannomas*
    - 50% of psammomatous melanotic schwannomas occur in patients with Carney syndrome
    - Most common sites are upper alimentary tract (esophagus and stomach) and paravertebral sympathetic chains
    - 10% malignant and fatal

Papillary Fibroelastoma

Clinical Manifestations

- A benign avascular papilloma of the endocardium
- Men and women affected equally; average age at diagnosis 60 years
- 3rd most common primary cardiac tumor (myxoma is 1st and sarcoma is 2nd)
- Most patients are asymptomatic
- Symptoms usually the result of emboli from lesions on left side of the heart (usually the mitral or aortic valves); eg, acute myocardial infarction, stroke, and renal vascular occlusion

Gross Pathology

- 90% occur on valve surfaces, usually away from the lines of closure; also occur on endocardial surface of both atria and ventricles
- Aortic valve most frequently involved
- Lesions on mitral and tricuspid valves tend to be on atrial side; lesions on aortic and pulmonic valves occur on either side with equal frequency
- 10% to 15% are multiple
- Characterized by a flowerlike appearance reminiscent of a sea anemone
- Gross appearance may be altered by the presence of attached, organizing thrombi
- Cystic foci may be evident on sectioning

Microscopic Pathology

- Characterized by narrow, long, and branching papillary fronds that resemble chordae tendineae; matrix consists of mucopolysaccharides, variable numbers of elastic fibers, and occasional spindle cells reminiscent of smooth muscle cells or fibroblasts
- Papillary surface covered by a single layer of endothelial cells

Special Stains

- Movat trichrome will highlight elastic fibers, smooth muscle cells, and fibroblasts in a mucopolysaccharide matrix

Immunohistochemistry

- Fibrin can be detected in papillary cores

Electron Microscopy

- Confirms the presence of mature collagen, longitudinally oriented irregular elastic fibers, and fibroblasts in connective tissue and matrix
- Surface endothelial cells are hyperplastic and contain numerous organelles and pinocytotic vesicles

Molecular Alterations

- None

Differential Diagnosis

- Lambl excrescences (thought to be organizing thrombi usually found along line of valve closure on the atrial surface; tend to be smaller and less gelatinous than papillary fibroelastoma); a papillary fibroelastoma may simply be a large Lambl excrescence
- Overgrowth by fibrin thrombi can obscure the underlying tumor, giving the lesion the appearance of marantic endocarditis

Treatment and Prognosis

- Surgical excision
- No reports of recurrence
- Death usually the result of embolization into the coronary arteries, cerebral vasculature, or peripheral arterial tree

Associations

- May be found in the setting of preexisting heart disease such as rheumatic valvular disease

Rhabdomyoma

Clinical Manifestations

- A congenital form of hamartoma
- Most common cardiac tumor of infancy and childhood
- Extremely rare in patients older than 10 years
- May occur as a sporadic lesion, in association with tuberous sclerosis, or in association with structural congenital heart disease
- Occasionally causes arrhythmias, cyanosis, right ventricular outflow track obstruction, and cardiac murmurs
- 50% of sporadic lesions solitary; tend to project into the ventricular lumen
- 50% of patients with cardiac rhabdomyoma have tuberous sclerosis; 100% of patients with tuberous sclerosis have cardiac rhabdomyomas; 90% of lesions in patients with tuberous sclerosis multiple; 85% of patients with multiple lesions have tuberous sclerosis
- Patients with tuberous sclerosis usually present with symptoms related to central nervous system lesions or fetal hydrops; cardiac lesions are usually asymptomatic (tend to be intramural do not result in obstruction of blood flow)

Gross Pathology

- Lesions tend to be firm, white, well circumscribed, and lobulated
- Can occur anywhere in the heart but are usually found in the ventricles; most commonly located in the left ventricle and the ventricular septum (30% involve the atrial wall or right ventricle)
- When multiple, may consist of miliary, 1-mm nodules (rhabdoymyomytosis)
- Sporadic lesions can be quite large (3 to 4 cm)

Microscopic Pathology

- Tumors generally well-demarcated from adjacent cardiac muscle
- Tumor cells are large and vacuolated with little cytoplasm; vacuolation the result of glycogen deposition
- Occasional spider cells may be scattered throughout; characterized by a centrally located nucleus and surrounded by a rim of cytoplasm that has radial extensions (myofibers) from the center of the cell to its periphery

Special Stains

- PAS strongly positive, confirming glycogen content of the tumor cells

Immunohistochemistry

- Tumor cells express myoglobin, desmin, muscle-specific actin, and vimentin
- Adult rhabdomyomas do not express myogenin

Electron Microscopy

- Tumor cells appear to be altered myocytes that contain abundant glycogen
- Tumor cells have cellular junctions that resemble intercalated disks that surround the periphery of the cell (differentiated myocytes have intercalated disks located exclusively at the poles of the cell)

Cardiac Tumors>Rhabdomyoma

Molecular Alterations

- Genes responsible for tuberous sclerosis on chromosomes 9q34 and 16p

Differential Diagnosis

- Histiocytoid cardiomyopathy
- Lipoma
- Granular cell tumor
- Glycogen storage disease

Treatment

- Surgical excision (particularly indicated in patients with single tumors)

Prognosis

- Spontaneous regression has been noted in tumors occurring in patients with tuberous sclerosis
- Associated arrhythmias and outflow obstruction seen with sporadic lesions primarily determine prognosis

Associations

- Tuberous sclerosis syndrome
  - A neurocutaneous syndrome characterized by cutaneous and neurologic manifestations (mental retardation and seizures) and tumors
  - Tubers (cerebral hemispheres)
  - Sclerosis (characterized by areas of decreased neurons and overgrowth of fibrillary astrocytes that may differentiate into malignant astrocytomas)
  - Cutaneous manifestations
    - Adenoma sebaceum (80%)
    - Ash-leaf spots (90%)
    - Shagreen patches (35%)
    - Café-au-lait spots (7%-16%)
    - Fibromas (trunk, gingivae, periungual region, hairline, and eyebrows)
    - Angiomas
  - Neurologic manifestations
    - Seizures (90%)
    - Mental retardation (60-70%)
  - Tumors
    - Retinal (50%-80%)
    - Nodular astrocytoma of retina or optic nerve
    - Hamartomas
    - Renal (50%-80%): Angiomyolipomas
    - Heart (50%): Cardiac rhabdomyoma
    - Cutaneous (20%): Subungual fibromas (Koenen tumors)
    - Intracranial (15%): Astrocytomas
    - Oral: Fibromas or papillomas
    - Other manifestations
      - Respiratory
      - Cystic or fibrous lesions in lungs
      - Musculoskeletal
    - Cystic changes and periosteal thickening of bones of hands and feet
  - Structural abnormalities of the heart
    - Hypoplastic left heart syndrome
    - Transposition of the great arteries
    - Ventricular septal defect
    - Endocardial fibroelastosis
    - Subaortic stenosis
    - Ebstein anomaly
    - Hypoplastic tricuspid valve
    - Double outlet right ventricle
    - Pulmonary atresia

Primary Cardiac Sarcomas

Clinical Manifestations

- All types of sarcomas have been described in the heart; all are very rare despite being the second most common primary heart tumor, after myxoma
- 50% located in left atrium
- Patients present with dyspnea secondary to venous obstruction or mitral stenosis
- No sex predilection
- Mean age at presentation 41 years
- Extremely rare in infants and children (childhood sarcomas are usually undifferentiated sarcomas, myxosarcomas, or rhabdomyosarcomas)
- Other symptoms include palpitations and symptoms related to pericardial effusion, congestive heart failure, chest pain, arrhythmias and/or cerebral embolism
- Tumors with fibrous, smooth muscle, and osteogenic differentiation often in the left atrial cavity; clinically mimic atrial myxomas

Gross Pathology

- Lesions tend to be large, bulky, infiltrative, nodular masses with irregular borders
- On sectioning, may be grossly mucoid or gelatinous (similar to a cardiac myxoma) or firm and white with areas of hemorrhage or calcification
- Usually confined to the heart at time of diagnosis (see angiosarcoma exception)

Clinical and Morphologic (Gross and Microscopic) Findings in Primary Cardiac Sarcomas

- Angiosarcoma
  - Most common
  - Peak incidence 4th decade; men and women affected equally
  - 80% arise in right atrium near atrioventricular groove and metastasize to lung early
  - Patients may present with hemorrhagic episodes, coagulopathy, anemia, recurrent or persistant hematomas or easy bruising
  - Usually a lobulated variegated dark gray to brown to black mass in right atrial wall
  - 65% well to moderately differentiated with well-formed irregular vascular channels lined by pleomorphic and atypical cells; remainder poorly differentiated and composed of anaplastic spindle cells
- Epithelioid hemangioendothelioma
  - Fewer than 5 reports
  - A vascular tumor composed of epithelioid cells arranged in short strands or solid nests; endothelial cells usually round to oval and contain small intracellular lumina
  - frequently infiltrate into muscular walls of vessels
- Pleomorphic malignant fibrous histiocytoma/undifferentiated pleomorphic sarcoma
  - Second most common malignant cardiac sarcoma in adults
  - Mean age 45 years
  - Men and women affected equally
  - Tends to be located on posterior wall or intratrial septum of the left atrium
  - Signs and symptoms include pulmonary congestion, mitral stenosis, and pulmonary vein obstruction
  - Usually a soft to firm, tan-white, polypoid endocardial based tumor; may extend into pulmonary veins and lung parenchyma; hemorrhage but no calcifications
  - Variably cellular storiform arrangement of spindled or epithelioid pleomorphic cells, some with abundant cytoplasm; many mitotic figures; osseous differentiation in 15%
- Fibrosarcoma and myxofibrosarcoma
  - 5% to 10% of all cardiac sarcomas
  - Most occur in left atrium; may occur in any chamber
  - May infiltrate pericardial space and mimic a mesothelioma

- Signs and symptoms include pulmonary congestion, mitral stenosis, and pulmonary vein obstruction
- Usually presents as a polypoid mass projecting into chamber; similar gross appearance to pleomorphic malignant fibrous histiocytoma except less hemorrhage, necrosis, and variegation
- Tumor cells are spindled and have darkly staining, spindled nuclei with tapered ends; a herringbone arrangement is typical (sweeping fascicles arranged at angles to one another); mitotic activity variable; in myxoid variant, cells tend to be more stellate or ovoid; pleomorphism and prominent vascularity both very unusual

■ Rhabdomyosarcoma

- Very rare
- Can occur anywhere in the heart; 50% in atria, 50% in ventricles
- Tends to be mural rather than intracavitary
- Occurs most frequently in children and young adults; mean age at presentation 20 years
- Most likely of all cardiac sarcomas to involve cardiac valves
- Tends to be bulky and invasive with a cut surface that resembles a myxoma with a mucinous or gelatinous texture; necrosis may be present
- Almost always of the embryonal type and consists predominantly of small round cells; may be well differentiated with readily identifiable tadpole-shaped rhabdomyoblasts (strap cells) or poorly differentiated with rare rhabdomyoblasts; rhabdomyoblasts contain glycogen and have abundant eosinophilic cytoplasm; cross striations may be visible
- Tumors histologically similar to sarcoma botryoides have been described
- Tumors with an alveolar pattern (characterized by a collagenous stroma and few rhabdomyoblasts) probably represent metastases

■ Leiomyosarcoma

- 10% of cardiac sarcomas
- No sex predilection
- Most occur between 40 and 50 years
- Most present with dyspnea; other symptoms include chest pain, cough, atrial arrhythmias, and hemoptysis
- Most arise on posterior wall of left atrium and invade pulmonary veins or mitral valve
- Tend to be firm, gray, fleshy, and have a broad base
- Tumor cells are spindled and arranged in bundles that intersect at 90 degree angles; nuclei usually have blunt ends (cigar-shaped); cytoplasmic glycogen and perinuclear vacuoles variably present; areas of necrosis and mitotitic figures usually easily found

■ Synovial sarcoma

- 5% of cardiac sarcomas
- Tend to arise in atria and on the pericardial surface
- Usually bulky and infiltrative; cut surface firm and white; necrosis and hemorrhage may be present
- A biphasic tumor (spindled and epithelial), but monomorphic, spindled variant especially common in heart
- Spindled tumor cells are small and compact with alternating cellular and edematous areas; lymphoid cells may be scattered about
- Epithelioid cells typically form clusters, nests, and occasionally glandlike spaces

Special Stains

■ PAS will highlight glycogen in rhabdomyoblasts

Immunohistochemistry

■ Role of immunohistochemistry inferred from its role in extracardiac soft tissue tumors

■ Angiosarcoma

- Most cells stain with factor VIII, CD34, and CD31 (most sensitive [90%])
- Cytokeratin and epithelial membrane antigen (EMA) may be focally or diffusely positive (epithelioid angiosarcoma)

■ Epithelioid hemangioendothelioma

- Usually cytokeratin negative
- Factor VIII-associated antigen present

- Pleomorphic malignant fibrous histiocytoma/undifferentiated pleomorphic sarcoma
  - Not helpful although most high grade, pleomorphic sarcomas show a reproducible line of differentiation
- Fibrosarcoma and myxosarcoma
  - Not helpful
- Rhabdomyosarcoma
  - Tumor cells typically positive for myogenin and desmin
- Leiomyosarcoma
  - Tumor cells positive for desmin and smooth muscle actin
  - Occasional aberrant expression of cytokeratin and EMA
- Synovial sarcoma
  - 60% to 70% of cases are immunoreactive for CD99 (product of MIC-2 gene)
  - Epithelial cells strongly express cytokeratin and EMA; some focal staining with these markers may be seen in spindled areas as well
  - Spindled cells express vimentin and occasionally smooth muscle actin
  - Both cell types negative for CD34

Electron Microscopy

- Angiosarcoma
  - Weibel-Palade bodies usually not demonstrable, but pinocytic vesicles and intermediate filaments may be seen
- Epithelioid hemangioendothelioma
  - Cells have characteristics of endothelial cells with basal lamina, pinocytotic vesicles, and occasional Weibel-Palade bodies
- Pleomorphic malignant fibrous histiocytoma/undifferentiated pleomorphic sarcoma
  - Confirms presence of undifferentiated, nonspecific fibroblasts, histiocytes, and primitive mesenchymal cells
- Fibrosarcoma and myxosarcoma
  - Tumor cells are fibroblasts with prominent rough endoplasmic reticulum and no myofilaments
- Rhabdomyosarcoma
  - Confirms presence of thick and thin filaments seen in normal striated muscle; abundant glycogen and mitochondria
- Leiomyosarcoma
  - Tumor cells have many of the same characteristics as normal smooth muscle cells but tend to be less well developed; pinocytotic vesicles and basal lamina are both prominent
- Synovial sarcoma
  - Biphasic tumors have epithelial cells, spindle cells, and transition forms
  - Epithelial cells may have microvilli and are arranged in clusters
  - Even lesions that appear to be monophasic will have areas of epithelial differentiation characterized by slitlike glandular spaces and microvilli
  - Spindle cells resemble fibroblasts with irregular nuclear membranes, marginated chromatin, and small nucleoli

Molecular Alterations

- No known familial induced cardiac sarcomas
- Angiosarcoma: TP53 tumor-suppressor gene in up to 50%
- Epithelioid hemangioendothelioma: None
- Pleomorphic malignant fibrous histiocytoma/undifferentiated pleomorphic sarcoma: RB1 gene implicated
- Fibrosarcoma and myxosarcoma: None
- Rhabdomyosarcoma: A mutation at the first base of codon 13 (G to A transition) at exon 1 of K-*ras*
- Leiomyosarcoma: None

- Synovial sarcoma: Reciprocal translocation t(X;18)(p11.2;q11.2) present in more than 90%; this translocation results in fusion of SS18 gene at chromosome 18q11.2 to 1 of 2 genes, SSX1 or SSX2, at Xp11.2

Differential Diagnosis

- Angiosarcoma
  - Unclassified spindle cell sarcoma
  - Fibrosarcoma
  - Pleomorphic malignant fibrous histiocytoma/undifferentiated pleomorphic sarcoma
  - Kaposi sarcoma
  - Pericardial angiosarcoma may resemble mesothelioma
- Epithelioid hemangioendothelioma
  - Adenocarcinoma
- Pleomorphic malignant fibrous histiocytoma/undifferentiated pleomorphic sarcoma
- Storiform-pleomorphic malignant fibrous histiocytoma (a diagnosis of exclusion)
  - Pleomorphic liposarcoma
  - Pleomorphic rhabdomyosarcoma
  - Metastatic pleomorphic carcinoma
  - Melanoma
  - Hodgkin disease (Leu-M1 staining of Reed-Sternberg cells helpful) and lymphoma
  - DFSP and benign fibrous histiocytoma
- Fibrosarcoma and myxosarcoma
  - Monophasic synovial sarcoma
  - Inflammatory myofibroblastic tumor
  - Myxoid variant must be distinguished from other myxoid sarcomas, such as pleomorphic malignant fibrous histiocytoma and leiomyosarcoma
- Rhabdomyosarcoma
  - Undifferentiated sarcomas
  - Metastatic small round cell tumors in children and young adults
- Leiomyosarcoma
  - Leiomyoma never reported to occur in the heart
- Synovial sarcoma
  - Mesothelioma and solitary fibrous tumor

Treatment

- Complete tumor excision (possible in fewer than 50%) with reconstruction using synthetic grafts as needed
- Tumor resection of rhabdomyosarcomas, even if palliative, often indicated; adjuvant chemotherapy may also be indicated; orthotopic heart transplantation also an option

Prognosis

- Most dead within 2 years
- Features associated with increased survival include left-sided tumor, a mitotic rate <10 per high-powered field and no necrosis
- Angiosarcoma: 80% present with metastatic disease; 10% survive longer than 1 year
- Epithelioid hemangioendothelioma: 10% of extracardiac hemangioendotheliomas recur; behavior in the heart unknown
- Pleomorphic malignant fibrous histiocytoma/undifferentiated pleomorphic sarcoma: Mean postoperative survival 5 to 18 months
- Fibrosarcoma and myxosarcoma: No difference in prognosis between cardiac fibrosarcoma and pleomorphic malignant fibrous histiocytoma
- Rhabdomyosarcoma: Mean survival rarely exceeds 12 months
- Leiomyosarcoma: Survival typically <1 year
- Synovial sarcoma: Survival typically <1 year

Associations

- Epithelioid hemangioendothelioma has been reported in association with myelodysplastic syndrome
- An association between cardiac synovial sarcomas and asbestos exposure has been reported

Cardiac Syndromes

Ehlers-Danlos Syndrome (EDS)

Clinical Manifestations

- A heterogeneous group of disorders resulting from defects in the synthesis or structure of collagen
- Different types of collagen (at least 14 genetically distinct collagen types have been identified) may be involved (see subsection on molecular alterations below)
- Most patients have manifestations of skin, ligament, and joint involvement; loss of tensile strength in the abnormal collagen results in hyperextensible skin and hypermobile joints
- Patients predisposed to joint dislocation
- Minor injuries can produce major wounds and surgical repair often quite difficult because of the lack of normal tensile strength of collagen
- Occasionally abnormal collagen can lead to catastrophic internal complications such as retinal detachment, diaphragmatic hernia, and rupture of intestine, larger arteries, and cornea
- Six variants
  - *Classic EDS (types I and II)*: Skin and joint hypermobility, atrophic scars, easy brusing
  - *Hypermobility EDS (type III)*: Joint hypermobility, pain, dislocations
  - *Vascular EDS (type IV)*: Thin skin, arterial, uterine, or intestinal rupture, bruising, small joint hyperextensibility
  - *Kyphoscoliosis (type VI)*: Hypotonia, joint laxity, congenital scoliosis, ocular fragility
  - *Arthrochalasia EDS (type VIIa, b)*: Severe joint hypermobility, skin changes. mild scoliosis, bruising
  - *Dermatosparaxsis EDS (type VIIc)*: Severe shin fragility, cutis laxa, bruising

Gross and Microscopic Pathology

- No characteristic gross or microscopic pathologic findings

Special Stains, Immunohistochemistry, and Electron Microscopy

- Not helpful

Molecular Alterations

- *Classic EDS (types I and II)*
  - Autosomal dominant pattern of inheritance
  - Mutations in genes for type V collagen (COL5A1 and COL5A2) detected in 30% to 50%
- *Hypermobility EDS (type III)*
  - Autosomal dominant
  - No known gene defects
- *Vascular EDS (type IV)*
  - Autosomal dominant
  - Abnormalities of type III collagen
  - Three distinct mutations affecting the COL3A1 gene for collagen type III
  - Mutations may involve rate of synthesis of pro-α1 (III) chains for collagen type III, the secretion of type III procollagen, and the synthesis of structurally abnormal type III collagen which involves a structural protein (rather than an enzyme protein)
- *Kyphoscoliosis EDS (type VI)*
  - Most common autosomal recessive form of disease
  - Results from mutations in the gene encoding lysyl hydroxylase, an enzyme necessary for hydroxylation of lysine residues during collagen synthesis
  - Collagen types I and III affected; collagen types II, IV, and V normal
- *Arthrochalasia EDS (type VIIa, b)*
  - Autosomal dominant
  - Mutations that affect 1 of the 2 type I collagen genes COL1A1 and COL1A2
  - Defect interferes with the conversion of procollagen to collagen
- *Dermatosparaxsis EDS (type VIIc)*
  - Autosomal recessive
  - Mutations in the procollagen-N-peptidase genes, essential for the cleavage of collagens

Differential Diagnosis

- None

Treatment

- None

Prognosis

- Particularly grim in patients with vascular EDS (type IV)

Associations

- None

Marfan Syndrome

Clinical Manifestations

- Characterized by abnormalities of cardiovascular system, eyes, and skeleton
- Cardiovascular involvement characterized by aortic root dilatation (40%), aortic dissections (35%), isolated mitral valve prolapse (20%), aneurysms of sinuses of Valsalva, and peripheral aneurysms
- Weakening of the media of the aorta predisposes to intimal disruption with subsequent intramural hematoma that may produce an aortic dissection; aortic dissections may extend from the root of the aorta down to the iliac arteries and rupture through the aortic wall (cause of death in 30%-45% of patients)
- Classic symptoms of progressive aortic dissection include sudden onset of severe pain, usually beginning in the anterior part of the chest, radiating to the back, and moving downward into the abdomen toward the pelvis
- Ocular changes
  - Usually characterized by bilateral subluxation or dislocation (usually outward and upward) of the lens of the eye (ectopia lentis); essentially pathognomonic of Marfan syndrome
- Skeletal abnormalities
  - Patients usually tall with long extremities and long tapering fingers and toes
  - Ratio of the upper portion of the body to the lower portion of the body significantly lower than normal for age, race, and gender
  - Lax joint ligaments of the hands and feet
  - Head usually long (dolichocephalic) with bossing of the frontal eminences and prominent supraorbital ridges
  - Various spinal deformities include kyphosis, scoliosis, or rotation/slipping of the dorsal or lumbar vertebrae
  - Chest frequently deformed by either pectus excavatum or carinatum

Gross Pathology

- Dilatation of mitral valve with prolapse characterized by elongated and redundant anterior and posterior leaflets (calcification present in 10%)
- Dilated proximal aorta with hematoma within the wall; a defect in the intima can often be identified in the proximal aorta in an area free of atherosclerotic plaque
- Propagation of intramural hematoma occurs for variable distances and may actually stop at a site where atherosclerosis begins

Microscopic Pathology

- Elastic tissue of the media fragmented with separation of the elastic and fibromuscular elements of the media by small cleftlike or cystic spaces
- Geographic foci show a disruption of the elastic pattern (often referred to as *cystic medial necrosis*) with the accumulation of mucopolysaccharide
- Advanced disease characterized by significant loss of elastic laminae
- Elastic tissue change not necessarily pathognomonic for Marfan syndrome
- No inflammation

Special Stains

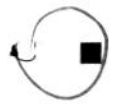

- Movat and elastic stains highlight fragmented nature of the elastin in the aortic wall

Immunohistochemistry

- Not helpful

Electron Microscopy

- Will confirm the fragmented nature of elastin and confirm that actual necrosis is not part of the pathologic process

Molecular Alterations

- Autosomal dominant
- A defect in extracellular glycoprotein, fibrillin 1 (*FBN1*), which is mapped to chromosome 15q21 (mutant *FBN1* disrupts the assembly of normal microfibrils)
- More than 500 distinct mutations have been identified involving the *FBN1* gene in patients with Marfan syndrome

Differential Diagnosis

- Aortic dissection secondary to atherosclerosis, syphilis, and trauma

Treatment

- Aortic replacement with or without aortic valve replacement

Prognosis

- Almost 50% of all deaths result from a ruptured aortic dissection

Associations

- None

Inflammatory Lesions

Myocarditis

Clinical Manifestations

- Most frequently (50%) result from infection with Coxsackieviruses A and B and other enteroviruses; less common viral agents include cytomegalovirus and human immunodeficiency virus (HIV)
- Other infectious agents include: chlamydiae, rickettsiae, various bacteria (eg, *Neisseria meningococcus*, *Borrelia burgdorferi*, and toxin from *Corynebacterium diphtheria*), fungi (*Candida*), protozoa (*Trypanosoma cruzi* [Chagas disease], toxoplasmosis), and helminths (trichinosis)
- May result from allergic reactions (hypersensitivity myocarditis), often to drugs such as methyldopa and sulfonamides
- Occasionally seen in association with systemic diseases of immune origin, for example, rheumatic fever and collagen vascular disease
- Sarcoidosis and rejection of a transplanted heart represent additional forms of myocarditis
- Clinical spectrum ranges from asymptomatic cardiac involvement, with complete resolution, to acute or late-onset congestive heart failure and sudden cardiac death; patients frequently present with sudden onset of congestive heart failure coupled with a recent history of a viral illness; others complain of rather nonspecific symptoms of fatigue, dyspnea, palpitations, precordial discomfort, and fever; clinical features may mimic an acute myocardial infarction
- 40% to 45% incidence of myocarditis in setting of a recent history of flulike febrile illness coupled with a recent onset of congestive heart failure, arrhythmias, or other conduction abnormalities
- Patients may develop a sudden systolic murmur secondary to mitral regurgitation resulting from dilation of the left ventricle (dilated cardiomyopathy)

Gross Pathology

- During the active phase of inflammation, heart may appear either normal or dilated with or without hypertrophy
- Ventricular myocardium often flabby and may be mottled, pale and contain minute foci of hemorrhage
- Mural thrombi may be present)

Microscopic Pathology)

- Characterized by a mononuclear, usually lymphocytic, inflammatory infiltrate with focal myocardial necrosis and/or degeneration adjacent to the inflammatory cells (Dallas criteria)
- *Presence of inflammatory cells in the myocardium without associated myocyte damage not sufficient for diagnosis*
- Myocyte damage defined as necrosis or myocyte vacuolization, latter characterized by irregular cell outlines and disintegration with lymphocytes or macrophages within the sarcolemma

- Inflammatory infiltrate may be focal or diffuse and consist of lymphocytes, eosinophils, neutrophils, giant cells, granulomas, or a mixture
- With persistent disease, endocardial, myocardial, perivascular, and interstitial fibrosis develop to a mild, moderate, or severe degree
- Three variants:
  - *Hypersensitivity myocarditis*: Interstitial infiltrates composed primarily of lymphocytes, macrophages, and numerous eosinophils that tend to aggregate around blood vessels
  - *Giant cell myocarditis*: Characterized by widespread inflammatory cellular infiltrate that contains multinucleated giant cells interspersed with lymphocytes, eosinophils, plasma cells, and macrophages
  - *Chagas disease*: Characterized by the presence of trypanosomes with accompanying inflammatory cells (neutrophils, lymphocytes, macrophages, and occasional eosinophils)

Special Stains

- Giemsa stain will highlight trypanosomes in myocarditis of Chagas disease

Immunohistochemistry

- Majority of T lymphocytes express major histocompatibility complex class II human leukocyte antigen (HLA-DR) molecules

Electron Microscopy

- Not helpful

Molecular Alterations

- None

Differential Diagnosis

- Organizing myocardial infarction (ischemic infiltrates often accompanied by hemosiderin deposits; endocardial and adjacent myocardial involvement common in myocarditis; ischemic myocardium often sharply demarcated from normal and subendocardium usually spared from ischemic injury)
- Hematologic malignancy
- Idiopathic dilated cardiomyopathy
- Previous biopsy site
- Differential diagnosis based on the nature of the myocardial inflammatory infiltrate
  - Lymphocytic infiltrate
    - Idiopathic
    - Viral
    - Toxic
    - Collagen vascular disease
    - Kawasaki disease
  - Neutrophilic infiltrate
    - Bacterial infections
    - Idiopathic (early)
    - Viral (early)
    - Pressor effect
  - Eosinophilic infiltrate
    - Hypersensitivity
    - Parasitic infestation
    - Hypereosinophilic syndromes
    - Idiopathic
  - Giant cell infiltrate
    - Idiopathic
    - Giant cell myocarditis
    - Sarcoidosis
    - Hypersensitivity
    - Rheumatic fever
    - Rheumatoid disease
    - Tuberculosis
    - Fungal infections

Treatment

- Identification and management of underlying etiologic agent when possible
- Cardiac support to include transplantation

Prognosis

- Idiopathic and occasional viral myocarditis may spontaneously resolve
- 10% of patients with Chagas myocarditis die during initial acute attack; others develop progressive signs of cardiac insufficiency over 10 to 20 years
- Patients with giant cell myocarditis have a particularly poor prognosis

Associations

- Approximately 65% of patients with Lyme disease (caused by the bacterial spirochete *Borrelia burgdorferi*) develop myocarditis

Comment

Persistent myocardial inflammatory lesions may be immunologically mediated through T-cell-dependent mechanisms; disease induced by a virus may be biphasic, consisting of an early virus-mediated myocardial infection. This infection is cleared by monocytes and the humoral immune system, but is followed by an immunologic phase mediated by T lymphocytes directed at an antigen resulting from the interaction between the virus and the myocardium

Vasculitis

Variants

- Large vessel vasculitis
  - Giant cell (temporal arteritis)
  - Takayasu arteritis
- Medium-sized vessel vasculitis
  - Polyarteritis nodosa
  - Kawasaki disease (mucocutaneous lymph node syndrome)
  - Granulomatous angiitis of CNS
  - Thromboangiitis obliterans (Buerger disease)
- Small vessel vasculitis
  - Wegener granulomatosis
  - Churg-Strauss syndrome (allergic granulomatosis)
  - Microscopic polyangiitis
  - Henoch-Schönlein purpura
  - Cutaneous leukocytoclastic vasculitis

Giant Cell (Temporal Arteritis)

Clinical Manifestations

- Most common of the vasculitides
- Typically occurs in patients older than 50 years
- Granulomatous inflammation of the aorta and its major branches with a predilection for the extracranial branches of the carotid artery (often the temporal artery)
- May involve the vertebral and ophthalmic arteries (involvement of the latter may result in blindness)
- Patients typically present with vague symptoms of fever, fatigue, and weight loss, and complain of headache, scalp tenderness, and jaw or tongue pain when chewing or talking
- Patient has a 90% chance of having disease if 3 of the following 5 diagnostic criteria are present:
  - 50 years of age or older
  - Recent localized headache
  - Temporal artery tenderness
  - Elevated erythrocyte sedimentation rate (50 mm/h)
  - Positive temporal biopsy
- Most patients experience unilateral facial pain or headache, most intense along the course of the supratemporal artery, which may be nodular and painful on palpation
- Ocular symptoms typically appear abruptly and vary from diplopia to transient or permanent loss of vision
- Involvement of visceral vessels may cause myocardial ischemia, gastrointestinal dysfunction, and neurologic symptoms
- 10% to 15% have some evidence of large vessel disease as manifested by diminished pulses, intermittent claudication, paresthesias, Raynaud phenomenon, and angina

Gross and Microscopic Pathology

- Nodular thickenings involving short segments of 1 or more affected arteries result in a slitlike orifice and thrombosis
- Two histologic patterns:
  - Granulomatous inflammation involving the inner half of the media centered on the internal elastic membrane and characterized by a marked mononuclear infiltrate, multinucleated giant cells of both foreign body and Langerhans type (present in 65%), and fragmentation of internal elastic lamina

- A nonspecific panarteritis consisting of a mixed inflammatory infiltrate of lymphocytes and macrophages admixed with some neutrophils and eosinophils (fibrinoid necrosis may be present); rare or no granulomas
- Healed disease characterized by collagenous thickening of the vessel wall
- Organization of a thrombus may give the artery the appearance of a fibrous cord

Special Stains

- Elastic tissue stains can confirm the presence of focal destruction of internal elastic lamina and intimal thickening characteristic of longstanding or healed arteritis

Electron Microscopy

- Not helpful

Molecular Alterations

- Giant cell (temporal) arteritis associated with certain HLA-DR antigens

Differential Diagnosis

- True vasculitis versus reaction to inflammation in surrounding tissue
- Self-limited, benign vasculitis versus systemic vasculitis
- Vasculitides involving small vessels have a considerable overlap in histologic appearance

Treatment

- Anti-inflammatory agents and corticosteroids

Prognosis

- Steroid therapy produces a rapid improvement in clinical symptoms but complete resolution of the histologic change does not typically occur
- Untreated patients may become blind
- Death may result from myocardial infarction, dissecting aneurysm of the aorta and cerebral infarction

Associations

- Polymyalgia rheumatica

Takayasu Arteritis

Clinical Manifestations

- Granulomatous inflammation of medium and large arteries
- Patients typically present with ocular disturbances and marked diminution of the pulses in the upper extremities ("pulseless disease")
- Primarily seen in women younger than 40 years
- As the pulses are lost in the upper extremities, patients experience coldness or numbness of the fingers
- Ocular disturbances include visual defects, retinal hemorrhages, and occasional total blindness
- Patients frequently hypertensive and may experience neurologic deficits such as dizziness, focal weakness, or even complete hemiparesis
- When more distal arteries involved, claudication dominant symptom
- Involvement of pulmonary arteries may cause pulmonary hypertension with subsequent development of cor pulmonale

Gross and Microscopic Pathology

- Aortic arch typically involved; 30% will have an involvement of the remainder of the aorta and its branches; aortic arch involvement typically results in markedly narrowed orifices of the arteries to the upper portion of the body; involvement of the aortic root may lead to dilatation of the aortic valve with subsequent aortic insufficiency
- Pulmonary arteries involved in 50%
- Both coronary and renal arteries may be affected and have vessels with irregularly thickened and wrinkled intima
- Early disease characterized by an adventitial mononuclear infiltrate with perivascular cuffing of the vasa vasorum; as disease progresses, an intense mononuclear infiltrate develops in the media, which may be accompanied by granulomatous changes to include giant cells and focal areas of medial necrosis
- Once disease has run its course or been treated, collagenous fibrosis with an accompanying lymphocytic infiltrate is present in all layers of the vessel wall (particularly the intima)

Inflammatory Lesions>Vasculitis: Takayasu Arteritis, Polyarteritis Nodosa

Special Stains

- Elastic tissue stains can confirm the presence of focal destruction of internal elastic lamina and intimal thickening characteristic of longstanding or healed arteritis

Electron Microscopy

- Not helpful

Differential Diagnosis

- True vasculitis versus reaction to inflammation in surrounding tissue
- Self-limited, benign vasculitis versus systemic vasculitis
- Vasculitides involving small vessels have a considerable overlap in histologic appearance

Treatment

- Associated renal vascular hypertension may be exacerbated if corticosteroids used
- Cytotoxic drugs are not typically used

Prognosis

- Course of disease often variable; some patients undergo rapid progression while others reach a quiescent stage after 1 or 2 years and experience long-term survival

Associations

- None

Polyarteritis Nodosa

Clinical Manifestations

- A necrotizing inflammation of medium-sized and/or small arteries
- Typically affects young adults; occasionally seen in children and the elderly
- Clinical course may be acute, subacute, or chronic; frequently characterized by long asymptomatic periods
- Pulmonary vasculature usually spared
- Vascular involvement may be quite widespread, resulting in various clinical signs and symptoms
- Patients typically complain of malaise, fever, and weight loss; hypertension develops quickly
- Lesions involving the mesenteric vessels often result in abdominal pain and gastrointestinal bleeding
- Diffuse muscular pain with or without peripheral neuritis (usually motor) may be present
- Involvement of medium-sized vessels in the kidney can be a major cause of death (small vessel involvement absent in the kidney so there is no glomerulonephritis)

Gross and Microscopic Pathology

- Distribution of lesions, in decreasing order of frequency: kidneys, heart, liver, gastrointestinal tract, pancreas, testes, skeletal muscle, nervous system, and skin
- Individual lesions often segmental and involve only a portion of the vessel's circumference leaving normal arterial wall adjacent to areas of inflamed arterial wall
- Involvement tends to occur at branching points and bifurcations
- Aneurysmal dilatation or localized rupture may occur at sites of involvement
- Acute disease characterized by transmural inflammation of the arterial wall (including adventitia) by heavy infiltrate of neutrophils, eosinophils, and mononuclear cells frequently accompanied by fibrinoid necrosis of the inner half of the vessel wall; thrombosis of lumen may be seen
- In later stages of the disease, the acute inflammatory infiltrate disappears, and is replaced by fibrous thickening accompanied by a mononuclear infiltrate; fibroblastic proliferation may extend to adventitia
- Long-standing disease characterized by marked fibrotic thickening of vessel wall without inflammation
- All stages of activity may coexist in different vessels or in the same vessel

Special Stains

- Elastic tissue stains can confirm the presence of focal destruction of internal elastic lamina and intimal thickening characteristic of longstanding or healed arteritis

Immunohistochemistry/Immunohistochemical Assay

- Patients with large vessel polyarteritis nodosa and patients with leukocytoclastic vasculitis associated with viral infections, particularly hepatitis, frequently have hepatitis B antigen (HBsAg) and HBsAg-anti-HBsAg immune complexes in the vascular lesions

Electron Microscopy

- Not helpful

Differential Diagnosis

- True vasculitis versus reaction to inflammation in surrounding tissue
- Self-limited, benign vasculitis versus systemic vasculitis
- Vasculitides involving small vessels have a considerable overlap in histologic appearance

Treatment

- Corticosteroids and cyclophosphamide (remission in 90%)
- Treatment of associated hypertension is required for a favorable prognosis

Prognosis

- Typically fatal if untreated
- Death may result from renal involvement as well as from vascular aneurysms or occlusions of major or visceral arteries (50%)

Associations

- 30% have hepatitis B antigen in their serum
- No association with ANCA

Kawasaki Disease (Mucocutaneous Lymph Node Syndrome)

Clinical Manifestations

- Most common cause of acquired heart disease in children in the United States
- Inflammatory disease of large, medium, and small arteries
- Coronary arteries frequently involved
- Typically seen in children and infants (80% younger 4 years)
- Tends to be self-limited
- Patients present with fever, conjunctival and oral erythema and ulceration, edema of the hands and feet, erythema of palms of hands and soles of feet, skin rash with desquamation, and enlargement of cervical lymph nodes
- 20% of patients develop cardiovascular signs or symptoms that vary from asymptomatic vasculitis of the coronary arteries to coronary artery atresia to frank aneurysm formation; coronary artery rupture or thrombosis with or without myocardial infarction or sudden death may occur

Gross and Microscopic Pathology

- Histologically similar to polyarteritis nodosa with necrosis and marked inflammation; fibrinoid necrosis less prominent
- Involvement of coronary arteries varies from mild changes limited to the intima to severe destruction of all components of the wall by a segmental necrotizing process with moderate fibrinoid changes and a dense inflammatory infiltrate
- Aneurysm formation may occur as the disease subsides during treatment and may be associated with thrombosis, rupture, and/or myocardial infarction
- Biopsies of involved (enlarged) cervical lymph nodes reveal obliteration of nodal architecture with depletion of lymphocytes, loss of follicular centers, vascular proliferation, increased numbers of histiocytes, small foci of necrosis in both the interfollicular and the follicular centers, and thrombi in small vessels; blood vessels may have concentric infiltrates of the adventitia by transformed lymphocytes and histiocytes

Inflammatory Lesions>Vasculitis: Kawasaki Disease (Mucocutaneous Lymph Node Syndrome), Granulomatous Angitis of CNS

Special Stains

- Elastic tissue stains can confirm the presence of focal destruction of internal elastic lamina and intimal thickening characteristic of longstanding or healed arteritis

Electron Microscopy

- Not helpful

Molecular Alterations

- Genetic susceptibility may be present in patients with Kawasaki syndrome

Differential Diagnosis

- True vasculitis versus reaction to inflammation in surrounding tissue
- Self-limited, benign vasculitis versus systemic vasculitis
- Vasculitides involving small vessels have a considerable overlap in histologic appearance

Treatment

- Aspirin to reduce the risk of coronary thrombosis
- Dipyridamole and intravenous gamma globulin may be of benefit

Prognosis

- 1% of patients die as a result of coronary involvement with either thrombosis or ruptured coronary artery aneurysm

Associations

- Mucocutaneous syndrome

Granulomatous Angitis of CNS

Clinical Manifestations

- Inflammatory disease of small and medium-sized arteries of meninges and cerebrum
- Patients present with various diffuse or focal neurologic symptoms and cognitive dysfunction
- Occasionally patients have a history of recent herpes infection or lymphoma

Gross and Microscopic Pathology

- Characterized by a marked mononuclear and giant cell infiltrate in arteries, arterioles, and veins of meninges and cerebrum
- Typically inflammatory infiltrates most pronounced in the cranial arteries with necrosis of the inner layers of the artery walls

Special Stains

- Elastic tissue stains can confirm the presence of focal destruction of internal elastic lamina and intimal thickening characteristic of longstanding or healed arteritis

Electron Microscopy

- Not helpful

Differential Diagnosis

- True vasculitis versus reaction to inflammation in surrounding tissue
- Self-limited, benign vasculitis versus systemic vasculitis
- Vasculitides involving small vessels have a considerable overlap in histologic appearance

Treatment

- Remission may occur with corticosteroids or cyclophosphamide

Prognosis

- Improvement typical with steroid and immunosuppressive therapy

Associations

- Amyloid angiopathy
- Recent herpes infection or history of lymphoma

Inflammatory Lesions>Vasculitis: Thromboangiitis Obliterans (Buerger Disease), Wegener Granulomatosis

Thromboangiitis Obliterans (Buerger Disease)

Clinical Manifestations

- Acute and chronic inflammation of medium-sized and small arteries that tends to involve the tibial and radial arteries of the extremities; cerebral vessels may be involved
- The inflammatory process may extend into adjacent veins and nerves
- Typically seen in men who are heavy smokers (less commonly seen in women who smoke)
- Onset typically before age of 35 years and often before the age of 20 years
- Vascular insufficiency: Early symptoms include superficial nodular phlebitis, cold sensitivity (Raynaud phenomenon) in the hands, and pain in the instep of the foot induced by exercise (instep claudication); patients tend to experience severe pain, even at rest (probably related to adjacent neural involvement); with progressive disease, ulceration of the toes and feet or fingers develops and may progress to gangrene

Gross and Microscopic Pathology

- Inflammation tends to be segmental with secondary extension to contiguous veins and nerves
- Acute and chronic inflammatory cells infiltrate arterial wall; vessel frequently thrombosed and may undergo organization and recanalization
- Thrombi often contain small microabscesses characterized by a central focus of neutrophils surrounded by granulomatous inflammation
- Internal elastic lamina usually preserved
- Usually no evidence of atherosclerosis
- Endstage disease characterized by fibrous obliteration of the vessel lumen with little associated inflammation

Special Stains

- Elastic tissue stains can confirm the presence of focal destruction of internal elastic lamina and intimal thickening characteristic of longstanding or healed arteritis

Electron Microscopy

- Not helpful

Molecular Alterations

- Increased prevalence of HLA-A9 and HLA-B5 in patients with thromboangiitis obliterans (Buerger disease)

Differential Diagnosis

- True vasculitis versus reaction to inflammation in surrounding tissue
- Self-limited, benign vasculitis versus systemic vasculitis
- Vasculitides involving small vessels have a considerable overlap in histologic appearance

Treatment and Prognosis

- Cessation of smoking may bring about a dramatic response
- Continued smoking usually leads to ulcerations followed by gangrene that frequently leads to amputation

Associations

- Cigarette smoking

Wegener Granulomatosis

Clinical Manifestations

- A necrotizing vasculitis involving small vessels
- Men more commonly affected than women; average age at diagnosis 40 years
- Characterized by a triad of clinical and pathologic findings:
  - Acute necrotizing granulomas of the upper respiratory tract (ear, nose, sinuses, throat), lower respiratory tract (lung), or both
  - Focal necrotizing or granulomatous vasculitis affecting small to medium-sized vessels (capillaries, venules, arterioles, and arteries) in the lung, upper airways, and various other sites
  - Renal disease in the form of focal or necrotizing, often crescentic, glomerulonephritis

Inflammatory Lesions>Vasculitis: Wegener Granulomatosis, Churg-Strauss Syndrome (Allergic Granulomatosis)

- Occasionally disease limited to the respiratory tract with sparing of the kidneys
- 95% present with bilateral pulmonary nodular and cavitary infiltrates, 90% with chronic sinusitis, 75% with mucosal ulcerations of the nasopharynx, and 80% with evidence of renal disease
- Other signs and symptoms include skin rash, muscle pain, articular involvement, mononeuritis or polyneuritis, and fever
- Cell-mediated immunologic mechanisms may be the underlying etiologic cause; 90% have circulating antibodies that recognize antigens in cytoplasmic granules of neutrophils (c-ANCA) in their serum (a reliable marker for disease activity)

Gross and Microscopic Pathology

- Upper respiratory tract lesions consist of inflammatory sinusitis secondary to mucosal granulomas and/or ulcerated lesions of the nose, palate, and/or pharynx that are rimmed by necrotizing granulomas and accompanying vasculitis
- Pulmonary lesions typically consist of focal necrotizing granulomas that may coalesce to produce a nodule with or without cavitation; granulomas in the lung characterized by a geographic pattern of necrosis rimmed by lymphocytes, plasma cells, macrophages, and variable numbers of giant cells; necrotizing or granulomatous vasculitis accompanies the granulomatous changes and may be found within, adjacent to, or separated from, the granulomas
- With time the granulomas undergo progressive fibrosis and organization

Special Stains

- Elastic tissue stains can confirm the presence of focal destruction of internal elastic lamina and intimal thickening characteristic of longstanding or healed arteritis

Immunohistochemistry/Immunohistochemical Assay

- Either c-ANCA or p-ANCA can be detected in patients with ANCA-associated small vessel vasculitis
- Patients with Wegener granulomatous typically positive for c-ANCA (anti-proteinase 3)

Electron Microscopy

- Not helpful

Differential Diagnosis

- True vasculitis versus reaction to inflammation in surrounding tissue
- Self-limited, benign vasculitis versus systemic vasculitis
- Vasculitides involving small vessels have a considerable overlap in histologic appearance
- Wegener granulomatosis may be difficult to differentiate from lymphomatoid granulomatosis and Churg-Strauss syndrome
- Churg-Strauss syndrome resembles eosinophilic pneumonia and Wegner granulomatosis

Treatment

- Immunosuppressive therapy (cyclophosphamide, prednisone, and occasionally antibiotics)

Prognosis

- Typically responds to immunosuppressive therapy with only occasional relapses

Associations

- None

Churg-Strauss Syndrome (Allergic Granulomatosis)

Clinical Manifestations

- Diagnosis requires presence of 4 of 6 features:
  - Asthma
  - Peripheral eosinophilia >10%
  - Mono- or polyneuropathy
  - Transient and fleeting pulmonary infiltrates
  - Paranasal sinus symptoms such as allergic rhinitis
  - Histologic evidence of perivascular eosinophilic infiltrates

Inflammatory Lesions>Vasculitis: Churg-Strauss Syndrome (Allergic Granulomatosis), Microscopic Polyangiitis

- Patients typically experience 3 phases of progression of disease:
  - Early: Symptoms of allergy, such as rhinitis, sinusitis, inflammatory nasal polyps, and asthma
  - Later: Tissue and peripheral blood eosinophilia
  - Last: Systemic vasculitis
- Pulmonary infiltrates in 90% during phases 2 and 3; 65% have skin and nerve involvement; 40% have gastrointestinal, cardiac, and renal involvement
- Patients ANCA positive; 70% perinuclear ANCA (p-ANCA) positive

Gross and Microscopic Pathology

- Pulmonary lesions characterized by granuloma formation with striking alveolar and interstitial eosinophilic infiltrate and eosinophilic vasculitis (involving arteries, capillaries, and veins)
- Most characteristic histologic finding is a small poorly formed granuloma (microgranuloma) composed of a bright red central body of necrosis that usually contain fragmented eosinophils and eosinophilic granular debris; palisading histiocytes and giant cells surround foci of fibrinoid material that often lie within or adjacent to small arteries or arterioles
- Other histologic features include fibrin-rich edema or lymphocyte infiltration, scattered isolated giant cells, sarcoidlike granulomas, and foci of fibrosis
- Eosinophilic microabscesses (containing Charcot-Leyden crystals) may be present
- Large bronchi may have changes of chronic asthma with eosinophils, mucous cell hyperplasia, and a prominent eosinophilic basement membrane
- Lesions in the upper airway typically characterized by edematous mucositis and rhinorrhea; ulcerating destructive lesions unusual
- Renal disease tends to be mild without crescents in the glomeruli or areas of fibrinoid necrosis

Special Stains

- Elastic tissue stains can confirm the presence of focal destruction of internal elastic lamina and intimal thickening characteristic of longstanding or healed arteritis

Immunohistochemistry/Immunohistochemical Assay

- Either c-ANCA or p-ANCA can be detected in patients with ANCA-associated small vessel vasculitis
- Patients with microscopic polyangiitis and Churg-Strauss syndrome typically positive for p-ANCA (anti-myeloperoxidase)

Electron Microscopy

- Not helpful

Differential Diagnosis

- True vasculitis versus reaction to inflammation in surrounding tissue
- Self-limited, benign vasculitis versus systemic vasculitis
- Vasculitides involving small vessels have a considerable overlap in histologic appearance
- Wegener granulomatosis may be difficult to differentiate from lymphomatoid granulomatosis and Churg-Strauss syndrome
- Churg-Strauss syndrome resembles eosinophilic pneumonia and Wegner granulomatosis

Treatment

- Corticosteroids and, occasionally, cytotoxic drugs if symptoms of systemic vasculitis present

Prognosis

- Patients typically experience a full recovery with steroid therapy
- Relapse may occur and is occasionally fatal

Associations

- Chronic asthma

Microscopic Polyangiitis

Clinical Manifestations

- A hypersensitivity reaction that primarily involves small vessels of skin, mucous membranes, lungs, brain, heart, gastrointestinal tract, kidneys, and muscle
- 90% have necrotizing glomerulonephritis
- Pulmonary involvement in the form of capillaritis common
- Typical clinical picture includes hemoptysis, hematuria, proteinuria, abdominal pain, gastrointestinal tract bleeding, and muscle pain or weakness

Inflammatory Lesions>Vasculitis: Microscopic Polyangiitis, Henoch-Schönlein Purpura

- If the lesions limited to skin, condition referred to as *cutaneous leukocytoclastic vasculitis*
- No immune deposits
- 80% of patients ANCA positive (usually p-ANCA)

Gross and Microscopic Pathology

- Lesions similar to those of polyarteritis nodosa except large muscular arteries not typically involved
- Affected vessels have segmental fibrinoid necrosis involving the media
- Occasionally the inflammatory infiltrate is limited to neutrophils, which tend to fragment along the vessel wall (leukocytoclasia)

Special Stains

- Elastic tissue stains confirm the presence of focal destruction of internal elastic lamina and intimal thickening characteristic of longstanding or healed arteritis

Immunohistochemistry/Immunohistochemical Assay

- Patients with microscopic polyangiitis and Churg-Strauss syndrome typically positive for p-ANCA (anti-myeloperoxidase)

Electron Microscopy

- Not helpful

Differential Diagnosis

- True vasculitis versus reaction to inflammation in surrounding tissue
- Self-limited, benign vasculitis versus systemic vasculitis
- Vasculitides involving small vessels have a considerable overlap in histologic appearance

Treatment

- Removal of the antigen causing the hypersensitivity reaction

Prognosis

- Patients with isolated cutaneous disease usually respond to removal of the causative agent
- Patients with systemic disease may progress to organ failure

Associations

- none

Henoch-Schönlein Purpura

Clinical Manifestations

- Typically seen in children between ages of 3 and 8
- A syndrome consisting of:
  - □ Purpuric skin lesions involving extensor surfaces of arms and legs as well as buttocks
  - □ Abdominal pain, vomiting, and intestinal bleeding
  - □ Nonmigratory arthralgia
  - □ Renal abnormalities
- 30% have a history of hypersensitivity secondary to hereditary influences; onset of disease frequently follows an upper respiratory tract infection
- 30% have renal signs and symptoms: gross or microscopic hematuria, proteinuria, and nephrotic syndrome
- Occasionally adults will develop a rapidly progressive form of glomerulonephritis with crescents
- IgA deposited in the mesangium of glomeruli in a pattern similar to that seen in IgA nephropathy (IgA nephropathy and Henoch-Schönlein purpura may be manifestations of the same disease)

Gross and Microscopic Pathology

- Skin involvement characterized by subepidermal hemorrhages as a result of a necrotizing vasculitis involving small vessels of the dermis
- IgA immune deposits present in small vessels
- Renal involvement varies from a mild focal mesangial proliferation to a diffuse mesangial proliferation to a typical glomerulonephritis with crescents
- Immunofluorescence done on a biopsy specimen from an involved kidney confirms the presence of IgA deposits and sometimes IgG and C3 in the mesangium

Special Stains

- Elastic tissue stains can confirm the presence of focal destruction of internal elastic lamina and intimal thickening characteristic of longstanding or healed arteritis

Immunohistochemistry/Immunohistochemical Assay

- IgA immune deposits can be found in the small vessels of patients with Henoch-Schönlein purpura

Electron Microscopy

- Not helpful

Differential Diagnosis

- True vasculitis versus reaction to inflammation in surrounding tissue
- Self-limited, benign vasculitis versus systemic vasculitis
- Vasculitides involving small vessels have a considerable overlap in histologic appearance

Treatment

- Management of renal manifestations if present

Prognosis

- Children have an excellent prognosis
- Patients with diffuse lesions or nephrotic syndrome have a poorer prognosis; renal failure tends to occur in those with crescentic lesions

Associations

- IgA immune deposits in small vessels

Cutaneous Leukocytoclastic Vasculitis

Clinical Manifestations

- A microscopic polyangiitis that involves arterioles, capillaries, and postcapillary venules in skin of lower leg; no associated systemic vasculitis or glomerulonephritis
- Classic clinical manifestation is palpable purpura
- Frequently patients have a history of exposure to an antigen such as drugs (penicillin), microorganisms (streptococci), heterologous proteins, or tumor antigens

Microscopic polyangiitis limited to skin

Gross and Microscopic Pathology

- Findings of microscopic polyangiitis confined to the dermis

Special Stains

- Elastic tissue stains can confirm the presence of focal destruction of internal elastic lamina and intimal thickening characteristic of longstanding or healed arteritis

Treatment

- Removal of offending antigen

Prognosis

- Excellent prognosis with removal of responsible antigen

Associations

- No immune deposits

References

Burke A, Virmani R. *Tumors of the Heart and Great Vessels: Atlas of Tumor Pathology, 3rd Series, Fascicle 16.* Washington, DC: Armed Forces Institute of Pathology, 1996.

Dabbs DJ. *Diagnostic Immunohistochemistry*. New York: Churchill Livingstone, 2002.

Kumar V, Abbas AK, Fausto N (eds.) *Robbins and Cotran Pathologic Basis of Disease. 7th ed.* Philadelphia: Elsevier Saunders, 2005.

Mills S, Carter D, Greenson JK, Oberman HA, Reuter V, Stoler MH (eds). *Sternberg's Diagnostic Surgical Pathology. 4th ed.* Philadelphia: Lippincott Williams & Wilkins, 2004.

Rosai J. *Rosai and Ackerman's Surgical Pathology. 9th ed.* St. Louis: Mosby, 2004.

Travis WD, Brambililla E, Muller-Hermelink HK, Harris CC (eds). *World Health Organization Classification of Tumours: Pathology and Genetics—Tumours of the Lung, Pleura, Thymus and Heart.* Lyon, France: IARC Press, 2004.

Chapter 2

Central Nervous System

Intraoperative Consultation

The 2 biggest challenges the pathologist faces during an intraoperative consultation on a central nervous system (CNS) lesion are the miniscule size of the specimen and the vast number of histologic patterns that might be encountered. In most instances the main role of the pathologist is to confirm whether adequate, diagnostic, non-necrotic tissue samples have been obtained. Sometimes a generic diagnosis will be enough to allow the operating surgeon to make decisions concerning the extent of resection based on a combination of gross findings such as anatomic site, size, and degree of circumscription. Classic examples that fall into this category are the gliomas. Astrocytomas, oligodendrogliomas, and mixed gliomas are all treated in a similar fashion; hence a more specific diagnosis is not usually required.

There are times when the pathologist must make a specific rather than a general diagnosis because that diagnosis will profoundly affect the operative treatment of the patient. Perhaps the most important, if not the most frequent, situation is one in which the patient is suspected of having a pilocytic astrocytoma. A pilocytic astrocytoma must be differentiated from a low-grade infiltrating glioma because it is treated with complete surgical resection whenever possible; infiltrating gliomas are treated with less than complete removal. Ependymoma must be differentiated from pilocytic astrocytoma in the spinal cord and from nonpilocytic astrocytoma

Generally accepted indications for intraoperative consultation include the following:

1. ***Confirming that sufficient diagnostic tissue has been obtained.*** It is important for both the surgeon and pathologist to realize that abnormal tissue does not always mean that a representative tissue sample has been obtained. For example, a biopsy specimen taken from the gliotic edge of an abscess may mimic a low-grade glioma. Whenever the entire surgical specimen is submitted for frozen section, additional tissue adjacent to the biopsy site should be submitted for permanent sections.
2. ***Helping the operating surgeon to determine the extent of resection in the case of certain neoplasms.*** High-grade astrocytomas, for example, are typically treated by wider resection than other neoplasms (eg, lymphoma).
3. ***Occasionally requiring a frozen section to determine immediate postoperative treatment.*** Confirmation of an abscess on frozen section will affect treatment literally within hours of the operation.
4. ***Determining the nature of an unexpected lesion at the time of resection of a large portion of brain.*** An example of this would be when a portion of the temporal lobe is removed in cases of epilepsy and a subtle neoplasm is found.

An intraoperative consultation to evaluate surgical margins after the resection of a glioma is of little practical value. The absence of identifiable neoplastic cells at a surgical margin in no way ensures against a tumor recurrence.

It can be of some help to the pathologist to know the incidence of the most common brain tumors as a function of location and age of the patient.

Astrocytomas, ependymomas, and oligodendrogliomas are the most frequent tumors in the cerebral hemispheres in children. In adults the most common tumors to occur in the cerebral hemispheres are astrocytoma, meningioma, metastatic carcinoma, and oligodendroglioma. Medulloblastoma, astrocytoma, and dermoid cyst are the 3 most common tumors to occur in the cerebellum of a child. In an adult, hemangiomas, metastatic carcinoma, astrocytoma, and medulloblastoma are most frequent in the cerebellum. Astrocytoma is the most common tumor to occur in the brainstem of both children and adults. Ependymoma and chorioid plexus papilloma are the 2 most common lesions to occur at the cerebellopontine angle in children. In adults the most common tumor to occupy the cerebellopontine angle is a schwannoma followed by meningioma, epidermoid cyst, choroid plexus papilloma, and glomus jugulare tumor. A craniopharyngioma is the most common tumor to occupy the sella turcica in a child; in an adult a pituitary adenoma is more common than a craniopharyngioma. Both children and adults develop germ cell tumors in this location. The suprasellar/third ventricle/optic chiasm region in a child is most frequently occupied by a pilocytic astrocytoma or an ependymoma. In an adult this area is more frequently involved with a meningioma or an astrocytoma. Pilocytic astrocytoma, oligodendroglioma, ependymoma, and colloid cyst also occur in this location in adults.

A number of specific clinical and pathologic issues represent potential pitfalls of an intraoperative consultation on a CNS lesion. Many of these problems can be avoided if the pathologist is aware of the results of the diagnostic studies that led to the operative procedure as well as the intraoperative findings.

1. ***Primary neoplasm versus metastatic neoplasm.*** The major problem in this area is differentiating a metastatic amelanotic melanoma from a high-grade glioma. Both lesions may have an infiltrating border, and amelanotic melanoma tumor cells on frozen section may have abundant eosinophilic cytoplasm that mimics the cytoplasm of a gemistocytic astrocytoma.
2. ***Recurrent glioma after irradiation therapy.*** Radiation induces necrosis, can induce marked nuclear atypia, and can stimulate the formation of markedly atypical reactive gliosis. All 3 of these features are present in high-grade gliomas. The necrosis seen in a glioblastoma multiforme (GBM) is usually surrounded by pseudopalisading tumor cell; this is not the case in radiation-induced necrosis. Radiation-induced atypia in normal tissue does not have the cellularity that is typically associated with a neoplasm. The vascular changes of irradiated tissue usually consist of fibrinoid necrosis, telangiectasis and fibrous thickening; the vascular changes of a high-grade glioma are those of endothelial proliferation with "glomeruloid" capillary structures and fibrinoid thrombi.
3. ***GBM by definition can have numerous histologic appearances.*** Necrosis can be quite extensive. The periphery of the lesion may mimic or actually be a low-grade glioma.
4. ***Non-neoplastic gliotic lesion versus low-grade astrocytoma.*** Astrocytomas and areas of gliosis are more cellular than normal brain. The determination of what constitutes hypercellularity is subjective at best. The presence of microcystic change is helpful because such a finding points strongly toward an astrocytoma. Microcystic change is rarely seen in gliosis.
5. ***Pilocytic astrocytoma.*** As mentioned earlier, pilocytic astrocytomas must be distinguished from other low-grade infiltrating gliomas. Pilocytic astrocytomas are characterized by spindled cells and microcystic change in the presence of Rosenthal fibers. Tumor cells may be pleomorphic. The cytoplasm of the tumor cells may be granular (occasionally best seen on cytologic preparations). In addition, pilocytic astrocytomas are more common in young patients, tend to have a cystic component, and are well-circumscribed.
6. ***Glioma versus primary CNS lymphoma.*** GBM and primary CNS lymphoma may appear quite similar on frozen section. They both may have foci of necrosis, be hypercellular, and have an infiltrating pattern. The vascular changes of a GBM are typically those of endothelial hyperplasia with glomeruloid changes; lymphomas tend to have an angiocentric pattern with infiltration of vessel walls by neoplastic lymphocytes.
7. ***Glioma versus infarct.*** Infarcts are characterized by the presence of shrunken brightly eosinophilic neurons that represent anoxic or ischemic changes. In addition, infarcts usually have a vascular proliferation that resembles that of granulation tissue.
8. ***Intraventricular tumors.*** Most are treated in the same way. The differential diagnosis includes ependymoma, meningioma, subependymoma, choroid plexus papilloma, and neurocytoma.
9. ***Tumors of the cerebellopontine angle.*** In an adult such a lesion is usually either a schwannoma or meningioma. Occasionally an exophytic pontine glioma may be present, and is an unexpected finding to the operating surgeon. Gliomas in this location are indistinguishable on imaging studies from the more common schwannoma or meningioma.
10. ***Pituitary lesions.*** Pituitary adenomas have a monomorphic population of cells. A normal pituitary has a variegated population of cells. The cells of an adenoma tend to have a sheetlike or papillary architecture with loss of the normal organoid pattern that is characteristic of a normal pituitary gland.

Craniopharyngiomas may cause a problem on frozen sections if a peripheral tissue specimen is obtained from the lesion. Tissue specimens taken from an area close to a craniopharyngioma may show marked gliosis with abundant Rosenthal fibers that can mimic an astrocytoma. In addition, nests of squamous cells typical of a craniopharyngioma may be present in reactive glial tissue near the lesion and mimic a well-differentiated metastatic squamous cell carcinoma.

Specimen Handling

Most neuropathologists prefer that cytologic preparations be made on all CNS lesions submitted for frozen section. Squashed and smear preparations are generally superior to touch preparations. High-quality cytologic preparations can be of benefit in establishing the proper diagnosis when the differential diagnosis includes primary glial neoplasm, metastatic tumor, and lymphoma. Tissue conservation is frequently a major priority for neuropathologists.

If the tissue specimen submitted is sufficient, it may be prudent to place a small portion in glutaraldehyde in anticipation of the need for electron microscopy.

Astrocytic Tumors

Anaplastic Astrocytoma

Clinical Manifestations

- An astrocytoma intermediate in differentiation between a well-differentiated fibrillary astrocytoma and glioblastoma multiforme (GBM)
- Most involve cerebral hemispheres
- Typically occur in 5th decade
- Lesions involving pons usually occur in children

Gross Pathology

- Usually produce an easily recognized mass; may be firm or soft
- Involvement of the cortex causes firmness, pallor, and expansion of overlying gyri

Microscopic Pathology

- Highly cellular lesions with nuclear atypia with or without mitotic figures
- Mirovascular proliferation is a typical feature (as it is with GBM)
- More cellularity, nuclear pleomorphism, and hyperchromasia of the neoplastic cells than in well-differentiated fibrillary astrocytoma, but less cellularity and necrosis than in GBM
- Mitotic figures usually present, but may be scant
- Microcysts rarely present (presence of microcysts usually indicates a more differentiated astrocytoma, a pilocytic astrocytoma, or oligodendroglioma)
- A gemistocytic component may be present
- Lesions with a significant gemistocytic component may have foci of glioblastoma

Special Stains

- Not helpful

Immunohistochemistry

- Tumor cells typically positive for both glial fibrillary acidic protein (GFAP) and S-100 protein
- Tumor cells express vimentin (little or no diagnostic significance)
- MIB-1(Ki67 antigen) often helpful

Electron Microscopy

- Astrocytes have cytoplasmic filaments and multidirectional processes

Molecular Alterations

- None

Differential Diagnosis

- Demyelinating lesions
- Progressive multifocal leukoencephalopathy (PML) especially in the setting of immunosuppression and acquired immunodeficiency syndrome (AIDS)
- Oligodendroglioma
- Astrocytic tumor of either lower (astrocytoma) or higher (glioblastoma) grade; anaplastic astrocytoma histologically lies between well-differentiated astrocytoma and glioblastoma

Treatment

- Surgical excision and radiotherapy
- Interstitial radiation for recurrent disease
- Chemotherapy seems to play more of a role in treatment than it does for glioblastoma

Prognosis

- Median survival following surgery and radiation approximately 2 to 3 years
- Favorable prognostic factors include young age, extensive resection, and little anaplasia

Associations

- None

Astrocytoma

Clinical Manifestations

- A diffusely infiltrative neoplasm of fibrillary astrocytes

- Tends to occur in young to middle-aged adults and involve the cerebral hemispheres
- Tends to involve the brainstem in children
- Typically produces nonspecific symptoms as a result of mass effect, seizures, and neurologic deficits; seizures are more common than functional deficits (result of parenchymal destruction)
- Neoplasms in the brainstem produce symptoms relative to involvement of cranial nerve nuclei and compression of sensory and motor tracts traversing the pons or medulla

Gross Pathology

- Initially, deep-seated neoplasm may not cause any gross abnormality
- Usually an ill-defined expansion of white matter, which may blur the typically well-demarcated gray-white junction
- More advanced lesions tend to expand white matter
- Cut surface reveals a variable texture; some are firm; others are soft (almost gelatinous)
- Intralesional cysts filled with clear fluid may be present
- Lesions of the brainstem are usually centered in the pons, which may undergo hypertrophy resulting in expansion of the pons posteriorly and superiorly toward the fourth ventricle, often resulting in obstruction of cerebrospinal fluid flow
- Lesions in the spinal cord characteristically produce an ill-defined fusiform enlargement

Microscopic Pathology

- Typically a hypercellular lesion with indistinct margins centered in white matter
- An infiltrative growth pattern overruns or incorporates preexisting axons, oligodendrocytes, and astrocytes
- Tumor cells usually irregularly distributed (in contrast to the ordered and regimented composition of normal white matter)
- There is marked variation in the amount and shape of tumor cell cytoplasm:
- Paucicellular lesions have tumor cells with scant cytoplasm (typically appear as "naked nuclei")
- Classic cellular lesions have short cellular processes (fibrillary astrocytoma)
- A minority have cells with abundant round eosinophilic cytoplasm (gemistocytic); such cells closely resemble reactive astrocytes (gemistocytic astrocytoma)
- Microcystic spaces consisting of round fluid-filled cavities characterize both gliomas of astrocytic and oligodendroglial type; microcyst formation usually indicates the presence of a well-differentiated or low-grade lesion
- Perivascular lymphocytes usually present particularly in tumors of the gemistocytic type; nuclei of small well-differentiated neoplasms tend to be round or oval with little hyperchromasia
- Nuclei in more typical astrocytomas tend to be elongated, irregular, and hyperchromatic
- Prominent nucleoli are very rare in fibrillary astrocytomas; small nucleoli are common in gemistocytic tumors
- Mitoses are never seen
- Microvascular proliferation absent
- Foci of cartilage rarely present
- Rosenthal fibers may be present at the periphery (more common in gemistocytic variant than in the diffuse or fibrillary variant); much more commonly found in pilocytic astrocytomas

Special Stains

- Mucicarmine can highlight the mucin content of microcystic spaces, but diagnosis is fairly straightforward on routine hematoxylin-eosin (H&E) staining

Immunohistochemistry

- Tumor cells of fibrillary astrocytomas have cytoplasmic positivity for GFAP; gemistocytic astrocytomas have cytoplasmic positivity for GFAP which is best appreciated at periphery
- Most tumor cells are reactive for S-100 protein, vimentin, and cytokeratin
- Ki-67 proliferation index usually $<2\%$

Electron Microscopy

- Most tumor cells show astrocytic differentiation with cytoplasmic filaments and multidirectional processes

- Gemistocytic cells have aligned subplasmalemmal filaments and jumbled filaments among organelles in the center of the cell body (correspond to the round eosinophilic cytoplasm seen on H&E)

Molecular Alterations

- Allelic loss on chromosome 17p or chromosome 10

Differential Diagnosis

- Reactive gliosis
- Demyelinating disease
- Cerebral infarct
- Oligodendroglioma
- Fibrillary astrocytic neoplasm of higher grade (anaplastic astrocytoma or glioblastoma multiforme)
- Pilocytic astrocytoma (pilocytic astrocytomas are more common than fibrillary astrocytomas in the optic nerve and the cerebellum; fibrillary astrocytomas are more common than pilocytic astrocytomas in the brainstem; pilocytic and fibrillary astrocytomas occur with equal frequency in the spinal cord)

Treatment

- Total surgical excision; residual disease requires radiation and chemotherapy

Prognosis

- Most patients dead within 10 years
- Tumors tend to progress to a higher grade with time
- Presence of gemistocytes is a poor prognostic sign (many feel that gemistocytic astrocytomas are anaplastic lesions)
- Younger patients with well-differentiated lesions tend to do better than older patients who seem to have a higher likelihood of progression to a high-grade malignancy
- Tumors diagnosed during the 2nd decade of life may remain stable for years
- Lesions in the brainstem frequently undergo malignant degeneration and most patients die within a year
- 5-year survival for lesions involving spinal cord may be as high as 50%

Associations

- None

Glioblastoma Multiforme

Clinical Manifestations

- Most common glioma
- In adults primarily affects cerebral hemispheres; in children primarily affects brainstem (same topographic distribution as diffuse or fibrillary astrocytomas)
- Rarely seen in spinal cord
- Cerebral lesions can occur at any age but usually after the 5th decade of life
- Most are solitary
- Typically present with the abrupt onset of neurologic deficits
- Produce symptoms by both mass effect and tissue destruction
- Occasionally acute hemorrhage will precipitate symptoms

Gross Pathology

- Surface of brain may show expansion of cortical gyri with irregular thickening and discoloration and abnormalities of surface vasculature
- Neoplasm typically has a surrounding gray fleshy rim of variable thickness and a necrotic core, and may be either diffusely infiltrative or fairly well-circumscribed
- Neoplasms tend to spread along compact fiber pathways (corpus callosum, optic radiation, anterior commissure, fornix, and subependymal regions)
- Tumors involving brainstem frequently extend along fiber pathways, that is, middle cerebellar peduncles

Microscopic Pathology

- Neoplasm typically represents a transition from a well-differentiated diffuse astrocytoma, but may appear without an obvious low-grade precursor lesion
- Neoplastic cells vary greatly in size, shape, fibrillary content, and extent of process formation
- Tumor cells tend to have pink cytoplasm, giving them an astrocytic quality

- Highly infiltrative lesions tend to be composed of uniform, small cells that occur in dense aggregates
- 2 most important histologic criteria for the diagnosis are microvascular proliferation, with or without glomeruloids and presence of necrosis
- Small foci of necrosis are frequently surrounded by a radially oriented collar of cells that are slightly smaller than the surrounding neoplastic cells (pseudo-palisading)
- Other tissue patterns include:
  - Tumors composed primarily of giant cells
  - Tumors with a fascicular pattern that resembles sarcoma
  - Tumors that are rich in lipid
  - Tumors that have epithelioid cells with discrete cell borders and resemble carcinoma

Special Stains

- Not helpful

Immunohistochemistry

- Typically tumor cells immunoreactive for GFAP (reactive astrocytes are strongly GFAP positive; tumor cells less so), vimentin, and cytokeratin
- Tumor cells are frequently positive for S-100 protein
- Ki-67 proliferative index usually over 20%

Electron Microscopy

- Obvious astrocytic cells have abundant intermediate filaments; undifferentiated tumor cells have few or no intermediate filaments
- Intracellular junctions tend to be poorly formed

Molecular Alterations

- Nonrandom loss of heterozygosity (LOH) on chromosome 10q
- CDKN2A deletions, PTEN alterations, and EGFR amplification in de novo glioblastomas
- p53 mutations are less common in primary (de novo) GBMs (approximatedly 25% vs 65%)
- Mutations in p53 seen in glioblastomas arising from lower grade astrocytoma

Differential Diagnosis

- Metastatic carcinoma
- Lymphoma

Treatment

- Radiation may have a profound or little therapeutic effect, but any response to radiation usually of short duration
- Recurrence typically appears in the margins of the original tumor bed, but may appear at sites well removed
- Surgical biopsy may need to be performed to establish diagnosis; most tumors are too advanced at the time of diagnosis for surgical excision
- Debulking may be worthwhile
- Recurrent neoplasm is usually treated with interstitial radiation; may extend survival by a year

Prognosis

- Median survival for patients with cerebral glioblastoma is approximately 12 months
- Children have a slightly better prognosis; elderly have a poor prognosis
- Tumors of the giant cell type have a slightly better prognosis
- Neoplasms of the brainstem have a poor prognosis

Associations

- None

Gliomatosis Cerebri

Clinical Manifestations

- A diffusely infiltrative glial tumor that may involve the supratentorial brain, posterior fossa, or intraspinal parenchyma
- Lesion tends to occupy most of a hemisphere and frequently both hemispheres and other adjacent structures in continuity

- Infiltrative component seems out of proportion to both degree of anaplasia of the tumor cells and the cellularity
- Affects patients of all ages

Gross Pathology

- Despite being widely invasive, the lesion often is not discernible on gross examination
- Occasionally a local mass effect will be present and cause neoplastic hypertrophy of affected regions

Microscopic Pathology

- A variably cellular neoplasm with a wide variety of histologic and cytologic features
- Tumor cells can appear quite benign with little or no cytoplasm or as frankly malignant fibrillary astrocytes
- Typically there is little destruction of preexisting parenchyma
- Neoplastic cells tend to accumulate around vessels (angiotropic) and neurons (perineuronal satellitosis), and in subpial and subependymal regions
- Focal areas of anaplastic transformation may be present
- Tumor cell nuclei vary from round to oval to elongated, and have moderately dense chromatin
- Mitotic figures infrequent; vascular proliferation infrequent
- Tumor cells may have discernible cytoplasm on H&E staining, but immunohistochemical stains usually required to see elongated cytoplasmic processes

Special Stains

- Not helpful

Immunohistochemistry

- Cytoplasmic processes of tumor cells occasionally positive for GFAP

Electron Microscopy

- Not helpful

Molecular Alterations

- None

Differential Diagnosis

- Fibrillary, diffuse, or ordinary astrocytoma
- Oligodendroglioma (nuclei tend to be round and have perinuclear halos; neither feature characteristic of tumor cell nuclei of gliomatosis cerebri)

Treatment

- Cannot be cured by surgical excision

Prognosis

- Clinical course quite variable
- Factors associated with more aggressive behavior include the presence of cytologic malignancy and high mitotic activity

Associations

- None

Gliosarcoma

Clinical Manifestations

- Approximately 2% of glioblastomas represent gliosarcoma subtype
- Lesions can occur anywhere in the brain, but tend to occur in the same sites affected by glioblastomas (cerebral hemisphere in adults and brainstem in children)

Gross Pathology

- Generally a discrete dense mass

Microscopic Pathology

- Characterized by the presence of a biphasic population of both malignant glial and malignant mesenchymal cells
- Mesenchymal or sarcomatous component can be quite variable, ranging from well-ordered, densely packed, long bundles of spindled cells arranged in a herringbone pattern typical of a well-differentiated fibrosarcoma to a disorganized and pleomorphic proliferation reminiscent of a malignant histiocytoma
- Usually the lesion has a sarcomatous center and a periphery that is more typical of a glioma; this arrangement suggests that the sarcoma arises as a secondary lesion in the proliferating vasculature of a high-grade glioma

- Mesenchymal cells are topographically related to blood vessels and appear to be arising from vascular or adventitial elements
- Glial component usually typical of a glioblastoma
- In time, the sarcoma component may overgrow the glioma component
- Other lines of mesenchymal differentiation may be present: cartilage, bone, chondroblastic osteosarcoma, smooth muscle, striated muscle, keratinizing squamous cells, and gland formation

Special Stains

- Reticulin and trichrome stains highlight a reticulin network that separates sarcomatous areas from glial areas

Immunohistochemistry

- Glial component immunoreactive for GFAP

Electron Microscopy

- Confirms presence of poorly differentiated cells and cells resembling fibroblasts, histiocytes, and myofibroblasts

Molecular Alterations

- Mutations in p53 may be present

Differential Diagnosis

- Glioblastoma

Treatment

- Surgical excision for accessible lesions

Prognosis

- Sarcomatous component may metastasize to extracranial sites
- Survival same as for glioblastoma
- Occasionally neoplasm will erode through skull and extend into adjacent soft tissue
- Patients younger than 45 years have better prognosis than elderly

Associations

- None

Infantile Desmoplastic Astrocytoma (Desmoplastic Cerebral Astrocytoma of Infancy)

Clinical Manifestations

- A supratentorial glioma typically located on the surface of a hemisphere
- Usually affects children during 1st year of life

Gross Pathology

- Lesion appears as large, firm, flat or globular, gray-white mass, often densely adherent to the surface of the brain, meninges, or dura
- Prominent cystic component may merge with a solid component

Microscopic Pathology

- A hypercellular mass of collagen-rich fibrotic tissue that gives the lesion an intense desmoplastic appearance
- Lesion typically well-demarcated from underlying brain but it will permeate brain along perivascular (Virchow-Robin) spaces
- Scattered elongated glial cells (reminiscent of fibroblasts) enmeshed in the dense collagenous stroma
- Occasionally glial cells arranged in a perivascular, pseudorosette pattern (reminiscent of an ependymoma)
- Focal areas of high cellularity with mitotically active cells with elongated hyperchromatic nuclei may be present (not considered malignant features)

Special Stains

- Trichrome stain highlights dense desmoplasia

Immunohistochemistry

- Neoplastic glial cells intensely positive for GFAP and are present in both desmoplastic and cellular areas

Electron Microscopy

- Astroglial and neuronal cell populations with variable numbers of fibroblasts
- Tumor cells have prominent nuclei with infolded nuclear membranes and variable nucleoli; abundant intermediate filaments

Molecular Alterations

- None

Differential Diagnosis

- Sarcoma
- Malignant glioma
- Gliosarcoma
- Gliofibroma

Treatment

- Total excision

Prognosis

- Long-term survival typical even in subtotally resected lesions

Associations

- None

Pilocytic Astrocytoma

Clinical Manifestations

- Arise anywhere in the neuroaxis
- More common in children and young adults
- Lesions involving the visual system can cause visual loss if arising on the optic nerve or can interfere with both visual acuity and hypothalamic-pituitary function if more centrally located
- Lesions in hypothalamus and region of third ventricle primarily affect children
- Lesions in cerebral hemispheres more common in older patients (young adults); can occur anywhere in the cerebral hemispheres
- Lesions arising in cerebellum have a deceptively circumscribed contour, but microscopically infiltrate surrounding cerebellar tissue; tend to present during the 2nd decade of life with symptoms of cerebellar dysfunction or obstruction of cerebrospinal fluid flow
- Rarely involve brainstem (fibrillary astrocytomas more common in this location)
- May involve spinal cord; patients tend to be younger and have a long history of symptoms

Gross Pathology

- Cerebellar lesions usually well-circumscribed and seem to expand rather than infiltrate; lesions at other sites less well-defined
- Cut surface gray-pink with mucoid degeneration and cysts; tumor may consist of a mural nodule in a large cyst
- Tend to break through pia and fill subarachnoid space

Microscopic Pathology

- Typically lesions consist of stellate astrocytes arranged in microcystic regions alternating with compact areas consisting of elongated and highly fibrillated cells (a biphasic combination of microcystic and compact areas)
- Cystic areas frequently contain brightly eosinophilic granular bodies
- Tumor cells may contain protein droplets and granular bodies, the former are eosinophilic hyaline globules; the latter are eosinophilic structures that are rounder and more finely granular than protein droplets (also seen in pleomorphic xanthoastrocytoma and ganglion cell tumors)
- Markedly hyalinized vessels may be present; suggestive of a vascular malformation
- Vascular proliferation common and may be quite prominent in the walls of cysts where they have a glomeruloid appearance
- Occasionally tumors have areas in which the nuclei are clustered together
- Tumors in the cerebellum and cerebrum often have multinucleated giant cells with peripherally oriented nuclei
- Solid areas may have a lobular appearance

Astrocytic Tumors>Pilocytic Astrocytoma

- Cells in the microcystic areas tend to have round nuclei while the cells in the more solid areas tend to have spindled nuclei
- Rosenthal fibers often seen in cellular areas especially in cerebellar lesions
- Perivascular irradiating processes reminiscent of an ependymoma may be present
- Occasionally prominent collagenous septa may be present
- Some neoplasms have a mucinous background instead of microcysts
- Tumor cell nuclei tend to be monomorphic with delicate chromatin (longstanding tumors may be more pleomorphic)
- Mitotic figures typically rare except in infants
- Tumors of cerebellum frequently have focal areas that resemble oligodendroglioma
- Tumor cells frequently extend into perivascular spaces

Special Stains

- Both protein droplets and granular bodies seen in neoplastic cells are periodic acid-Schiff (PAS) positive
- Rosenthal fibers appear bright red on Masson trichrome stain

Immunohistochemistry

- Tumor cells GFAP positive (cells in microcystic spongy tissue less strongly positive than those in more solid areas)
- Surface of a Rosenthal fiber immunoreactive for GFAP; body of a Rosenthal fiber reactive for $\alpha\beta$-crystallin
- Eosinophilic granular bodies reactive for GFAP, $\alpha\beta$-crystallin, ubiquitin, α_1-antichymotrypsin, and α_1-antitrypsin

Electron Microscopy

- Tumor cells from the densely cellular areas packed with intermediate filaments; tumor cells from microcystic zones contain few filaments
- Rosenthal fibers are nonfilamentous electron-dense masses surrounded by intermediate or glial filaments
- Granular bodies are intermediate, presumably glial, filaments

Molecular Alterations

- Trisomy 7 and 8 (30%)

Differential Diagnosis

- Fibrillary or diffuse astrocytoma (very important to distinguish pilocytic astrocytoma from fibrillary astrocytoma; former much less likely to invade or undergo malignant degeneration and is much more like to be resectable)
- Pleomorphic xanthoastrocytoma
- Ganglion cell tumor
- Dense chronic pilocytic gliosis

Treatment

- Surgical resection

Prognosis

- Neoplasms at any site typically grow slowly; incompletely resected tumors often grow little if at all
- Lesions involving anterior optic nerve, cerebrum, and cerebellum associated with an excellent prognosis
- Tumors in chiasmatic/hypothalamic region more likely to recur and result in a fatal outcome
- Lesions of spinal cord usually amenable to gross total surgical excision
- Tumors may undergo malignant degeneration as a function of time or as a result of previously administered radiotherapy

Associations

- 15% of patients with neurofibromatosis type 1 (NF-1) have multifocal pilocytic astrocytomas of optic nerve
- 30% of patients with pilocytic astrocytomas of optic nerve have NF-1

Pleomorphic Xanthoastrocytoma

Clinical Manifestations

- Typically affect adolescents and young adults who present with a long history of seizures
- Lesion frequently involves very superficial portion of the gyri of the temporal lobe; less frequently parietal region

Gross Pathology

- Typically a firm, well-circumscribed nodule or plaque overlying a cyst filled with clear fluid
- Occasionally appears to lie entirely outside brain parenchyma
- Usually well circumscribed, but deep portions often infiltrate adjacent brain
- On cut section, primarily yellow-orange with foci of hemorrhage

Microscopic Pathology

- A closely packed pleomorphic population of cells with abundant pink cytoplasm
- Pleomorphic cells vary in shape from round to spindled, and contain large, multilobed or multiple hyperchromatic nuclei
- Despite marked pleomorphism, few mitotic figures and absence of necrosis (presence of mitotic activity and necrosis indicate a malignant transformation)
- Cytoplasm frequently has a glassy or fibrillar "astrocytic" appearance; accumulation of lipid droplets in the cytoplasm gives tumor cells a vacuolated appearance, but a variable finding
- Neoplasm tends to mushroom from cortical surface, extend horizontally in the subarachnoid space, and surround cortical vessels in perivascular (Virchow-Robin) spaces
- Foci or diffuse areas of intercellular reticulin usually evident at low power
- Variable vascular hyalinization and foci of perivascular lymphocytic infiltrates common
- Cells from superficial portion of the lesion may contain eosinophilic granular bodies (a feature of slowly growing glial neoplasms including pilocytic astrocytoma and ganglion cell tumors). Cells deeper in the lesion (infiltrative portion) are typically less pleomorphic than those on the surface

Special Stains

- Reticulin stains highlight intercellular distribution of reticulin in nodular areas

Immunohistochemistry

- Both superficial and infiltrating components of tumor are immunoreactive for GFAP

Electron Microscopy

- Some tumor cells have intermediate filaments; others have occasional lysosomes or lipid droplets
- Lesions corresponding to granular bodies may be seen
- Typically there is little collagen

Molecular Alterations

- None

Differential Diagnosis

- Anaplastic fibrillary astrocytoma
- Glioblastoma with giant cells
- Malignant fibrous histiocytoma
- Pilocytic astrocytoma
- Ganglion cell tumor
- Hemangioma
- Vascular malformation (especially on imanging)

Treatment

- Gross total surgical removal
- Adjuvant radiotherapy of questionable benefit

Prognosis

- A less aggressive lesion)may undergo spontaneous transformation to an anaplastic neoplasm
- Lesions may recur and when they do they usually have increased cellularity and mitotic activity (malignant transformation)
- Recurrence is associated with rapid demise

Associations

- Rarely pleomorphic astrocytomas may be part of a combination tumor in which they form the glioma portion of a ganglioglioma

Subependymal Giant Cell Astrocytoma (Tuberous Sclerosis)

Clinical Manifestations

- Limited to the region of the foramen of Monro (midline channels connecting lateral ventricles to third ventricle)
- Present with clinical symptoms of increased intracranial pressure
- Usually seen in patients with tuberous sclerosis

Gross Pathology

- Typically arises in the wall of the lateral ventricle as a bulky, exophytic, smooth, domelike, broad-based mass that may cross the midline and produce marked dilatation of lateral ventricles
- Cut surface soft to firm, gray, and gritty (calcification)

Microscopic Pathology

- Usually demarcated or minimally infiltrative and characterized by marked microscopic variation
- Tumor cells have a somewhat vesicular or whorled appearance and appear to sweep from blood vessels in a perivascular pseudorosettelike manner
- Tumor cells have abundant glassy eosinophilic cytoplasm and eccentric nuclei; cytoplasmic processes arise from the cell surface opposite the nucleus (reactive astrocytes have a similar appearance but cellular processes are more symmetric and arise uniformly from the entire circumference of the cell)
- Tumor cells may be either multipolar or bipolar, and possess a very eosinophilic cytoplasm with a bluish tint (resemble neurons)
- Nuclei tend to have vesicular chromatin, distinct nucleoli, and occasionally intranuclear cytoplasmic inclusions
- Mitotic activity can be quite variable
- Calcospherites and vascular calcifications frequent
- Scattered mast cells usually present
- Vascular proliferation and necrosis both uncommon

Special Stains

- Large cells of tubers often weakly positive for PAS

Immunohistochemistry

- Tumor cells usually diffusely positive for S-100 protein and focally or weakly positive for GFAP
- Giant cell astrocytes positive for αβ-crystallin

Electron Microscopy

- Neoplastic cells have variable numbers of intermediate filaments
- Most cells lack features of neuronal differentiation, secretory granules, vesicles, and synapses, but cytoplasmic processes may contain microtubles

Molecular Alterations

- Genes responsible for tuberous sclerosis located on chromosomes 9q34 and 16p

Differential Diagnosis

- Gemistocytic astrocytoma

Treatment

- Surgical excision of as much of the neoplasm as possible, residual neoplasm grows slowly

Prognosis

- Long-term survival is excellent although recurrence can occur
- Malignant transformation to GBM unusual, unlike gemistocytic astrocytoma

Associations

- Tuberous sclerosis (Bourneville disease or epiloia): Clinical combination of cutaneous lesions, epilepsy (90%), and mental retardation (60%-70%)
  - *Cutaneous lesions* (adenoma sebaceum, subungual fibroma, shagreen patch, fibrous forehead plaques, patches of depigmentation, and café-au-lait spots similar to those of neurofibromatosis)
  - *Ocular lesions* include retinal astrocytic hamartomas (present in 50%)
  - *Visceral abnormalities* include renal angiomyolipoma, cardiac rhabdomyoma, pulmonary lymphangiomatosis, renal cortical cysts, renal cell carcinoma, splenic and hepatic angiomas, and fibrous dysplasia of bone

- *Intracranial lesions* include tubers, subependymal hamartoma, and giant cell astrocytoma
- Subependymal hamartoma probably a precursor lesion to giant cell astrocytoma
- Tubers are firm, pale, raised cortical lesions characterized by scattered large cells with large nuclei and glassy eosinophilic cytoplasm that have morphologic features of both astrocytes and neurons; typical cortical lamination disturbed; extensive gliosis and abundant calcospherites almost always present; reactive astrocytes tend to be concentrated in the superficial cortex and around blood vessels

Choroid Plexus Tumors

Choroid Plexus Papilloma and Carcinoma

Clinical Manifestations

- In children neoplasms typically arise in lateral ventricles and occasionally 3rd ventricle; in adults most often arise in 4th ventricle or its lateral recess
- Depending on location, neoplasm can obstruct cerebrospinal fluid flow and produce hydrocephalus
- Carcinomas usually invasive and may disseminate or metastasize

Gross Pathology

- Papillomas are well-circumscribed and lobular; often indent adjacent brain along a broad pushing front (no actual invasion); tend to have a cauliflowerlike surface and may be extensively calcified
- Carcinomas usually invasive and typically solid, fleshy, and hemorrhagic
- Both papillomas and carcinomas tend to be very vascular

Microscopic Pathology

- A wide morphologic spectrum of differentiation from well-differentiated papilloma to anaplastic carcinoma
- *Papillomas* are well-differentiated, with an orderly layer of columnar epithelium resting on a continuous basement membrane lining delicate fibrovascular stalks; neoplastic cells tend to be crowded and columnar, and display nuclear pleomorphism and hyperchromasia; not as "cobblestoned" as normal choroid plexus cells; stromal calcification (psammoma bodies) and xanthomatous change may be present
- *Atypical papillomas* are characterized by cytologic atypia, increased nuclear-cytoplasmic ratios, scattered mitotic figures, and nests of cells that penetrate the basement membrane into the underlying stroma
- *Carcinoma* characterized by an even greater degree of atypia and brisk mitotic activity; tumors are typically highly cellular with architecturally complex glands, cribriform arrangements, and poorly formed papillae
- *Undifferentiated tumors* characterized by sheets of neoplastic cells with no appreciable pattern

Special Stains

- None

Immunohistochemistry

- Most tumor cells of papillomas stain positively for cytokeratins, S-100 protein, and vimentin
- Occasionally tumor cells will be GFAP positive
- Tumor cells of carcinomas are cytokeratin positive, but have reduced positivity for S-100 protein
- Tumor cells of both papillomas and carcinomas are immunoreactive for prealbumin (transthyretin)

Electron Microscopy

- Papillomas resemble normal choroid plexus: Tumor cells sit on a basal lamina, contain intermediate filaments, have apical microvilli, scattered cilia, and lateral desmosomes
- Many of the features seen in papilloma are also seen in carcinoma

Molecular Alterations

- None

Differential Diagnosis

- Normal choroid plexus
- Papillary ependymoma
- Papilloma versus atypical papilloma versus carcinoma

- If choroid plexus carcinoma:
    - Embryonal tumors (especially medulloepithelioma)
    - Malignant ependymoma
    - Germ cell tumors (especially epithelial: embryonal carcinoma, endodermal sinus tumor, and immature teratoma)

Treatment

- Well-differentiated papillomas surgically resected
- Carcinomas treated with gross total resection with adjuvant radiotherapy and chemotherapy

Prognosis

- Papillomas can undergo malignant transformation
- Atypical papillomas can be treated with surgery and may act more like papillomas than carcinomas
- Carcinomas are likely to recur (usually within months), and tend to disseminate and may even metastasize outside the CNS

Associations

- None

Embryonal Tumors

Atypical Teratoid/Rhabdoid Tumor

Clinical Manifestations

- Affects infants and children; 95% <5 years at diagnosis
- Most patients are male
- Found in posterior fossa 50% (cerebellum, cerebellopontine angle, and/or brainstem), supratentorial 40% (cerebral or suprasellar), pineal 5%, spinal 2%, multifocal 2%
- Infants present with failure to thrive, lethargy, and vomiting
- Specific signs include paresis of cranial nerves VI and VII
- Computed tomography (CT) findings similar to medulloblastoma

Gross Pathology

- Gross findings similar to medulloblastoma
- Bulky, mass lesion with areas of hemorrhage and necrosis on cut section
- Mesenchymal areas appear firm and tan-white

Microscopic Pathology

- A malignant CNS tumor composed of rhabdoid cells, with or without areas resembling a classic primitive neuroectoermal tumor (PNET), epithelial tissue, and neoplastic mesenchyme
- 65% have a major small cell embryonal component, 30% a mesenchymal component in combination with rhabdoid cells with or without small cell embryonal areas, 25% have neoplastic epithelium
- Rhabdoid cells have a typical look with eccentric nuclei and prominent nucleoli; cytoplasm has fine granular homogeneous texture, or may contain a poorly defined denser pink body that resembles an inclusion; cell borders usually distinct; mitotic figures typically numerous; some rhabdoid cells are small and have a tapering cytoplasmic tail while others are very large and bizarre, and have >1 nucleus
- Mesenchymal areas have loose or compact arrangements of small spindle cells (the latter may resemble a sarcoma
- Epithelial component may have adenomatous pattern or resemble squamous epithelium
- Both areas of necrosis and hemorrhage common

Special Stains

- Not helpful

Immunohistochemistry

- Rhabdoid cells have prominent cytoplasmic staining for vimentin and express epithelial membrane antigen (EMA); smooth muscle actin (SMA) staining is not reliable; GFAP, neurofilament protein (NFP), and cytokeratin may be expressed; no expression for desmin or any markers for germ cell tumor
- Small embryonal cells may express vimentin, GFAP, NFP, and desmin
- Mesenchymal cells are vimentin positive and occasionally positive for SMA and desmin

- Epithelial cells express keratin
- MIB-1 shows growth fraction of up to 80%

Electron Microscopy

- Masses of intermediate filaments common

Molecular Alterations

- 90% have monosomy or deletion of chromosome 22

Differential Diagnosis

- Medulloblastoma

Treatment

- Too few cases

Prognosis

- 30% have metastases throughout CNS at presentation
- Most die within 1 year of diagnosis

Associations

- Relationship between intracranial atypical teratoid/rhabdoid tumors and renal or extrarenal rhabdoid tumor at a non-CNS site yet to be established

Medulloblastoma

Clinical Manifestations

- A small cell neuroectodermal cerebellar tumor
- More common in male than in female patients
- Second most frequent brain tumor in children (pilocytic astrocytoma first); represents 20% of all pediatric CNS neoplasms and 2% of all brain tumors
- Typically affects patients in the first 2 decades of life (mean age at presentation 7½ years)
- Symptoms usually a reflection of cerebellar dysfunction (gait disturbances, nystagmus, and dysmetria), increased intracranial pressure (headache, vomiting, and papilledema) or craniospinal dissemination

Gross Pathology

- Typically a fairly well-circumscribed mass in the vermis (midline of cerebellum); often arises from roof of 4th ventricle and compresses the cerebellar hemispheres
- Calcification uncommon
- Tumors often exit the cerebellum, invade the subarachnoid space, and spread a layer of neoplastic cells on the pial surface; from the subarachnoid space, the tumor can re-enter the cerebellum by way of perivascular (Virchow-Robin) spaces

Microscopic Pathology

- A broad range of histologic features result in several histologic subtypes:
- *Classic (undifferentiated) medulloblastoma*
  - 3 cytologic variants of tumor cells:
    - Cells with little or no discernible cytoplasm and round to slightly oval nuclei (resemble a small lymphocyte)
    - Cells with little cytoplasm and wedge-shaped nuclei in a faint fibrillary background
    - Frankly anaplastic or pleomorphic cells with vesicular chromatin, large nucleoli, and varying amounts of cytoplasm
  - Collagenous stroma may be present
  - Vascular endothelial proliferation present in 20%
  - Necrosis rarely extensive, but may be present as individual cell necrosis
  - Cytologic atypia and mitotic activity are quite variable
- *Medulloblastoma with neuronal/neuroblastic differentiation*
  - Characterized (in decreasing order of frequency) by nodular lucent foci, neuroblastic or Homer-Wright rosettes, mature ganglion cells, and large neoplastic cells with neuronal qualities
  - Nodular medulloblastomas represent a wide spectrum of tumors that vary both in degree and extent of nodular formation and cytologic differentiation
  - Cells in the nodular areas tend to have uniformly bland nuclei with little or no mitotic activity; background tends to be finely fibrillar; cells between the nodules have larger nuclei with coarse chromatin; these cells are typically more hyperchromatic and mitotically active than their intranodular counterparts (more well differentiated)

- A delicate rim of reticulum usually surrounds the nodules of tumor cells
- Tumors with neuroblastic differentiation classically have Homer-Wright rosettes; these tumors are more often diffuse than nodular
- Tumors with neuronal differentiation have ganglion cells (large vesicular nuclei with prominent nucleoli and abundant cytoplasm)

- *Medulloblastoma with glial differentiation*
  - Requires immunohistochemical stains to establish the diagnosis (focal immunopositivity for GFAP)
  - Glial differentiation may be present in many medulloblastomas; glial differentiation typically as isolated glial cells, multiple small cells with unexpected GFAP immunoreactivity or large regions with fibrillar cytoplasm
- *Desmoplastic medulloblastoma*
  - More frequent in adults
  - Typically located in 1 cerebellar hemisphere
  - Characterized by confluent islands of low cellularity in confluent areas of high cellularity and a dense reticulin framework

Special Stains

- Reticulin stains will highlight the presence of abundant reticulin in the internodular areas, its absence in the intranodular areas, and the dense reticulin network in the cellular areas of a desmoplastic medulloblastoma

Immunohistochemistry

- Tumor cells, regardless of pattern, exhibit some degree of immunoreactivity for synaptophysin and neuron-specific enolase (NSE)
- Glial cells in tumors with glial differentiation stain positively for GFAP (reactive astrocytes also GFAP positive)
- Ki-67 index approximately 15%

Electron Microscopy

- Uniform undifferentiated neuroepithelial cells with moderate nuclear pleomorphism, little cytoplasm, few organelles, and many cytoplasmic processes

Molecular Alterations

- 50% have isochromosome 17q (1 chromosome with 2 long arms of chromosome 17)
- Most have amplification of c-*myc*

Differential Diagnosis

- Ependymoma
- Pilocytic astrocytoma (cerebellar astrocytoma)
- Undifferentiated densely cellular malignant glioma (if GFAP staining negative, the lesion likely a medulloblastoma; if tumor cells GFAP positive, lesion could either be a medulloblastoma with glial differentiation or a malignant glioma)
- In infants a cerebellar lesion enters the differential: atypical teratoid rhabdoid tumor

Treatment

- Craniospinal radiotherapy

Prognosis

- 50% survive 5 or more years
- Most recurrences local
- Terminal neuraxis dissemination common
- Occasionally tumors metastasize to extracranial sites: bone, lymph nodes, and lungs
- Factors associated with less favorable prognosis include a high percentage of proliferating cells, nuclear atypia, high mitotic index, necrosis, and lack of cytoplasmic process formation
- Amplification of the c-*myc* oncogene associated with aggressive behavior

Associations

- Malignant rhabdoid tumor of the kidney and Wilms tumor
- *Gorlin syndrome*: An autosomal dominant disorder characterized primarily by skeletal anomalies (including craniomegaly), lamellar calcium deposition in the falx cerebri and diaphragma sellae, cutaneous epidermoid cysts, pits on the palms and soles, odontogenic keratocysts, calcifying ovarian fibromas, multifocal basal cell carcinomas occurring at an early age, medulloblastoma, and meningioma

- *Turcot syndrome*: Central neuroepithelial neoplasms and polyposis coli
- Patients with p53 germline mutations (not as frequent as glioma)
- *Coffin-Sinus syndrome*: Mental and growth retardation, joint laxity, and brachydactyly of 5th digit with absence of nail bed

Retinoblastoma

Clinical Manifestations

- Most common intraocular neoplasm of children
- Typically diagnosed between the ages of 16 months and 2 years
- Approximately 60% are sporadic; 40% are familial (a predisposition to tumor development transmitted as an autosomal dominant pattern)
- Bilaterality and earlier presentations characterize hereditary form of disease
- Usually presents as leukocoria (white pupillary reflex) or less often (35%) as strabismus (when the tumor involves the macula)
- May occur in the pineal gland in patients with bilateral disease

Gross Pathology

- Neoplasm tends to be gray/white with focal areas of necrosis and calcification
- May be endophytic (grow on inner surface of retina into vitreous), exophytic (grow on outer surface of retina toward choroid), or mixed endophytic-exophytic (most common)
- Neoplasm often extends into the vitreous or breaks through the retina to reach the subretinal space
- Advanced tumors penetrate the optic nerve head, enter the surrounding subarachnoid space, extend into orbital soft tissue, and metastasize to different sites
- 90% of familial cases are bilateral

Microscopic Pathology

- A densely cellular neoplasm with foci of necrosis often with areas of dystrophic calcification
- Nesting or trabecular masses of small round blue cells with hyperchromatic nuclei and scanty neoplasm
- Mitotic figures frequent
- Areas of photoreceptor differentiation result in the presence of Flexner-Wintersteiner rosettes; consist of small lumina circumscribed by neoplastic cells joined at their apexes to produce a form of internal limiting (basement) membrane; nuclei tend to be basally oriented at the periphery of the rosettes
- Homer-Wright rosettes may be present
- Hematoxyphilic deposits are frequently seen around blood vessel walls, particularly in necrotic areas (similar to the findings in pulmonary small cell carcinoma)
- Viable tumor cells surround dilated vessels
- Foci of benign cells with features of photoreceptors may be present; characterized by densely eosinophilic cytoplasmic processes that make rosettes

Special Stains

- Alcian blue and colloidal iron will highlight the presence of hyaluronidase-resistant acid mucopolysaccharide in lumina of Flexner-Wintersteiner rosettes

Immunohistochemistry

- Tumor cells are reactive for NSE, synaptophysin, S-100 protein, GFAP, myelin basic protein, and Leu-7

Electron Microscopy

- Cells of a Flexner-Wintersteiner rosette have features of photoreceptor cells

Molecular Alterations

- Retinoblastoma (*Rb*) gene located on chromosome 13 (13q14)
- Sporadic retinoblastoma is caused by a somatic mutation
- Hereditary retinoblastoma is caused by a germ cell mutation that results in inactivation of the Rb protein which probably functions as a negative regulator of cell growth (an example of the "2-hit" hypothesis)

Differential Diagnosis

- Flexner-Wintersteiner rosettes may be present in pineoblastoma and medulloepithelioma
- *Toxocara canis* endophthalmitis

Treatment

- Cases diagnosed early usually treated with conservative measures designed to preserve vision (unilateral radiation, cryopexy, or xenon arc photocoagulation)
- More advanced lesions treated with enucleation
- If tumor involves the optic nerve, irradiation of the orbit and systemic chemotherapy indicated

Prognosis

- 5-year survival for unilateral retinoblastoma is >90% and is only slightly less for bilateral disease
- Features associated with a less favorable prognosis include invasion of the optic nerve and through the optic coats
- Complete spontaneous regression may occur (more frequent in retinoblastoma than any other malignant neoplasm)

Associations

- Long-term survivors of the hereditary form of disease have an incidence of 25% of developing a second malignant tumor at 30 years: osteosarcoma most frequent
- Bilateral retinoblastomas associated with development of retinoblastoma in pineal gland (trilateral retinoblastoma)

Ependymal Tumors

Ependymoma

Clinical Manifestations

- Neoplasms of ependymal cells that arise throughout the neuraxis
- Intracranial tumors tend to occur in children; spinal lesions tend to occur in adults
- Intracranial lesions occur either in a supratentorial location or an infratentorial (4th ventricle) location and typically produce symptoms of increased intracranial pressure or local mass effect
- Tumors in posterior fossa tend to elevate intracranial pressure by obstructing flow of cerebrospinal fluid
- Intraspinal tumors lie in spinal cord or the filum terminale
- Lesions in spinal cord produce motor and sensory deficits
- Tumors arising in the filum terminale compress nerve roots and cause pain, lower extremity weakness, and sphincter dysfunction

Gross Pathology

- Tumors tend to be well-circumscribed and displace rather than infiltrate brain parenchyma
- Supratentorial intracranial lesions tend to intrude upon the ventricular system and appear as well-circumscribed, gray, fleshy mass
- Posterior fossa lesions arise from the floor of the 4th ventricle and fill it
- Intraspinal lesions tend to be well circumscribed, gray, soft, and noncalcified; a syrinx may be present in the adjacent cord
- Tumors arising in the filum terminale resemble delicately encapsulated soft, tan or gray mass

Microscopic Pathology

- Tumor cells tend to be uniform in size and shape, with round or oval nuclei that are uniformly and moderately hyperchromatic; nucleoli are distinct and small; cytoplasmic processes result in a fibrillary background and project toward blood vessels, forming pseudorosettes
- Increased nuclear-cytoplasmic ratio, brisk mitotic activity, and loss of pseudorosette pattern are features of malignancy (malignant lesions tend to lack significant nuclear pleomorphism)
- Variants
  - *Classic ependymoma*
    - Moderately cellular areas interspersed with areas of diminished cellularity
    - Cellular areas appear fibrillar and usually form perivascular zones in which tumor cell processes approach vessel walls (perivascular pseudorosette); perivascular pseudorosettes may be inconspicuous in areas of low cellularity

   - Occasionally tumors will have small glandlike structures with clearly defined central lumina (true ependymal rosettes); true ependymoma rosettes range from microscopic clusters of cells with indistinct lumina to large tubules or canals that are obviously epithelial in nature
   - Tumors with extensive and complex epithelial surfaces are referred to as *papillary ependymomas*
   - Tumors may occasionally have focal areas or be composed almost entirely of cells with uniform nuclear features and perinuclear halos (reminiscent of an oligodendroglial appearance); tumors composed almost entirely of these types of cells are referred to as *clear cell ependymoma*
- □ *Tanycytic type ependymomas* are composed of tumor cells with highly fibrillar processes that produce an appearance reminiscent of pilocytic astrocytoma
- □ *Myxopapillary ependymoma* is the characteristic lesion of the filum terminale; tends to have a pseudopapillary architecture, perivascular and intercellular mucin deposition, and elongated cells ; mucin is the most conspicuous diagnostic feature and is often confined to the walls of blood vessels; hyalinized vessels and hemosiderin almost always present
- □ *Anaplastic (malignant) ependymoma* characterized by increased cellularity, nuclear pleomorphism, conspicuous mitotic activity, and vascular proliferation; cells are polygonal and epithelial-like; necrosis prominent; no rosettes or pseudorosettes; diffusely invasive

Special Stains

- PAS or Alcian blue stains will highlight the mucin of myxopapillary tumors

Immunohistochemistry

- All ependymomas are immunoreactive for GFAP; reactivity is particularly prominent in perivascular pseudorosettes; true rosettes are typically GFAP negative
- Epithelial cells on surface of well-differentiated lesions are typically immunoreactive for epithelial markers such as EMA and cytokeratins

Electron Microscopy

- Neoplastic cells have intermediate filaments, are covered with microvilli and scattered cilia, and have complex intercellular junctions ("zipperlike" junctions that lack inserting)

Molecular Alterations

- Loss of chromosome 22 most frequent
- Chromosomes 9, 11, and 22 may have a role in pathogenesis

Differential Diagnosis

- If epithelial features are absent and there is a high degree of fibrillarity, astrocytoma or mixed glioma are major considerations
- Cellular lesions can be confused with medulloblastoma and central neurocytoma
- Myxopapillary ependymomas can be confused with schwannoma and paraganglioma
- Malignant ependymoma can resemble GBM

Treatment

- Complete surgical resection
- Recurrence rate approximately 45%

Prognosis

- Intramedullary tumors have best prognosis
- Patients younger than 5 years have worst prognosis
- 5% will undergo cerebrospinal dissemination if they recur
- Distant metastasis rarely occur (seem to be limited to tumors invading or arising within lumbosacral soft tissue)

Associations

- None

Subependymoma

Clinical Manifestations

- Arises in the walls of the ventricular system or (rarely) the parenchyma of the spinal cord
- Usually found incidentally at autopsy
- Rarely affects children
- Tumors in the posterior fossa can compress the brainstem, producing cranial nerve symptoms, dysfunction of the respiratory centers, or obstruction to flow of cerebrospinal fluid
- Tumors in the lateral ventricles usually asymptomatic
- Lesions in the spinal cord cause symptoms of a slowly enlarging intramedullary mass

Gross Pathology

- Tumors in the lateral ventricles arise from the anterolateral wall or the septum pellucidum and tend to be dome-shaped, sessile, or polypoid with a smooth surface
- Lesions in the posterior fossa arise from the floor of the 4th ventricle and are often multinodular and gritty
- Spinal tumors are usually discrete intramedullary masses
- Firm, lobulated, well-circumscribed, white nodule
- Junction between neoplasm and normal brain is typically very sharp

Microscopic Pathology

- Uniform population of ependymal cells in a densely fibrillar glial background
- Lesions in the lateral ventricles consist of sweeping highly fibrillar processes surrounding clustered nuclei; microcystic changes usually prominent
- Nuclear pleomorphism and occasional mitoses present in over 50%
- Necrosis is rare
- Hemosiderin deposits often present, especially in larger tumors
- Lesions arising in the 4th ventricle usually less microcystic and more fibrillar than those in the lateral ventricles; nuclei still clustered, but cells tend to be more uniform with fewer mitotic figures and less pleomorphism
- Lesions near the foramen of Monro tend to be more cystic (and have larger cysts)
- Spinal tumor histologically identical to intracranial tumor

Special Stains

- Not helpful

Immunohistochemistry

- Tumor cells are strongly immunoreactive for both S-100 and GFAP

Electron Microscopy

- Tumor cells have long processes filled with intermediate filaments
- Lesions in posterior fossa have typical features of ependymal differentiation (eg, long complex intercellular junctions, microvilli, and cilia)

Molecular Alterations

- Rare familial occurrence

Differential Diagnosis

- Posterior fossa tumors must be differentiated from ependymoma (subependymoma occurs in adults, is paucicellular, and has unique architecture of prominent nuclear clustering in highly fibrillar background)

Treatment

- Tumors arising from the septum pellucidum can usually be completely excised
- Tumors arising in the 4th ventricle are treated with gross total resection; there is no evidence that incomplete resection will result in recurrence

Prognosis

- One of the few gliomas considered benign

Associations

- Rhabdomyosarcomatous differentiation has been reported

Germ Cell Tumors

Clinical Manifestations

- Represents 1% of all brain tumors
- Usually develops during childhood or adolescence
- Typically arises in the midline in pineal (more common) or suprasellar region; 10% involve both regions
- Tumors involving pineal gland and basal ganglia more common in males; lesions in the suprasellar region more common in females
- Tumors have been associated with the production of α-fetoprotein, β-human chorionic gonadotrophin (hCG), and carcinoembryonic antigen (CEA)

Variants

- Lesions with one histologic pattern:
  - □ Common germinoma (seminoma)
  - □ Embryonal carcinoma
  - □ Yolk sac tumor (endodermal sinus tumor)
  - □ Teratoma (mature and immature)
  - □ Choriocarcinoma
- Lesions that contain 2 or more histologic patterns
  - □ Various combinations of any of the above to include immature teratoma with embryonal carcinoma or yolk sac carcinoma with germinoma

Germinoma

Gross and Microscopic Pathology

- Most frequent intracranial germ cell tumor (50%)
- Tends to occur in adolescents
- Usually well-circumscribed, solid, soft, and friable; necrosis and hemorrhage uncommon
- Similar to gonadal counterparts with 2 distinct cell types: large, neoplastic, polygonal, epithelioid cells with large round vesicular nuclei; nucleoli irregular and pleomorphic, with pale to clear cytoplasm (glycogen); and small lymphocytes occasionally associated with granulomatous inflammation (large epithelial cells tend to be poorly visualized on frozen section—look like ghosts of cells)
- Mitotic figures frequent
- Foci of necrosis may be present
- Syncytiotrophoblastic giant cells may be present

Differential Diagnosis

- Syncytiotrophoblastic cells may be seen in germinomas and immature teratoma as well as choriocarcinoma

Special Stains

- Tumor cells of a germinoma are PAS positive

Immunohistochemistry

- Tumor cells of germinomas are positive for placental alkaline phosphatase (PLAP) and CD117 (c-kit); syncytiotrophoblastic cells (if present) are hCG positive; cytokeratin usually negative

Electron Microscopy

- Germinoma tumor cells characterized by large eccentric nuclei with prominent, meandering nucleoli and cytoplasm with abundant rough endoplasmic reticulum and variable amounts of lipid and glycogen
- Yolk sac tumors have a pseudoglandular arrangement of cells with conspicuous endoplasmic reticulum and abundant glycogen; membrane-bound vesicles containing amorphous material present in both cytoplasm and in extracellular space

Treatment and Prognosis

- Germinomas usually curable (quite radiosensitive)

Associations

- Germinomas may occur in various dysgenic syndromes

Embryonal Carcinoma

Gross and Microscopic Pathology

- Rarely seen in its pure form (5% of all intracranial germ cell tumors)
- Usually fibrous, firm, and very vascular
- Characterized by large primitive-appearing epithelial (cuboidal to polygonal) cells that form cohesive sheets, thick cords, and glands; nuclei vesicular with prominent nucleoli
- Mitotic activity and foci of hemorrhage and necrosis common
- Rarely miniature embryos or embryoid bodies may be present

Differential Diagnosis

- Embryonal carcinomas and yolk sac tumors can resemble metastatic carcinoma and chorioid plexus carcinoma

Immunohistochemistry

- Embryonal carcinomas are typically positive for cytokeratin, PLAP (85 to 90%), and CD30 (80%) and negative for α-fetoprotein, CEA, and β-hCG

Electron Microscopy

- Yolk sac tumors have a pseudoglandular arrangement of cells with conspicuous endoplasmic reticulum and abundant glycogen; membrane-bound vesicles containing amorphous material present in both cytoplasm and in extracellular space

Treatment and Prognosis

- Germ cell neoplasms with an embryonal carcinoma, yolk sac carcinoma, or choriocarcinoma component tend to be highly malignant and frequently spread cerebrospinally

Associations

- None

Yolk Sac Tumor (Endodermal Sinus Tumor)

Gross and Microscopic Pathology

- Third most common (7%) germ cell tumor after germinoma and teratoma
- Rarely occurs in a pure form
- Characterized by cuboidal to columnar epithelial cells arranged in compact sheets, ribbons, cords, and/or papillae
- Schiller-Duval bodies may be present (characterized by epithelium covering blood vessels and projecting cytoplasm into clear spaces that are lined by similar-appearing epithelial cells)
- PAS-positive cytoplasmic and extracytoplasmic eosinophilic droplets typically present
- Characterized by the presence of syncytiotrophoblastic cells and cytotrophoblastic cells arranged in a bilaminar pattern and intimately associated with a sinusoidal vasculature
- Typically a component of embryonal carcinoma also present

Immunohistochemistry

- Yolk sac tumors are typically positive for α-fetoprotein (75% to 100%), CEA, and cytokeratin and negative for EMA and CD30

Electron Microscopy

- Tumor cells have short microvilli and tight junctional complexes with well-defined desmosomes
- Nests of cells often surrounded by a basement membrane

Treatment and Prognosis

- Germ cell neoplasms with a yolk sac carcinoma component tend to be highly malignant and frequently spread cerebrospinally

Associations

- None

Teratoma

Gross and Microscopic Pathology

- Usually large, well-circumscribed, and adherent to adjacent structures; cut surface often multicystic
- Characterized by tissues from each of the 3 germ cell layers
- Mature teratomas are fully differentiated
- Immature teratomas (more frequent) consist of fetal-appearing tissue consisting of developing neuroectodermal structures, retina, and chorioid plexus; mesenchymal elements consisting of a nondescript cellular or myxoid stroma, foci of cartilage, and bands of striated muscle; endodermal and ectodermal tissue characterized by the presence of skin and adnexa as well as respiratory tract, pancreas, and intestinal epithelium
- Occasional teratomas may contain both mature and immature elements
- Teratoma may be seen in association with a malignant germ cell component (especially germinoma and embryonal carcinoma)
- Conventional malignant tissue such as carcinoma or sarcoma may be present in a teratoma (eg, squamous cell carcinoma, adenocarcinoma, rhabdomyosarcoma)
- Typically a component of embryonal carcinoma or yolk sac tumor also present

Immunohistochemistry

- Epithelial component of teratomas is usually positive for CEA

Electron Microscopy

- Not helpful

Treatment and Prognosis

- Mature teratomas are benign and tend to be firm and well-demarcated hence relatively easy to completely excise; immature teratomas often are not easily resected despite being fairly well-circumscribed

Associations

- None

Choriocarcinoma

- Usually well-circumscribed and hemorrhagic
- Often associated with precocious puberty
- Characterized by the presence of syncytiotrophoblastic cells and cytotrophoblastic cells arranged in a bilaminar pattern and intimately associated with a sinusoidal vasculature
- Typically a component of embryonal carcinoma or yolk sac tumor also present

Immunohistochemistry

- Choriocarcinomas usually have PLAP, hCG, human placental lactogen, and creatine kinase-positive cells

Electron Microscopy

- Not helpful

Treatment and Prognosis

- Germ cell neoplasms with an embryonal carcinoma, yolk sac carcinoma, or choriocarcinoma component tend to be highly malignant and frequently spread cerebrospinally

Associations

- None

Neuronal Cell Tumors

Central Neurocytoma

Clinical Manifestations

- Usually present as an intraventricular mass near foramen of Monro; anterior portion of lateral ventricle, most frequent site (75%)—septum pellucidium region
- May obstruct flow of cerebrospinal fluid, resulting in symptoms of increased intracranial pressure (papilledema, headache, nausea, and vomiting)
- Typically occurs in young to middle-aged adults

Gross Pathology

- Usually a large well-circumscribed globular-shaped intraventricular mass that straddles the midline and is attached to ventricular wall

- Often calcified (occasionally extensively)
- Cut surface gray and gritty

Microscopic Pathology

- Typically a dense, uniform, and monotonous cellular neoplasm interrupted by irregular zones of fibrillarity
- Occasionally the cells have a streaming pattern (often in a single file)
- Tumor cell nuclei are monomorphic, have stippled chromatin, and small nucleoli
- Tumor cells are almost never multinucleated or pleomorphic
- Mitotic figures rare or absent
- Tumor cells frequently have perinuclear halos
- Focal areas of microcalcification (calcospherites) may be distributed throughout
- Structures resembling Homer-Wright rosettes and ganglion cells both rare
- Fibrillar zones often have a perivascular distribution

Special Stains

- Not helpful

Immunohistochemistry

- Tumor cells positive for synaptophysin (diffuse), NSE, and S-100 protein; usually negative for chromogranin
- Ki-67/MIB-1 positivity in <2%

Electron Microscopy

- Cytoplasmic processes containing microtubules make up the neuropil produced by neurocytoma cells
- Neurosecretory granules are usually seen within the cytoplasmic processes or in the perinuclear cytoplasm

Molecular Alterations

- None

Differential Diagnosis

- Oligodendroglioma
- Cellular ependymoma
- Neuroblastoma

Treatment

- Gross total resection; incomplete excision will result in recurrence (grows slowly)
- Incompletely excised lesions usually treated with radiation

Prognosis

- Excellent
- Despite intraventricular location spread by the way of cerebral spinal fluid is very rare
- Laterally located tumors may be high grade (anaplastic)

Associations

- Hormonal dysfunction (amenorrhea, giantism, and hypersecretion of vasopressin) seen in tumors of the septum pellucidum, third ventricle, and hypothalamus

Dysembryoplastic Neuroepithelial Tumor (DNT)

Clinical Manifestations

- Typically presents with chronic, intractable seizures of partial complex type
- Always supratentorial; temporal lobe most common site
- Usually becomes symptomatic during first 2 decades of life
- Usually presents as typical well-circumscribed "bubbles" within the parenchyma on magnetic resonance imaging

Gross Pathology

- Varies in size from a few millimeters to almost totally lobar in extent
- Some degree of gyral expansion with superficial blisterlike elevations on the cortical surface
- On sectioning, a mucinous texture with a nodular appearance, nodular areas tend to be located deep and at periphery

Microscopic Pathology

- Multiple intracortical nodules ranging from small foci of mild hypercellularity in a faintly basophilic background to large nodules that expand the entire cortical band
- Nodules contain abundant acid mucopolysaccharide
- Tumor cells closely resemble well-differentiated oligodendroglioma but tend to have a variable arrangement ranging from uniform masses with microcysts to a patterned targetoid appearance (architectural features that are not characteristic of oligodendroglioma)
- Neurons within tumor nodules tend to be well-differentiated and "swim" in the cystic fluid of clear spaces unaccompanied by tumor cells (perineuronal satellitosis not a feature)
- Cortex adjacent to nodules of tumor characterized by oligodendroglial hypercellularity and the accumulation of mucin; tumor cells penetrate the cortex and result in the isolation of neurons in pools of mucin
- Focal microcalcification may be present

Special Stains

- Alcian blue will highlight presence of acid mucopolysaccharide

Immunohistochemistry

- Neurons stain positively for synaptophysin and neurofilament protein
- Astrocytic component positive for GFAP

Electron Microscopy

- A heterogenous population of cells with both neuronal and oligodendroglial features

Molecular Alterations

- None

Differential Diagnosis

- Oligodendroglioma
- Ganglioglioma

Treatment

- Cure possible with subtotal resection
- No role for chemotherapy or radiation

Prognosis

- A slow growing lesion that is largely noninfiltrative

Associations

- Occasionally occur in patients with NF-1

Oligodendroglial Neoplasms

Gangliglioma and Gangliocytoma

Clinical Manifestations

- Well differentiated, slow-growing neuroepithelial neoplasm composed of neoplastic, mature ganglion cells, either alone (gangliocytoma) or in combination with neoplastic glial cells (ganglioglioma)
- Approximately 0.5% of all CNS tumors
- Age range 2 to 80 years; mean age in children approximately 10 years
- Most are supratentorial and involve temporal lobe; may occur throughout the CNS
- Symptoms vary by site; seizures most common presentation
- CT shows circumscribed solid mass or cyst with a mural nodule

Gross Pathology

- Tend to be solid or cystic without producing a mass effect
- Calcification may be present
- Necrosis and hemorrhage rare

Microscopic Pathology

- Gangliocytomas composed of irregular groups of large, multipolar neurons with dysplastic features
- Stroma consists of non-neoplastic glial elements and reticulin fibers, which are often perivascular
- Gangliogliomas have an additional neoplastic glial component consisting of astrocytes surrounded by a reticulin network
- Perivascular lymphocytic infiltrate is typically present
- Variants
  - *Papillary glioneuronal tumor*: Characterized by pseudopapillary appearance with single layer of pseudustratified, small, cuboidal cells around hyalinized blood vessels, associated with groups of neurocytes admixed with ganglion cells

- *Neoplasms containing small neurons ("neurocytes")*: Some similar to central neurocytoma, with or without focal differentiation into ganglion cells

Special Stains

- Reticulin stains will highlight the reticulin fibers in the stroma

Immunohistochemistry

- GFAP demonstrates the astrocytes in the neoplastic glial component of a ganglioglioma
- CD34 reactivity seen in 75% of gangliogliomas
- Ki67/MIB-1 stain only the glial component with values ranging from 1% to 3%

Electron Microscopy

- Neurons with dense core granules diagnostically useful

Molecular Alterations

- Abnormal karyotypes include a ring chromosome 1, trisomies of chromosomes 5 to 7, and deletion of chromosome 6

Differential Diagnosis

- May represent highly differentiated remnants of embryonal neuroblastomas or related primitive neuroectodermal tumors

Treatment

- Surgical resection

Prognosis

- Malignant change has been documented in gangliogliomas and invariably involves glial component

Associations

- Dyslastic gangliocytoma of cerebellum (Lhermitte-Duclos) seen in association with Cowden disease
- Small number associated with tuberous sclerosis
- One case report in a patient with NF-2

Oligodendroglioma

Clinical Manifestations

- Account for 5% of all intracranial neoplasms and 10%-20% of all gliomas
- Primarily involve the frontal lobes of cerebral hemispheres
- Multiple lobes involved in 50%; 20% bilateral
- Rarely in spinal cord
- Most patients present as adults between ages of 40 and 60 years with symptoms referable to an infiltrating expanding intracranial neoplasm; a long history of seizures common

Gross Pathology

- An infiltrating tumor that has a typically ill-defined border
- Usually visibly alters cerebral cortex as a result of extensive infiltration of gray matter; junction of gray and white matter may be effaced
- Tumors with a soft mucoid matrix may appear more clearly demarcated than tumors without this feature
- Areas of necrosis indicate malignancy

Microscopic Pathology

- A uniform, dense population of cells with similar nuclear size and shape
- Infiltrating cells tend to prefer cortical gray matter where they tend to form perineural satellitosis, accumulate in the subpial region, and aggregate around blood vessels (these secondary structures of Scherer are very typical of oligodendroglioma)
- Tumor cells frequently arranged in a columnar or palisading pattern; other patterns include prominent microcystic change, lobulation, and cell clustering
- Cells typically have clear perinuclear halos (a "fried egg" artifact created by autolytic absorption of water that occurs during delayed fixation); this diagnostic artifact is not always present (usually not present in specimens frozen before being embedded in paraffin)
- Calcification usually present either in the tumor itself or in the surrounding brain parenchyma

- Tumor nuclei tend to be round and uniform with little pleomorphism
- Density and distribution of nuclear chromatin varies according to histologic grade: higher-grade tumors have more dense and coarse chromatin than lower-grade tumors; high-grade tumors also have more prominent nucleoli and more mitotic activity
- Blood vessels tend to be arranged in a pattern resembling "chicken wire"
- Reactive astrocytes are typically a prominent feature and are evenly distributed throughout the lesion (appear as stellate cells with delicate nuclei, a moderate amount of eosinophilic cytoplasm, and long uniform radiating processes)
- Neoplastic cells with eccentric, hyaline, eosinophilic intracytoplasmic bodies are almost always present (except in highly differentiated lesions)
- Occasionally tumor cells will have cytoplasm filled with brightly eosinophilic skeins of fibrillar material, which form paranuclear whorls or encircle nuclei (mini-or microgemistocytes)
- *Malignant or anaplastic oligodendroglioma* are very cellular with marked nuclear hyperchromasia, conspicuous mitotic activity, and vascular proliferation; necrosis may be present; tumors tend to contain large numbers of neoplastic cells with astrocytelike cytoplasm and binucleate forms, but nuclei remain typical of oligodendrocytes

Special Stains

- Not helpful

Immunohistochemistry

- Leu-7 produces a pale membranous pattern of staining in oligodendrocytes
- Oligodendrocytes with prominent eosinophilic cytoplasm are strongly immunoreactive for GFAP (positivity usually confined to the globular inclusions and not the entire cytoplasm)
- Anaplastic lesions with prominent cytoplasm and short processes may be immunoreactive for GFAP (this finding makes the distinction between a malignant oligodendroglioma and glioblastoma quite difficult)
- Tumor cells positive for S-100 protein
- Reactive astrocytes strongly positive for GFAP

Electron Microscopy

- Neoplastic cells have round nuclei, empty cytoplasm (practically devoid of organelles), and short processes that contain microtubules
- Eosinophilic GFAP-positive cells contain many intermediate filament bundles

Molecular Alterations

- 50% to 60% have a genetic alteration of LOH on 19q
- Second most frequent alteration is LOH on short arm of chromosome 1

Differential Diagnosis

- Normal cerebral white matter
- Astrogliosis
- Ganglion cell tumor
- Demyelinating disease and infarction with a subsequent accumulation of macrophages (may closely resemble the cells of an oligodendroglioma)
- Diffuse or fibrillary astrocytoma
- Glioblastoma
- Gliomatosis cerebri
- Cells that resemble the tumor cells of oligodendroglioma are seen in ependymomas of the clear cell type, pilocytic astrocytomas, neuroblastic variants of medulloblastoma, and central neurocytoma
- Increased numbers of oligodendrocytes are often seen in association with gliosis
- Metastatic carcinoma (a major consideration in cellular oligodendrogliomas with desmoplasia)

Treatment

- Too infiltrative to be resectable
- Many respond favorably to chemotherapy
- Radiotherapy appears to have a role in partially resected neoplasms

Prognosis

- Most are associated with a fatal outcome
- Tumors with a genomic abnormality consisting of only a loss of chromosomes 1p and 19q respond well to chemotherapy and may be associated with long-term survival; tumors with intact 1p and 19q and amplification of EGF do not respond well to chemotherapy and are associated with a worse prognosis
- Extracranial metastases are rare
- Tumors tend to slowly progress and eventually undergo malignant degeneration

Associations

- None

Tumors of Meningothelial Cells

Atypical and Anaplastic (Malignant) Meningiomas

Clinical Manifestations

- Both atypical and malignant meningiomas more common in males
- 6% to 7% of meningiomas are atypical; 2% to 3% are malignant
- Typically affect adults in 6th decade (malignant) and 7th decade (atypical)

Gross Pathology

- Atypical lesions similar in appearance to meningioma; obvious parenchymal invasion evident in anaplastic lesions

Microscopic Pathology

- *Atypical meningioma*
    - Tumors characteristically hypercellular with tumor cells growing in a patternless manner with focal or geographic necrosis unrelated to vascular occlusion
    - Tumor cells typically small and have high nuclear-cytoplasmic ratios, coarse chromatin and prominent nucleoli (these features fall short of anaplasia)
    - Brisk mitotic activity usually present but varies from region to region
    - May have a broad attachment to the pial surface
- *Anaplastic (malignant) meningioma*
    - Characterized by hypercellularity, mitotic activity, necrosis, and cerebral invasion; usually induce significant edema in surrounding brain
    - Invasive (obviously malignant) meningiomas may have a broad histologic spectrum ranging from benign to atypical to anaplastic, but most are at least moderately anaplastic
    - There is a tendency for meningiomas to develop some atypia or anaplasia over time
    - May have a ragged, infiltrative junction at the cortical surface
    - True invasion is usually accompanied by marked reactive gliosis

Special Stains

- Not helpful

Immunohistochemistry

- Well-differentiated tumor cells have membranous staining with EMA and are always positive for vimentin
- Ki-67 index elevated

Electron Microscopy

- May be useful in establishing meningothelial nature of tumors with markedly anaplastic or sarcomatous components

Molecular Alterations

- LOH for loci on chromosome 22

Differential Diagnosis

- Primary meningeal sarcoma
- Metastatic carcinoma

Treatment

- Surgical resection with radiotherapy

Prognosis

- 50% of atypical meningiomas recur
- 100% of malignant lesions recur within 15 years

Associations

- None

Meningioma

Clinical Manifestations

- *Intracranial meningioma*
  - Most common location
  - Typically presents with the symptoms of an expanding intracranial mass: Focal neurologic deficits, increased intracranial pressure, and seizure
  - More common in females and blacks
  - May penetrate the calvarium and present as a scalp mass (frequently induce cranial hyperostosis)
- *Intraspinal meningioma*
  - Produce segmental neurologic deficits secondary to compression of spinal cord
  - Women much more frequently affected than men (10:1)
  - Most occur laterally or ventrally near the nerve root exit and are intradural and extramedullary; commonly occur in the cervicothoracic area; occurrence in the lumbosacral region rare
  - Rarely involve surrounding bone
- *Optic nerve sheath meningioma*
  - Most common extracranial site
  - Rarely affect children
  - Present clinically with visual loss, strabismus, or ptosis
- *Meningioma of ventricular system*
  - Lateral ventricle (usually left) most common site; also 3rd ventricle (15%) and 4th ventricle (5%)
  - Typically lies outside the dura
  - Can occur both intracranially and intraspinally
  - When intracranial often invade adjacent bone; intraspinal lesions rarely involve bone
- Ectopic meningioma
  - Sites include cranial bones, nasal and paranasal sinuses, neck, skin, lungs, mediastinum, and peripheral nerves

Gross Pathology

- Most are well-circumscribed, smooth, and soft and have a broad dural attachment
- Cut surface may be gritty secondary to calcification
- May be bright yellow if extensive amounts of lipid are present
- Tends to push rather than invade leptomeninges, resulting in a sharp anatomic plane between tumor and adjacent brain
- Recurrent tumors less well-circumscribed and tend to adhere to adjacent nerves and blood vessels

Microscopic Pathology

- A wide variety of histologic subtypes:
- *Meningotheliomatous (syncytial), transitional, and fibrous* characterize the classic meningioma; 2 or all 3 patterns often present in a single tumor
  - *Syncytial meningioma:* Characterized by lobules of tumor cells arranged in a sheetlike pattern with indistinct, interdigitating cell borders; tumor cells have round to oval nuclei, clumped chromatin, small solitary nucleoli, and nuclear-cytoplasmic invaginations (pseudoinclusions); scant fibrous tissue
  - *Fibrous meningioma:* May occur in a pure form; usually less cellular and consists of markedly elongated cells in a dense collagenous background; tumor cell nuclei tend to be elongated and hyperchromatic
  - *Transitional meningioma:* Consists of prominent lobules, whorls, collagenized blood vessels and psammoma bodies; center of a lobule may have a syncytial appearance while periphery appears fibroblastic with spindled tumor cells streaming out from the lobule

- Other meningioma variants
  - *Psammomatous meningioma*
    - Tumor with multiple psammoma bodies
    - Stroma may contain amyloid
    - Tends to involve spinal dura and olfactory groove
  - *Secretory meningioma*
    - Usually a syncytial or transitional meningioma with epithelial differentiation in the form of glandlike structures
    - Characterized by the presence of discrete, eosinophilic intracytoplasmic inclusions (pseudopsammoma bodies lack the calcification and whorled architecture of a true psammoma body)
  - *Microcystic meningioma*
    - Characterized by stellate tumor cells with large hyperchromatic, pleomorphic, but mitotically inactive nuclei in a loosely textured background with marked vascular hyalinization
    - Fluid-filled spaces surrounded by elongated cell processes give neoplasm a cobweb-like appearance
    - May be associated with a large intratumoral or peritumoral cyst
  - *Lymphoplasmacytic meningioma*
    - Characterized by an intense chronic lymphoplasmacytic inflammatory response; may be seen in association with any meningioma pattern (especially chordoid variant)
    - Russell bodies and germinal centers may be present
  - *Chordoid meningioma*
    - Characterized by cords or trabeculae of epithelioid cells in a mucinous background (reminiscent of a chordoma)
    - Prominent lymphoplasmacytic infiltrate may be present
  - *Metaplastic variants*
    - Characterized by the presence of mesenchymal elements such as fat, bone, cartilage, and xanthoma cells
    - Neoplastic cells may have a xanthomatous appearance or may contain lipid droplets (resemble adipocytes)
    - Metaplastic bone a more frequent finding than metaplastic cartilage
    - Myxoid change may be present resulting in widely separated aggregates of neoplastic cells
  - *Papillary meningioma*
    - Occur in pediatric age group
    - Characterized by pseudorosettes of neoplastic cells around blood vessels (the orientation of tumor cells to blood vessels similar to that of ependymomas)
    - Tumor cells uniform with nuclei typical of meningothelial cells
    - Mitotic figures may be present
    - Most aggressive of all of the subtypes of meningioma
  - *Additional rare meningioma variants*
    - Clear cell type: Tend to recur and seed the subarachnoid space; composed of clear (glycogen), polygonal cells; no whorls or psammoma bodies
    - Pseudoglandular type
    - Rhabdoid
    - Zellballenlike (reminiscent of paraganglioma)

Special Stains

- Pseudopsammoma bodies of secretory meningiomas and clear cells in clear cell variant PAS positive and diastase resistant

Immunohistochemistry

- Tumor cells will demonstrate a membranous pattern of staining with EMA; best seen in meningothelial and transitional variants
- All forms of meningioma stain diffusely with vimentin
- Occasional meningiomas reactive with S-100 protein
- Tumor cells surrounding pseudopsammoma bodies and the substance of pseudopsammoma bodies in secretory meningiomas are both positive for cytokeratins and CEA

Electron Microscopy

- Tumor cells usually have interdigitating processes, cytoplasmic intermediate filaments, desmosomes, and hemidesmosomes
- Pseudopsammoma bodies of secretory meningiomas consist of masses of minute vesicles and débris in an intracellular space; cells surrounding pseudopsammoma body have numerous short microvilli on their luminal surface

Molecular Alterations

- Monosomy 22 is most common cytogenetic finding in spontaneous meningiomas (70%-80%)
- Deletion of 22q; loss of genetic information on chromosome 22 may be responsible for the multiple meningiomas seen in the central form of neurofibromatosis (NF-2)

Differential Diagnosis

- Metastatic carcinoma to the dura
- Schwannoma (neurilemmoma)
- Glioma (oligodendroglioma, astrocytoma, or ependymoma)
- Meningeal hemangiopericytoma
- Capillary hemangioblastoma

Treatment

- Gross total surgical removal
- Recurrence may occur even after apparent total removal

Prognosis

- Largely dependent on location
- Chordoid, papillary, and clear cell variants tend to behave aggressively
- Death may result from the mass effect, destruction of brain parenchyma, or the development of bacterial meningitis as a result of defect in the skull or dura

Associations

- Other estrogen-dependent tumors including breast cancer and endometrial cancer
- Meningioma may be adjacent to or intermingled with a glioma (meningioma may actually induce the formation of the glioma)
- May result from cranial irradiation or trauma
- Meningioma may be a site for a metastatic carcinoma
- Chordoid meningioma associated with iron-refractory anemia and polyclonal gammopathy (Castleman syndrome)
- Multiple meningiomas seen in patients with NF-2 (see molecular alterations above)
- *Gorlin syndrome*: an autosomal dominant disorder characterized primarily by skeletal anomalies (including craniomegaly), lamellar calcium deposition in the falx cerebri and diaphragma sellae, cutaneous epidermoid cysts, pits on the palms and soles, odontogenic keratocysts, calcifying ovarian fibromas, multifocal basal cell carcinomas occurring at an early age, medulloblastoma and meningioma

Tumors of Pineal Gland

Pineoblastoma

Clinical Manifestations

- A highly malignant primitive small cell neoplasm with a tendency for local infiltration and cerebrospinal dissemination
- Represents 15% to 80% of pineal region neoplasms
- Tends to occur during the first 2 decades of life (median age, 18 years)
- May be more common in males than females
- May have a familial incidence

Gross Pathology

- Tends to be soft and infiltrate adjacent structures
- If neoplasm reaches the subarachnoid space or ventricular system, it spreads out as an opaque, gray, sheetlike infiltrate
- Cut surface often gelatinous and hemorrhagic

Microscopic Pathology

- Tumor cells have scant cytoplasm and small hyperchromatic, mitotically active nuclei

- Large rosettes characteristic of pineocytoma not present
- Retinoblastomalike differentiation may be seen; small fleurettes or Flexner-Wintersteiner rosettes
- Hemorrhage and necrosis common
- Cells containing melanin may be present
- Homer-Wright (neuroblastic) rosettes occasionally present

Special Stains

- Silver carbonate typically demonstrates short, blunt cellular processes

Immunohistochemistry

- Expression of retinal S-antigen is more common than in pineocytomas
- Fibrillar zones in rosettelike structures typically reactive for synaptophysin

Electron Microscopy

- Varying degrees of photosensory differentiation may be seen as polarization of cytoplasmic organelles, cilia, and annulate lamellae
- Differentiation to mesenchymal tissue such as striated muscle and cartilage and melanotic pigmentation may be evident

Molecular Alterations

- Deletion at chromosome 11q13 (characteristic of neuroblastomas) has been identified in congenital pineoblastoma

Differential Diagnosis

- Medulloblastoma
- Pineocytoma
- Intermediate pineal parenchymal tumor

Treatment

- Surgical excision

Prognosis

- Characterized by rapid recurrence and wide dissemination
- Survival rate rarely longer than 2 years

Associations

- May occur in the setting of bilateral retinoblastoma (trilateral retinoblastoma)

Pineocytoma

Clinical Manifestations

- Represents 5% to 30% of primary pineal tumors
- A well-differentiated neoplasm arising from pineocytes, cells that represent especially modified neurons related to retinal photoreceptors
- Typically affects adults (median age, 35 years)
- Occurs in the posterior 3rd ventricle

Gross Pathology

- Tends to displace rather than infiltrate surrounding structures
- On cut section, soft, homogeneous, and finely granular; occasional small foci of necrosis

Microscopic Pathology

- Mature tumor cells surround delicate, fibrillary continuous acellular zones (pineocytomatous rosettes)
- Rosettes vary from quite prominent to sparse and incomplete
- Rosettes do not wheel around a vessel and are larger and more irregular than Homer-Wright rosettes
- Fibrillarity of the rosette is produced by neoplastic cell processes that emanate from the cells that surround (palisade) the core
- Tumor cells tend to be better differentiated and have larger and paler nuclei than those seen in Homer-Wright rosettes
- Solid cellular areas frequently seen as sheets or ribbons between rosettes

- Rarely large, hyperchromatic, and/or multinucleated cells may be present
- Mitotic figures rare
- Focal areas of necrosis occasionally present

Special Stains

- Silver carbonate will demonstrate delicate argyrophilic clublike processes that project into the acellular regions of the rosettes

Immunohistochemistry

- Tumor cells typically immunoreactive for synaptophysin, NF, and retinal S-antigen
- Some tumor cells may be reactive for S-100 protein
- Reactivity for GFAP is limited to reactive or neoplastic astrocytes

Electron Microscopy

- Tumor cells have neurosecretory granules, microtubule and intermediate filament-containing processes, bulbous termination with dense core and clear vesicles
- Small, intertwined filaments are diagnostic

Molecular Alterations

- Loss of chromosome 22, deletions in the distal 12q region, and deletions or loss of chromosome 11

Differential Diagnosis

- Non-neoplastic pineal cyst
- Normal pineal gland (tends to be lobular; pineocytomas are patternless and form sheets rather than lobules)
- Pineoblastoma
- Intermediate pineal parenchymal tumor

Treatment

- Surgical excision

Prognosis

- A benign neoplasm with little tendency to invade surrounding brain or spread in the neuraxis

Associations

- None

Tumors of Uncertain Origin

Hemangioblastoma

Clinical Manifestations

- Represents 1% to 2% of all intracranial tumors
- Usually presents as a solitary sporadic lesion without extracerebellar stigmata or family history; may occur in the setting of von Hippel-Lindau disease
- Typically affects adults between the ages of 30 and 65 years (peak incidence, 35 to 45 years)
- Slightly more common in males than females
- Cerebellum most frequent site; tumors also arise in the medulla and spinal cord (particularly those associated with von Hippel-Lindau disease)
- 10% of patients present with polycythemia secondary to tumor production of erythropoietin

Gross Pathology

- Typically a highly vascular well-circumscribed, but unencapsulated nodule in the cerebellum that abuts the leptomeninges
- Cut surface dark red with a spongy or cystic texture; portions may appear yellow (secondary to the presence of lipid within stromal cells)
- Spinal lesions typically intramedullary, discrete, and border the leptomeninges

Microscopic Pathology

- Consists of large afferent and efferent blood vessels of various sizes and shapes and many small capillaries, all lined by a single layer of endothelium
- Stromal or interstitial cells (the principle component of the tumor) are large, polygonal, contain variable amounts of lipid and glycogen (the lipid is seen as clear cytoplasmic vacuoles), and lie packed between abundant capillary channels; the density and distribution of stromal cells vary throughout the neoplasm

- Considerable variation in cellular density with compact regions intermixed with large vessels and cystic spaces
- Two variants (cellular and reticular):
  - Cellular tumors have more stromal cells than vascular elements, resulting in large cellular lobules of tumor; stromal cells in cellular tumors tend to have large, hyperchromatic, round, and pleomorphic nuclei
  - Reticular tumors have prominent vasculature and few stromal cells evenly distributed around the capillary network; stromal cells in reticular tumors have smaller and more uniform nuclei
- Mitotic figures are rare
- Mast cells distributed uniformly throughout the neoplasm
- Foci of extramedullary erythropoiesis are occasionally present

Special Stains

- Toluidine blue will stain mast cells
- Reticulin stains will highlight the dense vasculature, particularly in the reticular variant

Immunohistochemistry

- Stromal cells always negative for factor VIII-related antigen (von Willebrand factor); also negative for *Ulex europaeus* lectin
- Occasionally stromal cells will be GFAP positive (even though they do not contain GFAP)
- Stromal cells are typically positive for NSE and negative for keratin and EMA
- Stromal cells and mast cells may be positive for erythropoietin

Electron Microscopy

- Stromal cells have variable amounts of glycogen and lipid, tend to be large, and lack specific organelles or cell attachments
- Endothelial cells line vascular channels
- Pericytes lie just outside basal lamina

Molecular Alterations

- Defective gene for sporadic as well as von Hippel-Lindau disease on short arm of chromosome 3

Differential Diagnosis

- If a biopsy of the wall of an accompanying cyst is performed, a cerebellar pilocytic astrocytoma becomes a consideration
- If a biopsy of cord parenchyma surrounding a spinal cord tumor is performed, an infiltrating fibrillary astrocytoma becomes a consideration
- If there is no accompanying cyst, metastatic clear cell carcinoma is a consideration (of particular importance because of the association of hemangioblastoma and renal cell carcinoma in von Hippel-Lindau disease)

Treatment

- Surgical excision
- Radiotherapy is used for unresectable or recurrent tumors of the medulla or high cervical spinal cord

Prognosis

- Benign tumors with a recurrence rate of 25%
- Recurrence may actually be a second primary lesion, particularly in the setting of von Hippel-Lindau disease

Associations

- *von Hippel-Lindau disease*: Multiple hemangioblastomas of the cerebellum, but also of the optic nerve and retina (40%); pheochromocytoma (40%); renal cysts and renal cell carcinoma (23%); cysts or cystadenomas of the pancreas (18%); bilateral papillary cystadenomas of the epididymis (3%); and aggressive papillary middle ear tumors

References

Burger PC, Scheithauer BW. *Tumors of the Central Nervous System: Atlas of Tumor Pathology, 3rd series. Fascicle 10.* Washington DC: Armed Forces Institute of Pathology, 1994.

Burger PC, Scheithauer BW, Vogel FS. *Surgical Pathology of the Nervous System and its Coverings. 4th ed.* New York: Churchill Livingstone, 2002.

Kleihues P, Cavenee WK (eds). *World Health Organization Classification of Tumours. Pathology and Genetics of Tumours of the Nervous System.* Lyon: IARC Press, 2000.

McLean IW, Burnier MN, Zimmerman LE, Jakobiec FA. *Tumors of the Eye and Ocular Adnexa: Atlas of Tumor Pathology, 3rd series, Fascicle 12.* Washington DC: Armed Forces Institute of Pathology, 1994.

Mills S, Carter D, Greenson JK, Oberman HA, Reuter V, Stoler MH (eds). *Sternberg's Diagnostic Surgical Pathology. 4th ed.* Philadelphia: Lippincott Williams & Wilkins, 2004.

Moss TM, Nicoll JAR, Ironside JW. *Intraoperative Diagnosis of CNS Tumors.* New York: Oxford University Press, 1997.

Rosai J. *Rosai and Ackerman's Surgical Pathology. 9th ed.* St. Louis: Mosby, 2004.

Chapter 3

Endocrine

Adrenal Gland

Adrenal Cortical Adenoma

Clinical Manifestations

- Most frequent endocrine abnormality is primary aldosteronism (Conn syndrome); Cushing syndrome is second
- Virilization and feminization are symptoms more frequently associated with malignancy
- More common in women than in men
- Equally distributed between the two adrenal glands

Gross and Microscopic Pathology

- *Adrenal cortical adenoma with Cushing syndrome*
  - Neoplasm typically unilateral, sharply circumscribed, encapsulated, weighs <50 g, and averages 3.5 cm in diameter
  - Cut surface usually uniformly yellow, but may have small foci of hemorrhage, lipid depletion, or increased lipofuscin (focal areas of dark discoloration)
  - May have a vague nodularity
  - Microscopically, tumor typically consists of pale staining, lipid-rich cells with uniform nuclei and optically clear cytoplasm arranged in a nested or alveolar pattern
  - Adenoma cells typically larger and are more pleomorphic than normal cortical cells
  - Cell borders tend to be distinct
  - Areas of lipid-poor cells with eosinophilic cytoplasm and prominent lipochrome pigment may be admixed with more typically lipid-rich cells
  - Nuclei usually single and round with chromatin that aggregates along the inner surface of the nuclear membrane giving the nucleus a vesicular appearance; a single small nucleolus typically present; nuclear pseudoinclusions may be present
  - Mitotic figures very rare
  - Adjacent cortex usually atrophic (glomerulosa not atrophic)
- *Pigmented ("black") adenoma*
  - Much more common in women than in men
  - Uncut surface is dark brown to black and gets darker after exposure to air
  - Microscopic architectural pattern similar to other adrenal cortical adenomas
  - Cells have compact, eosinophilic cytoplasm and contain brown or golden brown pigment distributed in the cytoplasm in such a way as to leave a halo around the nucleus; pigment most likely lipofuscin or maybe neuromelanin
- *Adrenal cortical adenoma with primary hyperaldosteronism (Conn syndrome)*
  - Typically unilateral and solitary; 5% bilateral
  - Typically sharply demarcated with a true capsule
  - Cut surface is uniformly yellow to orange
  - Larger tumors may have areas of hemorrhage or cystic degeneration
  - Tumor cells usually arranged in the typical nesting, alveolar, or trabecular patterns of an adenoma
  - Tumor cells do not necessarily resemble those of the zona glomerulosa (the region of the normal adrenal gland that produces aldosterone); cells of zona glomerulosa may be hyperplastic
  - Spironolactone bodies (eosinophilic, laminated intracytoplasmic inclusions) may be present in zona glomerulosa cells after treatment with spironolactone (an aldosterone antagonist)
  - 4 different cell types typically present:
    - Cells that resemble the zona fasciculata cells: Pale staining and lipid-rich
    - Cells resembling zona glomerulosa: High nuclear-cytoplasmic ratio with scant vacuolated lightly eosinophilic cytoplasm
    - Cells resembling zona reticularis (may have oncocytic features)
    - "Hybrid" cells with features similar to both zona glomerulosa and zona fasciculata

- *Adrenal cortical neoplasms with virilization or feminization*
  - More likely to be malignant than the other adrenal cortical neoplasms (especially if feminizing)
  - Neoplasm tends to be sharply circumscribed and encapsulated
  - Larger tumors may have focal areas of hemorrhage or necrosis
  - Tumor cells usually arranged in sheets and tend to resemble the cells of the zona reticularis with compact eosinophilic cytoplasm
- *Oncocytic adrenal cortical adenoma*
  - Tumor has the typical dark tan or mahogany brown appearance of an oncocytoma
  - Cells have abundant granular eosinophilic cytoplasm (secondary to the presence of abundant mitochondria)
  - Tumor cells tend to be lipid-poor
  - A marked degree of nuclear pleomorphism and nuclear pseudoinclusions may be present

Special Stains

- Lipid-rich tumor cells will stain with oil red O stain
- Pigmented adenomas have a positive argentaffin reaction with Fontana-Masson stain; they also stain positively with periodic acid-Schiff (PAS) and have a negative reaction with iron stains
- Spironolactone bodies in an aldosterone-producing cortical adenoma stain with Luxol fast blue

Immunohistochemistry

- Tumor cells are more likely to be positive for low-molecular-weight keratin than the tumor cells of an adrenal cortical carcinoma
- Tumor cells are less likely to be positive for vimentin than adrenal cortical carcinoma
- Tumor cells typically negative for epithelial membrane antigen (EMA) (in contrast to renal cell carcinoma, the primary consideration in the differential diagnosis)
- Tumor cells positive for inhibin

Electron Microscopy

- *Adrenal cortical adenoma with Cushing syndrome*
  - Adenoma cells resemble normal fasciculata or reticularis cells
  - Abundant pleomorphic intracytoplasmic lipid droplets
  - Nuclear pseudoinclusions represent an infolding of cell cytoplasm
  - Mitochondria may be numerous
- *Functional pigmented adenoma*
  - Cytoplasm with relatively few lipid droplets
  - Cytoplasm contains electron-dense granules of lipofuscin
  - No melanosomes or premelanosomes
- *Cortical adenoma with primary hyperaldosteronism*
  - A spectrum of lipid-rich to lipid-poor cells
  - Spironolactone bodies appear as a central core with electron-dense material surrounded by numerous smooth-walled circular membranes continuous with endoplasmic reticulum
- *Oncocytic adrenal cortical adenoma*
  - Cytoplasm contains numerous mitochondria
  - Nuclei contain pseudoinclusions

Molecular Alterations

- LOH at 11p15 and the P57 and IGF2 locus; overexpression of IGF2 and overexpression of FGFR at 7p12 have all been reported

Differential Diagnosis

- Adrenal cortical carcinoma
- Adrenal cortical hyperplasia
- Renal cell carcinoma
- If functional pigmented (black) adenoma:
  - Adrenal hematoma
  - Metastatic or primary melanoma

Treatment

- Surgical excision

Prognosis

- Benign cortical neoplasm

Associations

- Several inherited syndromes are associated with adrenal cortical adenomas: Carney complex, endocrine neoplasia type I (MEN 1), and McCune-Albright Syndrome
- May coexist with a myelolipoma

Adrenal Cortical Carcinoma

Clinical Manifestations

- A bimodal age distribution: 1st and 2nd decades and 5th decade
- More frequent in women than in men (1.5:1)
- Left adrenal gland involved more frequently than right
- Bilaterality extremely rare
- Incidence of metastasis at time of diagnosis approximately 70%
- Most common symptoms are flank pain or fullness; 30% have a palpable abdominal mass; other symptoms include weight loss, fever, hypoglycemia, and hypercalcemia
- 75% unassociated with any syndrome of hormone overproduction
- Patients may have Cushing syndrome, evidence of overproduction of sex steroid, or a combination of syndromes

Gross Pathology

- Typically a lobulated surface
- On sectioning, a nodular architecture with nodules ranging from yellow to brown (yellow associated with Cushing syndrome; brown associated with virilization or feminization)
- Focal areas of necrosis, hemorrhage, or cystic degeneration common
- Local invasion into adjacent structures may be evident

Microscopic Pathology

- The most common architectural pattern is patternless sheets of cells with a fine sinusoidal network
- Another frequent architectural pattern is one of broad trabeculae (10 to 20 cells wide) separated by delicate, wide sinusoids lined by small endothelial cells
- An insular or alveolar arrangement of cells may occur as a uniform finding or be admixed with the more common trabecular pattern
- Cells typically have well-defined cell membranes with cytoplasm that is compact and acidophilic; some cells contain lipid and are consequently pale on hematoxylin-eosin (H&E) staining
- Nuclear pleomorphism and hyperchromasia are usually present, but are not diagnostic for malignancy; nuclear pseudoinclusions may be seen; intracytoplasmic hyaline globules may be present (resemble those seen in pheochromocytomas)
- Mitotic figures common and atypical forms are usually present
- Criteria for malignancy include a mitotic rate of ≥5 per 50 high-powered fields (hpf), presence of atypical mitoses, and presence of invasion of venous structures; other histopathologic criteria include high (Furman) grade, diffuse architecture (>30% of tumor), necrosis and capsular invasion
- Vascular invasion characterized by the presence of aggregates of tumor within the lumens of veins
- Bands of fibrous tissue may traverse the tumor giving it an irregular lobulated appearance
- Foci of dystrophic calcification may be present
- Myxoid change in the stroma and the presence of lipomatous or myelolipomatous metaplasia may be evident
- If the adjacent cortex is atrophied it is likely that the neoplasm is producing cortisol with the resulting clinical manifestations of Cushing syndrome and/or virilization

Special Stains

- PAS with diastase will highlight the eosinophilic intracytoplasmic hyaline globules

Immunohistochemistry

- Tumor cells typically negative or weakly positive for cytokeratin (normal adrenal cortical cells are keratin positive and negative for EMA, CEA, and glycoprotein HMFG-2
- Variable staining for vimentin (usually positive)
- Tumor cells frequently positive for synaptophysin and inhibin-A, but always negative for chromogranin A. Chromogranin A is a reliable stain to discriminate adrenal cortical carcinoma from adrenal medullary tumor

Electron Microscopy

- Most tumor cells contain abundant smooth endoplasmic reticulum and short stacks of rough endoplasmic reticulum
- Presence of mitochondria variable; may be round, oval, or elongated
- Many tumor cells have short, broad microvillous cytoplasmic projections
- Glycogen deposits in 30%

Molecular Alterations

- Alterations on chromosomes 11p, 13q, and 17p with loss of alleles
- Overexpression of IGFB at 7p12 and of tumor suppressor genes p21 and p16 are frequent

Differential Diagnosis

- Benign cortical adenoma (see comment below)
- Hepatocellular carcinoma
- Renal cell carcinoma
- Metastatic carcinoma

Treatment

- Surgical excision—complete removal only chance for cure
- Palliation can be obtained with mitotane (mitotane is effective in controlling endocrine symptoms); approximately 30% of patients respond
- Some patients respond to the combination of mitotane in combination with cisplatin

Prognosis

- The most important pathologic prognostic factors are mitotic rate, tumor size, and the Ki-67 index
- 5-year survival rates are between 50% and 70%
- Spread may be local within the abdomen or via both lymphatic and vascular channels
- Metastasis occurs most commonly to liver, lung, retroperitoneum, and lymph nodes; metastasis to brain and skin are uncommon (poorly differentiated tumors may metastasize to skin)

Associations

- Rarely associated with hyperaldosteronism
- Occasionally associated with hypoglycemia, polycythemia, and inappropriate secretion of antidiuretic hormone
- Other associations:
  - *Li-Fraumeni syndrome* (kindreds predisposed to a characteristic wide variety of malignant tumors, including breast carcinoma and soft tissue sarcomas [2 most frequent], bone sarcomas, adrenal cortical carcinoma, brain tumors, and leukemia)
  - *Beckwith-Wiedemann syndrome* (characterized by enlargement of body organs, hemihypertrophy, renal medullary cysts, abnormally large cells in the adrenal cortex [adrenal cytomegaly], and an increased risk for the development of a Wilms tumor)

Ganglioneuroma

Clinical Manifestations

- Typically occurs in patients over the age of 7 years (an older age group than is seen with neuroblastoma)
- Most arise in posterior mediastinum; 2nd most common site is retroperitoneum, especially the presacral region
- Also reported in cervical and parapharyngeal areas, urinary bladder, prostate, and appendix
- Occurs in the gastrointestinal tract as a polypoid lesion
- Occasionally arises in the adrenal gland (<30%)

Gross Pathology

- Typically well circumscribed with an apparent fibrous capsule
- Tends to be firm and gray to yellow with a whorled appearance similar to a leiomyoma; calcifications may be detected on gross examination
- Raised, soft hemorrhagic areas may be present on cross section (may represent the presence of immature elements)

Microscopic Pathology

- Fibrous capsule that may be apparent on gross examination usually not evident on microscopic examination
- Tumor cells consist of a mixture of mature or almost mature ganglion cells and Schwann cells with variable amounts of collagen
- Schwann cell population predominates; typically arranged in small fascicles separated by a loose myxoid stroma
- Number of ganglion cells can vary from field to field and tumor to tumor; may be distributed diffusely or arranged in small clusters
- Aggregates of entrapped adipose tissue may be present, especially at the periphery
- Cellular atypia, mitotic activity, and necrosis typically absent
- Occasional ganglion cells may contain brown pigment (lipofuscin or neuromelanin—catecholamine products that have undergone auto-oxidation)
- Mast cells may be present (also seen in neurofibromas)
- Lymphocytes commonly present

Variants

- *Imperfect*: All stages of neuronal differentiation are present throughout the neoplasm (may be identical to a "differentiating neuroblastoma")
- *Immature or composite*: Typical appearance of a ganglioneuroma except for the presence of well-defined, cellular areas of neuroblastoma

Special Stains

- Not helpful

Immunohistochemistry

- Tumor cells stain for all neural markers

Electron Microscopy

- Tangled, unmyelinated cell processes in a maze of Schwann cells
- Ganglion cells contain large numbers of cytoplasmic organelles, including microfilaments and neurosecretory granules

Molecular Alterations

- None

Differential Diagnosis

- Neurofibroma
- Ganglioneuroblastoma

Treatment

- Complete surgical excision

Prognosis

- Malignant transformation to a malignant peripheral nerve sheath tumor may occur spontaneously or after irradiation for ganglioneuroblastoma or neuroblastoma

Associations

- Ganglioneuroma involving the adrenal gland may on rare occasions be masculinizing as a result of the presence of Leydig cells admixed with the more typical cells of a ganglioneuroma
- Rarely associated with hypertension, watery diarrhea (vasoactive intestinal peptide [VIP] present in cytoplasm of ganglion cells), and hypokalemia

Neuroblastoma and Ganglioneuroblastoma

Clinical Manifestations

- 4th most common malignant neoplasm of childhood (after leukemia, central nervous system tumors, and lymphoma)

Adrenal Gland>Neuroblastoma and Ganglioneuroblastoma

- Most common solid tumor in infants under the age of 1 year
- 80% are seen in children under the age of 4 years; median age at diagnosis 21 months
- Location typically parallels the distribution of the sympathic nervous system
- 70% occur in retroperitoneum (majority involve adrenal gland); ratio of adrenal to extraadrenal primary site approximately 2:1
- Also occurs in head and neck region, mediastinum, and pelvis
- Patients may present with diarrheal syndrome
- May have a familial incidence
- Most produce catecholamines; qualitative vanillyl-mandelic acid (VMA) can detect the presence of a neuroblastoma before the onset of symptoms
- Patients rarely hypertensive

Gross Pathology

- Vary in size from small-circumscribed mass to >10 cm
- Usually solitary; rarely bilateral
- Sectioning reveals a variety of appearances depending on the amount of stroma, hemorrhage, and/or necrosis
- Frequently lobular
- Calcification may be apparent and give the surface a gritty texture
- Adrenal primary tends to grow toward midline and may extend to contralateral gland; large lesions may invade adjacent viscera (eg, liver, kidney, and pancreas)

Microscopic Pathology

- Usually a lobular architecture that may be quite prominent with delicate, sometimes incomplete fibrovascular septa
- Hemorrhage, calcification, and necrosis frequently present
- Tumor cells may be arranged in a "zellballen," or organoid, configuration (similar to paraganglioma)
- Neuroblastoma cells typically arranged in sheets; small with hyperchromatic nuclei and little cytoplasm; may be closely packed together or separated by pink finely fibrillar material that represents neuritic cell processes; may be anaplastic with marked pleomorphism and hyperchromatic nuclei; nuclei typically round with evenly dispersed, stippled chromatin ("salt and pepper"); nuclei tend to be larger than the nuclei of mature lymphocytes
- Homer-Wright rosettes are present in 25% to 35% (tumor cells not related to blood vessels but are arranged around a central area filled with neuritic fibrillary material)
- Clusters of lymphocytes may be seen and may obscure the primary tumor in some areas
- Ganglion cell differentiation consists of cells with abundant eosinophilic cytoplasm, enlarged vesicular nuclei with coarsely clumped chromatin and prominent nucleoli, and distinct cell borders

Special Stains

- Metachromatic stains highlight Nissl substance in cells with ganglion cell differentiation

Immunohistochemistry

- Tumor cells are positive for NSE, chromogranin A, synaptophysin, and neurofilament proteins
- Tumor cells are always positive for norepinephrine and always negative for epinephrine
- S-100 protein will stain fibrovascular septa surrounding nodules of tumor cells (these cells occupy the same area that sustentacular cells occupy in paragangliomas)
- S-100 positive sustentacular cells often surround maturing ganglion cells

Electron Microscopy

- Nuclei have finely dispersed chromatin
- Tangled unmyelinated axons (neuritic processes) with dense-core neurosecretory-type granules and microtubules
- Glycogen present in 10%

Molecular Alterations

- Focal deletions in the short arm of chromosome 1 involving bands 1p36
- Abnormalities of chromosome 17 have been reported

- N-*myc* normally found on chromosome 2, may be translocated to short arm of chromosome 1 and become amplified

Differential Diagnosis

- Rhabdomyosarcoma
- Lymphoma
- Ewing sarcoma/primative neuroectodermal tumor
- Desmoplastic small round cell tumor
- Renal and extrarenal malignant rhabdoid tumor

Treatment

- Surgical excision with or without adjuvant chemotherapy
- Biopsy to establish diagnosis and obtain molecular studies followed by neoadjuvant chemotherapy with or without surgical resection

Prognosis

- Metastasizes widely by both lymphatic and vascular routes; bone marrow (80%) and bone (70%) most common sites
- Stage most important prognostic factor
  - Stage I: Tumor confined to area of origin with complete (microscopic) excision and negative ipsilateral and contralateral lymph nodes
    - 5-year survival rate of 90%
  - Stage IIA: Complete gross excision of unilateral neoplasm with negative ipsilateral and contralateral lymph nodes
    - 5-year survival rate of 70% to 80%
  - Stage IIB: Unilateral tumor with complete or incomplete gross excision with positive ipsilateral lymph nodes and negative contralateral lymph nodes
    - 5-year survival rate of 70% to 80%
  - Stage III: Neoplasm infiltrates across midline with or without regional lymph node metastasis or unilateral tumor with contralateral lymph node metastasis or midline tumor with negative ipsilateral and contralateral lymph nodes
    - 5-year survival rate of 40% to 70% (depending on completeness of surgical excision)
  - State IV: Tumor disseminates to distant lymph nodes, bone, bone marrow, liver, and/or other organs
    - 5-year survival rate of 60% in patients <1 year old; 25% if 1 to 2 years of age; and 10% if older than 2 years
  - Stage IV-S: A localized primary tumor (stage I or II) with dissemination limited to liver, skin, and/or bone marrow
    - 5-year survival rate of 80%
- Stroma-rich, well-differentiated tumors *without nodules* and stroma-rich, intermixed tumors *without nodules* have a favorable prognosis (100% and 90%, respectively)
- Stroma-rich *nodular* tumors have an unfavorable prognosis (20% survival)
- Stroma-poor tumors that are either differentiating or undifferentiated in *patients <1½ years old* with a mitosis-karyorrhexis index (MKI) of <200 have a favorable prognosis (85% survival); if the MKI is higher than 200, survival rate is 10%
- Stroma-poor tumors in *patients between the ages of 1½ and 5 years* that are undifferentiated have a poor prognosis regardless of the MKI (5% survival)
- Stroma-poor tumors in *patients between the ages of 1½ and 5 years* that are differentiating and have a MKI of <100 have a favorable prognosis (85% survival); if the MKI is higher than 100, the prognosis is poor (<5% survival)
- Stroma-poor tumors in *patients over the age of 5 years* have an unfavorable prognosis regardless of degree of differentiation or MKI (5% survival)
- Additional factors associated with a poor prognosis:
  - Patient older than 1 year
  - N-*myc* oncogene amplification (present in 25% to 30%)
  - Diploid karyotype
  - Decreased ratio of VMA to homovanillic acid

- Increased serum levels of NSE, ferritin, lactate dehydrogenase, chromogranin A, and creatine kinase BB
- Cytogenetic abnormalities of chromosome 1 (chromosome 1p deletion)

- Factors associated with an improved prognosis:
  - Patient under the age of 1 year
  - Lesions outside the adrenal gland
  - Presence of lymphocyte infiltration
  - Presence of S-100 protein–positive cells
  - DNA hyperdiploidy
  - Expression of *Trk* gene (encodes a nerve growth factor receptor); present in 90%
- Factors that do not significantly influence prognosis:
  - Sex
  - Lymph node status at time of diagnosis
  - Individual treatment modality
- 1% to 2% may spontaneously regress
- Reports of maturation into differentiated ganglioneuroma

Associations

- Beckwith-Wiedemann syndrome (exomphalos, macroglossia, gigantism)
- Hirschsprung disease
- Opsoclonus/myoclonus (probably paraneoplastic and autoimmune)
- Heterochromia iridis
- Horner syndrome (cervical or mediastinal tumor)
- Cushing syndrome
- Central hypoventilation syndrome ("Ondine curse")
- Late recurrence and death
- Watery diarrhea (secondary to the secretion of VIP): 5%-10%
- von Recklinghausen disease (neurofibromatosis)

Comments

- MKI is the number of mitotic figures and karyorrhectic nuclei per 5000 cells in randomly selected fields. Low index = lower than 100; intermediate index = 100 to 200, and high index = higher than 200.
- Undifferentiated tumors are composed almost entirely of immature neuroblasts and have <5% differentiating elements (characterized by cells with nuclear enlargement, nucleoli, eosinophilic cytoplasm, distinct cell borders and cytoplasmic processes)
- Differentiating tumors contain 5% or more differentiating elements

Pheochromocytoma

Clinical Manifestations

- Typically affects adults in the 5th decade of life
- Males and females generally affected equally
- Right adrenal gland involved more frequently than left
- The "10%" tumor:
  - 10% bilateral
  - 10% extra-adrenal (paraganglioma)
  - 10% malignant
  - 10% occur in childhood
  - 10% familial; 90% sporadic
- When sporadic, 95% solitary, 5% bilateral, and 5% to 10% extra-adrenal
- When familial, over 50% bilateral
- Most common clinical triad of symptoms: Hypertension, headaches, and diaphoresis
- Tumors may secrete epinephrine or norepinephrine or combinations of the 2 (norepinephrine usually predominates)
  - Tumors secreting norepinephrine are associated with sustained hypertension
  - Tumors secreting large amounts of epinephrine with norepinephrine are associated with paroxysmal hypertension
  - Tumors secreting epinephrine exclusively may cause hypotension

- Clinical diagnosis depends on presence of increased levels of urinary and plasma catacholamines and their metabolites

Variants

- Sporadic pheochromocytoma
- Familial pheochromocytoma

Gross Pathology

- Usually a round solitary mass that distorts the adrenal gland
- Typically measures 3 to 5 cm, but may be >10 cm
- On sectioning, sharply circumscribed with an apparent capsule (probably a pseudocapsule)
- Usually firm and gray-white to pink-tan with areas of hemorrhage
- Vascular structures may be present at periphery
- Areas of degenerative change, necrosis, fibrosis, and cystic change may be present particularly in the center of large tumors
- Dystrophic calcifications may be present
- May adhere to adjacent structures (local invasion is an indication of malignancy)
- May extend into the inferior vena cava
- Exposure of cut surface to air results in a darkening of the tumor secondary to the formation of yellow-brown adrenochrome or nonadrenochrome pigments (pigments similar to those produced when tumor immersed in potassium dichromate solutions)

Microscopic Pathology

- Typical architecture is an admixture of solid, alveolar (nesting or "zellballen"), and trabecular patterns
- Tumor cells tend to be large and polygonal and vary from lightly eosinophilic to amphophilic to basophilic with finely granular cytoplasm; occasionally cytoplasm is vacuolated
- Tumor cells may have either indistinct or well-defined cell membranes
- Nuclei of tumor cells are round or oval with coarsely clumped chromatin and prominent nucleoli and may contain "pseudoinclusions" (sometimes >1) which represent invaginations of cell cytoplasm
- Spindle cell patterns may be present (2%)
- Intracytoplasmic hyaline globules may be present
- Some areas of neoplasm may be markedly hyperchromatic and pleomorphic (no correlation to malignant behavior)
- Mitotic figures may be seen (do not necessarily indicate malignancy)
- Intercellular stroma may be sclerotic, contain amyloid, or have areas of myxoid change with foci of lymphocytic infiltration
- Stroma typically contains a prominent vascular component (capillary framework surrounds nests of tumor cells)
- Brown adipose tissue frequently present adjacent to neoplasm
- Areas of hemorrhage and/or necrosis may disrupt cellular architecture
- Composite pheochromocytoma: A pheochromocytoma with foci of neuroblastoma, ganglioneuroblastoma, ganglioneuroma, or malignant peripheral nerve sheath tumor (MPNST)

Special Stains

- Reticulin stains highlight the "zellballen" architecture or trabecular pattern
- PAS with diastase will demonstrate intracytoplasmic eosinophilic globules
- Cytoplasm of tumor cells is typically argyrophilic
- Grimelius stain highlights neurosecretory granules
- Fontana-Masson stain will confirm presence of melaninlike pigment in some tumor cells
- Congo red stain may demonstrate the presence of stromal amyloid

Immunohistochemistry

- Tumor cells negative for cytokeratin and positive for vimentin
- Tumor cells are immunoreactive for chromogranin A and synaptophysin
- Sustentacular cells surrounding the nests of "zellballen" strongly reactive for S-100 protein

Adrenal Gland>Pheochromocytoma

Electron Microscopy

- Tumor cells have variable numbers of rounded eccentric dense-core secretory-type granules with an enlarged peripheral clear zone
- Neurosecretory granules tend to be heterogenous with round, rod, oval, and comma shapes; norepinephrine-containing granules have very dense cores separated from their limiting membranes by a lucent halo; epinephrine-containing granules have a less dense core and are closely applied to their limiting membranes

Molecular Alterations

- Sporadic pheochromocytoma:
  - 10% have somatic mutation involving *ret* proto-oncogene
- Familial pheochromocytoma:
  - Loss of heterozygosity at chromosome 22q
  - RET proto-oncogene on chromosome 10q11.2 consistently expressed in multiple endocrine neoplasia (MEN) types IIa and IIb (also seen in papillary carcinoma of the thyroid)
  - Loss of heterozygosity at neurofibromatosis type 1 (NF-1) locus and loss of neurofibromin expression (chromosome 17)
  - *VHL* gene located on chromosome 3p
  - Loss of heterozygosity of the *SDHD* locus on 11q23 seen in 30% to 70%

Differential Diagnosis

- Pseudopheochromocytoma: Clinical differential diagnosis includes anxiety and psychiatric disorders, hyperthyroidism, hyperdynamic beta-adrenergic circulatory states, intracranial lesions, and ingestion of catecholaminergic drugs
- If tumor cells extensively vacuolated, may resemble adrenal cortical tumor

Treatment

- Surgical excision

Prognosis

- Excellent, with complete surgical excision
- If malignant, 5-year survival rates are approximately 45% to 55%; metastasizes most commonly to lymph nodes, bone, and liver

Associations

- Increased prevalence of periadrenal brown adipose tissue
- Sporadic pheochromocytoma
  - Catecholamine-associated cardiomyopathy (arrhythmias, cardiac failure, and sudden death)
  - Fibromuscular dysplasia
  - Renal artery stenosis
  - Multiple intracranial aneurysms
  - Cholelithiasis (~25%)
- Familial pheochromocytoma
  - MEN syndrome, type IIa and type IIb (30%-50%)
  - Tends to produce more epinephrine
  - May be associated with extra-adrenal paragangliomas
  - von Recklinghausen disease (~1%-5%)
  - von Hippel-Lindau disease (increased incidence of bilaterality; 10%-20%)
  - Sturge-Weber syndrome (questionable association)
- Carney triad:
  - Functioning extra-adrenal paraganglioma (pheochromocytoma reported)
  - Pulmonary chondroma
  - Gastric epithelioid leiomyosarcoma
- Composite pheochromocytoma may be seen in context of Verner-Morrison syndrome (watery diarrhea and hypokalemia)

- Other endocrine disorders associated with pheochromocytoma
  - Chemodectoma, bronchial carcinoid tumor, pituitary adenoma, parathyroid hyperplasia, and duodenal gastrin producing cells
  - Pituitary adenoma, parathyroid hyperplasia, and multiple functioning extra-adrenal paragangliomas
  - Medullary carcinoma of thyroid, multiple parathyroid adenomas, adrenal cortical adenoma, and small cell carcinoma of bronchus
  - Bilateral pheochromocytoma and pancreatic islet cell tumor
  - Familial pheochromocytoma and pancreatic islet cell tumor
  - Pituitary adenoma and pheochromocytoma
  - Pituitary adenoma, papillary thyroid carcinoma, bilateral carotid body paragangliomas, parathyroid hyperplasia, gastric leiomyoma, and systemic amyloidosis
  - von Recklinghausen disease, pheochromocytoma, jugulotympanic paraganglioma, and pulmonary paragangliomas
  - von Recklinghausen disease, pheochromocytoma, and duodenal carcinoid
  - Pheochromocytoma and papillary thyroid carcinoma

Extra-Adrenal Paraganglioma

Clinical Manifestations

- Typically distributed vertically along the paravertebral and para-aortic axis parallel to the distribution of the sympathetic nervous system (adrenal medulla is included; paragangliomas that arise in the adrenal medulla are referred to as *pheochromocytomas*)

Variants

- *Intra-abdominal (extra-adrenal)*
  - *Superior para-aortic (45%):* Typically located in the area of the adrenal gland, the hilum of the kidney, and the renal pedical
  - *Inferior para-aortic (30%):* Typically occurs below the kidneys and extends down the aorta to include the iliac vessels (most arise from the organs of Zuckerkandl); may have a midline location and actually lie over the aorta bifurcation
  - *Urinary bladder paraganglioma:* Usually located in the trigone; clinical symptoms include proximal (or sustained) hypertension and intermittent hematuria
  - Most occur between the ages of 20 and 50 years with an equal distribution in both sexes
  - Clinical symptoms reflect an excess of catecholamine secretion in up to 85% of patients
  - Typically solitary but may be multiple
  - Microscopically, tumor cells tend to have an anastomosing trabecular or a nested arrangement in a background of interconnecting fibrous trabecula with delicate vascular channels; individual tumor cells have abundant granular cytoplasm; intracytoplasmic hyaline globules may be present (less frequent than in pheochromocytoma); occasional bizarre nuclei; mitoses unusual; both argentaffin cells and argyrophilic cells are typically present; occasionally cells may be heavily pigmented (neuromelanin, a degradation product of catecholamine metabolism)
  - Tends to be the most aggressive of the paragangliomas with an incidence of malignancy of 15% to 50%
  - Also reported to occur in the kidney, urethra, prostate, spermatic cord, gallbladder, uterus, ovary, vagina, vulva, and hepatobiliary tree
- *Aorticopulmonary paraganglioma*
  - Arises near the base of the heart and great vessels; may be cardiac or extracardiac
  - More common in women than in men
- *Cardiac paraganglioma*
  - Arises within the pericardium, usually at the level of the atria
  - 50% have symptoms of excess catecholamine secretion
  - Average age at diagnosis 45 years
- *Extracardiac paraganglioma*
  - Occurs outside the pericardial cavity
  - Both intra and extracardiac paraganglioma associated with paragangliomas in other sites

- Reported in association with gastric epithelioid leiomyosarcoma and pulmonary chondroma *(Carney triad)*
- Typically round to oval and well-circumscribed
- Microscopically an organoid pattern of tumor cells with abundant granular cytoplasm; intracytoplasmic hyaline globules are rare (also true for all head and neck paragangliomas)
- Incidence of malignancy 15% to 20%; difficult to treat surgically as a result of involvement of vital adjacent structures

■ *Pulmonary paraganglioma*

- May not be a real clinical entity
- Tumors essentially impossible to distinguish from bronchial carcinoids
- Differential diagnosis for pulmonary paraganglioma includes:
  - Bronchial carcinoid
  - Carcinoid tumorlets: Peripheral location; usually associated with bronchial or bronchiolar epithelium
  - Minute meningothelial-like nodules: Seen with increased frequency in patients with heart failure, chronic bronchitis, emphysema, and pulmonary thromboemboli; no apparent relationship to paraganglia or paraganglioma; may be the explanation for the occasional appearance of a primary pulmonary meningioma

■ *Carotid body paraganglioma (chemodectoma)*

- Arises from chief cells within the carotid body paraganglia
- Affects men and women equally; typically present in 5th decade
- Usually presents as a painless, slow-growing mass at the angle of the mandible
- Occasionally causes bradycardia and syncopal episodes (carotid sinus syndrome)
- May be sporadic or familial; if familial may be bilateral, synchronous, or metachronous (30%); paragangliomas in other sites in the head and neck region are also common; bilateral or multicentric lesions in up to 5% to 10% of sporadic tumors
- On gross examination, tends to be a circumscribed with a fibrous pseudocapsule; cut surface may show a vascular network that is slightly retracted beneath the surface; tumors may not be particularly adherent to the adventia of the carotid artery or may be densely adherent to the adventitia and partially surround or completely surround 1 or both carotid vessels
- Microscopically, a uniform nesting arrangement of cells in a "zellballen" pattern; neoplastic chief cells have granular eosinophilic cytoplasm and indistinct cell borders; nuclear pseudoinclusions may be present; sustentacular cells present but constitute only a minor component of the neoplasm and are extremely difficult to identify in routine H&E sections; fibrosis may be so extensive that the nests of tumor cells are distorted and compressed; evidence of prior hemorrhage with the formation of fibrosiderotic nodules (Gamna-Gandy bodies) may be present as well as metaplastic bone
- Differential diagnosis includes hemangiopericytoma and hemangioendothelioma
- Treatment consists of complete surgical excision
- Carotid body tumors and other head and neck paragangliomas are rarely malignant (diagnosis of malignancy requires the presence of metastasis)

■ *Jugulotympanic paraganglioma*

- Typically arises in the region of the base of the skull and middle ear
- More common in women of an average age of 55 years
- Found with equal frequency on either side of the neck

■ *Tympanic paraganglioma*

- Typically located along the course of the Jacobson nerve (tympanic branch of cranial nerve X) in the middle ear
- Usually associated with tinnitus and may cause hearing loss
- May grow to fill the middle ear cavity and bulge into or through the tympanic membrane

- *Jugular paraganglioma*
  - Typically involves the lateral temporal bone at the base of the skull
  - May grow through the jugular foramen and project into the lumen of the internal jugular vein
  - Rarely functionally active with catecholamine production; norepinephrine and dopamine secretion have been reported
  - Microscopically, similar to paragangliomas in other sites in the head and neck region but tend to be more vascular with nests of cells that are less uniform and smaller; sclerosis may be a prominent feature; calcification may be present
  - Differential diagnosis includes middle ear adenoma, meningioma, metastatic renal cell carcinoma
  - Prognosis related to local aggressiveness with risk for bony destruction as well as intracranial extension and local recurrence; very rarely malignant
  - Treatment: Surgery with or without radiation; multiple reports of complete cure with radiation alone
- *Vagal paraganglioma*
  - Arises from paraganglia located in or adjacent to the vagus nerve
  - 3rd most frequent paraganglioma of the head and neck region
  - More common in women; usually diagnosed between the ages of 40 and 60 years
  - May produce various cranial nerve symptoms
  - Functional activity with catecholamine production has been reported (traction on the vagus nerve can lead to bradycardia and cardiac arrest)
  - Tends to have a fusiform or oval configuration and lie adjacent to the base of the skull
  - Microscopically a nested arrangement of tumor cells that may vary greatly in size; large ganglia typically present; stromal sclerosis often prominent (also prominent in jugulotympanic paragangliomas)
  - Rarely malignant
  - Treated with a complete surgical resection
- *Laryngeal paraganglioma*
  - Most present in the submucosa of the supraglottic larynx
  - Most common presenting symptom is hoarseness but dysphagia, dyspnea, stridor, dysphonia, hemoptysis, and a cervical mass are not uncommon presenting complaints
  - More common in women
  - Most arise on the right side of the larynx
  - Microscopically similar to other head and neck paragangliomas but less sclerotic than jugulotympanic or vagal paragangliomas
  - May invade locally; rarely malignant
  - Most important consideration in the differential diagnosis is an atypical carcinoid tumor; other considerations are melanoma (primary or metastatic) and hemangiopericytoma

Gross Pathology and Microscopic Pathology

- See specific variants above

Special Stains

- Stains for cytoplasmic argyrophilia will highlight individual tumor cells
- Reticulin stain will demonstrate the delicate fibrous septa that separate the trabeculae and nests of tumor cells
- Neuromelanin or lipofuscin will stain positively with Fontana-Masson silver stain

Immunohistochemistry

- Tumor cells invariably positive for neuron-specific enolase (NSE)
- Chromogranin and synaptophysin also typically positive
- S-100 protein will stain the sustentacular cells at the periphery of the trabeculae and nests of tumor cells

Electron Microscopy

- Dense-core neurosecretory granules with variable morphology; some neurosecretory granules have eccentric halos (norepinephrine-type); others are more uniform in size and shape (epinephrine-type)
- Large intracellular hyaline globules and large vacuolar spaces (probably lipid) may be present

Molecular Alterations

- Aortopulmonary paragangliomas have been reported in families (10% to 50%)
- Familial paragangiomas have been associated with germline mutations of *SDHD* (PGL1) on 11q23 (50%), *SDHB* (PGL4) on 1p36 (20%), and rarely of *SDHC* (PGL3) on 1q21

Differential Diagnosis

- See specific variants earlier in this section

Treatment

- Surgical excision

Prognosis

- Local invasion and metastasis indicate malignant
- If malignant with metastatic disease limited to lymph nodes 5-year survival is 80%; if distant metastases present, 5-year survival is 10%

Associations

- Urinary bladder paragangliomas have been reported in cases of von Recklinghausen disease, renal cell carcinoma, and polycystic kidney disease
- Carotid body paraganglioma seen in *Carney triad* (gastric epithelioid leiomyosarcoma, pulmonary chondroma, and functioning extra-adrenal paraganglioma) and in association with papillary carcinoma of the thyroid and hyperparathyroidism

Myelolipoma

Clinical Manifestations

- Most arise in the adrenal glands but may occur in the presacral region or the retroperitoneum
- Has been reported in the mediastinum, liver, stomach, leptomeninges, and lungs
- Rarely seen in patients under the age of 30 years
- Typically solitary and almost never bilateral
- Equal incidence in men and women
- Half are asymptomatic; other half may cause hematuria, hypertension, and rarely retroperitoneal hemorrhage

Gross Pathology

- Usually well circumscribed but not encapsulated
- Bright yellow to deep red or red brown depending on the amount of adipose and hematopoietic elements
- Vary from microscopic lesions to tumors that literally fill the abdomen

Microscopic Pathology

- A variable mixture of mature adipose with scattered islands of hematopoietic elements
- Hematopoietic elements typically have a complete spectrum of major cell lines with trilinear hematopoietic maturation
- Focal areas of calcification consisting of bony trabeculae may be present
- Large tumors often contain foci of necrosis, hemorrhage, and cyst formation

Special Stains, Immunohistochemistry, and Electron Microscopy

- Not helpful

Molecular Alterations

- None

Differential Diagnosis

- None

Treatment

- Simple surgical excision

Prognosis

- A benign lesion with no risk of malignant transformation

Associations

- May occur with an adrenal cortical adenoma or hyperplasia causing Cushing syndrome
- Seen in the adrenal gland of patients with Cushing disease (pituitary-dependent)
- Addison disease, virilism, and pseudohermaphroditism
- Occasionally seen in cases of congenital adrenal hyperplasia due to 21-hydroxylase and 17-hydroxylase deficiency
- Higher incidence in obese patients
- Occasionally associated with hypertension (may mimic a pheochromocytoma)
- Reported to occur in association with Castleman disease

Parathyroid Gland

Intraoperative Consultation

Most frozen section analyses are performed on patients with parathyroid disease to determine if the excised tissue is parathyroid tissue. The distinction between a parathyroid adenoma and a hyperplastic parathyroid gland cannot be made on pathologic examination and should not be attempted. Generally it is enough to provide the surgeon with the information that parathyroid tissue is present and whether it appears to be hypercellular. Even the distinction of hypercellular from normal can be difficult in light of the tremendous range of cellularity that can occur in normal parathyroid glands. Occasionally of equal importance to frozen section diagnosis is a determination of the weight of the excised parathyroid gland. The weight of the gland may a better indication of hypercellularity than microscopic examination. Glands weighing more than 80 to 100 mg (generally considered a borderline weight) are often hypercellular. How the surgeon proceeds with this information is largely determined by the intraoperative findings and the clinical setting in which the hyperparathyroidism has arisen. The increased use of intraoperative parathyroid hormone (PTH) assays are reducing the need for parathyroid frozen sections.

At times the simple diagnosis of parathyroid tissue can be quite difficult. Occasionally parathyroid glands have a prominent microfollicular pattern that is quite reminiscent of a microfollicular thyroid adenoma. Thyroid nodules can occur separate from the main thyroid gland, and a parathyroid gland with a follicular pattern may lie in the thyroid gland. Both of these situations can further complicate the diagnosis. Features of parathyroid tissue that help differentiate it from a microfollicular nodule of thyroid include the presence of solid or sheetlike patterns of growth somewhere in the nodule, various cell types (chief cells, clear cells, and oxyphil cells), circumscribed foci of oxyphil cells, and the presence of fat in the lesion.

Differentiating a parathyroid carcinoma from an adenoma may be quite difficult. Usually the operating surgeon suspects that he or she is dealing with a carcinoma and this clinical impression can be of significant help to the pathologist. Clues to the diagnosis of carcinoma include the presence of thick fibrous bands coursing through the gland, foci of necrosis, mitotic activity, diffuse nuclear atypia, and large nucleoli. Obviously invasion into adjacent soft tissue can by itself be diagnostic. It is important for the pathologist to realize that these features of malignancy are not always present in a parathyroid cancer. Malignant parathyroid tissue can appear quite benign on both frozen section and permanent section.

Specimen Handling

Parathyroid tissue is inked whenever there is a suspicion of malignancy. The specimen should be serially sectioned and submitted in its entirety.

Parathyroid Hyperplasia

Variants

- Primary chief cell hyperplasia
- Secondary chief cell hyperplasia
- Clear cell hyperplasia

Clinical Manifestations

- *Primary chief cell hyperplasia*

- Symptoms identical to those that occur in patients with parathyroid adenoma
- 20% have one of the MEN syndromes (90% MEN I; 30% to 40% MEN IIA; very rare in MEN IIB)

- *Secondary chief cell hyperplasia*
  - Typically seen in patients with chronic renal disease (increased secretion of PTH results from chronic persistent stimulation of parathyroids by low levels of ionized calcium in the blood)
  - Also seen in patients with dietary deficiency of vitamin D, abnormal vitamin D metabolism, or pseudohypoparathyroidism
  - Most patients experience symptomatic skeletal pain and deformities (osteitis fibrosa cystica and osteomalacia); others experience joint stiffness and pain secondary to periarticular deposits of calcium
  - Calciphylaxis characterized by ischemic necrosis of skin, muscles, and subcutaneous fat may develop
- *Clear cell hyperplasia*
  - Most patients have evidence of renal calculi or bone disease
  - No apparent familial incidence, hence no association with any of the MEN syndromes

Gross Pathology

- *Primary chief cell hyperplasia*
  - Typically all 4 glands variably enlarged and tan to red
  - Superior glands tend to be larger than inferior glands
  - Cut surface typically homogenous but cystic change may be present
- *Secondary chief cell hyperplasia*
  - Usually an inverse correlation between the size of glands and mean serum calcium level
  - All 4 glands tend to be relatively uniform in size
  - Glands tend to be yellow to tan to creamy grey
- *Clear cell hyperplasia*
  - Typically all glands are enlarged but with considerable variation in size
  - Glands tend to have an irregular shape with pseudopodal extensions into surrounding adipose
  - Superior glands are typically distinctly larger than inferior glands and usually are chocolate brown and may have foci of cystic change, hemorrhage, and fibrosis

Microscopic Pathology

- *Primary chief cell hyperplasia*
  - Characterized by a diffuse or nodular (occasionally glandular) arrangement of proliferating chief cells
  - Abundant stromal fat cells may be present
  - Variable numbers of oncocytic cells may be present
  - Occasional mitotic figures may be present and nuclei may demonstrate slight pleomorphism (usually not as extensive as seen in a typical adenoma)
  - Cystic change uncommon
- *Secondary chief cell hyperplasia*
  - Nests and cords of chief cells replace stromal fat cells and are architecturally arranged in diffuse sheets and occasionally in cords acinar or trabecular patterns
  - Advanced disease characterized by nodules of chief cells and oncocytes surrounded by a fibrous tissue capsule
  - Foci of fibrosis hemorrhage, chronic inflammation, and cyst formation may be present
  - Characteristic cell is large and vacuolated (glycogen) with a small, dense eccentric nucleus
- *Clear cell hyperplasia*
  - Cells typically polygonal with distinct cytoplasmic membranes; nuclei may be multiple and tend to be round to ovoid, moderately hyperchromatic, and contain an eccentrically located nucleolus
  - Nuclei tend to be located at the pole of the cell that is closest to the adjacent stroma and vessels

- Cells may have a glandular or tubular arrangement and occasionally they line cystic structures
- Cytoplasm tends to be clear and is filled with small vacuoles that contain moderate amounts of glycogen

Special Stains

- PAS will confirm the presence of glycogen in the vacuolated chief cells of secondary chief cell hyperplasia and clear cell hyperplasia

Immunohistochemistry

- Parathyroid cells stain for PTH

Electron Microscopy

- Cells of chief cell hyperplasia have focally complex interdigitations, secretory granules, and lipid droplets
- Cells of clear cell hyperplasia characterized by multiple cytoplasmic vacuoles (some represent Golgi vesicles and some contain PTH); cells generally have little endoplasmic reticulum and few secretory and prosecretory granules

Molecular Alterations

- MEN I the result of a single inherited locus on chromosome 11q13
- Gene for MEN IIA and MEN IIB syndromes linked to pericentromeric region of chromosome 10

Differential Diagnosis

- Normal parathyroid
- Adenoma

Treatment

- Chief cell and clear cell hyperplasia
    - Subtotal parathyroidectomy
- Secondary chief cell hyperplasia
    - Subtotal parathyroidectomy with approximately 50 mg of parathyroid tissue left in situ or implanted into the sternocleidomastoid muscle or a muscle of the forearm

Prognosis

- Recurrent hypercalcemia occurs in approximately 15% of patients undergoing subtotal parathyroidectomy for primary chief hyperplasia
- Patients with secondary hyperparathyroidism treated with subtotal parathyroidectomy and autotransplantation may experience either graft failure or insufficient graft function resulting in hypothyroidism or may develop recurrent hyperparathyroidism (chronic renal failure, the stimulus for parathyroid hyperplasia, is still present)
- Proliferation of autografted parathyroid tissue may rarely undergo malignant transformation

Associations

- *MEN I (Wermer syndrome):* Characterized by synchronous or metachronous hyperplasias, tumors, or both involving parathyroid glands, pancreatic islets, and the anterior pituitary gland; patients also have an increased incidence of bronchogenic and gastrointestinal carcinoids, adrenal cortical adenomas, and thyroid follicular neoplasms
- *MEN IIA (Sipple syndrome):* Characterized by medullary carcinoma of the thyroid, pheochromocytoma, and parathyroid hyperplasia
- *MEN IIB:* Characterized by pheochromocytoma, medullary carcinoma of thyroid, and ocular, oral, and gastrointestinal ganglioneuromatosis, megacolon, marfanoid habitus, pes cavus, and other skeletal abnormalities; parathyroid involvement has been reported but is extremely rare (may occur in patients with mixed MEN syndromes).

Parathyroid Adenoma

Clinical Manifestations

- Single most common cause of primary hyperthyroidism; 80% of patients with primary hyperparathyroidism have a single parathyroid adenoma
- Most occur during the 4th decade
- More common in women than in men (3:1)
- Most patients have elevated levels of serum calcium
- May be seen in patients with MEN I and MEN II syndromes (most parathyroid lesions in the MEN syndromes represent chief cell hyperplasia rather than adenoma)

Parathyroid Gland>Parathyroid Adenoma

- Few patients have a palpable mass
- 75% involve one of the inferior glands, 15% one of the superior glands, and 10% occur in an anomalous location (70% mediastinum, 20% within thyroid gland, remainder in soft tissue behind the esophagus or in the esophageal wall, pericardium, vagus nerve, and soft tissue adjacent to the angle of the jaw)

Gross Pathology

- 90% involve the upper or lower glands of the neck (lower glands more frequently involved)
- Typically encapsulated, with a thin fibrous capsule
- Larger tumors tend to be oval; occasionally tumors may be bilobed or multilobed
- Cut surface typically tan to orange to brown and soft (normal glands tend to be light brown or yellow)
- Foci of cystic change may be present and cysts may contain clear to brown fluid

Microscopic Pathology

- Typically composed of closely packed chief cells in various stages of their secretory cycles, arranged in cords and nests; may have a glandular or solid architecture; 50% to 60% have a rim of non-neoplastic chief cells
- Dominant cell type is the chief cell characterized by a polygonal shape with indistinct cell borders; neoplastic cells tend to have eosinophilic to clear cytoplasm (may appear vacuolated); clear cells typically contain abundant glycogen
- Neoplastic cell nuclei usually be round and centrally placed with dense chromatin and small nucleoli; occasionally cells are multinucleate
- Enlarged, hyperchromatic nuclei may be seen in 25% (not a criterion for carcinoma)
- Mitotic figures typically absent (if more than 1 mitosis per 10 hpf, consider the possibility of malignancy)
- Cystic structures surrounded by chief cells may be present and are typically filled with PAS-positive, eosinophilic material (quite reminiscent of thyroid colloid)
- Folliclelike or glandular structures may be present and may contain foci of calcification
- 3% consist predominantly of oncocytic cells (oncocytic adenoma)
- Stromal fat may be present
- Stroma typically sparse; occasionally adenomas contain large amounts of fibrous connective tissue similar to that seen in parathyroid carcinoma (represents degenerative changes)

Special Stains

- Eosinophilic material in cysts typically PAS-positive
- Congo red will confirm the presence of amyloid in some of the eosinophilic intraluminal material seen in folliclelike or glandular structures
- PAS stain will highlight the glycogen content of adenomas

Immunohistochemistry

- Eosinophilic material in cysts negative for thyroglobulin
- Neoplastic chief cells are typically positive for low-molecular-weight cytokeratins: 8, 18, and 19 and chromogranin

Electron Microscopy

- Cells show interdigitated plasma membranes and occasional lipid droplets and very few secretory granules
- Adenoma cells do not possess the normal secretory and synthetic functions typical of normal chief cells

Molecular Alterations

- Loss of heterozygosity at 1p36.3 (30 to 40%), 11q13 (20 to 30%), 6q22-23 (30%), 11p (27%), 9p (16%), and 3qcen-3q21 (10%)

Differential Diagnosis

- Parathyroid hyperplasia
- Parathyroid carcinoma
- Follicular lesions of the thyroid
- C-cell lesions of the thyroid

Treatment

- Surgical excision of the adenoma and biopsy of at least 1 additional normal-sized gland

Prognosis

- Recurrent hypercalcemia occurs in 3%

Associations

- Increased incidence in patients who have received ionizing irradiation to the neck region
- MEN I and MEN II

Parathyroid Carcinoma

Clinical Manifestations

- Represents 0.5% to 2% of all cases of primary hyperparathyroidism
- Affects men and women equally
- Most present with symptoms of hypercalcemia and have a serum calcium level in excess of 3.5 mmol/L (14 mg/dL) and concurrent markedly elevated levels of PTH
- Occasionally patients present with hypercalcemic crisis
- 60% to 65% have evidence of nephrolithiasis and bone disease (osteitis fibrosa cystica, subperiosteal bone resorption, and diffuse osteoporosis)
- 30% have a palpable neck mass

Gross Pathology

- Usually an ill-defined mass densely adherent to surrounding soft tissue and thyroid
- Rarely encapsulated; may be grossly indistinguishable from an adenoma
- Arises with equal frequency from upper and lower glands
- Cut section reveals grey to tan firm ill-defined lesion

Microscopic Pathology

- Classically contain thick fibrous bands (90%), increased mitotic activity (80%), and capsular and vascular invasion
- Thick fibrous bands characterized by a paucicellular collagenous tissue that divides the neoplasm into pleomorphic compartments; fibrous bands may extend directly from a thickened capsule into the parenchyma of the neoplasm
- Fibrous capsule of a carcinoma typically thicker than that of an adenoma
- Tumor cells usually arranged in a trabecular, rosette-like, or sheetlike pattern and are usually larger than normal chief cells and have uniform, round to oval nuclei; cytoplasm is usually clear to eosinophilic and granular (granular cytoplasm indicates possible oncocytic change)
- Mitotic activity must exceed 1 per 10 hpf (mitotic activity in this range may be seen in up to 15% of benign adenomas)
- Capsular invasion present in 60% to 65%
- Vascular invasion present in 10% to 15% and is usually seen in the thickened capsule (similar to criteria used to define vascular invasion in a follicular carcinoma of the thyroid; the tumor must not only be present in a vascular channel but must be at least partially attached to the vascular wall)

Special Stains

- Not helpful

Immunohistochemistry

- Tumor cells typically positive for PTH

Electron Microscopy

- Extensive interdigitations of plasma membranes
- Cytoplasm contains prominent stacks of granular endoplasmic reticula and occasional secretory granules

Molecular Alterations

- 30% are aneuploid

Differential Diagnosis

- Parathyroid adenoma
- Benign parathyroid tissue "seeded" into the operative field at the time of surgery for benign adenoma

- Follicular or medullary carcinoma of the thyroid (particularly if parathyroid carcinoma is nonfunctional)
- Oncocytic (Hürthle cell) carcinoma (parathyroid carcinoma with oncocytic features)

Treatment

- En bloc resection to include adjacent tissue (thyroid lobe, paratracheal soft tissue, lymph nodes, and ipsilateral thymus gland)
- Cervical lymph node dissection performed only with clinical evidence of node involvement
- Surgical excision of distant metastasis indicated when possible

Prognosis

- High probability of local recurrence
- Metastatic disease to regional nodes and distant sites may occur late
- Well-performed initial en bloc resection results in a 50% cure rate
- Typically recurs in 3 years
- 35% will ultimately develop metastasis (cervical lymph nodes 30%, lung 40%, and liver 10%)
- Tumor cells are not radiosensitive

Associations

- None

Pituitary Gland

Intraoperative Consultation

The primary role of the pathologist in evaluating pituitary lesions on frozen section is to determine the presence of an adenoma and to differentiate adenomatous tissue from normal pituitary. The cells of an adenoma tend to have sheetlike or papillary architecture and lack the normal organoid pattern that is characteristic of a normal pituitary. In addition, pituitary adenomas have a monomorphic population of cells whereas a normal pituitary has a variety of different cells.

The evaluation of a craniopharyngioma on frozen section can be more problematic. A tissue specimen taken from close to a craniopharyngioma may show marked astrogliosis with abundant Rosenthal fibers that can mimic an astrocytoma. In addition nests, of squamous cells typical of a craniopharyngioma may be present in reactive glial tissue and mimic a well-differentiated metastatic squamous cell carcinoma.

Specimen Handling

- Specimens are routinely submitted in their entirety.

Craniopharyngioma

Variants

- Adamantinomatous craniopharyngioma
- Papillary craniopharyngioma

Clinical Manifestations

- *Adamantinomatous*
    - Most frequent form; 5% of intracranial neoplasms in childhood
    - Typically presents during the first 2 decades of life as a calcified cystic suprasellar mass; 50% have an intrasellar component
    - Patients may present with complications such as hypopituitarism and visual abnormalities
    - Lesions occasionally rupture and spill their contents into the cerebral spinal fluid
- *Papillary*
    - Typically occurs in adults
    - Presents as solid, noncalcified mass, frequently in the 3rd ventricle

Gross Pathology

- *Adamantinomatous*
    - Lesion typically adheres to structures at the base of the brain and may indent the floor of the 3rd ventricle
    - Almost always cystic and filled with dark brown, machinery oil fluid; crystals of cholesterol and grey-yellow flecks of "wet keratin" float in the cystic fluid

- *Papillary*
  - Typically encapsulated solid mass (no cyst)
  - Tumor has a smooth surface and can be separated from surrounding brain tissue

Microscopic Pathology

- *Adamantinomatous*
  - Epithelial cells of a squamous nature form lobules grouped in a multinodular, cloverleaf pattern
  - Cells at periphery of lobules are columnar or polygonal and are palisaded; cells in the center are more loosely textured (stellate reticulum)
  - Cystic spaces filled with fluid or amorphous debris
  - Epithelial cells in cystic areas may not palisade
  - Nodules of plump, eosinophilic, keratinized cells (wet keratin)
  - Dystrophic calcification may be seen in nodules of wet keratin
  - Extensive fibrosis, chronic inflammation, and cholesterol clefts are typically present (especially in recurrent lesions)
  - Locally invasive with fingers of tumor projecting into adjacent part of the brain; marked gliosis rich in Rosenthal fibers surrounds these areas of infiltrating tumor
- *Papillary*
  - Solid sheets of well-differentiated squamous epithelial cells with prominent fibrovascular cores
  - Cellular sheets typically undergo dehiscence to form pseudopapilla
  - Goblet cells and ciliated cells may be present
  - Tumors do not have palisading cells, well-formed keratin pearls, nodules of wet keratin, inflammatory response, or cholesterol deposition

Special Stains

- Mucicarmine will highlight goblet cells occasionally seen in papillary lesions

Immunohistochemistry

- Epithelial cells stain positively for cytokeratins and EMA
- Focal staining for estrogen receptors not uncommon

Electron Microscopy

- *Adamantinomatous*
  - Epithelial cells contain bundles of tonofilaments and have well-formed desmosomes
  - Tumors cells adjacent to stroma have a basal lamina; tumor cells located internally or lining microcysts have microvilli and no basement membrane
- *Papillary*
  - Tumor cells have a high degree of squamous differentiation with desmosomes and bundles of tonofilaments

Molecular Alterations

- None

Differential Diagnosis

- *Adamantinomatous*
  - Papillary craniopharyngioma
  - Epidermoid cyst
  - Polycystic astrocytoma (areas adjacent to foci of invasion)
- *Papillary*
  - Adamantinomatous craniopharyngioma
  - Epidermoid and dermoid cyst

Treatment

- Surgical excision is the treatment of choice for both variants; total excision easier for papillary than adamantinomatous lesions
- Radiation is reserved for lesions that cannot be completely excised

Prognosis

- Adamantinomatous lesions more likely to recur than papillary lesions

- Most recurrences develop within 5 years of surgery
- Overall survival excellent for both variants

Associations

- None

Pituitary Adenoma

Clinical Manifestations

- Represents 10% to 20% of intracranial tumors
- Arises from cells of the adenohypophysis
- Most found within the confines of the sella turcica
- Vast majority are benign adenomas, but with a variable and unpredictable growth rate
- 70% have clinical and/or biochemical evidence of hormone production
- 10% to 20% exhibit suprasellar extension which is manifested by neurologic signs and symptoms usually related to compression of the optic nerves, optic chiasm (bitemporal hemianopsia), cavernous sinus, or oculomotor nerves
- Occurs more commonly in adults than in children
- Affects males and females equally
- Approximately 30% are endocrinologically silent
- Most adenomas in children and adolescents are functional
- Rarely multiple (~1%)

Gross Pathology

- Gray to red, soft and solid with cystic, hemorrhagic, and necrotic foci
- May be *enclosed* (encased in the dura of the sella), *invasive* (infiltrate the dura, floor of the sella, nasal sinuses, or other structures; seen in 20%-80% depending on tumor type), or *giant* (superior edge extends 20 mm above the jugum sphenoidal)
- If local invasion is present, it occurs in a lateral direction with penetration of the cavernous sinus
- Even invasive tumors tend to displace rather than actually infiltrate brain

Microscopic Pathology

- Tumor cells are usually round or polygonal with a round or oval nucleus and a variable amount of cytoplasm which may be basophilic, acidophilic, amphophilic, or chromophobic
- Cells tend to grow in a diffuse (solid), sinusoidal (trabecular), or papillary (pseudopapillary) arrangement; rarely grow in a glandular pattern
- Mitoses rare
- Occasional bizarre hyperchromatic nuclei with prominent nucleoli may be present, including giant and ring forms
- Foci of calcification present in 7% (primarily a finding in prolactin-secreting neoplasms)
- Deposits of endocrine amyloid may be present (primarily in prolactin-secreting tumors)

Variants

- *Prolactin cell adenoma*
  - □ Most common neoplasm arising in the adenohypophysis
  - □ Typically presents in women of childbearing age with galactorrhea-amenorrhea (Chiari-Frommel syndrome or Forbes-Albright syndrome)
  - □ Tumor tends to be chromophobic to slightly acidophilic, PAS-negative and often grow in a diffuse (occasionally papillary) pattern; 50% are invasive
  - □ Psammatomatous microcalcifications present in 10% to 20%
  - □ Amyloid frequently present
  - □ On electron microscopy, tumor cells are irregular and form intricate processes that interdigitate; rough endoplasmic reticulin is abundant and typically arranged in a whorled pattern (nebenkern); secretory granules are sparse
- *Growth hormone–producing adenoma*
  - □ Approximately 15% of all pituitary adenomas
  - □ Two variants:
    - Densely granulated adenoma corresponds to the classic acidophilic adenoma of acromegaly; cytoplasmic granules stain positively for eosin; lesions tend to be slow growing, well differentiated, and present in older patients; do not recur

    - Sparsely granulated adenomas are chromophobic and are characterized by eosinophilic paranuclear hyaline bodies (microfilaments); tend to be large at the time of presentation; occur in younger patients and tend to be more aggressive and invasive
  - May result in gigantism or acromegaly if functioning at a clinical level
  - Some secrete 2 or more hormones to include prolactin and thyroid-stimulating hormone
- Variants
  - Plurihormonal adenoma
    - Most produce both growth hormone (GH) and thyroid stimulating hormone (TSH); others produce TSH and prolactin (PRL) or GH, TRL and TSH
    - Most patients will present clinically with acromegaly
    - Tumors tend to be large and follow an aggressive clinical course
  - Mixed prolactin and growth hormone-producing adenomas:
    - 5% of pituitary adenomas
    - Adenomas that produce both growth hormone and prolactin tend to produce acromegaly as the dominant clinical feature
    - Usually more aggressive than pure growth hormone-secreting adenomas
    - Immunohistochemical stains confirm that both growth hormone-secreting cells and prolactin secreting cells are randomly arranged throughout the neoplasm
  - Acidophilic stem cell adenoma:
    - Neoplasms have ultrastructural features of both growth hormone and prolactin-producing cells
    - Tends to be fast growing and invasive
    - On electron microscopy, giant mitochondria, fibrous bodies, poorly organized rough endoplasmic reticulum, and primitive Golgi apparatus
    - Typically tumors are either nonfunctioning or cause hyperprolactinemia; rarely produce growth hormone
  - *Corticotroph cell (corticotropin [ACTH]-producing) adenoma*
    - Represents 7% to 15% of all pituitary adenomas
    - 15% invasive at time of surgery
    - 80% associated with Cushing disease; 15% Nelson syndrome; 10% hormonally silent
    - Most are amphophilic
    - Usually located in the central portion of the anterior lobe; rarely seen in the lateral lobes
    - Removal of hyperplastic adrenal glands in patients with Cushing disease (pituitary adenoma) may result in rapid enlargement of pituitary neoplasm that will have invasive tendencies (Nelson syndrome; caused by the loss of negative corticosteroid feedback resulting in rapid growth of a preexisting microadenoma)
    - Microscopically tumor cells typically arranged in a distinctive trabecular or sinusoidal pattern
    - Extratumoral pituitary cells usually have Crook's hyaline change (accumulation of cytokeratin microfilaments around nucleus resulting from glucocorticoid feedback on pituitary which acts to stop granule secretion)
    - On electron microscopy, secretory granules tend to be concentrated along the cell membrane or scattered in the cytoplasm and have a teardrop shape
    - Silent adenomas have a tendency to hemorrhage with sudden tumor expansion (pituitary apoplexy)
  - *Glycoprotein adenomas*
    - Hormone-producing cells are gonadotrophs and thyrotrophs
    - Adenoma of TSH cell type may be associated with hyperthyroidism or may arise in patients with longstanding hypothyroidism; least common pituitary tumor type; tends to have a sinusoidal growth pattern and are immunoreactive for TSH; most are chromophobic

- Adenomas of follicle-stimulating hormone (FSH)/luteinizing hormone (LH) cell type tend to grow slowly and be large at the time of presentation; cells tend to be elongated or polygonal and arranged in perivascular pseudorosettes; rarely associated with high serum levels of LH or FSH

□ *Null cell, non-oncocytic and null cell, oncocytic*

- Represents 20% of adenomas
- No biochemical or clinical evidence of hormone production
- Usually present as slow-growing sellar or parasellar neoplasms in elderly patients with progressive loss of vision and hypopituitarism
- Oncocytic change may affect more than 50% of cells; on electron microscopy, mitochondria occupy up to 50% of the cytoplasmic area and secretory granules are sparse

Special Stains

- Reticulin stains confirm lack of reticulin content in adenoma
- Basophilic adenomas (ACTH producing) usually strongly PAS positive

Immunohistochemistry

- Growth hormone, prolactin, ACTH, LH, FSH, TSH, and alpha subunit

Electron Microscopy

- See specific variants listed previously in this section

Molecular Alterations

- None

Differential Diagnosis

- Normal pituitary

Treatment

- Surgical excision
- Dopamine agonists (ie, bromocriptine) can control hyperprolactinemic symptoms and can lead to both a reduction in serum levels of prolactin as well as a reduction in the size of the tumor

Prognosis

- Depends on presence/absence of invasion
- Typical or invasive macroadenomas may give rise to a carcinoma

Associations

- 3% occur as one of the components of MEN I

Thyroid Gland

Intraoperative Consultation

There are 4 indications for intraoperative diagnosis for lesions of the thyroid gland:

- Determine the presence of a malignancy, and when possible, determine the specific type of malignancy. Well-differentiated carcinomas (papillary and follicular) are typically treated the same way, with the exception that papillary carcinomas involve thyroidectomy as well as the removal of clinically involved lymph nodes. Medullary carcinoma of the thyroid is usually treated with a formal central compartment lymph node dissection. Unless obvious papillary structures are present or a cytologic preparation is performed which confirms that a well-differentiated neoplasm is a papillary carcinoma, most well-differentiated carcinomas are described as follicular lesions and the final diagnosis is deferred to permanent sections.
- If well-differentiated thyroid carcinoma is seen in a cervical lymph node submitted for frozen section, the surgeon will remove all enlarged, clinically suspicious lymph nodes. The presence of medullary carcinoma in a lymph node will precipitate a formal lymph node dissection (usually central compartment).
- Occasionally a surgeon will encounter a thyroid that appears to be unresectable. An incisional biopsy of such a gland will be sent for frozen section to determine if the reason for unresectability is the result of the presence of an anaplastic carcinoma, malignant lymphoma, or sclerosing thyroiditis.

- The neoplasm in all lobectomy specimens in which a preoperative fine-needle aspiration biopsy revealed the presence of a Hürthle cell neoplasm or cellular/microfollicular neoplasm should be examined by frozen section. If an invasive follicular or Hürthle cell carcinoma is present, the surgeon will perform a total thyroidectomy. If the lesion is a papillary carcinoma, especially if it is larger than 1 cm and multifocal, or there is a clinical history of head and neck irradiation, a total thyroidectomy and lymph node "plucking" will be performed.

The diagnosis of medullary carcinoma on frozen section can be quite difficult and should be made with caution. The clinical and family history and pertinent laboratory data to include serum calcitonin levels are vital.

Frozen section diagnosis of papillary carcinoma may be quite difficult because well-formed papillary structures, psammoma bodies, nuclear clearing, and nuclear grooves may all be absent. Generally cytologic scrape preparations are far superior to frozen sections for demonstrating these classic cytologic features of a papillary carcinoma.

Minimally invasive follicular/Hürthle cell carcinoma is essentially impossible to differentiate from a follicular/Hürthle cell adenoma because the entire interface between the tumor and adjacent thyroid parenchyma (capsular area) must be examined before the absence of minimally invasive cancer can be ensured. The diagnosis in this setting is usually deferred to permanent section. The pathologic criteria used to differentiate a follicular adenoma from a minimally invasive follicular carcinoma are identical for Hürthle cell neoplasms.

A medullary carcinoma can be quite difficult to diagnose especially in the absence of an amyloid stroma. Medullary carcinoma of the thyroid can have various atypical patterns and consequently resemble papillary carcinoma, Hürthle cell tumor, follicular carcinoma, and lymphoma. In addition, giant cells may be present in a medullary carcinoma and give the lesion an appearance similar to that of anaplastic carcinoma of follicular origin. The mucinous and melanotic variant of medullary carcinoma can be confused with metastatic mucinous carcinoma and melanoma, respectively.

The frozen section diagnoses of poorly differentiated (insular) and anaplastic carcinoma are usually straightforward.

Intraoperative diagnosis of Hashimoto disease can be complicated by the presence of a malignant lymphoma or sclerosing mucoepidermoid carcinoma hidden in the changes of Hashimoto disease. In addition, a nodule of thyroid tissue separate from the main thyroid gland containing Hashimoto disease may be mistaken for metastatic carcinoma. It is important for the pathologist to always remember that a nodule of thyroid tissue unaccompanied by a main thyroid specimen is not an uncommon occurrence and the diagnosis of metastatic carcinoma should be made in this situation with great hesitancy.

Two classic metastatic lesions to the thyroid (renal cell carcinoma and metastatic melanoma) may be difficult to differentiate from clear cell follicular carcinoma and medullary carcinoma, respectively.

The 3 most frequent errors made by a pathologist in rendering an intraoperative consultation on the thyroid nodule include:

- Making the diagnosis of follicular variant of micropapillary carcinoma without a cytoscrape preparation
- Trying to distinguish between follicular/Hürthle cell adenoma and minimally invasive carcinoma
- Trying to distinguish a hyperplastic nodule from an adenoma

Specimen Handling

Thyroid lobes removed for the presence of a solitary nodule should be inked and serially sectioned. Whenever possible, the entire interface between the nodule and adjacent thyroid parenchyma should be submitted to ensure that the entire capsule can be microscopically evaluated.

Tumor-Like Conditions

Fibrosing (Riedel) Thyroiditis

Clinical Manifestations

- Typically presents as an ill-defined enlargement of the thyroid with associated severe dyspnea

- Typically affects adults and the elderly
- More common in women than in men
- No antecedent history of acute inflammation involving the thyroid
- On examination, thyroid feels extremely firm with apparent involvement of the adjacent soft tissues
- Most patients are euthyroid
- No drug association

Gross Pathology

- Extensive fibrosis involving most or the entire gland frequently in an asymmetric fashion
- Involved gland is rock hard and difficult to cut (surgeons describe it as having a woody consistency)
- Tissue planes between the gland and adjacent soft tissue are obliterated by extensive fibrosis
- Cut section characterized by complete obliteration of any recognizable thyroid architecture interspersed with areas having fairly normal thyroid architecture

Microscopic Pathology

- Extensive hyalinized (keloidlike) fibrous tissue destroys and replaces portions of the gland
- Fibrosis extends into adjacent soft tissue
- Lymphocytes and plasma cells permeate fibrous tissue; eosinophils may be present
- Usually an associated phlebitis, often with thrombosis involving veins encased in fibrous tissue
- Parathyroid glands may be encased in fibrous tissue (25%)
- An adenoma may be present in the center of a fibrotic area (25%)

Special Stains and Electron Microscopy

- Not helpful

Immunohistochemistry

- Plasma cells containing lambda light chains comprise more than 70% of the total immunocyte population
- Immunoglobulin (Ig) A–containing plasma cells make up 45% of the total

Molecular Alterations

- Familial cases with multifocal involvement documented

Differential Diagnosis

- Hashimoto thyroiditis, fibrous variant
- Spindle cell type of undifferentiated (anaplastic) carcinoma
- Desmoplastic reaction to papillary carcinoma
- Large cell lymphoma with sclerosis

Treatment

- Steroid therapy may be effective
- Most patients require a surgical intervention to relieve the compression symptoms in the neck and to rule out the presence of undifferentiated carcinoma (postoperative hypothyroidism rare)

Prognosis

- No reports of malignant transformation

Associations

- No relationship to Hashimoto thyroiditis or granulomatous thyroiditis
- May be a manifestation of a group of disorders characterized by retroperitoneal or mediastinal fibrosis, sclerosing cholangitis, or inflammatory pseudotumor of the orbit

Hashimoto Thyroiditis

Clinical Manifestations

- Typically a disease of women over the age of 40 years
- Usually presents as diffuse firm enlargement often with signs of tracheal or esophageal compression
- Initially associated with mild hyperthyroidism followed by hypothyroidism
- Most common presentation is that of an asymptomatic goiter usually of short duration
- Elevated serum levels of antibodies to thyroglobulin, thyroid peroxidase (catalyzes both tyrosine iodination and coupling of iodotyrosyl residues to form T_3 and T_4), TSH receptors (block action of TSH-causing hypothyroidism), and iodine transporter (mediates transport of iodine into thyroid)

Gross Pathology

- Gland is typically firm and symmetrically and diffusely enlarged
- Interlobular fibrosis makes the normal thyroid lobulation quite pronounced
- Cut surface has tan to yellow appearance

Microscopic Pathology

- Follicles tend to be small and atrophic
- Colloid is typically dense but may be absent
- Follicular cells are frequently metaplastic with oncocytic (Hürthle cell), clear cell, or squamous cell changes
- In the stroma and atrophic follicles, there is a dense lymphoid and plasmacytic infiltrate with large follicles complete with prominent germinal centers
- Interlobular fibrosis may be quite prominent (see associations later in this section)
- Follicular cells may be enlarged, overlap, and demonstrate nuclear clearing reminiscent of changes seen in papillary carcinoma
- Fibrosing variant (10%-15%) may have prominent aggregates of squamous cells with a mild nuclear atypia surrounded by a dense fibrous tissue
- Large intrathyroidal squamous lined cyst may develop (often closely resembles branchial cleft cyst)

Special Stains

- Not helpful

Immunohistochemistry

- Ratio of T to B cells (1:1) in the lymphocytic infiltrate can be confirmed on immunohistochemistry (T lymphocytes are usually of the suppressor type)
- Follicular cells reactive for cytokeratin (especially high molecular weight), S-100 protein, and HLA-DR
- Kappa light chain–containing plasma cells outnumber lambda light chain–containing cells 2 to 1
- IgA-containing plasma cells make up 15% of the immunocytic population

Electron Microscopy

- Mitochondria in cytoplasm of Hürthle cells

Molecular Alterations

- HLA-DR5 and HLA-DR3

Differential Diagnosis

- Subacute lymphocytic thyroiditis
- Papillary carcinoma
- Lymphoma
- Hürthle cell neoplasm
- Fibrosing variant may mimic Riedel thyroiditis

Treatment

- No treatment required for asymptomatic patients
- Thyroid hormone for symptomatic hypothyroidism
- Subtotal thyroidectomy for enlarged gland causing pressure symptoms

Prognosis

- Depends on the development of neoplasia (see associations below)

Associations

- Fibrous variant associated with lymphocytic infiltration in other organs (presumably on an autoimmune basis, eg, lymphocytic adrenalitis [Schmidt syndrome] and lymphocytic interstitial pneumonitis)
- Thyroid malignancy
  - Most common malignancy is lymphoma, B-cell type
  - Increased incidence of plasmacytoma
  - Increased incidence of mucoepidermoid carcinoma in fibrosing variant
  - Papillary carcinoma
  - Hürthle cell neoplasm

Thyroiditis

Variants

- Acute thyroiditis
- Granulomatous (De Quervain) thyroiditis
- Subacute lymphocytic thyroiditis

Clinical Manifestations

- *Acute thyroiditis*
  - Causative organisms include bacteria, fungi, and viruses
  - Usually seen in malnourished children, debilitated adults, or immunocompromised patients
  - May be seen after trauma especially in the setting of an open neck wound
  - Most present with painful enlargement of the thyroid
- *Granulomatous thyroiditis*
  - Probably has a viral etiology (see associations later in this section)
  - Typically presents in middle-aged women with a sore throat, painful swallowing, and tenderness
  - Fever and malaise usually present
  - During the initial stages of the disease, the serum levels of T3 and T4 are elevated, the TSH level is depressed, and radioactive iodine uptake is completely suppressed
- *Subacute lymphocytic thyroiditis*
  - Patients present with mild hyperthyroidism or enlarged thyroid or both
  - More common in women (especially postpartum) than men
  - Patients have elevated levels of antibodies to thyroglobulin and thyroid peroxidase
  - T3, T4, and TSH levels similar to those of granulomatous thyroiditis

Gross Pathology

- *Acute thyroiditis*
  - Gland usually appears normal but may have focal areas of softening secondary to suppuration
- *Granulomatous thyroiditis*
  - Typically an asymmetrically enlarged and firm gland
  - No adhesions between gland and surrounding soft tissue
  - Cut surface reveals irregular tan-white, poorly circumscribed nodules
- *Subacute lymphocytic thyroiditis*
  - Asymmetric gland with a vaguely nodular and white cut surface

Microscopic Pathology

- *Acute thyroiditis*
  - Acute inflammation with microabscess formation and tissue necrosis
- *Granulomatous thyroiditis*
  - Early in the course of the disease, inflammatory response consists of neutrophils (microabscesses may be present); later chronic inflammatory cells predominant with granulomas and foreign body giant cells
  - Follicular epithelium replaced by rim of giant cells admixed with macrophages (granulomas); giant cells contain ingested colloid
  - Patchy areas of central fibrosis
- *Subacute lymphocytic thyroiditis*
  - Multiple foci of aggregates of small lymphocytes with patchy disruption and collapse of thyroid follicles
  - Plasma cells and follicles with germinal centers are rare (presence suggests Hashimoto disease)

Special Stains

- Not helpful

Immunohistochemistry

- *Acute thyroiditis*
  - None
- *Granulomatous thyroiditis*
  - CEA-positive cells present in the center during the acute phase of disease
  - Reactivity for CA19-9 is found in the later stages of the disease

Electron Microscopy

- Not helpful

Molecular Alterations

- HLA-DR5 and HLA-DR3
- See associations later in this section

Differential Diagnosis

- *Acute thyroiditis*
  - A pyriform sinus fistula with secondary suppurative involvement of the thyroid
- *Granulomatous thyroiditis*
  - Tuberculosis
  - Sarcoidosis
  - Mycoses
  - Postoperative necrotizing granulomatous inflammation
- *Subacute lymphocytic thyroiditis*
  - Hashimoto thyroiditis

Treatment

- *Acute thyroiditis*
  - Antibiotics with surgical drainage of localized abscess
  - Cases resulting from pyriform sinus fistula require excision of the fistula
- *Granulomatous thyroiditis and subacute lymphocytic thyroiditis*
  - Subtotal thyroidectomy if symptomatic

Prognosis

- Granulomatous thyroiditis and subacute lymphocytic thyroiditis typically completely resolve

Associations

- *Acute thyroiditis*
  - See pyriform sinus fistula earlier in this section
- *Granulomatous thyroiditis*
  - Often follows infection involving the upper aerodigestive tract
  - Viral etiology not proven but there is a definite association with mumps, measles, influenza, coxsackievirus, mononucleosis, and adenovirus
  - Associated with HLA B_w35
- *Subacute lymphocytic thyroiditis*
  - HLA-DR3 and HLA-DR5
  - Family history of autoimmune thyroiditis

Graves Disease (Diffuse Toxic Goiter)

Clinical Manifestations

- Typically affects young adult women 7 times more frequently than men
- Presenting symptoms include muscle weakness, weight loss, exophthalmos, irritability, tachycardia, and increase in appetite (hyperthyroidism)
- Occasionally patients present in atrial fibrillation
- After longstanding disease patients may develop localized infiltrative dermopathy (pretibial myxedema), thyroid acropachy (swelling of the extremities and clubbing of the fingers and toes as a result of periosteal new bone formation), and infiltrative ophthalmopathy
- Represents the most common cause of hyperthyroidism in children
- Most common disease to cause clinically evident thyrotoxicosis (other causes include "toxic" follicular adenoma, "toxic" goiter, inappropriate TSH secretion, trophoblastic tumors, struma ovarii, and iatrogenic causes [ie, amiodarone-associated thyrotoxicosis; amiodarone contains 37% iodine by weight])

Pathogenesis

- Autoantibodies to TSH receptor: Long-acting thyroid stimulator binds to TSH receptor and stimulates thyroid hormone production
- Thyroid growth-stimulating immunoglobulins: Stimulate growth of thyroid follicular epithelium

- TSH-binding inhibitor immunoglobulins: Bind to TSH and prevent normal TSH-binding receptors while mimicking TSH function

Gross Pathology

- Typically diffusely and symmetrically enlarged without a nodularity
- Cut surface is "juicy" and uniformly red to brown; long-standing disease characterized by yellow, friable parenchyma

Microscopic Pathology

- Follicles with marked hypertrophy and hyperplasia with epithelium that is crowded, columnar, and has basally oriented nuclei and cytoplasm that may contain fat and glycogen
- Small papillae of follicular cells without fibrovascular cores may project into follicular lumina
- Colloid in the follicles is pale and finely vacuolated and typically demonstrates prominent scalloping where it abuts the epithelium
- Stroma may contain aggregates of lymph node tissue with or without germinal centers
- Oncocytic cells may be present (may be an indicator that the disease is evolving toward Hashimoto thyroiditis)
- Occasionally follicular cells are seen to have proliferated into adjacent perithyroid soft tissue
- Fibrosis unusual

Special Stains

- Not helpful

Immunohistochemistry

- Stromal lymphocytes CD4- and CD8-positive

Electron Microscopy

- Will confirm presence of immune complex in basement membrane of follicular epithelium

Molecular Alterations

- HLA-B8 and HLA-DR3
- Increased incidence in families (concordance rate of 60% in monozygotic twins)

Differential Diagnosis

- Nodular hyperplasia
- Papillary carcinoma

Treatment

- Medical suppression of hyperthyroid state with or without subtotal thyroidectomy
- Iodine administration causes involution of follicular epithelium and colloid accumulation by blocking thyroglobulin secretion
- Antithyroid medications (propylthiouracil, methimazole, and carbimazole)
- Radioactive iodine destruction of gland

Prognosis

- Incidence of carcinoma no greater than that found in normal glands
- If approximately 5 g of each lobe is left after subtotal thyroidectomy, most patients will become euthyroid

Associations

- Increased incidence after irradiation to the neck
- True thymic hyperplasia

Nodular Hyperplasia (Multinodular Goiter)

Clinical Manifestations

- Typically preceded by a transient phase of diffuse hyperplasia (diffuse nontoxic goiter)
- Most common thyroid disease in the United States with 3% to 5% of the adult population affected
- Most patients present with a large nodular gland that may distort the anterior neck and/or cause compression of the trachea; occasionally, the thyroid enlargement extends into the superior mediastinum
- Occasionally patients may experience a sudden enlargement and pain as a result of hemorrhage
- Most are euthyroid; when hyperthyroid, the condition is referred to as toxic nodular hyperplasia
- Two forms of disease:

- *Endemic goiter:* Deficient iodine ingestion that results in decreased thyroid hormone production which in turn leads to increased levels of TSH which produces a hyperplastic gland; initially the gland is characterized by tall follicular epithelium and small amounts of colloid (parenchymatous goiter); after some time the follicular component atrophies and increased amounts of colloid (colloid goiter) are seen
- *Sporadic nodular goiter:* More common than endemic in the United States; seen in late pubertal girls or young adult women

Gross Pathology

- Thyroid is enlarged, typically asymmetrical and nodular
- Thyroid capsule is usually intact
- Multiple nodules found on sectioning
- Focal areas of hemorrhage, calcification, and cystic degeneration often present

Microscopic Pathology

- Follicle morphology ranges from markedly dilated with a flat epithelium to small with tall columnar epithelium
- Some large follicles have aggregates of small active follicles ("Sanderson polster") at one pole that protrude into the lumen of the follicle; polsters typically covered with columnar epithelium while the follicle into which it protrudes is often lined with flattened epithelium
- Granulomatous inflammatory reaction may be seen near a ruptured follicle
- Foci of hemorrhage, fibrosis, and calcification are frequently encountered
- Osseous metaplasia occasionally seen
- Thickened arteries with calcified media may be seen at the periphery
- Inflammatory cells may be seen in the stroma
- Rarely follicular cells have a clear cell morphology
- Occasionally follicles composed predominantly or exclusively of oncocytic (Hürthle) cells

Special Stains

- Benign papillary formations typically stain negatively for Alcian blue (unlike the strong staining seen in papillary carcinoma)

Immunohistochemistry

- Papillary formations in nodular hyperplasia typically negative for EMA (unlike the strong staining in papillary carcinoma)

Electron Microscopy

- Not helpful

Molecular Alterations

- Several autosomal recessive conditions resulting in enzymatic defects that disrupt thyroid hormone synthesis and result in sporadic goiter
  - Iodine transport defect
  - Organification defect
  - Dehalogenase defect
  - Iodotyrosine coupling defect

Differential Diagnosis

- Papillary carcinoma (see special stains and immunohistochemistry earlier in this section)
- Follicular adenoma

Treatment

- Subtotal thyroidectomy

Prognosis

- No evidence of malignant transformation

Associations

- Hashimoto thyroiditis

Tumors

Follicular Adenoma

Clinical Manifestations

- Typically solitary
- Usually occurs in normal glands, but may be seen in glands with thyroiditis, nodular hyperplasia, and other lesions
- Women more commonly affected then men
- Most patients present with a painless mass that may cause tracheal compression
- Most are euthyroid; rarely associated with hyperthyroidism
- All except toxic variant are "cold" on isotopic scan

Gross Pathology

- Typically round or oval with a thin fibrous capsule
- Color ranges from gray to white to tan depending on cellularity, amount of colloid, and vascularity
- Areas of hemorrhage, necrosis, fibrosis and cystic degeneration may be present, especially in the center of the neoplasm

Microscopic Pathology

- An encapsulated mass of benign, uniform follicles, each surrounded by a basement membrane
- Fibrous capsule typically thin; interface between adenoma and capsule usually prominent
- Normal glandular tissue adjacent to the nodule often compressed and atrophic
- Center of nodule may contain a stellate fibrous scar, but fibrous septa coursing through the neoplasm are rare (should raise the possibility of a follicular variant of papillary carcinoma)
- Degenerative changes (hemorrhage, edema, myxoid change, fibrosis and hyalinization, calcification, and cystic change) may be present
- Common variants:
  - *Trabecular/solid variant*
    - Follicular cells grow in trabecular or solid pattern with few if any follicles
  - *Microfollicular variant*
    - Smaller than normal follicles with an increased ratio of cells to lumen and little colloid
  - *Normofollicular (simple) variant*
    - Follicles typically about the same size as the follicles in the non-neoplastic portion of gland
  - *Macrofollicular (colloid) variant*
    - Large follicles full of colloid (resemble hyperplastic nodules)
- Additional variants:
  - *Adenoma with bizarre nuclei*
    - Large irregularly shaped hyperchromatic nuclei that tend to occur in clusters; more common in adenomas than carcinomas
  - *Hyalinizing trabecular adenoma*
    - Neoplastic cells arranged in a trabecular or nesting pattern (similar to that seen in a paraganglioma) and surrounded by prominent hyaline; follicle formation unusual
    - Microscopically easily confused with papillary carcinoma because nuclear features similar to those of papillary carcinoma
    - Tumor cells positive for thyroglobulin and negative for calcitonin
  - *Adenolipoma*
    - Neoplastic follicles interspersed with islands of adipose tissue
  - *Adenochondroma*
    - Neoplastic follicles admixed with stroma consisting of lobules of mature cartilage
  - *Adenoma with papillary hyperplasia*
    - Follicles with short, blunt, nonbranching papillary formations with little or no fibrovascular core
    - Follicular cells tall with basally oriented nuclei and none of the cytologic features of a papillary carcinoma
  - *Toxic adenoma*
    - Approximately 1% of all thyroid adenomas
    - Cells lining follicles tend to be tall with a decreased nuclear-cytoplasmic ratio

Special Stains

- PAS or silver will highlight basement membrane material surrounding neoplastic follicles

Immunohistochemistry

- Neoplastic cells are positive for thyroglobulin but the staining is less intense than that seen in the adjacent normal gland
- Neoplastic cells uniformly positive for low-molecular-weight keratin and usually positive for vimentin
- Basement membrane material surrounding follicles positive for laminin and type IV collagen

Electron Microscopy

- Neoplastic cells similar to those of nodular hyperplasia and normal thyroid; few mitochondria, abundant dilated endoplasmic reticulum, and intertwining microvilli
- Follicular cells sit on continuous basement membrane

Molecular Alterations

- Expression of *ras*-oncogene p21 antigen is higher than in normal thyroid and lower than in carcinoma
- Aneuploid cell populations present in approximately 30%
- Gene for Cowden disease (see associations later in this section) localized to chromosome 10q22-23

Differential Diagnosis

- Dominant nodule in nodular hyperplasia
- Minimally invasive follicular carcinoma
- Encapsulated follicular variant of papillary carcinoma

Treatment

- Thyroid lobectomy (if lesion >4 cm then consider total thyroidectomy)
- Enucleation should never be performed

Prognosis

- A benign neoplasm

Associations

- Hyperfunctioning nodules may be more common in the setting of iodine deficiency
- May be seen concurrently with thyroiditis and nodular hyperplasia as well as other conditions of the thyroid
- Very common in patients with Cowden syndrome, characterized by follicular adenoma and carcinoma of thyroid, gastrointestinal polyps (hamartomas, inflammatory, ganglioneuromas, lipomas, and lymphoid), fibrocystic disease of the breast and breast cancer, facial trichilemmomas, papillomatosis of lips and oropharynx, multiple lipomas and hemangiomas, high arched palate, hypoplasia of the jaw, and central nervous system anomalies

Follicular Carcinoma

Clinical Manifestations

- 5% of all thyroid carcinomas
- More common in women than men
- Usually presents as a solitary "cold" nodule without cervical adenopathy

Variants

- Minimally invasive (grossly encapsulated)
- Widely invasive

Gross Pathology

- Minimally invasive tumors are typically round with a thick irregular capsule (capsule typically thicker and more irregular than that seen with a benign follicular adenoma); cut surface usually solid, light tan to brown and bulging; evidence of invasion into the capsule or blood vessels generally not discernible on gross inspection
- Widely invasive tumors have extensive areas of invasion and often lack any evidence of ever having been encapsulated

Microscopic Pathology

- Varies from well-formed follicles to predominantly solid growth pattern
- Cytoarchitectural features resemble those of a follicular adenoma
- More likely to have a solid, trabecular, microfollicular, or atypical pattern than benign adenoma
- Nuclei may have large nucleoli, and mitotic figures may be present
- Diagnosis of malignancy depends on unequivocal capsular and/or vascular invasion
- Diagnosis of capsular invasion requires penetration of the entire thickness of the capsule with clusters of follicular cells; clusters of follicular cells that have penetrated the capsule are typically covered by a new capsule at the point of penetration
- Vascular invasion requires the projection into the lumen of veins of unequivocal epithelial cells that result in either partial or complete occlusion of the vessel; epithelial cells should be attached to the vein wall and vein should be located within the capsule or immediately adjacent to it
- Microscopic features of the widely invasive cancer include a solid, nesting, or trabecular architectural pattern with increased numbers of mitotic figures, nuclear hyperchromasia, and focal areas of necrosis (features overlap with those of poorly differentiated (insular) carcinoma)

Special Stains

- Follicles typically surrounded by basement membrane that can be seen with PAS or silver stains

Immunohistochemistry

- Immunostains for endothelial cells (to establish the presence of a neoplasm within a vessel) are not particularly helpful
- Tumor cells are positive for low-molecular-weight keratin and usually vimentin

Electron Microscopy

- Follicular cells have no distinctive features that will separate them from a normal thyroid, hyperplastic thyroid or carcinoma

Molecular Alterations

- 60% have aneuploid cell populations
- Rearrangements of the peroxisome proliferators-activated receptor gamma (PPARγ) gene seen in 25% to 50%
- Point mutations of *RAS* genes seen in 20% to 50%

Differential Diagnosis

- Follicular adenoma
- Dominant nodule in a gland with nodular hyperplasia
- Follicular variant of papillary carcinoma
- Tubular (follicular) variant of medullary carcinoma

Treatment

- Thyroid lobectomy or subtotal thyroidectomy
- Total thyroidectomy with adjuvant radioactive iodine
- Metastatic disease typically treated with radioactive iodine if there is no residual thyroid in the neck
- Lymph node dissection not indicated

Prognosis

- Minimally invasive carcinoma has a prognosis as good as that of papillary carcinoma; (10-year survival > 80%)
- Widely invasive lesions have very poor prognosis (80% develop metastasis; tumor mortality of ~50%)
- Factors adversely affecting prognosis include: Multifocal disease, age more than 50 years, and the inability of the neoplasm to take up radioactive iodine

Associations

- Radiation exposure
- Iodine deficiency

Medullary Carcinoma

Clinical Manifestations

- Approximately 5% to 10% of all thyroid malignancies
- Occurs in either a sporadic (70%) or familial (autosomal dominant) setting (30%)

- Sporadic neoplasms are typically unilateral and slightly more common in women than men (usually middle age)
- Familial lesions occur in association with MEN IIA or MEN IIB (see associations later in this section)
- Tumors arising in the setting of MEN IIA or MEN IIB have an equal sex ratio, an average age of 20 years for MEN II and 15 years for MEN III, and are often multicentric and involve both lobes of thyroid
- Most patients present with a painless firm nodule: 50% have evidence of lymph node metastases at initial diagnosis; symptoms of medullary carcinoma occurring in a patient with MEN IIA may be masked by either the associated adrenal medullary lesion or parathyroid disease
- Familial lesions may present with various endocrinologically mediated symptoms, eg, watery diarrhea, carcinoid syndrome, and Cushing syndrome

Gross Pathology

- Generally well-circumscribed, but not encapsulated, and vary in size from barely detectable to complete replacement of the thyroid gland
- Usually firm and yellow with infiltrative borders
- Smaller lesions usually arise laterally at the junction of the upper and middle thirds of the thyroid lobes (areas of C-cell predominance)
- Sporadic tumors tend to be solitary; familial tumors often bilateral

Microscopic Pathology

- Typically a lobular, trabecular, insular (most common), or solid growth pattern
- Tumor cells may be round and/or polygonal or have a spindle shape; cytoplasm usually eosinophilic or amphophilic, but may be clear or contain mucin-containing vacuoles
- Tumor cell nuclei are round to oval with clumped or speckled chromatin and inconspicuous nucleoli; nuclei may contain cytoplasmic pseudoinclusions (similar to papillary carcinoma)
- Binucleated cells and giant cells may be present
- Mitotic activity unusual unless tumor very large
- Stromal amyloid present in approximately 80%; stroma also contains collagen and frequently areas of calcification
- Familial lesions typically have nearby foci of C-cell hyperplasia; sporadic tumors lack C-cell hyperplasia (C-cell hyperplasia can be nodular, defined as aggregates of at least 7 to 10 cells, or diffuse, defined as aggregates of 50 or more cells)
- Occasionally neoplasm associated with a prominent inflammatory infiltrate
- Variants of medullary carcinoma
  - *Papillary*: A papillary or pseudopapillary growth pattern
  - *Follicular*: Characterized by follicles, glands, or tubules lined by medullary carcinoma cells
  - *Encapsulated*
  - *Small cell*: Tumor cells small with hyperchromatic nuclei (reminiscent of pulmonary small cell carcinoma); marked mitotic activity and foci of necrosis
  - *Giant cell*: Large atypical cells morphologically similar to syncytiotrophoblastic cells admixed with more typical medullary cells
  - *Clear cell*: Characterized by cells with abundant clear cytoplasm (not mucin or glycogen)
  - *Oncocytic:* Characterized by cells with numerous mitochondria
  - *Squamous cell*

Special Stains

- Amyloid typically highlighted with Congo red
- 90% will demonstrate argyrophilia with a Grimelius stain
- Masson-Fontana argentaffin stain typically negative
- Tumor cells may be focally positive for PAS and Alcian blue
- Mucicarmine will highlight the presence of both extra- and intracellular mucin

Immunohistochemistry

- Tumor cells typically positive for low-molecular-weight cytokeratin, NSE, synaptophysin, chromogranin, and calcitonin (chromogranin more specific and more sensitive than calcitonin)

Thyroid Gland: Tumors>Medullary Carcinoma; Oncocytic (Hürthle Cell) Adenoma

- Small cell variant may be negative for calcitonin
- Essentially every tumor is positive for carcinoembryonic antigen (CEA; patients also have elevated levels of CEA in their blood)
- Amyloid deposits typically calcitonin positive
- 80% positive for *bcl*-2

Electron Microscopy

- Tumor cells have membrane-bound secretory granules (storage sites of calcitonin and other hormonal products)
- Amyloid has fibrillar structure

Molecular Alterations

- Gene for MEN IIA located near the centromere of chromosome 10
- Location of gene responsible for sporadic form of disease as well as for MEN IIB not identified
- Elevated levels of H-*ras* have been noted
- Germline *RET* mutations appear to be associated with both familial and sporadic tumors

Differential Diagnosis

- Papillary carcinoma (papillary or pseudopapillary variant of medullary carcinoma)
- Follicular carcinoma (follicular variant)
- Hyalinizing trabecular variant of follicular adenoma (encapsulated variant)
- Anaplastic carcinoma (giant cell variant)
- Lymphoma, metastatic bronchogenic oat cell carcinoma, and metastasis from bronchopulmonary or gastrointestinal carcinoids (small cell variant)
- Metastatic renal cell carcinoma (clear cell variant)
- Amyloid containing plasmacytoma
- Poorly differentiated (insular) carcinoma
- Intrathyroidal parathyroid adenoma

Treatment

- Total thyroidectomy with removal of lymph nodes from the central compartment of the neck

Prognosis

- Lesions arising in the setting of MEN IIB tend to be aggressive and metastasize early (5-year survival rate of 5%)
- Prognosis for sporadic lesions and those that arise in the setting of MEN IIA largely depends on the size of the neoplasm and the presence of metastasis; 60% to 70% survive 5 years; 40% to 50% survive 10 years
- Patients under the age of 40 years do significantly better than older patients, and women have a better prognosis than men
- Presence of nodal metastases correlates with size of primary tumor (20% incidence if tumor <0.7 cm; 80% incidence if tumor >1.5 cm)

Associations

- No association with history of head and neck irradiation
- Occasionally arises in the setting of Hashimoto thyroiditis
- Chronic hypercalcemia may predispose the patient to the development of medullary carcinoma
- MEN IIA
  - C-cell hyperplasia: Medullary carcinoma
  - Adrenal medullary hyperplasia: Pheochromocytoma
  - Parathyroid hyperplasia: Adenoma
- MEN IIB
  - C-cell hyperplasia: Medullary carcinoma
  - Adrenal medullary hyperplasia: Pheochromocytoma
  - Gastrointestinal and ocular ganglioneuromas
  - Marfanoid habitus
  - May be seen admixed with papillary carcinoma and/or follicular carcinoma

Oncocytic (Hürthle Cell) Adenoma

Clinical Manifestations

- More common in women than in men
- Mean age at diagnosis approximately 45 years
- Typically solitary
- May develop spontaneously or after fine-needle aspiration

Thyroid Gland: Tumors>Oncocytic (Hürthle Cell) Adenoma; Oncocytic (Hürthle Cell) Carcinoma

Gross Pathology

- Typically round or oval and completely encapsulated
- Cut surface solid, brown (mahogany), and bulging
- Foci of calcification, hemorrhage, cystic change, and central scarring may be present
- Occasionally the entire neoplasm is necrotic (a phenomenon that may develop spontaneously or be precipitated by fine-needle aspiration)

Microscopic Pathology

- Typically a follicular growth pattern, but may be trabecular or solid (a trabecular or solid growth pattern should raise the suspicion of malignancy)
- Colloid within follicles tends to be basophilic
- Psammomalike structures may be seen within colloid of follicles
- Nuclei typically vesicular and uniform but marked atypia with pleomorphism and hyperchromasia may be present (not an indication of malignancy)
- Coagulative necrosis may be present and occasionally involve the entire neoplasm
- Tumor cells may be round or polygonal with centrally located nuclei or columnar with either centrally or apically located nuclei

Special Stains

- Not helpful

Immunohistochemistry

- Neoplastic cells are positive for both keratin and thyroglobulin (intensity of staining less than in ordinary follicular cells)
- Immunostain for cytochrome C oxidase positive

Electron Microscopy

- Cytoplasm of neoplastic cells packed with large, pleomorphic mitochondria

Molecular Alterations

- Expression of p21 *ras*-oncogene consistently present

Differential Diagnosis

- Oncocytic carcinoma
- Oncocytic cells may be present in nodular goiter, chronic lymphocytic/Hashimoto thyroiditis, longstanding hyperthyroidism, and nodules and carcinomas

Treatment

- Thyroid lobectomy

Prognosis

- A benign neoplasm that does not recur or metastasize (assuming the benign nature of the neoplasm is established with extensive sampling)
- Size, nuclear atypia, multinucleation, cellular pleomorphism, mitoses, and histologic pattern do not predict clinical behavior

Associations

- None

Oncocytic (Hürthle Cell) Carcinoma

Clinical Manifestations

- Accounts for 2% to 3% of all thyroid carcinomas and 20% of all follicular carcinomas
- More common in women than men
- Mean age at diagnosis approximately 55 years (10 years older than for benign oncocytic adenoma)
- Does not take up radioactive iodine (cold on thyroid scan)

Gross Pathology

- Typically larger than benign oncocytic adenoma
- Typically solid and brown
- Rarely multiple
- Foci of necrosis, hemorrhage, and scarring more common than in oncocytic adenoma
- Minimally invasive lesions have a complete capsule; widely invasive lesions have either no capsule or a capsule obviously involved with tumor

Thyroid Gland: Tumors>Oncocytic (Hürthle Cell) Carcinoma; Papillary Carcinoma

- May invade surrounding thyroid in a pattern of sharply outlined nodules that connect to each other and to the main tumor mass

Microscopic Pathology

- Individual tumor cells resemble cells of a benign oncocytic adenoma
- Typically malignant tumor cells have less cytoplasm and consequently a higher nuclear-cytoplasmic ratio than those of a benign adenoma; tumor cells tend to be tall or columnar rather than round or polygonal (the latter more characteristic of benign oncocytoma)
- Scattered bizarre hyperchromatic nuclei may be present
- Increased numbers of mitotic figures typically present
- Psammomalike calcifications may be present within colloid
- Tumors tend to have a solid/trabecular architectural pattern (unlike the predominately follicular pattern of oncocytic adenoma)
- Diagnosis of carcinoma is based on the presence of invasion (capsular and/or vascular)
- A predominantly encapsulated lesion with foci of invasive tumor growth; blood vessels in the capsule will contain aggregates of tumor cells (usually quite prominent)
- Widely invasive carcinomas often lack a discernible capsule and invasion is obvious; invasive component rarely elicits a desmoplastic reaction (as seen with papillary carcinoma)

Special Stains

- None

Immunohistochemistry

- Tumor cells immunoreactive for both keratin and thyroglobulin (intensity of staining is less than in normal follicular cells)
- Immunostain for cytochrome C oxidase (an enzyme of the mitochondrial respiratory chain) positive

Electron Microscopy

- Features indistinguishable from those of an oncocytic adenoma; cytoplasm packed with mitochondria

Molecular Alterations

- Expression of p21 *ras*-oncogene typically present

Differential Diagnosis

- Benign oncocytic adenoma
- Oncocytoma of parathyroid
- Oncocytic variant of medullary carcinoma of thyroid

Treatment

- Total thyroidectomy
- Adjuvant suppression
- Radioactive iodine and external radiation of no therapeutic value

Prognosis

- 30% metastasize to lymph nodes
- 50% to 60% alive at 5 years
- Depends on degree of invasiveness and presence or absence of blood born metastasis and regional nodal metastasis
- Aneuploid tumors probably more aggressive than diploid tumors

Associations

- None

Papillary Carcinoma

Clinical Manifestations

- Most common thyroid cancer in the United States
- More common in women than in men
- Represents 90% of all thyroid cancers in children
- Typically presents as a hard nodule in the thyroid; cervical lymph nodes may be palpable (35%); may present with palpable cervical nodes and normal thyroid by palpation

Gross Pathology

- Typically invasive with ill-defined margins, but may be well-circumscribed (never encapsulated)
- Cut surface usually gray to white and granular (papillary formations); calcifications may be evident

- Necrosis rare
- Multicentric in approximately 20%

Microscopic Pathology

- Papillae consisting of a central fibrovascular stalk of loose connective tissue and variably sized thinned wall vessels covered by neoplastic epithelium
- Usually papillae are admixed with follicles that also have a neoplastic epithelium
- Nuclei of neoplastic cells tend to be round or oval and frequently have irregularities of the nuclear membrane consisting of indentations and folds (pseudoinclusions or grooves); a pseudoinclusion is an invagination of cytoplasm into the nucleus that results in an eosinophilic round structure with a sharply outlined border and a rim of compressed chromatin on one side; nuclear grooves tend to be oriented parallel to the long axis of the nucleus; nuclei tend to have an empty or cleared out appearance (devoid of chromatin) that is the result of the deposition of chromatin material along the inner wall of the nuclear membrane; the nucleolus also tends to be pushed up against the inner surface of the nuclear membrane (nuclei with this appearance are referred to as "Orphan Annie eyes")
- Tumor cell nuclei tend to be enlarged and overlap
- Mitotic figures usually absent
- Cytoplasm of tumor cells completely bland
- Tumor cells occasionally grow in solid or trabecular patterns
- Squamous metaplasia may be present (20% to 40%)
- Psammoma bodies present in 50% (more common in tumors with a predominantly papillary architecture); psammoma bodies tend to be located near the tips of papillary stalks
- Fibrous stroma typically present
- 30% show a prominent lymphocytic infiltrate
- Secondary cystic changes may be present
- Blood vessel invasion present in 5% to 10%

Special Stains

- Mucin stains frequently positive

Immunohistochemistry

- Tumor cells always positive for thyroglobulin, and low- and high-molecular-weight cytokeratin (normal thyroid follicular cells typically negative for high-molecular-weight cytokeratin)
- Both estrogen and progesterone receptors may be present in the nuclei of tumor cells
- Tumor cells frequently reactive for S-100 protein, EMA, and vimentin

Electron Microscopy

- Nuclei have dispersed chromatin, a folded nuclear membrane, and intranuclear cytoplasmic inclusions
- Cytoplasm contains abundant mitochondria, lysosomes, and filaments
- Apical surface has microvilli

Molecular Alterations

- Most are diploid (20% are aneuploid)
- Rearrangement of papillary thyroid carcinoma (PTC) *RET* oncogene on chromosome 10q11-q12, and *TRK*1 located on chromosome 1q22
- RAS mutation in 45% of follicular variant
- Point mutations of *BRAF* gene in up to 70%

Differential Diagnosis

- See variants later in this section

Treatment

- Thyroid lobectomy if the neoplasm is solitary and <1 cm
- Total thyroidectomy if the neoplasm is >1 cm, is multicentric, or there is a history of head and neck irradiation
- Lymph nodes are selectively removed if clinically involved; a radical neck dissection should not be performed
- If less than a total thyroidectomy is performed the remaining gland should be suppressed by suppressing the release of TSH
- Distant metastatic disease treated with radioiodine

Thyroid Gland: Tumors>Papillary Carcinoma

Prognosis

- Factors associated with a favorable prognosis include young age (<40 years), females, tumor <1.5 cm in diameter, solitary lesions, and absence of extrathyroidal extension and metastasis
- Factors associated with a worse prognosis include age over 40 years, male sex, tumors >1.5 cm, multicentricity, extrathyroidal extension, and distant metastases
- Regional lymph node metastases do not affect long-term prognosis
- Papillary carcinoma can progress to poorly differentiated (insular) or undifferentiated (anaplastic) carcinoma
- Death from typical papillary thyroid carcinoma uncommon
- Tall cell and columnar variants more aggressive

Associations

- Radiation exposure to the neck
- Lymphocytic/Hashimoto thyroiditis
- May appear in a familial setting
- Increased incidence in patients with ataxia-telangiectasia and MEN syndrome
- Seen in association with parathyroid tumors, carotid body tumors, adenocarcinoma of the colon, polyposis coli, Gardner syndrome, and Cowden syndrome

Variants

- *Papillary microcarcinoma*
  - A papillary carcinoma <1 cm in diameter
  - Reported incidence from 4% to 20% (autopsy series)
  - Typically has an irregular, stellate, and fibrous architecture with neoplastic elements at the periphery and entrapped in the center
- *Encapsulated*
  - 10% of all papillary carcinomas
  - Tumor completely surrounded by a fibrous capsule that is either intact or focally infiltrated by tumor
  - Involvement of cervical lymph nodes in over 25%
  - Differential diagnosis includes follicular adenoma and follicular carcinoma
- *Follicular*
  - May be diffuse or encapsulated
  - Papillary cancer with an almost exclusive follicular pattern
  - Follicles tend to be elongated with irregular epithelial lining with folds, ridges, and buds; colloid brightly eosinophilic and scalloped
  - Follicles may be large (macrofollicular variant)
  - Differential diagnosis includes nodular hyperplasia
- *Encapsulated follicular*
  - Papillary carcinoma with nuclear features typical of papillary carcinoma but architectural features of a follicular variant coupled with encapsulation
- *Solid/trabecular*
  - More common in cancers in the pediatric age group and in tumors of the diffuse sclerosing type
  - Microscopically consists of irregular fibrous trabeculae, occasional psammoma bodies, and clusters of lymphocytes
  - Typical nuclear features of papillary carcinoma always present
  - Differential diagnosis includes poorly differentiated or undifferentiated carcinoma
- *Diffuse sclerosing*
  - Diffuse involvement of 1 or both lobes
  - Numerous papillae in intrathyroidal lymph vessels; extensive squamous metaplasia; numerous psammoma bodies, marked fibrosis, and lymphocytic infiltration
  - High incidence of cervical lymph node involvement
  - More likely to metastasize to the lungs than conventional papillary carcinoma
  - Clinically mimics thyroiditis often resulting in a delay in diagnosis and treatment
  - Typically treated with total thyroidectomy and adjuvant radioactive iodine

- *Tall cell*
  - Approximately 10% of papillary thyroid carcinomas
  - Tends to occur in older patients and be >6 cm at presentation
  - Frequently demonstrates extrathyroidal extension and vascular invasion
  - Cells covering papillary stalks are twice as tall as they are wide and have abundant eosinophilic cytoplasm
  - Mitotic figures frequent
  - Nuclei may be hyperchromatic
  - An aggressive form of papillary cancer with a mortality rate of 25%
- *Columnar cell*
  - Marked by prominent nuclear stratification in cells covering papillary stalks
  - Nuclei may not have typical features of papillary carcinoma
  - Cytoplasm frequently clear with subnuclear vacuoles (reminiscent of POD#3 secretory endometrium)

Poorly Differentiated (Insular) Carcinoma

Clinical Manifestations

- Women slightly more commonly affected than men
- Average age at presentation 55 years
- A very rare neoplasm in the United States

Gross Pathology

- Cut surface typically solid and gray to white
- Foci of necrosis common
- Margin appears infiltrative and extrathyroidal extension may be present
- Most larger than 5 cm at diagnosis

Microscopic Pathology

- Round or oval well-defined nests (neuroendocrine or "carcinoidlike" growth pattern) of uniform small cells with round nuclei and little cytoplasm
- Typical pattern of growth is solid; microfollicles that contain dense colloid often present
- Mitoses always present
- An infiltrative growth pattern with blood vessel invasion
- Small foci of necrosis in the center of the islands; larger foci of necrosis spare nests of tumor adjacent to blood vessels
- Occasional tumors have well-defined nests and a solid growth pattern but consist of cells with papillary carcinoma nuclear features, follicular carcinoma architecture, or oncocytic cytoplasmic features

Special Stains

- Not helpful

Immunohistochemistry

- Tumor cells are negative for calcitonin and positive for keratin, thyroglobulin, and TTF1 thyroid transcription factor-1
- 80% express *bcl*-2
- p53 may be positive, but limited to areas of infiltrative growth

Electron Microscopy

- Not helpful

Molecular Alterations

- Mutations in p53 seen in 20% to 30%

Differential Diagnosis

- Medullary carcinoma and other neuroendocrine neoplasms
- Undifferentiated (anaplastic) carcinoma (especially when solid growth pattern predominates)

Treatment

- Total thyroidectomy and cervical lymph node dissection

Prognosis

- An aggressive neoplasm with frequent metastasis to both regional lymph nodes and distant sites (lung and bones)
- Prognosis between well-differentiated carcinoma and anaplastic carcinoma

Associations

- May coexist with or develop after well-differentiated carcinoma (papillary or follicular)

Undifferentiated (Anaplastic) Carcinoma

Clinical Manifestations

- Represents 10% of all thyroid carcinomas
- Typically occurs in the elderly (age at diagnosis between 60 and 65 years); rarely diagnosed before age 50 years
- More common in women than in men (3-4:1)
- Typically presents as a rapidly enlarging anterior neck mass
- 50% present with signs of neck compression (dyspnea, dysphagia, and hoarseness)
- A hard nodular thyroid on physical examination with palpable lymph nodes in 30%
- Patients typically euthyroid (even with extensive destruction of gland)

Gross Pathology

- Tumor typically replaces the thyroid, disrupts the capsule, and extends into adjacent soft tissues
- Cut section yellow to tan to white with foci of necrosis
- Foci of metaplastic cartilage may be visible

Microscopic Pathology

- Three morphologic patterns:
- *Squamoid*
  - Cells resemble nonkeratinizing squamous cell carcinoma and form distinct nests with irregular borders
  - Squamous pearls may be present
  - Small foci of mucin may be present
- *Spindle cell*
  - Indistinguishable morphologically from sarcoma; usually resembles storiform-pleomorphic form of malignant fibrous histiocytoma
  - Extensive areas of necrosis with palisading of tumor cells frequently present
  - Areas of myxoid change not uncommon
- *Large cell*
  - 80% have a history of goiter
  - Marked pleomorphism (greater than in either of the other 2 patterns)
  - Numerous giant cells with bizarre hyperchromatic and often multiple nuclei
- Mixtures of 2 or all 3 major patterns often seen
- Vascularization usually quite evident, with branching vessels similar in appearance to those seen in hemangiopericytoma
- Inflammatory cells usually scattered among the tumor cells
- Multiple mitotic figures, large foci of necrosis, and obvious invasion are common to all 3 patterns
- Osteoclast multinucleated giant cells admixed with the tumor cells in 10% (these cells are probably not neoplastic)
- Foci of neoplastic cartilage and bone may be present (especially in the spindle cell type)
- Well-differentiated lesions may be present at periphery (eg, goiter, follicular adenoma, papillary carcinoma, follicular carcinoma, and Hürthle cell carcinoma)

Special Stains

- Mucicarmine may highlight the mucin present in the squamoid areas

Immunohistochemistry

- Squamoid, spindle cell, and large cell variants all consistently express low-molecular-weight cytokeratin (most useful)
- High-molecular-weight cytokeratin and EMA only consistently stain epithelioid-looking areas

- Thyroglobulin of little use (only stains cells adjacent to preexisting thyroid or low-grade thyroid neoplasm)

Electron Microscopy

- Findings support the epithelial origin of this neoplasm

Molecular Alterations

- Expression of *ras*-oncogene p21 antigen is less than in other cancers arising from follicular cells
- Most cases are DNA aneuploid
- Mutations in p53

Differential Diagnosis

- Sarcoma (fibrosarcoma, malignant fibrous histiocytoma, malignant hemangiopericytoma, and angiosarcoma)
- Papillary carcinoma (solid variant)
- Poorly differentiated (insular) carcinoma
- Medullary carcinoma
- Lymphoma
- A metastatic tumor

Treatment

- Total surgical excision
- Suppression with radioactive iodine and adjuvant radiation therapy are both ineffective
- Occasionally neoadjuvant chemotherapy will convert an unresectable neoplasm to one that can be surgically excised

Prognosis

- Usually fatal (many dead within 6 months), but long-term survival has been reported, even in cases of widespread metastasis

Associations

- Pre-existing well-differentiated thyroid carcinoma (papillary or follicular)
- May arise in well-differentiated carcinomas treated with radioactive iodine or external irradiation
- May arise in a long-standing goiter

References

Asa SL. *Tumors of the Pituitary Gland: Atlas of Tumor Pathology, 3rd Series. Fascicle 22.* Washington DC: Armed Forces Institute of Pathology, 1998.

Dabbs DJ. *Diagnostic Immunohistochemistry.* New York: Churchill Livingstone, 2002.

DeLellis RA. *Tumors of the Parathyroid Gland: Atlas of Tumor Pathology, 3rd Series. Fascicle 6.* Washington DC: Armed Forces Institute of Pathology, 1993.

DeLellis R, Lloyd R, Heitz P, Eng C (eds). *World Health Organization Classification of Tumours: Pathology and Genetics of Tumours of Endocrine Organs.* Lyon: IARC Press, 2004.

Lack EE. *Tumors of the Adrenal Gland and Extra-Adrenal Paraganglia: Atlas of Tumor Pathology, 3rd Series, Fascicle 19.* Washington DC: Armed Forces Institute of Pathology, 1997.

Lloyd RV, Douglas BR, Young WF. *Endocrine Diseases: Atlas of Nontumor Pathology, 1st Series. Fascicle 1.* Washington DC: Armed Forces Institute of Pathology, 2002.

Mills S, Carter D, Greenson JK, Oberman HA, Reuter V, Stoler M*H (eds). Sternberg's Diagnostic Surgical Pathology. 4th ed.* Philadelphia: Lippincott Williams & Wilkins, 2004.

Rosai J. *Rosai and Ackerman's Surgical Pathology. 9th ed.* St. Louis: Mosby, 2004.

Rosai J, Carcangiu ML, DeLellis RA. *Tumors of the Thyroid Gland: Atlas of Tumor Pathology, 3rd Series, Fascicle 5.* Washington DC: Armed Forces Institute of Pathology, 1992.

Chapter 4

Breast

Intraoperative Consultation

Breast carcinomas, such as a large obvious carcinoma, multifocal carcinoma, or large ulcerated carcinoma, that can only be treated appropriately with mastectomy require an incisional biopsy and frozen section analysis if a preoperative core biopsy has not confirmed the presence of cancer. No other indications point to an intraoperative diagnosis on a breast mass detected on either mammography or physical examination.

There are several reasons to avoid doing frozen section analysis on breast lesions. Small lesions, if frozen in their entirety, may be difficult to interpret definitively even on permanent section because of artifacts that result from freezing and persist even after subsequent paraffin processing. In addition, small lesions may be difficult to interpret because they frequently represent low-grade carcinoma or benign lesions that may mimic an invasive carcinoma (eg, radial scar).

Biopsy specimens that do not contain a discrete lesion should not be frozen because no useful purpose can be served. A false-negative report based on frozen section diagnosis can be psychologically very traumatic. This scenario most frequently arises in the setting of a carcinoma in situ. In addition, frozen incidental atypical lesions can be irrevocably compromised to the point that a definitive diagnosis is impossible.

Frozen sections, however, do have a place in the evaluation of breast carcinoma. They may be useful to the surgeon in cases with suspicious sentinel lymph nodes. A pathologically confirmed positive sentinel node will allow a surgeon to immediately proceed to an axillary dissection, thus avoiding a second procedure

Several benign lesions are notoriously treacherous on frozen section and more often than not can lead the unwary pathologist to a false-positive diagnosis. These include radial scars, microglandular adenosis, adenosis tumor, fat necrosis, papillary lesions, pregnancy and lactational adenoma, phyllodes tumors, and granular cell tumor.

Specimen Handling

All breast biopsy specimens should be inked and if received oriented by the operating surgeon should be inked in different colors so that the orientation is preserved when the surgical margins are examined microscopically.

One inherent problem with inking breast specimens is the fact that ink can track into fissures and crevices in the specimen regardless of how carefully it is applied. This causes difficulty in the subsequent microscopic evaluation of surgical margins. The use of Bouins solution or acetone helps ink adhere to fat.

If after serial sectioning, an obvious lesion is noted, sections should be taken from all the inked surgical margins that appear anywhere close to the lesion. Biopsy specimens that do not have a grossly discernible lesion after serial sectioning should be submitted in their entirety.

Ideally, serially sections of breast parenchyma should be taken perpendicular to a plane that runs from the nipple through the lesion (perpendicular to the mammary ductal system).

Mastectomy specimens are typically inked in 2 or more colors to identify the different surgical margins. Generous samples should be taken of any obvious lesion or previous biopsy site . Sections should be taken from grossly uninvolved breast parenchyma from all quadrants distant from the lesion and from the closest surgical margin(s).

Benign Lesions

Fibrocystic Changes

Clinical Manifestations

- Affects approximately 30% to 35% of women between the ages of 20 and 45 years
- 75% of affected women between the ages of 35 and 40 years
- Usually multifocal and bilateral
- 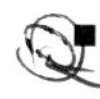 Women who have a history of taking oral contraceptive hormones less likely to development fibrocystic changes
- Three clinical stages of breast involvement:
  - Women in mid to late 20s experience premenstrual breast swelling or tenderness lasting approximately a week

- Multiple hard tender nodules and plaques up to 2 to 3 cm in diameter begin to develop as women enter their early 30s; premenstrual pain and tenderness may last for 2 weeks or more; condition known as "Schimmelbusch disease"
- Breast pain and tenderness become permanent and occasionally debilitating as women enter their 40s

- After menopause, fibrocystic changes and symptoms gradually disappear (women who take estrogen replacement therapy may continue to experience the symptoms)
- Estrogens stimulate proliferation of connective tissue with the development of fibrosis; the fibrosis causes obstruction of ductules that gradually dilate and become cystic as a result of persistent cyclic epithelial secretion

Gross Pathology

- Breast tissue contains several, small, randomly distributed blue-domed or clear cysts
- Large cysts (greater than 2 cm) less frequent

Microscopic Pathology

- Characterized by cystically dilated round to oval spaces lined by slightly attenuated epithelial and myoepithelial cell layers
- Stroma between lobules frequently sclerotic
- As cystic changes progress, smaller cysts coalesce and form larger cysts that continue to be lined by native, attenuated, epithelial and myoepithelial cells; metaplastic apocrine cells may be present
- When cysts rupture, an inflammatory response results and subsequent reparative changes cause additional fibrosis
- Microscopic expansion of lobules by an increased number of ductules or acini per lobule (adenosis) and a mild degree of epithelial hyperplasia (2-4 cells deep) both features of fibrocystic change

Special Stains and Electron Microscopy

- Not helpful

Immunohistochemistry

- Cyst fluid contains GCDFP-15; immunohistochemically this protein is seen in the cytoplasm of both benign and malignant apocrine epithelium

Molecular Alterations

- None

Differential Diagnosis

- Cystic lobular involution
- Duct ectasia (a disease of extralobular ducts)

Treatment

- Oral contraceptives, danazol, and tamoxifen all effective in reducing the progression and symptoms of disease
- Women with intractable systems and dense nodular breasts may be considered for bilateral subcutaneous mastectomy

Prognosis

- Fibrocystic changes involute and symptoms disappear with menopause

Associations

- Fibrocystic changes with apocrine cysts and mild epithelial hyperplasia (2-4 cells thick) do not represent an increased risk for the development of carcinoma
- Intraductal hyperplasia without atypia (more than 4 cells thick) associated with a slightly increased risk (1.5-2 times) for the development for carcinoma
- Atypical intraductal hyperplasia associated with a moderately increased risk (4-5 times) for developing invasive carcinoma

Microglandular Adenosis

Clinical Manifestations

- Most present with a palpable mass
- Seen in women between the ages of 30 and 80 (median 50) years
- No distinctive mammographic pattern
- May mimic carcinoma clinically and pathologically

Gross Pathology

- May appear as focal areas of irregular gray-white fibrous densities to irregularly circumscribed firm, rubbery mass
- Most approximately 3 to 4 cm in maximal dimension

Microscopic Pathology

- A haphazard scattering of round, glandlike structures in a hypocellular, fibrocollagenous, or fatty mammary stroma (an infiltrative growth pattern)
- Glandular units typically accompanied by a distinctive fibrocollagenous stroma that varies from densely collagenous to loose and hypocellular, courses between ducts and lobules, and extends into adjacent adipose tissue
- In some areas glands closely packed and in other areas widely separated; glands tend to be round or oval and have a flat to cuboidal epithelial lining with bland nuclei and abundant eosinophilic, clear, or amphophilic cytoplasm
- Epithelial cells with clear cytoplasm tend to be the dominant cell type within the epithelium (contain glycogen)
- Perineural or intravascular extension never present
- Differentiation from well-differentiated adenocarcinoma is based on the following characteristics of microglandular adenosis:
    - Thick basement membrane
    - Abundant cytoplasm
    - Characteristic inspissated eosinophilic secretory material
    - Rare mitotic figures

Special Stains

- Epithelial cells lining glands and luminal secretions PAS-positive and diastase resistant, and stain with mucicarmine and Alcian blue
- PAS stain will also highlight the presence of a well-formed basement membrane around tubules

Immunohistochemistry

- Epithelial cells in glandlike structures positive for cytokeratin, S-100 protein, and cathepsin D, and negative for EMA and estrogen and progesterone receptors
- Immunostains for muscle-specific actin typically confirm absence of a myoepithelial cell layer
- Basement membrane positive for laminin and type IV collagen

Electron Microscopy

- Single layer of epithelial cells without a surrounding myoepithelial cell layer in glandlike structures can generally be confirmed
- Basement membrane thick, multilayered, and surrounds glandlike structures
- Small intracellular cytoplasmic secretory granules may be seen in the luminal end of epithelial cells

Molecular Alterations

- None

Differential Diagnosis

- Tubular carcinoma (a myoepithelial layer absent in both tubular carcinoma and microglandular adenosis)
- Sclerosing adenosis (presence of a myoepithelial cell layer can be confirmed with muscle-specific actin)

Treatment

- Complete local excision

Prognosis

- This lesion has for years been considered benign, but it may recur and/or develop atypia if it is not completely excised. Some consideration is being given to the possibility that microglandular adenosis may be a form of low-grade carcinoma

Associations

- Carcinoma within microglandular adenosis in 20%

Sclerosing Adenosis

Clinical Manifestations

- Mimics infiltrating carcinoma on mammographic, gross, and microscopic examination
- Present in approximately 3% of breasts (autopsy series)
- Seen in approximately 12% of surgical specimens for benign disease and in 5% to 7% of surgical specimens for carcinoma
- May present as a palpable mass between the ages of 30 and 45 years
- May be painful
- Process tends to regress with menopause

Gross Pathology

- Often not visible on gross examination
- A nodule of sclerosing adenosis may appear as an irregular nodule of firm gray-white fibrous tissue with a rubbery consistency

Microscopic Pathology

- Typical lesion consists of a proliferation of densely packed ductules all of which have basal lamina and both an epithelial and myoepithelial layer; ductules tend to be elongated and distorted and have small compressed (slitlike) lumens as a result of being compressed by surrounding stroma; usually a lobulocentric arrangement; the lobulated arrangement of ductules the most important microscopic feature that distinguishes sclerosing adenosis from other histologically similar lesions
- Ductular proliferation a result of an increase in the number of ductules coupled with elongation of lobular structures and a proliferation of myoepithelial cells and stroma
- Caliber of proliferated ductules tends to be greater at the periphery of the lesion than at the center; this increased caliber may actually take on the appearance of cystic change
- Variable amounts of fibrosis present; when the fibrosis is minimal, the diagnosis is florid adenosis; when the fibrosis is more prominent, the diagnosis is sclerosing adenosis
- Microcalcifications common (50%) and often present in ductule lumens
- Epithelial cells tend to have a granular cytoplasm and may have features of apocrine metaplasia; myoepithelial cells usually appear vacuolated
- Occasionally the ductular elements invade nerves (2%)

Special Stains

- PAS will stain the basement membrane around ductules

Immunohistochemistry

- Muscle-specific actin will confirm presence of myoepithelial cells
- Laminin will confirm the presence of a basal lamina

Electron Microscopy

- Not helpful

Molecular Alterations

- None

Differential Diagnosis

- Tubular carcinoma
- Microglandular adenosis
- Radial scar

Treatment

- Local excision

Prognosis

- Relative risk for development of an invasive ductal carcinoma is approximately 1.7

Associations

- None

Radial Scar

Clinical Manifestations

- Typically occurs in women between the ages of 50 and 70 (mean 55) years
- May be present in as many as 30% of all women (autopsy series)
- 65% multicentric, 45% bilateral
- Seen more frequently in women with fibrocystic changes (45%) than in women with normal breasts (15%-20%)
- Mimics invasive carcinoma on mammography (a small spiculated structure)

Gross Pathology

- Most not visible on gross examination; usually incidental microscopic findings
- When visible, it mimics a carcinoma: a firm, stellate, or nodular appearance with central puckering

Microscopic Pathology

- Lesion consists of a fibroelastic core with radiating bands of fibrous connective tissue that contain lobules with the features of adenosis and ducts with papillary or diffuse intraductal hyperplasia
- Central portion characterized by fibrosis and elastosis that entrap haphazardly arranged, attenuated, and distorted ducts lined by epithelium and myoepithelium
- Fibrotic component characterized by dense bundles of collagen; elastotic component more basophilic and amorphous
- Periphery characterized by foci of sclerosing adenosis and fibrosis
- Early lesions tend to contain chronic inflammatory cells and reactive-appearing fibroblasts in their central areas without significant distortion of surrounding structures
- Older lesions tend to be densely hyalinized and fibroelastatic centrally
- Rarely an invasive carcinoma may be present in and around the fibroelastotic core
- Ductal dilatation with or without apocrine epithelium and squamous cell metaplasia may be present near the center

Special Stains

- Elastic stains highlight elastosis and confirm its condensation around encircled, attenuated ducts

Immunohistochemistry

- Smooth muscle actin will confirm presence of a myoepithelial cell layer around entrapped ductules

Electron Microscopy

- Confirms presence of both epithelial and myoepithelial cells in entrapped ductules (may be of use when presence of an associated invasive carcinoma suspected)
- A circumferentially distributed basal lamina can be confirmed

Molecular Alterations

- None

Differential Diagnosis

- Tubular carcinoma

Treatment

- Local excision

Prognosis

- A benign lesion associated with a 2-fold increased risk for the development of carcinoma (similar to the risk of florid hyperplasia)

Associations

- Usually seen in breasts with multiple foci of adenosis
- May occur in association with malignant lesions (intraductal carcinoma, lobular neoplasia, and invasive carcinoma)

Tubular Adenoma

Clinical Manifestations

- Tend to occur in young women of reproductive age
- Patients typically present with a well-defined, mobile mass without abnormality in overlying skin or nipple
- 25% experience tenderness to palpation
- 40% first note the presence of the nodule during pregnancy

Gross Pathology

- Typically well-circumscribed, firm, and solid with a homogenous tan to yellow cut surface

Microscopic Pathology

- Well-circumscribed with a delicate fibrous capsule
- Aggregates of compact, small, round tubules lined by both epithelial and myoepithelial cell layers
- Epithelial cells never atypical but may be mitotically active
- Epithelial cells not vacuolated and have no evidence of intracytoplasmic secretory material, but tubular lumens may contain eosinophilic secretory material; lumens rarely distended
- A paucicellular stroma separates the tubules and may be infiltrated by lymphocytes

- 20% have lactational and secretory changes

Special Stains, Immunohistochemistry, and Electron Microscopy

- Not helpful

Molecular Alterations

- None

Differential Diagnosis

- Adenosis and nodular adenosis (tubular adenoma at least 1 cm in size or encapsulated)

Treatment and Prognosis

- Total excision
- A benign neoplasm with no associated increased risk for the development of carcinoma

Associations

- May be seen in combination with a fibroadenoma (these 2 lesions may be related; tubular adenoma characterized by a prominent ductular component; fibroadenoma characterized by a predominant stromal component)

Malignant Intraductal Lesions

Intraductal Carcinoma (Ductal Carcinoma in situ [DCIS])

Clinical Manifestations

- May present as a palpable mass, Paget disease, or nipple discharge
- Frequently detected on mammography or incidentally at microscopic examination
- Lesions with comedonecrosis may be seen on mammography as dystrophic calcifications
- Average age at diagnosis 55 years
- Multicentric (foci of carcinoma in more than 1 quadrant) in approximately 30%

Gross Pathology

- Lesion not typically visible
- Lesions with comedonecrosis may be detected grossly by compressing the excised specimen and expressing soft thin cylinders of necrotic material from the cut surface
- Occasionally, periductal fibrosis may produce an area of firmness

Microscopic Pathology

- A proliferation of epithelial cells with morphologic features of malignancy that are confined to the duct system and do not demonstrate stromal invasion
- Proliferating epithelial cells may demonstrate various cytologic appearances from minimal atypia to highly anaplastic; typically ductal cells have a columnar shape and are larger, have more cytoplasm, and are more cohesive than lobular cells
- Extent of ductal involvement ranges from a localized area to widespread involvement of multiple terminal ductal-lobular units with extension into multiple major ducts in 1 or more segments
- An intact myoepithelial cell layer may be present around the duct wall; absence of a myoepithelial layer does not mean invasion has occurred (basement membrane may be intact)
- Typically DCIS will manifest distinctive patterns to include the following

Comedocarcinoma

- 45% to 65% of cases of DCIS
- Usually confined to 1 quadrant, but tends to be fairly extensive
- Characterized by presence of necrosis, cytologic atypia, and loosely cohesive cells
- Necrotic debris in the lumen consists of apoptotic and oncotic necrosis in various proportions
- Mitotic figures may be rare to abundant
- Periductal fibrosis and a periductal lymphoplasmacytic infiltrate usually present
- Myoepithelial cell layer usually retained, but may be attenuated or absent

Cribriform Variant

- A proliferation of a uniform population of cells that form round secondary lumens; cells surrounding lumens columnar with basally oriented nuclei and tend to form rigid arcades or "Roman bridges"
- Nuclei round to ovoid and evenly distributed with little overlap
- Cytologically cells vary from small and uniform (monotonous) with round nuclei and little cytoplasm to atypical cells with nuclear pleomorphism and small amounts of granular eosinophilic cytoplasm
- Mitotic figures rare
- Microcalcifications may be present in secondary lumens

Solid Variant

- Proliferating epithelial cells fill and occlude ductal lumens
- Cells tend to be round to polygonal and have distinctive cell borders that give the lesion a mosaic appearance

Micropapillary Variant

- Epithelial cells (similar to those of cribriform DCIS) form regularly distributed papillary tufts that project into the lumen and lack a fibrovascular core
- Areas of ductal wall between the epithelial tufts have 2 cell layers
- Luminal epithelial cells may be identical to those proliferating in the tufts or they may appear normal
- Myoepithelial cell layer usually intact
- Neoplastic cells may have some atypia and a hobnail appearance
- Occasionally, micropapillary pattern has features of cribriform pattern secondary to the formation of arcades and bridges
- More frequently multicentric (more than 1 quadrant) than any other type of DCIS

Apocrine Variant

- Usually multicentric (more than 1 quadrant)
- Proliferating cells have abundant granular, eosinophilic cytoplasm with moderate to severe atypia and central necrosis
- Apical snouts not always evident

Clinging Carcinoma

- Characterized by ducts that are lined by several layers of highly atypical cells or 1 or more layers of mildly atypical cells with lumens that are either empty or contain granular secretory material

- 3 grades of DCIS (grading based on the degree of nuclear atypia):
  - Grade I (low-grade): Cribriform and micropapillary patterns; a uniform population of epithelial cells that lack atypia; no necrosis; nuclei round to ovoid or spindled with smooth nuclear membranes and little pleomorphism; chromatin pattern diffuse; no nucleoli
  - Grade II (moderate grade):
    - Proliferating epithelial cells arranged in a solid, cribriform, or micropapillary pattern with central necrosis; no atypia
    - Epithelial cells with a cribriform, micropapillary, or solid pattern with cytologic atypia; no necrosis
    - Unusual variants (clear cell and spindle cell) with or without necrosis; nuclei tend to be round or ovoid with occasional clefts and may be twice the size of normal nuclei; chromatin tends to be coarse and nucleoli usually absent
  - Grade III (high-grade): Neoplastic cells display both cytologic atypia and necrosis or consist of purely signet ring cells; nuclei large and pleomorphic, and have markedly irregular membranes; chromatin tends to be vesicular or clumped; nucleoli often present, and may be multiple and large

Special Stains

- Not helpful

Immunohistochemistry

- Variable expression of estrogen receptor, p53, and *HER-2/neu* (*c-erbB-2*)
- *bcl-2* expression generally parallels that of estrogen receptor
- Estrogen receptor (ER) positivity present in 60% to 98% of low-grade DCIS; comedo-DCIS usually ER negative
- Progesterone receptor expression generally parallels ER expression
- Expression of p53 often present in high-grade DCIS
- Immunoexpression of *HER-2/neu* (*c-erbB-2*) less frequent in low-grade DCIS than in high-grade DCIS
- ER, progesterone receptor (PR), and *bcl-2* usually not expressed in apocrine cells; apocrine cells express androgen receptor
- E-cadherin expression typically positive (but reduced)

Electron Microscopy

- Many lesions prove to have basement membrane irregularity and foci of early invasion (neither finding may be evident on a routine hematoxylin-eosin (H&E) examination)

Molecular Alterations

- Loss of heterozygosity (LOH) on chromosome 17p (30%-50%); also chromosomes 1p, 3p, 6q, 7q, 11q, 16q, and others
- Allelic imbalance of *BRCA1* gene on chromosome 17q12-23 in 75%

Differential Diagnosis

- LCIS (almost indistinguishable from solid pattern of DCIS; E-cadherin typically negative in LCIS)
- Atypical intraductal hyperplasia
- Apocrine variant easily confused with apocrine metaplasia or hyperplasia seen in association with fibrocystic changes
- DCIS with microinvasion
- Invasive ductal carcinoma

Treatment

- Total mastectomy
- Lumpectomy with radiotherapy and adjuvant tamoxifen therapy
- Incidence of axillary node metastasis so low that axillary dissection not warranted
- Incidence of occult invasive carcinoma in women with DCIS ranges from 5% to 20%; axillary node involvement with metastatic disease occurs in 0% to 5% of this population
- Likelihood of occult invasion in nonpalpable lesions seems to be greatest for DCIS with comedonecrosis and is less likely with micropapillary or cribriform variants; more extensive surgical excision may be warranted for lesions with comedonecrosis
- Radiation therapy appears to reduce ipsilateral breast recurrence after lumpectomy by approximately 30%
- Most important determinant of recurrence is whether or not a complete excision of the lesion has been obtained at the time of initial surgery

Prognosis

- Risk of subsequent invasive carcinoma in contralateral breast approximately 3% to 5%
- Recurrence rate higher and recurrence occurs earlier following surgery for comedo type DCIS than for any of the other types

Associations

- Invasive carcinoma

Papillary Lesions

Variants

- Papilloma
- Papillomatosis
- Sclerosing papilloma
- Atypical papilloma
- Carcinoma arising in a papilloma
- Papillary Carcinoma

Microscopic Pathology

- Benign papillary lesions have a relatively uniform myoepithelial cell layer in the proliferating intraductal papillary lesion; carcinomas have an almost complete absence of a myoepithelial layer

Associations

- See sections on atypical intraductal hyperplasia and DCIS
- 20% to 40% of invasive carcinomas have a papillomatous lesion in surrounding breast tissue

Papilloma

Clinical Manifestations

- Typically solitary and arise from a major duct in a central subareolar location
- Close to 90% have a serous or serosanguinous nipple discharge
- Most diagnosed during fifth or sixth decade
- May occur in either men or women

Gross Pathology

- A soft friable papillary mass within a dilated duct
- Foci of hemorrhage may be present around the involved duct

Microscopic Pathology

- Characterized by epithelial fronds supported by a fibrovascular stroma in a dilated and sometimes cystic duct
- Epithelial cells line the luminal surface of the papillae and a myoepithelial cell layer is *always* present between the epithelial cells and the basement membrane
- Typically attached to duct wall at 1 or 2 places
- Metaplastic apocrine cells present in 20%
- 30% have areas of solid and cribriform epithelial hyperplasia without atypia
- Occasionally portions of a papilloma or the entire lesion may undergo hemorrhagic infarction (squamous metaplasia may be present in association with infarction)

Special Stains

- Not helpful

Immunohistochemistry

- S-100 and muscle-specific actin will confirm presence or absence of myoepithelial cells

Electron Microscopy

- Not helpful

Molecular Alterations

- All papillomas are monoclonal and the same allele of the X-chromosome–linked phosphoglycerokinase (PGK) gene is inactivated

Treatment

- Papilloma, papillomatosis, sclerosing papilloma, and atypical papilloma all treated with total excision

Prognosis

- A slight increased risk for the development of invasive carcinoma associated with both a papilloma and sclerosing papilloma (0.5%-8%)

Papillomatosis

Clinical Manifestations

- May be palpable, but usually small lesions, detected mammographically and associated with microcalcifications
- Patients typically younger than those with a solitary papilloma (median age 40 years)
- 30% have a nipple discharge
- *Typically involve multiple terminal ductal lobular units in the periphery of the breast*

Gross Pathology

- May present as a mass as a result of involvement of several duct systems or multiple foci of a single duct system

Microscopic Pathology

- Typically a simultaneous proliferation and protrusion of multiple papillae into the lumens of multiple terminal ductal lobular units

- Vast majority attached to duct wall diffusely at multiple places
- Lesions typically start as simple, nonbranching structures, which become progressively more architecturally complex and cellular with time
- Each papillary process has both an epithelial and a myoepithelial cell layer that overlies a distinct fibrovascular stromal core
- Some papillary fronds may have a proliferation of stratified spindle cells accompanied by focal loss of the myoepithelial cell layer
- Atypia may be present and typically appears as a proliferation similar to that seen in atypical intraductal hyperplasia
- 20% to 40% of malignant breast lesions (DCIS or invasive carcinoma) have areas of papillomatosis in the surrounding breast tissue

Special Stains

- Not helpful

Immunohistochemistry

- S-100 and muscle-specific actin will confirm presence or absence of myoepithelial cells

Electron Microscopy

- Not helpful

Molecular Alterations

- All papillomas are monoclonal and the same allele of the X-chromosome–linked phosphoglycerokinase (PGK) gene is inactivated

Differential Diagnosis

- Micropapillary DCIS

Treatment

- Papilloma, papillomatosis, sclerosing papilloma, and atypical papilloma all treated with total excision

Prognosis

- Papillomatosis often simultaneously associated with intraductal epithelial hyperplasia with or without atypia and DCIS
- Papillomatosis has a high incidence of recurrence and a 25% incidence of malignant transformation

Sclerosing Papilloma

Clinical Manifestations

- Most present with a mass that may be fixed to overlying skin
- Rarely patients experience pain or nipple discharge
- Median age at diagnosis 45 years
- May be solitary or multiple, grossly visible, or microscopic

Gross Pathology

- Rarely appears as an intracystic mass
- Usually presents as a solid, well-circumscribed mass varying in size from microscopic to 3.5 cm

Microscopic Pathology

- Characterized by an intraductal papillary proliferation with either focal or diffuse sclerotic changes
- Sclerotic areas typically contain distorted, entrapped tubules (mimic an invasive carcinoma)
- Myoepithelial cells present in the residual papillary processes and entrapped ductules and tubules
- Often the duct wall thickens, and occasionally the entire duct is surrounded by a band of sclerosing adenosis
- Sclerosis may be diffuse, resulting in a hyalinized nodule with scattered distorted ductules

Special Stains

- Not helpful

Immunohistochemistry

- S-100 and muscle-specific actin will confirm presence or absence of myoepithelial cells

Electron Microscopy

- Not helpful

Molecular Alterations

- All papillomas are monoclonal and the same allele of the X-chromosome–linked phosphoglycerokinase (PGK) gene is inactivated

Differential Diagnosis

- Sclerosing adenosis
- Invasive carcinoma

Treatment

- Papilloma, papillomatosis, sclerosing papilloma, and atypical papilloma all treated with total excision

Prognosis

- A slight increased risk for the development of invasive carcinoma associated with both a papilloma and sclerosing papilloma (0.5%-8%)

Atypical Papilloma

Clinical Manifestations

- May present as any of the papillary lesions described above

Gross Pathology

- May be indistinguishable from any of the papillary lesions described above

Microscopic Pathology

- Papillary processes contain focal areas that consist of a proliferation of monotonous cells identical to the cells of a low-grade, non-necrotic DCIS
- A myoepithelial cell layer may or may not be present
- These focal areas of proliferation occupy less than 1/3 of the lesion

Special Stains

- Not helpful

Immunohistochemistry

- S-100 and muscle-specific actin will confirm presence or absence of myoepithelial cells

Electron Microscopy

- Not helpful

Molecular Alterations

- All papillomas are monoclonal and the same allele of the X-chromosome–linked phosphoglycerokinase (PGK) gene is inactivated

Differential Diagnosis

- Intraductal hyperplasia
- Atypical intraductal hyperplasia
- DCIS
- Carcinoma arising in a papilloma

Treatment

- Papilloma, papillomatosis, sclerosing papilloma, and atypical papilloma all treated with total excision

Prognosis

- Atypical papilloma associated with a 4 to 5 times increased risk of the development of invasive carcinoma (similar to the risk for women with nonpapillary atypical hyperplasia)

Carcinoma Arising in a Papilloma

Clinical Manifestations

- May present as any of the papillary lesions described above

Gross Pathology

- May be indistinguishable from any of the papillary lesions described above

Microscopic Pathology

- Papillary processes consist of a proliferation of epithelial cells identical to the cells of a low grade, DCIS that occupy spaces between the papillary cores, that if seen in a single duct would qualify as DCIS

- Myoepithelial cell layer may or may not present, but at least 1/3 of the papillary fronds should show absence of the myoepithelial cell layer
- In the presence of necrosis, a highly atypical cell population, or a truly anaplastic cell population, the lesion qualifies as a carcinoma arising in a papilloma (even it occupies less than 1/3 of the lesion)

Special Stains

- Not helpful

Immunohistochemistry

- S-100 and muscle-specific actin will confirm presence or absence of myoepithelial cells

Electron Microscopy

- Not helpful

Molecular Alterations

- All papillomas are monoclonal and the same allele of the X-chromosome–linked phosphoglycerokinase (PGK) gene is inactivated

Differential Diagnosis

- Atypical papilloma
- DCIS

Treatment

- Carcinoma arising in a papilloma treated with total excision with a rim of uninvolved breast tissue

Prognosis

- Carcinoma arising in a papilloma frequently associated with the simultaneous presence of atypical hyperplasia and DCIS; all 3 lesions carry an increased risk for the development of invasive carcinoma

Papillary Carcinoma

Clinical Manifestations

- Represents approximately 2% of all breast carcinomas
- Almost always seen in female breasts but occasionally occurs in the male breast
- Nipple discharge occurs in 20% to 25% (usually blood-tinged)
- 90% palpable (typically in a central location)
- 25% to 30% present with skin dimpling, nipple retraction, or deviation
- Peripherally located lesions tend to be multifocal and may present as abnormal microcalcifications on mammography
- Central lesions usually seen mammographically as a well-circumscribed mass
- Most are in situ and noninvasive carcinomas (unequivocal stromal invasion occurs in a small minority and represent 1.5% to 2.5% of all invasive breast carcinomas)

Gross Pathology

- Centrally located lesions tend to be well-circumscribed, soft and friable, and may appear encapsulated; a papillary architecture may be detectable grossly; focal areas of hemorrhage may be present
- Multifocal peripheral lesions frequently not visible on gross examination

Microscopic Pathology

- A proliferation of papillary processes that protrude into a distended duct lumen and lack a myoepithelial cell layer
- *The complete absence of a myoepithelial cell layer is the single most important feature of a papillary carcinoma; its absence differentiates a carcinoma from a benign papillary lesion*
- Tumor cells typically uniform and monotonous and rarely show atypia
- Proliferating papillae may have various patterns: simple stratification of spindled epithelial cells, tufting (micropapillae), solid, or cribriform
- Epithelial cells, regardless of overall architectural pattern, tend to be closely packed together with hyperchromatic nuclei and a high nuclear-cytoplasmic ratio; cytoplasm usually amphophilic, but eosinophilic apocrine cells may be present
- Presence of mitotic figures typically correlates with degree of cytologic atypia

- Stroma tends to be quite delicate or absent (unlike the prominent fibrotic stroma that characterizes benign papillomas)
- Microcalcifications may be present (usually in the glandular portion of the lesion but occasionally in the stroma)
- Lesions with a solid, spindle cell growth pattern frequently produce intraluminal mucin, and occasionally small isolated papillary cell clusters can be found floating in this mucin
- Solid pattern may show a proliferation of cells so dense that the basic papillary nature of the neoplasm almost completely obscured; mucin production may be evident
- Invasion characterized by cells that have broken through the basal lamina and extend beyond the duct wall without a surrounding myoepithelial cell layer; invasive tumor cells may not necessarily be in continuity with intraluminal tumor cells; morphology of invasive foci may vary from tubular to ductal

Special Stains

- Mucicarmine, Alcian blue, and PAS stains highlight various types of mucin secretion when present

Immunohistochemistry

- Myoepithelial cells typically positive for actin and S-100 protein (S-100 protein positivity quite variable)
- Tumor cells show CEA positivity in 85% (CEA positivity never seen in benign papillomas)
- 70% to 75% of invasive lesions ER positive and HER-2/neu overexpressed (amplified) in <10%
- 10% to 15% p53 positive

Electron Microscopy

- Confirms absence or relative absence of myoepithelial cells
- Epithelial cells tend to have poorly formed microvilli and intracytoplasmic lumens

Noninvasive Lobular Carcinoma

Lobular Carcinoma In Situ (LCIS)

Clinical Manifestations

- Typically found as an incidental finding in a breast biopsy performed on a proliferative lesion
- Represents 30% to 50% of noninvasive carcinomas
- Rarely, if ever, produces a palpable mass
- Tends to be multifocal and multicentric (45% to 95%) and bilateral (50% to 60%)
- Patient has significant risk of developing an invasive carcinoma (not necessarily invasive lobular)
- May be found in association with ordinary invasive ductal carcinoma and other types of carcinoma as well as infiltrating lobular carcinoma
- Calcification may be present near LCIS but rarely found in the involved lobules themselves
- Average age at diagnosis 45 years

Gross Pathology

- Typically no grossly apparent alteration in breast parenchyma
- Abnormalities detected on gross examination of the breast are usually the result of coexisting benign proliferative lesions
- Extensively involved breast tissue may have a slightly granular appearance

Microscopic Pathology

- An epithelial proliferation in the lobule of a population of relatively uniform, loosely cohesive, small round cells with little cytoplasm and bland nuclei that typically lack nucleoli; intracytoplasmic lumens, mucous globules, and a signet ring cell appearance fairly common; cell margins usually indistinct
- Not infrequently, lobular cells deviate from "classic appearance" and show some variation in size and at times may develop abundant eosinophilic cytoplasm with apocrinelike features; these cells tend to have more pleomorphic nuclei that sometimes have prominent nucleoli; cells may be tightly packed together and coherent, loosely cohesive, or completely detached from each other (pleomorphic LCIS)

- Proliferating lobular cells typically cause expansion of acini and intralobular ductules; usually the entire lobule enlarged; occasionally only some acini in 1 lobule involved; at least 50% to 75% of 1 lobule must be involved to establish the diagnosis (specimens with smaller degrees of involvement represent atypical lobular hyperplasia)
- Intralobular and extralobular or terminal ductules as well as acinar units in the lobule usually involved; extralobular involvement present in 65% to 75%; native ductal epithelial cells usually completely replaced, but may be lifted off the underlying basement membrane by proliferating lobular cells (Pagetoid spread)
- Ductal involvement usually consists of neoplastic cells distributed in a continuous fashion along the ductal system; these cells undermine, displace, and flatten the normal ductal epithelium; as lobular cells proliferate beneath the epithelium, they form buds of neoplastic cells that project into the surrounding stroma adjacent to the duct; this gives the duct an architectural pattern resembling a clover-leaf
- Foci of necrosis and microcalcification rare
- A myoepithelial cell layer typically present but indistinct as a result of being displaced or disrupted; basement membrane surrounding acini also present (may be disrupted)

Special Stains

- PAS and reticulin stains can confirm presence of basement membrane around the acinar unit (may appear disrupted)

Immunohistochemistry

- Neoplastic cells usually positive for both estrogen and progesterone receptors
- Basal lamina surrounding acinar units positive for collagen type IV
- Tumor cells typically negative for *HER-2/neu* (C-*erb B-2*) overexpression
- Actin will confirm presence of myoepithelial cells
- Tumor cells negative for E-cadherin

Electron Microscopy

- Neoplastic cells show secretory activity (intracytoplasmic lumens with secretory droplets)
- Tumor cells have prominent Golgi apparatus and are attached to one another and to nearby epithelial cells by well-developed desmosomes
- Basement membrane is generally intact but may intrude between myoepithelial cells giving it a tortuous appearance; gaps may be present

Molecular Alterations

- Loss of heterozygosity (LOH reported at chromosome 16q, 16p, 17p, and 22q
- Expression of p53 rarely seen (of interest in light of the fact that LOH has been reported at 17p)
- E-cadherin lost (16q22)

Differential Diagnosis

- "Pseudolactational" hyperplasia
- Myoepithelial hyperplasia
- Clear cell change
- Atypical lobular hyperplasia
- Low-grade intraductal carcinoma (DCIS)

Treatment

- Clinical follow-up on a regular basis for life after diagnostic biopsy
- Total mastectomy
- Bilateral mastectomy
- If surgical treatment desired by the patient, all breast parenchyma should be removed because of the multicentric nature of the disease and the possibility of a coexistent occult invasive lesion (total mastectomy with removal of level I axillary lymph nodes [removal of level I required to ensure removal of all breast parenchyma])

Prognosis

- Ipsilateral carcinoma or contralateral carcinoma will develop in 20% to 25% of patients
- The risk of developing a carcinoma increases with time and exceeds the expected rate by 6 to 9 times; if a women has a positive family history of breast cancer, the risk is almost 15 times greater than the expected rate
- Most invasive carcinomas that develop in the setting of LCIS are invasive ductal carcinomas; 25% are invasive lobular carcinomas; fewer than 15% are histologically favorable lesions

Associations

- Multiple and varied benign lesions (eg, fibrocystic changes, fibroadenoma, adenosis, sclerosing adenosis, duct ectasia, cystosarcoma phyllodes)
- Increased risk of occult invasive carcinoma

Biphasic Tumors

Fibroadenoma

Clinical Manifestations

- Most common breast neoplasm in adolescents and young adult women
- Usually seen between ages of 20 and 30 years
- Presents as a solitary well-circumscribed, mobile, nonpainful mass
- 25% multiple in 1 or both breasts (synchronous or metachronous)
- More common in blacks than whites
- May increase in size during pregnancy
- Tends to regress after menopause
- Originates in the terminal duct/lobular unit and probably results from unopposed estrogenic stimulation
- Second most common lesion of the breast (fibrocystic disease first and carcinoma third)
- Mammographically appears as smooth, lobulated lesions frequently with a radiolucent surrounding halo; coarse calcifications may be present (usually in extensively hyalinized lesions)

Gross Pathology

- A well-circumscribed apparently encapsulated nodule
- Cut surface tends to bulge with a uniform grey-white, fleshy surface

Microscopic Pathology

- A biphasic tumor consisting of a proliferation of epithelial and mesenchymal elements
- *Pericanalicular pattern* characterized by proliferating stromal elements surrounding tubular epithelial structures in a random or concentric pattern
- *Intracanalicular pattern* characterized by proliferating stroma growing in a radial pattern perpendicular to the epithelial elements which are compressed into cleftlike structures
- Ducts usually lined by 2 cell layers: a luminal epithelial layer and an underlying or surrounding layer of myoepithelial cells; various metaplastic changes may be seen in the epithelium to include squamous, apocrine, and oncocytic
- Ductal epithelium may show various degrees of hyperplasia and atypia; myoepithelial cells may also become hyperplastic
- Majority have a pushing growth margin and a well-formed capsule
- Occasionally a focal phyllodes pattern may be present with leaflike processes protruding into dilated ductal spaces or cysts
- Most of the stroma consists of fibroblasts which are interspersed with collagen; hypercellularity may be focal or diffuse; myxoid or mucinous change and hyalinization may be present
- Rarely the stroma contains bundles of smooth muscle cells, benign multinucleated giant cells, and foci of chondroid or osseous metaplasia
- Fibrocystic changes, adenosis, and sclerosing adenosis may be present in a fibroadenoma
- Pregnancy and lactation may precipitate spontaneous infarction

Special Stains

- Reticulin stains highlight deposition of reticulin around ducts, confirming the concentric pattern of pericanalicular lesions and radial pattern of intracanalicular lesions

Immunohistochemistry

- Most stromal cells positive for smooth muscle actin (especially when the stroma is cellular or composed of myofibroblastic cells)
- Stromal cells with smooth muscle differentiation positive for desmin
- Stromal cells that are fibroblasts are CD34-positive
- Epithelial cell component positive for cytokeratin
- Estrogen and progesterone receptor positivity can be quite variable in the epithelial and stromal components; myoepithelial cells always negative for both receptors

Electron Microscopy

- Stroma consists of fibroblasts and myofibroblasts
- Ductal cells are epithelial and have an interrupted myoepithelial layer and a distinct surrounding basement membrane

Molecular Alterations

- A chromosomal abnormality probably present in 20% to 30%

Differential Diagnosis

- Phyllodes tumor
- Tubular adenoma
- Sclerosing lobular hyperplasia

Treatment

- Surgical excision

Prognosis

- No evidence of increased risk of malignant change to cystosarcoma after a local excision

Associations

- Myxoid fibroadenomas are associated with Carney syndrome (cardiac myxomas, cutaneous myxomas, myxoid fibroadenomas, spotty pigmentation and endocrine overactivity)
- No increased risk for the development of carcinoma
- Both carcinoma in situ and invasive carcinoma may arise within a fibroadenoma; lobular carcinoma in situ (LCIS) is most common noninvasive lesion to occur in this setting (50%)
- 20% of patients with carcinoma in situ within a fibroadenoma will have carcinoma in situ within adjacent breast tissue

Juvenile Fibroadenoma

Clinical Manifestations

- Most common breast lesion in adolescent girls
- In approximately 10%, the tumor rapidly enlarges, reaching massive size and stretching overlying skin and dilating superficial veins
- Most solitary, but successive and multiple lesions may occur

Gross Pathology

- Usually circumscribed, soft, and rubbery
- Cut surface may reveal slitlike spaces in an otherwise uniform, bulging, gray-white fleshy tumor

Microscopic Pathology

- Ducts engulfed by a pericanalicular (random or concentric) arrangement of cellular stroma
- Stroma usually much more dense and cellular than that seen in the adult type of fibroadenoma
- Myxoid degeneration and/or metaplastic change in stroma very unusual
- Epithelial component frequently hyperplastic with irregular tufts overlying stratified epithelium; appearance similar to the hyperplasia seen in gynecomastia; marked atypia may be present, reminiscent of intraductal carcinoma (a conservative interpretation warranted)

Special Stains, Immunohistochemistry, Electron Microscopy

- See fibroadenoma

Molecular Alterations

- None

Differential Diagnosis

- Benign phyllodes tumor (stroma more cellular, leaflike processes, and very rarely, a pericanalicular growth pattern)
- Juvenile hypertrophy

Treatment

- Local excision with preservation of as much breast tissue as possible to ensure normal breast development
- Long-term follow-up warranted when the ductal epithelium markedly atypical

Prognosis

- A benign lesion with no predisposition for development of carcinoma

Associations

- None

Phyllodes Tumor

Clinical Manifestations

- Represents fewer than 0.5% of all breast tumors and 2.5% of all fibroepithelial tumors
- Typically seen in women between 45 and 50 years (typically 15 to 20 years older than those with fibroadenoma)
- Rarely seen in the male breast, but has been reported in seminal vesicles and prostate
- Most patients present with a painless, small, hard, breast mass that may have been present for many years that suddenly started to enlarge
- Occasionally lesions become quite massive and actually displace the nipple, stretch the skin, and distend superficial veins; ulceration of overlying skin occasionally occurs (not an indication of malignancy)
- Regional lymphadenopathy seen in approximately 15% (usually due to reactive changes)
- Rarely bilateral
- Appears as a well-circumscribed, sometimes lobulated density on mammography

Gross Pathology

- Most well-circumscribed and solid with a fleshy, bulging gray-white or yellow cut surface; cystic areas usually present; small foci of hemorrhage and necrosis may be present in large lesions
- Leaflike processes may be visible

Microscopic Pathology

- Architecturally characterized by the formation of leaflike processes that protrude into cystic spaces
- Benign epithelial cells line ducts and slitlike spaces and cover leaflike process; consist of 2 cell types: luminal epithelial cells and surrounding myoepithelial cells
- Epithelial component may undergo hyperplasia, contain atypical cells, and/or undergo malignant change; myoepithelial hyperplasia usually accompanies any epithelial proliferation
- Stroma tends to be cellular (more cellular than in the typical fibroadenoma) and consists of spindle-shaped fibroblastic and myofibroblastic cells (atypical and multinucleated cells may be present); tend to condense around ("cuff") the glandular elements
- Stroma may have a predominance of myofibroblastic-appearing cells with foci of osseous and chondroid metaplasia (as well as lipoid, skeletal muscle, and smooth muscle differentiation)
- Malignant change characterized by stromal hypercellularity, atypical stromal cells, and >5 mitotic figures per 10 hpfs
- Malignant stroma most often fibrosarcomatous but other types of sarcoma (liposarcoma, chondrosarcoma, osteosarcoma, rhabdomyosarcoma, hemangiopericytoma, and pleomorphic malignant fibrous histiocytoma may be present); >1 type of differentiation may be seen in the sarcomatous component
- Occasionally sarcomatous changes proliferate to such an extent that the epithelial elements become inconspicuous
- Tumors classified as benign, low-grade (potential for local recurrence), and high-grade (potential to metastasize)
- Low-grade tumors have less than 5 mitotic figures per 10 hpfs, mild to moderate atypia, cellular stroma, and predominantly pushing margins
- High-grade tumors have a hypercellular stroma, 5 or more mitotic figures per 10 hpfs, moderate to severe stromal atypia, and infiltrating margins

Special Stains

- Not helpful

Immunohistochemistry

- Stromal cells stain positively for vimentin; most are positive for muscle-specific actin, and approximately 25% are positive for desmin
- Typically stromal cells negative for S-100 protein, cytokeratin, and EMA
- Tumors more frequently PR-positive than ER-positive

Electron Microscopy

- Stromal cells have features of fibroblasts and myofibroblasts unless a more specific type of sarcoma cell present

Molecular Alterations

- Some benign tumors show an interstitial deletion of the short arm of chromosome 3, del (3) (p12p14) and del (3) (p21p23)
- Malignant tumors tend to express p53; benign tumors do not

Differential Diagnosis

- Juvenile fibroadenoma
- Carcinosarcoma
- Metaplastic carcinoma (especially with a dominant spindle-cell growth pattern)
- Sarcoma (especially in tumors with extensive stromal overgrowth)

Treatment

- Wide local complete excision
- Mastectomy reserved for large tumors, tumors with infiltrating margins, and tumors with aggressive histologic features
- Total mastectomy performed for local recurrences of borderline and malignant lesions
- No role for axillary dissection; these neoplasms essentially never metastasize to lymph nodes

Prognosis

- 30% recur
- Malignant tumors metastasize hematogenously (usually lungs)
- Repeatedly recurrent tumors occasionally show progressive degeneration with the development of metastases

Associations

- LCIS, DCIS, and invasive carcinomas can all occur in a phyllodes tumor; the lesion most frequently seen in association with a phyllodes tumor is LCIS
- Squamous cell carcinoma may occur in a phyllodes tumor
- In situ and invasive carcinomas more likely to be in breast tissue near a phyllodes tumor than within the tumor itself

Infiltrating Carcinoma

Invasive Ductal Carcinoma

Clinical Manifestations

- Represents approximately 75% of all invasive carcinomas of the breast
- Diagnosis typically made in late 50s
- Patients present with either a palpable mass or a mammographic abnormality
- Rarely, patients present with skin fixation, edema ("peau d'orange"), nipple retraction or discharge, Paget disease, or ulceration of the overlying skin

Gross Pathology

- Various appearances including well-circumscribed or stellate
- Stellate lesions typically associated with extensive fibrosis ("scirrhous carcinoma")
- On cut section, stellate lesions usually have chalky, yellow to white streaks that radiate from center into surrounding breast tissue
- Focal areas of necrosis may be present and appear as soft, chalky white areas; cystic change rare

Microscopic Pathology

- Tumor cells usually arranged in irregular or rounded, solid aggregates admixed with single cells and cords that frequently appear as poorly formed tubules and have glandular lumens
- Tubules and clusters of cells do not have a surrounding basal lamina or myoepithelial cell layer
- Well-differentiated tumors composed of cells with small, round uniform nuclei that lack nucleoli, tend to form tubules and glands, and have little or no mitotic activity
- Poorly differentiated tumor cells have large pleomorphic nuclei with prominent nucleoli, grow in solid aggregates with little or no tubular gland formation, and have abundant mitotic activity

- Perineural invasion present in approximately 10%; more common in poorly differentiated neoplasms
- A dense lymphoplasmacytic infiltrate present in approximately 20% (lymphocytic component composed predominately of T lymphocytes, cytotoxic-suppressor type)
- Tumors typically graded on the amount of tubule formation, degree of nuclear pleomorphism, and mitotic activity (Bloom-Richardson)
- Poorly differentiated tumor cells may show phagocytic activity (engulfing red and white cells as well as other tumor cells)
- Stroma may be fibroblastic, collagenous, or elastotic
- Occasionally infiltrating ductal neoplasm accompanied by areas of LCIS
- A component of DCIS present in 80%
- DCIS may be found in or around the invasive component
- Abundant DCIS in the tumor associated with a high likelihood of having DCIS beyond the tumor margin and a multicentric carcinoma
- Patients with an extensive DCIS component have a high rate of local recurrence (up to 25%) if treated with breast-conserving surgery and radiation
- Invasive tumors associated with a prominent DCIS component seem to have a better prognosis and a decreased frequency of nodal metastasis

Special Stains

- Mucicarmine can help establish diagnosis of carcinoma when the differential diagnosis includes a melanoma

Immunohistochemistry

- 55% to 75% ER-positive; 35% to 70% PR-positive; poorly differentiated tumors less likely to be ER and PR-positive than well-differentiated tumors
- Approximately 15% ER-positive and PR-negative
- Overexpression of *HER-2/neu* oncogene in 25% to 30%
- Some vimentin positivity; correlates with histologic grade
- 45% positive for S-100 protein
- Tumor cells positive for E-cadherin
- Muscle-specific actin useful in proving absence of myoepithelial cell layer

Electron Microscopy

- Not helpful

Molecular Alterations

- Deletions of 1 or more gene segments suspected of containing tumor suppressor genes have been detected on multiple chromosomal arms (1p, 11q, 13q, 16q, and 18q)
- Mutations of the *ras* proto-oncogene present in 10% to 30%
- Increased amplification of c-*erbB-2* (*HER2/neu*) seen in 25% to 30%

Differential Diagnosis

- Pseudoinvasion (the result of artifactual disruption of epithelial-stromal interface of ducts involved by DCIS or papillary carcinoma)
- Metastatic melanoma a consideration if malignant ductal cells are large and have prominent nucleoli

Treatment

- Lumpectomy (excision of the primary tumor with 1 cm of adjacent normal breast tissue), axillary node dissection, and adjuvant radiation to the residual breast
- Modified radical mastectomy (removal of the entire breast to include levels I and II of the axilla) with or without immediate or subsequent reconstruction; postmastectomy radiation in high-risk patients (>4 positive axillary nodes and/or invasion of skin and/or muscle)
- Adjuvant hormonal therapy (lasting 5 years) given to all women with hormone receptor–positive tumor regardless of age, menopausal status, axillary node involvement, or tumor size
- Adjuvant polychemotherapy improves long-term, relapse-free, and overall survival in both pre and postmenopausal women regardless of nodal status

Prognosis

- Patients with tumors less than 1 cm without nodal metastasis have a 10-year disease-free survival rate of 90%
- Patients with tumors less than 2 cm in diameter with negative lymph nodes have a 10-year disease-free survival rate of 80%
- Patients with tumors greater than 2 cm and less than 5 cm with negative nodes have a 10-year disease-free survival rate of 70%
- Patients with tumors greater than 5 cm with negative nodes have a 10-year disease-free survival rate of 60%
- Presence or absence of axillary lymph node metastasis the single most important prognostic factor:
  - For tumors less than 2 cm with 1 to 3 positive axillary lymph nodes, 10-year disease-free survival rate is 75% (without adjuvant chemotherapy)
  - For tumors less than 2 cm with more than 4 positive axillary lymph nodes, 10-year disease-free survival rate is 50%
  - For tumors between 2 and 5 cm with less than 4 positive axillary nodes, 10-year disease-free survival rate is 40%
  - For tumors between 2 and 5 cm with more than 4 positive axillary lymph nodes, 10-year disease-free survival rate is 20%
- Women older than 50 years treated with tamoxifen have an approximate 20% improvement in 5-year survival rates
- Women younger than 50 years treated with a combination chemotherapy experience approximately 25% improvement in 5-year survival rates
- *HER2/neu* overexpression associated with significantly shorter disease-free and overall survival in node-positive women
- Presence of *HER2/neu* overexpression may have a role in identifying women with otherwise favorable tumors (small, low-grade, ER-positive, and node-negative) who are likely to experience an early recurrence

Associations

- See DCIS and LCIS

Invasive Lobular Carcinoma

Clinical Manifestations

- Represents 5% to 15% of all invasive breast carcinomas
- Usually occurs between the ages of 45 and 55 years; slightly more common in women over age of 75 years (10%) than in women under the age of 35 years (2%)
- Usually presents as an ill-defined, painless mass; may present as a vague thickening or nodularity
- Does not typically form calcifications but calcification may be present in a nearby proliferative lesion
- 15% to 30% multicentric
- Subsequent contralateral carcinoma develops in 10% to 15% (50% invasive)

Gross Pathology

- Lesion ranges from being grossly inapparent to diffusely involving entire breast; appears as an irregular firm to hard mass
- Occasionally on sectioning the neoplasm appears to contain innumerable fine, hard nodules that resemble tiny grains of sand (an appearance reminiscent of sclerosing adenosis)

Microscopic Pathology

- Architecturally characterized by loosely cohesive, small cells that form slender (1-cell-thick) cords ("Indian files") that invade stroma
- Tumor cells typically small and uniform with a thin rim of cytoplasm surrounding round or notched nuclei with inconspicuous or absent nucleoli; some cells have intracytoplasmic lumina containing sialomucins; cells with an increased luminal content often assume a signet-ring appearance
- Tumor cells diffusely infiltrate mammary stroma and often surround normal structures in a targetoid pattern
- Mitotic figures rare
- LCIS is present in 40% to 60%
- Other architectural patterns include solid, alveolar, pleomorphic, tubulolobular, and various combinations

- Solid variant characterized by closely packed lobular cells arranged in large nests or wide trabeculae separated by delicate vascular channels
- Alveolar variant consists of typical lobular cells that form rounded nests and islands of 20 or more cells separated by scanty stroma
- Pleomorphic variant has significant nuclear as well as cellular pleomorphism
- Tubulolobular variant combines features of a ductal and lobular carcinoma with an admixture of cords and tubules

Special Stains

- Mucicarmine and Alcian blue/PAS will highlight intracytoplasmic mucin in 50% to 60%

Immunohistochemistry

- Tumor cells positive for cytokeratin
- 70% to 90% ER-positive (this includes the classic form and all variants); 65% PR-positive
- 35% to 65% of neoplastic cells positive for CEA, and 60% for S-100 protein
- Tumor cells negative for E-cadherin

Electron Microscopy

- Some cells may have dense core "neurosecretory" granules (a small cell neuroendocrine carcinoma may be a variant of invasive lobular carcinoma)
- Some cells have a clear organelle-poor cytoplasm; others have an organelle-rich cytoplasm

Molecular Alterations

- 20% aneuploid

Differential Diagnosis

- Ductal carcinoma with lobular features
- Solid variant mimics lymphoma

Treatment

- Largely determined by stage
- Modified radical mastectomy often the treatment of choice (frequency of multicentricity); breast-conserving surgery with axillary dissection and primary radiation in appropriately selected cases has the same survival as a modified radical mastectomy

Prognosis

- 5-year and 10-year survival rates for node-negative women are 85% and 75%, respectively
- 50% of patients with positive lymph nodes and 15% of patients with negative nodes die of disease
- Presence of bilaterality does not affect prognosis unless the lesions are synchronous
- Variants of invasive lobular carcinoma may have a slightly worse prognosis than the classic lesion; pleomorphic variant has the worst prognosis
- Invasive lobular carcinoma more likely to metastasize to distant sites than invasive ductal carcinoma (bone, gastrointestinal tract, uterus, ovary, meninges, genitourinary tract, skin, and peritoneum)

Associations

- No association with Paget disease

Tubular Carcinoma

Clinical Manifestations

- Represents fewer than 2% of all breast carcinomas
- Median age at time of diagnosis mid to late 40s (slightly younger than average)
- Most present with a palpable mass that tends to be localized in the periphery
- 15% superficial and cause retraction of overlying skin
- 25% to 30% multicentric
- 15% to 40% bilateral
- 40% patients have a positive family history
- On mammography, lesions appear spiculated and may contain calcifications (features reminiscent of a radial scar)

Gross Pathology

- Typically spiculated or stellate with a scirrhous appearance
- Small lesions may simply appear as a gray to white chalky discoloration with induration and retraction
- Gross appearance similar to that of radial scar

Microscopic Pathology

- A haphazard proliferation of tubules in a reactive-appearing fibroblastic stroma
- Tubules tend to be angulated, oval, or elongated with open lumens, and are lined by a single layer of epithelial cells (no myoepithelial cell layer); may extend into adjacent adipose tissue and normal mammary structures
- Epithelial cells tend to be fairly homogeneous, cuboidal, or columnar with round or oval, hyperchromatic, basally oriented nuclei; nucleoli usually inconspicuous or absent; cytoplasm typically eosinophilic or amphophilic (rarely clear)
- Epithelial cells not particularly atypical and mitotic activity rare; apical snouts may be present
- Calcifications within lumens of malignant tubules or within stroma present in approximately 50%
- Ducts in the immediate vicinity may show an epithelial proliferation reminiscent of a low-grade DCIS (perhaps a precursor lesion to the invasive tubular carcinoma)
- LCIS is present in approximately 15%
- Intraductal carcinoma present in 75% (usually cribriform or micropapillary)
- Typically stroma appears reactive and fibroblastic, occasionally it is densely collagenous and/or elastotic
- If 25% of the tumor consists of another type of invasive cancer the lesion is referred to as "mixed" (ie, 75% of the cancer tubular and 25% infiltrating ductal types)
- Perineural invasion uncommon; angiolymphatic invasion almost never present

Special Stains

- Not helpful

Immunohistochemistry

- Actin will confirm the absence of a myoepithelial cell layer
- Laminin will confirm the absence or almost complete absence of a basement membrane around the tubules

Electron Microscopy

- Will confirm the absence of a myoepithelial cell layer and a basement membrane

Molecular Alterations

- LOH within the *ATM* gene

Differential Diagnosis

- Sclerosing adenosis (tubules with slitlike or round, partially obliterated lumens; myoepithelial cell layer present)
- Microglandular adenosis (tubules with round, open lumens filled with colloidlike material; no myoepithelial cells, but prominent basement membrane)
- Radial scar (tubules with epithelial and myoepithelial layers entrapped in collagenous/elastotic stroma)

Treatment

- Usually can be managed with conservative treatment: complete excision of the lesion with a 1-cm tumor-free margin (lumpectomy), level I and II axillary node dissection, and postoperative radiation to the breast
- In rare cases in which the lesion is very large relative to the size of the breast, modified radical mastectomy may be the treatment of choice

Prognosis

- Survival for pure tubular carcinoma much better than for infiltrating ductal carcinoma
- Survival for mixed tubular carcinomas better than for infiltrating ductal or lobular carcinoma
- Recurrence occurs in fewer than 5% of pure lesions and in up to 30% of mixed lesions
- 5-, 10-, and 20-year survival rates for pure tubular carcinoma are 95%, 85 to 90%, and 75%, respectively
- Long-term survival frequently occurs even with axillary metastasis (rarely >3 nodes involved)

Associations

- None

Mucinous (Colloid) Carcinoma

Clinical Manifestations

- Represents 1% to 6% of all breast carcinomas
- Generally diagnosed during early 60s (slightly older than for regular infiltrating carcinoma)
- Usually seen as a well-defined, lobular-shaped lesion on mammography; microcalcifications may be present

Gross Pathology

- A soft gelatinous and glistening neoplasm with pushing, bosselated margins

Microscopic Pathology

- Small clusters of uniform round cells with little eosinophilic cytoplasm floating in large pools of mucin
- Delicate bands of fibrovascular connective tissue may be evident within mucus lakes and often connect nests of tumor cells
- Clusters of tumor cells may be solid, form secondary lumens, or have a papillary appearance
- Atypia, mitotic figures, and signet-ring forms may be present
- Calcification rare (occasionally seen if a papillary pattern present)
- In situ disease present in 15%, usually in the immediate vicinity of the neoplasm
- Occasionally a mixed form of neoplasm will be present with features of a regular infiltrating ductal carcinoma adjacent to a mucinous lesion

Special Stains

- Generally of little help (both neutral and acidic mucopolysaccharides may be present)

Immunohistochemistry

- 45% to 75% are ER positive, 15% are PR positive

Electron Microscopy

- Tumor cells have microvilli, mucin vacuoles, round to pleomorphic dense core granules, and aggregates of intracytoplasmic filaments
- Mucin extracellular

Molecular Alterations

- Almost always diploid

Differential Diagnosis

- Other carcinomas associated with mucin production: signet-ring carcinoma, columnar mucinous carcinoma, and mucinous cystadenocarcinoma (all have intracellular mucin)
- Mucocele
- Myxoid fibroadenoma

Treatment

- Breast-conserving surgery (lumpectomy and radiation with axillary dissection) or modified radical mastectomy
- Tends to recur late (as long as 25 or 30 years after initial treatment)
- Lesions smaller than 4 cm rarely metastasize
- Factors associated with a more aggressive behavior and a decreased survival include increased cellularity, large size, and the presence of axillary lymph node metastasis

Prognosis

- Mucinous lesions tend to have low incidence of axillary lymph node metastasis and a favorable long-term prognosis

Associations

- Intraductal carcinoma (of any pattern) present in 15%, usually at the periphery of the lesion

Medullary Carcinoma

Clinical Manifestations

- Represents 5% to 7% of all breast carcinomas
- Mean age at diagnosis 50 years
- May be more common in young women with *BRCA1*-related hereditary breast cancer gene
- Tumor tends to present as a well-circumscribed soft palpable mass
- Overlying skin may be erythematous

- 10% to 15% bilateral (synchronous or metachronous)
- Multicentricity may be present in as many as 10%
- Resembles fibroadenoma on mammography
- Patients often have palpable axillary lymph nodes even without metastatic disease (a result of germinal center hyperplasia and sinus histiocytosis)

Gross Pathology

- Typically a round mass with a well-circumscribed margin (grossly resembles a fibroadenoma); may appear encapsulated
- Cut surface bulging and tan to gray-white with foci of necrosis and hemorrhage
- Larger tumors with central necrosis may have cystic degeneration

Microscopic Pathology

- Cancer consists of poorly differentiated cells with scant stroma and a prominent lymphoid infiltrate
- Classic features include:
  - A well-circumscribed lesion with round tumor cells with abundant cytoplasm and round, vesicular nuclei that contain 1 or more prominent nucleoli
  - Tumor cells grow in a syncytial pattern
  - Mitotic rate often high
  - A prominent lymphoplasmacytic reaction accompanies the neoplasm (this lymphoplasmacytic reaction must involve at least 75% of the periphery, be present diffusely in the supporting stroma of the tumor, and/or be diffusely admixed with carcinoma cells)
  - Nuclei very pleomorphic
- Foci of squamous metaplasia present in 10% to 15%
- Gland formation not present
- Central necrosis may be present
- Granulomatous reaction may be present
- In situ carcinoma occasionally present in adjacent breast tissue
- 10% to 15% contain foci of squamous metaplasia
- *Atypical medullary carcinoma*
  - Margin focally irregular or infiltrating
  - Mild lymphoplasmacytic infiltrate
  - Presence of conspicuous glandular or papillary growth
  - Neoplasms with more than 2 of the aforementioned features best classified as infiltrating duct carcinoma

Special Stains

- Not helpful

Immunohistochemistry

- Tumor cells typically positive for cytokeratin (AE1/AE3) and CAM5.2
- Tumor cells frequently positive for S-100 protein and vimentin
- Atypical nuclei of tumor cells immunoreactive for p53 (a feature generally associated with aggressive tumors
- Lymphocytes predominantly T lymphocytes
- Plasma cells primarily of IgG type
- 90% negative for estrogen and progesterone receptors

Electron Microscopy

- No specific findings diagnostic for medullary carcinoma
- Tumor cells tend to have well-developed Golgi complexes and contain numerous organelles; no secretory granules

Molecular Alterations

- Trisomy 18 (not unique to this variant of breast cancer)

Differential Diagnosis

- Typical medullary carcinoma should be differentiated from atypical medullary carcinoma; prognosis better for typical medullary carcinoma than for atypical; prognosis for both better than for infiltrating ductal carcinoma

Treatment

- Modified radical mastectomy or lumpectomy with level I and II axillary lymph node dissection and primary radiotherapy
- No indication for hormonal therapy if tumor hormone receptor negative

Prognosis

- 5- and 10-year disease-free survival rates for women with typical medullary carcinoma and negative nodes are 75% to 80% and approximately 60%, respectively
- 5- and 10-year survival rates are 55% and 40%, respectively, if lymph nodes involved
- 40% to 45% of women will have axillary lymph node metastasis at the time of diagnosis (incidence of axillary metastasis in other breast cancers at diagnosis is 65%)

Associations

- None

Metaplastic Carcinoma

A malignant neoplasm of the breast characterized by an admixture of adenocarcinoma with areas of benign or malignant, epithelial (squamous, spindle) and mesenchymal (chondroid, osseous) differentiation

Variants (Classification)

- *Squamous carcinoma*
    - Large cell (keratinizing or nonkeratinizing)
    - Squamous carcinoma with spindle cell metaplasia (with or without acantholytic features)
- *Adenosquamous carcinoma (adenocarcinoma with squamous differentiation)*
    - High-grade
    - Low-grade (including a syringomatous variant)
- *Adenocarcinoma with spindle cell metaplasia*
- *Carcinoma with chondroid differentiation*
    - Regular infiltrating duct or other types of carcinoma with focal chondroid differentiation
    - Chondroid carcinoma (epithelioid chondrosarcoma)
- *Carcinoma with osseous differentiation*

Clinical Manifestations

- *Squamous carcinoma*
    - Represents fewer than 1% of all breast carcinomas
    - Average age at diagnosis 55 years
- *Adenosquamous carcinoma (adenocarcinoma with squamous differentiation)*
    - Average age at diagnosis 55 years
    - Most present with a palpable breast mass (presentation essentially the same for infiltrating duct carcinoma)
- *Adenocarcinoma with spindle cell metaplasia*
    - May appear suddenly and grow rapidly
    - Usually has a smooth contour on mammography
- *Carcinoma with chondroid or osseous differentiation*
    - May be seen anytime from the early 30s to late 80s
    - May be quite large, displace the nipple, and ulcerate the overlying skin

Gross Pathology

- *Squamous carcinoma*
    - May be well-circumscribed or infiltrating
    - Usually contains cysts of various sizes
    - Cut surface may display a curvilinear pattern with small empty spaces
    - Focal areas of necrosis may be present
- *Adenosquamous carcinoma (adenocarcinoma with squamous differentiation)*
    - Cut surface may have pearly white nodules (a feature of localized keratinizing squamous carcinoma)
    - Usually about 2.5 cm in diameter and has ill-defined margins (occasionally well-circumscribed)
- *Adenocarcinoma with spindle cell metaplasia*

- May be circumscribed or irregular

■ *Carcinoma with chondroid differentiation*
- May resemble regular infiltrating ductal carcinoma or be well-circumscribed with areas of firm, glistening chondroid tissue
- May be quite large (up to 20 cm)

■ *Carcinoma with osseous differentiation*
- Cut section may reveal presence of tiny fragments of bone

Microscopic Pathology

■ *Squamous carcinoma*
- Tumor has no connection to overlying cutaneous squamous epithelium
- Tumor cells may be large and keratinizing, acantholytic, spindled, or any combination and typically proliferate around cystic structures
- Intracellular bridges, keratin pearls, keratohyaline granules, and focal areas of necrosis all common
- Cystic areas often lined by benign-appearing squamous but tongues of malignant tumor infiltrate surrounding stroma; cellular atypia increases with depth of infiltration
- Spindle cell metaplasia may be present in variable amounts; may be so extensive that foci of squamous epithelium difficult to find
- Acantholytic variant typically consists of an admixture of spindle cells and edematous-appearing squamous cells arranged in such a way that channels of various sizes give the tumor the appearance of a vascular lesion; these channels either empty or filled with amorphous mucoid material

■ *Adenosquamous carcinoma (adenocarcinoma with squamous differentiation)*
- An admixture of adenocarcinoma (usually an infiltrating duct carcinoma) and squamous carcinoma
- Proportion of 2 components very variable (often misdiagnosed as mucoepidermoid carcinoma)
- Squamous component may be spindled, but usually well-differentiated and of the keratinizing large cell type
- Often the central portion of the neoplasm has highly differentiated benign-appearing keratinizing squamous cells that become less differentiated and nonkeratinizing toward the periphery; peripheral area usually consists of poorly differentiated adenocarcinoma

■ *Adenocarcinoma with spindle cell metaplasia*
- Typically an intimate admixture of adenocarcinoma with spindle cells
- Tubules of adenocarcinoma appear to transform into a spindle cell population (tubules appear to be stretching out and merging with surrounding spindle cells) giving the appearance of a predominantly spindle cell tumor with well-formed ductal structures with either open or compressed lumens
- Adjacent foci of DCIS may also be spindled
- Spindle cells may be squamous epithelium or glandular epithelium (only electron microscopy can differentiate the 2)

■ *Carcinoma with chondroid differentiation*
- Carcinoma typically of the regular infiltrating ductal type
- More cellular regions of the neoplasm typically distributed at the periphery of areas of chondroid differentiation
- If there is an admixture of carcinoma with benign-appearing cytokeratin-positive chondrocytes, the lesion is referred to as *carcinoma with chondroid metaplasia*; if the carcinoma is admixed with chondrocytes that are clearly malignant and cytokeratin negative, the lesion should be called a *carcinosarcoma*

■ *Carcinoma with osseous differentiation*
- Carcinoma component usually infiltrating ductal carcinoma (mucinous carcinoma has been reported)
- A zone of reactive stromal cells usually separates the carcinoma from foci of metaplastic bone (occasionally little or no reactive stroma between the neoplasm and bone)

- Osteoblasts surround bone; osteoclasts less frequent
- If bone has the appearance of osteogenic sarcoma, neoplasm should be referred to as a *carcinosarcoma*

■ *Carcinoma with a spindle cell component*

- If spindle cells positive for cytokeratin and EMA on immunohistochemistry and electron microscopy, the spindle cells represent transformed epithelial cells and the lesion qualifies as a *metaplastic carcinoma*
- If spindle cells do not react with cytokeratin and EMAand do not have epithelial features on electron microscopy, they are mesenchymal in origin (they will be reactive for desmin, actin, and vimentin) and the lesion qualifies as a *carcinosarcoma*)
- In a lesion that is composed entirely of spindle cells (no recognizable squamous cell carcinoma or adenocarcinoma) if the spindle cells react with cytokeratin and EMA, they represent squamous cell carcinoma with spindle cell metaplasia, adenocarcinoma with spindle cell metaplasia, or myoepithelial carcinoma; only electron microscopy can differentiate among the 3

Special Stains

■ Mucin stains highlight presence of mucin in adenocarcinomatous components

Immunohistochemistry

■ *Squamous carcinoma*

- Squamous cells positive for cytokeratin
- Epithelial nature of spindle cells can be confirmed with cytokeratin (spindle cells of a reactive stroma stain negatively for cytokeratin and positively for actin, vimentin, and desmin)
- Rarely ER positive

■ *Adenosquamous carcinoma (adenocarcinoma with squamous differentiation)*

- Rarely ER or PR positive

■ *Adenocarcinoma with spindle cell metaplasia*

- Cytokeratin will confirm the epithelial nature of spindle cells; will also stain the adenocarcinoma component
- Immunostains do not reliably allow for the separation of spindle cell adenocarcinoma from spindle cell squamous carcinoma (both will be cytokeratin positive)

■ *Carcinoma with chondroid differentiation*

- Most tumor cells coexpress S-100 protein and cytokeratin
- Tumor cells negative for actin
- Almost invariably ER and PR negative

■ *Carcinoma with osseous differentiation*

- Almost invariably ER and PR negative

Electron Microscopy

■ *Squamous carcinoma*

- Tumor cells contain abundant tonofilaments and intracytoplasmic and intercellular desmosomes (confirming squamous nature of the cells)

■ *Adenosquamous carcinoma (adenocarcinoma with squamous differentiation)*

- Glandular cells have microvillous projections along the luminal surface
- Cells with squamous differentiation have abundant intracellular tonofilaments

■ *Adenocarcinoma with spindle cell metaplasia*

- Spindled adenocarcinoma cells have desmosomes and do not have tonofilaments; some have intracytoplasmic lumens (confirms their glandular nature)
- Spindled squamous cells have intracytoplasmic tonofilaments and desmosomes

■ *Carcinoma with chondroid differentiation*

- Cells with chondrocytic differentiation (short microvilli, abundant rough endoplasmic reticulum, a prominent Golgi apparatus, and rare lipid droplets)

    - Epithelial nature of the neoplasm confirmed by an abundance of tonofilaments and numerous well-developed desmosomes
- *Carcinoma with osseous differentiation*
    - Osseous areas appear to arise from stromal cells and do not represent transformation of the epithelial component

Molecular Alterations

- Both carcinomatous elements and spindle cell metaplastic elements may show LOH at NM23 (17q23) and INT-2 (11q13)

Differential Diagnosis

- *Squamous carcinoma*
    - Metastatic squamous carcinoma (most likely from the lung, esophagus, and uterine cervix)
    - Benign squamous metaplasia
- *Adenosquamous carcinoma (adenocarcinoma with squamous differentiation)*
    - Mucoepidermoid carcinoma
    - Infiltrating syringomatous adenoma
    - Adenocarcinoma with squamous metaplasia
- *Adenocarcinoma with spindle cell metaplasia*
    - Carcinosarcoma
- *Carcinoma with chondroid differentiation*
    - Carcinoma with chondrosarcoma (carcinosarcoma)
- *Carcinoma with osseous differentiation*
    - Carcinoma with osteosarcoma (carcinosarcoma)

Treatment

- Modified radical mastectomy
- Breast-conserving surgery (lumpectomy) and radiation with axillary lymph node dissection

Prognosis

- *Squamous carcinoma*
    - Generally similar to that of typical invasive ductal carcinoma
    - Acantholytic variant may be more aggressive (probably a more poorly differentiated tumor)
- *Adenosquamous carcinoma (adenocarcinoma with squamous differentiation)*
    - Prognosis dependent on degree of differentiation of the 2 components
    - Low-grade tumors treated appropriately have excellent long-term disease-free survival
    - High-grade lesions tend to be aggressive and lethal
- *Adenocarcinoma with spindle cell metaplasia*
    - Clinical behavior not well established
- *Carcinoma with chondroid differentiation or osseous differentiation*
    - 5-year survival rate approximately 60% to 70%
    - Slightly better prognosis than invasive ductal carcinoma

Associations

- May coexist with various benign lesions that produce a mass to include a fibroadenoma and papilloma

Comment

Carcinosarcoma is defined by the presence of unequivocal carcinoma admixed with unequivocal sarcoma (sarcomatous areas must be negative for epithelial antigens)

Apocrine Carcinoma

Clinical Manifestations

- Represents fewer than 1% of all mammary carcinomas
- Patients typically present with a mass, often in the upper outer quadrant
- Pain or nipple discharge uncommon presenting manifestations
- Peak age incidence 60s through 70s
- May occur in males
- Rarely bilateral

Gross Pathology

- Typically indistinguishable from infiltrating duct carcinoma
- Cut surface usually gray to white but may have a tan to brown appearance; may be cystic or solid

Microscopic Pathology

- Tumor cells appear as a solid, cellular mass arranged as tubules, cords, and/or sheets
- Cystic areas may be present
- Neoplastic cells tend to be large with abundant granular eosinophilic cytoplasm and have large, vesicular, pleomorphic nuclei, which tend to be located centrally (occasionally eccentrically) within the cell
- Nucleoli usually large, prominent, and eosinophilic
- Frequently tumor cells appear to contain intracytoplasmic lipid giving them the appearance of sebaceous cells
- When arranged in a glandular pattern with lumens, the tumor cells often appear to have apical cytoplasmic snouts along the luminal margin; sometimes a crescent-shaped concentration of eosinophilic granules will be present in the apical cytoplasm
- Intraductal apocrine carcinoma has an architectural appearance similar to that of nonapocrine intraductal carcinoma, including comedo (most common), micropapillary, solid, and cribriform patterns
- Lymphatic tumor emboli may be present adjacent to infiltrating neoplasm

Special Stains

- PAS with diastase, toluidine blue, and trichrome will highlight cytoplasmic granules within tumor cells
- Cytoplasmic iron granules may be present
- Most tumor cells negative for mucin

Immunohistochemistry

- Tumor cells tend to be positive for cytokeratins and CEA
- Tumor cells typically negative for S-100
- Apocrine cells (benign or malignant) almost always positive for monoclonal antibody B72.3
- Tumor cells typically negative for estrogen and progesterone receptors as well as *bcl-2* expression; 20% to 25% positive for androgen receptors
- Both benign and malignant apocrine cells tend to be strongly immunoreactive for gross cystic disease fluid protein 15 (GCDFP-15)

Electron Microscopy

- Carcinoma cells contain numerous organelles, including increased numbers of mitochondria, many of which have incomplete cristae
- Osmiophilic secretory granules and empty vacuoles often present

Molecular Alterations

- None

Differential Diagnosis

- Apocrine carcinoma of the axilla originating in axillary apocrine glands
- Mammary apocrine metaplasia seen in association with the epithelium of simple cysts, hyperplastic ducts, and other benign proliferative abnormalities (sclerosing adenosis, fibroadenoma, and papilloma)
- Oncocytic carcinoma (negative for GCDFP-15)
- Histiocytoid carcinoma
- Lipid-rich carcinoma
- Squamous carcinoma
- Granular cell tumor

Treatment

- Breast-conserving surgery with radiation and axillary dissection or modified radical mastectomy (same treatment options as with other invasive epithelial carcinomas of the breast)
- Androgens apparently increase the rate of gene transcription of GCDFP-15 while simultaneously inhibiting cell proliferation

Prognosis

- Similar to that of other infiltrating duct carcinomas

Associations

- Hamartomatous apocrine gland hyperplasia of the axillae

Vascular Lesions

Pseudoangiomatous Stromal Hyperplasia

Clinical Manifestations

- Presents in premenopausal women between the ages of 20 and 50 years
- May occur in the male breast
- May be multiple
- Usually presents as a firm, rubbery, painless unilateral mass

Gross Pathology

- Typically well-circumscribed, firm, and smooth; rarely nodular
- Cut surface homogeneous, tan-gray, and fibrous
- Cysts up to 1 cm in diameter may be present

Microscopic Pathology

- At low-power magnification, neoplasm appears to be a complex vascular proliferation in a densely collagenized (keloidlike) interlobular and intralobular stroma; slitlike spaces not true anastomosing vascular channels and almost invariably empty (represent separation of stromal cells in collagenized background); spindle cells at margins of these spaces resemble endothelial cells
- Nuclei of the endothelial-like cells never atypical and do not show any mitotic activity
- Focal areas of myofibroblastic hyperplasia may be present
- Round eosinophilic cytoplasmic inclusions similar to those seen in digital fibromas may be present

Special Stains

- Not helpful

Immunohistochemistry

- Spindled, endothelial-like cells that line spaces strongly immunoreactive for vimentin, actin, and CD34 and negative for cytokeratin, factor VIII–related antigen, and *Ulex europaeus*
- Stromal cells strongly positive for progesterone receptors and faintly positive for ERs (normal mammary stroma typically PR negative except during gestation)

Electron Microscopy

- Spindle cells that line spaces appear to be fibroblastic in nature with well-developed endoplasmic reticulum and prominent Golgi apparatus

Molecular Alterations

- None

Differential Diagnosis

- Low-grade angiosarcoma

Treatment

- Complete excision (incomplete excision predisposes to local recurrence)
- Recurrent lesions may require mastectomy

Prognosis

- No reports of a malignant transformation

Associations

- In women, 50% associated with proliferative fibrocystic changes; in men, 50% associated with gynecomastia

Mesenchymal Lesions

Myofibroblastoma

Clinical Manifestations

- Typically presents in men in their late 50s to early 60s
- Presents as a mobile, solitary, palpable, firm, nontender mass
- Rarely bilateral or multifocal
- A lobulated, well-delineated, and homogenous density without microcalcifications on mammography

Gross Pathology

- Typically located in breast parenchyma and ranges from 1 to 5 cm
- Usually well-circumscribed, nodular, round and slightly lobulated
- Cut surface gray to pink and may have myxoid appearance
- Cystic change and hemorrhage usually absent

Microscopic Pathology

- Usually a delicate fibrous capsule; rarely infiltrating
- Tumor cells tend to be fibroblastlike, uniform, bipolar, and oval to spindle-shaped; arranged diffusely or in short packets; and admixed with broad bands and ribbons of collagen; tumor cells do not mingle with adjacent breast parenchyma
- Nuclei oval to elongated and frequently grooved
- Mitotic figures rare
- Occasionally (15%) neoplasm has a diffuse increase in cellularity, but atypia and significant mitotic activity never present
- Mast cells often present
- Focal myxoid change and cartilaginous metaplasia may be present
- Occasionally focal or diffusely prominent vascularity present
- Neoplasm may be admixed with adipose tissue particularly if multifocal

Special Stains

- Not helpful

Immunohistochemistry

- A wide variation in reactivity to actin
- Tumor cells typically focally reactive for desmin, strongly and diffusely positive for vimentin, and occasionally positive for CD34 and S-100 protein

Electron Microscopy

- Tumor may be composed primarily of fibroblasts or myofibroblasts or an admixture of the 2
- Cells with myoid features contain characteristic myofibrils with dense bodies, basal lamina, and surface-oriented pinocytotic vesicles
- Cells with fibroblastic features lack myofibrils but contain abundant rough endoplasmic reticulum
- Thick bundles of collagen between tumor cells

Molecular Alterations

- None

Differential Diagnosis

- Fibromatosis (long, sweeping fascicles of thin fibroblasts)
- Nodular fasciitis
- Myoepithelioma
- Metaplastic carcinoma or sarcoma

Treatment

- Local excision

Prognosis

- Excellent (no reports of malignant transformation)

Associations

- None

Myoepithelial Lesions

Adenomyoepithelioma

Clinical Manifestations

- Typically seen in women between ages of 30 and 80 (median 60) years
- Not reported in men
- Women present with a palpable tumor that occasionally may be quite large and fungating
- Rarely tender
- Most located peripherally; 20% located centrally just beneath the nipple, of which 50% have a serous nipple discharge
- Stippled microcalcifications in a fairly discrete mass on mammography

Gross Pathology

- Usually sharply circumscribed, firm to rubbery, round, or multilobulated
- Cut surface uniform and predominantly solid and gray to pink, occasionally small cystic areas
- Hemorrhage rare (may be present in larger tumors)

Microscopic Pathology

- Three variants:
- *Tubular type*
  - Characterized by a proliferation of rounded tubules lined by both epithelial and myoepithelial cells
  - Despite gross appearance of encapsulation margin frequently shows the presence of tubules proliferating into adjacent breast parenchyma
  - Myoepithelial cells prominent and hyperplastic to the extent that they obliterate tubular lumens by compression
  - Mitotic figures may be present (up to 3 per 10 high-power fields [hpfs])
  - Mucinous apocrine metaplasia may be present in the epithelial elements
- *Lobulated type*
  - Composed of solid nests of clear, eosinophilic, or hyaline (plasmacytoid) myoepithelial cells that have proliferated around and compressed epithelial-lined spaces
  - Lesion typically surrounded by a thick fibrous capsule, and fibrous septa divide it into round nests or lobules
  - Myoepithelial cells may be clear or pink to amphophilic; focal aggregates of cells may have a "plasmacytoid" appearance with dense hyalinelike cytoplasm that pushes the nucleus to the side
  - Mitotic activity scant but usually present
  - Hyaline degeneration may be present centrally
  - Central necrosis or calcification present in 30%
  - Satellite nodules in adjacent breast parenchyma may be present
  - Epithelial cells tend to have sparse, darkly staining cytoplasm, and hyperchromatic nuclei
- *Spindle-cell type*
  - Composed of spindled myoepithelial cells admixed with a few epithelial-lined spaces
  - Spindle cells tend to form a solid mass that partially occludes entrapped ductlike structures; almost indistinguishable from a cellular leiomyoma especially when epithelial-lined lumens are inconspicuous (if epithelial cells cannot be identified, lesion classified as a *myoepithelioma*)
  - Intraductal epithelial component may appear papillary or solid and may extend into ducts outside the obvious lesion; apocrine metaplasia common

Special Stains

- Material within glands typically stains with periodic acid–Schiff (PAS) or mucicarmine

Immunohistochemistry

- Luminal epithelial cells intensely positive for cytokeratin and luminal surface of epithelial cells positive for carcinoembryonic antigen (CEA) and epithelial membrane antigen (EMA)
- Clear myoepithelial cells strongly positive for both actin and S-100, but positivity not as strong as in myoepithelial cells with a spindled morphology
- Normal myoepithelial cells more intensely positive for actin than proliferating myoepithelial cells
- Proliferating myoepithelial cells (particularly the spindled variant) more intensely reactive for S-100 protein than normal myoepithelial cells

Electron Microscopy

- Lesions contain both epithelial and myoepithelial components
- Clear and spindled myoepithelial cells have desmosomes and interdigitating cell processes; cytoplasm contains tonofilaments and pinocytotic vesicles
- Distinct basal lamina surrounds and interdigitates between myoepithelial cells

Molecular Alterations

- None

Differential Diagnosis

- Invasive ductal carcinoma (core biopsy)
- Myoepithelioma
- Malignant myoepithelioma (myoepithelial carcinoma)

Treatment

- Local surgical excision (incomplete excision may result in recurrence)

Prognosis

- A benign lesion not particularly related to the development of carcinoma

Associations

- Sarcoma, carcinoma, and carcinosarcoma may very rarely arise in an adenomyoepithelioma
- Either the epithelial or myoepithelial component may give rise to a carcinoma (typically the background lesion will retain the appearance of a benign adenomyoepithelial neoplasm)
- A sarcoma may arise from the supportive stroma or the myoepithelial cells

Myoepithelioma

Clinical Manifestations

- Very uncommon, especially in men
- May be hard, lobular and painful

Gross Pathology

- Cut surface uniform and predominately solid and gray to pink, occasionally small cystic areas
- Hemorrhage rare (may be present in larger tumors)

Microscopic Pathology

- Composed exclusively of myoepithelial cells (epithelioid and spindle myoepithelial cells)
- Spindle cells interlace and contain epithelioid myoepithelial cells arranged in a storiform pattern and are characterized by clear cytoplasm; fibrofatty tissue and collagen seen in the background
- May be composed entirely of spindled myoepithelial cells (also in a storiform pattern)

Special Stains

- Cells stain intensely with Masson's Trichrome

Immunohistochemistry

- Estrogen receptors and progesterone receptors may both be negative

Electron Microscopy

- Lesions contain both myoid and myoepithelial features
- Clear and spindled myoepithelial cells have desmosomes and interdigitating cell processes; cytoplasm contains tonofilaments and pinocytotic vesicles
- Distinct basal lamina surrounds and interdigitates between myoepithelial cells

Molecular Alterations

- None

Differential Diagnosis

- Spindle cell lesion may resemble fibrous histiocytoma, leiomyosarcoma, and metaplastic carcinoma
- Invasive ductal carcinoma (core biopsy)
- Adenoyoepithelioma
- Malignant myoepithelioma (myoepithelial carcinoma)

Treatment

- Local surgical excision (incomplete excision may result in recurrence)

Prognosis

- A benign lesion not particularly related to the development of carcinoma

Associations

- None

Malignant Myoepithelioma (Myoepithelial Carcinoma)

Clinical Manifestations

- Very uncommon, especially in men
- May be hard, multinodular and painful
- Usually solitary

Gross Pathology

- Usually well defined; may be obviously infiltrative so simply show some marginal irregularity
- Firm and rubbery often with foci of hyalinization
- Central foci of necrosis and/or hemorrhage may be present
- Vary in size from 1.0 to 20 cm

Microscopic Pathology

- Composed almost exclusively of infiltrating spindled myoepithelial cells dispersed in a collagenous stroma
- Spindled cells appear to arise from the myoepithelial cells of ductules usually entrapped at the infiltrating edge of the tumor
- Tumor cells often not particularily atypical
- Mitotic activity present but variable

Special Stains

- Cells stain intensely with Masson's Trichrome

Immunohistochemistry

- Neoplasic spindle cells intensely positive for muscle specific actin
- taining with CAM 5.2 often focal and no where near as intense as the staining seen with MSA
- ER and PR usually negative

Electron Microscopy

- Myoepithelial cells demonstrate both aggregates of myofibrils and dense core bodies

Molecular Alterations

- None

Differential Diagnosis

- Spindle cell carcinoma
- Fibromatosis
- Adenoyoepithelioma
- Myofibroblastic lesions

Treatment

- Complete surgical excision with uninvolved margins (incomplete excision may result in recurrence)
- Axillary nodes may be involved

Prognosis

- Reported survival up to 4 or 5 years

Associations

- None

Diseases of the Nipple

Paget Disease

Clinical Manifestations

- Represents 1% to 5% of all breast carcinomas
- May affect both men and women. No predilection for any age group age range 26 to 88 years
- Almost always unilateral
- Frequency of nipple involvement related to size of underlying carcinoma
- Initially nipple involvement is characterized by simple erythema and mild puritis; with progression nipple develops moist, scaling, eczematoid change that eventually evolves into an ulceration
- A solitary, painless mass is palpable in the underlying breast tissue in approximately 50%

Gross Pathology

- See nipple changes described before
- Underlying invasive adenocarcinoma indistinguishable from invasive carcinoma without associated nipple changes

Microscopic Pathology

- Characterized by presence of large, round to oval cells with abundant, pale, eosinophilic, or amphophilic cytoplasm with prominent round nuclei and distinct nucleoli scattered singly or in clusters in the surface epithelium of the nipple and areola
- An underlying carcinoma is present in 95% of cases; the majority are invasive ductal lesions but in situ carcinoma and invasive lobular, medullary, or papillary carcinomas may occur

Special Stains

- 50% to 60% of Paget cells are mucin- and PAS-positive

Immunohistochemistry

- Paget cells are positive for CEA, most cytokeratins (especially CAM 5.2) and EMA
- Cytokeratin 20 and high-molecular-weight cytokeratins typically negative
- Paget cells typically immunoreactive for GCDFP-15 and estrogen receptors
- Paget cells are negative for HMB-45
- Immunohistochemical profile for Paget cells is typically identical to that of the underlying carcinoma

Electron Microscopy

- Can confirm the presence of melanin pigment in Paget cells

Molecular Alterations

- None

Differential Diagnosis

- Melanoma (Paget cells can phagocytize melanin and mimic melanoma)
- Normal squamous epithelium with clear cells ("Toker's cells")
- Clear cell papulosis

Treatment

- Patients with a palpable underlying mass are generally treated with modified radical mastectomy
- Patients with small or noninvasive carcinomas can be treated with wide local excision of the nipple-areolar complex and underlying cancer (lumpectomy), axillary node dissection, and postoperative radiation therapy

Prognosis

- Axillary lymph node metastasis may be present without an underlying palpable mass
- Prognosis essentially depends on the presence and stage of underlying invasive carcinoma
- 5-year and 10-year survival rates for patients without a palpable mass are approximately 90% and 80%, respectively
- 5-year and 10-year survival rates for women with a palpable mass are approximately 40% and 25%, respectively
- 5-year and 10-year survival rates for patients with positive axillary lymph nodes are approximately 20% to 25% and 10%, respectively

Associations

- Reported in patients with Klinefelter syndrome
- Pemphigus vulgaris may coexist with Paget disease

Male Breast Lesions

Gynecomastia

Clinical Manifestation

- Generally involves both breasts, but usually more pronounced in one than the other
- May be reversible
- Nipple secretion rare
- Usually present as a retroareolar nodule or plaquelike induration
- An aching discomfort may be present
- 3 steroid-dependent age peaks; neonatal, adolescent (2nd to 3rd decade), and male climactic phase (6th to 7th decade)

Gross Pathology

- A non-neoplastic enlargement of the rudimentary duct system in the male breast with proliferalion of both ductal and mesenchymal tissue
- Usually a circumscribed enlargement that is dense and gray-white on cut surface

Microscopic Pathology

- Increased number of ducts lined by epithelial and myoepithelial cells
- Surrounding cellular stroma contains fibroblasts, myofibroblasts, admixed lymphocytes, and plasma cells
- Lobular structures very rare unless patient receiving exogenous estrogen

Special Stains

- Not helpful

Immunohistochemistry

- Elevated amounts of estrogen receptors and progesterone receptors seen in patients with Klinefelter syndrome, but not in others
- Gynecomastia induced by antiandrogen therapy may show strong focal positivity for PSA in both normal and hyperplastic duct epithelium; PSA phosphatase (PSAP) staining will be negative

Electron Microscopy

- Not helpful

Molecular Alterations

- See Klinefelter syndrome later in this book

Differential Diagnosis

- Metastatic carcinoma from prostate (PSAP will be positive)

Treatment

- May, and often does, regress
- Subcutaneous mastectomy (usually for cosnetic reasons)

Prognosis

- May recur
- No convincing evidence that gynecomastia is a precancerous lesion

Associations

- Frequent in Klinefelter syndrome
- Cirrhosis, endocrine tumors, and certain medications

References

Mills S, Carter D, Greenson JK, Oberman HA, Reuter V, Stoler MH (eds). *Sternberg's Diagnostic Surgical Pathology. 4th ed.* Philadelphia: Lippincott Williams & Wilkins, 2004.

Rosai J. *Rosai and Ackerman's Surgical Pathology.* 9th ed. St. Louis: Mosby, 2004.

Rosen PP. *Rosen's Breast Pathology.* 2nd ed. Philadelphia: Lippincott Williams & Wilkins, 2001.

Rosen PP, Oberman HA. *Tumors of the Mammary Gland: Atlas of Tumor Pathology, 3rd series, Fascicle 7.* Washington, DC: Armed Forces Institute of Pathology, 1993.

Tavassoli FA. *Pathology of the Breast. 2nd ed.* Stamford, Conn: Appleton & Lange, 1999.

Tavassoli FA, Devilee P (eds). *World Health Organization Classification of Tumours. Pathology & Genetics of Tumours of the Breast and Female Genital.* Lyon: IARC Press, 2003.

Chapter 5

Female Reproductive Tract

Intraoperative Consultation

The proper performance of an intraoperative consultation on a specimen taken from the female genital tract requires that the pathologist thoroughly understand the surgeon's operative plan. The pathologist should understand both the rationale and the indications for major surgical procedures performed for gynecological malignancy and understand the surgical and pathologic findings that will lead to either the performance of an extensive procedure or the abandonment of such a procedure.

The pathologist must always keep in mind that neoplasms that arise in the female genital tract may occur in any component of the Müllerian system. Pathologic findings of a particular distinctive Müllerian histology could have their origin in the ovary, endometrium, cervix, and fallopian tube, and may appear as synchronous, separate neoplasms. Different organs in the female genital tract may give rise to histologically identical neoplasms. This phenomenon requires that the primary site be known with as much certainty as possible before a diagnosis is rendered that will determine the type of operative procedure to be performed.

Finally it is important to always remember that the female genital tract may be the site of metastasis; this is particularly true of the ovary. Realizing that a given malignancy may represent a metastasis is important because such a diagnosis will usually result in the surgeon abandoning a procedure for a primary gynecologic malignancy in favor of an exploration for a primary neoplasm.

Errors in frozen section diagnosis on tissue specimens obtained from the female genital tract can be minimized if the pathologist adheres to a few simple principles:

1. Surgeon and pathologist both understand exactly what needs to be known for the determination of the appropriate operative procedure.
2. Difficult cases should be diagnosed in 1 of several broad categories: functional, inflammatory, vascular, neoplastic, or metaplastic. Often the operating surgeon only requires a broad classification of the neoplasm. Specific diagnosis is often unnecessary and may carry an unacceptable risk of error. Unequivocal diagnosis in a setting of any unusual process should be avoided.
3. Careful gross examination and appropriate sectioning obviously increases the likelihood that diagnostic material will appear in the frozen section.
4. Cytoscrape preparations may be a helpful adjunct to the frozen section.

The indications for intraoperative consultation vary somewhat depending on the area of the female tract being operated on.

Frozen sections on vulvar lesions are usually obtained to evaluate the adequacy of surgical margins in resected specimens. Intraoperative consultations of vaginal lesions include:

1. Assessment of surgical margins in resections for primary vaginal malignancy.
2. Suspected metastatic or recurrent malignancy arising from the cervix, endometrium, or ovary.
3. Discrete vaginal cysts or mass lesions.
4. Initial diagnosis of embryonal rhabdomyosarcoma in a pediatric patient (the frozen section report need only confirm the presence of a viable lesional tissue).

Most invasive carcinomas of the cervix are staged preoperatively; hence there is little need for an intraoperative evaluation, with the following exceptions:

1. The presence of metastatic disease in the peritoneal cavity, invasion of parametrial soft tissue, or possible nodal metastasis, the presence of which will result in the abandonment of a radical hysterectomy. Significant pathologic pitfalls in this clinical setting include the presence of ectopic decidua in pelvic or paraortic lymph nodes that may mimic squamous cell carcinoma. In addition, the presence of endometriosis or endosalpingiosis in a lymph node (a frequent finding during a frozen section evaluation of a lymph node in a patient with adenocarcinoma of the cervix) may mimic carcinoma.
2. Evaluation of vaginal margins for primary cervical squamous cell carcinoma.

A tissue specimen obtained from the uterus during curettage is submitted for intraoperative consultation in 1 of the following 3 clinical settings:

1. To rule out the presence of intrauterine gestation in cases in which the distinction between an intrauterine pregnancy and an ectopic pregnancy cannot be made on clinical grounds.
2. Curetting sample obtained from a patient with massive uterine bleeding in which intra-operative diagnosis might help in the immediate clinical decision-making process.
3. As a prelude to laparoscopic hysterectomy in which the uterus will be morcellated in the peritoneal cavity

Intraoperative consultation in a patient with endometrial carcinoma may be sought when the features that warrant a full staging procedure are either absent or equivocal. These features include the presence of a high-grade carcinoma, the presence of high-risk special variant carcinoma (eg, serous or clear cell), obvious adnexal involvement, grossly suspicious pelvic or periaortic nodes, and evidence of cervical involvement. Lymph node dissection may be performed if the pathologist can confirm the presence of extensive myometrial invasion, the presence of lower uterine segment involvement, and the presence of lymphatic or vascular space invasion.

Less common indications for a frozen section diagnosis involve operations for uterine mesenchymal neoplasms. Leiomyosarcomas and high-grade stromal sarcomas can be distinguished from their benign counterparts.

Specimen Handling

The surgical margins of all specimens of gynecologic malignancy should be inked and samples carefully taken from areas in which the neoplasm appears closest to the surgical margin. Samples of endometrial neoplasms should be taken from their point of deepest penetration into the myometrium. Sections should be taken from the area of the lower uterine segment closest to the neoplasm. Neoplasms arising in the cervix typically require the submission of the entire cervix and vaginal cuff sectioned vertically and circumferentially with a second set of circumferential, vertical sections taken from the adjacent lower uterine segment.

Cervix

Minimal Deviation Adenocarcinoma (Adenoma Malignum)

Clinical Manifestations

- Extremely well-differentiated adenocarcinoma with cells lining glands that lack cytologic features of malignancy
- Represents approximately 1% to 3% of adenocarcinomas of cervix
- Patients typically present with mucoid or watery vaginal discharge

Gross Pathology

- Cervix may be stenotic without an obvious mucosal abnormality; occasionally lesion either ulcerative or polypoid
- Cervix appears normal in early lesions, but eventually enlarges and assumes a barrel-shape

Microscopic Pathology

- Criteria for diagnosis include:
  - Cytologically bland, architecturally complex glands that vary in size and shape
  - Increased mitotic activity
  - Surface glands appear hyperplastic
  - An increased number of glands positioned deeper than normal in the region of the endocervix (normal glands seldom extend more than 5 mm below the endocervical surface)
  - Glands typically vary in size ranging from small and round to large, irregular, and distorted
  - Complex outlines and some element of desmoplasia usually present
  - Perineural invasion
  - Glands tend to be lined by a single layer of tall, columnar, cytologically bland cells that have basal nuclei that are slightly larger than normal endocervical nuclei; small nucleoli usually present

- Histologic variants
  - *Mucinous*: Most common form; glands lined by a single layer of columnar, mucin-producing cells that resemble the cells of the endocervix; glands often elongated or branching
  - *Endometrioid*: Tumor cells resemble those of proliferative endometrium or endometrial hyperplasia
  - *Clear cell*: Tumor cells with clear cytoplasm
  - *Nonspecific*: Glands tend to be small and uniform with large gaping lumens that often contain homogenous hyaline material

Special Stains

- Not helpful

Immunohistochemistry

- Focal staining with CEA may be present *(a well-differentiated cervical adenocarcinoma is more diffusely positive for CEA and all benign lesions are negative for CEA except microglandular hyperplasia)*

Electron Microscopy

- Not helpful

Molecular Alterations

- None

Differential Diagnosis

- Deeply positioned Nabothian cyst
- Nodular clustering of endocervical glands (tunnel clusters)
- Microglandular hyperplasia
- Mesonephric hyperplasia
- Adenocarcinoma in situ

Treatment

- Hysterectomy
- Intracavitary radiation usually not an option because diagnosis rarely made before hysterectomy

Prognosis

- Advanced disease often present as a result of tumor's tendency not to produce a visibly evident lesion, hence prognosis worse than that of other forms of cervical adenocarcinoma

Associations

- Mucinous form of minimal deviation adenocarcinoma may coexist with an ovarian neoplasm (usually a mucinous tumor and occasionally a sex cord tumor with annular tubules); the cervical tumor may occur before the development of the ovarian tumor or synchronously
- *Peutz-Jeghers syndrome*: Characterized by multiple (almost always <100) hamartomatous polyps scattered throughout the entire gastrointestinal tract (stomach [25%], small intestine [100%], and large intestine [30%]) with melanotic mucosal and cutaneous pigmentation of the lips, oral mucosa, face, genitalia, digits, palms, and soles; also associated with an increased incidence of other malignant neoplasms, including well-differentiated adenocarcinoma of the uterine cervix (adenoma malignum), carcinoma of stomach, small intestine, and colon, a distinctive ovarian neoplasm (sex-cord tumor with annular tubules), ovarian mucinous tumors, ovarian tumors of Wolffian origin (FATWO) breast carcinoma (often bilateral), and feminizing Sertoli tumors of the testis

Adenocarcinoma In Situ

Clinical Manifestations

- Glands or epithelium of endocervix replaced by cytologically malignant epithelial cells
- Represents 10% to 25% of all adenocarcinomas of the cervix
- Most patients asymptomatic
- Vaginal bleeding most common symptom (60%)
- Age at presentation usually between 35 and 40 years

Gross Pathology

- No obvious distinctive gross appearance
- Lesion usually lies anywhere in the transformation zone
- Usually multifocal; "skip lesions" as opposed to contiguous squamous lesions

Microscopic Pathology

- Involves surface endocervical glandular epithelium in the transitional zone
- Neoplasm extends along surface of endocervix and does not infiltrate underlying stroma, hence no desmoplasia
- Involved glands do not extend below the level of normal glands
- *Endocervical (mucinous) variant* (most common) characterized by cells that resemble those of the endocervix with basal nuclei and pale granular cytoplasm that contains mucin; tumor cells have markedly enlarged, crowded nuclei that are hyperchromatic and have coarse chromatin; prominent mitotic activity, and apoptotic cells both typical
- *Intestinal variant* characterized by presence of goblet cells with or without argyrophilic cells
- *Endometrioid variant* lacks both the goblet cells of intestinal variant and the clear light staining cytoplasm of endocervical variant; typically cells have scant cytoplasm and marked nuclear stratification (resemble malignant endometrial glands)
- *Adenosquamous*

Special Stains, Immunohistochemistry, and Electron Microscopy

- Occasionally tumor cells are positive for CEA, but not often enough to make this immunostain of diagnostic value

Molecular Alterations

- None

Differential Diagnosis

- Atypical hyperplasia
- Invasive adenocarcinoma
- Arias-Stella reaction
- Glandular atypia secondary to inflammation or radiation
- Microglandular hyperplasia
- Endometriosis
- Tubal metaplasia
- Mesonephric remnants

Treatment

- Hysterectomy (cone biopsy, even with clear margins, associated with recurrent adenocarcinoma in situ or invasive adenocarcinoma)

Prognosis

- Recurrence more likely after conization than hysterectomy
- A precursor to most forms of cervical adenocarcinoma

Associations

- CIN or invasive squamous cell carcinoma coexists with adenocarcinoma in situ in almost 65% of cases
- CIN I present in squamous epithelium adjacent to areas of adenocarcinoma in situ in 25%
- Approximately 90% contain HPV messenger RNA, usually types 16 and 18

Adenocarcinoma

Clinical Manifestations

- Accounts for 15% to 25% of primary invasive carcinomas of the cervix
- Women either asymptomatic or present with a watery or bloody vaginal discharge
- Typically diagnosed between the ages of 45 and 55 years
- At the time of diagnosis, 85% have disease limited to cervix (stage I) or extending into parametrium or upper vagina (stage II)

Gross Pathology

- 50% exophytic, polypoid, or papillary; 35% nodular, with diffuse enlargement or ulceration of the cervix; 15% have no visible lesion (carcinoma small or located high in endocervical canal)

Microscopic Pathology

- A variety of histologic patterns, several of which may be present in any given lesion
- *Mucinous adenocarcinoma*
  - Most common

- Three forms:
  - Cells resemble normal endocervix with pale granular cytoplasm and basal nuclei (*endocervical type*); may be entirely papillary or partly papillary
  - Cells resemble intestinal cells and line papillae or infiltrate in a manner similar to that of adenocarcinoma of the colon *(intestinal type*); epithelium tends to be pseudostratified and contains only small amounts of mucin, but may include goblet cells, Paneth cells, and/or argentaffin cells
  - *Signet-ring cell carcinoma*: usually a minor component mixed with endocervical or intestinal types

- *Endometrioid adenocarcinoma*
  - Usually resembles a typical adenocarcinoma in the endometrium and may even have areas of squamous differentiation and lack intracytoplasmic mucin (may be difficult to distinguish from endocervical type)
- *Adenosquamous carcinoma*
  - An adenocarcinoma with malignant squamous differentiation
  - Intracellular mucin almost always present
- *Glassy cell carcinoma* considered a variant of adenosquamous carcinoma; characterized by solid growth of large eosinophilic (glassy) cells with large nuclei with large eosinophilic nucleoli; stroma contains inflammatory cells with numerous eosinophils
- *Mucoepidermoid carcinoma*
  - A squamous cell carcinoma that contains mucin
- Microscopic grading
  - Well-differentiated: 90% or more of the lesion consists of glands or tubules (<10% does not make glands or tubules)
  - Moderately differentiated: 10% to 50% of the tumor does not make glands or tubules
  - Poorly differentiated: More than 50% of the tumor does not make glands or tubules
- Nuclear grading
  - Grade I: Cells with oval nuclei and finely dispersed chromatin
  - Grade II: Cells intermediate between grades I and III
  - Grade III: Cells with markedly enlarged nuclei with irregular, coarse chromatin and prominent nucleoli

Special Stains

- Mucicarmine will highlight the presence of mucin

Immunohistochemistry

- 75% of lesions contain carcinoembryonic antigen (CEA)-positive areas (CEA negative in normal endocervical mucosa and in most benign lesions of the cervix with the exception of microglandular hyperplasia which is always CEA-positive)
- CEA not specific enough to distinguish endometrial carcinoma from endocervical carcinoma
- HPV-18 predominant subtype

Electron Microscopy

- Not helpful

Molecular Alterations

- None

Differential Diagnosis

- Microglandular hyperplasia
- Hyperplasia of mesonephric remnants
- Adenocarcinoma in situ
- Metastatic adenocarcinoma
- Extension of endometrial adenocarcinoma

Treatment

- Small or early stage cancers treated with either radiation or hysterectomy
- Larger lesions generally best treated with hysterectomy

Prognosis

- Factors associated with a worse prognosis include:
  - Stage
  - Size
  - Histologic grade
  - Depth of invasion
  - Presence or absence of lymph node metastasis
  - High ploidy or aneuploid tumors
- Tumors associated with a better prognosis include:
  - High estrogen and progesterone receptor levels
  - Diagnosis before menopause
- 20% of patients with adenocarcinoma confined to cervix at surgery (stage I) will have lymph node metastasis
- Glassy cell variant of adenosquamous has a worse prognosis than standard adenosquamous

Associations

- Prior use of oral contraceptives, particularly those with a strong progestational component
- Obesity, hypertension, and nulligravidity (not as strong an association as with endometrial carcinoma)
- 60% associated with cervical intraepithelial neoplasia (CIN) or invasive squamous cell carcinoma
- 90% contain human papillomavirus (HPV) nucleic acid sequences (same proportion as seen in squamous cell carcinoma)
- Mucinous tumors of the ovaries

Squamous Cell Carcinoma

Clinical Manifestations

- Most common cancer (except skin cancer) in women worldwide
- Usually affects women between the ages of 45 and 55 years
- Most present with intermittent painless vaginal bleeding; may occur for the first time after sexual intercourse
- Occasionally patients complain of pain in the flank or the leg as a result of a tumor invasion into the pelvic wall or sciatic nerves
- Advanced disease with involvement of the bladder or rectum may be associated with dysuria, hematuria, rectal bleeding, or obstipation
- Lymphatic involvement may be manifested by either unilateral or bilateral lower extremity edema
- Tumor markers (carcinoembryonic antigen, cancer antigen 125, and subfraction of the TA-4 antigen) often elevated
- Squamous cell carcinoma antigen elevated in approximately 60% (rarely elevated in cases of adenocarcinoma)

Gross Pathology

- Neoplasm may involve either ectocervix or endocervix
- Infiltrative lesions may invade extensively throughout the cervical stroma, resulting in a very hard lesion with little obvious surface change
- Ulcerative lesions erode the cervix and appear as an obvious ulcer that may involve the cervix as well as the upper vaginal vault

Microscopic Pathology

- Microinvasive lesion characterized by irregular tongues of epithelium extending from the base of a high-grade squamous epithelial lesion (CIN III) for a distance of <3 mm
- Invasive lesions associated with a wide range in morphology:
  - Most composed of compact masses and nests of neoplastic squamous epithelium that show central keratinization or necrosis
  - Invasion may be present as cords and individual cells, which demonstrate a wide variation in size, shape, and amount of keratinization
- Typically tumor cells oval to polygonal with eosinophilic cytoplasm and sharp cell borders; intercellular bridges rarely apparent; nuclei may be uniform or pleomorphic, but usually have coarse chromatin
- Mitotic activity typically marked

- Subtypes
  - *Nonkeratinizing carcinoma*: Characterized by rounded nests of tumor cells that lack keratin pearls, but may have individual cell keratinization; cells tend to be uniform with indistinct cell borders and round or oval nuclei with coarse chromatin
  - *Keratinizing carcinoma*: Characterized by nests and cords of mature squamous cells and *keratin pearls* (a rounded nest of squamous epithelium in which the cells are arranged concentrically around a central focus of acellular keratin); cells tend to be large and eosinophilic with either large or pyknotic nuclei and prominent intercellular bridges
  - *Basaloid carcinoma*: Composed of small, oval-shaped, basaloid cells with scant cytoplasm that grow in nests and masses; nuclei tend to be hyperchromatic and mitotically active; necrosis frequent; must not be confused with *small cell neuroendocrine* (oat cell) carcinoma and *small cell, non-neuroendocrine* carcinoma
- Microscopic grading:
  - *Well-differentiated (grade I)*: Mature squamous cells, with abundant keratin pearl formation and few mitotic figures; nuclei tend to be uniform and cells have well-developed intercellular bridges
  - *Moderately differentiated (grade II)*: Cells with less cytoplasm and more indistinct cell borders; nuclei pleomorphic and mitotic activity increased over that seen in a well-differentiated tumor
  - *Poorly differentiated (grade III)*: Masses and nests of small, primitive oval cells with scant cytoplasm and hyperchromatic spindle-shaped nuclei with very high mitotic rates; little or no keratinization (neoplastic cells tend to resemble those seen in high-grade CIN)

Special Stains

- Not helpful

Immunohistochemistry

- Tumor cells immunoreactive for cytokeratin and involucrin
- *ras* oncogene product p21 localized at the cell membrane
- p16 useful to detect presence of HPV

Electron Microscopy

- Moderately and well-differentiated tumors do not have as well-developed intracytoplasmic tonofilaments, desmosomal-tonofilament complexes, and intracellular microvilli as well-differentiated lesions

Molecular Alterations

- Most are aneuploid; 20% to 40% diploid

Differential Diagnosis

- Squamous metaplasia (especially immature)
- Marked decidual reaction
- Placental-site nodules or plaques
- Clear cell adenocarcinoma (particularly when squamous cells contain glycogen)
- Small cell (undifferentiated) carcinoma of neuroendocrine type (especially important in the differential diagnosis of poorly differentiated or basaloid squamous cell carcinoma)

Treatment

- Stage I through stage IIA lesions treated with radical surgery or radiation
- Advanced disease (IIB tumor or greater) treated primarily with radiotherapy
- Radical hysterectomy performed for patients with stage IB or IIA disease (assuming the surgical margins will not be involved) and consists of wide excision of parametrial and paravaginal tissue with partial mobilization of bladder from the cervix and extensive dissection of the ureters with upper vaginectomy and pelvic lymphadenectomy

Prognosis

- Prognostic factors of significance include:
  - Depth of invasion
  - Presence or absence of vascular invasion
  - Greatest dimension of tumor

- Histologic grading and classification (keratinizing versus nonkeratinizing) not of prognostic significance
- 5-year survival rate for patients with tumors <2 cm is 90%; 5-year survival rate for patients with tumors ≥2 cm 65%
- Presence of positive lymph nodes has a profound effect on prognosis (negative nodes associated with 95% 5-year survival; ≥2 positive nodes associated with a 17% 5-year survival)
- Recurrence occurs in 10% to 20% of patients treated with radical hysterectomy (radiation has little role in treatment of recurrent disease)

Associations

- Risk increases with the number of sexual partners, the age at which sexual intercourse first occurs, and the promiscuity of the male partner
- Smoking a risk factor especially among women who have smoked continuously to the time of diagnosis
- HPV-16 and -18 found in 90% of patients with invasive squamous cell carcinoma; HPV-31, -33, -35, -51, -52, and -58 also associated with squamous cell carcinoma; (HPV-16, -18, -31, and -45 associated with 80% of all cervical carcinomas)
- Keratinizing squamous cell carcinoma strongly associated with HPV-16 (same association does not exist for nonkeratinizing squamous cell carcinoma)
- HPV-18 associated with both adenocarcinoma and poorly differentiated carcinoma and more frequent lymph node involvement than HPV-16

Trophoblastic Disease

Placental Site Trophoblastic Tumor

Clinical Manifestations

- A cellular mass in endometrium and myometrium that resembles the nonneoplastic trophoblastic infiltration of an implantation site
- Rarest form of gestational trophoblastic disease
- Typically occurs during reproductive years
- Most patients parous; a few have a history of a prior hydatidiform mole
- Antecedent pregnancy may be remote from presentation
- Serum hCG levels typically low
- Typically present with either amenorrhea or abnormal bleeding
- Uterus usually enlarged and frequently patient believes she is pregnant
- Perforation of the uterus may occur during curettage because of the tendency of these tumors to penetrate deeply into the myometrium

Gross Pathology

- Size varies from microscopic to large enough to distort the uterine fundus
- Tumor typically well-defined but may be poorly demarcated
- May project into uterine cavity or be confined to myometrium
- Tends to be soft and tan with areas of hemorrhage or necrosis
- May invade through uterine wall and extend onto serosal surface

Microscopic Findings

- Predominant tumor cell the intermediate trophoblast; cytotrophoblastic and syncytiotrophoblastic cells are minor components
- Typically large, polygonal, intermediate trophoblasts infiltrate myometrium and insinuate themselves between smooth muscle fibers at the interface between the tumor and myometrium; they also invade the walls of blood vessels from the outside and eventually replace the entire vessel wall; *fibrinoid material is deposited in the destroyed vessel wall*
- Tumor cells may be found singly or in large nests and may be spindle-shaped
- Various amounts of tissue destruction may be present
- Extensive deposits of fibrinoid material almost always present
- Chorionic villi always absent
- Decidua may be present in uninvolved endometrium
- Malignant features include: tumor cells with clear rather than amphophilic cytoplasm aggregating in large masses and sheets, extensive necrosis, and a high mitotic rate (≥5 mitotic figures per 10 high power fields). (Note: atypical mitotic figures can be seen in either benign or malignant tumors.)

Special Stains

- Not helpful

Immunohistochemistry

- Typically intermediate trophoblastic cells of a placental site trophoblastic tumor positive for hPL; very few positive for hCG
- Syncytiotrophoblastic giant cells almost always positive for hCG and occasionally positive for hPL
- All 3 trophoblastic cell types positive for cytokeratin
- Typically p63 negative

Electron Microscopy

- Confirms the presence of a predominant cellular population of intermediate trophoblastic cells
- Cells are mononucleate with complex cytoplasm that contains free ribosomes, partially dilated rough endoplasmic reticulum and glycogen
- Cell junctions and microvilli are present
- Bundles of intermediate filaments are found in a perinuclear location (a distinctive feature of the intermediate trophoblast)

Molecular Alterations

- None

Differential Diagnosis

- Choriocarcinoma
- Exaggerated implantation site
- Placental site nodule
- Epithelioid trophoblastic tumor (chorionic trophoblast) p63 positive
- Nontrophoblastic cancer:
    - Epithelioid leiomyosarcoma
    - Clear cell adenocarcinoma with minimal or no glandular differentiation
    - Extensively hyalinized squamous cell carcinoma of the cervix

Treatment

- Hysterectomy
- Malignant tumors do not respond to the multiagent chemotherapy used to treat choriocarcinoma

Prognosis

- Most benign
- 10% to 15% behave in a malignant fashion with rapid development of metastatic disease

Associations

- Reports of associated virilization
- May be associated with a unique form of renal disease characterized by the nephrotic syndrome
- Occasionally a focus of choriocarcinoma present within a placental site trophoblastic tumor

Partial Hydatidiform Mole

Clinical Manifestations

- Accounts for 25% to 45% of all molar pregnancies
- Typically occur between the 9th and the 34th week of pregnancy; average gestational age approximately 19 weeks
- Usually presents as abnormal uterine bleeding in women who are diagnosed as having a spontaneous or missed abortion
- Uterus usually of normal size or even small for the calculated gestational age
- Serum hCG levels are elevated, but the elevation is not as high as is typically seen with a complete mole

Gross Pathology

- Specimen typically consists of large hydropic villi admixed with more typical looking nonmolar placental tissue
- Fetus is almost always present (fetal death usually occurs at 8 to 9 weeks)

Microscopic Pathology

- A mixture of large edematous villi and normal-sized villi
- Degree of hydropic swelling less than that seen with complete moles
- Some hydropic villi contain a central, acellular cistern, but cisterns less prominent than in complete moles

- Chorionic villi frequently have a scalloped outline compared with the typically round and distended appearance of villi of a complete mole; this irregular outline of a partial mole results from infoldings of trophoblast into the villous stroma (often appear as inclusions)
- Villous stroma is often fibrotic and contains capillaries with fetal (nucleated) red blood cells
- Trophoblast that covers individual villi usually only minimally and focally hyperplastic; the overgrowth of trophoblast is circumferential rather than polar (as in complete mole)
- Cellular components of the trophoblast consist of cytotrophoblast and syncytiotrophoblast; intermediate trophoblastic cells rarely present
- Syncytiotrophoblastic cells usually from focal aggregates on the villous surface
- Fetal parts or amnion often present

Special Stains and Electron Microscopy

- Not helpful

Immunohistochemistry

- Partial moles show widespread and diffuse positive staining for hPL and PLAP and focal to moderate staining for hCG. Complete moles have widespread diffuse staining for hCG, moderately diffuse staining for hPL, and focal staining for PLAP)

Molecular Alterations

- Typically karyotypes show triploidy (69 chromosomes) with 2 paternal sets and 1 maternal chromosome complement
- When triploidy is present:
  - 70% have a complement that is XXY
  - 27% have a complement that is XXX
  - 3% have a complement that is XYY
- Egg is fertilized with a haploid set of chromosomes by either 2 sperms (each with a haploid set of chromosomes) or by a single sperm with a dipliod 46,XY complement
- 15% to 20% of triploid fetuses have a diploid 46,XX maternal genome and a haploid paternal set of chromosomes (digynic conceptus)

Differential Diagnosis

- Complete hydatidiform mole
- Invasive mole
- Nonmolar pregnancy, especially one with hydropic change (the trophoblastic proliferation seen in a nonmolar abortus is typically polar and characterized by growth arising from 1 pole of the villus; trophoblastic proliferation in a mole is more haphazard and circumferential; nonmolar pregnancies are not characterized by the formation of cisterns or the presence of atypia in the trophoblastic proliferation)

Treatment

- Evacuation with careful clinical follow-up of the serum hCG titers until they return to normal

Prognosis

- Gestational trophoblastic disease persists in 5% to 10% after evacuation (compared with 10% to 30% in complete moles)
- Development of a choriocarcinoma is extremely rare (occurs in 2% to 3% of complete moles)

Associations

- The higher the ratio of paternal to maternal chromosomes, the greater the molar change
- Complete moles typically have a 2:0 ratio of paternal to maternal chromosomes; partial moles typically have a 2:1 ratio

Complete Hydatidiform Mole

Clinical Manifestations

- Typically presents between the 11th and 25th week of pregnancy; average gestational age 16 weeks
- Characterized by uterine enlargement
- Often associated with severe vomiting (hyperemesis gravidarum), pregnancy-induced hypertension (usually doe not occur until the 3rd trimester in nonmolar pregnancies) and occasionally hyperthyroidism

Trophoblastic Disease>Complete Hydatidiform Mole

- Patients usually present with vaginal bleeding or passage of molar vesicles
- Occasionally ovarian enlargement secondary to multiple theca-lutein cysts (*hyperreactio luteinalis*) and pulmonary embolization may occur
- hCG level typically markedly elevated
- Pelvic ultrasound reveals a "snowstorm" appearance to the uterus

Gross Pathology

- Usually consists of 30 to 500 cm^2 of bloody tissue with grapelike, transparent vesicles 1 to 2 cm in diameter
- Suction curettage may make the gross diagnosis difficult because the procedure itself may disrupt most of the vesicles
- Floating a portion in water will reconstitute the vesicles

Microscopic Pathology

- Generalized hydropic villous change; almost all of the villi are edematous, but some may be small (average size 0.4 cm)
- Many have cisterns consisting of a central, acellular, fluid-filled space without mesenchymal cells
- A small rim of mesenchyme usually separates the cistern from the inner border of the surrounding trophoblast; the border of mesenchyme with acellular cistern is usually quite well-defined
- Villous stroma lacks both fibrosis and capillaries with fetal (nucleated) red blood cells
- Occasionally, focal areas of necrosis and calcification of villous stroma may be present
- Villous surface has some degree of circumferential, haphazard trophoblastic proliferation; the trophoblastic proliferation may affect almost all the villi in the specimen or may be minimal and focal
- Proliferating trophoblast is composed of all 3 cell types (syncytiotrophoblast, cytotrophoblast, and intermediate trophoblast)
- In addition to the trophoblast being hyperplastic there may be considerable atypia with nuclear enlargement, irregularity of the nuclear outline, and hyperchromasia; mitotic figures to include abnormal mitotic figures may be present
- Characteristically there is no evidence of the development of an embryo/fetus (no fetal parts or amnion present); villous stroma lacks the blood vessels that are a normal feature of embryogenesis

Special Stains and Electron Microscopy

- Not helpful

Immunohistochemistry

- Generally complete moles have widespread diffuse staining for hCG, moderately diffuse staining for hPL, and focal staining for placental alkaline phosphatase (PLAP)
- Syncytiotrophoblastic cells are positive for hCG, hPL, and PLAP
- Cytotrophoblastic cells are almost always negative for all 3 of these proteins
- Intermediate trophoblastic cells usually positive for hPL and negative for hCG

Molecular Alterations

- Most are diploid with a 46, XX karyotype; rarely triploid or tetraploid
- All chromosome complements are paternally derived
- Both X chromosomes result from duplication of a haploid sperm pronucleus in an empty ovum (an ovum that has lost its maternal chromosomal haploid set)
- Duplication of a 23,Y sperm results in a nonviable 46,YY cell
- 5% to 15% have a 46,XY chromosome complement, probably the result of an empty ovum being fertilized by 2 sperm pronuclei, 1 with an X and 1 with a Y chromosome

Differential Diagnosis

- Partial hydatidiform mole
- Invasive hydatidiform mole
- Early nonmolar pregnancy (swollen villi typically surrounded by attenuated trophoblast; when trophoblast proliferation is seen in an abortus it is typically polar and is characterized by a columnlike growth arising from only 1 pole of the chorionic villus)

Treatment

- Complete evacuation with careful monitoring of hCG titers to confirm their return to normal

Prognosis

- Persistent elevation of hCG titers after evacuation of complete moles indicates the presence of persistent gestational trophoblastic disease (gestational trophoblastic neoplasia) in 10% to 30%)
- 2% to 3% will develop choriocarcinoma

Associations

- The higher ratio of paternal to maternal chromosomes, the greater the molar change; complete moles typically have a 2:0 ratio of paternal to maternal chromosomes; partial moles typically have a 2:1 ratio

Invasive Hydatidiform Mole (Chorioadenoma Destruens)

Clinical Manifestations

- Hydropic chorionic villi found in myometrium or its vascular spaces or at distant sites (particularly vagina or lung)
- Usually arises in the setting of either a partial or complete mole
- Roughly 15% of hydatidiform moles evolve into invasive moles
- Extrauterine disease usually involves vagina, vulva, or lungs

Gross Pathology

- An irregular hemorrhagic lesion that invades myometrium; invasion may extend through the myometrium, perforate the serosa, extend into the adjacent broad ligament, and involve the adnexa

Microscopic Pathology

- Villi are typically enlarged but not as large as seen in the typical complete mole
- Amount of trophoblastic proliferation may be quite variable; at times it can be so pronounced that the underlying molar villus is obscured, leading to a misdiagnosis of choriocarcinoma
- Extrauterine disease characterized by the presence of molar villi in blood vessels without invasion of adjacent tissue (a phenomenon referred to as *deportation* rather than *metastasis*); occasionally no villi, just intermediate type trophoblastic cells

Special Stains

- Not helpful

Immunohistochemistry

- Staining pattern similar to that of complete moles (most are derived from complete moles):
  - ☐ Widespread diffuse staining for hCG, moderate diffuse staining for hPL, and focal staining for PLAP
  - ☐ Syncytiotrophoblastic cells typically positive for hCG, hPL, and PLAP
  - ☐ Intermediate trophoblastic cells usually positive for hPL and negative for hCG
  - ☐ Cytotrophoblastic cells almost always negative for hCG, hPL, and PLAP

Electron Microscopy

- Not helpful

Molecular Alterations

- Consistent with the type of mole from which the neoplasm arises (most are preceded by a complete mole)

Differential Diagnosis

- Noninvasive hydatidiform moles
- Choriocarcinoma
- Placenta increta or percreta

Treatment

- Chemotherapy

Prognosis

- Risk of the development of choriocarcinoma no greater than in noninvasive moles
- May regress spontaneously
- Pulmonary lesions (deportation) frequently regress after hysterectomy

Associations

- Complete mole

Choriocarcinoma (Gestational)

Clinical Manifestations

- May be associated with any form of gestation, but abnormal types of pregnancy more likely to be associated with choriocarcinoma (spontaneous abortion, ectopic pregnancy, and molar pregnancy)
- Abnormal uterine bleeding during the postpartum period a frequent presenting symptom; lesions confined to the myometrium may be asymptomatic
- Occasionally metastatic disease can be found without any detectable uterine tumor (presumed regression in the uterus after metastasis has occurred)
- Patients with metastatic disease may present with hemoptysis or hemorrhagic events in the central nervous system, liver, gastrointestinal tract, or urinary tract
- Symptoms of thyroxicosis may be present secondary to the thyrotrophic activity of human chorionic gonatropin (hCG)

Gross Pathology

- Usually a circumscribed, hemorrhagic mass
- Central portion usually hemorrhagic and necrotic with a thin rim of viable tumor at the periphery

Microscopic Pathology

- Typically a biphasic pattern of cytotrophoblast and syncytiotrophoblast or intermediate trophoblast and syncytiotrophoblast (syncytiotrophoblast always present; cytotrophoblast or intermediate trophoblast variably present)
- Nuclear pleomorphism, hyperchromasia, and prominent nucleoli prominent features of all cell types
- Extensive necrosis almost always present
- Vascular invasion usually prominent
- Chorionic villi never seen; their presence should rule out diagnosis of choriocarcinoma
- *Cytotrophoblastic cells*
    - □ Usually mononucleate small cells with scant pale cytoplasm that tend to be either granular or clear; mitotically active
    - □ Cell borders usually prominent
- *Syncytiotrophoblastic cells*
    - □ Multinucleate cells *without* mitotic activity (3 to 20 nuclei per cell)
    - □ Cytoplasm dense and stains deeply eosinophilic to basophilic
    - □ Cytoplasm may contain vacuoles and lacunae some of which contain red blood cells
- *Intermediate trophoblastic cells*
    - □ Share features of both cytotrophoblastic and syncytiotrophoblastic cells
    - □ Typically large and polyhedral with 1 nucleus and abundant eosinophilic to amphophilic cytoplasm without vacuoles
    - □ Cell membranes less distinct than cytotrophoblastic cell membranes

Special Stains

- None

Immunohistochemistry

- Syncytiotrophoblastic cells and intermediate trophoblastic cells typically stain intensely for β-hCG and are variably positive for human placental lactogen (hPL; a feature unique to a choriocarcinoma; rarely if ever occurs in other tumors)
- All 3 trophoblastic cell types are reactive for cytokeratin (both high and low molecular weight)

Electron Microscopy

- Cytotrophoblastic cells contain a single variably shaped nucleus and cytoplasm with few organelles; cells usually connected to each other by desmosomes with tonofilaments

- Syncytiotrophoblastic cells have irregular nuclei with dense heterochromatin; cytoplasm contains mitochondria, dilated smooth and rough endoplasmic reticulum, free ribosomes, vesicles, glycogen, and tonofilaments; thin microvilli cover plasma membrane
- Intermediate trophoblastic cells have a single nucleus and cytoplasm with dilated rough endoplasmic reticulum and few bundles of tonofilaments

Molecular Alterations

- Only of significance in tumors arising from molar pregnancies

Differential Diagnosis

- If cytotrophoblastic or intermediate trophoblastic cells predominate:
  - Poorly differentiated carcinoma
- If syncytiotrophoblastic cells are spindle-shaped:
  - Sarcoma
- Normal trophoblast of early gestation or hydatidiform mole
- Placental site trophoblastic tumor
- At metastatic sites:
  - Deported invasive mole (trophoblastic deportation syndrome)
  - Carcinoma with areas of choriocarcinomatous differentiation (seen in carcinomas of the gastrointestinal tract, urinary bladder, breast, liver, lung, and uterus)
  - Poorly differentiated carcinoma with tumor giant cells

Treatment

- Cytotoxic chemotherapy followed by hysterectomy

Prognosis

- Overall survival for all cases of persistent and metastatic gestational disease exceeds 90%
- Death from a choriocarcinoma usually results from a hemorrhagic event at a metastatic site or as a result of complications from irradiation and/or chemotherapy
- Lung metastases present in 90% of patients with extrauterine spread of disease
- 20% to 60% of patients have brain and liver metastasis
- 15% to 30% have vaginal involvement

Association

- 50% preceded by a hydatidiform mole (only 2.5% of hydatidiform moles are followed by choriocarcinoma)
- 25% follow an abortion
- 22% follow a normal pregnancy
- 2.5% follow an ectopic pregnancy
- Blood group A is more frequent; blood group O is less frequent

Uterus

Benign Lesions

Adenofibroma

Clinical Manifestations

- May be seen at any age but most frequently encountered in postmenopausal women
- Typically arise from the endometrium (10% originate in endocervix)

Gross Pathology

- Typically a broad-based polypoid mass with a villous surface
- On cut section, a spongy consistency with cystic spaces surrounded by white to tan, firm tissue

Microscopic Pathology

- Surface typically characterized by broad, club-shaped papillae of stroma covered by epithelium
- Epithelium may be mucinous, serous, endometrial (proliferative or secretory), flat, or cuboidal; various metaplastic changes may be present

- Stroma consists of bland cells that resemble fibroblasts, benign endometrial stromal cells, or a combination of both; usually hypocellular, mitotically inactive, and hyalinized
- Foci of smooth muscle may be present
- Cellularity of the stroma may vary from section to section
- Stromal cells do not condense around glandular structures (no cambium layer)
- Cystic spaces usually prominent

Special Stains, Immunohistochemistry, and Electron Microscopy

- Not helpful

Molecular Alterations

- None

Differential Diagnosis

- Endometrial polyp (papillary architecture of an adenofibroma and the regularity of the relationship between the epithelial and stromal components should make distinction from an endometrial polyp fairly straightforward)
- Adenosarcoma (stroma more cellular, atypical, mitotically active, and forms a cambium layer)

Treatment

- Hysterectomy

Prognosis

- Reports of myometrial invasion; no reports of metastasis

Associations

- Best considered as a mixed epithelial-nonepithelial tumor along with adenomyoma, adenosarcoma, and carcinosarcoma)

Adenomatoid Tumor

Clinical Manifestations

- An incidental finding in 1% of hysterectomy specimens
- Usually seen in women of reproductive age
- Almost always asymptomatic

Gross Pathology

- Typically resemble small leiomyomas but with a softer consistency, a yellow color, and ill-defined margins
- Usually found in the myometrium near the serosal surface (originate from serosa mesothelium) in the area of the cornua
- Extend toward the endometrium as they enlarge

Microscopic Pathology

- Typically an infiltrating adenoid or tubular lesion in the myometrium
- Infiltrative component may be quite small and focal or very extensive
- Lesion consists of anastomosing tubules or glandlike spaces of varying size and shape that are lined by cells that are flattened to cuboidal and lack nuclear atypia; mitotic figures rare
- Solid and cystic growth patterns also occur but much less frequently
- An angiomatoid configuration frequently present (may lead to a misdiagnosis of lymphangioma)

Special Stains

- Alcian-blue PAS with diastase will confirm presence of acid mucin

Immunohistochemistry

- Tumor cells are strongly reactive for keratin, epithelial membrane antigen (EMA), and calretinin and are negative for CEA and factor VIII-related antigen

Electron Microscopy

- Tumor cells have long slender microvilli, intracellular lumina, and bundles of intracytoplasmic filaments (all characteristic of mesothelial cells)

Molecular Alterations

- None

Differential Diagnosis

- Lymphangioma
- Adenocarcinoma (arising from the endometrium or metastatic to the uterus)
- Epithelioid leiomyoma

Treatment

- No specific treatment; almost always an incidental finding in hysterectomy specimen

Prognosis

- A benign neoplasm that behaves in a benign fashion despite its infiltrative characteristics

Associations

- None

Adenomyoma and Atypical Polypoid Adenomyoma

Clinical Manifestations

- An endometrial polypoid lesion with a stromal component that is largely or exclusively composed of smooth muscle
- Usually occurs in premenopausal women who present with abnormal uterine bleeding
- Typically a polypoid mass that often arises in the lower uterine segment or endocervix

Gross Pathology

- Typically pedunculated or sessile and sharply circumscribed from underlying myometrium or cervical wall

Microscopic Pathology

- *Adenomyoma* characterized by an admixture of benign endometrial glands without cytologic atypia or architectural complexity and a stroma that consists predominantly of benign-appearing smooth muscle and fibrous tissue
- Glands in an *atypical polypoid adenomyoma* exhibit architectural atypia and slight cytologic atypia similar to that seen in atypical hyperplasia of the endometrium
  - Stromal component consists of interlacing or whorling fascicles of smooth muscle that are cytologically benign (mitotic figures are occasionally seen in the stromal component)
  - Squamous or morular metaplasia is almost always found and may be extensive; areas of necrosis may be found in the areas of squamous or morular metaplasia but the cytology of the squamous component is always benign

Special Stains

- Not helpful

Immunohistochemistry

- Immunohistochemical stains for smooth muscle actin and desmin confirm the presence of smooth muscle in the stroma

Electron Microscopy

- Not helpful

Molecular Alterations

- None

Differential Diagnosis

- Invasive endometrial carcinoma
- Adenofibroma
- Adenosarcoma
- Carcinosarcoma

Treatment

- Typically cured with curettage

Prognosis

- Recurrence common if lesion incompletely excised
- Adenomyoma is a noninvasive, nonmetastasizing lesion not associated with malignant behavior

- Adenocarcinoma may arise in an atypical polypoid adenomyoma

Associations

- Seen in patients with Turner syndrome (especially in the setting of long-term estrogen therapy)
- Best considered as a mixed epithelial-nonepithelial tumor along with adenofibroma, adenosarcoma, and carcinosarcoma)

Adenomyosis ("Endometriosis Interna")

Clinical Manifestations

- Seen in 10% to 20% of hysterectomy specimens in the United States
- Typically seen in women during reproductive years
- Most common symptoms include abnormal menstrual bleeding, dysmenorrhea, and infertility
- May be completely asymptomatic

Gross Pathology

- Diffuse involvement produces a uterus that is symmetrically enlarged and soft with a globoid shape
- Focal involvement may mimic a leiomyoma
- Myometrium generally thickened and may have a bulging and trabeculated cut surface; condition may be visible as small soft gray or pink zones within the myometrium; small cysts occasionally visible

Microscopic Pathology

- Small or large islands of endometrial glands and stroma (basalis-type) in the myometrium and surrounded by hypertrophied bands of smooth muscle
- During pregnancy, decidual change may be present
- Foci of hemorrhage or hemosiderin pigment rarely present
- Generally accepted criterion for diagnosis requires presence of endometrial glands at least 0.2 cm (on half of a 40× field) below the endometrial-myometrial junction

Special Stains

- Not helpful

Immunohistochemistry

- Endometrial glands always positive for estrogen receptors and usually negative for progesterone receptors

Electron Microscopy

- Not helpful

Molecular Alterations

- None

Differential Diagnosis

- Normal uterus
- Low-grade endometrial stromal sarcoma (tends to infiltrate myometrium, usually does not have glands distributed throughout, and does not have surrounding hypertrophied smooth muscle)
- Hyperplasia
- Carcinoma (the most important differential diagnosis in adenomyosis)

Treatment and Prognosis

- Benign condition treated with hysterectomy if symptomatic

Associations

- Leiomyomata
- Endometriosis
- Endometrial carcinoma can arise in foci of adenomyosis

Endometrial Hyperplasia

Clinical Manifestations

- A benign proliferation of morphologically abnormal endometrial glands without evidence of cytologic atypia
- Term *atypical* used to describe hyperplasia in which proliferating endometrial glands have cytologic atypia
- Endometrial hyperplasia represents a continuous spectrum of proliferative disease that gradually increases in morphologic and clinical severity from simple to complex without atypia to simple to complex with atypia

- Women usually present with abnormal uterine bleeding in either premenopausal or postmenopausal years; hyperplasia rarely asymptomatic
- Uterus frequently enlarged

Gross Pathology

- Only typical abnormality is an increase in volume of endometrial tissue
- When visible, hyperplasia may be either diffuse or polypoid; almost always soft and velvety and very similar in appearance to normal secretory phase endometrium

Microscopic Pathology

- *Simple hyperplasia*
  - An increase in volume of both glandular and stromal elements
  - Number of glands relative to stroma increased but the glands themselves not particularly crowded together
  - In most cases, at least some glands cystically dilated and may be either round or have focal outpouchings
  - Glands lined by cells that resemble proliferative type epithelium; cells are columnar and have amphophilic cytoplasm and pseudostratified nuclei that are oval, smooth, have evenly distributed chromatin, and small nucleoli
  - Ciliated cell change may be present in glands on surface
  - Stroma consists of uniform, round, oval stromal cells with scant cytoplasm that are more densely packed than those seen in normal proliferative endometrium
  - Mitotic activity variable in both the glandular and stromal elements
- *Complex hyperplasia*
  - Architecturally complex glands with numerous lateral buds randomly distributed and closely packed together, often back-to-back with little intervening stroma
  - Cytologically, epithelium of glands identical to that of simple hyperplasia; the nuclei are uniform in size and shape, show normal polarity, and are not atypical; nucleoli tend to be inconspicuous
  - Mitotic activity variable
  - Stromal component much less prominent than in simple hyperplasia and stromal cells show marked spindling (may be a result of compression between adjacent glands); no fibrosis or necrosis
- *Atypical hyperplasia*
  - Architectural pattern may be simple or complex (vast majority are complex)
  - Papillary infoldings may be present in some glands; a cribriform or confluent pattern never present
  - Some or all of the hyperplastic endometrial glands lined by cytologically atypical epithelium
  - Atypical areas may be focal and found immediately adjacent to glands that are not atypical
  - Atypical cells tend to be enlarged; nuclear-cytoplasmic ratio is increased; nuclei large, hyperchromatic, and pleomorphic (tend to be more rounded than oval); nuclear membranes usually irregular and thick; nucleoli prominent
  - True nuclear stratification (2 to 4 cells thick) with loss of polarity usually present and often more marked than in complex hyperplasia without atypia
  - Mitotic activity variable
  - No stromal findings characteristic for atypical hyperplasia
  - Metaplastic changes may be present in any type of hyperplasia (particularly the morular variant of squamous metaplasia)

Special Stains, Immunohistochemistry, and Electron Microscopy

- Not helpful

Molecular Alterations

- None

Differential Diagnosis

- Differential diagnosis (benign lesions):
  - Disordered proliferative endometrium (focal areas of dilated or branched proliferative glands that do not meet quantitative criteria for simple hyperplasia)
  - Normal proliferative or secretory endometrium
  - Endometrial polyp
  - Endometrium with cystic atrophy
  - Endometritis
  - Atypical polypoid adenomyoma
- Well-differentiated adenocarcinoma

Treatment

- Suppression with progestational agents
- Atypical hyperplasia typically treated with hysterectomy

Prognosis

- Atypical hyperplasia probably represents a stage in the development of well-differentiated adenocarcinoma
- Simple or complex hyperplasia without atypia usually self-limited and spontaneously regresses (risk of progression to carcinoma 1% and 3% respectively)
- 60% of atypical hyperplasias regress; risk of progression to carcinoma 10% for simple atypical hyperplasia and 30% for complex atypical hyperplasia

Associations

- Obesity (Western diet)
- Nulliparity
- Diabetes mellitus
- Hypertension
- Functional ovarian tumors and stromal proliferations
- Exogenous estrogen administration
- 15% to 25% of uteri removed for atypical hyperplasia contain a well-differentiated adenocarcinoma

Endometrial Polyp

Clinical Manifestations

- Most likely arise from endometrial basalis as a result of estrogenic stimulation
- Most asymptomatic, but may be a cause of abnormal uterine bleeding
- Typically seen in perimenopausal women
- May cause infertility
- Large polyps, either sessile or pedunculated, that may be located anywhere in the endometrial cavity including the lower uterine segment

Gross Pathology

- External surface typically smooth, tan, and glistening
- Small granular erosions and foci of hemorrhage and necrosis may be present
- Typically solitary but may be multiple

Microscopic Pathology

- Typically pedunculated and extends above the endometrial surface
- Frequently will be in a different phase of the menstrual cycle than surrounding nonpolypoid endometrium
- Glands often sparse, irregularly distributed, dilated, and lined by atrophic, inactive, or weakly proliferative endometrium
- Stroma either focally or diffusely fibrotic; rarely cytologically atypical
- Various endometrial changes may be present: secretory changes (usually poorly developed), gestational changes, the entire spectrum of metaplastic changes, various forms of hyperplasia, carcinoma, sarcoma, and carcinosarcoma
- Variable amounts of smooth muscle may be admixed with stroma (if majority of the stroma is smooth muscle and epithelium is benign, the lesion is an *adenomyoma*; if the majority of the stroma is smooth muscle and epithelium is atypical, the lesion is an *atypical polypoid adenomyoma*)
- Large, thick-walled, coiled vessels usually found in the center

Special Stains, Immunohistochemistry, and Electron Microscopy

- Not helpful

Molecular Alterations

- None

Differential Diagnosis

- Cystic atrophy with fibrotic stroma containing cystically dilated glands lined by atrophic endometrial epithelium
- Normal proliferative endometrium
- Endometrial hyperplasia (polyps commonly misinterpreted as hyperplasia); endometrial polyps have a dense fibrotic stroma and thick-walled vessels
- Polypoid adenomyoma, adenofibroma, and adenosarcoma

Treatment

- Curettage cures most
- Larger polyps may be treated with hysterectomy

Prognosis

- Relationship of polyps to endometrial carcinoma unclear
- Malignant transformation of an endometrial polyp may occur in postmenopausal women receiving tamoxifen therapy

Associations

- 15% to 35% incidence of benign endometrial polyps in uteri with adenocarcinoma
- Polyps with foci of epithelial atypia associated with tamoxifen therapy

Intravascular (Intravenous) Leiomyomatosis

Clinical Manifestations

- A benign uterine smooth muscle proliferation extensively involving myometrial veins
- Symptoms most commonly related to decreased venous return to the right heart

Gross Pathology

- Convoluted masses of mature smooth muscle in the lumens of uterine veins
- Neoplasm may extend into broad ligament, pelvic veins, interior vena cava, and right heart
- Diagnosis requires the presence of wormlike intravascular masses of cytologically benign smooth muscle or the presence of microscopic intrusion of benign smooth muscle into vessels outside the confines of an otherwise unremarkable leiomyoma

Microscopic Pathology

- Smooth muscle neoplasm may be found exclusively in venous lumina, jointly in lumina, and in continuity with surrounding venous wall, or confined to the muscularis portion of vein walls
- Tumors found exclusively in venous lumina represent an extension of an ordinary leiomyoma into uterine veins
- Tumors in lumina and in continuity with surrounding vein wall or confined to vein wall are thought to originate from the smooth muscle in the vein wall
- Typically neoplasms have a lobulated architecture and are extensively hyalinized, hydropic, or both
- Mitotic figures rare or absent
- Any of the histologic variants of leiomyoma may be present: bizarre, cellular, epithelioid, myxoid, or lipoleiomyoma

Special Stains, Immunohistochemistry, and Electron Microscopy

- See section on leiomyoma

Molecular Alterations

- None

Differential Diagnosis

- Leiomyosarcoma with extensive vascular invasion
- Vascular invasion *within* a leiomyoma (leiomyoma with vascular intrusion)
- Low-grade endometrial stromal sarcoma (endolymphatic stromal myosis)

Treatment

- Lesions confined to the uterus cured by hysterectomy
- Lesions extending into pelvic veins and/or vena cava treated with hysterectomy and removal of the intravenous tumor

Prognosis

- A benign neoplasm with a propensity to recur
- If neoplasm has 2 to 5 mitotic figures per 10 hpf, it is considered to have an uncertain malignant potential

Associations

- None

Leiomyoma

Clinical Manifestations

- Most common neoplasm of the uterus
- Affects 20% to 40% of women over the age of 30 years; rarely seen in postmenopausal women or girls younger than 18 years
- Neoplasms appear to grow in response to female sex hormones
- Small tumors typically asymptomatic; large or multiple tumors may be associated with pain, menorrhagia or metrorrhagia, dysmenorrhea, urinary symptoms, or constipation
- May be a cause of infertility
- During pregnancy may be associated with abruptio placentae, intrapartum pain secondary to infarction, and premature labor; may grow rapidly and cause outlet obstruction or abnormal presentation

Gross Pathology

- Solitary or multiple, round, and well-circumscribed
- Cut surface reveals firm, gray-white lesion with whorled intersecting fascicles
- Submucous tumors lie immediately beneath the endometrium, subserous tumors project onto serosal surface, and intramural lesions entirely surrounded by myometrium
- Areas of degeneration characterized by foci of hemorrhage, hyalinization (smooth white depressed zones), foci of hydropic, mucoid, or mucinous change, necrosis, and calcification

Microscopic Pathology

- *Typical leiomyoma*
  - A mixture of bland smooth muscle cells, fibroblasts, and collagen
  - Smooth muscle cells usually arranged in whorled anastomosing fascicles separated by a fibrovascular stroma with focal hyalinization
  - Most smooth muscle cells tend to be small and have uniform nuclei that are spindled and cigar-shaped with blunt ends and inconspicuous nucleoli; nuclear chromatin tends to be fine and evenly distributed; mitotic figures rare and never atypical
  - Fairly inconspicuous blood vessels with thick walls irregularly distributed throughout lesion
  - Numerous microscopic variations from typical appearance of atypical leiomyoma:
    - *Hyalinization:* Typically occurs in the stromal component and results in separation of smooth muscle cells; can become so extensive that few residual identifiable smooth muscle cells remain
    - *Vascular leiomyoma:* Characterized by prominent blood vessel proliferation
    - *Neurilemmomalike leiomyoma:* Palisading nuclei of smooth muscle cells give the lesion the appearance of a schwannoma
    - *Myxoid leiomyoma:* Characterized by extensive myxoid change; degree of myxoid change can obliterate the benign smooth muscle nature of the neoplasm; differentiation from malignant counterpart (myxoid leiomyosarcoma) very difficult
- *Cellular leiomyoma*
  - Represents approximately 5% of all uterine leiomyomas
  - Tends to be more fleshy and less whorled than typical leiomyoma; characterized by significant increased cellularity over surrounding myometrium
  - Little or no mitotic activity and no nuclear atypia

Uterus: Benign Lesions>Intravascular (Intravenous) Leiomyomatosis; Leiomyoma

- *Hemorrhagic cellular leiomyoma*
  - Occurs almost exclusively in women taking oral contraceptives or who are pregnant
  - Characterized by discrete foci of hemorrhage
  - Mitotic activity may be increased in a narrow zone adjacent to the area of hemorrhage
  - Little or no nuclear atypia
- *Epithelioid leiomyoma*
  - Smooth muscle cells resemble epithelial cells with abundant eosinophilic cytoplasm
  - Tends to be more yellow and softer than a typical leiomyoma
  - Usually solitary and large
  - Tumor cells tend to be polygonal
  - Hyalinization frequently present
  - Three variants
    - *Leiomyoblastoma* characterized by round and polygonal tumor cells with granular eosinophilic cytoplasm and eccentrically located nuclei
    - *Clear cell leiomyoma* consists of round to polygonal cells with abundant clear cytoplasm; nuclei tend to be small and uniform
    - *Plexiform leiomyoma* characterized by tumor cells arranged in rows and columns separated by fibrous or hyalinized stroma; cells have little cytoplasm and indistinct cell borders
- *Bizarre (symplastic, pleomorphic, or atypical) leiomyoma*
  - Benign smooth muscle neoplasm with huge pleomorphic cells and extensive hyalinization
  - Symplastic changes usually focal and scattered throughout an otherwise typical leiomyoma
  - Giant cells may be mononuclear or multinucleate and often have large angular hyperchromatic nuclei with smudged chromatin
  - Intranuclear inclusions of cytoplasm commonly present
  - Cytoplasm tends to be abundant, eosinophilic, and somewhat granular
  - Mitoses almost always completely absent; if present they are never abnormal; if mitotic index 3 or more per hpf, consider malignancy
- *Lipoleiomyoma*
  - Resembles typical leiomyoma except for presence of benign-appearing fat cells intermixed with smooth muscle cells
  - Usually seen in postmenopausal women (may represent degenerative changes)

Special Stains

- Trichrome stains will highlight collagen fibers between smooth muscle cells and the brick-red, fibrillar cytoplasm of smooth muscle cells
- Reticulin stains confirm the presence of reticulin fibers surrounding individual smooth muscle cells

Immunohistochemistry

- Tumors typically positive for desmin, muscle-specific actin, and smooth muscle actin; cytokeratin and vimentin positivity may also be present
- Tumor cells usually positive for both estrogen and progesterone receptors

Electron Microscopy

- Confirms presence of smooth muscle differentiation, including the presence of myofilaments arranged longitudinally and parallel to the long axis of the cells, dense bodies associated with myofilaments, pinocytotic vesicles, and an incomplete basal lamina surrounding individual cells

Molecular Alterations

- None

Differential Diagnosis

- Myxoid leiomyoma:
  - Myxoid leiomyosarcoma
- Cellular leiomyoma:
  - Leiomyosarcoma

- Stromal nodule or low-grade endometrial stromal sarcoma
- Hemorrhagic cellular leiomyoma

- Epithelioid leiomyoma:
  - Metastatic carcinoma in myometrium
  - Clear cell adenocarcinoma of endometrium
  - Stromal nodule or uterine tumor resembling an ovarian sex cord tumor (plexiform variant)
  - Primary endometrial carcinoma
- Bizarre leiomyoma:
  - Leiomyosarcoma
  - Malignant fibrous histiocytoma

Treatment

- Local excision (myomectomy) or hysterectomy

Prognosis

- No evidence of malignant transformation, but some evidence that epithelioid leiomyomas, particularly leiomyoblastomas and clear cell leiomyomas, should be considered to be tumors of uncertain malignant potential

Associations

- None

Stromal Nodule

- Tend to be discrete, round, and are almost always confined to the myometrium
- Grossly resemble leiomyomas (tend to be softer and less likely to be white and have whorled configuration)
- Median diameter 4 to 6 cm

Microscopic Pathology

- A solitary, sharply circumscribed mass; small tumors may be completely embedded in endometrium; larger tumors usually involve myometrium
- No evidence of myometrial or angiolymphatic invasion
- Tumor cells closely resemble the stromal cells of normal proliferative endometrium; they are small and uniform without cytologic atypia and variable mitotic activity
- Tumors tend to be very vascular with vessels resembling spiral arterioles of the endometrium; vessels tend to be thin-walled, evenly spaced, and of uniform size and shape (loss of vascular uniformity more likely in low-grade endometrial stromal sarcoma)
- Tumor cells are often arranged around blood vessels in a whorling pattern
- Thick bands of collagen in areas of hyalinization may be present
- Areas of necrosis, cystic degeneration, foam cells, calcium deposits, and decidualization may be present, but are rare
- Foci of smooth muscle differentiation and/or epithelioid differentiation may be present

Special Stains

- Reticulin stains will demonstrate the presence of reticulin fibers surrounding individual tumor cells and will highlight the whorling pattern that typically surrounds blood vessels
- Trichrome stains will highlight the presence of hyalinized collagen that is frequently present in stromal nodules

Immunohistochemistry

- Tumor cells typically positive for vimentin and negative for EMA
- Occasionally some tumor cells positive for both desmin and muscle-specific actin, particularly in foci of epithelioid differentiation
- Focal areas of cytokeratin positivity may be present
- Stromal nodules are usually estrogen and progesterone receptor positive
- CD10 almost always positive

Differential Diagnosis

- The 3 types of endometrial stromal tumor must be differentiated from each other
- Stromal nodule and low-grade stromal sarcoma:
  - Hemangiopericytoma
  - Leiomyoma and leiomyosarcoma

- If glandular differentiation is present:
  - Carcinosarcoma
  - Adenosarcoma
  - Epithelioid leiomyoma
  - Metastatic carcinoma (particularly lobular carcinoma of the breast)
  - Malignant lymphoma/leukemia
  - Lymphangiomyomatosis
- High-grade endometrial stromal sarcoma:
  - Poorly differentiated sarcoma
  - Poorly differentiated carcinoma
  - Sarcoma arising in the endometrium but lacking endometrial stromal differentiation (undifferentiated endometrial sarcoma)

Treatment

- Hysterectomy

Prognosis

- Stromal nodules are typically benign; recurrence is extremely rare even if primary treatment is excision without hysterectomy

Associations

- None

Malignant Lesions

Endometrial Carcinoma

Clinical Manifestations

- Diagnosis usually made during perimenopausal and postmenopausal years
- Associated clinical findings include: obesity, nulliparity, late menopause, diabetes mellitus, hypertension, and history of exogenous estrogen administration
- Initial symptoms typically abnormal vaginal bleeding; pain often a late symptom
- Occasional patients are asymptomatic

Gross Pathology

- Tumors typically arise in the corpus; occasionally originate from the lower uterine segment
- Typically uterus slightly enlarged, but may be either normal or small
- Most often the neoplasm presents as a single dominant mass (occasionally it may be ≥2 separate masses or a diffuse thickening of the endometrial surface)
- Most have an exophytic component
- More common on the posterior wall than on the anterior wall
- External surface frequently shaggy with focally ulcerated areas
- Sectioning reveals a friable, soft, gray to white mass
- The greater the amount of tumor in the endometrial cavity, the greater the likelihood of myometrial invasion
- Myometrial invasion can be seen either as a pushing or an infiltrating border in the uterine wall
- Advanced disease frequently indicated by deep myometrial invasion and/or extension into the lower uterine segment and cervix

Microscopic Pathology

- *Endometrioid adenocarcinoma (endometrial adenocarcinoma, endometrioid type)*
  - Most common type (by far)
  - Diagnosis of adenocarcinoma (as contrasted to complex atypical hyperplasia) based on the presence of stromal invasion; stromal invasion characterized by glandular fusion (disappearance of endometrial stroma between adjacent glands), stromal fibrosis, or stromal necrosis
  - Glands typically small, round, and uniform, and easily distinguished from adjacent glands; occasionally a cribriform pattern may be present
  - Neoplastic cells that line glands usually fairly uniform in size, shape, and staining quality
  - Nuclei (especially in well-differentiated tumors) tend to be aligned in a single row with little or no stratification; when nuclei are oval the axis tends to be perpendicular to the basement membrane

Uterus: Malignant Lesions>Endometrial Carcinoma

- Mitotic activity can be quite variable
- Nucleoli generally present and often quite prominent
- Features of nuclear atypia consist of rounded nuclei, nuclear hyperchromatism, pleomorphism, nuclear clearing secondary to clumping of chromatin along inner surface of nuclear membrane, or any combination of these features
- International Federation of Gynecology and Obstetrics (FIGO) grading system grades carcinoma into 1 of 3 grades based on both architectural and nuclear features:
- Architecture Grade I: 95% of tumor forms glands (5% solid growth pattern)
- Architecture Grade II: 6% to 50% of the tumor has a solid growth pattern
- Architecture Grade III: More than 50% of the neoplasm has a solid growth pattern (areas of squamous differentiation and squamous morules do not count as solid areas)
- Nuclear Grade I: Oval, small, uniform nuclei with fine chromatin, small nucleoli, and few mitoses
- Nuclear Grade II: Features between grades I and III
- Nuclear Grade III: Enlarged, elongated, pleomorphic nuclei with irregular outlines, coarse chromatin, macronuclei and numerous mitoses
- If nuclear atypia out of proportion to the architectural grade, architectural grade raised by 1

- Variants of endometrioid adenocarcinoma (endometrial adenocarcinoma, endometrioid):
  - *Variant with squamous differentiation*
    - Neoplasm characterized by the presence of small or large foci of squamous (including morular) differentiation; criteria that suggest squamous differentiation include keratinization, presence of intercellular bridges, sheetlike growth pattern without gland formation or palisading, sharp cell margins, eosinophilic, dense or glassy cytoplasm, and a decreased nuclear-cytoplasmic ratio. Once presence of squamous differentiation identified, squamous cells must be classified as either benign (adenocarcinoma with squamous metaplasia) or malignant (adenosquamous carcinoma)
  - *Villoglandular variant*
    - Numerous villous fronds with delicate cores lined by cells with stratified nuclei perpendicular to the basement membrane
  - *Secretory variant*
    - Neoplasm composed of well-differentiated glands that resemble early to mid secretory endometrium (associated with a favorable prognosis)
  - *Ciliated cell variant*
    - Neoplasm largely composed of ciliated cells. Very rare
  - *Serous adenocarcinoma:*
    - Represents 5% to 10% of all endometrial carcinomas
    - An aggressive neoplasm that tends to invade myometrium early
    - Neoplasm tends to grow in complex papillary fronds that may be either broad or narrow and have a central, fibrovascular connective tissue core; single cells, small epithelial papillae and buds, and complex papilloglandular structures floating free in lumina are common (the latter may reduce the lumina to irregular slitlike spaces)
    - Psammoma bodies present in 30%
    - Foci of necrosis common
    - Tumor cells typically small and round and have pleomorphic nuclei with macronucleoli
    - Mitotic figures frequent
  - *Clear cell adenocarcinoma*
    - Represents 5% of all endometrial carcinomas
    - Usually diagnosed in postmenopausal women
    - Tumor cells are large and have clear cytoplasm (secondary to accumulation of glycogen)
    - Tumor cells frequently project into lumina in a hobnail pattern

- A dense hyalinized stroma may be present
- Extracellular (rarely intracellular) mucin may be present
- Neoplastic cells may grow in a solid, papillary, tubular, or mixed pattern

□ *Mucinous adenocarcinoma*

- Represents 5% to 10% of all endometrial carcinomas
- Most (at least 50%) tumor cells contain intracytoplasmic mucin
- 40% of typical endometrial adenocarcinomas have minor foci of mucinous differentiation

□ *Squamous cell carcinoma*

- Should only be diagnosed in the absence of cervical squamous cell carcinoma
- Neoplasm resembles squamous cell carcinoma found in other sites
- Tumor cells may be spindled (resemble sarcoma) or may be clear (resemble clear cell adenocarcinoma)
- Prognosis extremely poor

□ *Verrucous carcinoma* is a variant of squamous cell carcinoma characterized by a papillary architecture, bland cytologic features, and invasion on a broad pushing front

□ *Mixed carcinoma*

- A neoplasm with >1 cell type (often endometroid in combination with serous or clear cell); the 2nd, or minor cell type, must comprise at least 10% of the total volume of neoplasm

□ *Small cell carcinoma*

- Histologically similar to small cell carcinoma in other organs

□ *Transitional cell carcinoma*

- Usually admixed with an endometroid carcinoma and has a papillary architecture

□ *Undifferentiated carcinoma*

- No evidence of differentiation

Special Stains

- PAS will highlight the glycogen in the cytoplasm of the clear cell adenocarcinomas
- Mucicarmine stains will highlight the intracellular mucin of mucinous adenocarcinoma

Immunohistochemistry

- Tumor cells frequently coexpress cytokeratins and vimentin (endocervical carcinoma and metastatic adenocarcinoma frequently do not express vimentin)
- Tumor cells typically positive for CEA (tumor cells of endocervical origin also positive for CEA)
- Tumor cells typically positive for sex-steroid hormone receptors and receptor levels typically higher in well-differentiated tumors
- Serous carcinomas typically negative for both estrogen and progesterone receptors

Electron Microscopy

- Most useful in less well-differentiated neoplasms where nuclear pleomorphism and mitochondrial pleomorphism more prominent; in addition, junctional structures such as microvilli, cilia, and desmosomes generally reduced in number
- Electron microscopy can confirm presence of glycogen in clear cell variant and mucin in mucinous variant

Molecular Alterations

- Serous carcinomas are often aneuploid and demonstrate amplification of c-*myc* proto-oncogene

Differential Diagnosis

- Endometrial complex hyperplasia with and without atypia
- Normal menstrual endometrium
- Various reactive glandular atypias (endometritis and changes secondary to curettage or radiation therapy)
- Endometrial epithelial metaplastic changes
- Poorly differentiated adenocarcinoma with a significant solid component consisting of spindled cells and a malignant glandular component:

    - Carcinosarcoma (typically the malignant epithelial component of a carcinosarcoma is sharply demarcated from the malignant spindled stromal cells; carcinomas with spindle cell foci typically have a gradual transition from malignant glandular or squamous epithelium to malignant spindled stromal cells, with no intervening basement membrane or connective tissue)
- Poorly differentiated adenocarcinoma with a significant solid component consisting of spindled cells and no malignant glandular component:
    - Endometrial stromal sarcoma
    - Atypical polypoid adenomyoma
- Adenocarcinomas growing in a papillary pattern may be endometrioid, serous, or clear cell variant
- Clear cell adenocarcinoma may mimic the secretory variant of endometrial adenocarcinoma
- Mucinous adenocarcinoma of endometrium frequently shows endocervical differentiation (ER positive and p16 negative) and may be difficult to distinguish from adenocarcinoma arising from the endocervix (ER negative and p16 positive)
- Specific variants of endometrial carcinoma versus benign metaplastic change:
    - Secretory endometrial adenocarcinoma versus clear cell change
    - Ciliated cell endometrial carcinoma versus ciliary change
    - Adenocarcinoma with squamous metaplasia versus squamous metaplasia and morules in a proliferative or hyperplastic endometrium
    - Serous adenocarcinoma versus surface syncytial change and papillary proliferation
    - Clear cell adenocarcinoma versus Arias-Stella change
- Metastatic adenocarcinoma (benign endometrial glands tend to be preserved intact in large masses of tumor)

Treatment

- Extrafascial total abdominal hysterectomy and bilateral salpingo-oophorectomy with or without adjuvant radiation therapy for resectable disease
- Inoperable disease typically treated with radiation therapy alone
- Role of exploratory laparotomy with pelvic and paraortic lymph node dissection still debated; this approach may be reserved for patients with high risk factors such as high tumor grade, deep myometrial invasion, and/or extension into the lower uterine segment or cervix
- Chemotherapy as a form of primary treatment typically consists of progestational agents (low-grade tumors and progesterone receptor positive tumors most likely to respond)

Prognosis

- 5-year survival rates for stage I disease (tumor limited to the uterus) range from 80% to 95%
- 5-year survival rates for stage II (endocervical glandular involvement or cervical stromal invasion) range from 50% to 60%
- 5-year survival rates for clinical stage III (tumor that has invaded serosa and/or adnexa and/or is associated with positive peritoneal cytology, vaginal metastasis, or metastasis to pelvic and/or paraortic lymph nodes) range from 15% to 25%
- Microscopic features of prognostic significance include:
    - Tumor grade
    - Histologic type (serous, clear cell, squamous cell, and undifferentiated carcinomas have a poor prognosis)
    - Presence or absence and depth of myometrial invasion
    - Involvement of lower uterine segment
    - Myometrial lymphatic/vascular space invasion
    - Presence of hyperplasia in benign endometrium adjacent to the neoplasm associated with a more favorable prognosis
- Estrogen and progesterone receptor positive tumors tend to have a more favorable prognosis
- Presence or absence of squamous differentiation has no effect on prognosis
- Adenosquamous carcinomas have a worse prognosis than adenocarcinomas with squamous differentiation

Associations

- Increased incidence associated with unopposed exogenous estrogen by postmenopausal women
- Ovarian lesions associated with increased estrogen production and an increased incidence of endometrial carcinoma:
  - Polycystic ovaries
  - Stromal hyperplasia
  - Hyperthecosis
  - Granulosa cell tumor

Adenosarcoma

Clinical Manifestations

- Usually affects postmenopausal women
- More frequent than either adenofibroma or adenomyoma
- Most occur in uterus, but may occur in ovary or other sites

Gross Pathology

- Typically a polypoid mass arising from the endometrium; surface may be leaflike (phyllodeslike)
- Have been reported to arise in endocervix and in myometrium (presumably from foci of adenomyosis)
- Cut surface tends to be fleshy and multicystic; rarely foci of necrosis present; very similar to both adenofibroma and adenomyoma
- Myometrial invasion can be seen on gross examination
- May be multiple

Microscopic Pathology

- An admixture of benign epithelium with a sarcomatous stroma
- Surface of the neoplasm frequently has a papillary, leaflike appearance similar to a cystosarcoma phyllodes tumor of the breast
- Epithelial component consists of small glands, cystically dilated glands, or compressed slitlike glands lined by a benign proliferative-type endometrium; metaplastic change, eg, squamous metaplasia or eosinophilic cell change may be present
- Stromal component tends to be cellular and cytologically malignant, and consists of spindled or round cells that resemble endometrial stromal cells or fibroblasts; stromal cells coalesce in hypercellular cuffs around the epithelial component
- Nuclear atypia in the stromal component often mild to moderate (reminiscent of low-grade sarcoma)
- If stromal overgrowth occurs, sarcomatous component may take on the features of a high-grade sarcoma
- Mitotic rate in stromal component typically >20 mitotic figures per 10 hpf but may be as low as 2 or 3 per 10 hpf
- Foci of fibrosis, hyalinization, hemorrhage, and necrosis common
- Heterologous elements, particularly rhabdomyosarcoma and chondrosarcoma, may be present
- 25% invade myometrium; angiolymphatic space invasion may be present and typically consists of the sarcomatous component with or without accompanying glandular elements; distant metastases always purely sarcomatous
- Occasionally foci of sex cord–like elements may be present in stromal component (consist of solid nests, trabeculae, and solid or hollow tubules composed of benign-appearing epithelial-type cells that may have foamy cytoplasm)
- If more than 25% of the total tumor consists of pure sarcoma, diagnosis becomes *adenosarcoma with sarcomatous overgrowth*; degree of atypia and mitotic activity usually (not always) higher

Special Stains, Immunohistochemistry, and Electron Microscopy

- Not helpful

Molecular Alterations

- None

Differential Diagnosis

- Adenofibroma
- Carcinosarcoma
- Endometrial polyp
- Adenomyoma

Treatment

- Hysterectomy

Prognosis

- Both recurrence and metastasis may occur as long as five years after hysterectomy
- 10% to 25% of patients die of tumor progression
- Prognosis worse if sarcomatous overgrowth is high-grade or if there is a sarcomatous component

Associations

- Best considered as a mixed epithelial-nonepithelial tumor along with adenomyoma, andenfibroma, and carcinosarcoma)

Carcinosarcoma (Malignant Mixed Müllerian Tumor)

Clinical Manifestations

- Represents 2% to 3% of uterine cancers and is the most common of the mixed epithelial/nonepithelial endometrial tumors
- Typically occurs in older postmenopausal women
- Most present with abnormal vaginal bleeding
- Pelvic or abdominal pain may be present (secondary to extrauterine disease)

Gross Pathology

- Typically large, friable, soft, broad-based, and smooth polypoid neoplasms that completely fill the endometrial cavity, invade deeply into the myometrium, and may protrude through the external cervical os
- Cut surface usually fleshy, variegated, hemorrhagic, and necrotic
- Fragment of bones or cartilage may be recognized on sectioning

Microscopic Pathology

- Biphasic neoplasm with malignant epithelial and malignant nonepithelial elements
- Glandular (epithelial) component usually of endometrioid type, but may be any type of Müllerian carcinoma (mucinous, squamous, papillary, clear cell, undifferentiated, or any combination)
- Sarcomatous component may be either homologous or heterologous
    - *Homologous variant* typically contains a high-grade sarcomatous component that consists predominantly of spindled cells, round cells, or giant cells; may resemble a low-grade fibrosarcoma or leiomyosarcoma
    - *Heterologous variant* contains foci of rhabdomyosarcoma, chondrosarcoma, osteosarcoma, liposarcoma, or any combination
- Eosinophilic hyaline droplets usually present in stroma of both homologous and heterologous tumors

Special Stains

- PAS and α_1-antitrypsin will highlight eosinophilic globules

Immunohistochemistry

- Cytokeratins and EMA frequently positive in both epithelial and sarcomatous populations (perhaps in actuality the tumor is a metaplastic carcinoma)
- Myogenin will highlight presence of rhabdomyosarcoma cells
- S-100 protein will highlight presence of chondrosarcomatous differentiation

Electron Microscopy

- Distinct malignant stroma and malignant epithelial elements can usually be easily recognized, but often the 2 elements admixed

Molecular Alterations

- None

Differential Diagnosis

- Poorly differentiated endometrial carcinoma with spindle cell metaplasia
- Adenosarcoma
- Stroma with eosinophilic hyaline droplets easily confused with rhabdomyosarcomatous differentiation
- If heterologous elements present:
    - Foci of chondrosarcoma may resemble foci of squamous cell carcinoma

- Foci of benign chondroid, osseous, or fatty differentiation may be present in a typical endometrial carcinoma
- Chondrosarcoma, osteosarcoma, and liposarcoma (very rare)

Treatment

- Hysterectomy with staging with or without adjuvant radiation and chemotherapy
- Combination chemotherapy used for recurrent disease but never produces a cure

Prognosis

- 5-year survival rate ranges between 20% and 40% (recurrence rates very high)
- No apparent difference in survival in tumors with heterologous versus homologous elements

Associations

- Prior pelvic radiation
- Obesity, nulliparity, and diabetes mellitus (epidemiologic features also associated with endometrial carcinoma)
- May represent a complication of functioning ovarian lesions and exogenous estrogen therapy
- May arise in an endometrial polyp or an adenosarcoma

Endometrial Stromal Tumors

Variants

- Stromal nodule
- Low-grade endometrial stromal sarcoma (endolymphatic stromal myosis or stromatosis)
- High-grade endometrial stromal sarcoma

Clinical Manifestations

- Rarest primary neoplasms of the uterine corpus
- No known precursor lesions
- Most patients present with abnormal uterine bleeding; occasionally abdominal pain is a presenting symptom; rarely asymptomatic
- Median age of patients with low-grade tumors is approximately 40 years; median age of patients with high-grade sarcomas 60 years
- Uterus typically enlarged

Gross Pathology

- *Stromal nodule*
  - Neoplasms are typically soft and tan to gray to yellow
  - Usually solid with foci of necrosis, hemorrhage, or cystic change
- *Low-grade endometrial stromal sarcoma*
  - 50% are well-circumscribed; the remaining 50% have evidence of diffuse myometrial permeation
  - Occasionally multiple
  - May be confined to the myometrium; extrauterine extension evident in 30% to 35%
  - Vascular and lymphatic involvement common; vascular intrusion characterized as *wormlike*
- *High-grade stromal sarcoma*
  - May be a single polypoid mass, a grossly infiltrative mass, or multiple confluent nodules scattered throughout the myometrium
  - Endometrial involvement is almost always present
  - Foci of hemorrhage and necrosis fairly common
  - Frequently extends beyond uterus
  - Vascular and lymphatic invasion not typically evident on gross examination

Microscopic Pathology

- Cells that comprise *stromal tumors* resemble cells of normal proliferative endometrial stroma; endometrial stroma characterized by a monomorphous population of blunt, spindled or oblong cells with little cytoplasm and relatively small, uniform nuclei in an abundant reticulin matrix with a delicate arborizing vasculature that may contain some hyalinization
- *Low-grade endometrial stromal sarcoma*
  - Most common of the 3 variants

   - Cytologic and architectural appearance is identical to that of a stromal nodule except the border between the tumor and surrounding myometrium is infiltrative (pattern of infiltration usually consists of irregularly shaped tongues or islands of tumor cells randomly placed between bundles of smooth muscle) and foci of tumor are usually seen in angiolymphatic channels (vascular involvement is best seen at the periphery and is characterized by the presence of plugs of tumor cells in vascular and/or lymphatic spaces—the appearance is that of slitlike spaces around masses of tumor)
   - Typically minimal or no atypia and variable mitotic activity
   - Foci of foam cells, decidualization, calcification, cystic degeneration, hemorrhage, necrosis, epithelioid differentiation, and hyalinization may be present
- *High-grade endometrial stromal sarcoma*
   - An invasive neoplasm characterized by increased cellularity, pleomorphism, hyperchromasia, nuclear atypia, and high mitotic rate
   - Occasional cells are less atypical and more closely resemble cells of a stromal nodule or low-grade stromal sarcoma
   - Invasion occurs on a broad front as angular pointed proliferations
   - Small vascular channels course through the tumor but are less regularly distributed than those of low-grade endometrial stromal sarcoma
   - Focal areas of huge cells with bizarre solitary or multiple nuclei may be present
   - Foci of smooth muscle (leiomyosarcomatous) differentiation may be present
   - Angiolymphatic invasion is frequently present, but plugs of tumor in vessels and slitlike vascular spaces are rarely seen
   - Foci of necrosis frequent

Special Stains

- Reticulin stains will demonstrate the presence of reticulin fibers surrounding individual tumor cells and will highlight the whorling pattern that typically surrounds blood vessels
- Trichrome stains will highlight the presence of hyalinized collagen that is frequently present in stromal nodules

Immunohistochemistry

- Tumor cells typically positive for vimentin and negative for EMA
- Occasionally some tumor cells positive for both desmin and muscle-specific actin, particularly in foci of epithelioid differentiation
- Focal areas of cytokeratin positivity may be present
- Both stromal nodules and low-grade stromal sarcomas are usually estrogen and progesterone receptor positive
- CD10 almost always positive

Electron Microscopy

- Characteristics similar to normal stromal cells of proliferative-phase endometrium
- Foci of epithelial and smooth muscle differentiation can be confirmed

Molecular Alterations

- None

Differential Diagnosis

- The 3 types of endometrial stromal tumor must be differentiated from each other
- Stromal nodule and low-grade stromal sarcoma:
   - Hemangiopericytoma
   - Leiomyoma and leiomyosarcoma
- If glandular differentiation is present:
   - Carcinosarcoma
   - Adenosarcoma
   - Epithelioid leiomyoma
   - Metastatic carcinoma (particularly lobular carcinoma of the breast)
   - Malignant lymphoma/leukemia
   - Lymphangiomyomatosis

- High-grade endometrial stromal sarcoma:
  - Poorly differentiated sarcoma
  - Poorly differentiated carcinoma
  - Sarcoma arising in the endometrium but lacking endometrial stromal differentiation (undifferentiated endometrial sarcoma)

Treatment

- Low-grade and high-grade endometrial stromal sarcoma:
  - Total hysterectomy with bilateral salpingo-oophorectomy with surgical debulking of extrauterine tumor if appropriate and adjuvant progestational agents
- Nonhormonal chemotherapy and radiation not particularly effective

Prognosis

- Both low-grade and high-grade endometrial stromal sarcomas behave in a malignant fashion
- Low-grade stromal sarcomas have about a 50% recurrence rate, 5- and 10-year survival rates approach 90%
- Initial recurrence of low-grade stromal sarcoma tends to be in the pelvis (occasionally recurrence is first seen as a pulmonary metastasis)
- High-grade endometrial stromal sarcomas more likely recur as extrapulmonary, distant metastases, and most patients are dead in 3 years

Associations

- None

Leiomyosarcoma

Clinical Manifestations

- A malignant neoplasm with smooth muscle differentiation
- Represent 25% of all uterine sarcomas
- Usually presents as a rapidly enlarging uterine mass in postmenopausal women
- Occasionally patients present with symptoms of extrauterine extension or distant metastasis

Gross Pathology

- Usually solitary, large, and poorly circumscribed
- Cut surface reveals a soft fleshy neoplasm, a variegated color ranging from gray to yellow to pink, and foci of hemorrhage and necrosis
- Advanced lesions frequently exhibit gross evidence of extension beyond the uterine corpus
- Benign leiomyomas may also be present

Microscopic Pathology

- Tumor cells tend to be large and spindled with markedly atypical nuclei and many atypical mitotic figures; usually arranged in intersecting fascicles
- Nuclei tend to be vaguely cigar-shaped and have blunt or rounded ends with coarsely clumped chromatin and single or multiple prominent nucleoli
- Multinucleated giant cells frequently present (resemble osteoclasts)
- Small amounts of collagenous stroma may be present between tumor cells; foci of intratumoral hemorrhage and well-demarcated areas of coagulative necrosis (not to be confused with the hyaline necrosis seen as a degenerative change) usually prominent
- Margins may show focal infiltration of surrounding myometrium or extensive invasion of both myometrium and blood vessels
- *Diagnostic criteria for malignancy: Mitotic count of 10 per 10 hpf in a cellular neoplasm and/or more than 5 mitotic figures per 10 hpf in tumors with anaplasia, pleomorphism, giant cells, or an epithelioid pattern*
- Lower mitotic counts do not guarantee lesion benign and occasionally cytologically bland tumors have more than 5 mitotic figures per 10 hpf (especially in young women)
- Variants
  - *Epithelioid leiomyosarcoma:* Characterized by round or polygonal cells with abundant eosinophilic or clear cytoplasm
  - *Myxoid leiomyosarcoma:* Smooth muscle nature of neoplasm may be hidden by extensive myxoid change; mitotic figures typically rare (mitotic count is typically 0 to 2 per 10 hpf) and nuclear pleomorphism usually absent; classically areas free of myxoid change will be more atypical and mitotically active; these neoplasms tend to extensively infiltrate myometrium and myometrial blood vessels

Special Stains, Immunohistochemistry, and Electron Microscopy

- See section on leiomyoma

Molecular Alterations

- None

Differential Diagnosis

- Benign leiomyoma
- Intravenous leiomyomatosis
- High-grade endometrial stromal sarcoma
- Undifferentiated sarcoma
- Poorly differentiated or undifferentiated endometrial carcinoma
- Metastatic carcinoma to the uterus
- Malignant fibrous histiocytoma
- Rhabdomyosarcoma
- Metaplastic carcinoma or carcinosarcoma
- Smooth muscle tumors of uncertain malignant potential (see below)

Treatment

- Total abdominal hysterectomy with bilateral salpingo-oophorectomy
- No evidence that radiotherapy and single agent chemotherapy improves survival
- Multiagent chemotherapy that includes doxorubicin may improve survival

Prognosis

- 5-year survival rates range between 40% and 50% for stage I and II tumors
- Factors associated with a poor prognosis include high mitotic rate, marked anaplasia, vascular invasion, large tumor size, spread beyond the uterus, and advanced age

Associations

- None

Smooth muscle tumors of uncertain malignant potential

- Smooth muscle tumors with the typical histologic appearance of leiomyoma with any of the following are considered to be of uncertain malignant potential:
  - Cytologic atypia and 2 to 5 mitotic figures per 10 hpf
  - Hypercellularity, no atypia, and 5 to 10 mitotic figures per 10 hpf
  - 10 to 15 mitotic figures per 10 hpf, without hypercellularity or atypia
  - Infiltrating margins and 5 to 9 mitotic figures per 10 hpf
  - Any abnormal mitotic figures or areas of necrosis
- Tumors with an epithelioid pattern, bizarre (symplastic) pattern, vascular invasion within the tumor and 2 to 5 mitotic figures per 10 hpf
- Intravenous leiomyomatosis (vascular invasion outside the main neoplasm) with 2 to 5 mitotic figures per 10 hpf
- Parasitic leiomyoma (tumors detached from the uterus and attached elsewhere) with 5 to 9 mitotic figures per 10 hpf
- Tumors in any of these categories with <2 mitotic figures per 10 hpf are considered benign; tumors in any of these categories with more than 5 mitotic figures per 10 hpf are considered malignant

Vagina

Clear Cell Adenocarcinoma

Clinical Manifestations

- 50% of all clear cell adenocarcinomas involve the vagina, usually upper 3rd of anterior or lateral wall
- Age range 5 to 45 years, with a peak at 20 years (uncommon before age 15 years and after age 30 years)
- Most present with vaginal bleeding and discharge, but may be asymptomatic
- Cervix may be involved

Vagina>Clear Cell Adenocarcinoma

Gross Pathology

- Lesion may be polypoid, nodular, papillary, flat, or ulcerated

Microscopic Pathology

- Appearance similar to clear cell adenocarcinoma seen in cervix, endometrium, and ovary
- Predominant cell type is a hobnail cell with little cytoplasm and a bulbous nucleus that protrudes into glandular lumens
- Other cells have abundant intracytoplasmic glycogen (the clear cytoplasm of the clear cell)
- 3rd cell type may be flat with little or no atypia, bland nuclei, and scant granular eosinophilic cytoplasm
- Nonglycogenated cells that are neither flat nor hobnail have granular eosinophilic cytoplasm and may be admixed with the other 3 cell types
- Both clear cells and hobnail cells have considerable nuclear atypia (flat cells tend to be bland)
- Mitotic activity variable but usually fairly low
- Multiple histologic patterns:
  - *Tubulocystic*
    - Most common (60%)
    - Tubulocystic areas usually lined by any of the 4 types of cells (hobnail, clear, flat, or nonglycogenated)
  - *Papillary*
    - Least common (12%)
    - Psammoma bodies and intracellular hyaline bodies may be seen
    - Papillae usually lined by clear cells or hobnail cells
  - *Solid*
    - 20%
    - Usually composed of sheets of clear or eosinophilic cells

Special Stains

- PAS will highlight presence of glycogen

Immunohistochemistry

- Not helpful

Electron Microscopy

- All tumor cells, regardless of their light microscopy features, seem to be of the same basic type
- Most prominent feature is presence of abundant intracellular glycogen
- Tumor cells have short, blunt microvilli

Molecular Alterations

- Somatic mutation of microsatellite repeats

Differential Diagnosis

- Microglandular hyperplasia
- Arias-Stella phenomenon
- Metastatic renal cell carcinoma
- Endodermal sinus tumor

Treatment

- Early stage disease treated with radical hysterectomy, vaginectomy, and lymphadenectomy
- Radiotherapy effective for early stage disease but usually reserved for advanced-stage tumors

Prognosis

- 25% of patients experience recurrence
- Tumors that have invaded beyond 3 mm have a significant risk of having lymph node metastasis
- Factors associated with a favorable prognosis include:
  - Absence of symptoms at the time of detection
  - Age of 19 years or older
  - Small tumor size
  - Minimal invasion
  - Tubulocystic pattern
- 5-year survival rate almost 90% for patients with stage I disease
- Overall 5-year survival rate for all stages (combined) approximately 80%

- A higher tendency to spread beyond the abdominal cavity than either squamous cell carcinoma of the vagina or squamous cell carcinoma of the cervix

Associations

- *In utero exposure to diethyl stilbestrol (DES)*
- Factors associated with an increased risk with exposure to DES include:
  - Exposure prior to the 12th week of pregnancy
  - Maternal history of prior spontaneous abortion
  - Conception in the fall of the year
- Areas of adenosis found immediately adjacent to neoplasm in over 90% of cases (may be a precursor lesion)

Vulva

Aggressive Angiomyxoma

Clinical Manifestations

- Usually presents as a slowly enlarging, polypoid mass in the region of the vulva, vagina, perineum, inguinal region, or pelvic soft tissue
- Typically occurs in women between the ages of 25 and 60 years (may occur in men)
- In men usually occurs in the inguinal region along the spermatic cord or in the scrotum or pelvic cavity

Gross Pathology

- An infiltrative lesion that is uniformly rubbery and white or soft and myxoid or gelatinous
- Areas may appear partially encapsulated
- Tends to range in size from a few centimeters to over 20 cm (most ~10 cm)

Microscopic Pathology

- Majority of the tumor consists of small, bland fibroblasts and myofibroblasts with indistinct cytoplasm scattered throughout a myxoid stroma with few collagen fibers
- Neoplasm contains numerous capillaries and small to medium-sized arteries and veins with thick walls (hyalinized and hypertrophied) that are often grouped together; vessels may be dilated; extravasated red blood cells are usually present
- Foci of hemorrhage may be present
- Nuclear pleomorphism and mitotic figures are both typically absent
- Occasionally epithelial elements with mucin-secreting columnar cells forming small glandular structures may be present
- Neoplasm may invade muscle and entrap fat and nerves

Special Stains

- Not helpful

Immunohistochemistry

- Tumor cells are focally reactive to antibodies directed against vimentin, smooth muscle actin, muscle-specific actin, desmin, and keratin
- CD34, progesterone and estrogen receptors often positive
- Blood vessel endothelium positive for factor VIII and CD31

Electron Microscopy

- Tumor cells have a fibroblastlike and a myofibroblast-like morphology with delicate cytoplasmic processes that extend into the surrounding myxoid matrix

Molecular Alterations

- None

Differential Diagnosis

- Angiomyofibroblastoma (angiomyofibroblastoma is more circumscribed, blood vessels are not hyalinized and hypertrophied, plump stromal cells surround more numerous vessels, there is little stromal mucin, and extravasated erythrocytes are rare)
- Myxoma
- Myxolipoma
- Spindle cell lipoma
- Myxoid neurofibroma
- Myxoid leiomyoma

- Myxoid liposarcoma
- Botryoid rhabdomyosarcoma
- Myxoid malignant fibrous histiocytoma

Treatment

- Wide local excision
- No indication for lymphadenectomy

Prognosis

- An aggressive infiltrating neoplasm that does not metastasize
- Recurrence occurs in approximately 50%, usually in 3 to 4 years of excision

Associations

- None

Angiomyofibroblastoma

Clinical Manifestations

- Probably related to an epithelioid leiomyoma
- Develops slowly in subcutaneous tissues
- Typically presents as a polypoid, subcutaneous mass in the vulva; often diagnosed as a Bartholin cyst on physical examination
- Affects women from 3rd to 9th decade

Gross Pathology

- Lesion typically a well-circumscribed, tan, pink, or yellow mass in the subcutaneous tissue of the vulva or vagina (rare)
- Cut section resembles a leiomyoma or angiomyxoma; spongy with a variable firm to soft consistency

Microscopic Pathology

- Low-power appearance of alternating areas of hypercellularity and hypocellularity (stromal edema)
- Neoplasm characterized by prominent, occasionally ectatic vessels surrounded by eosinophilic, spindled, and epithelioid stromal cells that tend to blend with or fan out from the blood vessel walls
- Blood vessels neither hyalinized nor hypertrophied
- Occasionally tumor cells arranged in small chains, cords, or singularly in a matrix that may be myxoid, hyaline, or a combination of the two
- Epithelioid cells may have a spindled appearance and resemble conventional smooth muscle cells; a feature often seen at the periphery of the lesion

Special Stains

- Not helpful

Immunohistochemistry

- Tumor cells reactive for vimentin and desmin and occasionally for actin and CD34
- Cytokeratin and S-100 negative

Electron Microscopy

- Confirms the smooth muscle nature of epithelioid-appearing cells

Molecular Alterations

- None

Differential Diagnosis

- Aggressive angiomyxoma (aggressive angiomyxoma is not circumscribed; blood vessels tend to be hyalinized and hypertrophied; stromal cells fewer in number, less plump, and do not tend to surround vessels; there is abundant stromal mucin; extravasated erythrocytes are present)
- Leiomyoma
- Leiomyosarcoma

Treatment

- Wide local excision

Prognosis

- Recurrence rare, but will occur if lesion is incompletely excised
- No reports of metastases
- 1 report of sarcomatous transformation

Associations

- None

Paget Disease

Clinical Manifestations

- Usually presents as an intraepithelial adenocarcinoma arising from a multipotential cell in the epidermis, adnexa, or perineal mammarylike glands
- Less often presents as invasive carcinoma arising from an intraepithelial adenocarcinoma or pagetoid extension or metastasis from a nearby carcinoma (eg, cervix, Bartholin gland, urinary bladder, urethra)
- Extramammary Paget disease can develop anywhere along the milk line, from axilla to perineum
- Represents 2% of all vulvar neoplasms
- Most frequently diagnosed in white, postmenopausal women (7th decade)

Gross Pathology

- Usually presents on the labia majora as a granular, moist, red to pink lesion with irregular margins
- Foci of white hyperkeratotic epithelium usually present
- May be multifocal

Microscopic Pathology

- Paget cells are typically large with pale, finely granular amphophilic to basophilic cytoplasm; nuclei are round to oval vesicular with either finely granular or coarsely hyperchromatic chromatin; ≥1 prominent nucleoli are typically present; mitotic figures may be present as well as intracytoplasmic melanin
- Cells tend to be grouped predominantly in the basal and parabasal zones of the epithelium
- Occasionally gland spaces are present in groups of Paget cells
- Squamous epithelium acanthotic with hyperkeratosis and parakeratosis
- Dermal invasion (infrequent) characterized by nests, cords, and sheets of cells originating from the epidermal or adnexal component

Special Stains

- Paget cells contain neutral and acid mucopolysaccharide that may be highlighted with mucicarmine, PAS with diastase, aldehyde fuchsin, Alcian blue, and colloidal iron after hyaluronidase pretreatment

Immunohistochemistry

- Paget cells are typically positive for CEA, EMA, and low-molecular-weight cytokeratin (CEA is the most sensitive)
- Cells are negative for both S-100 and melanoma antigen (HMB-45)

Electron Microscopy

- Paget cells have features of apocrine or exocrine cells

Molecular Alterations

- None

Differential Diagnosis

- Superficial spreading melanoma
- Squamous intraepithelial neoplasia

Treatment

- Wide excision of the involved area down to underlying fascia or simple vulvectomy (recurrence rate may be as high as 30%-35%)
- If an underlying adenocarcinoma is present, radical vulvectomy with bilateral inguinal-femoral lymph node dissection

Prognosis

- Paget disease confined to the epithelium carries an excellent prognosis if treated with complete surgical excision
- An underlying adenocarcinoma carries a prognosis that is related to the stage of tumor and the status of regional lymph nodes (usually poor)—invasive anogenital disease is associated with an 85% incidence of lymph node metastases

Associations

- 30% associated with synchronous or metachronous carcinoma in genitourinary tract, gastrointestinal tract, or breast
- Paget disease of the vulva may be associated with an underlying adenocarcinoma of a Bartholin gland
- Paget disease of the perineum (perianal) is associated with a high frequency of rectal adenocarcinoma

Papillary Hidradenoma (Hidradenoma Papilliferum)

Clinical Manifestations

- Typically seen in white women
- Rarely seen before puberty (when apocrine gland development occurs)
- 80% located in the labia minora or labia majora
- Typically presents as an asymptomatic nodule that may or may not be associated with pruritis
- Occasionally lesions ulcerate and bleed and produce a watery fluid

Gross Pathology

- Typically a well-circumscribed subcutaneous nodule <1 cm in diameter
- Cut surface usually soft and gray to white to red; may be cystic or solid

Microscopic Pathology

- Usually well-circumscribed with a pseudocapsule
- Typically composed of complex tubules and acini lined by tall columnar cells that usually have basal nuclei and an apocrine appearance with an underlying layer of cuboidal cells that are smaller and lie along the basement membrane
- Some degree of nuclear pleomorphism may be present as well as mitotic figures

Special Stains

- Tubules and acini contain PAS-diastase–resistant secretions

Immunohistochemistry

- Tumor cells are CEA negative (cells of apocrine glandular origin are typically CEA negative while cells of eccrine sweat gland origin are typically CEA positive). Inner epithelial layer is EMA positive. Outer myoepithelial layer stains for myoepithelial markers (SMA, calponin)

Electron Microscopy

- Tumor cells contain secretory granules and lamellar bodies and show evidence of decapitation secretion, confirming their apocrine nature

Molecular Alterations

- None

Differential Diagnosis

- Skin appendage adenocarcinoma
- Metastatic carcinoma
- Endometriosis
- Ectopic breast tissue

Treatment and Prognosis

- Local excision
- A completely benign lesion with no tendency to malignant transformation

Associations

- Rarely in situ or invasive carcinoma (adenosquamous) may develop

References

Dabbs DJ. *Diagnostic Immunohistochemistry.* New York: Churchill Livingstone, 2002.

Kurman RJ (ed). *Blaustein's Pathology of the Female Genital Tract. 5th ed.* New York: Springer-Verlag, 2002

Kurman RJ, Norris HJ, Wilkinson E. *Tumors of the Cervix, Vagina, and Vulva; Atlas of Tumor Pathology, 3rd Series, Fascicle 4.* Washington DC: Armed Forces Institute of Pathology, 1992.

Mazur MT, Kurman RJ. *Diagnosis of Endometrial Biopsies and Curettings: A Practical Approach.* New York: Springer-Verlag, 1995.

Mills S, Carter D, Greenson JK, Oberman HA, Reuter V, Stoler MH (eds). *Sternberg's Diagnostic Surgical Pathology. 4th ed.* Philadelphia: Lippincott Williams & Wilkins, 2004.

Rosai J. *Rosai and Ackerman's Surgical Pathology. 9th ed.* St. Louis: Mosby, 2004.

Silverberg SG, Kurman, RJ. *Tumors of the Uterine Corpus and Gestational Trophoblastic Disease; Atlas of Tumor Pathology, 3rd Series, Fascicle 3.* Washington DC: Armed Forces Institute of Pathology, 1992.

Tavassoli FA, Devilee P (eds). *World Health Organization Classification of Tumours. Pathology and Genetics of Tumours of the Breast and Female Genital Organs.* Lyon: IARC Press, 2003.

Chapter 6

Ovary

Intraoperative Consultation

The essential role of surgery for ovarian carcinoma is to remove the primary lesion and as many metastases as possible without jeopardizing the patient's life. The chief role of the pathologist in the performance of a frozen section on an ovarian mass is to determine the presence of overtly malignant tumor, low malignant potential tumor, or surface epithelial malignancy. These diagnoses will lead to the performance of a surgical staging procedure.

The pathologist faces several major sampling pitfalls when performing a frozen section analysis on an ovarian mass. Large cystic lesions with scattered papillary projections may be problematic in terms of sampling. Even careful examination and sampling of solid and papillary areas may not yield a focus of low malignant potential tumor or even frankly malignant tumor that may subsequently be found with more extensive sampling for permanent sections.

All mucinous neoplasms are difficult to accurately diagnose on frozen section. Of all ovarian neoplasms, this group produces the highest discordance rate between frozen sections and permanent sections. Mucinous tumors tend to be very heterogenous and a single neoplasm may contain areas of benign mucinous cystadenoma, borderline mucinous tumor, and obvious carcinoma. All of these areas may, on gross examination, appear similar and the risk of sampling error is significant. Some mucinous tumors appear architecturally simple and cytologically bland and yet either present with or subsequently develop pseudomyxoma peritonei. Metastatic mucinous carcinoma from the gastrointestinal tract, pancreas, or biliary tract may mimic a primary ovarian carcinoma.

There are various findings on frozen section of ovarian neoplasms that mimic malignancy but are benign. Sections taken through the hilum of the ovary may reveal the presence of hilus cells around ovarian hilar nerves (a finding that mimics metastatic germ cell neoplasm) or rete ovarii embedded within fibrous tissue (may mimic metastatic carcinoma). Nests of stromal lutein cells, tangentially cut follicular structures, inclusion cysts on the surface, and decidual reaction may all mimic carcinoma. Endometriosis, especially with cytologic atypia, may mimic a primary endometrial or metastatic endometrial carcinoma.

Specimen Handling

The external surface of all ovarian neoplasms should be inked. All neoplasms with a cystic component should be sampled in areas in which the wall of the cyst contains papillary structures or areas of thickening. Extensive sampling of all solid areas is of paramount importance, particularly in lesions that are primarily cystic. One section is customarily taken for each centimeter of maximal diameter with emphasis on obtaining most of the sections from solid and papillary areas. Sections should also document tumor to fallopian tube and presence of surface involvement.

Germ Cell Tumors

Choriocarcinoma

Clinical Manifestations

- Pure ovarian tumors are very rare consisting of <1% of all malignant primitive germ cell tumors; most commonly seen as a component of a mixed germ cell tumor)
- Typically occurs in children and young adults and presents with an adnexal mass, pain, and occasionally hemoperitoneum (the clinical presentation often mimics that of an ectopic pregnancy)
- Serum levels of human chorionic gonadotropin (hCG) are elevated, resulting in isosexual pseudoprecocity in children and menstrual abnormalities, breast enlargement, androgenic changes, or any combination in adults

Gross Pathology

- Neoplasm is typically solid, friable and hemorrhagic
- Rarely bilateral

Microscopic Pathology

- Tumor cells represent a mixture of uninucleated trophoblastic cells with either scanty or abundant clear cytoplasm (cytotrophoblastic or intermediate trophoblastic cells, respectively) admixed with syncytiotrophoblastic cells in a background of massive hemorrhage
- Syncytiotrophoblastic cells typically contain eosinophilic cytoplasm with vacuoles and many dark nuclei; may form syncytial knots

- Foci may be poorly differentiated
- Neoplastic cells often aggregate around dilated vascular spaces; vascular invasion often prominent

Special Stains

- Not helpful

Immunohistochemistry

- Syncytiotrophoblastic cells are immunoreactive for cytokeratin, hCG, human placental lactogen and pregnancy-specific β-1 glycoprotein
- Cytotrophoblasts typically immunoreactive for cytokeratin
- Intermediate trophoblasts immunoreactive for cytokeratin, human placental lactogen, and β-1 glycoprotein
- Tumor cells may also be positive for placental-like alkaline phosphatase (PLAP), epithelial membrane antigen (EMA), neuron-specific enolase (NSE), α_1-antitrypsin, and carcinoembryonic antigen (CEA)

Electron Microscopy

- Not helpful

Molecular Alterations

- None

Differential Diagnosis

- Mixed malignant germ cell tumor that contain syncytiotrophoblastic cells (embryonal carcinoma, dysgerminoma, and yolk sac tumor)
- Poorly differentiated carcinoma of surface epithelial origin
- Metastatic gestational choriocarcinoma

Treatment and Prognosis

- Unilateral salpingo-oophorectomy with combination chemotherapy
- Ovarian choriocarcinoma of germ cell origin seems to be less responsive to chemotherapy than gestational choriocarcinomas
- Ovarian choriocarcinoma of germ cell origin is treated with combination chemotherapy
- Gestational choriocarcinoma is treated with single agent chemotherapy (methotrexate or actinomycin D)

Associations

- A component of 15% to 20% of mixed malignant germ cell tumors

Dysgerminoma

Clinical Manifestations

- Most common (~50%) malignant primitive germ cell tumor
- Represents 1% of all ovarian cancers; 5% to 10% of all ovarian cancers in first 3 decades of life
- Typically occurs in the 2nd and 3rd decades (rare under the age of 5 years or over the age of 50 years)
- Most patients present with signs and symptoms of an abdominal mass
- Vast majority of patients have an elevated serum level of lactic dehydrogenase (usually isoenzymes 1 and 2)
- Serum levels of AFP are rarely if ever elevated
- Very rarely (3%) patients have elevated levels of hCG resulting in isosexual precocity or menstrual irregularities
- 30% have extraovarian disease at presentation

Gross Pathology

- Usually solid with a smooth external surface
- On cut section neoplasm is lobulated, yellow-white-tan and has a soft fleshy consistency; focal areas of cystic degeneration, hemorrhage and necrosis may be present
- Contralateral ovary involved in 20%
- Calcification raises possibility of the presence of an underlying gonadoblastoma

Microscopic Pathology

- Tumor cells resemble primitive germ cells and tend to be arranged in solid, insular, trabecular, cordlike, and rarely, tubular patterns
- Tumor cells are relatively uniform and round with clear cytoplasm (glycogen-rich) and distinct cell membranes

- Nucleus tends to be central, large, and round or flattened with clumped chromatin and 1 or more prominent nucleoli
- Mitotic figures are typically numerous
- Stroma consists of variably sized fibrous bands that almost always contain mature lymphocytes (T-cell type) and occasionally lymphoid follicles
- Foci of a necrosis are frequently present
- Granulomas are present in 20% and may be the dominant microscopic feature to the point that they obscure the underlying neoplastic cells
- Syncytiotrophoblastic giant cells present in 3%
- Occasionally luteinized stroma cells may be admixed with the neoplastic cells

Special Stains

- PAS with and without diastase will confirm the presence of glycogen within tumor cells

Immunohistochemistry

- Tumor cells immunoreactive for PLAP and vimentin
- Tumor cells variably positive for lactic dehydrogenase, NSE, Leu-7, cytokeratin, desmin, and glial fibrillary acidic protein (GFAP)
- Tumor cells almost always negative for EMA and CEA
- If syncytiotrophoblastic giant cells present they are typically positive for both hCG and cytokeratin

Electron Microscopy

- Tumor cells typically have closely apposed cytoplasmic membranes, abundant cytoplasmic glycogen and display polarization of cytoplasmic organelles
- Nuclei have evenly dispersed chromatin
- Nucleolus is typically complex

Molecular Alterations

- None

Differential Diagnosis

- Yolk sac tumor (solid pattern)
- Embryonal carcinoma (solid pattern)
- Clear cell carcinoma (diffuse pattern)
- Large cell lymphoma

Treatment

- Unilateral salpingo-oophorectomy indicated for patients desiring preservation of reproductive function who have early stage disease; chemotherapy is reserved for recurrent disease
- Young patients with more advanced disease are treated with unilateral salpingo-oophorectomy and adjuvant combination chemotherapy
- Patients in whom preservation of reproductive function is not an issue are treated with bilateral salpingo-oophorectomy and hysterectomy with or without adjuvant chemotherapy according to stage
- Radiation therapy is used only in those patients who do not respond to chemotherapy

Prognosis

- Stage of disease is only significant prognostic factor
- Patients with stage I disease have a 5-year survival rate close to 100%
- Patients with higher stage disease or recurrent disease have a 5-year survival rate of 80% to 90%

Associations

- Neoplasm may arise in the setting of a phenotypic female with gonadal dysgenesis and a gonadoblastoma (usually in the setting of a Y chromosome)
- May be associated with ataxia-telangiectasia

Embryonal Carcinoma

Clinical Manifestations

- Usually a component of a mixed germ cell tumor; pure form represents fewer than 3% of malignant primitive ovarian germ cell neoplasms
- Much less common than yolk sac tumors
- 50% of patients are prepubertal; median age at diagnosis 12 years
- Most patients present with an adnexal mass; 50% have endocrine manifestations including isosexual pseudoprecocity, irregular bleeding, amenorrhea and hirsutism
- Serum hCG and AFP elevated in all patients

Gross Pathology

- Always unilateral
- Tends to be large (average 17 cm) with a smooth external surface
- Cut surface typically is variegated white to yellow to tan and solid with scattered small cysts containing mucoid material
- Foci of hemorrhage and necrosis are common
- Extraovarian spread found in 40% at initial surgery

Microscopic Pathology

- Tumor cells typically arranged in solid sheets and nests and often have areas of central necrosis, glandlike spaces, and papillae
- Tumor cells tend to be large and primitive with amphophilic and occasionally clear cytoplasm with well-defined cell membranes
- Nuclei tend to overlap and are round and vesicular with a coarse irregular nuclear membrane and 1 or more prominent nucleoli
- Mitotic figures, many of which are atypical, are easily identified
- Eosinophilic intracellular hyaline droplets (identical to those seen in yolk sac tumor) may be present
- Individual syncytiotrophoblastic giant cells are almost always present

Special Stains

- PAS will highlight hyaline droplets

Immunohistochemistry

- Cytoplasm of tumor cells positive for pancytokeratin, PLAP, and NSE
- 80% are positive for CD30 (Ber-H2, Ki-1)
- 30% to 50% are positive for AFP
- Tumor cells typically negative for EMA, CEA, and vimentin
- Syncytiotrophoblastic giant cells stain with β-hCG

Electron Microscopy

- Confirms the similar nature of the hyaline droplets to those seen in yolk sac tumor

Molecular Alterations

- None

Differential Diagnosis

- Dysgerminoma (characterized by a lymphocytic stroma and cells that are smaller and have smaller nuclei that are less variable and hyperchromatic than the cells of an embryonal carcinoma)
- Yolk sac tumor (cells of yolk-sac tumor tend to be smaller and less pleomorphic than those of embryonal carcinoma and are usually arranged in a distinctive reticular pattern; cells of embryonal carcinoma tend to grow in solid sheets and line glands and papillae; syncytiotrophoblastic giant cells very rarely present in yolk sac tumors)
- Juvenile granulosa cell tumor (characterized by folliclelike spaces, luteinized neoplastic cells, and absence of syncytiotrophoblastic giant cells; inhibin positive and AFP negative)
- Poorly differentiated adenocarcinoma and undifferentiated carcinoma
- Sertoli-Leydig cell tumor (SLCT; usually strongly positive for inhibin)

Treatment

- Unilateral salpingo-oophorectomy with excision of as much extraovarian tumor is possible and postoperative adjuvant combination chemotherapy

Prognosis

- 50% of patients with stage I disease survive 5 years (before the institution of adjuvant chemotherapy)
- Postoperative chemotherapy may be curative in some cases

Associations

- None

Polyembryoma

Clinical Manifestations

- Extremely rare
- Typically occurs in children or young adults who present with symptoms related to a pelvic mass
- Occasionally patients will have elevated levels of AFP and/or hCG

Gross Pathology

- Typically bulky tumors with a soft, spongy, or microcystic cut surface
- Foci of hemorrhage often present

Microscopic Pathology

- Many small structures resembling perfect or imperfect early embryos (embryoid bodies) scattered throughout a fibrous or edematous stroma
- Embryoid bodies typically consist of a thick germ cell disc with an amniotic cavity on 1 side and a yolk sac cavity on the other
- Syncytiotrophoblastic giant cells and mature and immature teratomatous elements (usually intestinal tissue or adult or embryonal hepatic tissue) usually present

Special Stains

- Not helpful

Immunohistochemistry

- Yolk sac component and hepatic elements positive for AFP and α_1-antitrypsin
- Syntrophoblastic giant cells positive for hCG

Electron Microscopy

- Not helpful

Molecular Alterations

- None

Differential Diagnosis

- None

Treatment

- Surgery and adjuvant chemotherapy

Prognosis

- A malignant germ cell tumor with the capacity to both metastasize and recur (either metastatic deposits or recurrent tumor may consist of mature teratomatous elements)

Associations

- None

Yolk Sac Tumor (Endodermal Sinus Tumor)

Clinical Manifestations

- Represents 20% of all malignant primitive germ cell tumors
- Tends to occur during the 2nd and 3rd decades of life; rare after age of 40 years
- Tumor usually grows very fast and most present with a large abdominal or pelvic mass and the sudden onset of abdominal pain (rupture of tumor)
- Almost all have an elevated serum AFP levels
- Extraovarian spread at time of diagnosis fairly common

Gross Pathology

- Typically large (average 15 cm) with a smooth and shiny external surface
- On cut section, neoplasms are typically solid and cystic; solid areas tend to be yellow or gray and friable
- Large areas of hemorrhage and necrosis are common
- Occasionally cut surface has a honeycomb appearance (characteristic of the polyvesicular-vitelline variant)
- Other germ cell elements (typically associated with a dermoid cyst) may be seen in as many as 15%
- Essentially never bilateral
- Involvement of the peritoneum and/or retroperitoneal lymph nodes evident in as many as 70% of cases

Microscopic Pathology

- Tumor cells usually arranged in a reticular pattern (giving the appearance of a loose network of communicating spaces and cysts)
- Tumor cells are typically primitive and have clear (glycogen or lipid) cytoplasm with nuclei that are hyperchromatic, irregular, and have prominent nucleoli
- Mitotic figures are typically numerous

Germ Cell Tumors>Yolk Sac Tumor (Endodermal Sinus Tumor)

- Reticular areas often (~75% of cases) contain *Schiller-Duval bodies* which are characterized by round or elongated papillae with fibrovascular cores containing a single vessel; these papillae are covered with primitive columnar cells and are found in spaces lined by cuboidal, flat, or hobnail cells
- Intracellular and extracellular hyaline bodies are often present and tend to be most numerous in reticular areas and in areas with a hepatoid pattern
- Linear, extracellular accumulations of (periodic acid-Schiff positive) basement membrane material, typically in the reticular and solid areas, present in 90% and represents "parietal" differentiation
- Several histologic variants
    - *Polyvesicular-vitelline*: Cysts lined by columnar, cuboidal, or flattened cells usually separated by a dense spindle-cell stroma; cysts may have eccentric constrictions
    - *Hepatoid*: Present in 15% to 50%; cells are large, polygonal, and have abundant eosinophilic cytoplasm with distinct cell borders; nuclei tend to be central with a single prominent nucleolus; hepatoid cells tend to grow in solid masses separated by thin bands of fibrous tissue and resemble hepatocellular carcinoma; hyaline bodies are usually very numerous
    - *Glandular*: Typically sparsely distributed in either the reticular or polyvesicular-vitelline areas
        - *Intestinal glandular variant:* Glands lined by pseudostratified columnar epithelium that may resemble mature enteric epithelium (may contain neuroendocrine, goblet and/or Paneth cells)
        - *Endometrioidlike variant:* Tubular glands and villi resembling endometrioid adenocarcinoma; glands often lined by cells with cytoplasmic vacuoles (resemble malignant secretory glands); nests of hepatoid cells (resemble squamous morules) and densely cellular, mitotically active, fibrous stroma may be present

Special Stains

- PAS with diastase will highlight hyaline bodies present in most yolk sac tumors

Immunohistochemistry

- 75% to 100% positive for AFP; staining is cytoplasmic and often weak and focal; hepatoid foci are usually strongly positive for AFP
- Intracellular and extracellular hyaline eosinophilic globules usually show negative immunoreactivity for AFP
- 50% positive for α_1-antitrypsin and PLAP
- Occasionally tumor cells positive for CEA (reactivity localized to cells and glands with enteric features)
- Tumor cells are typically strongly positive for cytokeratin and negative for EMA
- Tumor cells with a spindle cell morphology are typically positive for vimentin
- Tumor cells usually negative for CD30 (80% of embryonal carcinomas positive for CD30)

Electron Microscopy

- Confirms presence of round intracellular, nonmembrane-bound cytoplasmic inclusions (correspond to hyaline bodies seen on light microscopy)
- Basement membrane material is seen to be both intracellular and extracellular
- Hepatoid cells appear quite similar to the cells of hepatocellular carcinoma

Molecular Alterations

- None

Differential Diagnosis

- Clear cell carcinoma (age of patient most helpful in making differentiation)
- Endometrial adenocarcinoma, endometrioid type
- Hepatocellular carcinoma
- If neoplasm is predominantly hepatoid, the differential diagnosis includes steroid cell tumor; oxyphilic variant of clear cell carcinoma, metastatic melanoma, and metastatic hepatocellular carcinoma
- Dysgerminoma
- Embryonal carcinoma (cells of embryonal carcinoma are larger and more pleomorphic than the cells of a yolk sac tumor and usually line glands or papillae or grow in solid sheets)

- Juvenile granulosa tumor
- Small cell carcinoma of hypercalcemic type
- Sertoli-Leydig tumor

Treatment

- Unilateral salpingo-oophorectomy with excision of as much pelvic disease as possible with adjuvant combination chemotherapy

Prognosis

- Patients with stage I disease have survival rates of 70% to 90%
- Patients with higher than stage I disease have survival rates ranging from 30% to 50%
- Some evidence that patients with multiple histologic patterns have a better prognosis than patients with only 1 or 2 histologic patterns

Associations

- Dermoid cyst will be present in the opposite ovary in up to 5%
- May arise in patients with gonadal dysgenesis
- May occur in association with an endometrioid or mucinous ovarian tumor

Mixed Malignant Germ Cell Tumors

Clinical Manifestations

- Represent approximately 10% of malignant germ cell tumors

Gross Pathology

- Typically lobulated with a focally hemorrhagic cut surface

Microscopic Pathology

- A mixture of 2 or more types of germ cell neoplasia (dysgerminoma, yolk sac tumor, embryonal carcinoma, polyembryoma, choriocarcinoma, and/or immature teratoma)
- Dysgerminoma present in approximately 75%, yolk sac tumor in 65%, immature teratoma in 60%, embryonal carcinoma in 15%, and choriocarcinoma in 15%
- Most tumors contain only 2 components (most commonly dysgerminoma and yolk sac tumor)

Special Stains, Immunohistochemistry, and Electron Microscopy

- See individual germ cell tumors

Molecular Alterations

- None

Differential Diagnosis

- Thorough sampling will help ensure that all of the germ cell components are identified

Treatment and Prognosis

- Surgical excision with adjuvant chemotherapy
- Prognosis appears to be influenced by the nature of the malignant elements present as well as the quantity of the most malignant component (the most malignant component must account for more than 30% of the tumor volume)

Associations

- None

Gonadoblastoma

Clinical Manifestations

- Almost always occurs in patients with dysgenic gonads and intersex syndrome; 80% in phenotypic females, 20% in phenotypic males
- Patients typically have female internal genitalia that result from persistent Müllerian duct-derived structures
- 40% bilateral (frequency of bilaterality in phenotypic males slightly less)
- Gonads typically have the features of mixed gonadal dysgenesis (unilateral streak gonad or streak testis and contralateral testis or bilateral streak testis)
- Phenotypic females typically virilized
- Phenotypic males present under the age of 20 years with feminizing symptoms (gynecomatasia, hypospadias, and cryptorchidism)

Gross Pathology

- 25% are microscopic

- When visible on gross examination, usually brown to yellow to gray with a soft, fleshly consistency
- Cartilage-like areas and gritty calcifications may be present
- Areas of hemorrhage or necrosis may represent the presence of an invasive germ cell tumor

Microscopic Pathology

- Typically an admixture of germ cells resembling seminoma cells and small, immature Sertolilike cells arranged in round to irregularly shaped nests that contain hyaline deposits of basement membrane that are surrounded by sex cord cells
- Less often the sex cord cells are arranged peripherally around a nest of seminomalike cells or surround individual seminomalike cells in the nest (a pattern reminiscent of a primary ovarian follicle)
- Calcifications in 80%
- Leydiglike cells, with or without Reinke crystals in the periphery of 65%
- Typical invasive germ cell tumors may develop from a gonodoblastoma (the presence of coarse calcifications in an invasive germ cell tumor is an indication it likely arose from a gonadoblastoma)

Special Stains

- None

Immunohistochemistry

- Seminomalike cells stain for PLAP
- Sertolilike cells stain with cytokeratins and vimentin
- Basement membrane material stains with laminin
- Some of the sex cord cells stain with inhibin

Electron Microscopy

- Immature Sertoli cells may contain Charcot-Böttcher filaments

Molecular Alterations

- Y chromosome almost always present, usually as 45,X/46,XY mosaicism or 46,XY

Differential Diagnosis

- Dysgerminoma
- Sex cord tumor with annular tubules (SCAT)
- Unclassified germ cell sex cord-stromal tumors

Treatment and Prognosis

- Bilateral gonadectomy curative unless germ cell neoplasm present

Associations

- Approximately 50% incidence of progression to invasive germinoma (seminoma or dysgerminoma)
- 5% to 10% progress to embryonal carcinoma, yolk sac tumor, or teratoma
- Gonadoblastomalike foci present in 15% of normal fetuses and newborns

Sertoli-Stromal Cell Tumors

Sertoli Cell Tumor

Clinical Manifestations

- Represents 4% of Sertoli-stromal cell tumors
- Average age at diagnosis 30 years
- Usually nonfunctioning, but may be estrogenic, androgenic, or rarely progestogenic; tumors of the lipid-rich type may cause isosexual pseudoprecocity
- Tumors of oxyphil cell type seen in association with Peutz-Jeghers syndrome

Gross Pathology

- Always unilateral
- Average 9 cm in diameter and are typically lobulated, solid, and yellow or brown

Microscopic Pathology

- Lobules of round or elongated, hollow or solid tubules separated by variable amounts of fibrous stroma that may be hyalinized and contain rare Leydig cells
- Hollow tubules typically lined by cuboidal cells with moderate amounts of cytoplasm, which may be either densely eosinophilic or pale and vacuolated

- Solid tubules tend to contain closely packed cells with small nuclei with little cytoplasm or large cells with abundant eosinophilic cytoplasm (oxyphilic) or moderate to abundant cytoplasmic lipid (lipid-rich Sertoli cell tumor)
- Tumor cells are rarely atypical or mitotically active

Special Stains

- Oil red O will highlight cytoplasmic lipid in lipid-rich variant *(folliculome lipidique)*

Immunohistochemistry

- Tumor cells are typically reactive for cytokeratins and inhibin and negative for EMA

Electron Microscopy

- Confirms the tubular arrangement of the Sertoli cells which are characterized by the presence of interdigitating cell borders, basal lamina, cell junctions, and Charcot-Böttcher crystalloids

Molecular Alterations

- None

Differential Diagnosis

- Sertoli-Leydig cell tumor (SLCT)
- Low-grade endometrioid carcinoma
- Krukenberg tumor
- Carcinoid tumor with a solid trabecular pattern

Treatment

- Unilateral salpingo-oophorectomy

Prognosis

- 1 report of malignancy

Associations

- 2 Sertoli cell tumors have been reported in sisters with Peutz-Jeghers syndrome

Sertoli-Leydig Cell Tumor

Clinical Manifestations

- Represents fewer than 0.5% of all ovarian tumors
- 75% are younger than 30 years old; 10% are older than 50 years; the average age is 25 years
- Well-differentiated tumors occur at the average age of 35 years
- Retiform tumors occur at the average age of 15 years
- 30% of patients present with virilization (usually manifest by the onset of oligomenorrhea followed within months by amenorrhea)
- Women note the loss of secondary sex characteristics with atrophy of the breasts and disappearance of normal bodily contours; progressive masculinization is characterized by the appearance of acne, hirsutism, temporal balding, deepening of the voice, and enlargement of the clitoris
- Androgen secretion may result in erythrocytosis
- Symptoms of virilization are less frequent in the retiform variant and in variants that contain heterologous elements
- Patients usually have elevated levels of testosterone, androstenedione, and other androgens
- Urinary 17-ketosteroids are usually normal (in contrast to virilizing adrenal tumors)
- 50% of patients will have no endocrine manifestations and will present with abdominal swelling or pain
- Tumors rarely associated with estrogenic manifestations

Gross Pathology

- 98% are unilateral and rarely extend beyond the ovary
- Most often solid, lobulated, and yellow; may contain cysts filled with blood
- Poorly differentiated tumors tend to be larger than well-differentiated tumors and are more likely to have areas of hemorrhage and necrosis
- Tumors with heterologous elements or a retiform component are more likely to be cystic; tumors with a large heterologous mucinous component may closely resemble a mucinous cystic tumor
- Grossly visible polypoid excrescences may be seen within the cysts of retiform tumors (simulate serous papillary cystic tumors or a hydatidiform mole)

Subtypes (WHO classification)

- Well-differentiated SLCT
- SLCT with intermediate differentiation
- Poorly differentiated SLCT
- SLCT with retiform component
- SLCT with heterologous elements

Microscopic Pathology

- *Well-differentiated SLCT:*
  - Typically a predominantly solid or hollow tubular pattern
  - Hollow tubules are typically round or oval and small but may be dilated; occasionally simulate endometrial glands; usually lumens are empty but occasionally contain eosinophilic fluid
  - Solid tubules are often elongated and resemble prepubertal or atrophic testicular tubules
  - Cells that comprise the tubules tend to be cuboidal or columnar and have moderate to large amounts of cytoplasm that may be densely eosinophilic or vacuolated and lipid-rich
  - Nuclei of tumor cells are round or oblong without prominent nucleoli; nuclear atypia and mitotic figures rare
  - Stromal component consists of bands of fibrous tissue with variable conspicuous clusters of Leydig cells, 20% of which contain Reinke crystals
- *SLCT of intermediate differentiation*:
  - Sertoli and/or Leydig cells have variable degrees of immaturity
  - Aggregates of Sertoli cells are separated by a fibrous to densely cellular to edematous stroma that usually contains clusters of well-differentiated Leydig cells
  - Immature Sertoli cells have small, round, oval, or angular nuclei and are arranged typically in ill-defined masses that give the lesion a lobulated appearance
  - Sertoli cells may be arranged in solid and/or hollow tubules, nests, and short cords that resemble sex cords of embryonic testis
  - Small or large cysts with eosinophilic secretions giving the lesion a thyroidlike appearance may be present
  - Edema and Leydig cell aggregates are conspicuous in patients who are pregnant
  - Both Sertoli and Leydig cells may contain variable amounts of lipid that appears as small or large droplets in the cytoplasm
  - Differentiation that allows identification of Sertoli cell aggregates and Leydig cell aggregates is best seen at the periphery of the cellular lobules
- *Poorly-differentiated SLCTs:*
  - Cells are spindle-shaped and resemble cells of a fibrosarcoma, an undifferentiated carcinoma, or a primitive germ cell tumor
  - Usually lack the lobulation or orderly arrangement of Sertoli and stromal elements characterize intermediate differentiation
  - Mitotic rate usually exceeds 10 mitotic figures per 10 high power fields (hpf)
- *SLCT with a retiform component:*
  - Overall architectural pattern resembles that of rete testis; this pattern is present in 10% of SLCTs and when present is the predominant pattern in 50%
  - Retiform pattern has never been reported in association with well-differentiated tumors
  - Characterized by irregularly branching, elongated, narrow, slitlike tubules and cysts
  - Papillae or polypoid structures project into the lumens of the tubules and cysts giving the lesion a glomeruloid appearance
  - Most frequently the papillae are small and rounded and contain hyalinized cores; occasionally the papillae will be large and bulbous with edematous cores, or delicate and branching and lined by stratified cells that are reminiscent of a borderline or invasive serous tumor
  - Frequently the retiform variant contains columns or ribbons of immature Sertoli cells
  - The stroma in the retiform area may be hyalinized or edematous and either moderately or densely cellular

- *SLCT with heterologous elements*
  - Present in 20% of SLCTs and are typically confined to tumors with intermediate or poor differentiation
  - Most common (90%) heterologous elements consist of glands or cysts lined by moderately to well-differentiated gastric or intestinal-type mucinous epithelium (goblet cells, argentaffin cells, and occasionally Paneth cells)
  - Usually the mucinous epithelium appears benign, but occasionally may resemble a low-grade adenocarcinoma
  - Mucin often extravasates from glands or cysts into the adjacent stroma and may stimulate a giant cell reaction
  - Occasionally tumors with mucinous elements contain microscope foci of insular or goblet cell carcinoid
  - Stromal heterologous elements that include islands of cartilage and/or immature skeletal muscle present in 25%

Special Stains

- Grimelius stain can confirm the presence of argyrophil cells and a focus of carcinoid tumor in a Sertoli cell tumor with heterologous elements

Immunohistochemistry

- SLCTs are typically positive for α-inhibin (Leydig cells are more intensely positive than Sertoli cells)

Electron Microscopy

- Sertoli cells form tubular structures and are characterized by interdigiting cell borders, basal lamina, cell junctions, and rarely Charcot-Böttcher crystalloids
- Leydig cells contain smooth endoplasmic reticulum, lipid, lipofuscin, mitochondria with tubular cristae, and occasional Reinke crystals

Molecular Alterations

- Rare familial occurrence (some also have thyroid disease)

Differential Diagnosis

- Endometrioid carcinomas with sex cord-like differentiation
- Tubular Krukenberg tumor
- Carcinoid tumors with a trabecular pattern
- Struma ovarii with a tubular pattern
- Poorly differentiated lesions (especially those with few sex cord elements) may be mistaken for sarcoma or undifferentiated neoplasm
- SLCT with heterologous elements may resemble a teratoma or mucinous tumor
- Retiform SLCT may resemble yolk sac tumor, serous tumors, and malignant mixed müllerian tumors
- Retiform SLCT with sarcomatoid areas or heterologous areas containing skeletal muscle or cartilage may be misdiagnosed as malignant mesodermal mixed tumor

Treatment

- Young patients treated with unilateral salpingo-oophorectomy if tumor confined to 1 ovary
- Poorly differentiated tumors, tumors that contain heterologous elements, and tumors that have ruptured are typically treated with aggressive surgical resection and adjuvant chemotherapy
- Occasionally radiation therapy and combination chemotherapy may be of benefit

Prognosis

- Removal of the tumor typically results in the return of normal menses and some diminution in the excessive hair, but clitoromegaly and voice changes tend to persist
- Neoplasms are more likely to be clinically malignant if they are poorly differentiated and/or have heterologous elements
- Tumors with a retiform pattern are more likely to be malignant and have a worse prognosis
- Rupture of the neoplasm, particularly if it is of intermediate differentiation, is more likely to be associated with malignancy
- Tumors that present at a stage higher than stage I are almost always fatal

- Recurrence typically occurs early (65% of clinically malignant tumors recur within 1 year; recurrence is usually confined to the pelvis, but distant metastasis occur)
- Recurrent tumor is usually less differentiated than the original tumor and may resemble a soft tissue sarcoma

Associations

- Sarcoma botryoides of the cervix (rare)
- Thyroid disease (solitary or multiple adenomas or nodular goiter and occasionally Graves disease and carcinoma)

Sex Cord Tumor With Annular Tubules

Clinical Manifestations

- May present as a sporadic lesion or as an associated finding in patients with Peutz-Jeghers syndrome
- When the tumor occurs as a sporadic lesion:
    - Almost always presents as a palpable mass
    - Associated with estrogenic manifestations in 40%
    - Average age at diagnosis 34 years
    - 20% malignant
    - When the tumor occurs in association with Peutz-Jeghers syndrome:
    - Almost always an incidental finding
    - Average age at diagnosis 27 years
    - Always benign

Gross Pathology

- When sporadic, the lesion is almost always unilateral and on sectioning is typically yellow and solid
- When seen in association with Peutz-Jeghers syndrome the tumor is often bilateral (65%) and not recognized on gross examination (a tumorlet)

Microscopic Pathology

- Simple or complex annular tubules
- Simple tubules are ring shaped and the cells have nuclei that are oriented peripherally; the center of the tubule consists of hyaline basement membrane material; an intervening cytoplasmic halo forms the majority of the ring
- Complex tubules tend to be rounded structures consisting of intercommunicating rings surrounding multiple hyaline bodies
- Tumors in patients with Peutz-Jeghers syndrome often consist of multiple tumorlets varying from single tubules to clusters of tubules scattered throughout the ovarian stroma; occasionally islands of vacuolated sex cord cells distended with lipid may be present as well as foci in which the tubule pattern is replaced by a diffuse pattern; more than 50% have calcification (occasionally extensive) within tubules
- Tumors unassociated with Peutz-Jeghers syndrome may have extensive hyalinization of both the tubules and stroma; in addition areas of microfollicular granulosa cell tumor and well-differentiated Sertoli cell tumor may be present

Special Stains

- Not helpful

Immunohistochemistry

- Tumor cells typically reactive for inhibin

Electron Microscopy

- Bundles of Charcot-Bottcher filaments may be seen in the cells of the annular tubules (a finding consistent with Sertoli cell differentiation)

Molecular Alterations

- None

Differential Diagnosis

- Gonadoblastoma (typically seen in patients with a gonadal disorder and a Y chromosome)
- Sertoli cell tumor

Treatment

- Primary treatment is surgical

Prognosis

- 20% of tumors unassociated with Peutz-Jeghers syndrome are clinically malignant and metastasize by way of lymphatics; occurrences are usually late
- All tumors associated with Peutz-Jeghers syndrome are benign

Associations

- Peutz-Jeghers syndrome: Gastrointestinal hamartomatous polyposis, oral and cutaneous melanin pigmentation, occasionally adenoma malignum (minimal deviation adenocarcinoma) of the uterine cervix, and carcinoma of the gastrointestinal tract, pancreas, or breast

Sex Cord-Stromal Tumors

Adult Granulosa Cell Tumor

Clinical Manifestations

- 1% to 2% of all ovarian neoplasms
- 95% of all granulosa cell tumors
- Typically occur between the ages of 50 and 55 years
- Most common ovarian neoplasm to secrete estrogen; effect of the estrogen secretion typically seen in the endometrium as hyperplasia, often with foci of atypia, and occasionally (5%) as low-grade endometrial adenocarcinoma
- Women who present with hyperestrogenism typically have abnormal uterine bleeding or isosexual pseudoprecocity
- Usually women experience abdominal pain; 10% to 15% will present with an acute abdomen secondary to rupture of the neoplasm with a subsequent hemoperitoneum
- 80% to 90% are stage I at time of diagnosis

Gross Pathology

- 95% are unilateral
- The external surface is typically intact but may be disrupted
- Cut surface typically multicystic with interspersed yellow to white, soft to firm solid areas, and focal areas of hemorrhage and occasionally focal areas of necrosis
- Occasionally the entire neoplasm will be solid with areas of hemorrhage and, less frequently, areas of necrosis

Microscopic Pathology

- Granulosa cells grow in solid (diffuse), trabecular, insular, and follicular (macrofollicular and microfollicular) patterns; less frequent architectural patterns include macrofollicular, watered silk (undulating parallel rows of granulosa cells), and gyriform (zigzag arrangement of cords of granulosa cells); an admixture of patterns frequently present
- Microfollicular pattern consists of numerous small follicles reminiscent of the *Call-Exner bodies* of a graafian follicle; these follicles are typically separated by well-differentiated granulosa cells growing in a diffuse pattern and are filled with eosinophilic material and nuclear débris
- Granulosa cells tend to be haphazardly oriented, small with little cytoplasm, and have pale, uniform, oval to angular, and frequently grooved nuclei
- Mitotic rates vary, but mitotic activity is almost always present
- Stromal component usually scant, but may be fibrous; typically contains some cells resembling theca externa cells or luteinized theca interna cells
- Rarely encountered features include a predominance of hollow tubular or solid tubular patterns; focally luteinized granulosa cells, bizarre, large cells with hyperchromatic or multiple nuclei, foci of hepatic or sarcomatous differentiation, and areas reminiscent of poorly differentiated carcinoma

Special Stains

- Reticulin stains will reveal the presence of fibrils surrounding nests and solid areas of theca cells individually or in small groups; granulosa cells are not surrounded by reticulin in contrast to fibro-thecomas.

Immunohistochemistry

- Granulosa cells are typically positive for inhibin, vimentin, cytokeratin (punctate staining), S-100 protein, and smooth muscle actin
- Granulosa cells typically negative for cytokeratin-7 and EMA
- Stromal component may be focally positive for desmin

Electron Microscopy

- Granulosa cells have mitochondria with tubular cristae and abundant smooth endoplasmic reticulum

Molecular Alterations

- Consistent trisomy for chromosome 12

Differential Diagnosis

- Undifferentiated carcinoma
- Cellular fibroma and thecoma
- Small cell carcinoma of hypercalcemic type
- Endometrial stroma sarcoma
- Endometrial adenocarcinoma (especially diffuse, insular, or trabecular pattern)
- Call-Exner bodies of adult granulosa cell tumor may resemble the acini of a carcinoid tumor
- Gonodoblastoma
- Sex cord tumor with annular tubules
- Metastatic melanoma and metastatic breast carcinoma

Treatment

- Bilateral salpingo-oophorectomy with total hysterectomy
- If preservation of fertility is an issue, a unilateral salpingo-oophorectomy can be performed (careful examination of the other ovary must show no evidence of involvement; 5%-10% are bilateral)

Prognosis

- Characterized by slow growth and late recurrence (10+ years)
- Histologic pattern, grade, mitotic activity, and ploidy have little effect on prognosis of
- Stage I disease
- 10-year survival rate 85% to 95% for stage I; 25% to 50% for higher stages
- Recurrent disease is usually fatal
- Tumor >10 cm and/or rupture at time of diagnosis are poor prognostic indicators

Associations

- Endometrial hyperplasia and carcinoma (see clinical manifestations above)
- When present in children, 75% associated with isosexual precocity

Juvenile Granulosa Cell Tumor

Clinical Manifestations

- Represents fewer than 5% of all granulosa cell tumors
- More than 95% occur in the first 3 decades of life
- 80% of those that occur before puberty cause isosexual pseudoprecocity
- Postpubertal patients usually present with abdominal pain and or swelling that may be associated with menstrual irregularity and/or amenorrhea
- 6% present with an acute abdomen secondary to rupture with subsequent hemoperitoneum

Gross Pathology

- 2% bilateral
- Cut surface similar to that of adult granulosa cell tumor; typically an admixture of cystic and solid areas: The solid areas consist of yellow to gray tissue that may contain extensive areas of necrosis and hemorrhage
- Spread outside the ovary is unusual (2%) and when it occurs tends to be confined to the pelvis

Microscopic Pathology

- Typically a solid cellular neoplasm with foci of round to oval follicles; the proportion of follicles to solid areas varies greatly from tumor to tumor
- Follicles vary in size and shape (typically smaller than the macrofollicles occasionally seen in adult granulosa cell tumors but always larger than Call-Exner bodies)
- Follicles contain eosinophilic or basophilic secretions
- Neoplastic granulosa cells typically line follicles in variable numbers of layers and often blend into the more cellular areas between the follicles; neoplastic granulosa cells are typically round with abundant eosinophilic or vacuolated (luteinized) cytoplasm and a rounded hyperchromatic nucleus that is very rarely grooved

- Marked nuclear atypia in 10% to 15%
- Mitotic figures (sometimes atypical) frequent
- Thecal cells usually present and tend to be more spindled in shape than granulosa cells and contain moderate to large amounts of intracytoplasmic lipid (vacuolated cytoplasm)

Special Stains

- Mucicarmine will highlight the contents of the follicles

Immunohistochemistry

- Tumor cells positive for α-inhibin and negative for EMA

Electron Microscopy

- See adult granulosa cell tumor

Molecular Alterations

- Consistent trisomy for chromosome 12

Differential Diagnosis

- Adult granulosa cell tumor
- Malignant germ cell tumor (especially yolk sac tumor or embryonal carcinoma)
- Thecoma
- Surface epithelial-stromal tumors (especially clear cell, undifferentiated, and transitional cell carcinoma)
- Small cell carcinoma of hypercalcemic type
- Metastatic melanoma

Treatment

- Unilateral salpingo-oophorectomy (stage I)

Prognosis

- Survival rate higher than with adult granulosa cell tumor
- Most significant prognostic factor is stage
  - Stage I tumors typically behave in a benign fashion (97% survival)
  - Stage II tumors are typically fatal; recurrence tends to occur early (within 3 years of surgery)

Associations

- Ollier disease (enchondromatosis)
- Maffucci syndrome (endochondromatosis and hemangiomatosis)

Steroid Cell Tumors

Leydig Cell Tumor

Variants

- *Hilus cell hyperplasia or tumor*: Arises from Leydig cells in the hilum of the ovary, lies in the ovarian hilus, and is separated from the medullary stroma; more common
- *Leydig cell tumor*, non-hilar type: Originates from ovarian stromal cells and lies within ovarian stroma; very rare

Clinical Manifestations

- Represents approximately 20% of all steroid cell tumors
- Average age at diagnosis is 50 to 60 years
- 75% to 80% of patients will have hirsutism or virilization secondary to testosterone production (estrogenic manifestations rare)
- Androgenic changes typically develop slowly and are not as prominent as seen in SLCTs
- Patient may present with a palpable pelvic mass
- Almost always benign

Gross Pathology

- Typically <5 cm in diameter (mean diameter ~2.5 cm)
- Tends to be well-circumscribed, centered in the hilus, and ranges in color from red-brown to yellow to dark brown with foci of hemorrhage
- Typically centered in or near the ovarian hilum
- Rarely bilateral

Microscopic Pathology

- A diffusely arranged circumscribed mass of steroid cells
- Nuclei may cluster and be separated by eosinophilic areas devoid of nuclei
- Occasionally a prominent fibrous stroma gives the lesion a nodular appearance
- 30% will have vessels, the walls of which appear to contain fibrinoid material

- Tumor cells typically have round, hyperchromatic nuclei with a single prominent nucleolus; some pleomorphism may be present as well as bizarre nuclei; occasional nuclei contain pseudoinclusions of cytoplasm
- Tumor cells typically have abundant eosinophilic cytoplasm, which may contain lipid and/or lipochrome pigment
- Elongated eosinophilic crystals of Reinke must be present in the cytoplasm or nucleus of tumor cells to confirm the diagnosis (often very difficult to find)
- 30% have fibrinoid replacement of walls of moderate-sized vessels without an accompanying inflammatory infiltrate
- Mitotic figures rare
- Criteria for diagnosis of *hilus cell tumor*:
  - Hilar location
  - Background of hilus cell hyperplasia
  - Close association with nonmedullated nerve fibers
  - Fibrinoid degeneration of vessels within tumor
  - Uniform nucleus-free zone around blood vessels

Special Stains

- Oil red O may highlight the lipid content of some of the Leydig cells

Immunohistochemistry

- Tumor cells typically positive for inhibin

Electron Microscopy

- Reinke crystals are typically seen as rod-shaped when cut longitudinally and hexagonal when cut transversely; the inner portions of the crystal have a cross-hatched appearance

Molecular Alterations

- None

Differential Diagnosis

- Steroid cell tumor, not otherwise specified
- Stromal luteoma
- Sertoli cell tumor
- Oxyphilic clear cell carcinoma and oxyphilic endometrioid carcinoma
- Hepatoid yolk sac tumor
- Pregnancy luteoma

Treatment and Prognosis

- A benign neoplasm treated with unilateral oophorectomy

Associations

- May produce androgens resulting in hirsutism or virilization (75%)
- May produce estrogen

Steroid Cell Tumor, Not Otherwise Specified

Clinical Manifestations

- Represents approximately 60% of all steroid cell tumors
- Tends to occur in women in their mid-40s
- 40% associated with androgenic changes; 10% associated with estrogenic changes; occasionally associated with progestogenic changes
- Case reports of tumors producing cortisol with or without Cushing syndrome and aldosterone; also hypercalcemia, erythrocytosis, and ascites
- 5% bilateral

Gross Pathology

- Usually 3 to 10 cm, well-circumscribed, smooth or lobulated, and solid
- Cut surface yellow or orange (reflection of intracytoplasmic lipid) or red or dark brown to black (less intracytoplasmic lipid and more lipochrome pigment)
- Foci of necrosis, hemorrhage, and cystic degeneration may be present

Microscopic Pathology

- Typically a diffuse (occasionally nests or columns) arrangement of polygonal or round cells with distinct borders and moderate to abundant cytoplasm that is either eosinophilic and granular (lipid poor) to vacuolated (lipid rich) with a central nucleus containing a prominent nucleolus

- Stroma usually inconspicuous
- Intracytoplasmic lipochrome present in 50%
- Lipid content of the cytoplasm may be quite prominent giving individual cells a signet ring-like appearance
- Nuclear atypia and mitotic figures are both fairly unusual (when present tumor considered malignant)

Special Stains

- Oil red O will confirm the presence of intracytoplasmic lipid

Immunohistochemistry

- Tumor cells typically positive for α-inhibin
- Vimentin positive in 75%, CAM 5.2 positive in 45% (globoid paranuclear staining), AE1/AE3 positive in 40%
- EMA and S-100 protein positive in <10%
- Tumor cells are negative for CEA, chromogranin A, α-fetoprotein, and HMB-45

Electron Microscopy

- Confirms presence of lipochrome pigment and lipid in tumor cells

Molecular Alterations

- None

Differential Diagnosis

- Tumors containing oxyphil cells
- Luteinized granulosa cell tumor
- Sertoli cell tumor
- Oxyphilic clear cell carcinoma and endometrioid carcinoma
- Hepatoid yolk sac tumor, hepatoid carcinoma, and metastatic hepatocellular carcinoma
- Melanoma
- Oxyphilic struma ovarii
- Oxyphilic pituitary type tumor in dermoid cyst
- Primary paraganglioma
- Malignant mesothelioma
- Tumors containing clear cells
    - Clear cell carcinoma
    - Endometrioid carcinoma
    - Dysgerminoma
    - Brenner tumor
    - Yolk sac tumor
    - Melanoma
    - Renal cell carcinoma

Treatment

- Unilateral oophorectomy for stage IA
- Chemotherapy has not proven to be effective in high stage tumors or recurrent tumors

Prognosis

- Extraovarian spread is present at the time of initial surgery in 20%
- Most patients with Cushing syndrome have widespread intra-abdominal neoplasm
- Pathologic features associated with malignancy include:
    - Diameter >7 cm
    - 2 or more mitoses per 10 high-powered fields
    - Necrosis and hemorrhage
    - Grade II or III nuclear atypia

Associations

- See clinical manifestations earlier in this section

Stromal Tumors

Fibroma and Cellular Fibroma

Clinical Manifestations

- Represents 4% of all ovarian tumors
- Seen most frequently in middle age with the average patient being between 45 and 50 years at the time of diagnosis; 10% are seen in patients under the age of 30 years

- Meigs syndrome and Gorlin syndrome (see associations later in this section)
- 10% to 15% of tumors larger than 10 cm associated with ascites

Gross Pathology

- Approximately 10% bilateral; 75% bilateral if patient has Gorlin syndrome
- Sectioning reveals a solid, hard, flat, chalky white surface
- Areas of edema with cyst formation are fairly common (occasional tumors are predominantly edematous)
- Foci of hemorrhage may be present (more frequently a characteristic of cellular fibromas)
- Approximately 10% have areas of calcification (calcification almost always present in tumors from patients with Gorlin syndrome

Microscopic Pathology

- Typically intersecting bundles of spindle cells with little cytoplasm (occasionally storiform pattern) that produce collagen
- Hyaline bands or plaques and varying degrees of intercellular edema (sometimes with a myxoid appearance) often present
- Cytoplasm of the neoplastic spindle cells may contain small quanties of lipid or eosinophilic hyaline droplets
- Tumor cells show little or no atypia and mitotic figures are rare
- 10% are densely cellular (almost as cellular as a diffuse granulosa cell tumor) and are referred to as *cellular fibromas*; mitotic figures are more common in these lesions
- Occasional tumors will contain a minor component of a sex cord element (eg, granulosa cells, undifferentiated sex cord-type cells, or sertoliform tubules)

Special Stains

- Oil red O stain will confirm the presence of lipid in some of the tumor cells
- Reticulin-rich mesh surrounds individual cells

Immunohistochemistry

- Rarely immunoreactive for inhibin

Electron Microscopy

- Lack of cytoplasmic lipid helps differentiate fibroma cells from thecoma cells

Molecular Alterations

- None

Differential Diagnosis

- Thecoma
- Massive edema
- Fibromatosis
- Stromal hyperplasia
- Primary endometrioid stromal sarcoma or metastatic endometrial stromal sarcoma
- Krukenberg tumor

Treatment

- Oophorectomy

Prognosis

- Almost always benign
- Cellular fibromas, even when mitotic figures are present, have a low malignant potential but can recur in the pelvis or upper abdomen

Associations

- Meigs syndrome (seen in 1%): Ascites and pleural effusion accompanying an ovarian fibroma; the ascites and pleural effusion disappear on removal of the tumor
- Gorlin syndrome (nevoid basal cell syndrome): Multiple nevoid basal cell carcinomas, multiple jaw keratocysts, developmental defects of skeletal system (rib, vertebral and craniofacial), palmar and plantar pits (defective keratin production), epidermal inclusion cysts, ectopic calcification (falx cerebri, diaphragma sella), ovarian fibromas, medulloblastoma, meningioma and cardiac fibroma

Sclerosing Stromal Tumor

Clinical Manifestations

- Typically seen during the first 3 decades of life (average ages 25-30 years)
- Rarely associated with evidence of estrogen or androgen secretion
- Case reports of androgenic manifestations during pregnancy

Gross Pathology

- Sharply demarcated tumor that on cut section tends to be solid and white with areas of edema and cyst formation; rarely predominantly cystic
- Range in size from 10 to 20 cm
- Typically unilateral

Microscopic Pathology

- Cellular nodules separated by areas of acellular, densely collagenous, or edematous stroma
- Nodules of cells consist of a disorganized admixture of spindled fibroblasts producing collagen and rounded, vacuolated cells; variable amounts of sclerosis present
- Rounded, vacuolated cells contain lipid and have small, dark, eccentric nuclei (resemble signet ring cells)
- Prominent thin-walled ectatic blood vessels (reminiscent of those of a hemangiopericytoma) usually present within the cellular nodular areas
- If the tumor is functioning (and occasionally in nonfunctioning tumors) lutein cells resembling those of a luteinized thecoma may be present

Special Stains

- Oil red O stains confirm the presence of lipid in the rounded, vacuolated cells
- Reticulin mesh surrounds individual cells

Immunohistochemistry

- Occasionally immunoreactive for inhibin

Electron Microscopy

- Not helpful

Molecular Alterations

- None

Differential Diagnosis

- Fibroma and thecoma
- Krukenberg tumor
- Hemangiopericytoma

Treatment and Prognosis

- Oophorectomy
- Benign

Associations

- None

Thecoma

Variants

- Typical thecoma
- Luteinized thecoma

Clinical Manifestations

- Typical thecoma:
  - □ Most women present in their late 50s or early 60s; <10% present before age 30
  - □ Usually estrogenic with postmenopausal bleeding in 60%
  - □ Almost always unilateral (>95%)
  - □ Approximately 20% (in postmenopausal women) have a concurrent endometrial carcinoma
- Luteinized thecoma
  - □ 50% are estrogenic; 40% are nonfunctioning; 10% are androgenic
  - □ Tends to occur in younger patients than typical thecomas; 30% occur before age 30 years
  - □ Rarely bilateral

Gross Pathology

- On sectioning, a solid lobulated yellow or white mass
- Cystic changes and foci of hemorrhage and necrosis are occasionally present
- Foci of calcification may be present (thecomas with extensive calcification more likely in younger women)

Microscopic Pathology

- Sheets of ill-defined round or oval cells with abundant vacuolated cytoplasm (contain moderate to large amounts of lipid)
- Nuclei tend to be pale and vary from round to spindled with little or no atypia
- Mitotic figures are rare or absent
- Hyaline plaques are usually conspicuous and may be confluent
- Stroma may contain foci of calcification
- Reticulin fibrils typically surround individual tumor cells
- Lutein cells of a luteinized thecoma are present as single cells, as nests, or occasionally as large nodules and are almost always mitotically active; if Reinke crystals present the tumor is called a *stromal Leydig cell tumor*

Special Stains

- Oil red O stain demonstrates abundant intracytoplasmic lipid
- Reticulin stains highlight fibrils surrounding individual tumor cells

Immunohistochemistry

- Tumor cells stain positively for α-inhibin

Electron Microscopy

- Cytoplasmic lipid droplets

Molecular Alterations

- Tumors are usually aneuploid

Differential Diagnosis

- Fibroma
- Granulosa cell tumor
- An extensively luteinized thecoma may resemble a steroid cell tumor, stromal hyperthecosis, and a pregnancy luteoma

Treatment and Prognosis

- Oophorectomy
- Nearly always benign

Associations

- A luteinized thecoma characterized by a dense proliferation of plump spindle cells and focal differentiation into small lutein cells may be associated with sclerosing peritonitis
- 20% of thecomas associated with endometrial carcinoma (also associated with mixed müllerian tumors and endometrial stromal sarcomas)

Surface Epithelial-Stromal Tumors

Serous Tumors

Variants

- Benign (serous cystadenoma)
- Borderline (serous tumor of low malignant potential)
- Carcinoma (serous carcinoma)

Clinical Manifestations

- Approximately 30% of all ovarian neoplasms
- 60% are benign, 10% are borderline, and 30% are carcinomas
- Benign tumors most commonly occur in women during the reproductive ages
- Borderline tumors are rare before the age of 20 years; average age approximately 45 years
- Carcinoma is seen at an average age of 55 years (extremely rare before the age of 20 years); 80% associated with an elevated serum CA125
- Carcinomas occassionally associated with paraneoplastic endocrine abnormalities (secondary to the production of steroid hormones) and hypercalcemia (etiology currently unknown)

Gross Pathology

- Benign (serous cystadenoma)
  - 1 or multiple thin-walled cysts filled with watery fluid
  - Cyst lining may be smooth or have polypoid nodules typically composed of dense stroma that may be firm or soft
  - 10% to 20% bilateral
  - Serous surface papillary adenofibromas appear as nodules on the outer surface of 1 or both ovaries; usually limited in extent, but may be quite extensive
  - Serous adenofibromas and cystadenofibromas are usually hard white or yellow, solid, fibrosis tumors that contain glands or cysts filled with clear fluid; lining may have polypoid nodules
- Serous tumors of low malignant potential:
  - The lining of cyst(s) consist of extensive fine polypoid excrescences with or without similar papillary lesions on the surface of the ovary
  - Cystic fluid may be mucoid
  - Contain a white to yellow solid fibrous component
  - 70% confined to 1 or both ovaries (25%-30% bilateral); spread within pelvis in approximately 10%; spread to lymph nodes and/or upper abdomen in approximately 20%
  - Extraovarian spread more likely in tumors with exophytic (serosal) component (60%) than in tumors with no exophytic component (4%)
- Serous carcinoma
  - May be cystic with papillary excrescences or completely solid with or without a papillary surface
  - Occasionally the tumor is entirely exophytic (serous surface carcinoma), but more typically a portion of the underlying ovary will be replaced by neoplastic tissue
  - 65% bilateral (~25% of stage I tumors bilateral)
  - 15% confined to 1 or both ovaries; spread within pelvis in approximately 10%; spread to lymph nodes and/or upper abdomen in 55%; distant spread in 15% to 20%

Microscopic Pathology

- Benign tumors:
  - Cysts lined by epithelium similar to that of the fallopian tube (cells typically ciliated and lack nuclear atypia)
  - Occasionally cysts will be lined by a nonciliated cuboidal or columnar epithelium
  - Psammoma bodies may be present (usually inconspicuous)
  - Polypoid areas are usually composed almost entirely of stroma (may be dense and collagenous or edematous)
- Borderline tumors of low malignant potential (primary tumors):
  - Polypoid nodules and papillae arise from the lining of a cyst, the outer surface of the ovary or both
  - Cells that line cysts and comprise the epithelium of the papillae tend to be stratified and have mild to marked nuclear atypia and mitotic activity and occasional mitotic figures
  - Diagnosis of "borderline" typically based on 4 rather characteristic features:
    - (1) formation of cellular buds that appear to float in the intracystic fluid,
    - (2) cells with at least some degree of nuclear atypia,
    - (3) absence of "obvious" invasion of the stromal component of the ovary, and
    - (4) hierarchical branching
  - Tumor cells usually have little cytoplasm although the cells in the papillary buds may have prominent eosinophilic cytoplasm
  - Psammoma bodies may be present
  - At times there may be an extensive penetration of stroma by tubular structures and microcysts with papillae that do not produce a stromal reaction (without a stromal reaction this phenomenon should *not* be interpreted as invasion)
  - Occasionally sharply demarcated desmoplastic plaques may be seen on the outer surface of the ovary or on the inner (cystic) surface of the tumor; these features resemble non-invasive desmoplastic implants that can be seen in the pelvic peritoneum (these findings should *not* lead to the incorrect diagnosis of carcinoma)

- Borderline tumors of low malignant potential (microinvasion): One or more discrete foci of single epithelial cells and small clusters of epithelial cells most of which have abundant eosinophilic cytoplasm and borderline features within the stroma; no single area can exceed 10 square mm (a predictor of the appearance of invasive implants); stromal free papillae can be quite proliferative and are highly predictive of invasive implants
    - Psammoma bodies may be present
    - A stromal reaction characteristic of invasive carcinoma is absent
    - Vascular invasion present in approximately 10%
- Borderline tumors of low malignant potential (implants):
    - 65% of borderline serous ovarian tumors with an exophytic component will have peritoneal implants; neoplasms without an exophytic component will have peritoneal implants in <5%
    - 2 different types of implants:
        - Non-invasive (epithelial and desmoplastic type)
        - Invasive
    - Microscopic features of an implant should be evaluated independent of the associated ovarian neoplasm
    - Peritoneal implants may appear as benign foci of serous epithelium forming glands, cysts, and occasionally papillae with psammoma bodies (endosalpingiosis), as noninvasive deposits of borderline epithelium and stroma, and as invasive implants morphologically identical to serous carcinoma
- Carcinoma:
    - Characterized by high cellularity, nuclear atypia, cellular budding, and obvious stromal invasion
    - Neoplastic cells almost invariably have more pronounced nuclear atypia than is seen in borderline tumors
    - Typically the neoplasm appears malignant throughout all sections and only occasionally will have components that appear to be either benign or borderline
    - Papillae are almost always present (extent of papillae formation may be quite variable)
    - Solid proliferations of tumor cells with irregular slitlike spaces may be present (a characteristic of poorly differentiated tumors)
    - Other patterns include thin tubular glands lying in a dense collagenous stroma with or without large deposits of psammoma bodies; innumerable psammoma bodies within a dense fibrous stroma (*psammocarcinoma*); papillae lined by tumor cells lying in spaces without an endothelial lining; adenoid cystic carcinomalike component; foci of squamous differentiation; microcysts; multinucleated giant cells (reminiscent of syncytiotrophoblast cells); focal reticular pattern (similar to that of a yolk sac tumor)

Special Stains

- Cytoplasm of serous carcinoma cells frequently PAS positive and diastase resistant

Immunohistochemistry

- Serous carcinoma cells typically positive for Leu-M1, B72.3, BerEP4, CEA, CK7, EMA, and p53
- Tumor cells in borderline tumors may stain with S-100 protein
- 50% can be demonstrated to have receptors for estrogens, progesterone, and androgens

Electron Microscopy

- Not helpful

Molecular Alterations

- 65% of carcinomas are aneuploid
- p53 mutations common

Differential Diagnosis

- Benign tumors:
    - Epithelial inclusion cyst (epithelial inclusion cyst is ≤1 cm in diameter; serous cystadenoma is >1 cm)
    - Rete cystadenoma (characterized by hilar location and smooth muscle and hilus cells in walls)
    - Cystic struma ovarii
    - Endometrioid adenofibroma
    - Incidental warty excrescence on the surface of an otherwise normal ovary in an adult (tend to be multifocal and microscopic)

- Borderline tumors:
    - Mucinous borderline tumors (endocervical-like)
    - Retiform Sertoli-Leydig tumors
    - Serous tumor arising from an extraovarian site (particularly the peritoneum)
    - Implants of borderline serous tumors should not be confused with noninvasive implants from serous carcinoma
    - Florid mesothelial hyperplasia
- Carcinoma:
    - Endometrioid adenocarcinoma
    - Clear cell carcinoma with a papillary pattern
    - Retiform SLCTs
    - Primary ependymoma of the ovary
    - Malignant epithelial mesothelioma
- Secondary ovarian involvement by serous carcinoma arising in the fallopian tube, endometrium, or extraovarian peritoneum
    - Poorly differentiated carcinoma of the breast metastatic to the ovary

Treatment

- Benign tumors: Salpingo-oophorectomy with ovarian conservation of the opposite ovary if bilateral
- Borderline tumors: Hysterectomy and bilateral salpingo-oophorectomy with surgical staging
- Young woman who desire to preserve reproductive function can be treated with unilateral oophorectomy and careful followup with eventual likelihood of a residual salpingo-oophorectomy and hysterectomy
- Unilateral or bilateral cystectomy is associated with a recurrence in the residual ovarian tissue in 10% to 15%
- Postoperative adjuvant chemotherapy or radiation has not proven to be a benefit in stage II, III, and IV borderline tumors unless invasive peritoneal implants are present
- Carcinoma: Hysterectomy and bilateral salpingo-oophorectomy with staging to include lymph node sampling
- In young women who desire preservation of reproductive function treatment can consist of a unilateral oophorectomy if the lesion is low grade and unilateral

Prognosis

- Benign tumors:
    - Cured by salpingo-oophorectomy
- Borderline tumors:
    - Presence or absence of nuclear atypia, the DNA ploidy status, and the presence or absence of invasion in implants may have significant prognostic value
    - Survival rate approaches 100% for patients with stage I tumors
    - Five year survival for stage I, II, and III tumors is 90% to 95%
    - Patients with spread of tumor beyond the ovary may not die of their disease for more than 10 years (survival rate may drop from approximately 95% to 75% between 5 and 20 years)
    - Micropapillary pattern associated with a worse prognosis in stage II and III disease
    - Lymph node involvement probably does not affect survival
- Carcinoma:
    - 5-year survival: 75% (stage I); 55% (stage II); 25% (stage III); 10% (stage IV)

Associations

- Familial ovarian cancer seen in BRCA mutations

Mucinous Tumors

Variants

- Benign (mucinous cystadenoma)
- Mucinous tumor of low malignant potential(endocervical-like and intestinal-like)
- Carcinoma

Clinical Manifestations

- Typically the largest of all ovarian neoplasms (often >30 cm)
- Represents 10% to 15% of all ovarian neoplasms; 75% benign, 10% borderline, and 15% carcinoma

- Benign tumors usually diagnosed in women between 30 and 50 years
- Mucinous tumors of low malignant potential and carcinomas usually occur in older women; average age between 50 and 55 years
- Carcinomas have an elevated serum CA125 in 65% to 70%, CEA in approximately 85%, and carbohydrate antigen (CA19-9) in 85%

Gross Pathology

- *Benign (mucinous cystadenoma)*
  - Usually multilocular with thin walls; occasionally unilocular
  - Fluid may be thick to watery
  - 5% bilateral
- *Mucinous tumor of low malignant potential (endocervical-like and intestinal-like)*
  - 6% of intestinal-like borderline tumors and carcinoma are bilateral
  - 40% of endocervival-like borderline tumors are bilateral
- *Mucinous carcinoma (invasive)*
  - Foci of necrosis and/or hemorrhage are more common in carcinomas than in borderline or benign tumors

Microscopic Pathology

- *Benign (mucinous cystadenoma)*
  - Glands and cysts with an epithelial lining consisting of a single row of uniform mucin-filled columnar cells with basal nuclei (lining resembles endocervical endothelium)
  - Less commonly the lining resembles intestinal epithelium and contains of goblet cells, argyrophil cells, cells containing serotonin and peptide hormones, argentaffin cells and Paneth cells
- *Mucinous tumors of low malignant potential (endocervical-like and intestinal-like)*
  - Epithelial lining tends to be intestinal-like; a minority (~10%) will be completely devoid of intestinal-type epithelium (designated endocervical-like)
- *Intestinal-like mucinous borderline tumors* often lack papillae or have delicate branching papillae (filiform) that are lined by atypical epithelium that includes variable numbers of goblet cells and other cells characteristic of the epithelium of the gastrointestinal tract; often contain benign, borderline, and carcinomatous areas within the same tumor
- *Endocervical-like (Müllerian) mucinous borderline tumors* have an architecture similar to that of serous borderline tumors with large and small papillae with prominent cellular budding; papillae are lined by slightly atypical epithelial cells that may be up to 20 cells thick and contain abundant cytoplasmic mucin (some may be devoid of mucin and have eosinophilic cytoplasm instead); a diffuse acute inflammatory infiltrate is almost always present in the stroma; 30% will contain area(s) of endometriosis
- Extravasated pools of mucin frequently associated with histiocytes and a foreign body giant cell reaction are found in the stroma in 25% to 30% *(preudomyxoma ovarii)*
- *Mucinous carcinoma (invasive)*
  - Stromal invasion defined as either disorderly penetration of cyst wall or stromal component by carcinoma cells, with or without a stromal reaction
  - May have endocervical-like cells, intestinal-type cells, or both, but most frequently the cells are not classically endocervical or intestinal
  - Tumor cells may be arranged in cysts, glands, clusters, solid sheets, and individually and may resemble those of a well-differentiated endometrioid adenocarcinoma or a typical adenocarcinoma of the large intestine
  - Stroma usually resembles ovarian stroma but may be desmoplastic and/or extensively infiltrated by inflammatory cells
  - Extravasated pools of mucin are found in the stroma in 25% to 30% (frequently associated with histiocytes and a foreign body giant cell reaction)
- Mural nodules in mucinous tumors
  - Nodules in the walls of mucinous tumors may have histologic features markedly different from those of a mucinous tumor and are classified as:
    - Anaplastic carcinoma
    - Sarcoma of various histologic types
    - Carcinosarcoma
    - Sarcomalike nodules
    - Mixed nodules
    - Leiomyomas

Special Stains

- Not helpful

Immunohistochemistry

- Tumor cells express CEA, keratin, and EMA
- Typically negative for vimentin

Electron Microscopy

- Not helpful

Molecular Alterations

- Malignant tumors show K-*ras* (unlike serous tumors)

Differential Diagnosis

- Serous and endometrioid carcinomas with abundant luminal mucin
- SLCTs with heterologous mucinous epithelium
- Mucinous carcinoid tumor
- Metastatic adenocarcinoma from the gastrointestinal tract, biliary tract, pancreas, and uterine cervix

Treatment

- Stage I mucinous borderline tumors are treated with unilateral oophorectomy in patients who desire preservation of reproductive function (it is important to remember that approximately 40% of patients with endocervical-like mucinous borderline tumors will have bilateral disease)

Prognosis

- 5-year survival rate for stage I mucinous borderline tumors is almost 100%; 5-year survival for stage II is 90% to 100%; and for stage III 50%
- 5-year survival for stage I mucinous carcinoma is 85% to 90%, stage II 55%, stage III 20%, and stage IV 10%
- Mucinous tumors tend to recur late (survival rate drops from 95% to 87% if the follow-up period extends to 15 years)
- Presence of extraovarian spread (peritoneal implants or lymph node metastasis) in patients with endocervical-like mucinous borderline tumors has little prognostic significance
- Patients with mural nodules of anaplastic carcinoma usually have a rapidly fatal clinical course
- Patients with sarcomalike mural nodules do not appear to have a worse prognosis

Associations

- 5% of mucinous tumors develop an association with dermoid cyst
- Mucinous tumors may be associated with mucinous tumors of other organs (especially the appendix; an association that is almost always accompanied by *pseudomyxoma peritonei*)
- Mucinous ovarian tumors may be accompanied by mucinous adenocarcinoma of the cervix (especially adenoma malignum); an association that occurs in patients with Peutz-Jeghers syndrome
- May produce hormonal manifestations secondary to the secretion of steroid hormones, gastrin (Zollinger-Ellison syndrome), and carcinoid syndrome
- Endocervical-like mucinous borderline tumors are associated with endometriosis in the other ovary in 30% of cases and endometriosis in the same ovary in 20% of cases; intestinal-type mucinous borderline tumors are rarely associated with endometriosis
- Endocervical-like mucinous borderline tumors are essentially never associated with pseudomyxoma peritonei; pseudomyxoma peritonei is an associated finding in intestinal type mucinous tumors in 15% to 20%

Pseudomyxoma Peritonei

- Characterized by implantation of mucin-producing epithelial cells on the peritoneal surface and accumulation of mucin in the peritoneum
- May result from:
  - □ Rupture of a benign cystadenoma or cystadenocarcinoma of the appendix
  - □ Rupture of a benign mucinous tumor, mucinous tumor of borderline malignancy (intestinal type), or a mucinous carcinoma of the ovary
  - □ Invasion by a cystadenocarcinoma from another site
- When synchronous appendiceal and ovarian mucinous tumors are present, are they 2 independent primaries or is 1 the primary (either ovarian or appendiceal) and the other, a metastasis? Clinicopathologic studies favor intestinal (appendiceal) origin in most cases.

Endometrioid Tumors

Variants

- Benign (adenofibroma and cystadenofibroma)
- Low malignant potential
- Carcinoma

Clinical Manifestations

- All variants occur primarily in women in the peri-menopausal and postmenopausal age groups
- Most endometrioid tumors are carcinomas (benign and borderline tumors fairly rare)
- One of the most common primary neoplasms (nonendocrine) associated with endocrine manifestations (typically caused by the secretion of steroid hormones)
- Benign endometrioid tumors are associated with endometriosis in the same ovary or at another site in the pelvis in 25% to 30%
- Borderline endometrioid tumors are associated with endometriosis in 35% to 40%
- Endometrioid carcinoma is accompanied by ipsilateral ovarian endometriosis in 10% to 40% and by pelvic endometriosis in 10% to 30%; patients with an endometrioid carcinoma associated with endometriosis tend to be younger by 5 to 10 years than women without endometriosis
- -Serum CA125 elevated in 80% (Note: CA125 may be elevated in endometriosis, adenomyosis, and leiomyomas)

Gross Pathology

- Indistinguishable on gross examination from other surface epithelial-stromal neoplasms
- May have recognizable small foci of endometriosis or an endometriotic cyst
- Benign and borderline tumors tend to be predominantly solid but may contain variable numbers of cysts
- Benign endometrioid tumors (adenofibromas) and borderline tumors are almost always unilateral
- Endometrioid carcinomas may be solid or cystic
- Cystic carcinomas may have a thin soft papillary lining or a large fungating mass that protrudes into the lumen containing a chocolate-colored fluid
- Stage I endometrioid carcinomas are bilateral in 15% to 20% of cases

Microscopic Pathology

- Benign tumor (endometrioid cystadenofibroma)
  - Lined by stratified, nonciliated, non-mucin-containing epithelium
  - No endometrial-type stroma
- Benign tumor (endometrioid adenofibroma)
  - Irregularly shaped glands lined by stratified non-mucin-containing epithelium in a fibromatous stroma
  - Epithelium may be simple columnar, cuboidal or flat (resembles the epithelium of a serous adenofibroma)
  - Foci of squamous differentiation (morules) may be present
- Borderline tumors
  - Atypical or cytologically malignant endometrioid type cells arranged in aggregates or lining cysts or glands
  - "Obvious" stromal invasion is absent
  - Stromal invasion characterized by haphazard infiltration of stroma (usually accompanied by a stromal reaction) by glands or cysts or back-to-back arrangements of glands
- Carcinoma
  - Typically resemble endometrial adenocarcinoma of the uterine corpus
  - Invasive, round, oval, or tubular glands lined by stratified, non-mucin-containing epithelium usually with an orderly cribriform pattern of glandular differentiation
  - 30% to 50% will have foci of squamous differentiation; the squamous component may be either benign or malignant (adenoacanthoma or adenosquamous carcinoma respectively)

- *Various uncommon patterns may be present and represent pitfalls in the differential diagnosis*:
  - A villoglandular pattern
  - Sex-cord-like foci
  - Focal to abundant areas of spindle-shaped epithelial cells
  - Tumor cells with oxyphilic cytoplasm (may represent clear cell carcinoma0
  - Glands that resemble 16-day secretory endometrium
  - Neuroendocrine (argyrophil cells) (present in 10%)
  - Clear cell component (present in 20%-25%)
  - Epithelial islands and trabeculae reminiscent of a granulosa cell tumor
  - Luteinized cells throughout stroma

Special Stains

- Not helpful

Immunohistochemistry

- Tumor cells express EMA, CA125, and cytokeratin 7 (95% positive)

Electron Microscopy

- Not helpful

Molecular Alterations

- None

Differential Diagnosis

- Serous and mucinous neoplasms
- Endometrioid adenofibroma with squamous morular differentiation resembles as a Brenner tumor
- Secretory type endometrioid adenocarcinoma resembles a clear cell adenocarcinoma
- Granulosa cell tumor
- Sex cord-stromal tumor (Sertoli cell tumor or SLCT)
- If endometrioid carcinoma of the ovary is accompanied by endometrial adenocarcinoma of the uterine corpus:
  - May be synchronous occurrence of two primary neoplasms
  - May represent a metastasis from one organ to the other
- Extragenital metastatic carcinoma (especially from gastrointestinal tract

Treatment

- Similar to that of other ovarian epithelial cancers (serous and mucinous)

Prognosis

- 5-year survival for stage I, 75% to 80%; stage II, 60% to 65%; stage III, 25%; and stage IV, 5% to 10%

Associations

- Endometriosis in the same ovary or at any site in the pelvis all types of endometrial hyperplasia with or without atypia may be present in the foci of endometriosis
- Endometrial adenocarcinoma of the uterine corpus (usually synchronous but may be metachronous) present in up to 30% of ovarian endometrioid carcinomas

Clear Cell Tumors

Variants

- Benign
- Low malignant potential (rare)
- Carcinoma

Clinical Manifestations

- Benign and borderline clear cell tumors are rare (most are adenofibromas)
- Clear cell carcinoma accounts for 6% of all surface epithelial cancers
- Typical age range for clear cell carcinoma is 5th through 7th decades

Gross Pathology

- On cut section benign and borderline tumors usually adenofibromatous, but may have a spongelike appearance
- Benign and borderline tumors are essentially always unilateral
- Clear cell carcinomas are usually cystic (unilocular or multilocular) with 1 or more white to tan brown polypoid masses arising from the cyst wall and protruding into the lumen; lumen may contain serous or mucinous dark brown fluid
- Clear cell carcinomas rarely bilateral (2%)

Microscopic Pathology

- Benign clear cell tumors have totally benign appearing epithelium with no evidence of invasion
- Borderline tumors have atypical epithelium or frankly carcinomatous epithelium without invasion
- Clear cell carcinomas most frequently have a complex papillary pattern, but may be solid; tumor cells are usually round with clear cytoplasm, have eccentric nuclei and indistinct nucleoli, and are usually hobnailed; may be arranged in solid nests or line cysts, tubules and papillae—all patterns may be present in same tumor
- Papillae of a clear cell carcinoma are usually multiple and complex and contain densely eosinophilic hyaline basement membrane material that actually expands the core of the papillae
- Psammoma bodies may be present
- Oxyphilic cells may be a major component of a clear cell carcinoma and are typically seen lining glands or growing in nests and solid masses
- Hyaline bodies present in 25%

Special Stains

- PAS with diastase confirms the presence of glycogen within the clear tumor cells

Immunohistochemistry

- Not helpful

Electron Microscopy

- Cells have short blunt microvilli on the luminal surface
- Glycogen is seen in the cytoplasm

Molecular Alterations

- None

Differential Diagnosis

- Serous carcinoma
- Endometrial carcinoma, secretory variant
- Germ cell tumors, especially dysgerminoma and yolk sac tumor
- Juvenile granulosa tumor
- Krukenberg tumor (especially when signet-ring cells constitute a major proportion of the neoplasm)
- Metastatic renal cell carcinoma
- Oxyphilic tumors (primary or metastatic)

Treatment

- Benign and borderline tumors: Salpingo-oophorectomy
- Carcinoma:
  - Stage I: Bilateral salpingo-oophorectomy with total hysterectomy
  - Stage II and III: Removal of as much tumor as surgically possible by adjuvant chemotherapy

Prognosis

- Benign and borderline tumors have a benign clinical course
- 5-year survival for stage I, 70%; stage II, 55%; stage III, 15%; and stage IV, 4%
- Survival rates similar to those for undifferentiated carcinoma (worse than for other epithelial neoplasms)

Associations

- Ovarian tumor most likely to be associated with ovarian and/or pelvic endometriosis and paraendocrine hypercalcemia
- Ipsilateral ovarian endometriosis in approximately 25%
- A component of endometrioid carcinoma in 20% to 25%
- Sweet syndrome (acute febrile neutrophilic dermatosis)

Transitional Cell Tumors

Variants

- Benign Brenner tumor
- Borderline Brenner tumor (atypical proliferating)
- Malignant Brenner tumor
- Transitional cell carcinoma

Clinical Manifestations

- May represent an incidental finding in a patient with a mucinous cystic tumor or a dermoid cyst
- Occasionally associated with endocrine manifestations (estrogenic or rarely androgenic); the stromal component of the tumor may secrete steroid hormones
- Benign tumors have peak incidence at age 50 years; borderline and malignant tumors peak at about age 60 years
- Occasionally associated with estrogenic or androgenic manifestations

Gross Pathology

- Benign Brenner tumor:
  - Typically small; 30% microscopic 50% <2 cm
  - 5% to 10% bilateral
  - Typically a sharply circumscribed, solid, firm, white or pale yellow, nodular neoplasm with a smooth or slightly bosselated external surface
  - Multiple tiny cysts may be present throughout as well as flecks of calcification; rarely lesion consists of a large cyst
  - In approximately 25%, another ovarian neoplasm present; 65% are mucinous tumors (almost always benign); remainder serous cystadenomas and dermoid cysts
- Brenner tumor of borderline malignancy
  - Usually cystic and uni- or multilocular
  - Cystic areas may have papillary or polypoid masses arising from the cyst walls and protruding into lumen
  - Almost always unilateral
- Malignant Brenner tumor:
  - Typically have both solid and cystic areas with the cystic areas containing papillary or polypoid masses or solid nodules in their walls
  - Calcifications present in 50%
  - 10% to 15% bilateral
- Transitional cell carcinoma:
  - Resemble malignant Brenner tumor except no calcifications
  - 15% bilateral

Microscopic Pathology

- Benign Brenner tumor
  - Transitional cells arranged in round or oval nests (occasionally trabeculae) in a prominent fibrous stroma
  - Tumor cells have pale cytoplasm and oval nuclei that are frequently grooved
  - Nests of tumor cells may be either solid or have a central cavity filled with dense eosinophilic material; occasionally a transitional cell nest with a cavity will be lined by mucinous, ciliated, serous or undifferentiated glandular epithelium
  - Pure mucinous glands and cysts may be present (metaplastic Brenner)
  - 30% will have spicules of calcification that tend to be located near nests of transitional cells
  - Foci of squamous differentiation may be present in transitional cell nests
- Borderline Brenner tumor
  - Characterized by papillae lined by proliferating transitional-type cells that protrude into lumen of a cyst
  - Mucin-containing cells may be present
  - Criteria for diagnosis: the presence of atypical or frankly carcinomatous transitional cells without stromal invasion

- Malignant Brenner tumor
  - Malignant-appearing transitional cells or squamous cells, with or without the presence of mucinous cells, that clearly invade cyst wall and/or adjacent stroma, usually in a background of benign or borderline tumor
- Transitional cell carcinoma
  - Tumor cells have the characteristics of malignant transitional cells (in most cases at least grade II and usually grade III)
  - 2 characteristic patterns: Intracystic papillary and nests of transitional cells separated by fibrous stroma (may occur together)
  - In 50% small pools of mucin surrounded by glandular epithelium may be present
  - In most cases the transitional cell elements will be mixed with other types of surface epithelial carcinoma (typically serous type)

Special Stains

- Not helpful

Immunohistochemistry

- Tumor cells frequently positive for serotonin
- Tumor cells usually negative for cytokeratin-20 (urothelial tumors are usually positive for cytokeratin-20)

Electron Microscopy

- Tumor cells resemble the transitional cells of the urinary tract

Molecular Alterations

- None

Differential Diagnosis

- Benign Brenner tumor:
  - Insular granulosa cell tumor
- Insular carcinoid
  - Endometrioid adenofibroma with squamous differentiation
- Brenner tumor of borderline malignancy, malignant Brenner tumor and transitional cell carcinoma:
  - Metastatic transitional cell carcinoma of urothelial origin
  - Granulosa cell tumor (either adult or juvenile) with a papillary-cystic pattern
  - Undifferentiated carcinoma

Treatment

- Benign and borderline Brenner tumors are treated with conservative surgery
- Malignant Brenner tumors are managed similarly to other epithelial-stromal malignancies
- Transitional cell carcinomas are treated with surgery and adjuvant chemotherapy

Prognosis

- Borderline Brenner tumors do not metastasize
- Malignant Brenner tumors have an excellent prognosis when confined to the ovary, but extraovarian spread present at time of diagnosis in 20%
- Transitional cell carcinomas have a worse prognosis than malignant Brenner tumors and have an overall 5-year survival rate of 35%
- 5-year survival for stage I malignant Brenner tumor, 85% to 90%; 5-year survival for stage I transitional cell carcinoma, 40% to 45%
- Patients with metastasis composed solely or primarily of transitional cell carcinoma probably respond to chemotherapy better than patients with other forms of metastatic epithelial ovarian carcinoma

Associations

- Synchronous with other ovarian neoplasms (see above)

Teratomas

Carcinoid Tumors

Variants

- Insular carcinoid
- Trabecular carcinoid
- Strumal carcinoid
- Goblet cell (mucinous) carcinoid

Clinical Manifestations

- 85% to 90% associated with other teratomatous components; 10% to 15% pure
- Insular carcinoid
  - Most common primary ovarian carcinoid tumor
  - Patients range in age from 30 to 80 years
  - 30% present with symptoms of carcinoid syndrome (flushing, diarrhea, murmur of pulmonary stenosis or tricuspid insufficiency, and peripheral edema)
  - Patients with carcinoid syndrome are almost always over the age of 50 years and have large tumors
  - Urinary 5-hydroxyindole acetic acid (5-HIAA) usually elevated
  - Tumor typically confined to the ovary at the time of initial surgery
- Trabecular carcinoid
  - Typically diagnosed between the ages of 30 and 60 years
  - Presenting symptoms are typically those of a slow-growing pelvic mass
  - Not associated with carcinoid syndrome
- Strumal carcinoid
  - Typically occurs between the ages of 30 and 60 years
  - Patients present with symptoms of a pelvic mass
  - Only 1 reported case of the carcinoid syndrome
- Goblet cell (mucinous) carcinoid
  - May have spread beyond the ovary at the time of initial surgery
  - Not associated with carcinoid syndrome

Gross Pathology

- Insular carcinoid
  - Typically a small nodule that protrudes into the lumen of a dermoid or mucinous cyst
  - On sectioning a solid, firm, tan or yellow fibrous nodule; may be cystic (rarely)
  - Unilateral
  - 15% of contralateral ovaries will contain a dermoid cyst, mucinous tumor, or Brenner tumor
- Trabecular carcinoid
  - Similar to insular carcinoid
  - Unilateral
  - Contralateral ovary may contain a dermoid cyst
- Strumal carcinoid
  - Typically an easily recognized combination of thyroid and carcinoid components in varying proportions
  - May appear as a solid nodule protruding into the cavity of a typical appearing dermoid cyst
- Goblet cell (mucinous) carcinoid
  - On sectioning, a solid cream-colored surface that resembles other ovarian carcinoid tumors
  - May occur in a pure form or in association with a mature teratoma or epidermoid cyst

Microscopic Pathology

- Insular carcinoid
  - Masses and nests of tumor cells separated by fibromatous stroma cells are round and uniform and have nuclei with stippled chromatin
  - Mitotic activity is very rare or absent
  - Cells at the periphery of a nest usually have abundant cytoplasm that may contain red or orange or brown argentaffin granules
  - Glandular lumens may contain eosinophilic material that may undergo psammomatous calcification
- Trabecular carcinoid
  - Tumor cells arranged in long, wavy, parallel ribbons usually separated by thin fibromatous stroma
  - Cells tend to be columnar and have abundant eosinophilic cytoplasm that usually contains argyrophilic granules; nuclei are oblong, contain finely dispersed chromatin, and are oriented perpendicularly to the axis of the ribbon
  - Mitotic figures are occasionally present
  - Other teratomatous elements are almost always present
- Strumal carcinoid
  - Typically the 2 components (thyroid and carcinoid) are intimately admixed but 1 component may predominate

- In 50% the carcinoid component has a trabecular pattern
- Thyroid component usually resembles normal thyroid or follicular adenoma; colloid in the thyroid follicles may contain calcium oxalate crystals
- Small foci of glands or cysts lined by mucinous epithelium present in 50%

- Goblet cell (mucinous) carcinoid
  - Acini and nests of goblet cells and argyrophil cells resembling glands with small or inconspicuous lumens floating in pools of mucin (reminiscent of mucinous or goblet cell carcinoid of appendix)
  - Stroma is fibrous and may be scanty or abundant
  - Occasionally hybrid cells containing both mucin and granules may be present
  - Foci of goblet cell carcinoid tumor may be seen in a strumal carcinoid tumor

Special Stains

- Argentaffin and argyrophilic stains highlight the presence of intracytoplasmic granules

Immunohistochemistry

- Insular carcinoid
  - Tumor cells positive for NSE, serotonin, and chromogranin
- Trabecular carcinoid
  - Tumor cells are immunoreactive for chromogranin and synaptophysin
  - In 50% the presence of 1 or more peptide hormones can be demonstrated: Somatostatin, glycogen, pancreatic polypeptide, vasoactive intestinal peptide, neurotensin, enkephalin, calcitonin, corticotropin, and peptide YY
- Struma carcinoid
  - Cells of the carcinoid component are immunoreactive for NSE, chromogranin, synaptophysin, serotonin, and prostatic acid phosphatase
  - In approximately 40%, the carcinoid cells immunoreactive for 1 or more peptide hormones
  - Strumal component (and occasionally foci within the carcinoid component) immunoreactive for thyroglobulin
- Goblet cell (mucinous) carcinoid
  - Occasional cells may be reactive for CEA, pancreatic polypeptide, serotonin, gastrin, and chromogranin

Electron Microscopy

- Insular carcinoid
  - Pleomorphic, reniform, or dumbbell-shaped dense core granules present within the cytoplasm of tumor cells
- Trabecular carcinoid
  - Dense core granules tend to be small, round, and uniform
- Strumal carcinoid
  - Carcinoid cells contain uniform, round, dense core granules
  - Follicles are lined by neuroendocrine type cells and/or by cells typical of thyroid epithelium
  - Hybrid cells with ultrastructural features of both thyroid and carcinoid may be present
- Goblet cell (mucinous) carcinoid
  - Dense core granules may be present

Molecular Alterations

- None

Differential Diagnosis

- Insular carcinoid
  - Metastatic insular carcinoid (usually ileal in origin)
  - Microfollicular granulosa cell tumor
  - Strumal carcinoid
  - Brenner tumor
- Trabecular carcinoid
  - Metastatic carcinoid tumor (typically from the hindgut)
  - Strumal carcinoid
  - SLCT

- Strumal carcinoid
  - If thyroid component scant, confusion with trabecular carcinoid may occur
- Goblet cell (mucinous) carcinoid
  - Goblet cell carcinoid metastatic from the appendix
  - Krukenberg tumor
  - Mucinous tumors

Treatment

- Insular carcinoid
  - Hysterectomy and bilateral salpingo-oophorectomy
  - Postoperative course monitored by urinary 5-HIAA levels
- Trabecular carcinoid
  - Hysterectomy and bilateral salpingo-oophorectomy
- Strumal carcinoid
  - Hysterectomy and bilateral salpingo-oophorectomy
- Goblet cell (mucinous) carcinoid
  - Hysterectomy and bilateral salpingo-oophorectomy with staging if extraovarian spread is present (more likely with this carcinoid than any of the others)
  - The appendix should be removed at the time of oophorectomy

Prognosis

- Insular carcinoid
  - Benign clinical course; recurrence very rare
- Trabecular carcinoid
  - No reports of death secondary to a metastatic disease although peritoneal implants occur
- Strumal carcinoid
  - Benign clinical course; neoplasm rarely extends beyond the ovary
- Goblet cell (mucinous) carcinoid
  - Risk of extraovarian spread is greater than in any of the other types of primary carcinoid tumor

Associations

- Insular carcinoid tumor may be seen mixed with a trabecular carcinoid tumor; this pattern may be associated with hyperinsulinemic hypoglycemia
- Trabecular carcinoid tumor may be associated with chronic constipation (inhibitory effect on gastric motility of peptide YY)
- Strumal carcinoid tumor has been reported in association with hyperinsulinemic hypoglycemia and cutaneous melanosis; also reported in association with multiple endocrine neoplasia , type 2A (Sipple syndrome)
- Goblet cell (mucinous) carcinoid tumor may occur as part of a mature teratoma or epidermoid cyst

Immature Teratoma

Clinical Manifestations

- A germ cell neoplasm consisting of 2 or 3 germ cell elements (ectoderm, mesoderm, endoderm)
- Immature tissue (usually immature neuroepithelium) must be present to warrant the diagnosis
- Represents only 3% of all ovarian teratomas but are 3rd most common primitive germ cell tumor
- Most frequently seen in young adults and children (median age 18 years)
- Usually present as a painful abdominal or pelvic mass
- 65% will have an elevated level of α-fetoprotein
- 30% have spread beyond the ovary at the time initial diagnosis (usually peritoneal implants)

Gross Pathology

- Typically large (median 18 cm), smooth, glistening, well-encapsulated mass that is predominantly solid on sectioning
- Small cysts (and rarely large cysts) that contain mucin, serous fluid, or hemorrhagic fluid may be present
- Elements of a typical dermoid cyst can be identified in 25%
- Solid areas (usually neural) tend to be soft, gray to pink, and fleshy with focal areas of hemorrhage and/or necrosis

Microscopic Pathology

- Immature element usually consists of neuroectodermal tissue (in the form of primitive neuroepithelial rosettes and tubules, mitotically active glia, and sometimes areas that resemble glioblastoma or neuroblastoma)
- Immature elements of epithelium (both ectodermal and endodermal) and mesenchymal tissue (cartilage and skeletal muscle) are common; diagnosis of "immature" requires presence of embryonic tissue, not simply fetal-type tissue
- Grade (based on amount of immature tissue [usually neural] present):
    - Grade 1: Embryonal neural tissue in <1 low-power field (×40) in any slide
    - Grade 2: Embryonal neural tissue in 1 to 4 low-power fields in any slide
    - Grade 3: Embryonal neural tissue in >4 low-power fields in any slide
- Peritoneal implants (peritoneal gliomatosis) or nodal metastases tend be composed of immature glial tissue (rarely consist of mature glial tissue); mature epithelial elements, mature cartilage, or foci of endometriosis may be admixed with glial elements

Special Stains

- Not helpful

Immunohistochemistry

- Neuroectodermal tissue is reactive for GFAP, NSE, and S-100 protein
- If hepatic tissue, yolk sac-like vesicles, and intestinal-type epithelium are present, α-fetoprotein may be expressed
- Syncytiotrophoblastic elements are immunoreactive for hCG

Electron Microscopy

- Not helpful

Molecular Alterations

- Trisomy, tetraploidy, and mosaicism seen in 7% of all teratomas

Differential Diagnosis

- Cerebellar differentiation may resemble neuroepithelium
- Mature solid teratoma
- Typical dermoid cyst with microscopic foci of immature neural tissue
- Malignant mesodermal mixed tumor with heterologous elements
- Neuroectodermal tumor

Treatment

- Unilateral salpingo-oophorectomy with excision of as much extraovarian tumor as possible
- Patients with stage II or III disease and patients with metastasis of immature elements receive combination chemotherapy; chemotherapy typically results in disappearance of high grade metastases but leaves behind mature metastases that may continue to grow

Prognosis

- Sustained remission in 90% to 100% treated with surgery and combination chemotherapy
- Presence of peritoneal gliomatosis *not* associated with an adverse prognosis

Associations

- Increased incidence of immature teratoma in patients with a dermoid cyst (especially if dermoid cysts are bilateral, multiple, or have ruptured)
- Opposite ovary contains a dermoid cyst or other benign tumor in 10%

Mature Cystic Teratoma (Dermoid Cyst)

Clinical Manifestations

- Most common ovarian neoplasm
- 80% occur during the reproductive years
- Represents 50% of ovarian neoplasms in women under the age of 20 years and 65% of ovarian neoplasms in children under the age of 15 years
- 25% are asymptomatic; remainder present as abdominal or pelvic mass with or without pain

- May present as a result of a complication:
  - Torsion with infarction, perforation, hemoperitoneum or autoamputation (5%-15%)
  - Bacterial infection (2%)
  - Perforation (more likely during pregnancy) resulting in a localized or generalized granulomatous peritonitis or a fistula to an adjacent hollow viscus (urinary bladder, vagina, or bowel) or through the anterior abdominal wall (1-2%)
- 50% associated with elevated serum CA19-9; 35% associated with elevated serum CEA

Gross Pathology

- Most <15 cm in diameter with a white to gray smooth external surface
- 15% are bilateral
- On cut surface, one or multiple cysts with a lining reminiscent of skin filled with yellow to brown sebaceous material and hair
- Rounded or polypoid masses attached to the internal surface of the cyst (mamillae) protrude into the lumen and are usually composed of fat (Rokitansky protuberances)
- Teeth are present in 30% (within the cyst wall or free within a cyst cavity or in a rudimentary mandible or maxilla)
- Bone, cartilage, mucinous cysts, adipose, thyroid (20%) and brain tissue may be present as well as partially developed organs (intestine, skull, vertebrae, extremity buds, external genitalia and eyes)

Microscopic Pathology

- All 3 germ cell layers typically present; ectodermal tissue usually predominates; the cyst lining usually composed of epidermis and underlying skin appendages
- Neuroectodermal elements (glia and peripheral nerve) as well as foci of cerebrum, cerebellum and choroid plexus are usually present
- Mesodermal elements consist of smooth muscle, bone, teeth, cartilage, and fat
- Endodermal elements usually consist of respiratory and gastrointestinal epithelium as well as thyroid and salivary gland tissue
- Neuroendocrine cells can be found in the respiratory and intestinal epithelium
- Tissue often arranged in an organoid fashion
- Mitotic figures are almost never seen

Special Stains

- Not helpful

Immunohistochemistry

- Different germ cell elements can be confirmed with immunohistochemical stains
- Neuroendocrine cells may be immunoreactive for a wide variety of hormones (glucagon, gastrin, secretin, insulin, somatostatin, and pancreatic polypeptide)
- The presence of anterior pituitary gland (a rare finding in teratomas) can be confirmed with positivity for growth hormone, prolactin, and/or thyroid-stimulating hormone

Electron Microscopy

- Not helpful

Molecular Alterations

- None

Differential Diagnosis

- Immature teratoma

Treatment

- If patient premenopausal, surgical resection with conservation of ovarian tissue the treatment of choice
- If patient perimenopausal or postmenopausal, unilateral salpingo-oophorectomy is indicated

Prognosis

- Clinically benign (even if microscopic foci of immature tissue present)
- 1% to 2% may contain an adult-type of malignancy (malignant transformation); 80% of these malignancies are squamous cell carcinomas (typically invasive); well differentiated neoplasms are associated with 75% to 80% survival; poorly differentiated neoplasms and sarcomas typically die of tumor

Associations

- 5% to 10% of contralateral ovaries contain a yolk sac tumor or immature teratoma
- Coombs positive autoimmune hemolytic anemia (disappears with removal of tumor)
- Erythrocytosis secondary to secretion of erythropoietin (very rare)
- Ruptured dermoid associated with peritoneal melanosis (focal or diffuse peritoneal tan to black staining) or tumorlike nodules
- 1% to 2% of mature teratomas contain an adult-type cancer; in patients older than 70 years the incidence is 15%; grossly malignant areas usually appear as a cauliflowerlike mass that protrudes into cystic cavity; 80% are squamous cell carcinomas (remainder are adenocarcinoma and variants and various sarcomas)

Mature Teratoma, Solid

Clinical Manifestations

- Seen in the same age group as patients with immature teratoma (young adults and children: median age 20 years)
- Patients almost *never* postmenopausal
- Typically present with an abdominal or pelvic mass

Gross Pathology

- Similar to immature teratoma except the soft gray to pink, fleshy solid areas typical of neural tissue are much less common

Microscopic Pathology

- Mature elements of all 3 germ cell layers present
- Predominant element may be well-differentiated neural tissue (glia)
- Small foci of hepatic, renal, or retinal tissue may be present as well as squamous respiratory and intestinal-type epithelium
- Mitotic activity usually absent
- Mature peritoneal glial implants (peritoneal gliomatosis) may be present

Special Stains

- Not helpful

Immunohistochemistry

- Epithelial and neural markers can confirm the presence of these elements

Electron Microscopy

- Not helpful

Molecular Alterations

- Trisomy, tetraploidy, and mosaicism may be present

Differential Diagnosis

- Immature teratoma (the presence of *any* immature tissue justifies the diagnosis of immature teratoma)

Treatment

- Salpingo-oophorectomy with removal of all surgically accessible tumor

Prognosis

- A benign tumor associated with a benign clinical course even in the presence of mature implants

Associations

- None

Struma Ovarii

Clinical Manifestations

- A monodermal teratoma the predominant or sole component of which is thyroid tissue
- Most frequently diagnosed during the 5th decade of life
- Patients usually present with signs and symptoms of a pelvic mass; 30% have ascites
- 30% have ascites and pleural effusion (Meigs syndrome)
- 5% will have evidence of excess thyroid hormone production and occasionally oophorectomy will be followed by compensatory hypertrophy of the thyroid gland with or without thyrotoxicosis
- 5% to 10% malignant

Gross Pathology

- Cut section reveals obvious reddish or greenish brown, solid, gelatinous tissue characteristic of thyroid
- Occasionally the gross appearance is a unilocular or multilocular cyst with gelatinous or mucoid contents

Microscopic Pathology

- All types and patterns of thyroid tissue may be present: Normal, macrofollicular, microfollicular, pseudotubular, trabecular, and solid adenomas and carcinoma
- Neoplastic thyroid cells tend to appear bland without significant nuclear atypia
- Mitotic figures may be present but are rare
- Colloid within follicles often contains birefringent calcium oxalate crystals
- Oxyphil cells or clear cells may be present (occasionally predominate)
- Struma may be sole component or may associated with another tumor, eg, dermoid cyst, mucinous tumor, carcinoid tumor, or Brenner tumor

Special Stains

- Not helpful

Immunohistochemistry

- Tumor cells reactive for thyroglobulin

Electron Microscopy

- Confirms the neoplastic cells to be thyroid follicular cells

Molecular Alterations

- None

Differential Diagnosis

- Struma with a predominance of oxyphilic or clear cells may be confused with clear cell carcinoma, oxyphilic cell tumors metastatic melanoma, hepatocellular carcinoma, carcinoma of breast, large cell carcinoma of lung, and carcinoid tumor; hepatoid yolk sac tumor; luteinized granulosa cell tumor; steroid cell tumor; paraganglioma, and malignant mesothelioma and metastatic renal cell carcinoma
- Sertoli cell tumor
- Granulosa cell tumor
- Metastatic follicular carcinoma of the thyroid

Treatment

- Benign struma is treated with oophorectomy
- Malignant struma is treated with oophorectomy and removal of as much extraovarian tumor as possible
- Malignant struma with extraovarian spread can be treated with radioactive iodine (^{131}I)

Prognosis

- Typically a benign clinical course even when atypical or malignant microscopic features present
- Factors associated with an increased likelihood of recurrence (may be late) include:
    - Large tumor
    - Adhesions
    - Ascites
    - Solid microscopic pattern
- Presence of peritoneal implants does not necessary imply a worse prognosis and long term survival is likely

Associations

- Contralateral ovary may contain a dermoid cyst or another struma
- 30% of strumas associated with a serous cystadenoma (possibly a serous cyst lined by cells that resemble thyroid epithelium)

Miscellaneous Tumors

Small Cell Carcinoma, Hypercalcemic Type

Clinical Manifestations

- Diagnosed between the ages of 2 and 45 years (mean 24 years)
- Rarely bilateral (<1%) unless familial in which bilaterality approaches 100%
- 65% to 70% have paraendocrine hypercalcemia

Gross Pathology

- Typically large, solid, and lobulated
- Cut section cream-colored and fleshy with foci of hemorrhage and necrosis
- Cystic degeneration common
- 50% have spread beyond the ovary at the time of surgery

Microscopic Pathology

- Most commonly a diffuse arrangement (occasionally insular, nested, cords, or trabeculae) of small, closely packed epithelial cells with scant cytoplasm and small, round, or oval nuclei with a single small nucleolus
- Mitotic figures frequent
- Folliclelike structures containing eosinophilic fluid and lined by tumor cells present in up to 80%
- 50% of neoplasms will have foci in which the neoplastic cells have abundant eosinophilic cytoplasm; these larger cells have a larger and less hyperchromatic nucleus with a more prominent nucleolus
- 10% have foci of mucinous glands lined by benign or atypical epithelium
- Stroma is usually inconspicuous but may be prominent, edematous, hyalinized, or myxoid

Special Stains

- Mucicarmine stain will highlight atypical mucinous cells lining mucinous glands when they are present

Immunohistochemistry

- Tumor cells variably positive for vimentin, cytokeratin, and EMA

Electron Microscopy

- Tumor cells have an epithelial appearance and contain abundant dilated rough endoplasmic reticulum
- No dense core granules

Molecular Alterations

- Rarely familial
- Tumor cells diploid

Differential Diagnosis

- Primary ovarian tumors with small round cells
- Granulosa cell tumor (adult or juvenile)
- SLCT
- Melanoma
- Small cell tumor, pulmonary type
- Primitive neuroectodermal tumor
- Metastatic tumors with small round cells
- Melanoma
- Lymphoma and leukemia
    - Embryonal and alveolar rhabdomyosarcoma
    - Desmoplastic small round blue cell tumor
- Small cell carcinoma pulmonary type
- Merkel cell tumor
- Ewing sarcoma

Treatment

- Bilateral oophorectomy with postoperative radiation
- High-stage tumors are treated with intensive chemotherapy and radiation

Prognosis

- 30% with stage IA will have a disease-free survival of up to 6 years
- Patients with higher stage disease typically die within 2 years
- Factors associated with a better prognosis in stage IA disease include:
    - Normal preoperative calcium level
    - Tumor <10 cm
    - Absence of large cells
    - Patient age >30 years

Associations

- None

Small Cell Carcinoma, Pulmonary Type

Clinical Manifestations

- Very rare (<15 reported cases)
- Average age at diagnosis 55 to 60 years
- Approximately 50% bilateral
- Most have spread beyond the ovary at the time of diagnosis

Gross Pathology

- Typically large (10-15 cm) and solid
- A minor cystic component may be present

Microscopic Pathology

- Tumor cells tend to grow in sheets, islands, and trabeculae
- Tumor cells are usually small to medium-sized, round or spindled, and have little cytoplasm, a hyperchromatic nucleus with stippled ("salt and pepper") chromatin and an inconspicuous nucleolus
- Most contain a differentiated epithelial component (endometrioid carcinoma, focus of squamous differentiation, cyst lined with atypical mucinous cells, or Brenner tumor)

Special Stains

- Argyrophilic stains may highlight the presence of argyrophil cytoplasmic granules

Immunohistochemistry

- Most tumor cells variably immunoreactive for keratin, EMA and NSE; staining for chromogranin and Leu-7 less likely
- Tumor cells typically negative for vimentin

Electron Microscopy

- No reproducible data

Molecular Alterations

- Majority probably aneuploid

Differential Diagnosis

- Small cell carcinoma, hypercalcemic type
- Metastatic tumor from lung or other sites
- Primary and metastatic ovarian tumors with small cells (adult granulosa cell tumor, poorly differentiated SLCT, melanoma, peripheral neuroectodermal tumor, embryonal rhabdomyosarcoma, lymphoma, Merkel cell tumor, neuroblastoma, and Ewing sarcoma)

Treatment and Prognosis

- Surgical resection; most dead within 1 year

Associations

- A Brenner tumor may be present in the same ovary

References

Clement PB, Young RH. *Atlas of Gynecologic Pathology.* Philadelphia: WB Saunders Co, 2000.

Dabbs DJ. *Diagnostic Immunohistochemistry.* New York: Churchill Livingstone, 2002.

Hendrickson MR (ed). *Surface Epithelial Neoplasms of the Ovary: State of the Art Reviews.* Philadelphia: Hanley & Belfus, Inc, 1993.

Mills S, Carter D, Greenson JK, Oberman HA, Reuter V, Stoler MH (eds). *Sternberg's Diagnostic Surgical Pathology. 4th ed.* Philadelphia: Lippincott Williams & Wilkins, 2004.

Rosai J. *Rosai and Ackerman's Surgical Pathology. 9th ed.* St. Louis: Mosby, 2004.

Scully RE, Young RH, Clement PB. *Tumors of the Ovary, Maldeveloped Gonads, Fallopian Tube, and Broad Ligament; Atlas of Tumor Pathology, 3rd Series, Fascicle 23.* Washington DC: Armed Forces Institute of Pathology, 1996.

Tavassoli FA, Devilee P (eds). *World Health Organization Classification of Tumours. Pathology and Genetics of Tumours of the Breast and Female Genital.* Lyon: IARC Press, 2003.

Chapter 7

Gastrointestinal Tract

Intraoperative Consultation

A request for intraoperative consultation involving the gastrointestinal (GI) tract is typically submitted in 1 of 3 clinical situations:

1. To evaluate the adequacy of surgical margins. Usually surgical margins for neoplasm can be evaluated with a gross examination, but occasionally a frozen section examination may be required. This is most commonly encountered when an esophagectomy or a low anterior sigmoid resection has been performed for carcinoma. If the proximal surgical margin of the esophagus or the distal surgical margin of the rectum is positive, an additional resection may be required.
2. Despite a multitude of technological advances involving imaging techniques, endoscopic procedures, and fine-needle aspiration, occasionally intraoperative consultation is requested to render a diagnosis that could not be established preoperatively. The most frequent clinical situation in which this occurs is when surgery is being performed emergently for bleeding, perforation, or obstruction and a possible neoplasm is encountered. Establishing a diagnosis of malignancy in this clinical setting has obvious important immediate surgical management implications.
3. To provide staging information in the case of malignancy. Occasionally lesions that preoperatively appear to be localized turn out on exploration to represent more advanced disease. Frozen section diagnosis on lesions distant from the main neoplasm may have an influence on the procedure performed.

A request for intraoperative consultation during an esophagectomy usually involves evaluation of the proximal surgical margin. Appropriate evaluation requires inking and sampling the entire circumference with full-thickness sections taken parallel to the margin. The inked margins are placed deepest in the block. A focus of cancer anywhere in the block is close enough to recommend additional resection. If cancer is found at the proximal margin, an attempt should be made to differentiate between direct extension and lymphatic permeation. Further resection is justified if direct extension of neoplasm is present, but not if lymphatic permeation is present. One pitfall the pathologist faces in the evaluation of any surgical margin is the fact that radiation and chemotherapy can induce microscopic changes that can be easily confused with malignancy. These changes can appear in the epithelium, the connective tissue, or within submucosal glands. The differentiation between atypical epithelium secondary to radiation and dysplasia/carcinoma in situ may be quite difficult. Radiation effect is typically characterized by a low nuclear-cytoplasmic ratio, the absence of full thickness changes, and the absence of mitotic figures. Before rendering a diagnosis that could potentially represent reactive changes rather than carcinoma the pathologist should determine for certain whether the patient has undergone preoperative radiation and/or chemotherapy.

Gastrectomy specimens taken for resections performed either electively or emergently to evaluate for ulcer disease warrant a frozen section of the ulcer to determine the presence of malignancy. The treatment of benign gastric ulcers and malignant gastric ulcers may be quite different particularly in an emergent setting such as hemorrhage or perforation. Gastrectomy for malignancy may be accompanied by a request for intraoperative consultation concerning the adequacy of surgical margins. The most treacherous tumor to evaluate intraoperatively is the poorly differentiated carcinoma with a diffusely infiltrating pattern (signet ring carcinoma). This neoplasm can spread beyond the grossly visible and palpable lesion and can generate very subtle findings on frozen section. Interpretation of this particular neoplasm represents the vast majority of false-negative diagnoses rendered intraoperatively on tissue specimens from the gastrointestinal tract. Additional false-negative diagnoses may be the result of the fact that this particular neoplasm may have "skip" areas at its advancing edge. Metastatic lobular carcinoma of the breast may mimic a primary signet ring cell adenocarcinoma of the intestine.

Ischemic enteritis involving the small intestine does not require intraoperative consultation. The sites of resection are best determined by the operating surgeon. The presence of mucosal ischemic changes at a surgical margin has little clinical significance.

Occasionally a frozen section request is made during resection for a mass involving the appendix. The reason for the request is to determine if simple appendectomy is adequate treatment. The most common mass lesions of the appendix include carcinoid tumor, mucinous cystadenoma, mucinous cystadenocarcinoma, colonic-type adenocarcinoma, and endometriosis. Each of these lesions may present with

Intraoperative Consultation

symptoms of acute appendicitis and as a consequence represent incidental findings at the time of surgery for what may otherwise appear to be a straightforward diagnosis. Obviously the treatment for endometriosis involving the appendix is radically different from that of adenocarcinoma. One neoplasm that appears to arise exclusively in the appendix is a microglandular goblet cell carcinoma (goblet cell carcinoid). On frozen section it is difficult to differentiate this lesion from a signet-ring cell carcinoma. The distinction is important, because the treatment can be radically different, particularly if the carcinoid tumor is small, does not extend beyond the muscularis propria, and/or is located at the tip of the appendix. If the appendix is enlarged as a result of distension of the lumen by mucous (mucocele), 3 possibilities exist: 1 is non-neoplastic and 2 are neoplastic. A non-neoplastic mucocele results from proximal obstruction of the lumen; the epithelial lining is normal. Mucinous cystadenoma and mucinous cystadenocarcinoma represent fairly common causes of neoplastic mucocele. The former is usually often associated with intraperitoneal mucin. If peritoneal mucin is abundant (pseudomyxoma peritonei), the lesion is more likely a cystadenoma. If there is no extra-appendiceal component, an intraoperative consultation will be required. A benign mucinous cystadenoma is treated with simple appendectomy (assuming a tumor-free margin). A cystadenocarcinoma requires a right hemicolectomy with the removal of as much of the mucinous material from the abdomen as possible. Female patients with a mucinous neoplasm of the appendix should be carefully explored for the possibility of a mucinous carcinoma involving the ovary. A frozen section of any ovarian lesion found in this setting may be requested for definitive diagnosis.

Segmental resections of the colon for neoplasm may require an intraoperative evaluation of the distal margin, if it is within 3 cm of the tumor.

Endometriosis involving the GI tract usually involves the rectosigmoid colon. An incisional biopsy of the colon involved by endometriosis may reveal the presence of glands in a distorted muscularis propria, findings quite reminiscent of an adenocarcinoma.

In the setting of Hirschsprung disease, particularly when a resection is performed as an emergency procedure for acute obstruction, intraoperative consultation is requested to determine the presence or absence of ganglion cells. The surgeon's ability to determine the correct level for a diverting colostomy, which represents the first stage of the surgical management, is dependent on this information. A bowel with ganglion cells cannot be distinguished from a bowel without ganglion cells by means of a gross examination, particularly in the newborn. Ganglion cells are typically easy to identify in older children, but in neonates ganglion cells tend to be quite immature and difficult to identify. Immature ganglion cells lack the characteristic cytologic features of more mature cells. They tend to have little cytoplasm, lack an eccentrically placed prominent nucleus and have inconspicuous nucleoli. Often the frozen section diagnosis is based on architectural features such as the formation of neural units between the 2 layers of muscularis propria. These neural units are characterized by peripherally oriented, small cells that often form a horseshoe or elongated organoid structure. The absence of ganglion cells when accompanied by hypertrophy of nerve fibers is a feature that can be quite helpful in supporting the diagnosis of short-segment aganglionosis. Hypertrophied nerves are not present in long-segment disease.

Crohn disease and ulcerative colitis involving the colon rarely require an intraoperative consultation unless an unexpected malignancy is encountered or there is some question as to which type of inflammatory bowel disease is present. In the setting of equivocal preoperative findings, a definitive intraoperative diagnosis may be required. The creation of an ileal pouch is contraindicated in the presence of Crohn disease; it is usually the procedure of choice in ulcerative colitis. The adequacy of the surgical margin is not an issue; the presence of microscopic inflammatory bowel disease at a margin is of little clinical significance.

Typically GI stromal tumors should not be submitted for frozen section diagnosis. It is often impossible to determine on frozen section if a stromal tumor is benign or malignant based on morphologic features alone. Sampling issues also play a role. The extent of resection is a decision that should be made by the operating surgeon.

The diagnosis of lymphoma involving the GI tract should not be made intraoperatively. Lymphoma cannot be distinguished from undifferentiated carcinoma or a benign lymphoproliferative lesion. The presence of lymphatic tissue and the possibility of a lymphoproliferative disorder can be determined by frozen section, but the final diagnosis should be deferred. If lymphoma is suspected, a lymphoma workup is performed.

Specimen Handling

Resection specimens of the esophagus, stomach, small bowel, and colon for malignancy are generally handled in the same fashion. Proximal and distal margins of resection should be identified, inked, and submitted as sections taken parallel to the margin either circumferentially or at the margin closest to the neoplasm. A section of the neoplasm itself should be taken where it appears to penetrate the wall at its deepest extent and submitted. The esophagus and rectum do not have a peritoneal covering hence the adjacent soft tissue of these specimens should be inked and soft tissue from the area closest to the neoplasm submitted. An accompanying lymphatic tissue specimen should be carefully examined and all lymph nodes should be submitted and identified as to their relationship to the neoplasm.

Colon resections for chronic inflammatory disease should be extensively sampled at least every 10 cm from the proximal margin to the distal margin regardless of the gross appearance of the mucosa.

Esophagus

Adenocarcinoma

Clinical Manifestations

- Represents approximately 35% of all primary esophageal malignancies and 80% of all carcinomas in lower 1/3 of the esophagus
- Appears to have same etiologic factors as Barrett mucosa (reflux and increased alcohol and tobacco consumption)
- Affects men more frequently than women (3 to 7:1)
- Much more common in whites than in blacks; opposite true for squamous cell carcinoma of the esophagus
- Clinical symptoms essentially the same as those for Barrett esophagus: regurgitation, heartburn, dysphagia, and pain with swallowing
- With more advanced disease, patients experience progressively worsening dysphagia with or without associated weight loss

Gross Pathology

- 80% originate in the distal 1/3
- Gross and endoscopic appearance varies from a slight mucosal irregularity or plaque to a large exophytic, fungating, or deeply ulcerated mass
- Most tumors flat and ulcerated; 30% polypoid or fungating
- Does not typically infiltrate diffusely but may occasionally be multifocal
- Salmon-pink mucosa of Barrett esophagus may be present in adjacent mucosa

Microscopic Pathology

- Typically arise from dysplastic epithelium in the setting of Barrett mucosa, but Barrett epithelium may be absent (presumably replaced by the carcinoma)
- Architectural spectrum identical to that of adenocarcinoma of the stomach
- Most tumors are of the intestinal type and may include all of the mature and immature cell types found in the normal esophagus, stomach, or intestine to include endocrine cells, Paneth cells, and squamous epithelium
- Most well to moderately differentiated
- Poorly differentiated lesions typically composed of sheets of uniform epithelial cells containing large vesicular nuclei with prominent nucleoli and often have little in the way of glandular differentiation; tumors tend to be diffusely infiltrative and consist of poorly formed tubules, signet ring cells, and a desmoplastic stroma
- Vascular and perineural invasion frequent
- Presence of mucin can be quite variable and may be present intracellularly, in neoplastic glands, or as extracellular pools; a tumor must be more more than 50% mucinous to be considered mucinous adenocarcinomas

Special Stains

- Mucicarmine will highlight the presence of mucin if it is not readily apparent on hematoxylin-eosin (H&E)

Immunohistochemistry

- Tumor cells may be CEA positive

Electron Microscopy

- Not helpful

Molecular Alterations

- Barrett esophagus without neoplasia express the *MUC2* gene but not the *MUC1* gene
- c-*myc* expression typically present
- H-*ras* gene consistently expressed in both high-grade dysplasia and carcinoma
- *TP53* mutations in 60%

Differential Diagnosis

- Well-differentiated adenocarcinoma may be extremely difficult to differentiate from high-grade dysplasia or carcinoma in situ
- Differentiating high-grade dysplasia from carcinoma on biopsy may be very difficult; cytologic features usually identical in both; invasion must be present to diagnosis carcinoma
- Poorly-differentiated adenocarcinoma may be difficult to distinguish from poorly differentiated squamous cell carcinoma; if Barrett mucosa present, lesion more likely to be an adenocarcinoma

Treatment

- Typically a transhiatal or transthoracic esophagectomy

Prognosis

- Most important prognostic factors include depth of invasion, presence of positive lymph nodes, and overall size
- Survival approximately 90% to 100% for tumors that do not penetrate the muscularis propria
- Survival approximately 45% when the muscularis propria penetrated
- Survival 15% to 25% if neoplasm extends beyond muscularis propria
- Involvement of adjacent organs associated with a 0% survival
- Adenocarcinoma may spread proximally with submucosal lymphatics
- Tumors in the lower 1/3 may metastasize to intraabdominal lymph nodes

Associations

- Barrett mucosa with dysplasia

Comments

Adenocarcinoma of the esophagus can arise in settings unassociated with Barrett esophagus.

Adenocarcinoma can arise from foci of heterotopic gastric mucosa (inlet patch). Foci of ectopic gastric mucosa are present in the esophagus in 3% to 4% of patients undergoing endoscopy; the microscopic incidence is probably higher. Intestinal metaplasia may occur in these areas of ectopic gastric mucosa and carcinoma can arise in these areas as well. Patients typically present with dysphagia. The neoplasm tends to be friable and ulcerated and microscopically resembles a typical adenocarcinoma of the stomach or esophagus. Most arise in the upper 1/3 and are separated from the gastric cardia by a segment of normal squamous epithelium.

Adenocarcinoma can arise in submucosal esophageal glands and their ducts. These lesions appear to be adenoid cystic carcinomas and tend to be very aggressive and rapidly fatal.

Barrett Mucosa and Barrett Dysplasia

Clinical Manifestations

- Normal stratified squamous epithelium that lines the entire esophagus is partially or completely replaced at the lower esophageal sphincter by columnar epithelium that extends for variable distances in a cephalad direction
- Most common predisposing factor chronic (acid or alkaline) gastroesophageal reflux

Esophagus>Barrett Mucosa and Barrett Dysplasia

- Barrett esophagus occurs in 10%-20% of patients with prolonged gastroesophageal reflux
- Incidence of dysplasia in Barrett mucosa varies from 15%-20%
- Incidence of adenocarcinoma at the time of diagnosis of Barrett esophagus 5%-10%
- Barrett esophagus with dysplasia present in 90% of adenocarcinomas
- Barrett esophagus usually diagnosed between ages of 40 and 60 years and frequently associated with heavy cigarette smoking and alcohol abuse
- Most patients asymptomatic; when symptomatic, regurgitation, heartburn, dysphagia, and odynophagia most common complaints

Gross Pathology

- Barrett mucosa usually seen in association with a sliding hiatal hernia
- Typically the gross or endoscopic appearance consists of a segment of red, velvety mucosa that extends in tongues from the esophageal gastric junction into the more proximal esophagus as an irregular, circumferential band that displaces the squamocolumnar junction cephalad; this metaplastic epithelium frequently described as being salmon-pink; in addition whitish squamous islands may be seen more proximally in a distal esophagus; ulcerations may be present anywhere in these areas of metaplastic change

Microscopic Pathology

- Columnar epithelium, typically accompanied by underlying mucous glands, replaces the normal squamous epithelium in the distal esophagus in the region of the esophageal sphincter
- Metaplastic epithelium characterized by various cells to include goblet cells, gastric and intestinal (both small bowel and colonic) columnar cells, intermediate cells (characterized by features of both gastric and intestinal cells), Paneth cells, and endocrine cells
- In the area of lower esophageal sphincter, pancreatic acinar metaplasia may be present in up to 10%
- Presence of goblet cells is the most important diagnostic feature of Barrett esophagus
- Metaplastic epithelium of Barrett mucosa identical to intestinal metaplasia of the incomplete type (type II and type III) in the stomach
- Mucosal surface typically flat and composed of pits or cryptlike structures typical of those of the stomach but occasionally may have a villiform surface (especially in areas of erosion with regeneration)
- Surface epithelium lined by a combination of goblet cells and columnar cells; goblet cells usually contain acidic mucin consisting of admixtures of sialomucins and lesser amounts of sulfomucins; columnar cells may appear as normal gastric foveolar cells, intestinal absorptive cells, or gastric mucous neck cells
- Metaplastic mucous glands usually lie between the metaplastic epithelium and the muscularis mucosae; occasionally these glands "infiltrate" the bands of muscle of the muscularis mucosae and mimic invasive carcinoma
- Barrett mucosa rarely associated with intense inflammatory infiltrate of mononuclear cells, but occasionally inflammation can be quite intense and *H pylori* organisms can be found in the esophagus of patients with Barrett mucosa in cardiac type mucosa

Barrett Dysplasia

- Characterized by a combination of cytologic and architectural abnormalities that usually involve the entire thickness of the mucosa and/or the surface and superficial portion of the glandular crypts
- Dysplastic glands usually have a normal configuration but may show some distortion consisting of budding, branching, crowding, and irregular shapes with papillary extensions into adjacent lumina
- Occasionally a villous architecture may be present as well as cystic dilatation of mucosal glands
- Dysplastic cells typically depleted of mucin and have prominent cytoplasmic basophilia
- 2 types of dysplasia may occur:
  - Dysplastic cells mimic adenomatous change elsewhere in the GI tract and is characterized by nuclear crowding, nuclear stratification, enlarged, elongated and hyperchromatic nuclei, inconspicuous nucleoli, and increased numbers of atypical mitotic figures
  - Dysplastic cells display a loss of polarity but are not stratified; nuclei occupy the basal half of each cell and tend to be round, elongated, pleomorphic, and vesiculated with chromatin lying against the inner surface of the nuclear membrane; nucleoli usually prominent

Esophagus>Barrett Mucosa and Barrett Dysplasia

- 3 grades of dysplasia
  - Low-grade: Characterized by mild architectural changes with little glandular distortion but some degree of crypt branching; cytologic changes less severe with nuclei that are smaller, less hyperchromatic, and generally polarized
  - High-grade: Characterized by marked glandular distortion with branching, complex budding, a cribriform pattern, and occasionally a villiform surface; nuclei tend to be pseudostratified and actually reach the luminal surface of the crypt; basal polarity lost; nuclei large and pleomorphic; bizarre chromatin patterns usually present
  - Indefinite for dysplasia: Cytologic changes that fall short of low-grade dysplasia but typically include a moderately distorted architecture, numerous dystrophic goblet cells, reduced amounts of mucin production, increased cytoplasmic basophilia, some nuclear abnormalities to include increased numbers and stratification; mitotic figures are normal

Special Stains

- Acidic mucins of goblet cells (sialomucins and sulfomucins) stain positively for Alcian blue at a low pH (2.5)
- Alcian blue can be useful in confirming that isolated goblet cells represent a short segment of Barrett mucosa rather than eccentric gastroesophageal junction
- PAS-Alcian blue will stain acid mucin blue and neutral mucins red-purple

Immunohistochemistry

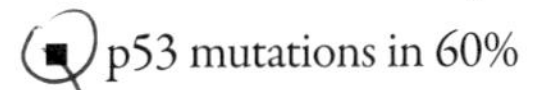

- p53 mutations in 60%

Electron Microscopy

- Not helpful

Molecular Alterations

- Point mutations affecting the *APC* suppressor gene have been seen in both adenocarcinoma and squamous cell carcinoma of the esophagus
- c-*myc* expression present in all grades of dysplasia and carcinoma
- H-*ras* gene consistently expressed in high grades of dysplasia and carcinoma (absent in nondysplastic epithelium)

Differential Diagnosis

- Congential islands of ectopic gastric mucosa (usually of the fundic type)
- Architecturally distorted dysplastic glands may resemble a superficial invasive adenocarcinoma
- Regenerative or reactive epithelial change the most difficult condition to differentiate from dysplasia

Treatment

- Acid suppression with an antireflux procedure can probably reduce the incidence of development of Barrett mucosa in patients with intractable reflux disease
- Patients with biopsy-proven Barrett mucosa with low-grade dysplasia or changes indefinite for dysplasia should undergo frequent endoscopic followup
- Patients with high-grade dysplasia should be considered for esophagectomy
- Low-grade dysplasia typically treated with antireflux measures and repeat biopsies at 6-month intervals for at least 2 years
- Typically biopsies showing high-grade dysplasia are repeated immediately and if confirmed are frequently treated with a transhiatal esophagectomy

Prognosis

- Development of esophageal columnar dysplasia appears to be directly related to prolonged gastroesophageal reflux complicated by Barrett esophagus
- Presence of high-grade dysplasia felt to be a precursor lesion for the development of adenocarcinoma
- Factors that may be responsible for the transformation of squamous epithelium to Barrett mucosa to dysplasia to carcinoma most likely multifactorial and include hereditary factors, infections with *H pylori*, and continued reflux injury
- Reports (sporadic) that Barrett esophagus can regress; to date there is no solid proof that high-grade dysplasia ever regresses
- Risk of developing carcinoma sometime during the lifetime of a patient with Barrett mucosa is 5% to 10% after 50 years of age

Associations

- Adenocarcinoma

Gastroesophageal Reflux

Clinical Manifestations

- Classic symptoms include a substernal burning sensation (heartburn) that tends to radiate toward the mouth
- Occasionally heartburn will be associated with an acid or bitter taste that usually occurs within 1 hour of a meal and is worse when the patient is supine or bends over; heartburn often associated with regurgitation (described by the patient as the sudden appearance of acid or bitter taste in the mouth; may awaken patient from sleep as a result of coughing or strangling often with secretions on the pillow)
- Some patients complain of *water brash*, the sudden filling of the mouth with clear, slightly salty fluid (secretions from the salivary glands that occur by reflex stimulation secondary to acid irritation of the distal esophagus)
- Other less characteristic symptoms include unexplained chest pain, chronic hoarseness, "nonallergic" asthma, chronic hiccups, and dysphagia
- Symptoms typically relieved by the ingestion of some form of antacid
- Development of reflux esophagitis in a patient with gastroesophageal reflux depends on:
    - Volume of refluxed gastric acid (determined by the amount of gastric secretion, efficiency of gastric emptying, and the presence of duodenogastric reflux)
    - Potency of refluxed material (may include pancreatic and biliary secretions as well as acid and pepsin)
    - Efficiency of esophageal clearing of refluxed material (gravity, peristalsis, saliva, and normal esophageal sphincter relaxation with swallowing)
    - Resistance of esophageal squamous epithelium to injury
- At the cellular level, squamous epithelium exposed to gastric and/or biliary contents undergoes increased cellular desquamation and increased epithelial cell turnover; if injury occurs faster than it can be repaired, an inflammatory infiltrate of the epithelium with or without erosion and ulceration may result

Gross Pathology

- Low-grade changes: Normal to slightly erythematous squamous mucosa in the distal esophagus
- High-grade changes: Vary from mild erythema to frank ulceration
- Barrett esophagus: Typically described as salmon-colored tongues or islands extending in a cephalad direction from the esophagogastric junction for various distances

Microscopic Pathology

- Low-grade changes: Widening of the basal zone of epithelium, increased numbers and elongation of vascular papillae, dilated vessels ("lakes") at the top of papillae, loss of longitudinal orientation of surface epithelial cells as a result of the presence of immature cells at the surface, increased mitotic figures, presence of balloon cells in the midzone of the squamous epithelium (balloon cells are enlarged translucent squamous epithelial cells that contain plasma proteins and result from epithelial injury with subsequent increased permeability of the cell membrane), increased mitotic figures in the epithelium, and presence of polymorphonuclear leukocytes (neutrophils and eosinophils) in the epithelium
- High-grade changes: A marked increase in neutrophils in the epithelium as well as in the lamina propria (eosinophils may predominate), edema (characterized by widening of intercellular spaces with some loss of epithelial cohesion), epithelial destruction (characterized by erosion, acute ulcer, or active chronic ulcer), and inflammatory polyps with granulation tissue
- Barrett esophagus
    - A metaplastic columnar-lined mucosa that has replaced the original squamous-lined mucosa
    - Cells that constitute the epithelium of Barrett mucosa include intestinal-type goblet cells, gastric-type columnar mucous-containing cells, columnar epithelial cells with a brush border and no mucous vacuoles (similar to small-intestinal absorptive epithelial cells), Paneth cells, parietal cells, chief cells, and neuroendocrine cells
    - Architecture of Barrett mucosa can include glands with deep and shallow pits similar to gastric mucosa and villous structures similar to small-intestinal mucosa

- Lamina propria of all types of Barrett mucosa may have varying degrees of congestion, edema, acute and chronic inflammation, and fibrosis
- Acute inflammation involving the epithelium often accompanied by reactive epithelial changes that can be easily misinterpreted as dysplasia
- A distinctive-type Barrett mucosa is occasionally encountered and is characterized by villous structures and cryptlike glands with an epithelium that is composed primarily of columnar mucous cells with interspersed goblet cells (a mucosa that is indistinguishable from incomplete intestinal metaplasia seen in the stomach); in addition, absorptive cells, Paneth cells, and endocrine cells may be present

Special Stains

- Distinctive-type Barrett mucosa: Columnar mucous cells stain with PAS confirming presence of gastric-type mucin; goblet cells stain with PAS, Alcian blue, and mucicarmine
- Cardiac-type Barrett mucosa: Mucous-containing epithelial cells stain with Alcian blue, confirming the presence of intestinal-type mucin

Immunohistochemistry and Electron Microscopy

- Not helpful

Molecular Alterations

- None

Differential Diagnosis

- True gastric cardiac or fundic mucosa
- Embryonic ciliated cell rests
- Tracheobronchial remnants
- Gastric heterotopia (ectopia)

Treatment

- Medical management of reflux consists of agents that block acid production and/or neutralize acid
- Once diagnosis of Barrett mucosa established, routine periodic surveillance indicated
- Development of high-grade dysplasia in Barrett mucosa a consideration for esophagectomy

Prognosis

- Entirely dependent on the development of dysplasia and/or adenocarcinoma

Associations

- Barrett mucosa, dysplasia and adenocarcinoma
- When adenocarcinoma arises in the site of Barrett mucosa, the surrounding mucosa typically shows changes of dysplasia; a dysplasia-carcinoma sequence is well established in association with Barrett mucosa
- Squamous carcinoma may occur in patients with Barrett mucosa
- Dysplasia in Barrett mucosa characterized by abnormalities in mucosal architecture and epithelial cells; architectural changes include presence of bizarrely shaped glands and villiform structures (resemble adenomas in other sites of the GI tract); epithelial cell changes include depletion of cytoplasmic mucin; hypercellularity with stratified, enlarged, hyperchromatic, and pleomorphic nuclei that have lost their polarity and have an abnormal distribution of chromatin and prominent nuclei
- It may be difficult to distinguish dysplasia present in Barrett mucosa complicated by the presence of reactive changes that are almost always present in the setting of active inflammation
- In the evaluation of Barrett mucosa, the following classification scheme typically used:
  - Negative for dysplasia
  - Indefinite for dysplasia
  - Positive for dysplasia: Further classified as low-grade or high-grade; the criteria for separating low-grade from high-grade is based on:
    - Severity of mucosal architectural abnormality
    - Epithelial cellularity
    - Extent of stratification of nuclei
    - Degree of loss of cellular polarity
    - Prominent nuclear enlargement, irregularity, pleomorphism, hyperchromatism, and nucleolar enlargement
- 35% to 50% of patients with high-grade dysplasia on biopsy will have an established adenocarcinoma at the time of esophagectomy

Squamous Cell Carcinoma

Clinical Manifestations

- 3 times more common in men than women
- Worldwide, the highest incidence is in northern China, northern Iran, along the Caspian Sea, and the Transkei region of South Africa

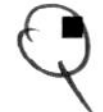

- Risk factors:
  - N-nitrosamines
  - Alcohol and tobacco: Alcohol and tobacco may have synergistic effects; alcohol may modify the absorption or metabolism of tobacco-specific carcinogens
  - Dietary factors: Pickled vegetables and moldy food, smoked meat and fish, dried vegetables, and a diet low in β-carotene, vitamin A, B complex, C, and E
  - Infectious agents: Human papilloma virus (HPV) induces papilloma formation in the esophagus (esophageal carcinomas generally not associated with papillomas)
  - Radiation and thermal injury
- Tumors most commonly located in the middle 1/3 of the esophagus; least commonly in the upper 1/3
- Early-stage disease typically asymptomatic
- Dysphagia most common presenting symptom of advanced disease

Gross Pathology

- Early squamous cell carcinoma, 4 types:
  - Plaque-type (most common): Flat sessile lesion with a coarsely granular, white surface with or without superficial erosions; cut surface reveals a thickened zone along the surface
  - Erosive type: Well demarcated and slightly depressed with a granular surface
  - Papillary type: Well demarcated and elevated above surrounding mucosa with a polypoid or papillary appearance
  - "Occult type" (least common): Typically a pink or congested surface that is flat and in continuity with normal surrounding mucosa
- Advanced squamous cell carcinoma, 3 types:
  - Fungating type: Most common; may be flat, nodular, or polypoid and protrude into the lumen causing partial or complete obstruction; may be ulcerated; usually does not involve the entire circumference
  - Ulcerative type: Represents 25%; ulcerated area usually depressed and shaggy with a slightly elevated peripheral margin that overhangs the edge of the ulcerated area; lateral spread may be extensive and characterized by a nodular appearance with an overlying intact mucosa; may be complicated by fistula formation
  - Infiltrating type: Represents 15%; characterized by intramural infiltration and a small shallow ulcerated surface; involved portion of esophagus tends to be rigid and stenotic
- Cut surfaces of all advanced carcinomas reveal a homogeneous gray to white hard tissue that disrupts the mucosa and infiltrates the esophageal wall; areas of necrosis may be present and are usually characterized by a white or yellow discoloration

Microscopic Pathology

- *Early squamous cell carcinoma*
  - Plaque type: 45% intramucosal; 35% submucosal; 20% intraepithelial
  - Erosive type: Usually intraepithelial or intramucosal
  - Papillary type: More than 50% submucosal; remainder intraepithelial or intramucosal
  - Occult type: Always intraepithelial
- *Intraepithelial carcinoma* characterized by malignant squamous cells involving the entire thickness of the squamous epithelium; the underlining basement membrane intact (squamous cell carcinoma in situ); neoplastic cells irregularly arranged, large, and pleomorphic and tend to have hyperchromatic nuclei; mitoses present
- *Intramucosal carcinoma* characterized by the infiltration of small groups of carcinoma cells or single cells through the basement membrane into the lamina propria, but not beyond; interface between epithelium and stroma typically irregular

- *Submucosal carcinoma* characterized by carcinoma cells that have penetrated the muscularis mucosa and extended into the submucosa (they do not reach the muscularis propria); invasive area typically shows continuity with intraepithelial component; changes of chronic inflammation usually surround the invasive component
- *Advanced squamous cell carcinoma*
  - Well-differentiated tumors contain few basal cells; tumor cells disorganized, round or polygonal and have oval to round nuclei with prominent nucleoli; some degree of maturation evident and keratin production ("keratin pearls") always present; mitoses uncommon
  - Moderately differentiated tumor, characterized by tumor cells that tend to be small and more pleomorphic than those of well-differentiated lesions; focal areas of keratin formation may be seen; mitoses frequent; tumor cells may form sheets and clusters or may be arranged in trabecular pattern
  - Poorly differentiated tumors contain many basal cells; tumor cells very pleomorphic with variable amounts of cytoplasm and bizarre nuclei with prominent nucleoli; keratin not present; tumor cells may be round, polygonal or spindled and do not resemble normal squamous cells; tumors that are composed predominantly of spindle cells are considered to be *spindle cell carcinomas or sarcomatoid carcinomas*; tumor necrosis and mitotic figures both frequently present
  - HPV-type changes or koilocytosis frequently seen
  - Foci of glandular differentiation present in as many as 20% as well as small foci reminiscent of small cell undifferentiated carcinoma
  - Variants:
    - *Verrucous carcinoma*: Surface of these neoplasms has papillary projections; deeper portion is composed of islands of acanthotic squamous epithelium that compresses or infiltrates the underlying esophageal wall; malignant nature of the neoplasm best determined by the markedly atypical features of the squamous cells in the basal layer
    - *Basaloid squamous cell carcinoma:* Characterized by solid sheets or islands of tumor cells surrounded by a basal lamina (closely resembles basal cell carcinoma of the skin); tumor cells tend to be small with little cytoplasm and are similar to the cells in the basal layer of squamous epithelium; peripheral palisading prominent; mitoses frequent; focal areas of necrosis may be present; neoplasm may closely resemble adenoid cystic carcinoma of the salivary gland
    - *Spindle cell carcinoma and carcinosarcoma*: Characterized by malignant squamous cells admixed with malignant spindled cells; neoplasms tend to be polypid; bone, cartilage, and muscle tissue may be present; inflammatory cells typically admixed with the neoplasm and surround it

Special Stains

- Not helpful

Immunohistochemistry

- Epithelial nature of spindle cells in carcinosarcoma variant can be confirmed with cytokeratin
- Cytokeratin 14 and 19 will stain the peripheral neoplastic basal cells and the basal cells of normal squamous mucosa in the basaloid carcinoma variant
- ~25% have deletion of A, B, or H blood group antigens
- Some react for human chorionic gonadotropin (even in the absence of morphologically demonstrable trophoblastic differentiation)

Electron Microscopy

- Confirms that spindle cell carcinoma (carcinosarcoma) can be divided into 2 groups:
  - Epithelial nature of the squamous cell carcinoma can be proven as well as the mesenchymal nature of the spindle cell component (a true carcinosarcoma)
  - Both the squamous cells and malignant spindle cells have epithelial characteristics (sarcomatoid carcinoma)

Molecular Alterations

- Amplification and overexpression has been found for oncogenes c-*myc*, c-*fos*, c-*ras*, c-*sis*, c-*raf*, cyclin D1, c-*erb*-B, *hstl*, and *int*-2
- Suppressor genes showing inactivation, mutation or loss of heterozygosity include *p53*, *rb*, *APC*, *MCC*, *DCC*, and *MTS-1*

Differential Diagnosis

- Papilloma
- Poorly differentiated lesions may be difficult to distinguish from adenocarcinoma, melanoma, large cell lymphoma, and sarcoma
- Sarcomatous component of carcinosarcoma may be indistinguishable from leiomyosarcoma and other sarcomas

Treatment

- Esophagectomy, irradiation, and chemotherapy either alone or in various combinations
- External radiation, intraluminal brachytherapy, and chemoradiotherapy

Prognosis

- Level of differentiation adds little prognostic information
- 5-year survival rate for tumors confined to the lamina propria or submucosa approximately 85%; tumors confined to esophageal wall without lymph node metastasis 45%; tumors confined to the esophageal wall or tumors that invade adjacent structures with lymph node metastasis 25%; tumors with distant metastasis 5% to 10%
- Factors that adversely affect prognosis include depth of invasion, size of primary neoplasm, and presence of lymph nodes with metastasis

Associations

- Synchronous tumors may be present in up to 30% (especially likely in alcoholics)
- Associated carcinomas include squamous cell carcinoma of the head and neck, gastric carcinoma, and primary carcinoma of the lung
- Squamous cell carcinoma present in approximately 1% of patients with hiatus hernia
- Esophageal stricture secondary to ingestion of lye or caustic liquids usually during childhood (up to 4%)
- Achalasia (an esophageal motility disease characterized by inability of lower esophageal sphincter to relax and inability of body of esophagus to undergo peristalsis)
- Plummer-Vinson syndrome (iron deficiency anemia, stomatitis, and dysphagia); esophagus may have webs; carcinomas develop in the pharynx and cervical esophagus in 1% to 2%
- Celiac disease

Stomach

Non-Neoplastic

Autoimmune Gastritis

Clinical Manifestations

- Used to be known as type A chronic gastritis or chronic fundic gastritis
- Typically occurs in elderly women
- Primarily involves the fundic corpus mucosa (in longstanding cases, inflammatory lesions may spread into the antrum)
- Results from antibodies against parietal cell membranes, intrinsic factor, and gastrin receptor
- Clinical manifestations result from loss of parietal cells in the specialized glands of the corpus-fundic region which leads to achlorhydria and loss of intrinsic factor (located in parietal cell membranes)
- Loss of intrinsic factor results in impaired absorption of vitamin B_{12} in the ileum, which eventually leads to pernicious anemia
- Achlorhydria results in sustained stimulation of gastrin by endocrine cells (G-cells) in the antrum; since there are few to no parietal cells, hypergastrinemia results; as a side effect the gastrin stimulates endocrine cells in the gastric body; if the condition persists, small indolent carcinoid tumors (multiple hyperplastic nodules of G-cells) begin to develop in the body
- Diagnosis based on the finding of achlorhydria, both basal and stimulated, and an abnormal Schilling test result, which can be corrected by the addition of intrinsic factor

Gross Pathology

- Endoscopic findings may be completely unremarkable with normal folds
- Atrophic mucosa flat with few or no folds and prominent vascularity (prominent vascularity the result of submucosal vessels that can be seen through the unusually thin mucosa)
- In the antrum, hyperplasia of endocrine G-cells may result in multiple small nodules that can be visualized endoscopically
- Occasionally antral mucosa may be atrophic with widespread inflammatory changes (either the result of extension of fundic disease into the antrum or the simultaneous coexistence of chronic fundic and chronic antral gastritis)

Microscopic Pathology

- Unequivocal diagnosis can only be made on mucosal biopsy of the gastric body or fundus where there is gastritis and parietal and chief cell destruction; the antrum should be normal
- Early in the course of disease an increased number of mononuclear inflammatory cells (primarily lymphocytes and plasma cells) infiltrate upper part of the lamina propria beneath the surface epithelium and between the gastric pits of the body; damage to superficial mucosal epithelium generally minimal and patchy; no significant inflammation in the antrum
- As disease progresses, the mononuclear cell infiltrate extends into the lower part of the mucosa and centers around the fundic glands with progressive destruction of these specialized glands throughout the body and fundic region
- Eventually the fundic mucosa is replaced by a mixture of pyloric or intestinal glands (pyloric and intestinal metaplasia); foveolar hyperplasia and pancreatic metaplasia may also develop (metaplasia and atrophy only occur in the body and fundus)
- Patients are hypoacidic as a result of the loss of parietal cell mass; this loss of acid stimulates antral G-cells to produce abundant gastrin (this G-cell stimulation never progresses in gastrinomas)
- Multifocal gastric enterochromaffin cell-like (ECL) cell hyperplasia, micronests, and multifocal carcinoid tumors develop in the atrophic and metaplastic gastric body as a side effect of the gastrin stimulation (hyperplastic ECL cells only present in atrophic fundic glands and pyloric metaplastic glands; never in intestinal metaplastic glands)
- Other changes in the antrum include patchy areas of chronic inflammation; intact pyloric glands; *H pylori* rarely seen even when active inflammation present (probably the result of the achlorhydria)

Special Stains

- Presence of intestinal metaplasia can be confirmed with PAS reaction for neutral glycoproteins, Alcian blue at pH 2.5 for sialomucins and other slightly acidic mucosubstances, and Alcian blue at pH 1.0 and metachromatic stains for strongly acidic mucins

Immunohistochemistry

- Chromogranin will react with ECL cell hyperplasia in the body
- Chromogranin will stain a normal number of G-cells in the antrum
- Gastrin will not stain the hyperplastic neuroendocrine cells in the body
- Gastrin will stain the G-cells in the antrum

Electron Microscopy

- Not helpful

Molecular Alterations

- None

Differential Diagnosis

- Mild superficial chronic inflammation with rare foci of acute inflammation and intestinal metaplasia may be seen as a normal finding in the elderly and in patients with late-stage chronic antral gastritis
- Atrophy of fundic mucosa may occur in areas overlying mural tumors or adjacent to foci of helminthic infection
- Extensive foveolar cell hyperplasia that leads to enlarged rugae and an overall thickening of the mucosal surface raises a differential diagnosis of hyperplastic polyps, adenoma, tumor infiltration (carcinoma and lymphoma), and Menetrier disease

Treatment

- Administration of vitamin B_{12}

Prognosis

- Increased risk for development of adenocarcinoma (1%-3%)

Associations

- Affects 25% of patients with dermatitis herpetiformis (gluten restriction does not reverse gastritis)
- Intestinal metaplasia may undergo dysplastic alterations and progress to adenocarcinoma (incidence of adenocarcinoma in this setting <3%)
- Thyroiditis and hypothyroidism
- Diabetes mellitus
- Adrenal insufficiency
- Sjögren disease
- Myasthenia gravis

Comments

- *Changes in the body in patients with autoimmune gastritis*
  - ☐ Loss of parietal cells
  - ☐ Intestinal and pyloric metaplasia
  - ☐ Negative staining with chromogranin
  - ☐ Enterochromaffin cell hyperplasia positive of chromogranin
- *Changes in antrum in patients with autoimmune gastritis*
  - ☐ Antrum usually normal
  - ☐ No intestinal metaplasia
  - ☐ Neuroendocrine cell positive for gastrin
  - ☐ No neuroendocrine cell hyperplasia on chromogranin stain

Helicobacter pylori Gastritis

Clinical Manifestations

- Type B or environmental form of chronic gastritis caused by bacteria (primarily *H pylori*)
- Prevalence increases with age and almost universally presents in patients older than 40 years
- Only rarely do patients develop active disease or atrophy
- Episodes of active disease characterized by abdominal pain, vomiting, and occasional bleeding

Gross Pathology

- Endoscopic findings range from essentially normal to frank ulceration in stomach and/or duodenum

Microscopic Pathology

- Gastric microorganisms (*H pylori*) present in 75% to 85% of patients with active disease, but in only 5% of patients with inactive disease
- Organisms present in antrum in 75% of patients with chronic peptic ulcers involving either the stomach (60%) or duodenum (95%)
- Organisms typically found on the surface and in the lumina of gastric pits in the mucous coat over the intercellular junctions of gastric mucous cells
- Bacteria not commonly found in the gastric corpus-fundus or in the duodenum
- When organisms seen in the duodenum they are confined to areas of gastric mucus cell metaplasia (perhaps a specific receptor in such cells bind the organism to the cell surface)
- Active phase of chronic antral gastritis characterized by presence of neutrophils in the mucous neck region of the gastric pits (mucous neck region hyperplastic as a result of repairing dying cells)
- Areas of intestinal metaplasia may be present but are rarely involved with active inflammation (metaplastic epithelium may be resistant to the destructive effect of the organisms)
- Active (acute) inflammation quickly evolves into chronic inflammation
- Early stages of chronic antral gastritis (without activity) characterized by an expansion of the upper lamina propria with a mononuclear inflammatory infiltrate with some accompanying foveolar hyperplasia

- As the disease progresses the inflammation extends into the lower part of the lamina propria and there is partial loss of pyloric glands and endocrine cells; lymphoid follicles appear and the mucosa is replaced by intestinal metaplasia
- Persistent foveolar hyperplasia may lead to the formation of localized hyperplastic polyps or to a diffuse thickening of the mucosal surface

Special Stains

- Warthin-Starry, Gram, Giemsa, and Dieterle stains can all facilitate the identification of organisms

Immunohistochemistry

- Antibodies to *H pylori* will identify the organisms

Electron Microscopy

- *H pylori* have 4 flagella at 1 pole
- *H pylori* partially enveloped by the surface membranes of gastric mucus cells

Molecular Alterations

- None

Differential Diagnosis

- Allergic gastritis
- Proximity to chronic peptic ulcer
- Gastritis secondary to *Gastrospirillum hominis (Helicobactor heilmanni)*

Treatment

- Eradication of organisms with antibiotics coupled with proton pump inhibitor

Prognosis

- Largely dependent on complications of gastric or duodenal ulcer

Associations

- Induction of gastric lymphoid tissue as a result of chronic *H pylori* infection may be a precursor to gastric lymphoma of the B-cell type that arises from mucosa-associated lymphoid tissue
- Gastric carcinoma

Comments

Helicobacter heilmanis can infect adults and children (<1%) and produce a mild form of gastritis. Organisms have a "corkscrew" shape and are usually found lying free in lumen or in gastric pits and necks of pyloric glands; they are rarely attached to epithelium

Multifocal Atrophic Gastritis

- Intestinal metaplasia (no matter how limited or small the focus) is the result of mucosal injury
- Atrophic gastritis is defined as a patch of metaplasia accompanied by a reduction in the number of adjacent or underlying glands
- Patches of metaplasia may be seen in otherwise normal stomachs as well as in *H pylori* gastritis (chronic active gastritis) and in chronic fundic gastritis (autoimmune gastritis)

Gross Pathology

- Metaplasia is a microscopic diagnosis
- Its presence can be surmised in cases in which chronic or chronic active gastritis are endoscopically diagnosed

Microscopic Pathology

- Typically seen in both the antrum and the body and increases in quantity in direct relation to the duration of chronic gastritis
- Early mild disease tends to result in metaplastic cells largely confined to the upper part of the foveolae or pits and may involve only 1 or a few pits; tends to be focal and merges with gastric mucus cells on the epithelial surface of the foveolae
- Advanced cases more frequently associated with atrophic forms of chronic gastritis and characterized by metaplastic cells that extend to the base of the mucosa and actually occupy the entire mucosal thickness
- 3 types:
  - *Complete (mature) intestinal metaplasia* (type I): Resembles small intestine with straight intestinal crypts lined by absorptive cells with a well-formed brush border, goblet cells that secrete sialomucins, and sometimes Paneth cells tend to be concentrated in the base of glands; not precancerous

- *Incomplete (immature) intestinal metaplasia* (type II): Characterized by architectural distortion, with irregular crypts lined by goblet cells that secrete sialomucins and columnar cells with varying degrees of differentiation that contain a mixture of neutral mucins and sialomucins; no Paneth cells; precancerous
- *Incomplete (immature) intestinal metaplasia* (type III): Characterized by extensive architectural distortion with tortuous and branched crypts lined by undifferentiated columnar cells that are large and pleomorphic and have hyperchromatic nuclei (resemble low-grade dysplasia) and goblet cells that secrete sialomucins or sulfomucins

- Intestinal-type endocrine cells present in all forms of intestinal metaplasia

Special Stains

- Normal surface and foveolar mucous cells stain strongly with PAS and are negative for acid substances, except for a faint staining with Alcian blue at pH 2.5 in the lower part of the gastric pits in the proximal part of stomach
- Goblet cells of the normal small intestine and in complete (mature) intestinal metaplasia (type I) stain faintly with PAS and strongly with Alcian blue at pH 2.5
- Goblet cells of the normal colon and in incomplete (immature) intestinal metaplasia (type II) stain strongly with Alcian blue at both pH 2.5 and pH 1.0

Immunohistochemistry

- Not helpful

Electron Microscopy

- Will confirm presence of brush border of small intestinal absorptive type cells in complete (type I) metaplasia

Molecular Alterations

- None

Differential Diagnosis

- Complete intestinal metaplasia versus incomplete intestinal metaplasia
- Etiology of chronic gastritis with or without activity

Treatment

- Treat underlying chronic (active) gastritis

Prognosis

- Type II (incomplete) has a strong association with subsequent development of adenocarcinoma
- Type I (complete) does not represent a risk factor for the development of gastric carcinoma

Associations

- Chronic active gastritis
- Autoimmune chronic atrophic gastritis

Neoplastic

Adenocarcinoma

Clinical Manifestations

- Incidence of gastric cancer has declined over 20 years between 1973 and 1993 by 25% and the mortality has decreased by 35%
- More common in men than women (ratio of 2:1)
- Primarily affects the elderly; when individuals under the age of 35 years, they are more likely to be women (ratio of 3:1)
- In the United States the incidence of gastric carcinoma twice as frequent in the black population as in the white population
- A higher incidence in patients with blood type A, patients with a family history of gastric cancer, and patients with pernicious anemia
- Most patients present with nonspecific symptoms such as epigastric discomfort and dyspepsia
- Occasionally patients present with anemia (occult blood in the stool more common than massive bleeding)

- Patients with advanced disease typically experience profound weight loss
- Occasionally patients present with free perforation, hypoglycemia, granulocytosis, pneumatosis cystoides, thrombocytopenic purpura, and immune complex disease, microangiopathy, and hepatic failure secondary to intrasinusoidal metastasis
- Approximately 50% involve the pyloric mucosa, 25% the fundic mucosa, 25% both areas; 30% arise in the cardia

Gross Pathology

- 5 types (Borrmann classification)
  - Superficial carcinoma (Borrmann type 0 carcinoma, early carcinoma): 6%
  - Polypoid carcinoma (Borrmann type 1): 7%
  - Fungating carcinoma (Borrmann type 2): 35%
  - Ulcerative carcinoma (Borrmann type 3): 25%
  - Diffusely infiltrative carcinoma (Borrmann type 4) linitis plastica carcinoma: 25%
- Early superficial gastric carcinoma (carcinoma confined to mucosa and submucosa regardless of the presence of lymph node metastases):
  - Type I (elevated type): A nodular lesion that typically has an irregular surface with crevices between papillary projections
  - Type IIa (superficial, elevated type): Lesion is slightly elevated and approximately twice the thickness of normal mucosa
  - Type IIb (superficial, flat type): The level of the carcinoma is approximately the same as that of the surrounding mucosa
  - Type IIc (superficial, depressed type): Lesion characterized by a shallow depression; most frequent
  - Type III (excavated type): Deep ulcerlike lesion surrounded by a narrow rim of carcinomatous epithelium at the ulcer border; frequency of <1%
- Advanced gastric carcinoma (cancer that has invaded beyond the muscularis propria):
  - Polypoid carcinoma: A broad-based nodular neoplasm without gross ulceration
  - Fungating carcinoma: A nodular neoplasm that has a large ulcer at the dome; the bottom of the ulcer crater rests on the tumor mass and is above the level of the surrounding gastric wall
  - Ulcerated carcinoma: A penetrating ulcerated lesion with a slightly elevated tumor mass at the periphery of the ulcer; tumor cells are present in both the base as well as the margins; lesion most likely to resemble a benign ulcer
  - Diffusely infiltrative carcinoma: Infiltrates throughout the gastric wall without forming a mass or becoming ulcerated; the resulting diffuse thickening of the gastric wall has led to the term "linitis plastica"; prominent fibrosis is usually present

Microscopic Pathology

- Many cell types can be identified in gastric carcinoma:
  - Mucous cells (the majority of which are goblet cells and secrete intestinal acidic mucins) present in glandular carcinomas (gastric type mucous cells rare in glandular carcinoma)
  - Nonmucous tumor cells tend to be immature absorptive cells (have a distinct striated border)
  - Pyloric gland cells, endocrine cells, Paneth cells, parietal cells, pepsinogen-secreting cells, chief cells, and squamous cells
- Occasionally neoplasms (particularly solid carcinomas) will be composed of sheets of poorly differentiated or undifferentiated cells
- Amount of fibrous stroma varies from tumor to tumor; stroma typically most prominent in infiltrative carcinomas; occasionally stroma has a prominent lymphocytic infiltrate (especially in some solid undifferentiated carcinomas)
- World Health Organization (WHO) classification:
  - Adenocarcinoma
  - Intestinal type: Consists of glands of varying degrees of differentiation (associated with *Helicobacter pylori* infection)
  - Diffuse type: Composed of single neoplastic cells or small nests diffusely infiltrating through gastric

wall; typically occurs in the gastric body and in younger patients

- Tubular adenocarcinoma: Most common; a glandular lesion in which glands form branching tubules; lumens of these tubules vary in size and may actually appear cystic; most of the tumor cells of the absorptive type with scattered goblet cells; nuclei tend to be round or irregular with a coarse chromatin pattern
- Papillary adenocarcinoma: A glandular neoplasm characterized by prominent intraglandular foldings and projections with cuboidal or tall columnar cancer cells that line bands of interstitial tissue; tumor cells usually of the absorptive type with scattered goblet cells; nuclei typically round or irregular with a coarse chromatin
- Mucinous adenocarcinoma: Approximately 10%; characterized by excessive production of mucin which ruptures cells and glands and forms pools in the stroma; if mucin occupies >50% of the area of the tumor, the term *mucinous adenocarcinoma* appropriate
- Signet-ring cell carcinoma: Tumor cells distended by intracytoplasmic mucin that compresses the nucleus against the cell wall giving it a crescentic shape; tumor cells infiltrate individually; little gland formation
- Adenosquamous carcinoma: Adenocarcinoma admixed with malignant squamous cells
- Squamous cell carcinoma: Extremely rare; 50% arise in the antrum; usually large and ulcerated
- Small cell carcinoma: Typically an ulcerated mass composed of small cells with hyperchromatic nuclei and little cytoplasm (similar to small cell carcinoma of lung); foci of adenocarcinoma or squamous cell carcinoma may be present; tumor cells contain neurosecretory granules
- Undifferentiated carcinoma: Characterized by no specific evidence of differentiation either structurally or functionally; typically have a prominent lymphocytic infiltrate and may be related to Epstein-Barr virus

Special Stains

- PAS with diastase, PAS-Alcian blue, and mucicarmine stains will highlight the mucinous nature of signet-ring cells which may be otherwise difficult to identify on routine H&E staining

Immunohistochemistry

- Epithelial nature of these neoplasms confirmed by cytokeratin and epithelial membrane antigen (EMA) positivity
- Most are CEA positive
- Small cell carcinomas positive for chromogranin and neuron-specific enolase (NSE); negative for CEA and EMA

Electron Microscopy

- Will demonstrate presence of neurosecretory granules in small cell carcinoma variant

Molecular Alterations

- Oncogenes K-*sam*, c-*met*, c-*erbB*-2, *ras*, and c-*myc* have all been identified
- Expression and mutation of tumor suppressor gene p53
- Chromosomal loss of heterozygosity in chromosomes 7p, 17p, 1q, and 5q
- Germline mutations in the E-cadherin/*CDH1* gene occur in familial gastric cancer; penetrance of the gene 70% to 80%

Differential Diagnosis

- Primary gastric lymphoma
- Metastatic tumor
- Direct extension of pancreatic or esophageal adenocarcinoma
- Undifferentiated carcinoma may resemble poorly differentiated carcinoma, small cell carcinoma, lymphoma, leukemia, and poorly differentiated sarcoma

Treatment

- Surgical resection

- Advanced neoplasms treated with postoperative adjuvant chemotherapy and radiotherapy
- Preoperative neoadjuvant chemotherapy for locally advanced cancer may produce enough remission that an unresectable tumor can become resectable (40% to 60%)
- Postoperative immunochemotherapy followed by multidrug chemotherapy may have a role in improving 5-year survival

Prognosis

- Surgical resection for cure only possible in ≤50%
- 5-year survival rate after "resection for cure" approximately 30%
- 5-year and 10-year survival rates for early cancer without lymph node metastasis as high as 95%; 5-year survival for patients with early cancer with positive lymph nodes as high as 50%

Associations

- Precancerous conditions:
  - Adenoma (cancer develops in approximately 40%)
  - Hyperplastic polyp (carcinoma occurs in 2% or less)
  - Chronic gastric ulceration secondary to *H pylori* infection: presence of *H pylori* probably more significant than the actual presence of an ulcer
  - Chronic atrophic gastritis: 3 patterns:
    - *Autoimmune type*, involving acid secreting mucosa (body and fundus) and associated with pernicious anemia (cancer develops more frequently in this type)
    - *Hypersecretory type*, involving pyloric mucosa
    - *Environmental type*, involving multiple areas at random but most frequently the junctional zone between the antrum and body
- Intestinal metaplasia; carcinoma often develops in areas of intestinal metaplasia and the risk of gastric carcinoma appears to be proportional to the amount of metaplasia
- 3 types of intestinal metaplasia:
  - Type I: Mature or complete intestinal metaplasia. Resembles normal small intestinal mucosa, with straight crypts lined by absorptive cells with well formed microvilli, goblet cells and occasional Paneth cells; not a precancerous lesion
  - Type II: Immature or incomplete intestinal metaplasia. Goblet cells present but no Paneth cells; mucous cells immature with short, blunted microvilli and no digestive enzymes and contain acidic glycoproteins (mucins); most gastric carcinomas arise in areas of incomplete metaplasia
  - Type III: Intestinal metaplasia with extensive architectural distortion. Columnar cells tend to be undifferentiated with large, irregular hyperchromatic nuclei; risk of gastric cancer may be highest
- Gastric remnant: Neoplasm typically develops 15 to 25 years after initial resection and is often located at the anastomosis; may be more common after a Billroth II than after a Billroth I
- Immunodeficiency disorders: Common variable immunodeficiency, x-linked immunodeficiency, and infantile x-linked agammaglobulinemia
- Synchronous carcinomas: Present in 8% to 9% of early gastric cancers and approximately 5% of advanced cancers
- Hereditary tumor syndromes associated with an increased risk for development of gastric cancer:
  - Familial diffuse gastric carcinoma
  - HNPCC
  - Familial adenomatous polyposis (FAP)
  - Li-Fraumeni syndrome
  - Peutz-Jegherrs syndrome
  - Hyperplastic gastric polyposis

Fundic Gland Polyp

Clinical Manifestations

- Majority seen in middle-aged woman
- No specific association with other primary gastric diseases
- May be sporadic or associated with familial adenomatous polyposis

Stomach: Neoplastic>Fundic Gland Polyp; Gastric Leiomyoma

- Represents one of the most common gastric polyps (along with hyperplastic polyps)
- Found in 1% to 2% of routine upper gastrointestinal tract endoscopic examinations
- Women outnumber men 5 to 1
- Both sporadic and FAP-associated polyps can increase, decrease or remain constant in number

Gross Pathology

- Typically small; rarely bigger than 1 cm, sessile and dome-shaped
- May be single but are often multiple
- Often appear as clusters of small, mostly sessile lesions with a glassy transparent appearance
- Restricted to the body and fundus of the stomach (within the acid-secreting area)
- They do not arise in the duodenum

Microscopic Pathology

- Fundic gland polyps and changed induced by proton pump inhibitors overlap (the former, of course, is associated with an endoscopic lesion)
- Microcysts vary in size and are present at different levels of the gastric glands and are admixed with normal glands; they consist of a localized hyperplasia of the deep epithelial compartment of the oxyntic mucosa, especially of the mucous neck cells
- Disordered glandular architecture with budding and tortuosity is a conspicuous feature
- The microcysts are often interconnected and lined by parietal cells chief cells
- Dysplasia can be seen in a sporadic fundic gland polyp, but is distinctly unusual (<1%); however dysplasia may be present in 40% to 45% of FGPs in patients with FAP

Special Stains, Immunohistochemistry, and Electron Microscopy

- Not helpful

Molecular Alterations

- Same as those of FAP when associated with that condition (APC gene 5q21)
- β-catenin mutations seen in sporadic polyps

Treatment and Prognosis

- Typically innocuous and require little more than polypectomy
- It is important to realize that dysplasia (usually low-grade) of foveolar and surface epithelium can occur, usually in FAP patients

Associations

- Tend to be more common in individuals with the hereditary flat adenoma syndrome
- There is an increased frequency of epithelial neoplasms in the colon
- Usually no associated inflammation; a low prevalence with associated *H pylori* infection
- Never been reported to progress to gastric adenocarcinoma, but adenocarcinoma has been reported in patients with fundic gland polyps
- Increased risk for duodenal polyposis (>300-fold); these duodenal lesions typically are periampullary and represent either an adenoma or a carcinoma

Gastric Leiomyoma

Clinical Manifestations

- Typically too small to cause symptoms
- Most are confined to the cardia

Gross Pathology

- Tends to be well-circumscribed but lacks a fibrous capsule
- Typically occurs in the muscularis propria, but may arise within the muscularis mucosa
- Often multiple

Microscopic Pathology

- Typically composed of bland, mature, usually hypertrophied smooth muscle cells arranged in whorls and fascicles (cells identical to those seen in uterine leiomyomas)
- Tumor cells have eosinophilic, fibrillary, and often clumped cytoplasm
- Occasional focal atypia and mitotic figures present

Special Stains

- Not helpful

Immunohistochemistry

- Tumor cells reactive for desmin, muscle-specific actin, and smooth muscle myosin
- Tumor cells are negative for CD34 and CD117 (c-kit)

Electron Microscopy

- EM confirms the mature nature of the smooth muscle cells; cells contain prominent cytoplasmic filaments, subplasmalemmal linear densities, rows of pinocytic vesicles, and basal lamina

Molecular Alterations

- None

Differential Diagnosis

- GI stromal tumor (GIST)

Treatment

- Local excision

Prognosis

- Excellent unless large enough to cause obstruction which is associated with an inherent morbidity and mortality

Associations

- None

Gastrointestinal Stromal Tumors (GISTs)

- Mesenchymal tumors of stomach, small intestine, colon, and rectum

Clinical Manifestations

- Both benign and malignant variants tend to occur between the 5th and 8th decades of life
- Stomach:
  - 60% to 80%
  - Men and women affected equally

- 70% benign; 30% malignant
- Represents 2% to 3% of malignant gastric tumors
- Most common clinical manifestation is upper GI bleeding (50%); patients also present with pain similar to that of an ulcer; this symptom is more common with malignant than benign lesions; 25% complain of anorexia, nausea, and vomiting
- A palpable abdominal mass present in 10% of benign tumors and in up to 30% of malignant tumors
- Weight loss more frequently associated with malignant tumors than benign
- Endoscopically, both benign and malignant lesions appear as smooth masses that protrude into the lumen and are covered by intact (occasionally ulcerated: 20% to 30%) mucosa

- Patients with Carney triad (see below) are nearly all women
- Small intestine:
  - 20% to 30%
  - Men affected slightly more often than women
  - Sarcomas represent approximately 15% of small intestinal malignancies
- Colon and rectum:
  - <10%

Gross Pathology

- Gross appearance fairly similar at all locations
- Both benign and malignant lesions tend to be situated in the submucosa and the muscularis propria
- Larger tumors extend into the perigastric tissues and may take on a dumbbell shape with the bulbous components in the submucosa and the subserosa with the constricted area in the muscularis propria
- Occasional tumors are almost entirely extramural with a thin attachment to the outer layer of muscularis propria
- Cut surface flat, granular, and contains conspicuous vessels, foci of hemorrhage, cystic degeneration, and necrosis
- Benign and malignant tumors may appear quite similar, but larger malignant lesions often have large, firm, and white homogeneous areas that resemble sarcomas seen in soft tissue

- Tumors may appear well circumscribed and encapsulated but lack a fibrous capsule; typically the tumor is at least partially enveloped by muscularis propria
- Local invasion rare
- Stomach:
  - 50% of benign spindle cell tumors and 30% of epithelioid malignant tumors arise in the proximal part of the stomach (fundus and cardia); 50% of benign epithelioid cell tumors and 25% of epithelioid sarcomas arise in the antrum
- Small intestine:
  - Evenly distributed throughout small intestine
- Colon and rectum:
  - Most are malignant

Microscopic Pathology

- 3 morphologic variants similar throughout GI tract
- Majority are spindle cell tumors that may have various histologic patterns, but often resemble smooth muscle tumors; may resemble nerve sheath tumors
- *Common benign spindle cell stromal tumors* (previously designated cellular leiomyoma and leiomyoma with regimentation):
  - Tumor cells tend to be arranged in whorls and fascicles some of which interlace in either a storiform or herringbone pattern; occasionally spindle cells form palisades reminiscent of those seen in schwannomas (tumors with this palisade appearance have been referred to as *leiomyomas with regimentation*)
  - Tumor cells are long and spindled with abundant, fibrillar, eosinophilic cytoplasm; tend to be of uniform size and shape; rarely pleomorphic
  - Nuclei are elongated and may vary in shape from straight to wavy with either blunt or tapered ends
  - Many cells contain single perinuclear vacuoles, which indent the nucleus at one end giving the nucleus a "torchlike" appearance
  - Mitotic figures may be present but are rare
- *Benign epithelioid cell tumors* (previously designated epithelioid leiomyoma, leiomyoblastoma, bizarre smooth muscle tumor)
  - Typically lobulated
  - Tumor cells tend to be round with an epithelioid appearance
  - Cells have pale cytoplasm that tends to be adherent to and aggregate near the nuclei with peripheral clearing; occasionally the area of cytoplasmic clearing (an artifact of fixation) is eccentric and appears to push the nucleus to one side resulting in a cell that resembles a lipoblast or signet-ring carcinoma cell
  - Tumor cells are occasionally densely eosinophilic without cytoplasmic clearing
  - Nuclei tend to be round and dense with small nucleoli
  - Neoplasm may have zones of liquefaction or hyalinization; in these areas the epithelioid-appearing cells may be pleomorphic and accompanied by multinucleated giant cells and cells with a single, large, bizarre nucleus
  - Mitotic figures rare
  - Occasionally tumors consist of a mixture of epithelioid cells and plump spindle cells
  - Epithelioid lesions in small intestine, colon, and rectum
  - Eosinophilic, extracellular, collagen, globoid lesions (skeinoid fibers) may be seen in benign small intestinal GISTs
- *Sarcomas* (previously designated leiomyosarcomas)
  - In general, the cells of these malignant tumors are smaller, more densely crowded, and have more mitoses than their benign counterparts; cells may be predominantly epithelioid, spindled, or a combination of the two
  - Tumor cells tend to be arranged in large sheets
  - Tumors composed of spindle cells tend to have vesicular nuclei
  - Mitotic figures are generally conspicuous (5/50 hpfs)
  - The larger the tumor, the more likely it will be malignant

- Tumors that are predominately epithelioid often have lobules or geographic areas with different patterns: eg, epithelioid cells arranged in acinuslike clusters resembling carcinoma cells or tiny spindle cells arranged in tight palisades; tumors with a mixture of pattens are frequently surrounded by an acid mucopolysaccharide-rich stroma
- Cellular and nuclear pleomorphism is relatively rare (pleomorphism is more often seen in benign epithelioid cell tumors)
- Epithelioid cell variants of malignant tumors often have lobules of cells that are histologically identical to a benign epithelioid cell tumor

Special Stains

- Reticulin stains will highlight the delicate reticulin fibers that surround individual epithelial cells and clusters of epithelial cells in benign tumors

Immunohistochemistry

- Stomach
  - Nearly all (>90%) tumor cells stain for c-*kit* (CD117) (see Comment later in this section)
  - 70% to 80% positive for CD34 (usually a membrane pattern
  - 30% to 40 % positive for α-smooth muscle actin
  - Usually negative for desmin and S-100 protein
  - Smooth muscle markers may or may not stain the tumor cells; staining with muscle markers does not correlate with ultrastructural evidence of smooth muscle differentiation and does not necessarily mean the tumor is a leiomyoma; strong and diffuse staining with desmin and smooth muscle actin with negative staining with c-*kit* required to diagnose leiomyoma
- Small intestine
  - Essentially always c-*kit* (CD117) positive
  - Usually positive for CD34
  - 30% to 50% positive for α-smooth muscle actin
  - Almost always negative for desmin and S-100 protein
- Colon and rectum
  - c-*kit* (CD117) positive
  - Most CD34 positive
  - Occasionally smooth muscle actin positive; desmin negative

Electron Microscopy

- Cells of GISTs are largely undifferentiated
- Occasional tumor cells will show smooth muscle differentiation while others will show differentiation characteristic of Schwann cells
- Ultrastructural findings are identical in both benign and malignant tumors

Molecular Alterations

- Both benign and malignant tumors show losses in chromosomes 14 and 22

Differential Diagnosis

- Fibromatosis
- Schwannoma (positive for S-100; negative for desmin, smooth muscle actin, and c-*kit*)
- Solitary fibrous tumor/hemangiopericytoma
- Glomus tumor (positive for smooth muscle actin; negative for keratins)
- Leiomyoma and leiomyosarcoma (see Immunohistochemistry earlier in this section)
- Arrangement of epithelioid cells in epithelioid cell tumors dictates the differential diagnosis:
  - Epithelioid cells arranged in strands may resemble signet ring cell carcinomas
  - Epithelial cells arranged in small clusters or nests may resemble adenocarcinoma and carcinoid tumor

Treatment

- Gross total surgical removal with a narrow rim of uninvolved tissue
- Adjuvant chemotherapy with the tyrosine kinase inhibitor imatinib mesylate (STI-571, Gleevec or Glevic; Novartis, Basel, Switzerland) used in nonresectable and metastatic disease

Prognosis

- Most dependant on mitotic rate, size of the tumor, depth of invasion, and presence or absence of metastasis
- Other factors associated with malignancy include high cellularity and nuclear DNA measurements (aneuploid sarcomas are more aggressive than diploid sarcomas)
- S-100 positivity and CD34 negativity both associated with malignant behavior
- Expression of desmin and smooth muscle actin frequent in benign tumors
- All sarcomas have metastatic capability; favored metastatic sites include peritoneal surfaces, liver, and retroperitoneal soft tissue; lymph node metastasis rare (5%); extraabdominal metastasis (lung or bone) occurs in 10%
- Highly cellular spindle cell sarcomas are the most aggressive and have the poorest survival rate (10% at 10 years)
- Epithelioid cell sarcomas of Carney triad (see associations below) are rarely fatal

Associations

- Carney triad:
  - Epithelioid cell gastric sarcoma: Usually multifocal; small discrete nodules (occasionally a large single mass); usually a pure epithelioid cell population with small densely packed, uniform cells that have clear peripheral cytoplasm; cells have less cytoplasm than benign tumors and have more mitotic figures; architectural arrangement may be organoid with nests of tumor cells separated by fine fibrovascular septa (may resemble neuroendocrine tumors); metastatic risk is low
  - Pure cartilaginous pulmonary chondromas
  - Functioning extraadrenal paragangliomas that are often multifocal and cause hypertension
- Gastric tumors also linked to neurofibromatosis type I

Comments

- Several tumors, some of which are in the differential diagnosis of GIST, can be c-*kit* (CD117) positive: Small cell carcinoma, melanoma, angiosarcoma, germ cell tumor, Ewing/primary neuroectodermal tumor, perivascular epithelioid cell tumor (angiomyolipoma), myeloid sarcoma, and fibromatosis
- Other mesenchymal tumors of stomach:
  - GI autonomic nerve tumor
  - Leiomyomyoma and leiomyosarcoma
  - Glomus tumors
  - Schwannomas
  - Lipoma
  - Granular cell tumor
  - Kaposi sarcoma
- Other mesenchymal tumors of small intestine:
  - Leiomyoma and leiomyosarcoma
  - Angiosarcoma
  - Kaposi sarcoma
- Other mesenchymal tumors of the colon and rectum:
  - Kaposi sarcoma and angiosarcoma
  - Lipomas
  - Neurofibromas and schwannomas
  - Leiomyoma

Glomus Tumor

Clinical Manifestations

- Most common vascular tumor in the stomach of immunocompetent patients
- Seen with equal frequency in adult men and women
- Symptoms include pain, nausea, vomiting, and bleeding; occasionally asymptomatic

Gross Pathology

- Typically a solitary, circumscribed, intramural nodule ranging in size from 2 to 2.5 cm located with the muscularis propria of the gastric antrum
- Lesions more than 4 cm may be ulcerated

Microscopic Pathology

- Glomus cells are modified smooth muscle cells; they are uniform, round or epithelioid with pale amphophilic to slightly eosinophilic cytoplasm and uniform, round nuclei with coarse chromatin; they tend to cover dilated, irregularly shaped thin-walled vessels in thick layers, nests, strands, and/or sheets
- Tumors typically located in the muscularis propria, which becomes hypertrophied and collagenized at the margins of the neoplasm, giving the impression of a pseudocapsule; mucosa is never infiltrated
- Stroma is frequently hyalinized and small aggregates of glomus cells may be found entrapped in hyalinized areas
- Basement membrane material and reticulin surrounds individual glomus cells

Special Stains

- PAS or toluidine blue will highlight a "chicken-wire" network of basal lamina material encircling individual glomus cells
- Reticulin stains will highlight the reticulin surrounding individual tumor cells

Immunohistochemistry

- Basement membrane material can be demonstrated with either laminin or collagen type IV
- Tumor cells stain for vimentin and smooth muscle actin

Electron Microscopy

- Confirms the smooth muscle nature of glomus cells

Molecular Alterations

- None

Differential Diagnosis

- Epithelioid cell stromal tumor
- Carcinoid
- Lymphoma

Treatment

- Local excision

Prognosis

- Occasional reports of malignancy (probably represents leiomyosarcoma, epithelioid type)

Associations

- Glomus cell tumors have been reported in the esophagus and small intestine

Hyperplastic Polyp

Clinical Manifestations

- Among the most common gastric epithelial polyps (constituting from 50-90%)
- A range from a few millimeters to many centimeters
- Frequently arise at a site of or bordering an ulcer or erosion and likely represent excessive regeneration following mucosal damage (sometimes they have been referred to as regenerative polyps)

Gross Pathology

- Smooth surface or slightly lobulated, oval or hemispherical in shape
- Surface often eroded
- Most are sessile but larger polyps may be pedunculated
- May be single or multiple
- Can occur anywhere in the stomach, although most commonly in the antrum on a background of *H pylori* gastritis
- When multiple (20%), they may be widely scattered or confined to one area (may be concentrated at the junction of the body and the antrum

Microscopic Pathology

- Characteristically composed of hyperplastic, elongated, and dilated foveolae with an edematous, inflamed stroma
- Foveolae are generally lined with mature gastric mucin cells
- True dysplasia is extremely uncommon (<4%)
- Hyperplastic and elongated foveolae may produce intraluminal infolding and apparent branching and cystic dilatation is almost always present in the deeper parts of the polyp

- Small groups of pyloric type glands may be present under the proliferating foveolae
- Intestional metaplasia may be present but is rarely conspicuous and is usually focal and of the incomplete type
- Bundles of smooth muscle fibers growing into the polyp from muscularis mucosa are often seen and the lamina propria is often edematous and infiltrated by plasma cells, lymphocytes, eosinophils, mast cells, and macrophages
- Lymphoid aggregates with germinal centers may be present
- If the lesion is eroded, there is often a fibrinopurulent exudate with acute inflammatory cells and proliferating capillaries just under the focus of erosion; this phenomenon is usually associated with regenerative changes, including mitoses; the individual cells may appear quite atypical (pseudocarcinomatous)

Special Stains and Immunohistochemistry

- Strongly positive for vimentin
- Smooth muscle in the stroma will stain with muscle specific actin
- Stain negatively for epithelial and lymphoid markers (probably a reactive fibroblast or myofibroblast)

Electron Microscopy

- Not helpful

Molecular Alterations

- p53 expression has been identified in focal areas of dysplasia in hyperplastic gastric polyps and is associated with malignant transformation
- A point mutation in codon 12 of the K-*ras* oncogene has been reported in hyperplastic polyps with focal high-grade dysplasia

Differential Diagnosis

- Polypoid gastritis
- Polypoid foveolar hyperplasia
- Endoscopically may be confused for a carcinoma especially when large
- Generalized gastric mucosal hyperplasia (Ménétrier disease) and/or inflammation (Cronkhite-Canada syndrome)
- Hamartomatous polyps and syndromes involving the stomach (Peutz-Jeghers syndrome)

Treatment and Prognosis

- Considered to be non-neoplastic lesions
- When a hyperplastic polyp is removed, adjacent surrounding flat mucosa should be biopsied (see association with adenocarcinoma below)
- It is important to remember the association between hyperplastic polyps and autoimmune gastritis; autoimmune gastritis is suggested histologically when biopsies show inflammation in the body, glandular atrophy and intestinal metaplasia; in addition, immunostains for chromogranin and gastrin on biopsies of the body and antrum may be helpful (see Autoimmune Gastritis)

Associations

- Adenocarcinomas are occasionally reported to occur within one of these polyps but this is unusual (<1%)
- Associated with a wide range of background gastric mucosal abnormalities (rarely arise in a normal stomach)
- Strongly associated with atrophic gastritis of either the autoimmune or *H pylori* associated types
- Tend to be a response to a variety of injuries
- Patients with a hyperplastic polyp are at increased risk (up to 6% for a synchronous or metachronous adenocarcinoma)
- *H pylori* organisms are a usual associated finding
- Examples of epithelial dysplasia and malignant change are being increasingly reported (1-2%)
- Hyperplastic polyp may be seen in up to 20% of patients with gastric cancer elsewhere in the stomach

Inflammatory Fibroid Polyp

Clinical Manifestations

- Typically occurs in distal stomach or pylorus (*Vanek polyp*) and terminal ileum (have been found in the esophagus, colon, and more proximal part of small intestine)
- Gastric lesions typically asymptomatic (primarily because of their small size) but gastric outlet obstruction may be a presenting symptom)
- Terminal ileal lesions may present with bowel obstruction secondary to intussusception
- Typically diagnosed in 6th decade of life
- Men slightly more commonly affected than women

Gross Pathology

- Gastric inflammatory fibroid polyp:
  - Typically found just proximal to and occasionally overlying the pyloric sphincter musculature
  - Tend to be sessile but may be pedunculated
  - Average about 1.5 cm
  - Occasionally have overlying ulcers
- Ileal inflammatory fibroid polyp:
  - Typically larger than gastric counterpart
  - Usually extensively ulcerated

Microscopic Pathology

- Gastric inflammatory fibroid polyp
  - Composed of plump spindle cells and inflammatory cells (usually eosinophils)
  - Tends to fill superficial submucosa and have a very well-defined lower border deep in the submucosa
  - Typically infiltrates the base of the mucosa where it separates the glands and spreads apart the bundles of muscularis mucosa
  - Tumor cells rarely involve muscularis propria
  - Spindle cells and eosinophils tend to form concentric layers around small, thin-walled vessels resulting in a perivascular orientation of the neoplastic cells
- Ileal inflammatory fibroid polyp
  - Neoplasms look like excessive granulation tissue and tend to have an edematous stroma (more edematous than gastric counterpart); they tend to be transmural, fill the submucosa, replace the muscularis propria, and extend into the subserosa
  - Vessels tend to be more elongated than rounded and lack the prominent perivascular laminations characteristic of the gastric lesions
  - Cell population tends to be more stellate than spindled and the inflammatory component consists of a mixture of plasma cells, lymphocytes, and eosinophils
  - Occasionally numerous mitoses and prominent nuclear hyperchromatism present near the center of the polyp (may resemble sarcoma)
  - Inflammatory fibroid polyps in the esophagus tend to look like those in the terminal ileum; lesions in the colon tend to look like those in the stomach

Special Stains and Immunohistochemistry

- Not helpful

Electron Microscopy

- Stellate (ileal) and spindle (gastric) cells have features of fibroblasts and myofibroblasts
- A population of macrophages also easily identified

Molecular Alterations

- None

Differential Diagnosis

- Ileal lesions may resemble sarcoma (see microscopic pathology)
- GIST
- Fibromatosis

Treatment

- Simple excision

Prognosis

- Related solely to presence or absence of complications (usually obstruction)

Associations

- Gastric lesions may be encountered in the setting of atrophic gastritis and pernicious anemia, gastric adenomas, and/or carcinoma
- Ileal lesions have no known associations

Mucosa-Associated Lymphoid Tissue Lymphoma (MALToma)

Clinical Manifestations

- Typically referred to as low-grade extranodal marginal zone B-cell lymphoma of mucosa-associated lymphoid tissue (MALT)
- Arise within organized lymphoid tissue in gastric mucosa
- Usually acquired in response to *H pylori* infection
- The majority are restricted to the gastric wall at the time of presentation
- Low-grade MALT lymphoma is the commonest form of lymphoma in the stomach
- Males more commonly affected than females
- Approximately 40% of all non-Hodgkin lymphomas arise at extranodal sites; the GI tract is the most common extranodal site
- The majority of patients are over the age of 50
- *H pylori* organisms are present in 90% of cases limited to mucosa and submucosa, in 75% when the deep submucosa is involved and are present in 50% of cases in which there is extension of the lymphoma beyond the submucosa
- Patients often present with a long history of dyspepsia, nausea and vomiting; high-grade lesions may present as a palpable mass in the epigastrium and may cause weight loss

Gross Pathology

- The tumor predominantly involves the mucosa and submucosa but may spread into the muscularis propria and less commonly into the submucosa
- Local lymphoid involvement may occur

Microscopic Pathology

- Normal gastric mucosa contains scattered lymphocytes and plasma cells but does not have organized lymphoid tissue
- The initial change that occurs in the development of primary gastric lymphoma is the acquisition of organized lymphoid tissue from which the lymphoma can develop; as noted this can be associated with an infection by *H pylori* and its also seen in cases of infection with *H heilmannii*
- The lamina propria is expanded with small uniform cells some of which appear to have a "halo" around them
- The lymphocytes may infiltrate the muscularis mucosae (physiological lymphoid collections do not infiltrate the muscularis mucosa)
- The classic "lymphoepithelial lesion" in which lymphocytes are seen in residual gland epithelium is not always present, but represents a pathonomonic finding when it is present
- *H pylori* gastritis may be seen in the background
- One particular feature of low-grade MALT lymphoma is the stomach is multifocality; there may be one dominant lesion, but additional small foci of lymphoma are often present remote from the main mass
- The histopathology of low-grade MALT lymphoma closely resembles the physiological appearance of gut lymphoid tissue
- Reactive lymphoid follicles with germinal centers are a prominent feature but between these follicles there are interspersed sheets of marginal zone cells; these cells have small to intermediate sized nuclei and show prominent grooves with moderate amounts of cytoplasm
- The lymphoid cells may be relatively monotonous or show a fair degree of pleomorphism
- Prominent plasmacytoid features may be present in 30%
- The infiltrate usually contains transformed cells that are morphologically similar to that of follicular center cell blasts (centroblasts); these transformed cells are usually diffusely admixed with smaller lymphoid cells
- The neoplastic marginal zone cells often infiltrate gastrointestinal epithelium creating the highly distinctive *lymphoepithelial lesion*, in which the marginal zones displace and destroy epithelium
- The epithelium of a lymphoepithelial lesion shows a striking eosinophilic change as they are destroyed

Immunohistochemistry and Special Stains

- CD20 or 79a, CD3, CD43, cytokeratin and sometimes κ and λ light chains will show a predominance of B-cells with scattered T-cells; B-cells may co-express CD43; cytokeratin is useful in demonstrating lymphoepithelial lesions; if plasma cell differentiation prominent then light chain restriction may be helpful
- Reactive lymphoid follicles and germinal centers are almost always part of the lymphoma and are characterized by having margins of the germinal centers infiltrated and obscured by the neoplastic cells, thereby producing a moth-eaten appearance in the germinal center (eventually the lymphoid follicle will be completely overrun and destroyed by the lymphoma)
- Cells do not express CD10, CD5, and cyclin D-1
- Cells usually positive for bcl-2 protein
- CD23 or CD35 can demonstrate underlying follicular dendritic cells

Electron Microscopy

- Not helpful

Molecular Alterations

- The genetic abnormaly of t(11;18) may be associated with a lack of response to *H pylori* eradication
- *p53* and *bcl-2* overexpression are features of high-grade transformation
- Translocation t (11;18) (q21;q21) has been seen in a significant number of low-grade MALT lymphomas (this translocation is less common in high-grade lesions)

Differential Diagnosis

- MALT lymphomas may have prominent numbers of plasmacytoid cells may result in a misdiagnosis (these plasma cells usually have pronounced entercytoplasmic immunoglobulin that actually pushes the nucleus to one side of the cell; the plasmacytoid cells in a MALToma may resemble signet ring cells of a diffuse-type gastric adenocarcinoma
- Florid gastritis
- Reactive infiltrate (in gastritis, the infiltrate surrounding the lymphoid follicles in the lamina propria tends to be plasma cell predominant; in MALT lymphoma this infiltrate contain a dominant population of "centrocyte-like cells"
- Follicular lymphoma
- Mantle cell lymphoma

Treatment and Prognosis

- 70% to 80% of patients will experience long term remission if *H pylori* organisms are eliminated; the MALTomas most likely to respond to the eradication of *H pylori* are those located superficially within the gastric mucosa
- Low-grade lymphomas can recur following *H pylori* eradication, but these recurrences are fairly rare and often regress spontaneously
- MALT lesions progress slowly and may be present after the initiation of treatment to eradicate the *H pylori* organisms
- Distant spread of disease is distinctly uncommon but spread to the marginal zone of the spleen may occur
- Low-grade lymphoma should be treated with antibiotic therapy for *H pylori*
- Cases that do not respond to antibiotic therapy might benefit from local radiotherapy
- Advanced cases can be treated with chemotherapy
- Stage is the most important determinant of long-term prognosis
- *H pylori* eradication produces tumor regression between in 60% to 90% of cases
- 90% 5-year survival rate and 75% 10-year survival rate

Associations

- There are several reports of synchronous and metachronous coexistence of primary malignant lymphoma and adenocarcinoma
- Epstein-Barr virus is not associated with a low-grade lymphoma and is only seen in some high-grade lymphomas

Comment

- High-grade primary lymphoma may outnumber low-grade tumors. The diagnosis of high-grade MALT type malignant lymphoma can be difficult and is generally based on a *predominance* of blast cells
- Tumor cells typically express CD20 and often lack other lymphocytic markers
- Transformed high-grade lymphoma demonstrates the same immunoglobulin gene rearrangements as its low-grade component

Neuroendocrine Tumors

Clinical Manifestations

- Clinical symptoms typically dominated by the underlying etiology (autoimmune gastritis, MEN type I, or Zollinger-Ellison syndrome [ZES])
- Diagnosis based on the fact that most tumor cells show:
    - Strong argyrophilia by both the Grimelius and Sevier-Munger technique
    - Absent reactivity for argentaffin or diazonium tests for serotonin
    - Positive immunoreactivity for chromogranin A
    - Usually no immunoreactivity for other hormonal products
- 3 variants:
    - Type I: Associated with diffuse chronic atrophic gastritis restricted to body/fundus (type A or autoimmune); 70% occur in women and typically diagnosed in 7th decade; usually coupled with achlorhydria with or without pernicious anemia
    - Type II: Associated with hypertrophic, hypersecretory gastropathy with high levels of serum gastrin usually in conjunction with MEN type I and ZES; relatively rare (approximately 6%); seen with equal frequency in both sexes and tends to occur in the 5th decade
    - Type III: Sporadic; not associated with any specific gastric pathology; presents as either a mass with clinical features similar to carcinoma (hemorrhage, obstruction, or metastasis) or as an endocrinopathy if it produces hormonal products (may differ from ordinary carcinoids by producing 5-hydroxytryptophan rather than serotonin); usually seen in gastric mucosa without any evidence of gastritis; represents approximately 14% of cases; more common in men than women; typically presents in the 6th decade; usually neither hypergastrinemia nor gastrin-dependent neuroendocrine cell hyperplasia present

Gross Pathology

- Tumors associated with autoimmune atrophic gastritis tend to be multiple, small, and limited to the mucosa and submucosa of the gastric fundus; almost always benign; most <1 cm in diameter
- Tumors associated with MEN and the ZES usually multiple and multicentric; may metastasize to local lymph nodes
- Sporadic tumors are usually solitary and more common than MEN and ZES-associated tumors

Microscopic Pathology

- Autoimmune-chronic diffuse atrophic gastritis-associated tumors (Type 1)
    - Tumor cells typically arranged in ribbon or trabecular patterns with occasional rosettes; insular pattern (characteristic of carcinoids in the small intestine and proximal colon) usually absent
    - Individual tumor cells tend to be bland, round, or polygonal with ill-defined cellular borders, little atypia; nuclei centrally located and have finely stippled chromatin and a small eccentric nucleolus; no mitoses
    - When invasion present, typically limited to the mucosa or submucosa
- MEN and ZES-associated tumors (Type II):
    - Neuroendocrine cell-like hyperplasia and dysplasia usually seen in surrounding normal (nontumor) mucosa
    - Histology always bland with no mitoses; quite similar to that of autoimmune-atrophic gastritis associated tumors
- Sporadic tumors (Type III):
    - 50% have moderate cellular atypia with nuclear pleomorphism, prominent nucleoli, hyperchromasia, and significant numbers of mitoses

- Tumors tend to grow in solid aggregates and trabeculae
- Mean diameter usually >3 cm
- Invasion frequently present (in the muscularis propria in 75% and in the serosa in 55%)
- High incidence of distant metastasis
- An "atypical carcinoid syndrome" with red cutaneous flushing (rather than cyanotic flushing) without diarrhea usually seen in the presence of liver metastasis secondary to the production of histamine and/or 5-hydroxytryptophan

Special Stains

- Tumor cells are usually argyrophilic (Grimeliusand Sevier-Munger technique)

Immunohistochemistry

- Tumor cells stain for chromogranin A
- 50% stain for synaptophysin
- Usually no significant immunohistochemically identifiable hormone product present but scattered cells may show secretory products such as serotonin, PP, histamine, gastrin, and rarely corticotropin, epinephrine, and parathyroid hormone–related protein

Electron Microscopy

- Tumor cells show vesicular granules containing a markedly dense core, often with a coarsely granular substructure

Molecular Alterations

- None

Differential Diagnosis

- Poorly differentiated adenocarcinoma
- Lymphoma
- Mesenchymal neoplasm
- Glomus cells of the stomach

Treatment

- Multiple small lesions <1 cm in diameter can often be removed endoscopically
- Multiple lesions resulting from hypergastrinemia (autoimmune atrophic gastritis) regress with antrectomy
- Surgical excision of gastrin-producing tumor in patients with MEN type I syndrome and ZES
- Solitary lesions (unassociated with atrophic gastritis and endocrine cell hyperplasia) treated with aggressive surgical excision

Prognosis

- Lesions associated with autoimmune chronic atrophic gastritis and MEN and ZES will essentially disappear with the abolishment of the associated hypergastrinemia
- Tumors associated with autoimmune chronic atrophic gastritis can metastasize (although rarely) but no tumor-related deaths have been reported
- Tumors associated with MEN and ZES may cause death, usually as a result of coexisting (often aggressive) gastrin-producing tumor in the pancreas or duodenum
- Sporadic tumors may be lethal in light of their high metastatic potential

Associations

- Autoimmune-atrophic gastritis (see above)
- MEN type I and ZES (see above)

Small Intestine

Non-Neoplastic

Acute Self-Limited Enterocolitis

Clinical Manifestations

- Patients typically present with an acute episode of bloody diarrhea
- Sigmoidoscopic examination at the time symptoms first appear most often consistent with inflammatory bowel disease
- Symptoms typically resolve within 2 weeks and follow-up sigmoidoscopic examination findings are normal

- Enteric pathogens recovered in 50%
- "Pathogens" include *Campylobacter, Salmonella, Shigella, Yersinia,* and *Escherichia coli* 0157:H7

Gross Pathology

- Findings typically limited to first 4 days after onset of symptoms and include mucosal edema, superficial ulcers, and/or increased friability

Microscopic Pathology

- Findings at time of peak activity (0-4 days after onset of bloody diarrhea):
  - Mucosal edema, particularly in upper 1/3 of the mucosa
  - Superficial mucosal injury with thin layer of neutrophilic exudate
  - Cryptitis (neutrophils in crypt epithelium), crypt ulcers (loss of crypt epithelium), and crypt abscesses (neutrophilic exudate within dilated crypts; cryptitis and crypt abscesses frequently present in crypts that are small, atrophic, and thin-walled
  - Partial loss of intracellular mucin in cells of crypt epithelium
  - A generalized increase in the cellularity of the lamina propria with groups of neutrophils and occasional lymphocytes, plasma cells, and eosinophils
  - No crypt distortion (defined as branching, dilated, abnormal-shaped crypts, and loss of crypt parallelism)
  - No basal plasmacytosis (defined as increased numbers of plasma cells in lower one-fifth of the mucosa)
- Findings at time of partial resolution (5-9 days after onset of bloody diarrhea):
  - Slight mucosal edema
  - Surface and crypt epithelial regeneration (regenerating epithelial cells characterized by large nuclei with ≥1 irregular nucleoli, decreased mucin content, and increased numbers of mitotic figures)
  - Focal cryptitis and/or crypt abscesses
  - Moderate increase in cellularity of lamina propria with eosinophils, plasma cells, lymphocytes, and occasional neutrophils
  - No crypt distortion
  - No basal plasmacytosis
- Findings at later stages of resolution (9 days or more after onset of bloody diarrhea):
  - No mucosal edema
  - Some continued epithelial regeneration
  - Occasional lymphocytes in crypt epithelium
  - Slight increase in cellularity of lamina propria (plasma cells, lymphocytes, and eosinophils; no neutrophils)
  - No crypt distortion
  - No basal plasmacytosis
  - Biopsy findings may be normal
- At no time during a course of acute self-limited colitis is there evidence of significant crypt distortion (abnormal shapes, branching, or loss of parallelism) or plasmacytosis in the lower 1/5 of the mucosa; *the absence of crypt distortion and basal plasmacytosis are the most useful diagnostic criteria for differentiating acute self-limited colitis from ulcerative colitis*

Special Stains

- Special stains for microorganisms not especially helpful

Immunohistochemistry and Electron Microscopy

- Not helpful

Molecular Alterations

- None

Differential Diagnosis

- Ulcerative colitis (features most useful in distinguishing a first attack from acute self-limited colitis are absence of crypt distortion and absence of lamina propria plasmacytosis in the latter)
- Crohn colitis

Treatment and Prognosis

- Typically self-limited with complete resolution within two weeks
- Potential for dehydration must be appreciated

Associations

- None

Celiac Disease

Clinical Manifestations

- A systemic autoimmune disease induced by gluten proteins found in wheat, barley, and rye
- Primarily consists of injury to the small intestine
- Often presents with gastrointestinal distress or diarrhea of the malabsorption type, but may be essentially asymptomatic with slight iron deficiency anemia
- Commonly presents in children but many patients are first recognized during adolescence, during adult life, and even in old age
- Clinical presentation may be subtle and not related to the gastrointestinal tract
- Sites of extraintestinal injury include the skin (dermatitis herpetiformis), joints (rheumatoid arthritis), and the uterus (dysmenorrhea and deep dyspareunia)
- When undiagnosed may cause growth retardation and has been associated with fetal loss, infertility, and osteoporosis
- Recommended tests include anti-tissue transglutaminase or anti-endomyosial test (both are IgA-based tests); may yield false-negative results in patients with IgA deficiency

Microscopic Pathology

- Subtle lesions usually display only intraepithelial lymphocytosis that is either similar in density or more prominent in the tips of the villi than in the bases (in a normal small bowel biopsy, the number of intraepithelial lymphocytes decreases in the tips of the villi when compared to the bases)
- The fundamental process is a gluten-induced enteropathy that results in damage to enterocytes produced by breakdown products of gluten, and the failure of cell replication by the crypt zone to keep pace with this damage
- The earliest changes tend to be an increase in the number of intraepithelial T-lymphocytes (in the small intestine the upper limit of normal is 40 lymphocytes per 100 enterocytes)
- Lamina propria is usually expanded as a result of increased numbers of plasma cells; these plasma cells are usually responsible for producing the IgA antibodies to gliadin, to endomysium and to tissue transglutaminase (all important serological markers)
- Mast cells, basophils, and eosinophils are also increased in the lamina propria; the number of eosinophils does not reach that seen in protein allergies
- Neutrophils and histiocytes are not a typical inflammatory component

Special Stains

- Not helpful

Immunohistochemistry

- CD3 may be useful in helping to count the number of intraepithelial lymphocytes; more than 95% are CD3 and CD2 positive
- As the crypt zone cannot keep pace with the increased rate of loss of damaged surface enterocytes, the villi shorten in height and appear to increase in width; these changes are accompanied by an increase in the length of the crypts which is the result of increased mitotic activity
- Patients with refractory celiac disease typically have T-cells that are CD3 positive and CD8 negative; celiac disease that responds to dietary therapy typically has CD3 and CD8 positive T-cells

Electron Microscopy

- A reduction in the number and size of microvilli that are short, irregular in shape and may be fused together
- Pinocytic vesicules decrease in number
- The basement membrane is disrupted and increased in width and in density
- The vascular endothelial cells appears swollen

Molecular Alterations

- T-cell receptor (TCR-*g*) gene rearrangements seen in refractory sprue (see Associations below)

Differential Diagnosis

- Diseases that may produce flat duodenal mucosa include dermatitis herpetiformis, cow's milk protein intolerance (pediatric), giardiasis, peptic duodenitis, Crohn disease, small bowel bacterial overgrowth (usually anaerobes), eosinophilic gastroenteritis, radiation enteritis, tropical sprue, severe malnutrition, lymphoma, GVHD, hypogammaglobulinemia/ common variable immunodeficiency syndrome, and autoimmune enteropathy

Treatment and Prognosis

- 98% experience a beneficial effect of gluten withdrawal from the diet
- Certain human leukocyte antigens (HLA) are associated with an increased risk for the development of celiac disease (HLA-DQ2 and HLA-DQ8); increased risk is also associated with type I diabetes, children with Down syndrome and in individuals with iron deficiency anemia
- Some patients respond briefly to gluten-free diet then become refractory (a condition termed "refractory sprue")
- Some patients with refractory sprue develop collagenous sprue which is associated with a poor prognosis and may be terminal

Associations

- Dermatitis herpetiformis
- Collagenous sprue may be associated with T-cell lymphoma
- 60-80% of all patients with dermatitis or herpetiformis have a true gluten-induced enteropathy which responds to gluten withdrawal
- Microscopic colitis (lymphocytic and callagenous)
- Increased frequency of carcinoma in the GI tract
- Patients with celiac disease also have increased numbers of relatives with enteropathy
- Enteropathy-associated lymphoma

Crohn Disease

Clinical Manifestations

- More common in Western developed countries
- More frequent in the White population and in Jewish people
- A familial history in 3% to 11%
- Peak incidence in the 3rd decade; occasionally seen in both children and the elderly
- Males and females affected equally
- A slightly lower frequency than ulcerative colitis
- Patients with involvement of the ileum who experience an acute attack frequently present with signs and symptoms that mimic acute appendicitis
- More typically ileal involvement causes fever, crampy abdominal pain (often from obstruction), and watery diarrhea (usually the result of the toxic effects of unabsorbed bile salts on colonic mucosa)
- More extensive small bowel disease may result in development of an abdominal mass and/or sepsis (the latter secondary to localized perforations with sinus tracts and fistula between adjacent viscera and/or skin)
- Malabsorption may be a significant feature particularly in preadolescence when normal maturation may be affected
- Disease involving the colon usually presents in a similar fashion to ulcerative colitis with the acute onset of purulent diarrhea and rectal bleeding
- 20% to 25% of patients will have perianal disease (fistulae and abscesses); 5% will present with perianal disease
- Patients usually experience periods of relapses and remissions interspersed with periods of recurrences; recurrences usually indicate extension and worsening of the disease

Gross Pathology

- At initial presentation small intestine alone involved in about 45%, small intestine and colon in about 35%, and colon alone in 15% to 20%
- Most cases that involve the small intestine affect the terminal ileum with or without extension to the ileocecal valve
- 5% of patients with involvement of terminal ileum will eventually develop involvement of the proximal ileum and jejunum by either direct extension or over skip areas
- When colon involved, the right side affected more commonly than the left; rectum usually normal
- 50% of patients with Crohn disease of the colon will have proctitis with or without continuous disease into the left colon (this particular distribution similar to ulcerative colitis)
- Occasionally Crohn disease (with or without gross involvement of the small or large intestine) may

present with lesions in the oral cavity, esophagus, stomach, and proximal duodenum

- Early lesions appear endoscopically as multiple small aphthous ulcers surrounded by a slightly raised edematous and inflamed mucosa
- As the disease progresses, larger ulcers coalesce and extend over variable lengths of bowel in a longitudinal or serpiginous fashion
- Ulcers separated by patches or segments of normal mucosa that give the mucosal surface a cobblestone-like appearance
- Ulcers tend to penetrate deep into the submucosa; 65% associated with inflammatory fissures or sinus tracts that extend well into muscularis propria
- Sinus tracts can extend through the bowel wall resulting in localized perforation or external abscess formation (free perforation with peritonitis unusual because the inflammatory process results in the formation of adhesions between the involved loops of intestine, other intraabdominal organs, or the abdominal wall)
- Fistulas present in 35% and connect diseased segments of bowel to other segments of bowel, the urinary bladder, and the abdominal wall
- Deep ulcers and fistula usually result in a marked submucosal fibrosis which leads to stricture formation
- Adipose tissue adjacent to areas of inflammation tends to wrap itself around the external surface of the bowel in a "protective fashion" and may actually obscure the serosa surface
- Disease involving terminal ileum is generally characterized by marked stenosis, muscular hypertrophy, "fat wrapping," and fistula formation with or without abscesses
- Disease involving colon does not result in as much thickening of the bowel wall as seen in small bowel disease and the mucosal ulceration may be slightly more superficial and oriented longitudinally with intervening inflammatory pseudopolyps (findings similar to those of ulcerative colitis with the differential diagnosis resting on the demonstration of definite skip areas or coexisting involvement of the terminal ileum)

Microscopic Pathology

- Earliest lesions represent aphthous ulcers that are fairly superficial (limited to the mucosa and submucosa) with a nonspecific inflammatory reaction at the ulcer's edge; initially there is prominent edema and neutrophilic infiltration followed by the appearance of granulation tissue and mononuclear inflammatory cells
- More advanced lesions characterized by a sharp demarcation between the edge of an ulcer and adjacent normal mucosa
- Proliferation of small lymphoid nodules some with germinal centers occurs in the submucosa but may involve any layer of the bowel wall
- Prominent dilatation of lymphatics usually evident in submucosa and submucosa usually considerably expanded by fibrosis often accompanied by proliferation of nerves
- Muscularis propria variably hypertrophied and foci of inflammation usually seen in the muscularis propria as well as serosa
- Ulcers and fistula tracts that extend deep into the bowel wall typically lined with chronic inflammatory cells and resemble granulation tissue; foreign body–type giant cells may be seen but well-formed granulomas rarely present
- Disease involving small intestine has more extensive submucosal fibrosis, neuroproliferation, and muscular hypertrophy than colonic disease; regenerating mucosa characterized by a reduction in the number of villi, hyperplasia of Paneth cells, and presence of pyloric gland metaplasia
- Disease involving the colon characterized by less submucosal fibrosis and muscular hypertrophy; ulcers that tend to be relatively shallow and limited to the mucosa or upper submucosa (similar to the findings in ulcerative colitis except that even in areas of superficial ulceration there is usually some inflammation in the muscularis propria and serosa)
- Chronic disease characterized by crypt deformity, a marked increase in mononuclear inflammatory cells and eosinophils in the lamina propria, a villiform mucosal surface, and the presence of increased numbers of Paneth cells in the crypt epithelium (only the presence of skip areas reliably distinguishes the chronic form of Crohn disease from the chronic form of ulcerative colitis)

- Epithelioid cell granulomas (the pathognomonic feature of Crohn disease) seen in 50% of resected specimens; may be found in any portion of the bowel wall (most common in submucosa) and in areas distant from ulceration
- Well-formed granulomas composed of enlarged macrophages and giant cells admixed with other inflammatory cells (plasma cells and eosinophils); no necrosis unless the granuloma located in the serosa; resemble granulomas of sarcoidosis (may even contain Schaumann bodies)
- Granulomas of Crohn disease must be differentiated from the granulomatous response to a ruptured crypt of other inflammatory conditions or to foreign material

Special Stains and Immunohistochemistry

- Not helpful

Electron Microscopy

- Scanning EM confirms that the earliest lesion is a tiny erosion in the mucosa overlying normal mucosal lymphoid tissue

Molecular Alterations

- None

Differential Diagnosis

- Small intestinal disease:
  - Lymphoma
  - Ischemic disease
  - Chronic granulomatous infections (tuberculosis, *Yersinia*, *Histoplasma*, and *Anisakiasis*)
- Colonic disease:
  - Right-sided involvement: Tuberculosis, amebiasis, and infection due to *Clostridium histolyticum*
  - Segmental disease: Ischemic colitis, diverticula disease, and neoplasm
  - Left-sided disease: Ulcerative colitis, vasculitis, reactions to drugs, ischemic colitis, and acute infections (*Campylobacter*, *Chlamydia*, *Shigella*, and *Clostridium difficile*)

Treatment

- Medical management includes nutritional support, antiinflammatory and immunosuppressive agents (corticosteroids and 6-mercaptopurine), and antibiotics for secondary infections
- Surgery usually reserved for complications and intractable disease and limited to conservative resections of involved intestine (once patient has undergone a surgical resection, there is a recurrence rate of approximately 5% per year with recurrences tending to appear at the site of previous surgery

Prognosis

- Disease associated with multiple relapses; with each operation the risk that another operation will be necessary continues to increase
- Overall mortality approximately twice that of the general population

Associations

- *Perianal disease*
  - Occurs in 20% to 25% of patients with either small or large bowel disease
  - First manifestation of disease in 5% (may precede development of intestinal disease by 2 to 3 years)
  - Characterized by multiple complex fissures and perianal abscesses
  - Adjacent rectum may be inflamed or normal
- *Toxic megacolon*
  - Less common than in ulcerative colitis (probably secondary to the fibrosis that is so characteristic of Crohn disease)
  - May be further complicated by development of ischemic necrosis with perforation and peritonitis
- *Secondary infections*
  - *C difficile* may be responsible for a relapse of disease
  - Opportunistic infections (herpes and cytomegalovirus) may develop as a result of immunosuppressive or antiinflammatory therapy

- *Colitis cystica*
  - Glandular tissue that traverses the muscularis mucosa and lies within the submucosa as a consequence of regeneration
- *Extraintestinal manifestations of disease*
  - Uveitis, polyarthritis, ankylosing spondylitis, erythema nodosum, and pyoderma gangrenosum (conditions similar to those seen in ulcerative colitis)
  - Nutritional deficiency can result from fatty changes in the liver
  - Other hepatic changes include chronic pericholangitis, sclerosing cholangitis, increased risk for the development of bile duct carcinoma, and increased incidence of gallstones
- *Dysplasia*
  - Epithelial dysplasia often present in mucosa adjacent to a carcinoma in either the small or large intestine involved by Crohn disease
  - Other histologic features of dysplasia in Crohn disease identical to those of ulcerative colitis
- *Carcinoma*
  - Patients with chronic Crohn disease of the small intestine have a 20-fold increased incidence of carcinoma in the area of involvement
  - Overall incidence of carcinoma in the colon approximately 3%
  - Development of a carcinoma directly related to duration of disease and may be more likely in patients who experience an onset of symptoms prior to age 30 years
  - Incidence of carcinoma in Crohn colitis less than in ulcerative colitis
  - Carcinoma tends to occur in younger patients (10 years younger than the average population) and more frequently multiple
  - Carcinoma typically presents as advanced disease; 30% well-differentiated and mucinous

Microvillous Inclusion Disease

Gross and Microscopic Pathology

- Primarily involves the small intestine (duodenum, jejunum, and ileum), colon, and gastric antrum
- Characterized by a diffuse villous atrophy with little or no crypt hyperplasia, and *no inflammatory reaction*
- Increased crypt cell apoptosis
- Intact crypts appear shortened or slightly dilated, but the enterocytes typically retain their columnar shape
- Enterocytes have no surface microvilli or are shortened and disorganized; cytoplasmic inclusions consisting of variably sized vesicular bodies, targetoid microvillous inclusions, and some lysosome-like structures lie close to the apical surface or deep in the supranuclear cytoplasm; these inclusions give the apical cytoplasm a bubbly vacuolated appearance
- Nearby goblet cells and Paneth cells are normal by both light microscopy and ultrastructurally

Special Stains

- PAS or alkaline phosphatase will demonstrate the apical, supranuclear inclusions in the cytoplasm of the enterocytes; PAS will also confirm the discontinuous brush border over the apices of atrophic residual villi

Immunohistochemistry

- Carcinoembryonic antigen (CEA) and CD10 stain the apical enterocytes that contain the fragmented brush border

Electron Microscopy

- Intracytoplasmic vesicles lined by microvilli
- Poorly developed brush border microvilli of intestinal epithelium

Molecular Alterations

- Autosomal recessive

Differential Diagnosis

- Celiac disease

Treatment and Prognosis

- Without small bowel transplantation or life-long parenteral nutrition, patients almost always die before the age of 18 months (sepsis, liver failure, and dehydration)
- Patients with late on-set disease do somewhat better than those with congenital disease

Associations

- None

Whipple Disease

Clinical Manifestations

- A systemic disease that may involve joints, skin, nervous system, eye, skeletal and cardiac muscle, serosal membranes, lung, kidney, liver, spleen, and lymph nodes
- Causative agent a small rod-shaped bacterium, *Tropheryma whipplei*
- Patients usually present with the signs and symptoms of malabsorption

Gross Pathology

- Mucosal folds thickened and have a patchy coating of granular, whitish material (secondary to the accumulation of chyle in the lymphatics of the lamina propria)
- More normal-appearing areas of reddish mucosa interspersed between thickened folds

Microscopic Pathology

- Villi usually rounded and somewhat flattened or blunted
- Extracellular accumulations of lipid present in lamina propria and lymphatic channels
- *Sine qua non* the presence of numerous macrophages in the lamina propria with a basophilic, stippled cytoplasm
- Typically the normal inflammatory component of the lamina propria reduced but neutrophils occasionally present

Special Stains

- PAS with diastase will demonstrate presence of rods and granules in macrophages and the lamina propria
- Iron stains will highlight hemosiderin-laden macrophages deep in the lamina propria and lipofucin in cells of muscularis mucosa

Immunohistochemistry

- Not helpful

Electron Microscopy

- Rod-shaped bacteria easily seen both in macrophages and extracellularly
- Macrophage granules are membrane-bound phagosomes that contain bacteria in various stages of digestion
- Confirms the bacteria have an inner membrane that is responsible for the PAS-positive material that makes up the macrophage granules
- Confirms presence of rod-shaped intracellular bacteria in other cell types to include epithelium, fibroblasts, endothelium, leukocytes, lymphocytes, mast cells, and smooth muscle cells

Molecular Alterations

- None

Differential Diagnosis

- *Mycobacterium avium-intracellulare* infection
- *T whipplei* can be detected through use of PCR

Treatment

- Antibiotics

Prognosis

- Antibiotic treatment results in cure

Associations

- Patients with Whipple disease may have innate defects in cell-mediated immunity
- A rare cause of amyloidosis

Neoplastic

Neuroendocrine Tumors—Duodenum

Clinical Manifestations

- 3% of all GI neuroendocrine tumors
- Usually associated with carcinoid syndrome
- May present with bleeding and/or a polypoid growth
- Most occur in 1st or 2nd portion of duodenum; may be multicentric; usually small (<1 cm)
- Endocrine hyperfunction resulting from duodenal and some upper jejunal endocrine tumors causes symptoms of the Zollinger-Ellison syndrome (ZES): hypergastrinemia, gastric acid hypersecretion, and fulminant ulcer diathesis
- Lesions located in duodenal bulb often "nonfunctioning"; may be a result of the small well-differentiated nature of the neoplasms that arise in this location; they produce milder peptic ulcer disease than usually seen in ZES caused by gastrinomas in the pancreas or elsewhere in the duodenum
- Tumors associated with ZES tend to occur earlier (mean age 40 years) than nonfunctioning tumors (mean age 65 years)
- Tumors associated with the ZES more likely to be infiltrative and metastasize than the nonfunctioning tumors

Gross Pathology

- Both functioning and nonfunctioning tumors appear as small (<1 cm) slightly polypoid lesion
- 5 subgroups:
  - *Gastrin-producing (G-cell) tumor*: Most common (65%); lymph node metastases in 30% at time of diagnosis
  - *Somatostatin-producing (D-cell) tumor*: 30% associated with von Recklinghausen disease; somatostatin usually strongly expressed, but somatoststin syndrome (hyperglycemia, cholelithiasis, and constipation) rare
  - *Serotonin/calcitonin-producing tumor*: Hepatic metastases may cause carcinoid syndrome
  - *Poorly differentiated neuroendocrine tumor*: Usually in periampullary region; prognosis very bad (survival 6 months to a 1½ years)
  - *Gangliocytic paraganglioma*: Rarely recur; considered benign

Microscopic Pathology

- Tumor cells tend to be uniform with scant cytoplasm; usually arranged in broad gyriform trabeculae and vascular pseudorosettes
- Multifocal, intraepithelial growths that form chains or micronodules of endocrine cells occasionally with mild atypia in direct continuity with the main tumor have been found deep in the crypts of intestinal mucosa adjacent to gastrin cell tumors (microscopic evidence to support the impression these tumors arise from differentiated intraepithelial endocrine cells)
- 5 subgroups:
  - *Gastrin-producing (G-cell) tumor*: Mixture of growth patterns
  - *Somatostatin-producing (D-cell) tumor*: Characterized by pseudo-acini with psammoma bodies
  - *Serotonin/calcitonin-producing tumor*: Typically type A growth pattern
  - *Poorly differentiated neuroendocrine tumor*: Usually in periampullary region; prognosis very bad (survival 6 months to a 1½ years)
  - *Gangliocytic paraganglioma*: An admixture of ganglion cells and endocrine cells (pancreatic polypeptide and somatostatin-positive cells) in a stroma of S-100–positive spindled cells; rarely recur; considered benign

Special Stains

- Not helpful

Immunohistochemistry

- Tumor cells positive for chromogranin and synaptophysin
- Functioning gastrin tumors positive for gastrin (nonfunctioning tumors negative)

- Somatostatin (inhibits gastrin release from gastrinoma) frequently present in nonfunctioning tumors and occasionally present in gastrin-producing tumors

Electron Microscopy

- Presence of dense core neurosecretory granules throughout cytoplasm of tumor cells confirms neuroendocrine nature of these tumors

Molecular Alterations

- None

Differential Diagnosis

- Grossly polypoid neoplasms can resemble ectopic pancreas, ectopic gastric mucosa, and an inflammatory polyp

Treatment

- Local surgical excision or pancreaticoduodenectomy depending on extent of disease

Prognosis

- Nonfunctioning tumors tend to be benign
- Tumors associated with the ZES have a low-grade malignant potential especially if they arise in sites where gastrin cells are not normally present (jejunum or pancreas)
- 25% to 50% of duodenal lesions associated with ZES have metastases in regional lymph nodes
- Presence of lymph node metastasis has little influence on survival
- Incidence of lymph node metastasis in patients with primary pancreatic versus primary duodenal gastrinomas essentially identical, but frequency of metastases to liver much greater in patients with pancreatic gastrinomas than in patients with duodenal gastrinomas (50% versus 5%)
- Overall malignancy rate of gastrin-producing duodenal tumors (associated with ZES) ranges from 40% to 55%; overall malignancy rate of pancreatic gastrinomas associated with ZES 70%
- 10-year survival rate of patients with duodenal gastrinomas approximately 95%, and of patients with pancreatic gastrinomas approximately 60%

Associations

- MEN and ZES(see above)
- von Recklinghausen disease

Colon/Rectum

Non-Neoplastic

Collagenous Colitis

Clinical Manifestations

- Typically seen in middle-aged and older women (rarely seen in men)
- Usually presents with a gradual onset of watery diarrhea and cramping abdominal pain
- Diarrhea may progress in severity or remit and recur and persist for several years
- Many patients are misdiagnosed clinically as having irritable bowel syndrome or a psychosomatic disorder

Gross Pathology

- No gross abnormalities endoscopically or radiologically

Microscopic Pathology

- Marked deposition of subepithelial collagen
- Collagen deposition limited to region just beneath surface epithelium and is irregular and encircles superficial capillaries in the lamina propria; thickened membrane measures from 15 to 65 μm (normal basement membranes measures 3 to 5 μm), is limited to the surface area (does not extend downward to involve the basement membrane region of the underlying crypts), and contains increased numbers of fibroblasts and eosinophils
- Typically there is an increase in plasma cells and eosinophils in the superficial lamina propria and a patchy increase in lymphocytes in the surface epithelial layer
- Occasionally small foci of epithelial degeneration and Paneth cell metaplasia may be present
- Findings of chronic colitis (granulomas, crypt distortion, atrophy, and/or a villiform surface) are absent
- Lesion not uniform throughout colon (rectum usually less involved)

Special Stains

- Thickened collagen deposition can be highlighted with the use of trichrome stains

Immunohistochemistry

- Not helpful

Electron Microscopy

- Basement membrane has normal dimensions and appearance; the thickening is due solely to deposition of mature collagen of type I and III in the subadjacent tissue

Molecular Alterations

- None

Differential Diagnosis

- Lymphocytic colitis
- Inflammatory bowel disease
- Acute colitis
- Solitary rectal ulcer syndrome
- Ischemia
- Amyloidosis
- Radiation colitis
- Hyperplastic polyp
- Celiac sprue

Treatment and Prognosis

- 80% to 90% of patients respond to therapy with sulfasalazine and corticosteroids
- Bismuth
- May spontaneously resolve

Associations

- Autoimmune diseases (thyroid disease, rheumatoid joint disease, pernicious anemia, small bowel villous atrophy, iritis, and myasthenia gravis)
- May have a (coincidental) association with adenocarcinoma of colon and Crohn disease
- May coexist with celiac disease
- Nonsteroidal antiinflammatory drugs may play a role in etiology

Graft-Versus-Host Disease (GVHD)

Clinical Manifestations

- Small intestine more frequently involved than esophagus, stomach, or colon
- Seen in children with severe combined immunodeficiency and in patients who have received allogenic bone marrow transplantation
- Acute disease produces diarrhea and abdominal pain
- After 3 months, 10% of patients develop chronic disease and experience dysphagia, reflux esophagitis, diarrhea, malabsorption, and/or abdominal pain

Gross Pathology

- Esophageal involvement is typically manifest by the presence of mucosal ulcerations
- Depending on the stage and severity of disease, gastric mucosa may appear normal, somewhat atrophic, or denuded
- Small intestine may the most severely affected portion of the GI tract by acute GVHD but is rarely involved by chronic GVHD

Microscopic Pathology

- Changes in the esophagus consist of a necrotizing and desquamative esophagitis primarily in the proximal esophagus; apoptosis of individual squamous cells and inflammation in the epithelium are additional typical findings (identical findings are seen in cutaneous GVHD)
- Early changes in the stomach consist of isolated epithelial cell necrosis in the neck cells of the pits with associated karyorrhexis debris and dilatation of pits or glands ("exploding crypt cell")
- Involvement of the colon and rectum by acute GVHD produces the same microscopic findings that are seen in the small intestine; most sensitive indicator is presence of apoptotic bodies in crypt bases
- Grading of acute GVHD:
  - Grade I: Apoptosis (single cell necrosis characterized by formation of apoptotic body, a collection of eosinophilic globules and nuclear debris)
  - Grade II: Apoptosis accompanied by crypt abscesses

  - □ Grade III: Total necrosis of individual crypts
  - □ Grade IV: Total denudation of areas of bowel
- Chronic GVHD is characterized by submucosal fibrosis, mucosal calcification, and focal fibrosis in the lamina propria
- Cytomegalovirus colitis may be present

Special Stains, Immunohistochemistry and Electron Microscopy

- Not helpful

Molecular Alterations

- None

Differential Diagnosis

- Bowel injury secondary to chemotherapy (cytotoxic drugs) and irradiation
- Severe immunodeficiency and T-cell defects
- Acquired immunodeficiency syndrome (AIDS)
- Grade IV disease is indistinguishable from typhlitis and ischemic bowel disease
- Grade II disease may be indistinguishable from changes produced by a sodium phosphate bowel preparation

Treatment

- Immunosuppression and corticosteroids

Prognosis

- Approximately 10% of patients with acute GVHD progress to chronic GVHD (chronic GVHD tends to spare the small intestine and colon)

Associations

- Cytomegalovirus colitis may appear identical to acute GVHD and may coexist with acute GVHD
- GVHD-like colitis has been reported as a complication of a malignant thymoma

Hirschsprung Disease (Congenital Aganglionic Megacolon)

Clinical Manifestations

- Most common motility disorder of the newborn; estimated incidence of 1 in 5,000 live births
- A congenital disease that primarily affects the neonate but occasionally symptoms do not become manifest until childhood or adult life
- 80% occur in males with the exception of total colonic aganglionosis in which the sex distribution is approximately equal
- Typically presents as constipation or intestinal obstruction beginning at birth
- 80% of cases diagnosed within 1st year of life
- Patients usually experience vomiting and progressive abdominal distention secondary to dilatation and hypertrophy of the colon proximal to the narrowed segment
- Occasionally alternating constipation and diarrhea associated with failure to thrive and anemia
- Symptoms result from absence of ganglion cells in the intermuscular Auerbach, deep submucosal Henle, and submucosal Meissner plexuses
- Lack of ganglion cells results in an absence of intrinsic nonadrenergic inhibitory innervation with the persistence of extrinsic parasympathetic cholinergic and sympathetic adrenergic innervation; this imbalance results in an inability of the aganglionic colon or sphincters to relax

Variants

- *Short-segment disease*
  - □ 90% of cases
  - □ Aganglionosis extends from rectum to splenic flexure
  - □ More common in men than women with ratio of approximately 5:1
- *Long-segment disease*
  - □ Aganglionosis extends from rectum to cecum
- *Total colonic aganglionosis*
  - □ Approximately 10% of cases
  - □ Involvement of the entire colon to include occasional involvement of the ileum, jejunum, and on rare cases the stomach

Colon/Rectum: Non-Neoplastic>Hirschsprung Disease (Congenital Aganglionic Megacolon)

- *Ultrashort segment disease*
  - Aganglionosis involving the distal 1/3 of rectum (considered as achalasia of the anal sphincter)
  - Diagnosis usually based on manometric measurements rather than histologic findings

Gross Pathology

- Affected colon segment usually narrowed (occasionally normal in diameter); transition zone between the aganglionic segment and the normal ganglionic bowel funnel-shaped distal to the proximal distended colon or small intestine
- Internal sphincter usually involved
- Zonal or skip aganglionosis rare

Microscopic Pathology

- Ganglion cells normally present at intervals of approximately 0.1 cm and occur in clusters of 1 to 5
- Ganglion cells tend to be polygonal and have abundant amphophilic cytoplasm and a round eccentric nucleus with a prominent nucleolus (the latter less obvious on frozen section)
- In the rectum there is typically a hypoganglionotic zone extending from the dentate line proximally for 0.5 to 1 cm; biopsy specimens should be obtained 2 to 3 cm above the dentate line
- Ganglion cells of Meissner plexus may be difficult to identify in the neonate; they are immature, small, have little cytoplasm and lack an obvious nucleolus; architecturally tend to be arranged in a horseshoelike garland around small nerves
- If ganglion cells not identified in the submucosal Meissner plexus, a full-thickness rectal biopsy may be necessary; ganglion cells in the intermuscular Auerbach plexus more numerous and larger
- Typically there is an increase in number and size of parasympathetic nerve fibers in the muscularis mucosae and the lamina propria (hypertrophied nerve trunks characteristically present in short-segment Hirschsprung disease and absent in long-segment disease and in the neonate)

Special Stains

- Acetylcholinesterase stains may be of use in rectal suction biopsies; in patients with Hirschsprung disease, these stains will demonstrate hyperplasia of parasympathetic fibers in the lamina propria and muscularis mucosa; normally patients have few or no positively staining nerve fibers; the stain must be performed on frozen tissue and is technically difficult to perform

Immunohistochemistry

- Ganglion cells stain positively for NSE, cathepsin D, and protein gene product (PGP) 9.5

Electron Microscopy

- Not helpful

Molecular Alterations

- An approximate 4% familial occurrence
- Mothers with Hirschsprung disease have a higher incidence of affected children than fathers with the disease (probably an autosomal recessive and sex-linked trait)
- In cases of short-segment disease, the risk to a brother of an affected man is approximately 6%; the risk to a sister of an affected man is approximately 1%; the risk to a brother of an affected woman is 8% and the risk to a sister of an affected woman is 3%
- In cases of long-segment disease, the risk to a brother of an affected man is 7% and the risk to a sister of an affected man is 10%; the risk to a brother of an affected woman is 18% and the risk to a sister of an affected woman is 9%
- Mutations, deletions, and point mutations have been localized to chromosome 10q11.2 involving the receptor tyrosine kinase gene *RET* (mutations in the *RET* gene also responsible for multiple endocrine neoplasia (MEN) IIa and IIb and familial medullary carcinoma of the thyroid)
- A second locus of Hirschsprung disease has been mapped to chromosome 13q22 in a group of inbred Mennonite kindred

Differential Diagnosis

- Intestinal neuronal dysplasia (hyperganglionosis) characterized by hyperplasia of myenteric plexus, increased acetylcholinesterase activity in nerves of the lamina propria and submucosa, and increased numbers of ganglion cells with formation of giant ganglia
- Meconium ileus

Treatment

- Initial operative procedure consists of a suction rectal biopsy to confirm the presence of aganglionosis accompanied by a proximal colostomy (in the case of short-segment disease) or ileostomy (in the case of long-segment disease); the presence of normal ganglionic bowel at the colostomy site is typically established with frozen section at the time of this first procedure
- Definitive operation involves removing the aganglionic segment of bowel and reestablishing intestinal continuity with either a J-pouch or endorectal pull-through

Prognosis

- Resection of the aganglionic segment under frozen section control should result in a cure

Associations

- Down syndrome (2%-6%)
- Congenital muscular dystrophy
- Cleft palate
- MEN IIa and IIb
- Congenital central hypoventilation syndrome (Ordine curse in Haddad syndrome)
- Neuroblastoma
- Pheochromocytoma
- Colonic atresia
- Cartilage-hair hypoplasia
- Tetrasomy 9p and 9q with Dandy-Walker cyst
- Midline field defects similar to those in Toriello-Carey syndrome
- Infantile osteopetrosis
- Smith-Lemli-Opitz syndrome
- Goldberg-Shprintzen syndrome
- Aarskog syndrome
- Cytomegalovirus genomes present by PCR in up to 9% of cases

Ischemic Colitis

Clinical Manifestations

- Patients typically present with abdominal pain out of proportion to findings on physical examination, diarrhea, and passage of blood per rectum
- Severity of symptoms vary depending on duration of ischemic episode and depth of involvement
- Transient ischemic episodes typically produce superficial necrosis and spontaneously heal with no significant sequelae
- More prolonged episodes of ischemia produce necrosis that may extend to the muscularis propria; recovery usually characterized by the development of prominent submucosa fibrosis with stricture
- Prolonged acute ischemia that results in a transmural necrosis of bowel wall can lead to perforation, peritonitis, sepsis, and a high mortality rate

Gross Pathology

- Endoscopic findings include patchy erythema, friable mucosa, erosions, and/or ulcers
- Pseudomembranes may be present
- Polyps or mass lesions (secondary to marked submucosal edema) not uncommon (responsible for the "thumbprinting" seen on barium enema)

Microscopic Pathology

- Mild cases characterized by necrosis of superficial mucosa with sloughing of epithelial cells from both surface and upper portions of crypts (bases of crypts remain undamaged), edema of the lamina propria, and ballooning capillaries with sludging of red blood cells; a superficial zone of hemorrhage typically present in the area of necrosis
- More severe cases characterized by full-thickness necrosis of mucosa with extension into deeper layers
- Capillary thrombi may be prominent

- Inflammatory cells (mostly neutrophils) may be present but are not as prominent as in acute self-limited colitis unless a superimposed infection present
- Submucosa typically markedly edematous, contains deposits of hemosiderin, and may produce a polyp or a mass
- Foci of regenerative epithelium may be present
- Some degree of fibrosis and dense hyalinization in the lamina propria typically present
- Atrophic crypts (microcrypts) frequently present
- Pseudomembranes tend to diffusely involve the mucosal surface (unlike the patchy distribution of pseudomembranes seen in *C difficile* colitis)

Special Stains

- Trichrome stains confirm presence of hyalinization in lamina propria

Immunohistochemistry and Electron Microscopy

- Not helpful

Molecular Alterations

- None

Differential Diagnosis

- *C difficile* colitis
- Hemorrhagic enterocolitis secondary to verotoxin-producing *E coli* 0157:H7
- Ulcerative colitis
- Crohn colitis
- Radiation colitis
- Uremic colitis

Treatment

- Varies from supportive care for transient ischemia that results in simple mucosal loss to emergency surgery for transmural infarction

Prognosis

- Depends on duration and extent of ischemic episode; superficial mucosal ischemia self-limited and heals without sequelae; ischemia extending to muscularis propria usually results in stricture formation with stenosis; transmural ischemia leads to perforation peritonitis sepsis and death depending on timing of surgical intervention and the extent of infarcted intestine

Associations

- Hypoperfusion most commonly the result of cardiac failure or arrhythmia, digitalis toxicity, shock, and septicemia
- Arterial embolus
- Arterial thrombosis (usually in the setting of atherosclerosis)
- Venus thrombosis (usually in the setting of intraabdominal sepsis)
- Arteritis, amyloidosis, thromboangiitis obliterans
- Volvulus and hernia (internal, inguinal, or ventral)
- Young people taking nonsteroidal antiinflammatory drugs
- Young women taking birth control pills

Lymphocytic (Microscopic) Colitis

Clinical Manifestations

- Typically affects middle-aged women
- Occasionally seen in men and younger patients
- Predominant symptom is watery diarrhea (secondary to a decrease in the active and passive absorption of sodium and chloride)
- Patients occasionally present with anemia, hypokalemia, and hypoproteinemia

Gross Pathology

- No gross abnormalities by endoscopy or radiology

Microscopic Pathology

- Classically affects the entire colon and is characterized by a diffuse increase in lymphocytes and plasma cells in the upper lamina propria
- Surface epithelium tends to be flatter than normal and contains increased numbers of apoptotic bodies
- Eosinophils usually prominent: Neutrophils may invade epithelium of upper parts of tubules

- Increased numbers of intraepithelial lymphocytes throughout tubules (a feature of more longstanding disease)
- No crypt deformity, gross inflammatory destruction of epithelium, lymphoid nodules, or significant thickening of collagen band beneath surface epithelium

Special Stains, Immunohistochemistry, and Electron Microscopy

- Not helpful

Molecular Alterations

- None

Differential Diagnosis

- Collagenous colitis
- Inflammatory bowel disease
- Acute colitis
- A mucosal prolapse syndrome (solitary rectal ulcer syndrome)
- Ischemic bowel disease
- Amyloidosis
- Resolving infectious colitis

Treatment and Prognosis

- 80% to 90% respond to therapy with sulfasalazine and corticosteroids

Associations

- Autoimmune disease (thyroid disease, rheumatoid arthritis, myasthenia gravis, and celiac sprue)

Ulcerative Colitis

Clinical Manifestations

- Most common cause of chronic colitis in United States
- May affect people of all ages; peak incidence in 3rd decade of life (a second smaller peak in the 6th to 7th decades)
- Slightly more common in women than men
- Significantly more common in people from Western developed countries, Caucasians and Jews
- 1% to 2 % of cases familial
- A lower incidence in people who smoke cigarettes
- A lower incidence in people who have had an appendectomy
- Immune mechanisms may play a role in etiology
- Symptoms typically appear suddenly and include crampy abdominal pain, tenesmus, and diarrhea that may be slightly mucoid to frankly bloody
- Serum levels of antineutrophil cytoplasmic antibodies (p-ANCA) elevated
- 90% of patients present with disease confined to the rectum and sigmoid colon (50% of these will eventually develop more extensive disease)
- Periods of remission and relapse characteristic; relapses often associated with proximal extension of disease
- 15% of patients with rectal disease develop perianal complications
- Disease remains limited to rectum in 5% to 10%; recurrence extension into the sigmoid and descending colon occurs in 35%; eventually proximal transverse colon and right colon become involved in 50%
- Skip areas of normal colon within an inflamed segment are never present (focal areas of healing may resemble skip areas)
- Occasionally a small patch of cecum or the appendix may be involved without apparent involvement of the right colon
- Terminal ileum (distal 10 cm) may be dilated, especially in cases of pancolitis

Gross Pathology

- Early changes consist of a diffuse erythema with patchy areas of hemorrhage that with time progress to friability and eventually ulceration
- Rectum and colon involved in a continuous fashion with a sharp demarcation between normal and inflamed mucosa
- Advanced lesions show extensive ulceration with undermining of intact/inflamed mucosa, resulting in mucosal bridges

- Ulcerations tend to be superficial and expose underlying relatively normal muscularis propria
- With time, gross examination shows evidence of repair, with formation of inflammatory polyps (pseudopolyps); inflammatory polyps represent a combination of elevated intact mucosa next to an ulcerated area, intense inflammation, and mucosal repair
- Presence of pseudopolyps good indicator of chronic disease (not specific for ulcerative colitis; also seen in Crohn disease and ischemic colitis)
- Pseudopolyps may persist after the ulcerating and inflammatory acute disease has resolved
- Inactive or quiescent disease does not have any ulcers but may have inflammatory pseudopolyps and flattening of the haustral markings on the mucosal surface
- Recurrent disease, especially when severe, may be associated with pronounced dilatation and thinning (megacolon)
- Longstanding disease with multiple episodes of inflammation interspersed with periods of quiescence may lead to shortening of the colon and stricture formation

Microscopic Pathology

- Acute phase of disease characterized by marked edema and infiltration of the mucosa with neutrophils, plasma cells, and increased numbers of eosinophils together with degeneration of both surface and crypt epithelia
- Neutrophils are typically present both in lamina propria and damaged epithelium; the injury to crypt epithelia ranges from the simple presence of neutrophils to denudation of epithelial cells to complete destruction leaving a pool of luminal neutrophils (crypt abscess)
- Features of epithelial regeneration (elongation and palisading of nuclei with central, large nucleoli and numerous mitotic figures) usually present; goblet cell component lost
- More severe disease characterized by erosions and ulcerations limited to upper submucosa; extension of inflammation into submucosa unusual
- Giant cells may be present in inflamed mucosa and poorly formed granulomas may surround a crypt abscess
- Disease in remission (quiescent colitis) characterized by mucosal changes consisting primarily of abnormal architecture with extensive budding and branching of crypts, atrophy, loss of crypts (shortening and separation from the muscularis mucosa), and a villouslike transformation of the mucosal surface; quiescent disease also characterized by an increase in mononuclear inflammatory cells and eosinophils in the lamina propria particularly between the crypts and the muscularis mucosa; regenerating tubules do not extend to the muscularis mucosa ("crypt shortfall")
- Persistent ulceration coupled with regeneration results in formation of pseudopolyps consisting of granulation tissue with a pseudomalignant histologic appearance secondary to the presence of large pleomorphic spindled cells with large ganglion cell-like nuclei)
- Paneth cells may appear in the crypt epithelium (a metaplastic change of more significance when seen on the left side of the colon than the right, because Paneth cells are a normal inhabitant of crypt epithelium in the cecum and ascending colon)
- Less common features of chronic disease include hyperplasia of the endocrine cell population of the crypts, pyloric gland metaplasia (classically associated with Crohn disease but may be seen in chronic ulcerative colitis as well), squamous metaplasia, fibrosis of the lamina propria, and lymphoid follicles or nodules at the base of the mucosa (usually in association with increased numbers of inflammatory cells in the same region)

Special Stains and Immunohistochemistry

- Not helpful

Electron Microscopy

- May be helpful in cases of suspected dysplasia; dysplastic epithelium has a reduction in the density and size of surface cells and their microvilli

Molecular Alterations

- If dysplasia present, there appears to be an early appearance of mutations of p53 and loss of heterozygosity of other gene products

Differential Diagnosis

- Acute infections:
  - *Campylobacter* and *Chlamydia* (may be associated with the presence of granulomas)
  - *Shigella*
  - *C difficile*
- Amebic colitis (*Entamoeba histolytica*)
- Ischemic colitis
- Reactions to drugs
- Vasculitis
- Crohn disease

Treatment

- Medical therapy includes sulfasalazine derivatives (ie, 5-aminosalicylic acid) and corticosteroids (administered as an enema in the rectum or orally) with or without antibiotics
- Intractable disease and disease with complications treated with surgery; complete proctocolectomy with or without a primary reconstruction of the GI tract (ileal reservoir and ileal anal anastomosis)

Prognosis

- Generally excellent
- Death usually related to megacolon with perforation and sepsis or carcinoma

Associations

- *Toxic megacolon*
  - Usually associated with a severe episode of active disease either at initial presentation or with recurrence
  - Perforation with generalized peritonitis a significant life-threatening event
- *Secondary infections*
  - *Salmonella* and *C difficile* most common infectious to complicate ulcerative colitis
- *Colitis cystica*
  - Results from downward growth of dilated colonic glands into submucosa and occasionally muscularis propria
  - Lesions may be associated with inflammatory pseudopolyps and mimic histologic features of adenocarcinoma
- *Extraintestinal manifestations*
  - Present in 30% of patients with ulcerative colitis and may be the result of circulating immune complexes
  - Conditions include uveitis, polyarthritis, ankylosing spondylitis, erythema nodosum, pyoderma gangrenosum, and sclerosing cholangitis
  - Patients with sclerosing cholangitis at an increased risk to develop bile duct adenocarcinoma
- *Non-Hodgkin colonic lymphoma and extraintestinal non-Hodgkin lymphoma* both associated with long-standing ulcerative colitis
- *Dysplasia*
  - 90% of patients with ulcerative colitis and carcinoma have foci of dysplasia elsewhere in the colon
  - May be seen as a gross lesion (dysplasia-associated lesion or mass)
  - When a mass is present, dysplastic epithelium tends to be most prominent in the base of the crypts
- *Carcinoma*
  - Incidence a reflection of both extent and duration of disease
  - Disease extending to hepatic flexure and beyond associated with an incidence of approximately 15%; disease limited to the left side of colon associated with an incidence of approximately 5%
  - 1% to 2% annual increase in incidence of carcinoma after 10 years of extensive disease
  - Cancer in the setting of ulcerative colitis tends to occur in a younger population (10 years less than seen in cases of sporadic colon cancer)
  - Neoplasms tend to occur in areas of prior inflammation

- □ Majority of symptomatic cases present with a stenotic or occluding lesion (typical adenoma-carcinoma sequence not usually evident)
- □ 35% to 40% of carcinomas well-differentiated or mucinous
- □ An inflammatory polyp rarely the site of either dysplasia or a carcinoma

Solitary Rectal Ulcer Syndrome (SRUS)

Clinical Manifestations

- Prolapse intestinal mucosa may be found at the margin of a colostomy, at the apex of a prolapsing hemorrhoid, adjacent to any polypoid lesion of the large intestine and at the margin of a colonic diverticulum
- The best recognized site of mucosal prolapse is the anterior wall of the rectum where it is called the solitary rectal ulcer syndrome
- Usually presents in young adults of either sex who may have a variety of symptoms of anal rectal disease; rectal bleeding is the most common, but other symptoms involve passage of mucous, perineal pain and tenesmus
- Mucosal prolapse occurs during excessive straining at defication a situation which is compounded by trauma and ischemia that may eventually lead to ulceration and/or the formation of a polyp
- The straining that leads to the mucosal prolapse results from an abnormality the puborectalis muscle and the external anal sphincter which undergo inappropriate contraction rather than relaxation during straining

Gross Pathology

- The ulcers are not always "solitary"; sometimes there is more than one ulcer and occasionally no ulcerations are present
- Tend to be quite distinctive
- Are situated on the anterior or anterior lateral walls of the rectum
- Tend to be flat and well-demarcated with an irregular shape often covered with a white exudate

Microscopic Pathology

- The earliest and most significant change is the obliteration of the laminal propria by fibrosis and smooth muscle that extend toward the lumen from a thickened muscularis mucosa
- If the specimen is cut tangentially, mucosal glands may be seen within a muscle and can give the false impression of an invasive carcinoma
- Superficial mucosal erosion, irregularity of crypts with metaplastic-like changes in the epithelium and depletion of goblet cells are all typically present
- The crypts are often diamond-shaped
- Occasionally the lesion will be covered by a "cap" of granulation tissue
- If an ulcer is present, it is invariably superficial, never penetrates beyond the submucosa; the floor of the ulcer is covered by necrotic cells and overlying organizing granulation tissue
- In some cases there is misplacement of mucous-filled glands lined by normal colonic epithelium into the submucosa at the edge of the ulcer (another feature that may be mistaken for an adenocarcinoma); this phenomenon has been described as *localized colitis cystica profunda*

Special Stains

- Mucins typically are predominately sialomucinans rather than normal sulphomucins

Immunohistochemistry, Electron Microscopy

- Not helpful

Molecular Alterations

- None

Differential Diagnosis

- Can be confused clinically and histologically with carcinoma of the rectum
- When "localized colitis cystica profunda" is present it should not be confused with an inverted hamartomatous polyp of the rectum
- Similar prolapse findings of the anterior rectal mucosa without ulceration and may be seen in the "descending perineum syndrome" where the

perineum descends; a condition seen more frequently in women than in men and may result from perineal damage at childbirth or some other pelvic injury

- Mucosal prolapse changes adjacent to a carcinoma are identical to those of isolated mucosal prolapse and may mimic a Puetz-Jeghers polyp
- Distorted and inflamed mucosa may resemble inflammatory bowel disease

Treatment and Prognosis

- Benign but frequently quite chronic
- No treatment is entirely satisfactory, but am increase in dietary fiber usually recommended
- Local excision may prove curative

Associations

- None

Comment

- A polypoid variant of the solitary rectal/mucosal prolapse syndrome is the *inflammatory cloacogenic polyp.* These polyps occur at the anorectal transition and thus have both squamous and columnar mucosa. They are covered with a combination of colorectal and transitional zone epithelium; the superficial ulceration and adjacent epithelium show a regenerative hyperplasia that mimics an adenoma; the lamina propria contains increased amounts of smooth muscle. Prolapsing hemorrhoids may show similar epithelial changes.

Neoplastic

Adenocarcinoma

Clinical Manifestations

- Signs and symptoms:
  - □ Abdominal pain or cramping (80%)
  - □ Change in bowel habits (65%)
  - □ Hematochezia (55%)
  - □ Weight loss (40%)
  - □ Anemia (25%)
  - □ Intestinal obstruction (10%)
  - □ Symptoms related to metastasis (5%-10%)
  - □ Palpable abdominal mass
- Distal colon and rectal lesions typically present with fresh blood in the stool, a change in bowel habits, tenesmus, and genitourinary symptoms
- Lesions in right colon typically present with anemia, weight loss, and a palpable mass
- Lesions in the left colon more common in men than in women and are 3 times more likely to have synchronous adenomas
- Lesions in right colon more likely to have carcinoid and mucinous components
- Majority of lesions located in the sigmoid colon and rectum (over the course of the past 40 years there seems to be an increase in the incidence of carcinoma in the cecum and ascending colon and a decrease in the incidence of carcinomas in the distal or left colon)
- Complications:
  - □ Obstruction and perforation (perforation associated with a localized abscess in approximately 60% and generalized peritonitis in 40%)
  - □ Blood loss (massive rare; anemia common, especially in right-sided lesions)
  - □ Superimposed infection (promotes necrosis and may contribute to perforation and fistula; in addition infection may spread to other organs)
  - □ Lower urinary tract involvement (obstruction, gross hematuria, or neurogenic bladder)
  - □ Metastasizing mucin-producing tumors may cause a coagulopathy
  - □ Microangiopathic hemolytic anemia
  - □ Dermatomyositis
  - □ Extrahepatic obstructive jaundice
  - □ Nodular intraabdominal panniculitis

Gross Pathology

- Synchronous lesions occur in 3% to 8%; metachronous lesions in 2% to 3 %

Colon/Rectum: Neoplastic> Adenocarcinoma

- Tumors in the right colon tend to be polypoid and fungating and rarely involve entire circumference of the bowel wall (hence these lesions rarely present with intestinal obstruction, unless the ileocecal valve involved)
- Tumors in the left colon typically ulcerative and fungating and more likely to involve entire circumference of colon wall (hence left-sided lesions more likely to present with signs and symptoms of obstruction or impending obstruction)
- Carcinomas complicating inflammatory bowel disease usually flat and may not be evident on gross or endoscopic examination
- Polypoid tumors tend to arise from a preexisting adenoma and form an exophytic intraluminal mass with little or no ulceration; may have a nodular, lobulated, or papillary surface
- Fungating tumors tend to be polypoid with prominent ulceration; typically a raised or rolled border in which adenomatous epithelium may be present; ulceration can be extensive enough to destroy much of the tumor
- Ulcerative lesions tend to be more common in the left colon than the right and usually infiltrate deeply and thicken the colon wall in a circumferential manner, producing a nodular mass that narrows the involved segment; ulcerated surface usually even with or below the adjacent normal mucosal surface

Microscopic Pathology

- 85% well to moderately differentiated; remainder poorly differentiated or almost completely undifferentiated
- 2 basic patterns of growth:
    - *Expanding:* Characterized by aggregates of tumor that consist of interconnecting glands within a network of fibrous tissue; usually polypoid or fungating
    - *Infiltrative:* Characterized by narrow tubular glands with few connections that invade the colon wall individually or in single groups; tubules produce little fibrosis and are typically surrounded by acellular collagenous tissue; usually ulcerative or infiltrative
- With the exception of signet-ring cell carcinoma, diffuse infiltration of the colon wall by individual cancer cells relatively rare
- Cell type:
    - Most carcinoma cells are columnar and some contain small globules of mucin in the apical cytoplasm; intraluminal secretions usually contain predominantly sulfomucin with minor amounts of sialomucin; neutral mucins rarely present; goblet cells rare
    - Endocrine cells: Mostly argyrophilic (occasionally argentaffin); most commonly seen in nonmucinous carcinomas (rarely found in mucinous or undifferentiated lesions)
    - Paneth cells
- Endocrine cells, Paneth cells, columnar, and goblet cells all derived from the same stem cells in the intestinal crypt
- Variants:
    - *Mucinous adenocarcinoma*
        - Mucus forms pools in connective tissue that surrounds malignant glands
        - 50% or more of the tumor mass must consist of mucus
        - If 25% of the lesion consists of mucus, it is considered as having a "mucinous component"
        - 5% to 15% of colonic carcinomas mucinous; an additional 5% have a mucinous component
        - Most arise from adenomas and consist of tubular structures
        - More often seen in right colon and rectum than elsewhere
        - Tends to be diagnosed at a more advanced stage and consequently have a worse prognosis than more typical adenocarcinoma
        - May have a familial incidence
    - *Signet-ring carcinoma*
        - 0.2% to 1% of all colonic carcinomas
        - Mucus intracellular rather than extracellular as in mucinous lesions

- Tumor cells shaped like signet rings with an eccentric crescent-shaped nucleus that is pushed to the cell wall by intracytoplasmic mucus
- Cells tend to infiltrate the colon wall individually or in small groups
- Diffuse infiltration produces a linitis plastica type of appearance
- Prognosis poor

□ *Carcinomas with DNA mismatch repair deficiency (microsatellite unstable)*

- DNA mismatch present in 10% to 15%; most of these are sporadic (90%); remainder familial (see section on hereditary nonpolyposis colorectal cancer [HNPCC] below)
- Female predominance (4:1) especially after the age of 70 years
- Most (90%) sporadic cancers located in right colon; 50% of all right-sided cancers in women older than 70 years
- May be multiple and tend to be polypoid or exophytic
- Often show mucinous or signet ring cell morphology with microglandular differentiation; tumor-infiltrating lymphocytes (5 per 10 high-power fields [hpf]) commonly present
- Associated with improved survival

Special Stains

- Periodic acid–Schiff (PAS)–Alcian blue may confirm presence of mucin

Immunohistochemistry

- Staining for carcinoembryonic antigen (CEA) present in essentially 100% (CEA positivity also seen in carcinomas of stomach, pancreas, small intestine, and extraintestinal sites such as lung, breast, ovary, cervix, and endometrium)
- Cell proliferation can be documented with proliferating cell nuclear antigen , Ki-67, or MIB-1 (cell proliferation may not be a major risk factor for carcinoma)
- *bcl*-2 can be expressed immunohistochemically in 98% of adenomas and 55% of carcinomas
- p53 expressed in 43% of adenomas and 75% of carcinomas (there seems to be an increased expression of *bcl*-2 early and of p53 late in the evolution of the adenoma carcinoma sequence)

Electron Microscopy

- Microvilli not particularly common but cells contain dense core microfilaments that extend as long rootlets into a clear zone of apical cytoplasm (these long rootlets are a marker for colon adenocarcinoma)
- Electron microscopy (EM) helpful in recognizing special cell types (ie, endocrine cells) that may be present

Molecular Alterations

- One of the earliest events leading to formation of colonic carcinoma is the activation of mitogen-activated protein (MAP) kinases which are responsible for relaying information (proliferation, differentiation, or programmed cell death) to the nucleus
- MKP-1, which regulates MAP activity, overexpressed
- p53 mutations the most common genetic alteration seen in carcinoma of the colon and rectum; deletions of chromosome 17p (which contains gene for p53 found in 75%)
- DCC (***d***eleted in ***c***olorectal ***c***ancer) located on chromosome 18q 21.2
- 10% to 15% are microsatellite unstable secondary to promoter methylation and silencing of transcription of *hMLH1*
- APC/β-catenin inactivation initiates the process of epithelial dysplasia in the base of crypts upward towards the luminal surface

Differential Diagnosis

- Adenoma
- Stricture secondary to diverticular disease, inflammatory bowel disease, or chronic ischemia

Treatment

- Surgical resection (approximately 85% can be resected for cure, 10% either unresectable or can only be resected for palliation; 5% completely inoperable)
- Postoperative adjuvant radiation has a role in controlling local recurrence and may improve survival

Colon/Rectum: Neoplastic>Adenocarcinoma

- Preoperative radiation used to improve resectability of rectal cancer
- Patients with advanced cancer may experience some response to chemotherapy using 5-fluoruracil (5-FU) alone or in combination with interferon
- Combination of 5-FU and levamisole (an immunostimulant) may be a benefit
- Liver metastasis treated surgically and carries a 5-year survival rate of up to 45%
- Arterial infusion of 5-FU into liver provides some partial remission and prolongs survival

Prognosis

- Stage of tumor at time of diagnosis most important (Astler-Coller modification of Dukes classification: A: lesion confined to mucosa, B1: lesion does not penetrate muscularis propria, B2: lesion extends through bowel wall, C1: a B1 lesion with positive nodes, C2: a B2 lesion with positive nodes, D: presence of distant metastasis)
- Signet-ring cell carcinoma with an infiltrative pattern has the worse prognosis
- 5-year survival rate 10% or better for patients with diploid tumors than for aneuploid tumors (75% versus 65%)
- A lack of expression of *bcl*-2 associated with both larger tumors and a shortened survival
- p53 overexpression associated with a lower survival rate than p53 negative tumors (only applies to stage III tumors)
- Carcinomas with a K-*ras* have a worse prognosis than those without this mutation
- Expression of DCC inversely related to survival in patients with stage II and stage III carcinomas

Associations

- Precancerous conditions:
  - Adenomas and adenomatosis: Incidence of carcinoma in an untreated adenoma 2.5% in 5 years, 8% in 10 years, and 25% in 20 years; <10% of adenomas develop carcinoma in a lifetime
  - Hyperplastic polyps: May become adenomatous
  - Hamartomatous polyposis: Not considered premalignant; patients with Peutz-Jeghers have an increased incidence of small intestinal carcinoma; patients with juvenile polyposis syndrome have an increased incidence of colonic carcinoma
  - Inflammatory bowel disease (ulcerative colitis and Crohn disease): Incidence of colorectal cancer in ulcerative colitis approximately 1% after 10 years of colitis, 5% to 6% at 20 years, and 10% to 15% at 30 years (incidence rate higher in patients who have sclerosing cholangitis); incidence of colon carcinoma in Crohn disease related to duration of disease, presence of a fistula and/or stricture, and disease in the right colon
  - Infestation with *Schistosoma japonicum*: carcinoma often multicentric
  - Familial adenomatous polyposis: An autosomal dominant disease; patients have a germline deletion or mutation of the adenomatous polyposis coli (*APC*) gene on chromosome 5q21; similar genetic lesions present in patients with Gardner syndrome and Turcot syndrome
- HNPCC: An autosomal dominant disease
  - Tumor DNA of affected patients have widespread instability in short repeat sequences, termed *microsatellite instability*, detected as extra bands on polymerase chain reaction (PCR)–amplified short repetitive segments of DNA; DNA instability is present in most of the adenomas that develop in patients with this syndrome
  - Disease not associated with a mutation or allelic loss of *APC* gene; genetic abnormality involves a germline mutation of at least 6 genes in the DNA mismatch repair system; overall risk of developing a colon cancer 80% in these patients; multiple lesions common (synchronous in 20% and metachronous in 25%)
  - *Lynch syndrome*
    - *Type I:* Familial incidence of colon cancer unassociated with cancers of other organs
    - *Type II (cancer family syndrome):* Familial incidence of colon cancer associated with cancers of other organs—endometrium, ovary, and pancreas
  - 75% to 80% of HNPCC families have abnormalities on chromosome 2p and 3p which relate to mutations in the mismatch repair genes h*MSH2* (40% of NHPCC cases), h*MLHI*, *hMLH6*, *PMS1*, and *PMS2*; these mutations result in loss of stability of the DNA
  - Hyperplastic gastric polyps (approximately 20%)
  - Gastric adenoma (4%)
  - Coexisting carcinomas in other parts of the digestive tract: Ampulla Vater, gallbladder, appendix, and squamous carcinoma of the anus

Intestinal Polyps

Adenomatous Polyp (Tubular Adenoma)

- Distributed rather regularly throughout the large intestine, with 40% found in the right colon, 40% in the left colon, and 20% in the rectum
- Blacks have a lower prevalence than whites, and a predominance of right-sided lesions
- A familial predisposition has been detected and found to result from an inherited autosomal dominant gene for susceptibility
- Most are asymptomatic
- On gross examination, most measure under 1 cm in diameter; may be sessile or pedunculated, and single or multiple; when multiple, they have a tendency to cluster; when pedunculated, they may have short or a long stalk attached by a narrow base; when sessile; they may be protruding, flat, or depressed
- Microscopically, number of glands and cells per unit area is increased compared with normal mucosa; epithelial cells are crowded and contain large hyperchromatic nuclei that are stratified in the cell with an increased number of mitoses, some of which may be atypical; mucin production is highly variable but usually decreased; the basement membrane is not thickened; the changes first affect the superficial portion of the glands
- Immunohistochemically, CEA, *p53,* and B-catenin localization is often seen in the highly atypical areas
- Focal areas of villous configuration are not infrequent; the incidence of villous configuration is related to the size of the polyp, reaching 76% in lesions larger than 1 cm in diameter; polyps with adenomatous and villous components in equal amounts are referred to as *villoglandularpolyps* or *tubulovillous adenomas*
- Degree of atypia seen in adenomatous polyps is related to increasing age, number of polyps per patient, size of the polyps, and presence of villous changes
- Occasionally, clusters of atypical glands in an adenomatous or villoglandular polyp are seen beneath the muscularis mucosa (pseudoinvasion) and may lead to mistaken diagnosis of malignant transformation; features that characterize pseudocarcinomatous invasion include:
  - □ Cytologic features of the misplaced glands are similar to those in the surface
  - □ Glands are surrounded by inflamed loose stroma and scattered bundles of muscularis mucosae, instead of the desmoplastic reaction associated with carcinoma
  - □ There are abundant hemosiderin granules around the neoplastic glands; some of these glands may become cystic, rupture, and result in the formation of mucin lakes (may resemble the overall appearance of a localized form of colitis cystica profunda); adenocarcinoma in this setting will frequently show increased staining of the submucosal epithelium for matrix metalloproteinase-1 (MMP-1) and p53 and will show decreased staining of the submucosal epithelium for membranous E-cedherin and decreased or irregular collagen deposition surrounding the submucosal glands
- Rarely, adenomatous polyps may exhibit morular formation (focal squamous metaplasia), a minor component of Paneth cells, and a population of endocrine cells; less frequent phenomena are the occurrence of focal malakoplakia in the stroma of the polyp, the development of osseous metaplasia, or the presence of metastases from another site within the polyp

Ganglioneuroma

- May occur in the small and large intestine as either solitary lesions or, more commonly, as multiple lesions (ganglioneuromatosis)
- Ganglioneuromatosis may be associated with von Recklinghausen disease and MEN type IIB
- Lesions may be polypoid and histologically consist of a proliferation of ganglion cells and Schwann cells
- In MEN type IIB, the ganglioneuromatosis may consist of a marked accentuation of both the submucosal and myenteric nerve plexuses

Hamartoma (Peutz-Jeghers Polyp)

- A hamartomatous lesion that can occur in the stomach, small intestine, and colon
- Usually seen as a component of the Peutz-Jeghers syndrome (an autosomal dominant disorder consisting of hamartomatous polyps associated with mucocutaneous pigmentation and, in women with ovarian sex cord tumors with annular tubules and breast cancer)
- May develop in patients without Peutz-Jeghers syndrome
- 2 long-term follow-up studies indicate that patients with Peutz-Jeghers syndrome have an increased incidence of both GI and non-GI malignancy; there is some controversy as to whether the GI malignancies actually arise from Peutz-Jeghers polyps

- On gross examination, they vary in size from <l to 3.5 cm in diameter; may be sessile or pedunculated; identical to the more common adenomatous polyp
- Microscopically, the basic architecture is that of glandular epithelium resting on a branching smooth muscle framework that arises from the muscularis mucosae; the polyp has a "Christmas tree" or arborescent appearance; the bands of smooth muscle fibers tend to be thick in the center of the lesion and thinner at the periphery; intermingling of glands and smooth muscle may lead to a mistaken diagnosis of carcinoma; the epithelial component resembles the normal epithelium of the intestinal area from which the polyp arises; in the small intestine, the epithelium consists of goblet and absorptive cells with a normal component of endocrine and Paneth cells; in the large intestine, the epithelium is predominately of the goblet-cell type, often with branching crypts lined by hypertrophic goblet cells; polyp may be associated with mucosal glands and mucinous cysts deeply embedded in the submucosa or beyond (enteritis cystica profunda)
- Areas of hyperplastic polyp-type epithelium may be noted in these polyps; rarely areas of adenomatous and carcinomatous transformation can be found; when adenomatous changes occur, they do so on the surface of the polyp and not in the crypts

Juvenile Polyp

- Occur mainly in the first 2 decades of life
- Usually solitary and localized chiefly to rectum
- A polyposis syndrome exists and may be limited to the colon or may be associated with polyps in the small intestine and stomach; associated intestinal and extraintestinal congenital defects (such as malrotation of the gut, mesenteric lymphangioma, hypertelorism, hydrocephalus, tetralogy of Fallot, and coarctation of the aorta) have been reported; an increased risk for developing intestinal and gastric cancer
- On gross examination, mainly pedunculated and rarely sessile; usually under 3.0 cm in diameter; have a smooth glistening surface and are red-tan to red in color; on cut section cystic filled spaces are easily appreciated
- Microscopically, consist of cystically dilated and tortuous glands in an inflamed stroma; glands are made up of well-formed mucus-secreting cells that may become flattened and attenuated; in approximately 45% of cases there are pink regenerative epithelial cells similar to those seen in hyperplastic polyps; the stroma usually contains acute and chronic inflammatory cells and granulation tissue; when dilated glands rupture into the stroma, there may be a foreign-body giant cell reaction; occasional areas of osseous metaplasia

Lymphoid Polyp

- Benign lesion that occurs mainly in the rectum
- Occur in all age groups and may be found incidentally or may cause symptoms such as bleeding, discomfort, or prolapse
    - 80% are sessile; 20% are pedunculated
    - 80% are solitary
- Microscopically, consist of prominent lymphoid follicles with active germinal centers located in the mucosa and submucosa
- Local excision is curative; spontaneous regression has been noted
- Cases of multiple lymphoid polyposis have been reported, primarily in children
- Lymphoid polyposis of the terminal ileum has been seen in patients with FAP coli and Gardner syndrome

Hyperplastic Polyp

- A benign epithelial proliferation located predominantly in the rectum; also commonly found in the sigmoid colon; less commonly found in the more proximal large intestine
- Incidence increases after the age of 40 years
- Vast majority 3 to 6 mm in size
- Not considered premalignant
- On gross examination, tend to be small, dome (convex)-shaped structures that are the same color as, or paler than, the surrounding mucosa; often sit on the crest of a mucosal fold; occasionally may be pedunculated and mimic adenomas
- Microscopically, at low power, well-oriented specimens tend to have a serrated or "saw-tooth" appearance not unlike secretory endometrium; when biopsy material is cut tangentially, the crypts assume a "star-shaped" appearance; lesions consist of mixtures of absorptive and goblet cells, with the former usually predominating; in both cell types, the nuclei are basally located and bland; occasionally, the nuclei may be stratified and show nucleoli (these features are more common in the larger polyps); the columnar cells have a distinct eosinophilic cytoplasm with a well-defined brush border; the subepithelial collagen layer along the luminal surface may also

be thickened; mitotic figures are limited to the lower 2/3 of the crypt and are never seen at the surface; in well-oriented material, the basal portions of the crypts of hyperplastic polyps tend to show cellular crowding and an increased mitotic rate compared with normal surrounding mucosa; the muscularis mucosae often shows a characteristic splaying, with muscle fibers extending into the mucosa and surrounding individual crypts (may give the false impression of invasion of glands into the submucosa, "pseudoinvasion")

- Occasional polyps (admixed type)) show features of both adenoma and hyperplastic polyps, consisting of either a small focus of adenoma in a hyperplastic polyp or an adenoma with a small focus of hyperplastic polyp; adenomatous change is closely associated with large (>1.0 cm) hyperplastic polyps
- Mixed hyperplastic adenomatous polyps *(serrated adenoma)* are characterized by low-power serrated or saw-tooth glandular pattern similar to classic hyperplastic polyp; at high-power, these polyps show goblet cell immaturity, upper zone mitoses, prominence of nucleoli, and absence of a thickened surface subepithelial collagen layer; the epithelial cells show cytologic changes that are between those of classic hyperplastic polyp and classic adenoma

Inflammatory Fibroid Polyp

- Benign tumor masses occurring in the small intestine, stomach, and less commonly, in the large intestine
- Range in size from 1.5 to 13 cm (3.0 to 4.0 cm average) and are polypoid with a broad base
- Limited mainly to the submucosa but can infiltrate the muscularis propria and serosa
- Gross appearance tan, gray, or yellow; overlying mucosa may be ulcerated
- Microscopically, mesenchymal lesions with an inflammatory infiltrate and a variable vascular component; fibroblasts may be spindle-shaped or stellate with indistinct basophilic cytoplasm; in some areas, the lesions may be sparsely cellular with a prominent myxoid component; the inflammatory infiltrate consists of eosinophils, lymphocytes, plasma cells, macrophages, and mast cells (the eosinophils may vary in number from few to many); the vascular component may be prominent
- Other terms used to describe inflammatory fibroid polyps include eosinophilic granuloma, submucosal fibroma, hemangiopericytoma, inflammatory pseudotumor, and fibroma

Inflammatory Polyp

- May be secondary to inflammatory disease of the intestine
- Seen in 10% to 20% of ulcerative colitis and may also occur in Crohn disease, ischemic disease, amebiasis, and schistosomiasis; also seen adjacent to ulcers and at surgical anastomotic sites In ulcerative colitis and Crohn disease, the polyps are simply raised tags of mucosa and/or submucosa

Sessile Serrated Adenoma (SSA)

- Tend to have a sessile configuration
- More prominent in the right colon
- Characterized by features similar to a those of serrated adenoma, which include serration, architectural distortion, occasional small areas with superficial cytologic dysplasia, and eosinophilic change
- A major diagnostic feature of an SSA is that it is more disorganized that a conventional hyperplastic polyp; the proliferative zones are not in the base of the crypt, but higher in the crypt (1 side of the crypt may have a proliferative zone that is higher than the other side of the crypt or only 1 side of the crypt may be involved); the normal proliferative zone at the base of the crypt is replaced by mature cells with goblet cells or gastric foveolar cells
- The most important architectural features of SSA include the presence of crypts that seem to grow parallel to the muscularis mucosa, often creating an inverted Tor L-shaped crypt; crypts also tend to branch and are often dilated; serration is also present at the base of the crypts; SSAs are much more architecturally disorganized than conventional hyperplastic polyps but the surface epithelium of a traditional serrated adenoma and a sessile serrated adenoma can be quite similar; if there is strikingly eosinophilic cells with pseudostratified central nucleoli and dysplasia, the possibility of serrated adenoma should be considered.
- Mitoses in the upper 1/3 of the crypts along with nuclear atypia are common
- Unlike traditional serrated adenomas, uniform cytologic dysplasia is not a characteristic of a SSA
- SSAs show decreased staining for hMLH1 and hMSH2 suggesting that these lesions may be precursors to some colorectal adenocarcinomas, particularly those that are microsatellite instable (MSI)
- At least 6% (and probably more) of adenocarcinomas have an adjacent SSA that may have a transition zone of more typical adenoma between the SSA and the carcinoma

- Some cases of SSA have areas of adenoma (this transition is more common than the transition of a SSA to traditional serrated adenoma [TSA])
- Despite the link between SSA and adenocarcinoma with microsatellite instability, the rate and incidence of progression to carcinoma is unknown.

Traditional Serrated Adenoma (TSA)

- A morphologic subtype of adenoma with features of *uniform dysplastic epithelium* and a growth pattern similar to that of a hyperplastic polyp
- An adenoma with a serrated configuration should be regarded as a conventional adenoma until natural history is fully known
- 5% or less of all adenomas
- May be sessile or pedunculated, but tends to be pedunculated.
- Slightly more common in the left colon
- The surface epithelial cells are columnar with prominent eosinophilic cytoplasm and elongated hyperchromatic, mildly pseudostratified, centrally placed nuclei (these changes are similar to those seen on the surface of a SSA); serration is typically confined to the upper 1/2 to upper 1/3 of crypts and can be quite variable; the lower 1/3 of the crypts remain narrow and are lined with proliferative cells; mitosis may be present but is not common

Giant Condyloma (Verrucous Carcinoma)

- Giant condyloma and verrucous carcinoma are not exactly identical but share several etiological, pathological and clinical features
- More formally referred to as giant condyloma of Buschke and Loewenstien
- A rare penial or vulvar lesion which presents as a large warty cauliflower-like growth
- Characteristically penetrates and burrows into deeper tissues
- Similar lesions may rarely occur in the perianal and anal rectal region
- Tumors may become ulcerated and complicated by the formation by fistula tracts
- Locally aggressive lesion, very limited metastatic potential, node metastasis have been described when the lesion undergoes transformation to a conventional squamous cell carcinoma
- Total excision is typically curative (may require an abdomino-perineal excision)
- Typically insensitive to radiotherapy
- Microscopic features are similar to those of typical anal wart to include the presence of vacuolated cells; the major difference is the presence of endophytic or downward growth by giant condyloma
- *The advancing tongues of epithelium are bulbous and pushing and have an intact basement membrane*
- HPV type 6 and 11 can be found in giant condyloma, verrucous carcinoma and simple viral warts
- Progression to dysplasia and squamous cell carcinoma has been documented

Multiple Polyp Syndromes

Cowden Disease (Multiple Hamartoma Syndrome) 10q23.3

- Named for family of index patient (Rachel Cowden)
- An autosomal dominant disorder associated with hamartomatous colonic and small intestinal polyps (35%), facial trichilemmomas (85%), acral keratosis and oral mucosal papillomatosis, usually benign fibromas (85%); breast cancer (35%), and thyroid cancer (10%-15%)
- Additional extraintestinal manifestations include lipomas (40%), hemangiomas (20 to 25%), neuromas (10%), benign thyroid lesions, colloid goiter and adenoma (60%), and several congenital abnormalities, including high arched palate (15%), and adenoid facies (10%), female patients have an increased incidence of fibrocystic changes in the breast (65%) and ovarian cysts (25%)
- The most common GI lesion is a hamartomatous polyp characterized by distorted, inflamed, non-neoplastic mucosa which is mildly fibrotic and has extensive splaying of the muscularis mucosae in the center (polyp microscopically reminiscent of the polyp of the solitary rectal ulcer syndrome)
- GI polyps of Cowden disease have no malignant potential
- PTEN mutation in Cowden disease

Cronkhite-Canada Syndrome

- A nonhereditary GI polyposis associated with alopecia, nail atrophy (thinning and splitting), and macular hyperpigmentation of the face
- 80% present after 50 years of age; 60% are men
- Clinical symptoms include diarrhea, weight loss, abdominal pain, and complications of malnutrition
- Polyps typically sessile and occur in the stomach (most frequent), small intestine, colon, and rectum
- Microscopically, these polyps are identical to juvenile polyps, with tortuous and cystically dilated glands filled with inspissated mucus in an edematous stroma; lamina propria is hypercellular with increased numbers of inflammatory cells, including eosinophils and mast cells, fibroblasts, and smooth muscle from the muscularis mucosa
- In the Cronkhite-Canada syndrome, the nonpolypoid intervening mucosa contains cystically dilated glands and an inflammed, edematous lamina propria, whereas in patients with juvenile polyps, the intervening mucosa is histologically normal
- Areas of hyperplastic polyp-type epithelium may be noted in these polyps; rarely areas of adenomatous and carcinomatous transformation can be found; when adenomatous changes occur they do so on the surface of the polyp and not in the crypts; occasional cases of colorectal adenocarcinoma have developed in patients with this syndrome

Devon Family Syndrome

- Index family from Devon, England
- Characterized by multiple inflammatory polyps in the ileum (most common) and occasionally the gastric antrum
- Ileal lesions may present with intussusception
- No extraintestinal manifestations
- No association with carcinoma in the GI tract

Familial Adenomatous Polyposis (FAP)

- Autosomal dominant with a high degree of penetrance
- Responsible gene localized to chromosome 5q21 and the *APC* gene
- K-*ras* mutations are found in 25% of the polyps (a frequency similar to that seen in sporadic cases)
- Polyps become manifest in the 2nd decade of life
- On gross examination, the bowel is studded with adenomatous polyps ranging from very slight elevations of normal mucosa to relatively large polypoid masses; may be flat or depressed
- A minimum of 100 polyps is needed to make the diagnosis
- Polyposis can involve other portions of the GI tract (stomach, small bowel, colon, and rectum)
- If left untreated, 1 or more carcinomas of the large intestine will develop in every instance; carcinomas occur an average of 20 years earlier than ordinary colorectal carcinomas
- Prophylactic colectomy should be performed at 20 to 25 years of age at the latest when the diagnosis is established during adolescence and at the time of diagnosis in patients with no family history of disease (new mutation)
- Carcinomas may develop in other organs such as gallbladder, thyroid, adrenal gland
- Other associations include hepatoblastoma, MEN, nasopharyngeal angiofibroma, medulloblastoma, and lymphoid polyps of the terminal ileum
- A variant known as *hereditary flat adenoma syndrome* is associated with flat polyps (rather than elevated) that usually number <100, exhibit a right-sided predominance, occur at a later age than classic FAP, and give rise to deeply invasive carcinomas (probably a variant of Lynch syndrome); other associated conditions include fundic gland polyps of the stomach and adenomas and carcinomas of both the stomach and duodenum

Familial Juvenile Polyposis

- Loss of SMAD4 on chromosome 18q21.1
- Most occur in children below the age of 5 years
- Juvenile polyps seen throughout the GI tract, but 80% occur in the colon and rectum
- Some polyps have combined juvenile and adenomatous features
- Associated with the development of adenomatous polyps and adenocarcinoma of the large bowel, duodenum, stomach, or pancreas (50% lifetime risk for developing colorectal cancer, usually at an early age)

Gardner Syndrome

- Autosomal dominant with variable expression

- A variation of FAP
- Affected patients have coexisting somatic and germ line mutations of the *APC* gene, suggesting that inactivation of both alleles of this gene is involved in their development
- Intestinal polyps identical to those in FAP are seen in association with multiple osteomas (particularly of mandible, skull, and long bones), epidermal cysts, and fibromatosis (most of the fibromatoses are intraabdominal and develop after surgical intervention)
- Adenomatous polyps may also be present in the stomach and small intestine as well as the colon
- Potential for development of large bowel carcinoma as high as for FAP
- Patients also at risk for development of carcinomas of small bowel, particularly in the periampuallary area
- Other associations include abnormalities of dentition, such as unerupted and supernumerary teeth, benign lymphoid polyposis of the terminal ileum, and congenital hypertrophy of retinal pigment epithelium resulting in solitary or multiple oval pigmented lesions in 1 or both eyes

Hereditary Nonpolyposis Colorectal Cancer (HNPCC)

- Also known as Lynch syndrome I and II
- An autosomal dominant disease caused by mutations in 1 of at least 4 DNA mismatch repair genes

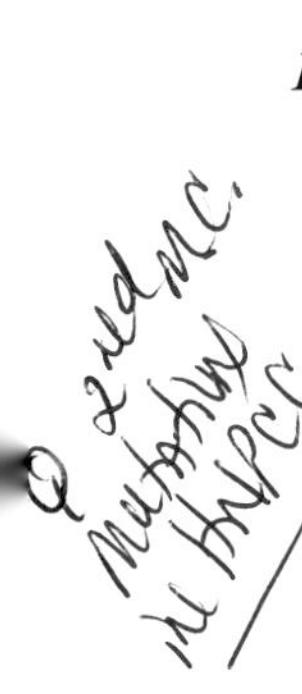

- 75% to 80% of HNPCC families have abnormalities on chromosome 2p and 3p which relate to mutations in the mismatch repair genes *MSH2* (40% of HNPCC cases), *MLHI*, *PMS1*, and *PMS2*; these mutations result in loss of stability of the DNA
- Tumor DNA of affected patients has widespread instability in short repeat sequences, termed microsatellite instability, detected as extra bands on PCR-amplified short repetitive segments of DNA; DNA instability is present in most of the adenomas that develop in patients with this syndrome
- Patients still develop cancer through progression of adenoma to malignancy, but lack diffuse polyposis seen in FAP; incidence of polyps probably equal to that seen in patients with sporadic colorectal cancer, but once a polyp develops there appears to be an increased rate of tumor progression
- May be the most common form of familial colon cancer and accounts for 5% to 10% of all colorectal carcinomas
- Characterized by a relatively young age at diagnosis (~45 years), first cancer usually in the right colon (~75%), and a high incidence of multiple cancers (synchronous in ~18% and metachronous in ~25%)
- Colon cancers tend to be mucinous and poorly differentiated
- 50% risk of developing adenocarcinoma in first-degree relative of an affected patient
- Two major variants of HNPCC:
  - *Lynch syndrome I* (hereditary site-specific colorectal cancer):
    - An increased incidence of multiple colon carcinomas that occurs 2 to 3 decades earlier than typically seen
    - Cancers have a predilection for proximal colon (65%-75%)
  - *Lynch syndrome II* (cancer family syndrome):
    - All the features of Lynch syndrome I plus the early onset of carcinoma at other sites (endometrium, ovaries, pancreas, bladder, larynx, brain, and stomach)
- A variation (of Lynch syndrome) is represented by colorectal carcinoma–prone families who have right-sided flat adenomas; the number of adenomas is intermediate between that in FAP and classic Lynch syndrome; most carcinomas are right-sided and occur at a later age than seen in FAP and classic Lynch syndrome

Intestinal Ganglioneuromatosis

- May occur in the small and large intestine as either solitary lesions or, more commonly, as multiple lesions (ganglioneuromatosis)
- Ganglioneuromatosis may be associated with von Recklinghausen disease and MEN type IIB
- Microscopically, characterized by multifocal proliferation of ganglion cells, axons, dendrites, and supporting Schwann cells in any layer of the bowel wall; resulting nodules may project into lumen as a polyp, may be entirely intramural, or project from the serosal surface
- No significant association with GI malignancy, although scattered reports of malignant peripheral nerve sheath tumor in patients with von Recklinghausen disease
- In MEN type IIB, the ganglioneuromatosis may be associated with a marked accentuation of both the submucosal and myenteric nerve plexuses

- Rare association with juvenile polyposis and Cowden disease

Muir-Torre Syndrome

- Colorectal carcinoma (often multiple) associated with genitourinary tumors, multiple sebaceous tumors (yellow facial papules), and keratoacanthomas
- May occur in members of a cancer family; mutations in both *MLH1* and *MLH2* have been reported (may be a variant of HNPCC)

Multiple Hyperplastic Polyposis Syndrome

- Pure hyperplastic polyps do not become malignant
- Polyps in this syndrome tend to be large and sometimes accompanied by adenocarcinoma

Oldfield Syndrome

- Typically diagnosed in 5th decade
- Multiple adenomatous polyps throughout GI tract, especially colon; associated with multiple sebaceous cysts

Peutz-Jeghers Syndrome

- Autosomal dominant (variable penetrance); mutation of serine threonine kinase (STK11) on chromosome 19q13.3
- Usually diagnosed in 3rd decade; men more commonly affected than women
- Symptoms include diarrhea, weight loss, abdominal pain, and complications of malabsorption
- Polyps tend to be large and pedunculated
- Characterized by multiple (almost always <100) hamartomatous polyps scattered throughout the entire GI tract (stomach 25%, small intestine 95%, colon 25%, and rectum 25%) with melanotic mucosal and cutaneous pigmentation of the lips, oral mucosa, face, genitalia, digits, palms, and soles
- Microscopically, Peutz-Jeghers polyp characterized by an arborizing network of connective tissue and a well-developed smooth muscle arising from the muscularis mucosae, extending into the polyp, and covered with glandular epithelium rich in goblet cells; the epithelial component resembles the normal epithelium of the intestinal area from which the polyp arises
- Adenomatous polyps with a marked degree of atypia and a potential to progress to adenocarcinoma may coexist with Peutz-Jegher polyps in either the small intestine or colon
- Increased risk for the development of adenocarcinoma of the stomach, small bowel, and colon; reports of carcinoma arising within a Peutz-Jeghers polyp
- 10% of small intestine lesions have areas of pseudo-invasion characterized by the presence of herniated mucinous glands and cysts in the muscularis mucosae and deeeper (enteritis cystica profunda)
- Increased incidence of other malignant neoplasms, including well-differentiated adenocarcinoma of the uterine cervix (adenoma malignum), pancreatic carcinoma, a distinctive ovarian neoplasm (sex-cord tumor with annular tubules), ovarian mucinous tumors, breast carcinoma (often bilateral), and feminizing Sertoli tumors of the testis
- Associated abnormalities include cerebral and pulmonary arteriovenous malformations, cardiac anomalies, polydactyly, malrotation, and cranial malformations

Ruvalcaba-Myhre-Smith Syndrome

- Probable autosomal dominant
- Hamartomatous intestinal polyposis associated with macrocephaly, mental deficiency, unusual craniofacial appearance, and pigmented macules on shaft and glans of penis
- Polyps identical to juvenile polyps (may be a variant of juvenile polyposis)

Turcot Syndrome

- Probably a recessive pattern of inheritance
- Characterized by a combination of adenomatous colonic polyposis and tumors of the central nervous system
- Patients with FAP tend to develop medulloblastomas
- Patients with HNPCC tend to develop high-grade gliomas
- Malignant potential of colon polyps probably the same as in FAP
- Brain tumors are associated with a high mortality; patients may die of central nervous system lesions before intestinal carcinoma develop

Neuroendocrine Tumors—Small Intestine, Appendix, and Colon

Clinical Manifestations

- Tumors almost exclusively composed of serotonin-producing enterochromaffin cells and represent almost all the endocrine tumors that arise in the ileum, appendix, and Meckel diverticulum; represent the majority of those arising in the jejunum and cecum; represent a minority of those that occur in the duodenum, stomach, distal colon, rectum, pancreas, biliary tract, and lung
- *Small intestine*
  - May be an incidental finding and asymptomatic
  - Patients with metastatic disease nearly always symptomatic; intermittent intestinal obstruction and/or the "carcinoid syndrome", with cutaneous flushing, diarrhea, fibrous thickening of the endocardium and valves of the right heart
  - Men and women affected equally
- *Appendix*
  - More common in women than men (3:1)
  - Usually (80%) <1 cm; often discovered incidentally at time of pelvic surgery or surgery for symptoms of acute appendicitis
  - Carcinoid syndrome very unusual (its presence associated with widespread metastasis predominantly to the liver or retroperitoneum)
  - Represent 75% of all benign and malignant tumors of the appendix
- *Colon*
  - Patients typically present with symptoms similar to those of colon carcinoma: abdominal pain, diarrhea, rectal bleeding, and palpable abdominal mass
  - Average age approximately 60 years
  - Carcinoid syndrome seen in fewer than 5%
  - Most occur in right colon and tend to be larger than the carcinoids seen in the small intestine, appendix, and rectum
  - Frequently malignant with evidence of local spread in 45% and distant metastasis in 40%

Gross Pathology

- *Small intestine*
  - Multiple in 40%
  - Typically a deep mucosal or submucosal, pale yellow nodule with an intact or slightly eroded overlying mucosa; most larger than 2 cm
  - Deep invasion of muscular wall with involvement of the peritoneum frequently present
  - Considerable fibroblastic or desmoplastic reaction present in adjacent mesentery, which may cause kinking and/or obstruction
  - Adjacent (underlying) muscularis propria frequently markedly hypertrophied
- *Appendix* (70%)
  - Usually small and located at the tip of the appendix (70%)
  - Lymph node metastasis rarely present (an incidence between 2% and 9%; metastases only occur in tumors >2 cm)
- *Colon*
  - Midgut enterochromaffin cell (ECC)-derived
  - Most aggressive GI neuroendocrine tumor
  - More common in women then men
  - 65% arise in cecum and right colon
  - Lesions tend to average 5 cm
  - Patients present with nausea, vomiting, and weight loss, and/or abdominal mass
  - Carcinoid syndrome in 5%

Microscopic Pathology

- 4 growth patterns:
  - Type A: Tubular or nested; tumor cells grow without intervening stroma, into large or small islands or nests; peripheral palisading may be discernable; pattern most often seen in ECC tumors
  - Type B: Trabecular; cells grow may grow in long cords that are only 1-cell thick and look like long ribbons or festoons or grow in short cords; amount of styroma very variable

- Type C: Acinar; small polygonal cells form glandlike lumina and may contain secretions and psammoma bodies; true glands do not occur
- Type D: Cells have typical neuroendocrine nuclear features but do not have an organized growth pattern; nuclear-cytoplasm ratio high and nuclei hyperchromatic; Type D pattern typically associated with a poor prognosis

- *Small intestine*
  - ECC derived
  - Most produce serotonin and substance P
  - Tumor cells typically organized in closely packed solid or rounded nests (insular) with peripheral palisading (typically a type A growth pattern)
  - Occasionally the tumor will have rosette-type, glandlike structures within solid areas
  - In areas of deep invasion, tumor may take on a trabecular pattern or may be arranged in cords
- *Appendix*
  - Tumors probably arise from subepithelial neuroendocrine complexes
  - Schwann-like (sustentacular) cells an important component (these cells are lacking in both small intestinal and colonic neuroendocrine tumors both of which are thought to arise from intraepithelial endocrine cells rather than from subepithelial neuroendocrine complexes)
  - 3 histologic types of appendiceal neuroendocrine tumors
    - *ECC-derived*: Type A growth pattern usually predominates with a type B pattern at the periphery; tumor cells arranged in solid nests with some peripheral palisading; tend to invade serosa, lymphatics, and nerves; histologic and cytologic appearance essentially identical to that seen in small intestinal tumors; tumor cells arranged in solid nests with some peripheral palisading 70% located in tip, 20% in midportion, and 10% in base
    - *Appendiceal neuroendocrire tumors with mucin production*: Goblet cell carcinoid characterized by cells with a mixture of all normal crypt elements (goblet cells, Paneth cells, and ECC cells); cytologic features bland; minimal nuclear atypia and no mitotic figures; tend to invade serosa, lymphatics, and nerves. A small subset of mucinous appendiceal neuroendocrine tumor have focal histologic features of pure conventional glandular differentiation and/or true signet ring cell differentiation with cytologic features of malignancy; tend to have large mucin pools, gland formation with cribriforming, solid sheets, and signet ring cells with atypical nuclei; Most aggressive carcinoid tumor to involve the appendix
    - *Enteroglucagon or L Cell*: May be composed of neuroendocrine cells that produce glicentin-related peptides (enteroglucagons) and PP and PYY; these tumors most closely resemble neuroendocrine tumors found in the rectum; composed of small acini or tubules dispersed in a loose fibrous stroma that often whorles around teardrop-shaped tubules
- *Colon*
  - ECC-derived tumors have histologic and cytologic features identical to those of small intestinal neuroendocrine tumors to include the absence of S-100–positive sustentacular cells
  - High-grade neuroendocrine tumor (small cell carcinoma)

Special Stains

- Mucin stains will demonstrate mucin in goblet cells
- Most tumor cells intensely argyrophilic

Immunohistochemistry

- Most enterochromaffin cells in small intestine produce serotonin and are positive for synaptophysin and chromogranin
- Substance P and other tachykinins will highlight tumor cells of midgut neuroendocrine tumors (foregut neuroendocrine tumors tend not to be reactive for substance P)
- L-cell tumors of the appendix express enteroglucagon, peptides YY and PP, but not chromogranin

- S-100 protein will demonstrate the Schwann-like (sustentacular) cells in appendical tumors
- Colon tumors tend to stain in a fashion similar to small intestinal tumors

Electron Microscopy

- Tumor cells have medium-sized, rod to pyriform, heavily osmiophilic dense-core granules

Molecular Alterations

- Small intestinal tumors are typically DNA diploid or tetraploid

Differential Diagnosis

- Adenocarcinoma
- Lymphoma
- Mesenchymal neoplasm

Treatment

- Surgical excision
- Carcinoid tumors located at the base of the appendix, are >2 cm, or show features of malignancy, and are typically treated with right colectomy with removal of mesenteric lymph nodes

Prognosis

- *Small intestine*
  - 5-year survival rate approximately 65%; 10-year survival rate approximately 45%
  - Incidence of metastasis 2%, 50%, and 80% in tumors smaller than 1 cm, 1 to 2 cm, and more than 2 cm, respectively
  - Patients without liver metastases have a 5and 10-year survival rate of 70% and 60% respectively; patients with liver metastases have a 5and 10-year survival rates of 35% and 15%, respectively
  - Extraabdominal metastases very rare (<1%)
- *Appendix*
  - Incidence of metastases ranges between 1.5% and 10% and is the sole determinant of prognosis
  - 5-year survival rate 95%
- *Colon*
  - 5-year survival rate 25%; 10-year survival rate 10%

Associations

- See carcinoid syndrome above

Neuroendocrine Tumors—Rectum

Clinical Manifestations

- Represents 1% to 2% of all rectal tumors and 10% to 25% of all GI endocrine tumors
- Typically single; 2% to 5% multiple
- Average age at diagnosis 50 years
- Most asymptomatic; symptoms include constipation, rectal bleeding, change in bowel habits, and pain
- No definite hyperfunctional syndrome has been identified
- Carcinoid syndrome rarely occurs (these tumors do not typically produce serotonin; they produce glucagon, insulin, glicentin, somatostatin, serotonin, endorphins, enkephalins, and pancreatic peptide (PP) and pancreatic peptidelike peptide with N-terminal tyrosine amide (PYY) –related hormonal peptides, or a combination of 2 or more peptides

Gross Pathology

- Usually appears as small (<2 cm), yellow, submucosal nodule with an intact overlying epithelium; may be polypoid
- Small lesions freely moveable; larger lesions tend to be fixed to rectal wall and can invade directly into bladder
- Typically located between 4 and 13 cm above the dentate line; 85% located on either anterior or lateral rectal wall

Microscopic Pathology

- Derived from hindgut enteroglucagon or L cells
- Tumor cells tend to be arranged in ribbons (type B pattern) with or without irregular trabeculae and rosettes; areas of solid nestlike structures rare
- Criteria for malignancy include size >2 cm, invasion of muscularis propria, 2 or more mitoses/10 hpf, and DNA aneuploidy

Special Stains

- Tumors often negative for silver stains
- Rarely argentaffinic; usually argyrophilic

Immunohistochemistry

- Tumor cells typically stain positively for synaptophysin and chromogranin
- Approximately 30% show some immunoreactivity for serotonin
- Most somatostatin positive
- 80% to 100% show immunoreactivity for prostatic acidic phosphatase and vimentin (not typical findings in other GI neuroendocrine tumors)

Electron Microscopy

- Tumor cells contain round to atypical angular dense core secretory granules that fill the basal cytoplasm

Molecular Alterations

- Metastatic lesions tend to be aneuploid

Differential Diagnosis

- Poorly differentiated carcinoma
- Lymphoma
- Mesenchymal tumors

Treatment

- Tumors <1 cm in diameter can be treated by either fulguration or wide full-thickness excision
- Tumors between 1 and 2 cm are treated by wide local excision
- Tumors >2 cm that have invaded the muscularis externa treated with radical excision (low anterior sigmoid resection or abdominal-perineal resection)

Prognosis

- 5-year survival rate 75%
- Tumors >2 cm have 60% to 85% incidence of metastases; tumors 1 to 2 cm 10% to 15%; tumors <1 cm <2%

Associations

- Multiple rectal-type neuroendocrine tumors may be seen in the large intestine of patients with either ulcerative colitis or Crohn disease

References

Dabbs DJ. *Diagnostic Immunohistochemistry.* New York: Churchill Livingstone, 2002.

Day D, Jass JR, Price AB, et al (eds). *Morson and Dawson's Gastrointestinal Pathology. 4th ed.* Malden, Blackwell Publishing, 2003

Fenoglio-Preiser CM. *Gastrointestinal Pathology: An Atlas and Text. 2nd ed.* Philadelphia: Lippincott Williams & Wilkins, 1999.

Hamilton SR, Aaltonen LA (eds). *World Health Organization Classification of Tumours. Pathology and Genetics of Tumours of the Digestive System.* Lyon: IARC Press, 2000.

Lewin JJ, Appelman HD. *Tumors of the Esophagus and Stomach: Atlas of Tumor Pathology. 3rd Series, Fascicle 18.* Washington DC; Armed Forces Institute of Pathology, 1996.

Mills S, Carter D, Greenson JK, Oberman HA, Reuter V, Stoler MH (eds). *Sternberg's Diagnostic Surgical Pathology. 4th ed.* Philadelphia: Lippincott Williams & Wilkins, 2004.

Ming S, Goldman H. *Pathology of the Gastrointestinal Tract.* 2nd ed. Baltimore: Williams & Wilkins, 1998.

Montgomery EA. *Biopsy Interpretation of the Gastrointestinal Tract Mucosa.* Philadelphia, Lipppincott, Williams & Wilkins, 2006.

Odze RD, Goldblum JR, Crawford JM. *Surgical Pathology of the GI Tract, Liver, and Pancreas.* Philadelphia: WB Saunders Co, 2004.

Rosai J. *Rosai and Ackerman's Surgical Pathology. 9th ed.* St. Louis: Mosby, 2004.

Whitehead R. *Mucosal Biopsy of the Gastrointestinal Tract: Volume 3—Major Problems in Pathology. 5th ed.* Philadelphia: WB Saunders Co, 1997.

Chapter 8

Liver, Gallbladder, and Extrahepatic Bile Ducts

Intraoperative Consultation

There are 5 generally accepted indications for intraoperative consultation on a liver specimen:

- The unexpected finding of a liver nodule during abdominal surgery for disease unrelated to the liver.
- The presence of a second, unexpected lesion in a planned hepatic resection for neoplasm. The rendering of an intraoperative consultation in this setting may dramatically change the extent or result in abandonment of the originally planned hepatic resection.
- Evaluation of the adequacy of surgical margins of resected specimens for either primary hepatic malignancy or metastatic disease.
- To provide a definitive diagnosis for a hepatic lesion that could not be diagnosed preoperatively. The intraoperative determination of benign versus malignant will obviously dictate the subsequent course of the procedure.
- Frozen section examination of a portion of donor liver to ensure its adequacy for transplantation.

Nodules in the liver that are found as incidental findings during abdominal surgery are generally submitted for frozen section diagnosis. These lesions include benign cysts, localized scars secondary to old granulomatous disease, biliary hamartomas, bile duct adenomas, metastatic carcinomas, focal nodular hyperplasia, and hepatocellular carcinoma.

A major problem faced by the pathologist in this clinical setting is to make the distinction between a bile duct hamartoma or bile duct adenoma and metastatic well-differentiated adenocarcinoma. Hamartomas typically consist of multiple small (occasionally dilated) ductular structures lined by uniform cuboidal or flattened epithelial cells with bland nuclei and moderate to scant cytoplasm. These structures may contain inspissated bile and are typically separated by a fairly acellular dense connective tissue stroma. Bile duct adenomas appear similar to bile duct hamartomas except that the ductules tend to be smaller (occasionally without a lumen) and are quite uniform and closely packed with little intervening stroma. Well-differentiated adenocarcinomas tend to have infiltrating margins, irregularly shaped glands, nuclear atypia, and mitotic activity.

Focal nodular hyperplasia is not an uncommon intraoperative finding, and on frozen section the normal hepatic acinar structure is lacking; eg, both portal tracts and hepatic veins are absent. The diagnosis is based on the presence of dense, fibrous, collagenized septa that contain eccentrically thickened and occasionally narrow blood vessels and bile ductules at the parenchymal interface; these septa divide the lesion into lobules that resemble cirrhosis. The presence of small ductules in the lesion differentiates focal nodular hyperplasia from adenoma, which does not contain these structures. The distinction between hepatocellular adenoma and focal nodular hyperplasia on intraoperative frozen section biopsy may be important if the lesion is an adenoma and the surgeon plans to resect. The surgical margins can be assessed with a gross examination. Patients with primary malignant tumors of the liver, including hepatocellular carcinoma, cholangiocarcinoma, epithelioid hemangioendothelioma, and pediatric neoplasms such as hepatoblastoma and undifferentiated (embryonal) sarcoma that are unresectable or unsuitable for transplantation, are generally treated with transarterial chemoembolization, percutaneous ethanol injection, or cryosurgery. In any of these situations, the diagnosis should be confirmed with frozen section analysis before the placement of the appropriate medical device.

The most common clinical situation is one in which the malignant hepatic neoplasm has been diagnosed preoperatively. The role of the pathologist in that situation is simply to evaluate the adequacy of surgical margins. The goal of the surgeon is to obtain at least a 1 cm margin of normal tissue. A false-negative margin has major adverse implications to the patient, particularly if the lesion is small and potentially curable. The pathologist must take great care to serially section the lesion in continuity with its adjacent inked surgical margin to ensure an accurate report.

If a preoperative diagnosis has not been made on a potentially malignant neoplasm, a frozen section will be requested to provide a definitive diagnosis. Frozen section evaluation of a hepatocellular carcinoma can be particularly problematic, and have the following pitfalls:

- If the section is cut too thickly there will be an apparently increased nuclear density and increased nuclear-cytoplasmic ratio that will result in a benign lesion having the appearance of a well-differentiated hepatocellular carcinoma.

- The presence of fatty change, particularly if it is extensive, can result in some alteration in the architecture of the liver cell plates, producing trabeculae that are 3 or 4 cells thick (a characteristic of hepatocellular carcinoma).
- Hepatocellular carcinomas with little cytologic atypia may be extremely difficult to differentiate from an adenoma, regenerative cirrhotic nodule, and normal liver. If the issue cannot be resolved intraoperatively, a deferred diagnosis is appropriate even when such a deferral may result in a patient having to undergo a second surgical procedure.

The distinction of a cholangiocarcinoma from a metastatic adenocarcinoma can be quite difficult, but fortunately from a pathologist's perspective, the most important issue is the adequacy of surgical margins. Whether a lesion is a cholangiocarcinoma or a metastasis can usually be determined clinically either during the preoperative or postoperative workup. Benign glandular structures in the wall of a large bile duct can mimic a well-differentiated adenocarcinoma. Factors that favor a benign finding include clustering of glandular structures into vague nodules and bland cytologic features. Problem cases are best approached by simultaneously freezing both a portion of known neoplasm as well as the surgical bile duct margin so that the known malignant cells can be compared with the cells in the ductular structures in the bile duct wall.

Frozen section diagnoses of specimens taken from a donor liver are performed to determine the presence of fatty change, ischemic necrosis, chronic viral hepatitis, and malignancy. Frozen sections are routinely requested to evaluate a donor liver to determine if it is functionally compromised and to avoid transplanting a malignancy. The presence of significant steatosis or the presence of focal ischemic necrosis indicates an increased risk of significant hepatic dysfunction and graft failure. Donor livers from patients with hepatitis C and no evidence of clinical disease that are destined for a recipient with hepatitis C should be evaluated by frozen section analysis to determine the extent of inflammation and fibrosis. The surgeon then must decide on the appropriateness of proceeding with transplantation.

The presence of an incidental mass in a donor liver always requires a definitive diagnosis. Any malignancy or a hepatic adenoma is a contraindication for transplantation whereas focal nodular hyperplasia, hemangioma, or biliary hamartomas can be transplanted with impunity.

Specimen Handling

Explanted livers should first be examined in the area of the porta hepatis to determine the patency of the hepatic artery, portal vein, and common hepatic duct. The specimen is then serially sectioned perpendicular to its long axis (sagittal plane) at approximately 0.5 to 1 cm intervals working from one of the lateral edges toward the middle. It is important to realize that a wire meshwork shunt may be present and when encountered should be blocked out and removed. All dominant or suspicious nodules are sectioned as well as normal parenchyma and the gallbladder. In cases of chronic cholestatic disease, sections should be taken near the hilum.

Livers resected for end-stage liver disease are typically sliced at 1 cm intervals. Particular attention should be given to any nodules, cirrhotic or otherwise, that differ in color and consistency from their neighbors. In livers without neoplasm, sections should include hepatic parenchyma taken at least 1 cm from the capsule. A section of hilar structures to include the bile duct, portal vein, and hepatic artery should be taken. In cases of cholangitis, multiple sections of both hilar ducts and peripheral ducts should be obtained.

Livers resected for neoplasm require a minimum of 4 sections to include the interface between the neoplasm and adjacent liver parenchyma. At least 1 section should be taken at the point where the neoplasm most closely approximates the capsule and a section should be taken at the margin if the tumor is within 2 cm of the margin. Additional sections should be taken of uninvolved hepatic parenchyma.

Non-Neoplastic Diseases

Alcoholic Liver Disease

Clinical Manifestations

- Patients may be asymptomatic or show any of the broad range of signs and symptoms associated with chronic alcohol consumption

Gross Pathology

- Liver may appear normal on gross examination, demonstrate fatty change, or be frankly cirrhotic

Microscopic Pathology

- *Alcoholic fatty change*
  - Typically consists of large fat vacuoles in hepatocytes in acinar zone 3
  - Fatty change tends to progress outward from perivenular regions toward the portal tracts as severity of steatosis increases
  - Occasionally an acute fatty liver will be characterized by finely vacuolated hepatocytes in the perivenular areas (alcoholic foamy degeneration) often accompanied by the more common large fat droplets elsewhere; megamitochondria (round or spindle-shaped cytoplasmic inclusions) present in vacuolated perivenular hepatocytes
  - Areas of canalicular cholestasis, foci of liver cell necrosis, and formation of delicate collagen fibers in areas of fatty change often present
  - Occasional Mallory bodies may be present, but inflammatory infiltrates usually absent
- *Alcoholic hepatitis and fibrosis (steatohepatitis)*
  - Characterized by liver cell damage, inflammation, and fibrosis that begins near terminal hepatic venules
  - Almost all acini affected
  - Fatty change usually present (but not always)
  - Liver cell damage seen as ballooning; affected cells tend to be round rather than polygonal and have abundant pale-staining cytoplasm, with or without fat vacuoles; megamitochondria and Mallory bodies may be present
  - Mallory bodies are clumps, strands, or perinuclear rings of dense material composed largely of intermediate filaments of cytoskeleton (found in both bile duct epithelium and hepatocytes); may be present in conditions other than alcoholic hepatitis (other forms of steatohepatitis)
  - Mallory hyaline tends to be centrilobular and is chemotactic for neutrophils
  - Canalicular cholestasis may be seen
  - Inflammatory infiltrate usually consists of neutrophils but lymphocytes and macrophages also present; neutrophils found among or even within damaged hepatocytes
  - Fibrosis a constant feature of alcoholic hepatitis and typically is seen as pericellular (perisinusoidal) fibrosis around individual ballooned hepatocytes in zone 3
  - Fibrosis typically persists even after alcoholic hepatitis resolves
  - As fibrosis develops in the areas of the terminal hepatic venules, the vein walls thicken (perivenular fibrosis) and may represent the initial changes of developing cirrhosis
  - Occasionally perivenular fibrosis results in narrowing or occlusion of terminal hepatic venules producing the clinical features of veno-occlusive disease
  - Liver cell destruction and fibrosis at times are so extensive that large fibrous scars in the perivenular areas will develop with fibrous bridges linking these scars to portal tracts
- *Cirrhosis*
  - Alcoholic cirrhosis is the end result of alcoholic hepatitis
  - Alcoholic hepatitis evolves into cirrhosis by the contraction of fibrous bridges linking perivenular to portal areas; surviving hepatic parenchyma regenerates to form small nodules that frequently manifest some fatty change
  - As cirrhosis progresses, the nodule size increases and with time the features of an alcoholic etiology may disappear
  - Chronic hepatitis (viral or alcoholic) can contribute to the formation of cirrhosis and are characterized by the presence of hepatocyte necrosis adjacent to portal tracts (piecemeal necrosis) and portal and acinar lymphocytic infiltrates
- *Other significant syndromes and lesions in the alcoholic liver*
  - *Chronic hepatitis*: Characterized by portal lymphoid follicles or aggregates and lymphocytic infiltration of portal tracts and acini (hepatitis C)
  - *Extensive perivenular necrosis:* Seen in alcoholics taking therapeutic doses of acetaminophen

- *Fetal alcohol syndrome*: Children of alcoholic mothers may have fatty liver with both perisinusoidal and portal fibrosis
- *Chronic alcoholic pancreatitis*: Multiple strictures of the pancreatic duct system and bile duct obstruction with cholestasis with or without cholangitis; biliary cirrhosis often develops; fibrosis develops primarily in a portal distribution
- *Hepatocellular siderosis*: Occasionally seen in alcoholics; never of the magnitude seen in genetic hemochromatosis
- *Hepatocellular carcinoma*: Longstanding alcohol use may promote the development of hepatocellular carcinoma in hepatitis B virus (HBV) carriers and in patients with chronic hepatitis C

Special Stains

- Trichrome stains will highlight megamitochondria (seen as red, spherical, fairly sharply outlined cytoplasmic inclusions) and Mallory hyaline (which will stain blue and have an indistinct outline)
- Reticulin and trichrome stains will outline pericellular fibrosis in the area of the central veins characteristic of steatohepatitis

Immunohistochemistry

- Mallory bodies will stain with ubiquitin and p62

Electron Microscopy

- May confirm the presence of megamitochondria in vacuolated perivenular hepatocytes of alcoholic foamy degeneration
- Confirm that Mallory bodies consist largely of intermediate filaments of cytoskeleton; usually seen as clusters of randomly oriented filaments, bundles of parallel filaments or granular nonfilamentous material

Molecular Alterations

- None

Differential Diagnosis

- Viral hepatitis (viral hepatitis typically causes collapse of preexisting connective tissue rather than the formation of new collagen)
- Chronic venous congestion (characterized by perivenular and pericellular fibrosis similar to that of alcoholic liver disease; differential diagnosis may be quite difficult in the absence of liver cell ballooning and Mallory bodies)
- Chronic cholestasis, Wilson disease, hypervitaminosis A, methotrexate therapy, and nonalcoholic steatohepatitis are all associated with hepatocellular ballooning, Mallory bodies, neutrophils, and fibrosis

Treatment

- Most hepatic changes in the alcoholic, with the exception of well-established cirrhosis, will regress with the cessation of alcohol
- Cirrhosis with end-stage liver disease treated with hepatic transplantation

Prognosis

- 90% of patients with alcoholic cirrhosis who continue to drink will be dead within a year

Associations

- Presence of HLA antigen (antigens A1, A9, A28, and Bw35 are associated with a significantly increased risk for the development of alcohol-associated cirrhosis)
- Increased susceptibility to viral hepatitis (see above)

α_1-Antitrypsin (A1-AT) Deficiency

Clinical Manifestations

- Over 30 variants identified and assigned a protease inhibitor (PI) designation
- A1-AT produced in the liver; 1 of the body's major inhibitors of several proteolytic enzymes
- There are over 70 alleles of the α_1- antitrypsin (RAT) gene; two of these alleles determine an individual's phenotype
- Most common phenotype PIMM is associated with normal serum levels of A1-AT
- Individuals who are heterozygous (PiMZ) have moderately reduced serum levels of A1-AT
- Individuals who are homozygous (PiZZ) have profoundly reduced levels of A1-AT
- Children who are homozygous develop neonatal cholestasis with jaundice, hepatomegaly, and elevated

liver function test results; their clinical course varies from gradual resolution to development of a chronic cholestatic syndrome with a paucity of bile ducts and eventually cirrhosis

- Adults (usually over the age of 50 years) who are homozygous typically present with pulmonary emphysema or liver disease (complications of portal hypertension or hepatic failure); occasionally asymptomatic

Gross Pathology

- Liver may appear normal to obviously cirrhotic

Microscopic Pathology

- Hepatocytes contain intracytoplasmic eosinophilic globules
- Eosinophilic globules in a noncirrhotic liver are most evident in the periportal region; in the cirrhotic liver they are most evident at the periphery of parenchymal nodules
- Areas of hepatocellular degeneration, giant cell formation, cholestasis, portal fibrosis, cholangitis, and cirrhosis may be present (especially in infants)
- Liver cell dysplasia present in up to 90% in patients with well-developed cirrhosis
- Histologic picture in adults includes chronic active hepatitis with portal and periportal inflammation, piecemeal necrosis, and varying amounts of fibrosis; cirrhosis usually present

Special Stains

- Periodic acid-Schiff (PAS) will highlight the intracytoplasmic globules of A1-AT

Immunohistochemistry

- Eosinophilic intracytoplasmic globules stain positively for A1-AT

Electron Microscopy

- Granular, proteinaceous material in dilated sacs of endoplasmic reticulum

Molecular Alterations

- Globules accumulate in hepatocytes as a result of a structural change in the glycoprotein which is encoded by the mutant Z gene; an abnormal folding of the protein as a result of the substitution of lysine for glutamic acid at position 342 results in a failure of endoplasmic reticulum to secrete A1-AT with its resulting accumulation in hepatocytes

Differential Diagnosis

- Neonatal hepatitis
- Biliary atresia
- Chronic active hepatitis
- Cirrhosis

Treatment

- Liver transplantation

Prognosis

- Increased risk of hepatocellular carcinoma (may be significant only in men)
- Patients who are homozygous run a risk of liver disease (ranging from cholestasis to advanced cirrhosis to liver failure and death); this risk is 65% in infants

Associations

- Emphysema (A1-AT is capable of degrading structural proteins in numerous organs to include both the lung and liver)

Autoimmune Hepatitis

Clinical Manifestations

- Primarily affects young women (female-to-male ratio 8:1) between ages of 15 and 35 years
- Viral serologic markers absent unless the disease superimposed on viral hepatitis
- Serum IgG levels elevated

- Types of autoimmune hepatitis (each characterized by a different antibody pattern):
  - Type 1: Previously called lupoid hepatitis; most common (80% of cases); characterized by the presence of antinuclear antibodies (ANA), and/or antismooth muscle antibodies (SMA), hypergammaglobulinemia and concurrent autoimmune disorders, usually seen in women between ages of 10 and 20 years and between 45 and 70 years; 25% have cirrhosis at time of presentation
  - Type 2: Characterized by liver-kidney microsome type 1 antibodies (anti-LKM1); ANA and smooth muscle antibodies negative; more common in children (2 to 14 years); tends to progress rapidly to cirrhosis
  - Type 3: Antibodies against soluble liver antigen/liver pancreas (anti-SLA/LP); 35% will have antismooth muscle antibodies and antimitochondrial antibodies; no anti-ANA or LKM1

Gross Pathology

- Liver may appear normal to frankly cirrhotic on gross examination

Microscopic Pathology

- Appearance similar to that of chronic hepatitis with a dense uniform periportal infiltrate (especially in untreated patients) of lymphocytes (T-helper/inducer cells predominate) and plasma cells (plasma cells may occur in clusters); lymphoid follicles may be present (much less often than in hepatitis C)
- Plasma cells typically abundant at interface and throughout lobule, but having few in the inflammatory infiltrate does not preclude the diagnosis
- Eosinophils may be present
- Hepatocyte swelling, pyknotic necrosis, and interface hepatitis also characteristic
- Hepatocellular ballooning, architectural disruption, and cell drop out primarily in centrilobular areas
- Areas of bridging necrosis, piecemeal necrosis, and rosette formation common with increasing severity of disease
- Multinucleated giant hepatocytes may be present

Special Stains

- Trichrome

Immunohistochemistry and Electron Microscopy

- Not helpful

Molecular Alterations

- HLA DR3 and DR4 independent risk factors for type 1 autoimmune hepatitis

Differential Diagnosis

- Hepatitis C (major difference is large numbers of plasma cells seen in autoimmune hepatitis)
- Hepatitis B (plasma cells may be present)
- Primary biliary cirrhosis (PBC)
- Primary sclerosing cholangitis (PSC)
- Autoimmune hepatitis can be distinguished from PBC and PSC by preservation of bile ducts; serologic testing (positive ANA and negative hepatitis C virus [HCV] and HBV) helpful in distinguishing autoimmune hepatitis from viral hepatitis

Treatment

- Type 1 responsive to low-dose steroid administration
- Type 2 not responsive to steroids
- Immunosuppressive therapy may reduce the severity of the inflammatory component as well as reduce the amount of fibrosis, but development of cirrhosis cannot be prevented
- Liver transplantation

Prognosis

- An aggressive hepatitis with recurring bouts of hepatic injury that progresses to cirrhosis within 6 months if not treated

Associations

- HLA haplotypes A1, B8, and DR3
- Other forms of autoimmune disease present in 60%:
  - Rheumatoid arthritis
  - Thyroiditis
  - Sjögren syndrome
  - Ulcerative colitis

Overlap (Variant) Syndromes

- *Autoimmune hepatitis—PBC overlap variant*: Disproportionate alkaline phosphatase elevation, antimitochondrial antibodies (AMA), cholangitis (lymphoid, granulomatous), hepatic copper deposition, improvement with corticosteroids
- *Autoimmune hepatitis—PSC overlap variant*: Cholestatic laboratory features, cholangitis (lymphoid, fibrous obliterative), abnormal cholangiogram, inflammatory bowel disease, resistant to corticosteroids
- *Autoimmune hepatitis—chronic viral hepatitis C overlap variant*: Smooth muscle antibodies and/or ANA of 1:320 or more, moderate to severe interface hepatitis, lobular hepatitis, and/or portal plasma cell infiltrate

Cirrhosis

Clinical Manifestations

- Results from hepatocellular damage followed by regeneration and fibrosis
- Typically cirrhosis develops in the setting of a persistent damaging agent such as alcohol, chronic hepatitis B infection, or continued deposition of iron or copper
- Patients usually present in the 4th to 6th decades; patients with chronic active hepatitis or Wilson disease can present in late adolescence
- Men are more commonly affected than women if the etiology is hemochromatosis or hepatitis B
- Primary biliary cirrhosis predominantly a disease of women
- Sex incidence is approximately equal in postnecrotic or cryptogenic cirrhosis
- Men may slightly outnumber women when alcohol is the etiologic agent
- Patients present with various signs and symptoms to include generalized malaise, abdominal pain, loss of libido, jaundice, fluid retention, gastrointestinal hemorrhage, spider nevi, Dupuytren contracture, gynecomastia, testicular atrophy, hepatosplenomegaly
- Symptoms of advanced disease consist of liver failure, ascites, edema, variceal bleeding, and secondary infections

Etiology

- Viral hepatitis (B, C, D)
- Alcohol
- Biliary disease
- Metabolic diseases
  - Hemochromatosis
  - Wilson disease
  - A1-AT deficiency
- Venous outflow obstruction
- Drugs and toxins
- Autoimmune disease
- Cryptogenic (cause unknown)
- Nonalcoholic steatohepatitis (NASH)

Pathogenesis

- Cirrhosis is a diffuse nodulation of the liver that results from fibrous bands that subdivide the liver into regenerating nodules
- Fibrous bands of cirrhosis represent collagen (type I and III collagen) deposited in all portions of the hepatic lobule
- Deposits of collagen result in disruption of blood flow and impair diffusion of solutes between hepatocytes and plasma
- Ito cells (vitamin A fat-storage cells) become activated, lose their retinyl ester stores, transform into fibroblastlike cells, acquire contractile properties similar to those of myofibroblasts and synthesize collagen
- Stimuli for the deposition of fibrous tissue (collagen) may be related to several factors:
  - Chronic inflammatory conditions
  - Inflammatory mediators may link hepatic inflammation and fibrosis
  - Other factors, such as Kupffer cells, stimulate Ito cells
  - Disruption of normal extracellular matrix may lead to the transformation of Ito cells into collagen-forming cells

Gross Pathology

- A nodular liver with nodules <0.3 cm with delicate fibrous bands (micronodular cirrhosis) or nodules >0.3 cm with wide fibrous bands (macronodular fibrosis)

Microscopic Pathology

- Two basic criteria for the diagnosis: *nodularity and fibrosis*
- Other criteria that suggest the possibility of cirrhosis include:
  - Fragmentation at the time of biopsy or during processing is characteristic of cirrhosis
  - Abnormal structure: Nodules cored out of connective tissue by the biopsy procedure retain a thin layer of connective tissue that is adherent to the nodular margin
  - Approximation of portal tracts and terminal venules and increased numbers of venules in relation to the number of portal tracts
  - Presence of septa linking terminal hepatic veins to portal tracts
  - Hepatocellular changes: Occasionally hepatocytes in cirrhotic livers are normal
  - Regeneration is indicated by thickening of liver cell plates; widespread presence of double-cell plates indicate active growth
  - Hepatocytes in hyperplastic areas contain little or no lipofuscin pigment even in the central zones (adjacent to terminal venules)
  - Adjacent populations of hepatocytes may grow at different rates with resulting different cell and nuclear characteristics (pleomorphism); responsible for a distorted reticulin pattern
    - Reticulin fibers often arranged in abnormal patterns as a result of different rates of growth in different areas of the liver
  - Occasionally hepatocytes from cirrhotic livers will show a degree of structural atypia that warrants the designation "dysplasia"
    - Large cell dysplasia characterized by enlarged hepatocytes with hyperchromatic, pleomorphic nuclei with prominent nucleoli; typically the nuclear-cytoplasmic ratio is normal or only slightly increased; large cell dysplasia is mainly found in patients with HBV infection
    - Small cell dysplasia is characterized by smaller than normal hepatocytes with an increased nuclear-cytoplasmic ratio; may be a marker for the eventual development of hepatocellular carcinoma

Special Stains

- Reticulin

Immunohistochemistry

- Hepatitis B surface antigen can be demonstrated in cases of cirrhosis secondary to hepatitis B

Electron Microscopy

- Not helpful

Molecular Alterations

- None

Differential Diagnosis

- Nodular regenerative hyperplasia (nodularity secondary to regeneration but little or no fibrosis)
- Congenital hepatic fibrosis (intact acinar architecture with ductal plate malformations)
- Chronic hepatitis with fibrosis and structural abnormalities
- Well-differentiated hepatocellular carcinoma

Treatment

- Liver transplantation for impending hepatic failure (end-stage liver disease)

Prognosis

- With fully developed cirrhosis, approximately 50% will survive 1 year and 10% will survive 6 years
- 5-year survival for cryptogenic cirrhosis approximately 25%

- 5-year survival for alcoholic cirrhosis and active hepatitis approximately 50%
- 5-year survival for cirrhosis secondary to hemochromatosis 70%
- All forms of cirrhosis, regardless of etiology, have an improved survival if the underlying etiology is treated

Associations

- Hepatocellular carcinoma (cirrhosis of any disease etiology associated with an increased risk for the development of hepatocellular carcinoma)

Graft-vs-Host Disease (GVHD)

Clinical Manifestations

- Seen in patients who have received a bone marrow transplant
- Early after transplantation most clinical manifestations of disease related to opportunistic infections especially with fungal elements and cytomegalovirus (CMV) and to drugs used in cytoreductive therapy (may cause veno-occlusive disease or nodular regenerative hyperplasia)
- Manifestations of GVHD usually do not become apparent until at least 20 days after transplantation

Gross Pathology

- Liver parenchyma usually appears fairly normal

Microscopic Pathology

- Acute disease characterized by presence of a sparse lymphocytic infiltrate in the portal tracts with bile duct damage and endothelialitis (lymphocytic infiltrate in venous endothelium)
- Bile duct damage characterized by vacuolated or acidophilic cytoplasm, individual cell loss, pleomorphic nuclei with multilayering, and eventually complete loss of ducts; lymphocytes almost invariably present in the epithelial layer
- Amount of bile duct damage may be quite variable and is often present in many inflammatory conditions (it is generally felt that if more than 50% of the bile ducts are damaged it is presumptive evidence of GVHD in the proper clinical setting)
- Endothelialitis is characterized by lymphocytic infiltration of portal veins or central vein endothelium (damage to central vein endothelium characterized by lifting of the endothelium off its underlying basement membrane)
- Frequently there is associated hepatocellular damage characterized by ballooning degeneration and/or focal necrosis with scattered dead hepatocytes throughout the lobule
- Venous occlusion by loose or mature connective tissue common
- Chronic GVHD occurs after the 100th posttransplant day and is characterized by prominent portal lymphocytic infiltrates associated with the loss of interlobular bile ducts (vanishing bile duct syndrome) and portal fibrosis; cirrhosis may eventually develop

Special Stains, Immunohistochemistry and Electron Microscopy

- Not helpful

Molecular Alterations

- None

Differential Diagnosis

- Other causes of loss of bile ducts include longstanding biliary obstruction, primary biliary cirrhosis, primary sclerosing cholangitis, idiopathic adult ductopenia, reaction to certain medications (eg, amoxicillin/clavulanate potassium [Augmentin]), arterial ischemia, and chronic allograft rejection; hepatocellular damage (with the exception of piecemeal necrosis) typically not present in these conditions
- Most inflammatory conditions of the liver (especially viral hepatitis and drug hepatitis) are typically associated with hepatocellular damage (findings of extensive hepatocellular damage with little bile duct damage, probably not GVHD; findings of little hepatocellular damage with extensive bile duct damage, probably GVHD)

Treatment and Prognosis

- Acute disease treated with immunosuppressive therapy (methotrexate and cyclophosphamide)

- Chronic disease treated with combinations of prednisone and either cyclophosphamide or azathioprine
- Patients susceptible to a wide variety of opportunistic infections during first 90 days; interstitial pneumonia with or without CMV in 30%—mortality high

Associations

- Bone marrow transplantation

Congenital Hepatic Fibrosis

Clinical Manifestations

- Patients typically present between 1 and 2 years with an enlarged and hard liver
- May present with signs and symptoms of portal hypertension, particularly during adolescence
- Hepatocellular function almost always normal

Gross Pathology

- Typically liver enlarged and may appear cirrhotic (depending on stage of disease)

Microscopic Pathology

- Islands of normal liver parenchyma with normal vascular relationships separated by narrow and broad septa of dense mature fibrous tissue containing elongated or cystic, anastomosing biliary channels
- Biliary channels tend to be concentrated at the periphery of the fibrous bands but occasionally 2 sets of ductlike structures can be identified, 1 lying centrally within a fibrous septum and the other closer to the parenchyma
- Lumens of biliary structures may contain inspissated bile
- Portal vein branches may be small and inconspicuous
- No necrosis, inflammation, hepatocellular regeneration (regenerative nodules), or neocholangiogenesis (all of which are features of cirrhosis)
- Histologic evidence of cholangitis, other types of inflammation, or cholestasis may be present (coexisting Caroli disease should be considered)

Special Stains

- Trichrome and reticulin stains will highlight the fibrous septa

Immunohistochemistry, Electron Microscopy, and Special Stains

- Not helpful

Differential Diagnosis

- Cirrhosis

Treatment

- Patients have normal liver function test results; only long-term risk is development of portal hypertension which may require a shunting procedure

Prognosis

- Other than the development of portal hypertension, there is no evidence that this condition limits life expectancy

Associations

- Frequently associated with abnormalities in the kidneys or pancreas (primarily cystic changes)
- Slight increased risk (<5%) for development of hepatocellular carcinoma
- Congenital dilatation of intrahepatic bile ducts (Caroli disease)

Cystic Fibrosis

Clinical Manifestations

- Most common autosomal recessive disorder among whites (1 in 2,000 to 1 in 4,500)
- Liver involvement appears to be age-dependent; present in 40% of affected adolescents
- May present as neonatal cholestasis (secondary to bile duct obstruction by viscous bile) or intestinal obstruction (secondary to meconium)

Gross Pathology

- Hepatic changes range from essentially normal to mild steatosis to cirrhosis

Microscopic Pathology

- Steatosis most common hepatic lesion (usually macrovesicular without a zonal pattern)
- Most reliable diagnostic features include areas of stellate scarring (focal biliary fibrosis) with proliferating, dilated, bile ducts filled with inspissated eosinophilic material (may be quite focal and easily missed on biopsy)
- Bile duct cells may appear degenerated or necrotic
- Chronic inflammatory portal infiltrate
- Neocholangiogenesis (bile duct proliferation)

Special Stains

- PAS will highlight inspissated material in bile ductules

Immunohistochemistry

- Not helpful

Electron Microscopy

- Filamentous material in bile ducts

Molecular Alterations

- Cystic fibrosis gene is located on chromosome 7
- Most common mutation is a deletion of 3 nucleotides coding for phenylalanine at position 508, known as *delta F508*
- Mutations result in defective processing of the cystic fibrosis transmembrane conductance regulator (CFTR), which serves as a chloride channel

Differential Diagnosis

- During infancy histologic findings are those of neonatal hepatitis (canalicular cholestasis, hepatocyte injury, and giant, multinucleated hepatocytes)

Treatment

- Supportive care

Prognosis

- Death usually the result of pulmonary infections

Associations

- Disease may evolve into secondary biliary cirrhosis

Fatty Liver

Clinical Manifestations

- Steatosis (fatty change) a result of accumulation of triglycerides in hepatocytes
- May be asymptomatic or present with hepatomegaly
- Elevated serum aminotransferases, alkaline phosphatase, and/or gamma glutamyl transpeptidase may be present
- Most common etiologies include alcohol, obesity, diabetes, and malnutrition

Gross Pathology

- Liver may be yellow/orange and be enlarged
- Obvious cirrhosis may be present

Microscopic Pathology

- *Macrovesicular steatosis*
  - Most common form
  - Hepatocytes contain large single fat vacuoles that displace nuclei to 1 side
  - Fatty changes typically involve liver cells in acinar zones 2 or 3 but with time progress to involve all 3 zones
- *Microvesicular steatosis*
  - Finely divided fat droplets occupy hepatocyte cytoplasm
  - Nucleus tends to remain in a central position
  - Fat accumulation in the pericentral region (acinar zone 3) a feature of alcoholism, obesity, diabetes, and corticosteroid therapy
  - Fat accumulation in periportal regions (zone 1) seen in kwashiorkor, acquired immune deficiency syndrome (AIDS), and in patients receiving total parenteral nutrition
  - Occasionally a focus of fat accumulation will be seen in a subcapsular location in an otherwise normal or slightly fatty liver (may be confused with a neoplasm)
  - Rupture of a hepatocyte filled with fat will induce an inflammatory response, which will appear as a

focal accumulation of macrophages and neutrophils or the formation of a lipogranuloma (usually results in focal fibrosis of little clinical significance)

- In alcoholics, steatosis may be associated with steatohepatitis, portal fibrosis, and cirrhosis

- *Steatohepatitis*
  - Typically localized to acinar zone 3
  - Characterized by liver-cell ballooning, intracytoplasmic accumulations of Mallory hyaline, and inflammatory infiltrates (predominantly neutrophils) and both perivenular and pericellular fibrosis
  - When features of steatohepatitis present in alcoholics, the condition is referred to as *alcoholic* steatohepatitis
  - When the features of steatohepatitis present in nonalcoholics (such as obesity or diabetes) the condition is referred to as *nonalcoholic* steatohepatitis
  - Alcoholic and nonalcoholic steatohepatitis are almost identical:
    - Nonalcoholics may have more pronounced fatty change
    - Mallory hyaline more plentiful in alcoholics
    - Neutrophils present in greater numbers in alcoholics
  - Portal fibrosis and cirrhosis may complicate both the alcoholic and nonalcoholic liver

Special Stains

- Reticulin stains and trichrome stains will highlight perivenular and pericellular fibrosis characteristic of steatohepatitis
- Oil Red O stains on frozen material may be required to identify trace amounts of finely divided microvesicular fat

Immunohistochemistry

- Not helpful

Electron Microscopy

- Mallory hyaline seen as bundles of intermediate filaments of cytoskeleton

Molecular Alterations

- None

Differential Diagnosis

- Fatty liver with macrovesicular fat:
  - Alcohol
  - Obesity
  - Diabetes mellitus
  - Corticosteroids
  - Malnutrition
  - Chronic hepatitis C
- Fatty liver with microvesicular fat:
  - Fatty liver of pregnancy
  - Reye syndrome
  - Tetracycline and valproate toxicity
  - Alcoholic foamy degeneration
  - Jamaican vomiting sickness
  - Total parenteral nutrition
  - Wolman disease
  - Cholesterol ester storage disease
- Steatohepatitis:
  - Alcohol
  - Obesity
  - Diabetes
  - A complication of intestinal bypass, gastric partitioning, and extensive intestinal resection
- Glycogen vacuolation of hepatocyte nuclei:
  - Diabetes mellitus
  - Normal finding in children
  - Wilson disease

Treatment

- Management of underlying etiology frequently results in resolution unless well-established cirrhosis present

Prognosis

- Largely depends on etiology

Associations

- See above

Hemochromatosis

Clinical Manifestations

- Screening accomplished by determining a serum ferritin, transferrin saturation, serum iron concentration, and total iron-binding capacity
- Biochemical determination of hepatic iron concentration in unfixed tissue standard for quantitating hepatic iron content (normal <1,000 µg/g of dry weight of liver; values >22,000 µg/g of dry weight of liver associated with development of cirrhosis)
- Variants:
    - *Genetic (hereditary) hemochromatosis*
        - Patients with fully developed disease have micronodular cirrhosis (100%), diabetes (75%-80%), and skin pigmentation (75%-80%)
        - Progressive accumulation of iron in liver, heart, pancreas, and other organs
        - A combination of clinical, biochemical, genetic, and historical information necessary to make an accurate diagnosis
    - *Neonatal hemochromatosis*
        - Characterized by enhanced intestinal iron absorption leading to parenchymal cell iron overload
        - Patients present early in life with signs of hepatic fibrosis and cirrhosis
    - *Secondary hemochromatosis*
        - Generally seen in patients with thalassemia and other hematologic disorders
        - Source of excess iron usually easily identified
        - Anemia associated with ineffective erythropoiesis
        - Alcoholic cirrhosis, chronic hepatitis, status post portacaval shunt, and porphyria
        - Increased oral intake and parenteral iron overload (eg, iron pots to ferment alcoholic beverages in South Africa "bantu siderosis")
        - Congenital transferrinemia

Gross Pathology

- Depending on stage of disease, liver may be normal, fibrotic, or frankly cirrhotic
- Early stage of genetic hemochromatosis characterized by portal tracts expanded by fibrous tissue but with overall preservation of acinar architecture and vascular relationships

Microscopic Pathology

- *Genetic hemochromatosis*
    - First abnormality the appearance of stainable iron in periportal hepatocytes
    - As iron stores increase, portal tracts become fibrotic and slender fibrous septa develop
    - Expanded portal tracts contain iron-laden macrophages and proliferating bile ductules, but little portal inflammation
    - Hepatocyte damage minimal even with extensive parenchymal siderosis
    - In very advanced disease, iron overload results in foci of sideronecrosis consisting of eosinophilic necrotic hepatocytes in close association with clusters of macrophages
    - As hemosiderosis advances, a sequential gradient of iron staining extends from zone 1 to zone 2 to zone 3
    - Within individual hepatocytes iron tends to be deposited in pericanalicular granules that outline the bile canalicular system
    - Cirrhosis gradually develops
- *Neonatal hemochromatosis*
    - Characterized by extensive hepatocellular necrosis, giant cell formation, siderosis, fibrosis, and nodule formation in both fetal life and early perinatal period

- *Secondary hemochromatosis*
  - Iron present in both hepatocytes and macrophages
  - Often a lymphocyte infiltration of portal tracts, septa, and sinusoids which is more pronounced than in genetic hemochromatosis
  - Focal hepatocellular damage may be present and probably represents transfusion related hepatitis (hepatitic C)

Special Stains

- Iron stains readily demonstrate the presence of iron in both hepatocytes and macrophages
- Trichrome stains highlight the periportal and septate fibrosis as it develops during the course of the disease

Immunohistochemistry and Electron Microscopy

- Not helpful

Molecular Alterations

- *Genetic hemochromatosis*
  - Abnormal gene *(HFE)* located on the short arm of chromosome 6 in proximity to the polymorphic major histocompatibility (MHC) class 1 (most common mutation is cysteine-to-tyrosine substitution at amino acid position 282)
  - A heterozygote frequency of 1 in 10; a homozygote frequency of 2 to 3 in 1,000
- *Neonatal hemochromatosis*
  - An autosomal recessive disorder
- *Secondary hemochromatosis*
  - No molecular alterations

Differential Diagnosis

- Cirrhosis secondary to excess iron (iron in both fibrous bands and bile ducts) versus iron accumulation as a secondary event during the development of cirrhosis for some other reason (iron in regenerative nodules and not in fibrous bands)

Treatment

- Periodic (weekly or twice-weekly) phlebotomies
- Liver transplantation

Prognosis

- Development of cirrhosis is associated with a decreased life expectancy and an increased risk for the development of hepatocellular carcinoma
- Proper treatment prior to the development of fibrosis will prevent the development of cirrhosis and markedly reduce the risk of hepatocellular carcinoma
- Most manifestations of disease will improve or disappear with treatment with the exception of diabetes, testicular atrophy, and articular chondrocalcinosis
- Iron-chelating agents can be used in patients with hemochromatosis secondary to chronic anemia (when phlebotomy not feasible)

Associations

- Increased risk for the development of hepatitis B and hepatitis C
- Increased incidence of hepatocellular carcinoma (risk 20%-25% in untreated patients)

Neonatal Hepatitis

Clinical Manifestations

- A general term that designates hepatocellular cholestasis occurring during infancy
- Represents a large and varied group of nonobstructive disorders that have some common clinical and histologic features
- Condition best considered as a characteristic but nonspecific reaction of the newborn liver to various different insults
- Accounts for more than 35% of all cases of neonatal cholestasis
- Etiology usually unknown, but established causes include:
  - Infectious agents, eg, CMV, rubella, herpes simplex, *Toxoplasma gondii,* varicella, coxsackievirus, echo virus, human immunodeficiency virus, *Treponema pallidum* (particularly gram negative)
  - Metabolic disorders
  - A1-AT deficiency
  - Niemann-Pick type C disease

- Neonatal hypopituitarism
- Inborn errors of bile acid synthesis
- Depletion of mitochondrial DNA

- Typically seen in premature males with low birth weights
- Approximately 15% occur in patients with affected siblings
- Patients typically present with jaundice that begins several weeks after birth, hepatomegaly, and splenomegaly
- Conjugated hyperbilirubinemia, serum transaminase and alkaline phosphatase levels elevated

Gross Pathology

- Liver may appear normal or show evidence of irregular collapse and fibrosis

Microscopic Pathology

- Low-power examination reveals the presence of lobular disarray with giant multinucleated hepatocytes (the latter represent the most conspicuous microscopic feature of the disease)
- Overall lobular architecture is intact despite disordered and disorganized liver cell plates
- Hepatocytes often enlarged and swollen
- Multinucleated hepatocytes contain 3 or 4 and occasionally as many as 10 nuclei; cytoplasm tends to be granular and contain a brown pigment that may be bilirubin, hemosiderin, or lipofuscin; tend to be located near the center of the lobule
- Nuclei of giant hepatocytes may either cluster in the center of the cell or be dispersed at the periphery of the cell
- Focal areas of necrosis and acidophilic bodies are seen scattered throughout the lobule
- Hepatocyte injury may lead to irregular collapse with subsequent focal intralobular fibrosis
- Canalicular cholestasis is usually prominent and may be associated with the formation of cholestatic liver cell rosettes
- Lobular inflammation may be present but is usually not particularly prominent; neutrophils may accumulate around necrotic giant liver cells
- A mild inflammatory infiltrate is seen in the portal tracts, and occasionally ductular proliferation is present (never to the degree seen in biliary atresia)
- Foci of extramedullary hematopoiesis and iron deposition often present
- In the healing phases of the disease with the resolution of cholestasis, giant hepatocytes disappear
- Progressive disease is associated with portal fibrosis, changes of chronic cholestasis and the eventual development of cirrhosis
- CMV infection characterized by nuclear and cytoplasmic viral inclusions primarily in biliary epithelial cells
- Herpes simplex infection characterized by irregular zones of coagulative-type necrosis with viral inclusions in viable hepatocytes at the margins of the areas of necrosis
- A1-AT deficiency characterized by PAS-positive globules in periportal hepatocytes
- Metabolic conditions (eg, galactosemia and tyrosinemia) characterized by fatty change and prominent cholestatic rosettes

Special Stains

- Iron deposition within hepatocytes can be confirmed with iron stains
- PAS may highlight the presence of A1-AT globules in appropriate cases

Immunohistochemistry

- CMV and herpes simplex virus may be detected

Electron Microscopy

- Not helpful

Molecular Alterations

- Some etiologies such as A1-AT have specific molecular alterations

Differential Diagnosis

- Biliary atresia (typically associated with less hepatocyte damage, giant cell formation, and inflammation and more prominent ductular proliferation and portal fibrosis than neonatal hepatitis)

- Paucity of interlobular bile ducts (characterized by reduction in the number of small intrahepatic bile ducts); *Alagille syndrome* (loss of small intrahepatic bile ducts associated with abnormal facies, vertebral anomalies, and various other abnormalities) is most common cause

Treatment

- Patients should be tested for A1-AT levels, to include phenotyping
- TORCH (toxoplasmosis, rubella, CMV, and herpes simplex virus) titers should be obtained
- Supportive medical management and nutritional support

Prognosis

- Recovery is typical in sporadic cases; jaundice resolves over a period of weeks to months
- 5% to 25% of patients may die from liver failure or sepsis sometime during the 1st year
- 5% to 10% develop chronic liver disease to include cirrhosis
- Familial cases have a worse prognosis with recovery in 25% and death within the 1st year in 60%
- Factors associated with a poor prognosis include family history, marked or prolonged jaundice, and peak serum bilirubin level in excess of 15 mg/dL

Associations

- See etiologic conditions in clinical manifestations

Primary Biliary Cirrhosis

Clinical Manifestations

- Probably an autoimmune disease of uncertain etiology characterized by lymphocyte-mediated injury or destruction of biliary epithelium
- Typically presents in middle life; occasionally seen in young adults and the elderly
- Women much more frequently affected than men (10:1)
- Typically an insidious onset (50%-60% asymptomatic at diagnosis); puritis most common presenting symptom
- Jaundice tends to be a late manifestation of disease
- Laboratory studies typically reveal presence of an elevated alkaline phosphatase and presence of antimitochondrial antibodies; most significant antibody is antibody against the M2 antigen, part of the pyruvate dehydrogenase complex of mitochondria (present in 90%)
- Other antimitochondrial antibodies associated with primary biliary cirrhosis include anti-M4, anti-M8, and anti-M9
- 6% of patients will be antimitochondrial antibody negative, but 95% of these will be ANA or antismooth muscule antibody positive

Gross Pathology

- Hepatic appearance ranges from essentially normal to obvious cirrhosis

Microscopic Pathology

- 4 histologic stages of disease
  - *Florid duct lesion (chronic nonsuppurative destructive cholangitis)*: Septal and interlobular bile ducts mainly affected; epithelium of affected ducts becomes irregular and hyperplastic (crowded and stratified nuclei) and is infiltrated with lymphocytes; basement membrane disrupted; inflammatory infiltrates seen around or to one side of duct and may consist of lymphocytes (which may form germinal centers) as well as a mixture of plasma cells, eosinophils, and neutrophils; epithelioid cell granulomas may be present; typically an absence of ducts in a significant number of portal tracts; sites of former ducts marked by small aggregates of lymphocytes and/or remnants of PAS-positive material; slight disruption of limiting plate; canalicular cholestasis not a feature of early stage primary biliary cirrhosis
  - *Ductular proliferation and periportal hepatitis*: Bile duct damage is less dramatic and there is ductular proliferation accompanied by fibrosis at the periphery of portal triads; the necroinflammatory process extends from the portal tracts into adjacent parenchyma resulting in a periportal interface necrosis that may resemble the lesion of chronic hepatitis; at this stage the changes of chronic cholestasis, with swollen rarefied periportal hepatocytes and the accumulation of copper, begin to appear

- *Scarring; bridging and septal fibrosis*: Combination of cholestatic and hepatitic processes with a progressive decrease in bile duct numbers and increased portal-septal fibrosis; lymphocytes form bridgelike extensions into acini and may indicate the subsequent development of fibrous septa; centrally there is chronic inflammation and fibrosis with clear margins ("halo" effect)
- *Cirrhosis*: Septa extend from portal tracts to portal tracts and to terminal hepatic veins (fully developed cirrhosis); a typical biliary pattern, in which nodules have irregularly shaped "jigsaw puzzle" shapes

- Occasionally portal tracts may simply have a relatively mild "nonspecific" portal inflammation and actual bile duct lesions or granulomas may not be readily apparent
- Loss of bile ducts leads to a chronic form of cholestasis characterized by swollen hepatocytes, intracellular or canalicular bile staining, Mallory hyaline formation (tends to be periportal and lack the associated neutrophilic infiltrate more typical of alcoholic hepatitis), and an accumulation of copper; bile plugs, and lipid-laden macrophages may be seen in either a diffuse or localized (xanthoma) distribution

Special Stains

- Special stains for copper (rhodamine) may confirm its accumulation in hepatocytes (characteristic of chronic cholestatic conditions)
- PAS will highlight the disrupted and fragmented basement membrane surrounding injured/destroyed ducts

Immunohistochemistry

- Cytokeratin 7 will identify bile duct epithelium in the presence of extensive injury

Electron Microscopy

- Activated lymphocytes with pseudopods closely apposed to damaged biliary epithelial cells

Molecular Alterations

- None, but 1% to 6% have an affected family member

Differential Diagnosis

- Primary sclerosing cholangitis (may be impossible to differentiate from PBC on histology alone)
- Chronic hepatitis C (this distinction may be difficult in that piecemeal necrosis and bile duct injury are features of both, especially hepatitis C and stage 1 and 2 of PBC)
- Idiopathic ductopenia
- GVHD
- Sarcoidosis
- Drug injury

Treatment

- Some symptomatic relief with ursodeoxycholic acid (especially in early disease)
- Liver transplantation only effective therapy for advanced disease

Prognosis

- Cirrhosis and end-stage liver disease will inevitably develop without transplantation
- Survival ranges from 6 to 12 years (median 5-year survival rate 65%)
- Hepatocellular carcinoma may occur as a terminal complication (usually develops several years after the onset of cirrhosis)

Associations

- Sjögren syndrome or the "sicca complex" (dry eyes and mouth)
- CREST syndrome: Calcinosis cutis, Raynaud phenomenon, Esophageal dysfunction, Sclerodactyly, and Telangiectasia)
- As seen in other cholestatic syndromes, patients may develop progressive bone loss (osteoporosis)
- Autoimmune thyroiditis
- Rheumatoid arthritis
- Renal tubular acidosis
- Celiac disease
- HLA-DR8
- PBC-AIH overlap syndrome: Approximately 20% of patients with PBC lack antimitochondrial antibodies or have features of both conditions in various combinations

Primary Sclerosing Cholangitis

Clinical Manifestations

- Affects men more frequently than women
- Usually diagnosed between ages of 25 and 45 years
- Patients typically present with jaundice, vague right upper quadrant discomfort, pruritus, weight loss, generalized malaise, and occasionally fever
- Late in the course of the disease, signs of portal hypertension and liver failure may appear
- 10% to 30% asymptomatic
- Most common abnormality of liver function test is elevation of the alkaline phosphatase level
- No specific abnormality of immunoglobulins or autoantibodies; hypergammaglobulinemia in 30%; 80% have serum antineutrophil antibodies, but so do most patients with PBC

Gross Pathology

- A spectrum of changes from near normal to frank cirrhosis depending on duration of disease
- A diffuse thickening of bile duct walls with strictures and saccular dilations as a result of dense fibrosis that may affect any part of the biliary tree to include the gallbladder; both extrahepatic and large intrahepatic ducts involved in 85%; involvement often centered at bifurcation of hepatic ducts

Microscopic Pathology

- Histologic findings may be very heterogenous and not always diagnostic
- Ductal epithelium typically intact with diffuse thickening of the bile duct wall as a result of dense fibrosis associated with a mild mixed inflammatory infiltrate (sometimes containing eosinophils, especially early in course of disease)
- Portal granulomas distinctly unusual
- Fibrous obliteration of ducts with replacement of duct segments by solid cords of connective tissue
- Biopsy specimen taken proximal to a stricture reveals changes of bile duct obstruction or cholangitis
- Biopsy specimen from site of stricture reveals periductal edema, concentric fibrosis, ductal proliferation, portal inflammation, and atrophy with ductopenia
- Loss of bile ducts the most common finding in small portal tracts (60%); periductal fibrosis is the most common finding in medium-sized portal tracts (fibrosis has a lamellar pattern reminiscent of an "onion-skin")
- Portal tracts usually contain a mixture of inflammatory cells (lymphocytes, plasma cells, and occasional neutrophils and eosinophils)
- Liver lobules usually not affected until late in disease when changes of chronic cholestasis become common

Special Stains

- PAS with diastase highlights presence of regular or irregular thickening of basement membrane material around both scarred and unscarred ducts
- Copper stains usually positive

Immunohistochemistry

- Ductal epithelium can be identified with cytokeratins AE1, 7, and 19

Electron Microscopy

- Not helpful

Molecular Alterations

- None

Differential Diagnosis

- Primary biliary cirrhosis (PSC tends to have less of an inflammatory infiltrate and be less fibrotic than PBC and florid duct lesions are not seen)
- Chronic active hepatitis
- Intrahepatic artery chemotherapy (floxuridine)
- Chronic large duct obstruction
- Langerhans cell histiocytosis
- Infectious cholangiopathy (CMV and cryptosporidium) in patients with AIDS

Treatment

- Liver transplantation for end-stage liver disease

Prognosis

- Cirrhosis and end-stage liver disease inevitably develop without transplantation
- Median survival 10 to 12 years; 65% to 85% survive 5 years
- Increased risk for development of cholangiocarcinoma and adenocarcinoma of the gallbladder in approximtely 15%

Associations

- HLA-DRw52a antigen
- Riedel thyroiditis
- Retroperitoneal or mediastinal fibrosis
- Orbital pseudotumor
- Crohn disease (10%)
- Ulcerative colitis (70%-75% of patients with PSC have VC; 2%-7% of patients with ulcerative colitis have PSC)
- HLA-B8, -DR3, and -DR2
- Cholangiocarcinoma (may arise from dysplastic ductal epithelium) and gallbladder carcinoma

Veno-Occlusive Disease

Clinical Manifestations

- Clinical presentation may be acute with a sudden onset of jaundice, hepatomegaly, abdominal pain, ascites, and rarely hepatic failure (associated with bone marrow transplant or hepatic irradiation)
- Occasionally clinical manifestations present more gradually with jaundice, hepatomegaly, and evidence of portal hypertension (gradual onset of symptoms more typical in renal transplant recipients)
- Serum levels of aminotransferases, bilirubin, and a lkaline phosphatase all mildly to moderately elevated

Gross Pathology

- Liver typically appears normal

Microscopic Pathology

- Initial event appears to involve damage to endothelium of the central vein, or centrilobular sinusoids; this damage leads to localized activation of coagulation cascade with intramural and adventitial deposition of fibrin followed by a fibrotic response that leads to fibrous occlusion of the vascular lumen with a resulting increase in sinusoidal pressure
- Most prominent pathologic findings found in the central and sublobular veins is an edematous proliferation of loose connective tissue that thickens the subintimal zone and produces a concentric or eccentric luminal narrowing
- Vascular thrombosis and infiltration of inflammatory cells in the fibrous proliferation are not features of early disease, although occasional red blood cells may be trapped within fibrous tissue
- As the disease progresses, the subintimal fibrosis becomes more densely fibrotic and begins to grow into small vascular channels; perivenular fibrosis, pericellular fibrosis, and central to central fibrous bridges develop with the eventual appearance of cirrhosis
- In the last stages of disease the affected veins disappear into the centrilobular fibrous scar and cannot be readily discerned on routine H&E
- Other changes in hepatic lobule may accompany the vascular changes to include hepatocyte hypertrophy (characterized by thickened hepatic plates primarily in the periportal region) and changes similar to those of nodular regenerative hyperplasia (characterized by the development of ill-defined regenerative nodules)

Special Stains

- Trichrome will highlight subintimal proliferation of fibrous tissue in early stages of disease and will help identify affected veins that become incorporated into centrilobular fibrous scarring in the later phases of disease

Immunohistochemistry and Electron Microscopy

- Not helpful

Molecular Alterations

- None

Differential Diagnosis

- Early disease may be difficult to distinguish from sinusoidal congestion of any cause
- Later-stage disease can be seen as a consequence of any chronic outflow obstruction
- Fibrous obliteration of central veins is commonly seen in alcoholic hepatitis and in cirrhosis of several different causes

Treatment

- Removal of the offending agent before disease develops

Prognosis

- 50% of patients with pyrrolizidine alkaloid-associated disease undergo complete resolution, 20% die, and 30% develop chronic disease
- Disease complicating bone marrow and renal transplantation has a morality rate of up to 50%
- Supportive therapy consists of antithrombotic therapy, portacaval shunt, and liver transplantation

Associations

- Pyrrolizidine alkaloid ingestion (toxins found in many plants, folk remedies, and dietary supplements made from alkaloid-containing plants)
- Cytotoxic chemotherapeutic agents (azathioprine, 6-mercaptopurine, cyclophosphamide, mitomycin C, busulfan, carmustine, doxorubicin, and intra-arterial floxuridine)
- Bone marrow transplant recipients may develop veno-occlusive disease as a result of alkylating agents administered during conditioning
- Azathioprine used in renal transplantation
- Hepatic irradiation
- Hypervitaminosis A, arsenic poisoning, and thorotrast exposure

Viral Hepatitis

Clinical Manifestations

- *Hepatitis A*
    - RNA virus (hepatovirus genus of picornavirus family)
    - Incubation period approximately 4 weeks.
    - Early antibody response: IgM-anti-hepatitis A virus (HAV) (appears within several months; rarely as long as 6-12 months)
    - Diagnosis of acute hepatitis A infection made on the basis of a high titer of anti-HAV of IgM class, diagnosis of *history* of hepatitis A infection based on high titers of anti-HAV of IgG class
    - During convalescence: the predominant antibody is IgG-anti-hepatitic A virus (HAV) (persists indefinitely and provides immunity to reinfection)
    - HAV does not cause chronic hepatitis or a carrier state
- *Hepatitis B*
    - DNA virus (hepadnavirus)
    - Three antigens:
        - Protein on surface of virion; hepatitis B surface antigen (HBsAg)
        - Protein on surface of nucleocapsid core: Hepatitis core antigen (HBcAg)
        - A second nucleocapsid protein: Hepatitis Be antigen (HBeAg)
    - HBsAg appears first (before the onset of symptoms) and increases from one to two months and then becomes undetectable
    - Anti-HBs becomes detectable after HBsAg disappears and remains indefinitely but is not detectable for weeks to months after HBsAg disappears; this interval referred to as "window period" during which anti-HBc and anti-HBe are only markers of disease; if anti-HBs is never produced then HBsAg may not be cleared; if HBsAg is not cleared but HBeAg is cleared then the patient becomes an asymptomatic carrier; if HBsAg is not cleared but HBeAg persists then patient becomes a chronic carrier who has progressed to chronic active hepatitis (anti-HBc is present in both these conditions)
    - HBcAg is not detectable after HBV infection (it is sequestered within the viron)
    - Anti-HBc is detectable within 1 to 2 weeks of the appearance of HBsAg and precedes the appearance of anti-HBs by weeks to months; anti-HBc of the IgM class predominates for the first 6 months after acute infection; anti-HBc of the IgG class predominates after 6 months
    - HBeAg appears concurrently with HBsAg; in self-limited HBV infections HBeAg disappears before the disappearance of HBsAg
    - Anti-HBe becomes detectable only after HBeAg disappears

- *Hepatitis C*
  - RNA virus
  - Hepatitis C RNA virus can be detected within days of exposure to HCV by molecular amplification by polymerase chain reaction
  - No immunity after HCV infection
  - Diagnosis of hepatitis C based on presence of anti-HCV in serum
  - A proportion of patients with hepatitis C have anti-HBc of the IgG class in their blood (hepatitis B and hepatitis C are transmitted by comparable routes)
- *Hepatitis D*
  - A defective RNA virus that coinfects with and requires the helper function of HBV
  - Hepatitis D virus can infect simultaneously with HBV or superinfect after the person is already infected with HBV
  - Duration of hepatitis D virus infection determined by the duration of the HBV infection
  - Hepatitis D virus infection cannot outlast HBV infection
  - Diagnosis of acute hepatitis D infection based on presence of anti-HDV and HBcAg (IgM anti-HBc in coinfection)
- *Hepatitis E*
  - Single-stranded RNA virus (calicivirus)
  - Waterborne (India, Asia, Africa, and Central America)
  - Both IgM anti-HEV and IgG anti-HEV can be detected after acute infection, but both fall rapidly to very low levels within 9-12 months

Gross Pathology

- Normal to cirrhotic

Microscopic Pathology

- *Acute Viral Hepatitis*
  - Acute disease characterized by hepatocellular necrosis, portal and lobular lymphocytic infiltrates, and regenerative activity
  - Hepatocyte damage can be seen as ballooned cells that appear swollen and have granular, pale-staining cytoplasm or as acidophilic degeneration characterized by densely eosinophilic pleomorphic cells with concave borders (acidophil or Councilman bodies)
  - Inflammatory infiltrate predominantly composed of small lymphocytes often with some intermixed eosinophils, neutrophils, plasma cells, and macrophages; infiltrate most prominent in portal tracts and may spill over into periportal parenchyma; in the lobule small inflammatory infiltrates are typically found in areas of hepatocellular necrosis
  - Syncytial giant hepatocytes may be present
  - The combination of hepatocyte swelling, hepatocyte shrinkage, apoptosis, and cell drop out together with regenerative hyperplasia results in a disarray of hepatic cell plates that is a helpful diagnostic feature
  - Majority of hepatocyte injury present in zone 3 near the terminal hepatic venules
  - Some degree of cholestasis typically present and results from damage to bile secretory and contractile functions of hepatocytes
  - Occasionally in acute hepatitis, necrosis of hepatocytes is so extensive that necrotic bridges link portal tracts to terminal hepatic venules ("bridging hepatic necrosis"); indication of severe hepatitis associated with early death or the development of chronic liver disease
  - Occasionally patients with acute hepatitis will develop confluent necrosis which extends throughout an entire acinus (panacinar necrosis); a pattern typical of clinically fulminant, coma-producing hepatitis; these areas of necrosis are characterized by collapsed stroma, inflammatory cells, and macrophages
  - Occasionally hepatocyte necrosis may be in a periportal distribution accompanied by a substantial portal inflammatory infiltrate (may coexist with other patterns of necrosis); the periportal lesion closely resembles the piecemeal necrosis of chronic hepatitis
  - *Acute hepatitis A*
    - Histologic picture of perivenular cholestasis with little liver cell damage or inflammation (easily mistaken for other causes of cholestasis)

- Hepatitis with periportal necrosis and dense portal infiltrate which includes abundant, often aggregated plasma cells
- Extensive microvesicular fatty change may be present
- Fibrin-ring granulomas may be present

□ *Acute hepatitis B*

- Lymphocytes and macrophages sometimes lie in close contact with hepatocytes (peripolesis) or invaginate into them (emperipolesis)
- Liver cells and their nuclei may have a moderate degree of pleomorphism
- Hepatitis B core and surface antigens are rarely identifiable early in an acute attack but recurrence of HBV infection after transplantation will reveal the presence of antigens in large amounts
- Prominent ballooning degeneration in zone 3 (more characteristic of acute hepatitis B then hepatitis C or A)

□ *Acute hepatitis C*

- A prominent lymphocyte infiltration of portal tracts and sinusoids in the absence of severe liver cell damage (the histologic picture reminiscent of infectious mononucleosis)
- Lymphoid follicles and bile duct damage often present within weeks of the onset of symptoms
- Features of cholestasis and fatty change are usually seen
- Fulminant hepatitis with multiacinar necrosis is rarely seen

□ *Acute hepatitis D*

- Coinfection or superinfection with hepatitis D virus alters the course of hepatitis B, encouraging chronicity and enhancing severity
- Histologic changes include microvesicular fatty change, few lymphocytes and abundant macrophages in parenchyma and marked portal inflammation
- Hepatitis D antigen can be seen as finely granular eosinophilic inclusions in hepatocyte nuclei

□ *Acute hepatitis E*

- Histologic changes similar to hepatitis A with prominent cholestasis and predominantly a portal and periportal inflammatory infiltrate

■ *Chronic Viral Hepatitis*

□ Portal changes of chronic hepatitis

- Majority of portal tracts infiltrated by inflammatory cells
- Portal tracts may contain short fibrous scars that extend variable distances
- Inflammatory infiltrate consists primarily of lymphocytes, which may aggregate into follicles with or without germinal centers (especially in chronic hepatitis C); may be completely confined to the portal tract leaving an intact limiting plate of hepatocytes or the portal tracts may be enlarged by the inflammatory process with extension of inflammatory cells into the acini with concomitant hepatic necrosis
- Plasma cells may be present
- Interlobular bile ducts may show focal abnormalities such as swelling of part of the wall, vacuolation of epithelial cells, and infiltration by lymphocytes (as seen in acute hepatitis)

□ Parenchymal changes of chronic hepatitis

- Necrosis of hepatocytes results from extension of inflammatory infiltrate from the portal tract into the lobule (piecemeal necrosis), the defining lesion of chronic active hepatitis
- Deep in the acini there may be focal areas of necrosis with or without bridging
- Bridging necrosis usually accompanied by piecemeal necrosis
- Fatty changes typically mild
- Cholestasis very uncommon
- Severe intra-acinar necrosis often accompanied by formation of small hepatitic rosettes in the inflammatory tissue (probably represent a form of regeneration)
- Multinucleated giant hepatocytes reminiscent of neonatal hepatitis may be seen

□ Continued interface hepatitis and necrosis result in the deposition of fibrous tissue; portal tracts first to exhibit increased fibrosis; with time, periportal fibrosis develops which is followed by linking of fibrous septa between lobules (bridging fibrosis); continued loss of hepatocytes and fibrosis eventually results in cirrhosis

- Chronic hepatitis B and D
  - Hepatitis B surface antigen can be seen in hepatocytes as eosinophilic ground-glass areas bordered by a characteristic pale-staining halo
  - Hepatocyte nuclei containing hepatitis B core antigen particles have a pale, eosinophilic appearance ("sanded")
  - Hepatocytes often have marked pleomorphism
  - Typically there is close contact between hepatocytes and lymphocytes
  - Lymphoid follicles occasionally present in portal tracts (less common and less prominent than in hepatitis C)
- Chronic hepatitis C
  - An early prominent periportal inflammation followed by the presence of acinar lesions, which consist predominantly of lymphocytes, which may form aggregates or follicles, some of which have prominent germinal centers
  - Changes within the acini include acidophilic degeneration of hepatocytes and the formation of acidophil bodies
  - Macrovesicular fatty change is more common than in the other forms of chronic hepatitis
  - Sinusoids may be focally or diffusely infiltrated by lymphocytes
  - Scattered hepatocytes may be abnormally acidophilic and have scalloped outlines

Special Stains

- Reticulin stains confirm areas of hepatocyte collapse as well as outline lymphoid follicles
- Trichrome stains confirm presence of fibrosis
- PAS with diastase demonstrate enlarged aggregated Kupffer cells that tend to accumulate in zone 3 in acute hepatitis
- Elastic stains reveal presence of elastic fibers in recently formed bridges

Immunohistochemistry

- Not particularly useful in diagnosis of acute viral hepatitis, with exception of hepatitis D
- HCV antigens can be detected by immunohistochemistry (not a practical routine procedure)
- Both hepatitis B core and surface antigens are readily demonstrable with immunostains in chronic disease (rarely seen during an acute attack)

Electron Microscopy

- Ground-glass hepatocytes of hepatitis B result from a cytoplasm rich in endoplasmic reticulum and HBV surface material

Molecular Alterations

- None

Differential Diagnosis

- Inflammation confined to portal tracts:
  - Resolving acute hepatitis
  - Nonspecific inflammation near a focal lesion
  - Primary biliary cirrhosis
  - Lymphoma
- Acute hepatitis must be differentiated from chronic hepatitis
  - Elastic bridges characteristic of acute disease; fibrous septa characteristic of chronic disease
  - Cholestasis more common in acute disease; not found in chronic hepatitis
- Primary biliary cirrhosis
- Primary sclerosing cholangitis
- A1-AT deficiency
- Wilson disease
- Lymphoma, especially low grade
- Loss of small and medium-sized bile ducts indicates biliary tract disease rather than chronic hepatitis

Treatment

- Hepatitis C: Combination interferon-α and ribavirin will clear HCV RNA in approximately 50% and result in sustained response in 30% to 70%
- Patients with actively replicating hepatitis B infection and decompensated cirrhosis treated with lamivudine
- End-stage liver disease best treated with orthotopic liver transplant

Prognosis

- Extent of fibrosis most significant prognostic factor
- Possible clinical course following acute viral hepatitis:
  - Complete resolution (normal liver)
  - Death in acute phase
  - Posthepatitic scarring
  - Chronic virus carrier state without significant disease
  - Chronic hepatitis
  - Cirrhosis
  - Hepatocellular carcinoma (develops on the basis of cirrhosis in patients with HBV or HCV; occasionally seen in patients with HBV without cirrhosis)
- Incidence of fulminant hepatitis following acute infection:
  - Hepatitis A: 0.2%
  - Hepatitis B: 0.2% to 1%
  - Hepatitis C: 0.2% to 1%
  - Hepatitis D:
    - Coinfection: 1% to 10%
    - Superinfection: 5% to 20%
  - Hepatitis E: 0.2% to 1%
- Incidence of chronic hepatitis following acute infection:
  - Hepatitis A: No
  - Hepatitis B: 1% to 10%
  - Hepatitis C: 50% to 70%
  - Hepatitis D:
    - Coinfection: 2% to 5%
    - Superinfection: 40% to 70%
  - Hepatitis E: No
- Development of fulminant hepatitis as a sequela of viral hepatitis associated with a 5% to 20% survival rate

Associations

- Celiac disease may be associated with changes in the liver of chronic hepatitis

Wilson Disease (Hepatolenticular Degeneration)

Clinical Manifestations

- A defect in the ability of the liver to excrete copper into bile; copper accumulates in liver and other organs (brain, cornea, kidneys, striated muscle, bones, and joints)
- Patients typically present during the 2nd to 4th decades of life; younger patients tend to present with evidence of chronic liver disease (eg, chronic active hepatitis and cirrhosis) and/or various neurologic, psychiatric, and hematologic abnormalities
- Occasionally fulminant hepatic failure the first manifestation of disease
- Screening procedures include slit-lamp examination for Kayser-Fleischer rings and serum ceruloplasmin levels
- Serum levels of ceruloplasmin low in 85% to 95% (typically <20 mg/dL)
- Increased urinary copper excretion (typically in excess of 30-50 μg/24 hours)
- When families screened for Wilson disease, hypoceruloplasminemia found in 10%

Gross Pathology

- Findings range from a slightly enlarged liver to frank cirrhosis

Microscopic Pathology

- Earliest hepatic changes tend to be nonspecific and include cellular ballooning, macrovesicular or microvesicular steatosis, glycogenated nuclei, acidophilic bodies, and mild portal lymphocytic inflammation; Kupffer cells may be enlarged and contain hemosiderin
- More severe changes include aggregates of liver cell necrosis, cholestasis, extensive macrovesicular fatty change, and a pattern of chronic active hepatitis
- Advanced disease marked by fibrosis or macronodular cirrhosis often with Mallory hyaline; intracellular accumulation of copper may be visible in periportal hepatocytes
- End-stage disease characterized by confluent hepatocyte necrosis and collapse

Special Stains

- Rhodamine or Timm silver stain will highlight cytoplasmic copper

Immunohistochemistry

- Not helpful

Electron Microscopy

- Microvesicular steatosis, glycogen in nuclei, and copper deposits
- Mitochondria enlarged with increased matrix density and crystalline inclusions; cristae swollen and separated by cyst-like dilatations filled with flocculent material

Molecular Alterations

- Condition transmitted as autosomal recessive trait
- Defective gene located on chromosome 13q-14.3, which encodes a P-type ATPase that transports copper

Differential Diagnosis

- Patients with chronic cholestasis (particularly primary biliary cirrhosis) will have increased hepatic copper concentration and increased urinary copper excretion
- Decreased levels of ceruloplasmin occasionally seen in patients with fulminant hepatic failure of any etiology

Treatment

- Chelating agents (penicillamine trientine and zinc acetate) usually effective in arresting disease and preventing its development in siblings
- Established disease can be treated successfully with liver transplantation

Prognosis

- Untreated disease will eventually progress to fibrosis or cirrhosis, liver failure, and death

Associations

- None

Tumors and Tumorlike Conditions

Angiomyolipoma

Clinical Manifestations

- Benign tumor composed of variable admixtures of adipose, thick-walled vessels, and smooth muscle (spindled or epithelioid)
- Age range 30 to 70 years; mean of 50 years
- Men and women affected equally
- Occasionally associated with tuberous sclerosis

Gross Pathology

- Usually solitary; 60% in right lobe; 30% in left lobe; rarely multiple
- Well-demarcated but not encapsulated
- Cut surface yellow or yellow-tan depending on amount of fat

Microscopic Pathology

- An admixture of adipose tissue, thick-walled, occasionally hyalinized blood vessels, and smooth muscle; variants include lipomatous, myomatous, angiomatous, pelioid, and inflammatory pseudotumorlike types
- Smooth muscle cells may be arranged in a solid or trabecular pattern; cells may be spindled, polygonal, epithelioid in shape, and have clear (empty or glycogen-rich), oncocytic, or rhabdoid cytoplasm; nuclei of spindle cells elongated with blunt ends (cigar-shaped); larger, more epithelioid smooth muscle cells have perinuclear condensation of cytoplasm around large, hyperchromatic nuclei with prominent nucleoli
- Fat cells usually mature; lipoblasts rare
- Vessels tend to be tortuous, and have thick, hyalinized walls; vessels usually surrounded by mantels of smooth muscle cells
- Rich capillary network present throughout the tumor
- Extramedullary hematopoiesis may be present (a minority of cases)

Special Stains

- PAS with diastase may highlight eosinophilic globules

Immunohistochemistry

- Smooth muscle cells stain with antibiodies against desmin and smooth muscle actin
- Smooth muscle cells contain melanin and consequently stain for melanoma markers HMB-45 and Melan-A

Electron Microscopy

- Confirms smooth muscle nature of epithelioid cells with glycogen

Molecular Alterations

- Small number associated with tuberous sclerosis

Differential Diagnosis

- Microscopic appearance may be quite varied (see Microscopic Pathology above) and may mimic several malignant tumors to include leiomyosarcoma, malignant fibrous histiocytoma, and hepatocellular carcinoma

Treatment

- Surgical excision

Prognosis

- Completely benign

Associations

- Immunostaining pattern (HMB-45 and Melan-A) suggests tumor belongs to a group of perivascular epithelioid cell tumors (PEComas): lymphangiomyomatosis, clear cell "sugar" tumor of lung, and pancreatic and cardiac rhabdomyoma

Angiosarcoma

Clinical Manifestations

- Most common primary malignant mesenchymal neoplasm of adult liver
- Represents fewer than 0.5 % of all primary hepatic malignancies
- Typically presents in the 6th to 7th decade of life; male to female ratio 3-4:1
- Rare in children (may occur in association with infantile hemangioendothelioma)
- Most patients present with abdominal pain, fatigue, weight loss, and/or abdominal mass
- Intraabdominal bleeding in 30%, thrombocytopenia in 50%

Gross Pathology

- Typically multicentric in both lobes
- Tumor foci vary in size and have ill-defined borders and a spongy consistency
- On cut surface, an admixture of gray-white solid nodules with large blood-filled spaces
- Uninvolved liver usually normal; if cirrhotic suspect exposure to thorotrast, vinyl chloride, or arsenic

Microscopic Pathology

- Malignant endothelial cells tend to be plump, somewhat spindled, and pleomorphic with hyperchromatic nuclei and variably sized nucleoli
- Cytoplasm tends to be eosinophilic and pale; cell borders poorly defined
- Endothelial cells with more prominent cytoplasm and prominent nucleoli as well as bizarre giant tumor cells and nodules of spindle cells that mimic fibrosarcoma may be seen
- Mitotic activity prominent
- Tumor cells typically grow in 1 or more layers along sinusoids that line thickened hepatic cords
- Hepatocellular rosettes with bile plugs (a feature of cholestatic change) may be evident
- As sinusoids are obliterated by tumor, hepatocytes atrophy and are replaced by fibrous tissue; variably sized cavernous cavities filled with blood and lined by tumor cells usually develop
- Tumor invasion of portal or hepatic veins a frequent finding
- Extramedullary hematopoiesis frequently present
- Tumor cells may demonstrate phagocytic activity

Special Stains

- Tumors arising in childhood may have foci of spindled cells that contain PAS-positive intracytoplasmic globules that simulate the findings in Kaposi sarcoma

Immunohistochemistry

- Tumor cells immunoreactive for endothelial markers CD34, CD31, factor VIII-related antigen, and *Ulex europaeus* lectin
- Malignant endothelial cells occasionally cytokeratin positive

Electron Microscopy

- Tumor cells contain Weibel-Palade bodies

Molecular Alterations

- A p53 mutation (A:T to T:A transversion) present in 50% of vinyl chloride associated cases (not seen in sporadic forms of disease or in disease related to thorotrast exposure)

Differential Diagnosis

- Includes many reactive, inflammatory, congestive, and fibrosing disorders of the liver
- Hepatocellular carcinoma
- Kaposi sarcoma
- Endothelioid hemangioendothelioma
- Metastatic angiosarcoma to liver cannot be distinguished from primary angiosarcoma of liver

Treatment

- No treatments have proven effective; but rare instances of some response to cytotoxic chemotherapy or irradiation

Prognosis

- Most patients dead within 6 months of diagnosis
- At the time of death, approximately 60% have metastatic disease (usually lung, lymph nodes, spleen, and bone marrow)

Associations

- 25% to 45% have an associated etiologic agent or condition:
  - Thorotrast
  - Vinyl chloride monomer
  - Inorganic arsenic
  - Androgenic steroids
  - Copper sulfate
  - Estrogenic steroids
  - Phenelzine
  - Radiotherapy
  - Chemotherapeutic agents
  - Cirrhotic stage of hereditary hemochromatosis

Bile Duct Adenoma (Peribiliary Gland Hamartoma)

Clinical Manifestations

- 85% solitary; 15% multiple
- Typically asymptomatic

Gross Pathology

- Resemble metastatic carcinoma
- A well-circumscribed (not encapsulated) white mass located just beneath the capsule often with a central depression
- Cystic change rare
- 60% <0.5 cm; 40% between 0.5 and 2 cm

Microscopic Pathology

- Composed of a compact proliferation of small, well-formed ducts embedded in a sclerotic or edematous stroma of mature fibrous tissue that may contain chronic inflammatory cells, foci of calcification and granulomas
- Ducts tend to be small, numerous, and without lumina; typically not dilated and do not contain bile
- Cells lining ducts are cuboidal and have more cytoplasm and paler nuclei than cells of normal interlobular ducts
- Cells contain intracytoplasmic mucin but no bile
- No pleomorphism, hyperchromasia, mitoses, or angiolymphatic invasion
- Stroma may contain inflammatory cells, lymphocytes that tend to form small clusters, or follicles

Special Stains

- Mucicarmine or Alcian blue will confirm presence of intracytoplasmic mucin
- Trichrome will demonstrate collagenous nature of stroma

Immunohistochemistry and Electron Microscopy

- Not helpful

Molecular Alterations

- None

Differential Diagnosis

- Bile duct microhamartoma
- Metastatic adenocarcinoma
- Intrahepatic cholangiocarcinoma

Treatment

- None required
- Frequently excised for frozen section because of their gross resemblance to a metastatic carcinoma

Prognosis

- Benign with no evidence to date that malignant transformation ever occurs

Associations

- None

Bile Duct Microhamartoma (von Meyenburg or Moschowitz Complex)

Clinical Manifestations

- Typically asymptomatic
- May arise as a result of focal hepatic ischemia that causes aberrant development or remodeling of embryonic bile ducts
- Typically found incidentally and do not cause symptoms or abnormalities of liver function

Gross Pathology

- Typically visible on the surface of the liver as a well circumscribed 1 to 2 mm white nodule
- Usually multiple (≥4 in 20%)
- Cut section gray to white or green
- Almost always <0.5 cm

Microscopic Pathology

- Rounded, circumscribed nodule of ductlike structures in or adjacent to a portal tract
- Multiple, interconnected, ectatic, branched, or angulated biliary channels lined by a single layer of bland, cuboidal, or flattened epithelium in a densely fibrous tissue stroma
- Lumens of biliary ducts irregularly dilated and sometimes contain eosinophilic material or inspissated bile
- Cellular atypia not a feature
- Stroma lacks significant numbers of inflammatory cells

Special Stains and Immunohistochemistry

- Not helpful

Electron Microscopy

- Confirms the normal cytologic appearance of ductal cells

Molecular Alterations

- None

Differential Diagnosis

- Metastatic adenocarcinoma
- Bile duct adenoma
- Congenital hepatic fibrosis

Treatment

- None required
- Frequently excised at the time of surgery for frozen section diagnosis because of gross resemblance to metastatic carcinoma

Prognosis

- Benign

Associations

- Portal hypertension
- Autosomal dominant polycystic kidney disease
- Caroli disease
- Congenital hepatic fibrosis

Bile Duct Carcinoma—Intrahepatic (Cholangiocarcinoma)

Clinical Manifestations

- Patients present with vague right upper quadrant pain with or without hepatomegaly and jaundice

Gross Pathology

- Usually a multicentric neoplasm with a gross appearance reminiscent of metastatic disease
- May appear as a massive, solitary mass, a multinodular mass, or diffuse (many nodules all <1 cm in diameter throughout the liver)
- Lesions tend to be gray-white and firm and have infiltrative margins; may have a cystic component
- Intraductal lesions are variably sized, multifocal, pink to white, papillary excrescences within a dilated duct
- Usually a noncirrhotic liver

Microscopic Pathology

- A mucin-secreting adenocarcinoma with a fibrous stroma
- Heterogeneity of neoplastic epithelial cells can be seen in the same gland; may be cuboidal or columnar and have a papillary pattern
- Tumor cells have basophilic or clear cytoplasm, uniform round nuclei, and inconspicuous nucleoli; intracytoplasmic mucin always present
- No bile production
- Tumor cells may have adenosquamous, squamous, mucinous, and anaplastic morphology
- Tumor tends to infiltrate between hepatocyte plates and duct walls
- Stroma usually arranged circumferentially around neoplastic glands
- Mucin production may be abundant and is often accompanied by the formation of signet ring cells
- Intraneural and perineural invasion common (80%)

Special Stains

- Mucicarmine and Alcian blue will highlight the presence of mucin

Immunohistochemistry

- Tumor cells reactive for cytokeratins 7 and 19 and epithelial membrane antigen (EMA)
- Tumor cells have cytoplasmic and luminal positivity for polyclonal antibody to CEA (CEA positivity is not canalicular which is characteristic of hepatocellular carcinoma)
- 10% to 20% express p53

Electron Microscopy

- Not helpful

Molecular Alterations

- A high incidence of *ras* gene mutations

Differential Diagnosis

- Metastatic adenocarcinoma (cholangiocarcinoma more likely to have free stromal mucin, small groups or single cells in a fibrous stroma, and an admixture of normal ductal structures and malignant cells in a ductlike structure)
- Hepatocellular carcinoma (acinar type)
- Epithelioid hemangioendothelioma
- Bile duct adenoma
- If cystic component present: cystadenocarcinoma

Treatment

- Surgical resection or transplantation

Prognosis

- Mean survival <2 years

Associations

- Predisposing factors include:
  - Dilated intrahepatic ducts (Caroli disease and choledochal cysts)
  - Congenital hepatic fibrosis
  - Parasitic infestation with liver flukes (*Clonorchis sinensis* or *Opisthorchis viverrini*)
  - Exposure to thorotrast and anabolic steroids
  - Hepatolithiasis (Japan)
  - Ulcerative colitis with primary sclerosing cholangitis
  - Hereditary hemochromatosis
- May arise in bile duct microhamartomas
- No direct relationship with cirrhosis

Echinococcal Cyst (Hydatid Cyst)

Clinical Manifestations

- Rare in the United States; fairly frequent in Sicily, Turkey, South America, Iceland, Australia, and New Zealand
- Caused by larval or cystic stage (metacestode) of the dog tapeworm (definitive hosts include dogs, wolves, cats, and other carnivores)
- 4 species have been identified:
  - *Echinococcus granulosus* (by far the commonest)
  - *Echinococcus multilocularis*
  - *Echinococcus obligartharus*
  - *Echinococcus padagonicus*
- Most common sites of involvement are the liver (67%), brain, and lung; also reported to involve the spleen, soft tissue, bone, breast, heart, and spinal extradural space
- Diagnosis made by hydatid serology; reliable antibody detection tests exist for *E multilocularis* and *E granulosus*
- Asymptomatic until they reach 10 cm in diameter
- When the cyst is viable, skin and complement fixation tests are usually positive and blood eosinophilia is frequently present; once the parasite dies with collapse of the cyst wall and subsequent calcification, skin test is of little value and eosinophilia disappears

Gross Pathology

- Cysts of *E granulosis* (cystic hydatid disease)
- Cysts tend to be filled with clear fluid, solitary, unilocular, and white
- Majority involve the right lobe of liver
- May be subcapsular and pedunculated
- Cysts can rupture into the abdomen or into the gallbladder or through the diaphragm into the pleural space
- Viable cysts are filled with a colorless fluid that contains daughter cysts and brood capsules with scolices
- Occasionally daughter cysts are present outside the fibrous laminar layer of the cyst, referred to as extracapsular or satellite cysts
- Cysts of *E multilocularis* (alveolar hydatid disease) simulate malignant neoplasm or cirrhosis
- Numerous small, irregular cysts, all <2 cm in diameter
- Border with uninvolved liver appears infiltrative

Microscopic Pathology

- Cysts of *E granulosis*
  - Wall has 3 layers:
    - Germinal layer (innermost) contains nuclei and gives rise to brood capsules; the future heads of the adult tapeworm (protoscolices) develop within brood capsules; a protosolex consists of a double row of refractile, birefringent, acid-fast hooklets and 4 round suckers; daughter cysts are detached brood capsules; calcification in the germinal layer indicates that the cyst is dead
    - Laminated membrane (middle layer) is avascular, eosinophilic, refractile, and chitinous and does not contain nuclei
    - Advential layer (outer; pericyst) consists of dense fibrovascular tissue with variable numbers of inflammatory cells
  - Adjacent liver parenchyma often shows changes of pressure atrophy with a moderate portal infiltrate with increased numbers of eosinophils
- Cysts of *E multilocularis*
  - A thin, laminated wall
  - Germinal layer absent or very attenuated; forms small vesicles that invade adjacent structures, result in an infiltrative multilocular fibrotic mass that has the capability of metastasizing
  - Inner portion may be necrotic
  - Calcification in 70%
  - Brood capsules and protoscolices seen in <10%

Special Stains

- Laminated (middle) chitinous layer stains strongly with PAS, Gomori methenamine silver, and Best carmine

Immunohistochemistry and Electron Microscopy

- Not helpful

Molecular Alterations

- None

Differential Diagnosis

- Nonparasitic cysts

Treatment

- Percutaneous or open aspiration of cyst with injection of hypertonic 20% saline (scolices and cysts should be destroyed within 10 minutes) followed by repeat aspiration
- Plane of dissection used to excise a cyst is the laminated, chitinous layer; the adventitial (outer layer of the cyst) should be left intact
- Cysts localized to the lateral segment of the left lobe can be removed with simple segmentectomy
- Cysts that are secondarily infected or are associated with a persistent biliary fistula best treated with resection
- Disease resulting from *E multilocularis* requires complete surgical excision

Prognosis

- Unilocular cysts appropriately treated have an excellent prognosis
- If spillage occurs at the time of aspiration, recurrence rate will be as high as 50%
- Infection with *E multilocularis* a serious and progressive disease and will result in death unless radical hepatic resection eliminates all disease

Associations

- None

Embryonal Sarcoma (Undifferentiated Sarcoma)

Clinical Manifestations

- 3rd most common hepatic malignancy in children
- Represents 6% of all childhood hepatic tumors
- Peak incidence 6 to 10 years
- Slightly more common in boys than girls
- Most present with abdominal swelling or pain of short duration

Gross Pathology

- Usually large (10-20 cm) and well demarcated, but not encapsulated
- Tends to occur in right lobe
- Cut surface variegated with areas of solid gray-white interspersed with foci of cystic degeneration, hemorrhage, and necrosis
- May grow into the inferior vena cava and extend into right atrium and present as an intracardiac tumor

Microscopic Pathology

- Characterized by malignant stellate or spindle-shaped cells closely packed in sheets or fascicles or scattered loosely in a mucopolysaccharide myxoid stroma
- Tumor cells usually very pleomorphic and have hyperchromatic nuclei with inconspicuous nucleoli; cell borders indistinct
- Bizarre giant cells may be present
- Variably sized intracellular and extracellular eosinophilic globules typically present
- Fibrous pseudocapsule may surround tumor
- Bile ducts (often dilated) and hepatocytes often entrapped in the periphery of the tumor
- Hematopoietic activity in 50%
- Focal areas of hemorrhage and/or necrosis often present

Special Stains

- PAS with diastase will highlight intracellular and extracellular eosinophilic globules

Immunohistochemistry

- Inconsistent positivity for histiocytic markers, desmin, vimentin, and cytokeratin
- Intracellular and extracellular eosinophilic globules variably stain for A1-AT, α_1-chymotrypsin, and albumin; always negative for α-fetoprotein

Electron Microscopy

- Features suggest pleomorphic malignant fibrous histiocytoma
- Eosinophilic globules are pleomorphic, and vary in density; may represent apoptotic bodies phagocytosed by tumor cells
- Fibroblastic, myofibroblastic, lipoblastic, rhabdomyoblastic, or leiomyoblastic differentiation occasionally present

Molecular Alterations

- None

Differential Diagnosis

- Embryonal rhabdomyosarcoma
- Mesenchymal hamartoma

Treatment

- Complete surgical excision with or without preoperative or adjuvant chemotherapy

Prognosis

- Most dead within 1 year of diagnosis, but some live 5 or more years
- Overall survival approximately 20%

Associations

- May arise from a mesenchymal hamartoma
- Single report of prenatal exposure to phenytoin

Hepatocellular Carcinoma

Clinical Manifestations

- More common in men than in women particularly when associated with cirrhosis (in normal liver, men and women affected equally)
- More common in all African countries south of the Sahara and in Southeast Asia
- Patients typically present with abdominal pain and right upper quadrant fullness or mass
- Occasionally presenting features are indistinguishable from those of cirrhosis
- Most arise in the setting of preexisting cirrhosis and grow as 1 or more relatively large nodules (nodular type) or numerous smaller nodules (diffuse type)
- Tumors that arise in the normal liver usually grow as a single homogenous mass that occasionally has satellite nodules
- Serum levels of α-fetoprotein are elevated in 40% to 75%

Gross Pathology

- Usually a nodule with a distinct fibrous capsule and/or fibrous septa
- Lesions smaller than 1.5 cm usually have indistinct borders
- Nodules typically bulge from the cut surface and are gray-white, green, or yellow
- Larger tumor nodules contain many of the gross features of small nodules with the addition of obvious foci of hemorrhage and necrosis
- Larger nodules also may have obvious evidence of portal vein, hepatic vein, and bile duct invasion; occasionally there is involvement of the inferior vena cava; tumor may extend into the right atrium

Microscopic Pathology

- Smaller tumors tend to be better differentiated than larger tumors; as a hepatocellular carcinoma enlarges, moderate to poorly differentiated foci tend to appear in the center of the nodule with a peripheral component of well-differentiated tumor that decreases in size as the nodule of tumor enlarges
- Foci of steatosis (40%) and occasional Mallory hyaline (2% to 25%) may be seen
- Tumor cells tend to resemble normal hepatocytes and are typically arranged in thin trabeculae (≤3 cells thick) outlined by vascular channels (sinusoids) lined by endothelium (endothelial lining a very helpful diagnostic feature on fine-needle aspirates)
- Bile in neoplastic cells or tubular lumina is pathognomonic for hepatocellular carcinoma (only seen in 30% and very rarely seen in poorly differentiated lesions)
- Tumor cells typically have a polygonal shape, abundant finely granular eosinophilic cytoplasm with distinct cell membranes and an increased nuclear-cytoplasmic ratio compared with normal; nucleus usually has coarse chromatin and a thickened or irregular nuclear membrane; nucleoli are often prominent; intranuclear cytoplasmic invaginations are common

- Cytologic variants
  - Pleomorphic (giant cell):
    - Fewer than 1% of all hepatocellular carcinomas
    - Hyperchromatic multinucleated giant cells predominate
    - Cellular discohesion is typical
  - Clear cell:
    - The dominant feature in 5% to 16%
    - Tumor cells have prominent clear cytoplasm (cytoplasmic glycogen and/or fat lost during processing)
    - Nuclear features are frequently quite bland and differentiation from metastatic renal, adrenal, or ovarian carcinoma may be impossible on histologic criteria alone
  - Oncocytic:
    - Markedly eosinophilic and coarsely granular cytoplasm (mitochondria)
  - Sarcomatoid (spindle cell, pseudosarcomatous):
    - Spindle-shaped cells are reminiscent of a fibrosarcoma or malignant fibrous histiocytoma
- Well-differentiated hepatocellular carcinoma:
  - Tumor cells with little nuclear atypia and an increased nuclear-cytoplasmic ratio arranged in thin trabeculae not >3 hepatocytes thick; fatty change is typically present; differentiation from a benign adenoma may not be possible without finding areas of more poorly differentiated neoplasm; most common type of differentiation in tumors <2 cm in maximum diameter
- Moderately differentiated hepatocellular carcinoma:
  - Tumor cells are arranged in a trabecular pattern that is more than 3 cells thick; tumor cells tend to be larger and have distinct nucleoli and more abundant eosinophilic cytoplasm than normal or well-differentiated hepatocytes; pseudoglandular structures and bile are frequently seen; giant tumor cells may be present; the most common type of differentiation in tumors >2 cm
- Poorly differentiated hepatocellular carcinoma
  - Tumor cells larger with hyperchromatic nuclei; tend to be arranged in compact (solid) patterns with very little trabecular formation and little or no bile; pleomorphism is typically prominent and areas of spindle cells and small cells may be seen; the hepatocellular nature of the neoplastic cells may not be obvious
  - Tumor typically induces little in the way of stroma; significant fibrosis seen in only 5%
  - Vascular lakes (resemble peliosis hepatis) may be present
  - As tumor progresses from small to advanced disease the extent of sinusoidal capillarization (endothelial lining of vascular spaces) increases
- Histologic patterns:
  - Trabecular (sinusoidal, platelike)
    - Typically present in all hepatocellular carcinomas
    - Trabeculae of variable thickness surrounded by sinusoids lined by flattened endothelial cells and macrophages (Kupffer cells)
    - Little or no reticulin framework
  - Compact (solid)
    - 5% to 15%
    - Adjacent trabeculae fuse to form sheets that compress sinusoids making them inconspicuous
  - Pseudoglandular (acinar, adenoid)
    - The dominant pattern in 5% to 10%
    - May be mistaken for adenocarcinoma (primary or secondary)
    - Spaces represent dilated bile canaliculi lined by cells with cytologic features of malignant hepatocytes
    - Bile and/or eosinophilic, hyaline, PAS-positive diastase-resistant material may be found in lumens
  - Fibrolamellar
    - 1% to 5%
  - Sclerosing
    - 1% to 2%

Special Stains

- Reticulin stains confirm the paucity of reticulin, especially in early lesions
- Iron stains may reveal the presence of intracellular accumulations of iron in hereditary hemochromatosis (seen only in normal hepatocytes; almost never seen in malignant hepatocytes)
- PAS positive diastase resistant intra- and extracellular eosinophilic hyaline globules easily identified (see section on immunohistochemistry)
- Rhodamine stain for copper positive in 40%
- Absence of mucin in hepatocytes confirmed by mucicarmine stain (stain will be positive in foci of cholangiocarcinoma)

Immunohistochemistry

- Endothelial cells lining vascular channels (sinusoids) between tumor trabeculae positive for factor VIII-related antigen, CD34, and *Ulex europaeus*
- Polyclonal carcinoembryonic antigen will confirm the presence of bile canaliculi in 70% to 80% (most useful immunohistochemical marker)
- Both intra- and extracellular eosinophilic hyaline globules may have immunoreactivity for α-fetoprotein, A1-AT, or α_1-antichymotrypsin
- Tumor cells are typically positive for cytokeratins 8 and 18 and hepatocyte antigen (Hep Par 1)

Electron Microscopy

- Hepatocytes irregularly sized with 1 side covered by cells with endothelial features and a sinusoidal space; cytoplasm contains mitochondria, lipid, Golgi complex; intercellular lumens with microvilli (counterpart of canaliculi in normal liver)

Molecular Alterations

- Trisomy 1 and 8
- Multiple chromosomal aberrations, including losses and gains at 1q, 4q, 8q, 16p, and/or 17p

Differential Diagnosis

- Hepatocellular tumors
  - □ Focal nodular hyperplasia
  - □ Nodular regenerative hyperplasia
  - □ Hepatocellular adenoma
  - □ Macroregenerative (dysplastic) nodule
- Neuroendocrine tumors
- Clear cell carcinoma
- Renal cell carcinoma (non-clear cell type)
- Squamous cell carcinoma
- Melanoma
- Angiomyolipoma (especially if there is a prominent epithelioid component)
- Prostate adenocarcinoma
- Angiosarcoma
- Adenocarcinoma (primary [cholangiocarcinoma] or metastatic)
- Poorly differentiated carcinoma

Treatment

- Surgical excision when possible
- Palliation can be obtained with percutaneous ethanol injection, cryoablation, and transcatheter arterial chemoembolization
- Hepatic transplantation (usually limited to solitary lesions ≤5 cm or multiple lesions, none >3 cm)

Prognosis

- 5-year survival rate after resection approximately 20% to 30%
- Survival better in noncirrhotic patients with tumors <5 cm (5-year survival >50%)
- Recurrence rate following surgery ranges from 50% to 80%
- Factors affecting prognosis include:
  - □ Tumor size, number, and location
  - □ Presence or absence of vascular invasion
  - □ Presence or absence of cirrhosis
  - □ Distance of neoplasm from resection margin (≥1 cm)
  - □ Presence or absence of tumor capsule and capsular invasion
  - □ Degree of hepatocellular differentiation

Associations

- Hepatocellular carcinoma may be seen concurrently with cholangiocarcinoma (5%)
- Chronic hepatic injury
  - □ Cirrhosis most common
  - □ Chronic hepatitis less common (hepatitis B a greater risk factor than hepatitis C)

- Specific etiologies associated with a high risk (>15%) for the development of hepatocellular carcinoma include: HBV, HCV, hereditary hemochromatosis, hereditary tyrosinemia, porphyria cutanea tarda, hypercitrullinemia, and membranous obstruction of the inferior vena cava
- Etiologies associated with an intermediate risk (~5%-15%) for the development of hepatocellular carcinoma include: alcohol, A1-AT deficiency, types I and III glycogen storage disease, and autoimmune hepatitis
- Etiologies associated with low risk (<5%) for development of hepatocellular carcinoma include: PBC, PSC, hereditary fructose intolerance, paucity of bile ducts, progressive intrahepatic cholestasis (Byler disease), congenital hepatic fibrosis, biliary atresia, Wilson disease, oral contraceptives, anabolic-androgenic steroids, cardiac cirrhosis, exposure to aflatoxin B, (only in regions with high incidence of hepatocellular carcinoma)
- Sclerosing variant frequently associated with hypercalcemia

Fibrolamellar Hepatocellular Carcinoma

Clinical Manifestations

- Typically arises in a noncirrhotic liver (90%)
- Tends to affect young patients usually in the 3rd decade of life (<20% over the age of 40 years)
- Men and women affected equally
- Typically present with vague symptoms of right upper quadrant pain or fullness
- Occasionally gynecomastia or symptoms of the Budd-Chiari syndrome may be present
- Serum levels of α-fetoprotein elevated in about 10% to 15%

Gross Pathology

- Most tumors arise in the left lobe; both lobes may be involved
- Tend to be firm, tan-white, gray, or brown
- Focal bile staining and foci of necrosis or hemorrhage may be present
- Typically large, solitary and well-circumscribed
- Tend to bulge from the cut surface and are divided into multiple nodules by radiating fibrous septa which frequently coalesce in the center to form a stellate scar (this same pattern may be present in metastases)
- Adjacent non-neoplastic liver usually appears normal

Microscopic Pathology

- Neoplastic cells are large and polygonal with abundant granular eosinophilic cytoplasm, clearly defined cell borders, and large vesicular nuclei with a prominent nucleolus
- Tumor cells tend to be separated into nests, columns, or sheets by parallel, hyalinized bands of acellular collagen that often contain small, thick-walled arteries
- Focal areas of nuclear pleomorphism and a trabecular or adenoid pattern, more typical of a conventional hepatocellular carcinoma, may be present
- Mitotic figures infrequent
- Areas of necrosis and foci of vascular invasion frequent
- Eosinophilic hyaline globules and pale bodies (ground-glass cells) often present (50%)
- Usually cytoplasmic bile and copper present (features of cholestasis); occasionally intracytoplasmic fat and Mallory hyaline present

Special Stains

- Eosinophilic hyaline globules can be seen with PAS with diastase (occasionally negative)

Immunohistochemistry

- Tumor cells typically positive for A1-AT and HepPar 1 (hepatocyte antigen) and rarely positive for α-fetoprotein
- Tumor cells typically cytokeratin positive and share the same immunoprofile as tumor cells in hepatocellular carcinoma
- Pale bodies (ground glass cells) are immunoreactive for fibrinogen
- Cytokeratins 7 and 20 usually both negative
- Polyclonal CEA will show canalicular or apical staining

Electron Microscopy

- Tumor cells are packed with mitochondria (hence the oncocytic morphology)
- Eosinophilic, ground glass inclusions contain fibrinogen and may be associated with intracytoplasmic luminal bile canaliculi or rough endoplasmic reticulum

Molecular Alterations

Rate of allelic loss less than that of usual hepatocellular carcinoma

Differential Diagnosis

- Focal nodular hyperplasia
- Usual and scirrhous hepatocellular carcinoma
- Cholangiocarcinoma
- Adenosquamous/squamous carcinoma with sclerosis
- Metastatic tumors
- Neuroendocrine tumors (usually metastatic)

Treatment

- Neoplasm more frequently resectable than usual hepatocellular carcinomas
- Transplantation is treatment of choice for unresectable lesions
- When possible isolated metastases resected

Prognosis

- Patients have a better prognosis than those with the usual form of hepatocellular carcinoma even when the tumor is found in a noncirrhotic liver
- Metastatic disease typically involves abdominal lymph nodes, peritoneum, and lung
- Overall 5-year survival rate 25% to 30%; 5-year survival rate for resectable lesions ranges from 55% to 75%

Associations

- None

Infantile Hemangioendothelioma

Clinical Manifestations

- Most common mesenchymal liver tumor in childhood; a benign vascular proliferation
- Represents 15% to 20% of all primary pediatric hepatic neoplasms
- Patients almost always under the age of 6 months
- Girls affected twice as often than boys
- Patients typically present with an abdominal mass; other symptoms include high output cardiac failure, severe thrombocytopenia, and bleeding diathesis secondary to platelet sequestration (Kasabach-Merritt syndrome)
- Spontaneous rupture may occur

Gross Pathology

- Solitary or multiple tumor nodules ranging in size from <0.5 to 15 cm
- Solitary lesions tend to occur in right lobe, multiple lesions usually scattered throughout both lobes
- Tumor nodules tend to be circumscribed but not encapsulated
- Smaller lesions usually red to tan, soft, and spongy; larger nodules usually variegated with a red to brown periphery and a gray to white, scarred, umbilicated center with focal areas of hemorrhage and calcification (vascular nature of lesion may not be grossly apparent)

Microscopic Pathology

- Border of neoplasm infiltrative in approximately 35%
- Tumors composed of capillarylike vascular channels lined by plump endothelium that in time undergo progressive maturation scarring and involution
- In central portions of the lesion, there may be cavernous foci, fibrous stroma, intravascular thrombosis, and foci of dystrophic calcification
- 2 histologic subtypes:
  - Type I: An orderly proliferation of small, capillarylike, slightly irregular, and dilated bloodless vascular structures lined by a continuous layer of bland endothelial cells with round to oval nuclei; vascular channels separated by a loose connective tissue; mitoses rare; hepatocytes and small bile ducts may be found admixed with blood vessels and at the periphery of the lesion; foci of extramedullary hematopoiesis present in vascular lumina in 60%; most have areas of regressive change consisting of thrombosis, fibrosis, myxoid change, and calcification; regressive changes are particularly prominent in larger lesions
  - Type II: Characterized by poorly formed, irregularly shaped branching vascular structures lined by large hyperchromatic and pleomorphic endothelial cells; mitotic activity often pronounced; many consider type II change to represent a low-grade angiosarcoma

Special Stains

- Not helpful

Immunohistochemistry

- Cytokeratin will demonstrate infiltrative border of the tumor by highlighting entrapped hepatocytes and bile ducts
- Tumor cells will show positive staining for factor VIII-related antigen and *Ulex europaeus* I lectin

Electron Microscopy

- Endothelial nature of tumor cells confirmed by the presence of Weibel-Palade bodies

Molecular Alterations

- None

Differential Diagnosis

- Angiosarcoma
- Mesenchymal hamartoma

Treatment

- Solitary, surgically accessible lesions resected
- Steroids, radiotherapy, arterial embolization, and transplantation have all been successful

Prognosis

- Spontaneous regression tends to occur after 6 to 8 months
- Factors associated with a poor prognosis include presence of congestive heart failure and jaundice at time of presentation and presence of multiple nodules without evidence of cavernous differentiation
- Presence of type II change with increased mitoses does not necessarily indicate a poorer prognosis, most pursue a benign course

Associations

- 40% to 55% of patients have cutaneous, cavernous type hemangiomas as well as hemangiomas of other organs (lung, gastrointestinal tract, pancreas, and thymus)
- Reports of angiosarcoma development even after regression

Epithelioid Hemangioendothelioma

Clinical Manifestations

- Second most common primary hepatic sarcoma of adults
- May be seen anywhere from the 2nd to the 8th decade of life, but usually middle age (mean 47 years)
- Women more commonly affected than men (1.5 to 1)
- Etiology uncertain, but there may be some relationship to oral contraceptive use
- Patients frequently present with abdominal pain or weight loss; 50% asymptomatic
- An incidental finding in 40%

Gross Pathology

- 80% consist of multiple nodules varying in size from 1 to 12 cm distributed throughout both lobes
- When nodules are small they mimic cirrhosis
- On cut surface of nodules often gritty, white to gray to tan and firm with ill-defined margins (vascular nature inapparent)

Microscopic Pathology

- Typically a zonal pattern; 3 zones each with characteristic microscopic findings;
  - □ Zone 1 (peripheral or periportal): A cellular sinusoidal proliferation of tumor cells (often in clumps) with residual intact hepatocytes and scanty myxoid stroma; portal tracts may appear normal at low power but small aggregates of tumor cells may be found in portal vein branches
  - □ Zone 2 (mid zone): Consists of atrophic hepatocyte plates, few bile ductules, and increasing quanties of variably inflamed, paucicellular, myxochondroid stroma that becomes progressively sclerotic and occasionally calcified toward zone 3
  - □ Zone 3 (central or perivenular): Partial or total luminal obliteration of terminal hepatic venules and larger hepatic vein branches by fibrous, hyalinized, and often calcified stroma with rare tumor cells that usually have a stellate or spindled shape
- Tumor cells best seen in the zone 2 where they are arranged as single cells, short single-file cords, or nests embedded in a myxohyaline matrix

- 2 different types of tumor cells typically present:
  - Dendritic cells:
    - Spindle-shaped or stellate cells with eosinophilic cytoplasm and branching processes that appear to connect adjacent cells
    - Nuclei vesicular, occasionally grooved, and contain small nucleoli
  - Epithelioid cells:
    - More rounded than dendritic cells and have a more eosinophilic cytoplasm
    - Nuclei generally round with mild to moderate atypia and prominent eosinophilic nucleoli
    - Mitoses may be present but usually inconspicuous
    - Cells often have 1 or more prominent intracytoplasmic vacuoles ("blister cells"); these vacuoles vary in size and represent incipient vascular lumina; may contain erythrocytes

Special Stains

- Mucin stains are always negative (the cytoplasmic vacuoles in the endothelial cells are easily confused with signet ring cell carcinoma)
- Trichrome and/or elastic stains may be required to identify central hepatic veins in sclerotic zone 3

Immunohistochemistry

- Neoplastic cells typically positive for factor VIII-related antigen as well as CD34 and other endothelial markers
- Tumor cells negative for CEA
- Approximately 15% of tumors will be positive for cytokeratin (in addition, trapped hepatocytes or bile ductules will be positive for cytokeratin)
- 25% show positivity for smooth muscle actin

Electron Microscopy

- Confirms the presence of Weibel-Palade bodies in tumor cells
- Tumor cells also contain numerous intermediate filaments (account for the epithelioid appearance)

Molecular Alterations

- None

Differential Diagnosis

- Metastatic carcinoma (signet ring cell type)
- Scirrhous cholangiocarcinoma
- Hepatocellular carcinoma
- Neuroendocrine neoplasms
- Sclerosing hemangioma
- Scar
- Collapsed fibrotic hepatic parenchyma
- Granulation tissue
- Cirrhosis
- Veno-occlusive disease
- Leiomyosarcoma
- Chondrosarcoma

Treatment

- Resection or transplantation

Prognosis

- Clinical course unpredictable; some patients survive for decades while others die within months of diagnosis
- Tumor cellularity seems to be the only histologic feature of prognostic significance
- Approximately 50% have extrahepatic disease (lung, omentum, mesentery, or lymph node)

Associations

- None

Hepatoblastoma

Clinical Manifestations

- Most common primary hepatic neoplasm in children
- Represents 50% of all primary hepatic malignancies
- Twice as common in boys as in girls
- Occurs almost exclusively in children younger than 5 years (70% <2 years; 90% <5 years)
- Approximately 5% will have signs of disease at birth; most present with abdominal mass
- Serum α-fetoprotein level elevated in 90%

Gross Pathology

- Typically a solitary, tan-green mass that may be either smooth or lobulated
- On cut section, neoplasm may be either solid and/or partially cystic
- Most occur in right lobe and average 10 to 12 cm in diameter
- May be partially encapsulated
- Foci of calcification, necrosis, and hemorrhage may be present (usually seen in tumors with a prominent mesenchymal component)
- In approximately 10%, gross evidence of portal or hepatic vein invasion may be present

Microscopic Pathology

- 3 types: Epithelial, mixed epithelial-mesenchymal, and anaplastic (undifferentiated)
- 6 histologic patterns:
  - Epithelial type—fetal (31%)
  - Epithelial type—embryonal (19%)
  - Epithelial type—macrotrabecular (3%)
  - Epithelial type—small cell undifferentiated (3%)
  - Mixed epithelial mesenchymal type—nonteratoid (34%)
  - Mixed epithelial mesenchymal type—teratoid (10%)
- Epithelial cells are typically arranged in irregular lobules separated by septa of collagenous tissue
- Foci of extramedullary hematopoiesis may be found in sinusoids of either fetal or embryonal patterns (especially fetal pattern)
- Occasionally foci of rhabdoid-type cells or multinucleated giant cells containing human chorionic gonotrophic may be seen
- *Fetal pattern*
  - Most closely resembles normal hepatocytes with light and dark zones secondary to presence of glycogen and fat, respectively
  - Hepatocytes are similar in size to (may be slightly smaller than) those of adjacent normal liver
  - Nuclear-cytoplasmic ratio low; nucleoli inconspicuous
  - Tumor cells tend to be uniform and polygonal with distinct cell borders and little pleomorphism
  - Mitoses are rare
  - Tumor cells arranged in trabeculae that are 2 or 3 cells thick, separated by sinusoids lined by endothelial cells
  - Portal tracts, bile ducts, and bile ductules all absent
- *Embryonal pattern*
  - Less differentiated, poorly cohesive cells arranged in sheets, ribbons, acini, papillary formations, pseudorosettes, and trabeculae
  - Vascular lakes (pelioid foci) may be present as well as numerous mitoses and foci of necrosis
  - Embryonal cells have ill-defined cell borders, tend to have a more basophilic cytoplasm, and a higher nuclear-cytoplasmic ratio than fetal cells; frequently pleomorphic
  - Nuclear chromatin coarser and nucleoli are more prominent than in fetal cells
- *Macrotrabecular pattern*
  - Cells arranged in trabeculae 10 or more cells thick
  - Cells may be fetal, embryonal, or hepatocellular carcinomalike with abundant eosinophilic cytoplasm
- *Small cell undifferentiated pattern*
  - Discohesive sheets of uniform small cells with scanty cytoplasm
  - Tumor cells have indistinct cell borders, oval hyperchromatic nuclei, and occasional prominent nucleoli
  - Mitotic activity is typically brisk
  - Hyalinized septa may course through the tumor cells; occasionally the stroma is mucoid
  - The diagnosis of the small cell variant requires the presence of other patterns of hepatoblastoma
- *Mixed epithelial and mesenchymal pattern:*
  - A variable mixture of epithelial (fetal and embryonal) and mesenchymal (primitive and undifferentiated) cell types

- Primitive mesenchymal component usually located near neoplastic epithelial components and consists of oval to spindle-shaped cells with little cytoplasm
- Fibrous septa, myxoid change, and osteoid may be present
- Presence of osteoid may be a more frequent finding after treatment with chemotherapy
- Mixed pattern may have teratoid features (10%; keratinized squamous epithelium, intestinal epithelium, skeletal muscle, mature bone and cartilage, melanin pigment, and neuroectodermal structures) or no teratoid features (34%)
- Tumors in combination with either yolk sac tumor or teratoma have been reported

Special Stains

- Not helpful

Immunohistochemistry

- Prominent endothelial cells seen in the fetal pattern stain with CD34
- Primitive mesenchymal cells and osteoblastlike cells in mixed pattern cytokeratin positive
- Tumor cells typically stain for α-fetoprotein
- Tumor cells may also stain for A1-AT, cytokeratin, vimentin, and CEA
- Fetal and embryonal cells may be focally immunoreactive for chromogranin
- Embryonal cells stain positively for cytokeratins 8, 18, and 19
- Fetal cells stain positively for cytokeratins 8 and 18 and are only weakly positive for cytokeratin 19

Electron Microscopy

- Not helpful

Molecular Alterations

- Trisomy 2 and trisomy 20
- Abnormalities of chromosome 11; loss of heterozygosity at 11p15.5
- Overexpression and mutation of p53 may be present

Differential Diagnosis

- Metastasis from neuroblastoma, lymphoma, rhabdomyosarcoma, and Wilms tumor (differential particularly difficult if hepatoblastoma has primarily an epithelial, small cell, undifferentiated pattern)
- Hepatocellular carcinoma
- Undifferentiated (embryonal) sarcoma
- Metastatic or primary hepatic germ cell tumor
- Malignant rhabdoid tumor

Treatment

- Surgical excision when possible
- Treatment with chemotherapy often results in a marked improvement in resectability (>90%)
- If a tumor is unresectable at initial surgical exploration and then becomes resectable after chemotherapy, adjuvant radiation administered after the second operation
- Unresectable tumors limited to the liver often best treated with liver transplantation

Prognosis

- Fetal type has best prognosis
- Some evidence that small cell undifferentiated pattern and macrotrabecular pattern have a slightly worse prognosis
- Presence of osteoid or other mesenchymal components in a mixed neoplasm may be associated with a better prognosis
- 60% to 70% of patients with resectable tumors (even after chemotherapy) experience long-term survival
- Recurrences typically occur within 3 years
- Metastatic disease primarily involves lymph nodes and lung and present at the time of death in up to 50%

Associations

- Precocious puberty as a result of human chorionic gonatropin production by the tumor
- Familial adenomatous polyposis (~1% develop hepatoblastoma)
- Maternal exposure to certain metals, petroleum products, paints and pigments may be important etiologic factors
- No association with risk factors for hepatocellular carcinoma

Hepatocellular (Liver Cell) Adenoma

Clinical Manifestations

- 95% occur in women
- Pathogenically related to the use of oral contraceptives (85% to 90%)
- 70% solitary
- May occur in patients with sex hormone imbalance resulting from use of anabolic/androgenic steroids
- Multiple lesions occasionally seen in patients taking anabolic/androgenic steroids
- May present with rupture with intraperitoneal hemorrhage

Gross Pathology

- Usually a well-defined (not encapsulated) nodule of a different color than surrounding normal liver
- May be pedunculated
- Cut surface variegated with tan (normal), yellow (necrotic), white (infarcted), and red (hemorrhagic) foci
- No central scar (as seen in nodular hyperplasia)
- Focal nodular hyperplasia may be present
- No fibrosis or cirrhosis in surrounding hepatic parenchyma

Microscopic Pathology

- Well-differentiated hepatocytes with abundant pale eosinophilic granular cytoplasm arranged in sheets and cords interspersed with thin-walled blood vessels; no acinar architecture
- Large arteries with intimal thickening, accumulation of mucopolysaccharide, and thickening of internal elastic lamina present at periphery of tumor
- Regular septa, portal tracts, and bile ducts are absent
- Tumor cell nuclei are round and bland; no mitotic figures
- Small liver cell rosettes (pseudoglands) with an empty or bile-filled central lumen may be seen (typical of a cholestatic liver)
- Foci of fat or areas of steatohepatitis with Mallory hyaline may be present
- Degenerative changes of dilated, blood-filled sinusoids, areas of focal necrosis and hemorrhage, areas of scarring with hemosiderin-laden macrophages from old hemorrhages, apoptotic bodies, and a myxoid stroma may all be present
- Reticulin is normal or reduced depending on the amount of necrosis and/or hemorrhage

Special Stains

- Reticulin stains confirm normal amounts of reticulin except in areas of necrosis or hemorrhage
- PAS confirms presence of intracellular glycogen

Immunohistochemistry

- Tumor cells negative for α-fetoprotein
- CD34 staining focal and weak (unlike the diffuse and widespread staining of sinusoids in hepatocellular carcinoma)

Electron Microscopy

- Tumor cells contain mitochondria with paracrystalline inclusions, Mallory hyaline, and increased glycogen

Molecular Alterations

- None

Differential Diagnosis

- Hepatocellular carcinoma (adenoma and carcinoma may coexist in the same liver)
- Macroregenerative nodules in cirrhosis
- Focal nodular hyperplasia

Treatment

- Complete excision

Prognosis

- Some risk of rupture and intraperitoneal hemorrhage particularly in those associated with the use of oral contraceptives
- Probably a precursor lesion to hepatocellular carcinoma

Associations

- Oral contraceptive steroids
- Noncontraceptive estrogens
- Sex hormone-producing ovarian tumors
- Anabolic/androgenic steroids
- Familial diabetes mellitus
- Type Ia glycogenosis
- Type III glycogenosis
- Hurler disease
- Hereditary tyrosinemia
- β-thalassemia with secondary iron overload
- Severe combined immunodeficiency
- Familial adenomatous polyposis
- Untreated lesions that spontaneously develop in children may eventually become to hepatocellular carcinoma

Mesenchymal Hamartoma

Clinical Manifestations

- Most likely represents a developmental anomaly resulting from aberrant formation of primitive portal mesenchyme coupled with secondary degenerative changes
- Typically seen in children <2 years of age (median age 10 months)
- Represents approximately 6% of all pediatric hepatic neoplasms
- Slightly more frequently in boys than in girls
- Usually presents with progressive abdominal extension or palpable abdominal mass; occasionally patients experience abdominal pain, respiratory distress, and failure to thrive

Gross Pathology

- Typically a solitary mass in the right lobe well demarcated from adjacent liver
- Range from 3 cm to as much as 30 cm in diameter
- 20% pedunculated
- Cut surface typically consists of multiple cysts of varying diameter; cysts filled with clear or mucoid fluid and have a ragged internal surface; tissue surrounding cyst yellow to gray and myxoid with white, fibrous bands
- Foci of necrosis, calcification, and hemorrhage usually absent
- May appear to have an infiltrative border and satellite lesions may be present

Microscopic Pathology

- Typically an admixture of immature mesenchymal tissue with bland stellate or spindle cells dispersed in edematous myxoid stroma that contains various amounts of collagen, bile ducts, blood vessels, and hepatocytes
- Grossly visible cysts scattered through the lesion represent collections of fluid in the stroma
- Stroma contains numerous thick-walled veins and foci of extramedullary hematopoiesis (90%)
- Bile ducts in stroma appear to be branching or cystically dilated and are encircled by a cuff of mesenchymal tissue; bile duct epithelium may be atrophic, hyperplastic, or inflamed
- Small cords of unremarkable hepatocytes without a recognizable lobular arrangement may be interspersed throughout, but usually best seen at periphery as thin compressed strips
- At periphery small portal-based tumor nodules may extend into adjacent normal hepatic parenchyma

Special Stains

- Trichrome stain will highlight collagen in mesenchyme, especially around bile ducts

Immunohistochemistry

- Stromal cells (mesenchyme) positive for vimentin
- Bile ducts positive for cytokeratin
- Muscle markers, muscle-specific actin, desmin, and myoglobin, may show some positivity
- α-fetoprotein and A1-AT both negative

Electron Microscopy

- Confirms features of myofibroblasts in spindle cells (may be helpful in the differentiation from embryonal rhabdomyosarcoma)

Molecular Alterations

- A balanced translocation involving chromosomes 11 and 19 with a breakpoint at 19q13.4

Differential Diagnosis

- Vascular malformation

Treatment

- Complete surgical excision is the preferred treatment
- Long-term favorable outcome can also be achieved with incomplete excision or marsupialization

Prognosis

- Recurrence rare even after only partial removal
- Generally excellent (most mortality associated with operative complications; 5%-10%)

Associations

- Very rare association with undifferentiated sarcoma

Focal Nodular Hyperplasia

Clinical Manifestations

- 80% asymptomatic; abdominal mass in 10% to 15%
- 70% to 80% solitary
- Adults affected more commonly than children (4:1)
- Typically diagnosed during the 3rd to 5th decades
- 80% to 95% occur in women of reproductive age
- 10% to 15% occur in children
- Pediatric cases more likely to be multiple

Gross Pathology

- Subcapsular depressed white area of fibrosis with broad strands of fibrosis radiating from the center to the periphery in a stellate configuration
- Nodules well demarcated from normal, surrounding hepatic parenchyma and protrude from surface
- <5% pedunculated
- Foci of hemorrhage or necrosis unusual (unless patient taking oral contraceptives)
- No bile staining

Microscopic Pathology

- Hepatocyte nodules well demarcated from normal hepatic parenchyma and contain parenchymal elements (including endothelial cells and Kupffer cells), but lack classic lobular architecture; central veins are markedly reduced in number or absent
- Features of cholestasis (eg, pseudoxanthomatous change, ballooning hepatocytes, intracellular copper, Mallory hyaline, and small foci of bile pigment) usually present in hepatocytes adjacent to septa (probably related to the absence of normal interlobular bile ducts)
- Fibrous/fibromyxoid septa divide the lesion into lobules that resemble cirrhosis; septa contain large, eccentrically thickened, and occasionally narrowed blood vessels, small proliferating bile ductules primarily localized to the periseptal parenchymal interface (region of the limiting plate), a paucity of interlobar bile ducts and portal vein branches, and a predominately lymphocytic infiltrate

Special Stains

- PAS will highlight Mallory hyaline

Immunohistochemistry

- A1-AT may highlight the presence of hyaline globules in hepatocytes near septa
- p53 immunoreactivity absent

Electron Microscopy

- Not helpful

Molecular Alterations

- *ras* oncogene product p21 may be present

Differential Diagnosis

- Normal liver
- Hepatocellular adenoma
- Cirrhosis
- Hepatocellular carcinoma, fibrolamellar variant

Treatment

- None required except cessation of oral contraceptives
- Frequently biopsies performed because of gross resemblance to metastatic carcinoma

Prognosis

- Benign; no reports of malignant transformation

Associations

- If multiple, may be associated with:
  - Vascular anomalies (hepatic hemangioma, telangiectasias of the brain, berry aneurysm, dysplastic systemic arteries, portal vein atresia)
  - Central nervous system neoplasms (meningioma, astrocytoma)
  - Hemihypertrophy
- Oral contraceptives may promote growth, but do not induce formation
- Portal hypertension

Nodular Regenerative Hyperplasia

Clinical Manifestations

- A diffuse nodularity of liver parenchyma without accompanying fibrosis
- Typically seen in adults between the ages of 50 and 70 years
- Affects men and women equally
- Most cases are asymptomatic and not associated with clinical disease
- Symptomatic patients present with hepatomegaly and splenomegaly; 40% to 60% have evidence of portal hypertension with esophageal varices and ascites
- Rarely nodules can rupture and produce hemoperitoneum
- Condition appears to arise from disturbed hepatic circulation, most likely involving occlusion of the portal vein branches; size and distribution of nodules determined by the size of the occluded vessel
- Serum alkaline phosphatase level usually mildly to moderately elevated; serum α-fetoprotein level typically normal

Gross Pathology

- Multiple pale or tan nodules scattered throughout the liver that resemble either metastatic disease or cirrhosis
- Capsular surface finely granular
- Nodules measure between 1 and 3 mm in diameter; occasionally much larger
- Nodules tan to white and separated by congested internodular liver parenchyma
- Larger nodules may be hemorrhagic or infarcted (rare)

Microscopic Pathology

- Nodules of hyperplastic hepatocytes that appear to be arising from the periportal region; larger nodules develop as small nodules coalesce
- At low power there is variable orientation of the liver cell plates in the nodules
- Nodules surrounded by regions of internodular hepatocyte atrophy with sinusoidal congestion and dilatation or compression of central veins
- Intranodular hepatocyte plates tend to be 1 to 2 cells thick and show very little pleomorphism
- Almost no fibrosis
- Hepatocytes that comprise the nodules typically similar to those in the surrounding parenchyma; as nodules enlarge, their hepatocyte population tends to show clear or vacuolated (fat/glycogen) cytoplasm
- Cholestasis rarely present
- Lipofuscin absent within nodules but may be present in the internodular atrophic hepatocytes
- Portal vein branches may have variable degrees of narrowing and show evidence of sclerosis with or without thrombosis or even complete obliteration

Special Stains

- Reticulin stains highlight collapse of reticulin and atrophy of hepatocytes at periphery of nodules and thickening of hepatocyte plates within the nodules

Immunohistochemistry

- Regenerative hepatocytes stain for A1-AT

Electron Microscopy

- Not helpful

Molecular Alterations

- None

Differential Diagnosis

- Cirrhosis (no fibrosis in nodular regenerative hyperplasia)
- Hepatocellular carcinoma
- Focal nodular hyperplasia

Treatment

- Management of associated conditions (see associations later in this section)

Prognosis

- Hepatic decompensation rarely occurs
- Development of hepatocellular carcinoma extremely rare

Associations

- Immunologic disorders: Connective tissue diseases (rheumatoid arthritis, systemic lupus erythematosus, progressive systemic sclerosis), glomerulonephritis, cryoglobulinemia, common variable immunodeficiency, autoimmune hemolytic anemia, myasthenia gravis, hyperthyroidism and hypothyroidism, and idiopathic thrombocytopenic purpura
- Neoplastic disorders: Myoproliferative disorders, lymphoproliferative disorders, primary and secondary hepatic carcinomas, and multiple myeloma
- Drugs and toxins: Azathioprine, chemotherapeutic agents, arsenic, vinyl chloride, corticosteroids, anabolic steroids, and contraceptive steroids
- Vascular disorders: Obliterative portal venopathy, extrahepatic portal vein thrombosis, arteritis, veno-occlusive disease, peliosis hepatis, and primary pulmonary hypertension
- Transplantation: Kidney, bone marrow, liver, and heart
- Miscellaneous disorders: Primary biliary cirrhosis and chronic liver disease (precirrhotic), diabetes mellitus, generalized mastocytosis, sarcoidosis, tuberculosis

Gallbladder and Extrahepatic Bile Ducts

Adenomyoma and Adenomyomatosis

Clinical Manifestations

- Usually asymptomatic
- If gallstones present, signs and symptoms of acute or chronic cholecystitis may be present

Gross Pathology

- Diffuse disease characterized by a gallbladder wall thickened to up to 5 times normal with a velvety mucosal surface
- Localized disease tends to be confined to the fundus where nodules of mucosa vary in size from 0.5 to 2.5 cm and have a gray-white cut surface, often with multiple cysts
- Occasionally nodules are unencapsulated and may be found entirely within the subserosa

Microscopic Pathology

- Extension of surface epithelium into and through thickened gallbladder muscular layer (Rokitansky-Aschoff sinuses)
- 2 variants:
  - Generalized (cholecystitis glandularis proliferans—adenomyomatosis)
  - Segmental or localized (adenomyoma)
- Glands lined by columnar or cuboidal epithelium are embedded in bundles of smooth muscle and may contain inspissated bile
- Surface epithelium may have a papillary configuration and does not always communicate with underlying glands
- Typically the nuclei of the glandular epithelium are benign looking, although at times they may have the appearance of reactive atypia
- Occasionally frank dysplasia or adenocarcinoma may coexist
- Coexisting chronic cholecystitis present in up to 80%

Special Stains, Immunohistochemistry, and Electron Microscopy

- Not helpful

Molecular Alterations

- None

Differential Diagnosis

- Adenocarcinoma of the gallbladder

Treatment

- Cholecystectomy

Prognosis

- Benign condition that appears to be acquired and seems to represent "diverticular disease" (extensions of surface epithelium protruding into and beyond a thickened gallbladder muscle)

Associations

- Areas of high-grade dysplasia and carcinoma may be seen in otherwise unremarkable foci of adenomyomatosis

Bile Duct Carcinoma—Extrahepatic

Clinical Manifestations

- Patients typically present in their 7th or 8th decade (rarely seen before age of 40)
- Males slightly more frequently affected than females
- May be seen in patients with ulcerative colitis, primary sclerosing cholangitis, and choledochal cysts (usually presents 20 years earlier in this subset of patients)
- Vast majority present with jaundice; other symptoms include epigastric pain, weakness, and puritis
- Hepatomegaly a common physical finding

Gross Pathology

- 70% are perihilar (involve hepatic duct bifurcation, Klatskin tumor); 30% distal (involve distal extrahepatic or intrapancreatic portion of the bile duct)
- Sclerosing lesions that typically appear as gray to white, circumferential ductal thickenings (may resemble nonneoplastic stricture); proximal and distal margins usually very indistinct; extension along duct wall and beyond duct wall into adjacent structures frequently present
- Nodular lesions tend to be more circumscribed, firm, gray to white, more than 2 cm in diameter, and frequently project into the duct lumen while simultaneously extending through the duct wall
- Papillary lesions usually friable and gray to pink; may be multifocal and may appear to be noninvasive

Microscopic Pathology

- 90% to 95% are pure well to moderately differentiated adenocarcinomas
- Tumor cells tend to be cuboidal or columnar and have vesicular nuclei with prominent nucleoli
- Well-differentiated lesions have obvious gland formation with mucin in tumor cells and within glandular lumina; may be extremely difficult to differentiate from normal glands; malignant glands may be widely dispersed with the only evidence of malignancy being a desmoplastic response or the presence of perineural invasion (75%-80%)
- Papillary tumors have a complex architecture with intestinal- or biliary-type epithelium and some cytologic atypia
- Tumors may have small cell, signet ring cell, spindle cell, giant cell, and squamous cell features; occasionally undifferentiated
- Lymphatic and venous invasion, necrosis, and a chronic inflammatory infiltrate may all be present
- Foci of high-grade dysplasia or carcinoma in situ may be found in ducts distant from the primary neoplasm

Special Stains

- Mucicarmine and Alcian blue will confirm the presence of intracellular and intraluminal mucin

Immunohistochemistry

- Tumor cells have cytoplasmic and luminal positivity for polyclonal antibody to CEA (CEA positivity is not canalicular as it is in hepatocellular carcinoma)
- Neuroendocrine cells present in intestinal-type epithelium are positive for neuron-specific enolase, synaptophysin, and chromogranin
- 65% stain positively for p53 protein

Electron Microscopy

- Not helpful

Molecular Alterations

- Mutations in codon 12 of K-*ras* gene may be present (not specific for carcinoma; may also be present in hyperplastic ductal lesions in the pancreas)

Differential Diagnosis

- Sclerosing cholangitis (particularly if the biopsy sample is taken from the proximal segment of the extrahepatic bile duct)
- Primary neoplasm arising in the pancreas, liver, ampulla, duodenum, gallbladder, stomach, or colon extending into the extrahepatic bile ducts
- Metastatic disease from breast, ovary, colon, or kidney
- Intraductal spread of hepatocellular carcinoma, intrahepatic cholangiocarcinoma, and metastatic colon carcinoma, and metastatic renal cell carcinoma

Treatment

- Tumors involving the confluence of the extrahepatic ducts resected with biliary continuity reestablished with a Roux-en-Y choledochojejunostomy; even if not resectable for cure, biliary flow should be reestablished
- Distal lesions (if resectable) are usually treated with pancreaticoduodenectomy
- Adjuvant radiotherapy of little value

Prognosis

- 10% to 35% of patients with resectable perihilar tumors survive for 5 years
- Resectable distal tumors more likely to be resectable for cure (5-year survival rate of 30%)
- Papillary lesions more likely to be only superficially invasive and hence have a better prognosis

Associations

- Primary sclerosing cholangitis in the setting of chronic ulcerative colitis
- Choledochal cyst
- *Clonorchis sinensis* and *Opisthorchis viverrini* infestation
- Cystic fibrosis
- Familial adenomatous polyposis
- Chronic typhoid carrier state
- Biliary giardiasis
- Thorotrast exposure
- 30% have cholelithiasis; 10% have choledocholithiasis

Biliary Cystadenocarcinoma

Clinical Manifestations

- Accounts for 1% of all primary malignant carcinomas in the liver
- Usually develops as a complication of an antecedent biliary cystadenoma
- Men and women affected equally
- Age range at presentation 45 to 70 years

Gross Pathology

- Cystic with solid areas

Microscopic Pathology

- Lining epithelium frequently demonstrates a complex tubulopapillary growth pattern with invasive glands
- Solid areas may be present
- Adenosquamous, pure squamous, hepatoid, oncocytic, and spindle cell features may be present
- 30% have dense, spindle cell, ovarianlike stroma (only women)
- 50% have foci of benign cystadenoma (almost always women)
- Stromal invasion is definitive evidence of adenocarcinoma; diagnosis of carcinoma can be made in the absence of stromal invasion when there is high-grade dysplasia (carcinoma in situ) or complex architecture

Special Stains

- Mucin stains can highlight the mucinous nature of the epithelial tumor cells

Immunohistochemistry

- Focal areas of smooth muscle actin and vimentin positivity can be seen in the areas of ovarianlike stroma

Electron Microscopy

- Not helpful

Molecular Alterations

- None

Differential Diagnosis

- Metastatic disease from similar neoplasms arising in the pancreas, ovary, or appendix

Treatment

- Complete surgical excision

Prognosis

- 50% survive 4 years
- Presence of an ovarianlike, spindle cell stroma associated with a more favorable prognosis

Associations

- None

Biliary Cystadenoma

Clinical Manifestations

- Represents 5% of all solitary cysts of liver
- 95% develop in women
- Mean age at diagnosis 45 years
- Patients typically complain of abdominal pain, abdominal mass, and occasionally jaundice
- Serum levels of CA 19-9 usually elevated

Gross Pathology

- Tends to be multilocular (occasionally unilocular)
- 85% intrahepatic; remainder occur in common bile duct, hepatic ducts, cystic duct, and gallbladder
- Intrahepatic lesions tend to be encapsulated and solitary; range in size from 1.5 to 20 cm
- Cyst fluid usually clear and mucinous, but may be brown, serous, bilious, gelatinous, or hemorrhagic
- Internal surfaces usually smooth with few trabeculations or polypoid cystic projections
- Intracystic gallstones may be present
- Nodules of solid tissue may be present (a finding that should raise the suspicion of malignancy)

Microscopic Pathology

- *Mucinous type*
  - A 3-layered structure: epithelial lining, cellular ovarianlike stroma, and outer hyalinized, fibrous layer
  - Lining epithelium resembles biliary or gastric foveolar cells and tends to have basally oriented nuclei and apical mucin; in areas it may be flattened, denuded, or pseudostratified
  - Foci resembling squamous cells may be present
  - Intestinal metaplasia (goblet cells and occasionally Paneth cells) present in 20%; neuroendocrine cells present in 30%
  - Areas of dysplasia may be present (raising the possibility of a borderline malignancy)
  - In 80% there is a dense subepithelial spindle cell stroma that resembles normal ovarian stroma (only seen in female patients); this spindle cell stroma may be quite focal and may contain areas of both smooth muscle and mature adipose
  - A focal, linear, hyalinized collagenous zone frequently present between epithelium and dense stroma (reminiscent of collagenous zone in collagenous colitis)
  - Outer or adventitial capsular layer consists of dense collagen and separates the cystadenoma from surrounding liver parenchyma; frequently contains blood vessels and anomalous bile ducts
  - Foamy histiocytes, multinucleated giant cells, hemosiderin-laden macrophages, and cholesterol may be present throughout
- *Serous type*
  - Small cystic spaces lined by flat, bland cells with clear (glycogen) cytoplasm
  - No dense spindle-cell stroma

Special Stains

- Mucicarmine will highlight the mucinous nature of the lining epithelium of mucinous type

Immunohistochemistry

- Epithelial cells positive for cytokeratin, EMA, CEA, and CA19-9
- Spindle cells of ovarianlike stroma typically estrogen and progesterone receptor positive
- Focal areas of immunoreactivity for muscle specific actin and vimentin may be seen within the dense spindle cell stroma

Electron Microscopy

- 3 cell types in stroma: undifferentiated mesenchymal cells, fibroblasts, and myofibroblasts
- Epithelial cells have luminal microvilli and mucin droplets

Molecular Alterations

- None

Differential Diagnosis

- Hepatitic metastasis from similar neoplasms arising in the pancreas, ovary, or appendix
- Choledochal cyst (never multiloculated)
- Retention cyst of periductal gland etiology

Treatment

- Complete excision

Prognosis

- A benign neoplasm
- Malignant transformation not reported in extrahepatic lesions even when dysplastic epithelium present

Associations

- May coexist with an identical lesion in the pancreas

Gallbladder Carcinoma

Clinical Manifestations

- Most common malignant tumor of biliary tract
- Found in 1% to 2% of cholecystectomies (more frequently found during open cholecystectomy than laparoscopic cholecystectomy)
- 90% of patients over the age of 70 years; a focus of invasive carcinoma present in 10% of gallbladders removed in patients over age of 65 years
- Affects women more frequently than men (2-3:1)
- Cholelithiasis present in 70% to 90% (risk of carcinoma in a patient with cholelithiasis <1%)
- Symptoms typically similar to those of benign disease until invasion occurs; invasive disease characterized by pain, jaundice, anorexia, and weight loss
- Disease inoperable at the time of diagnosis in 50%
- Serum levels of CEA and CA19-9 frequently elevated

Gross Pathology

- Most appear as infiltrating gray to white mass
- Occasionally large, bulky, intraluminal polypoid lesion may be present
- Most originate from the fundus (60%); 30% arise in the body and 10% in the neck
- Extension into adjacent liver present in 80%

Microscopic Pathology

- Tumor cells may resemble biliary, gastric foveolar, or intestinal epithelium
- Most are well to moderately differentiated adenocarcinomas (75%); degree of differentiation determined by percentage of tumor-containing glands (well: 95%; moderate: 40%-95%; poor: 5%-40%)
- Superficial portion of the tumor may be more well-differentiated than deeper areas
- Tumor cells columnar with eosinophilic, slightly granular cytoplasm and round or oval basal or centrally located nuclei with vesicular or coarsely granular chromatin; scattered goblet cells frequently present
- Foci of squamous differentiation present in 5% to 10%
- Choriocarcinomalike foci may be present
- Mitotic activity quite variable

- Papillary lesions frequently show some degree of intestinal differentiation with goblet cells, Paneth cells, and neuroendocrine cells
- Other histologic variants include: mucinous (4% to 7%) and signet-ring cell (3%)
- Rare variants include: adenosquamous, clear cell, squamous, and small cell
- Undifferentiated carcinoma (sarcomatoid, pleomorphic, giant cell, or spindle cell) represents 5% to 10% of cases; cells typically large, pleomorphic, polygonal, or spindle-shaped

Special Stains

- Mucicarmine or Alcian blue may be helpful in establishing presence of mucin in some tumor cells and in neoplastic glands

Immunohistochemistry

- Tumor cells typically cytokeratin, EMA, CEA, and tumor-associated antigen CA19-9 positive
- Well-differentiated tumors often have positive nuclear staining for p53 protein

Electron Microscopy

- Findings resemble normal gallbladder epithelium with the exception of no basal cells
- Tumor cells contain mucin and are covered by microvilli that project into gland lumina
- Focal intestinal metaplasia can be identified in 30%

Molecular Alterations

- K-*ras* codon 12 mutation
- p53 protein expression
- APC gene mutation
- Amplification of *c-erb*-2 gene in 30%-45%

Differential Diagnosis

- Cribriform, clear cell, and pseudoangiosarcomatous variants (all very rare) may resemble metastatic breast cancer, metastatic renal cell carcinoma, and primary clear cell squamous cell carcinoma or angiosarcoma, respectively
- Cholesterolosis may resemble signet-ring cell carcinoma

Treatment

- Cholecystectomy with wedge liver resection (extended cholecystectomy) and en bloc removal of regional nodes and resection of extrahepatic bile duct
- Adjuvant chemotherapy and radiotherapy of little value

Prognosis

- Tumor confined to gallbladder: 10-year survival rate 35%; regional disease: 10-year survival rate <10%
- Disease confined to mucosa typically usually cured with simple cholecystectomy
- 50% to 80% of patients have positive regional lymph nodes at time of presentation
- 5-year survival 35% for papillary carcinoma and 10% to 15% for adenocarcinoma

Associations

- Porcelain gallbladder (diffuse calcification) 10% to 25%
- Mirizzi syndrome (impaction of stone in gallbladder neck or cystic duct with extrinsic compression or obstruction of adjacent common bile duct, causing jaundice)
- Abnormal choledochopancreatic junction (union of pancreatic and common bile ducts outside wall of duodenum) with or without a choledochal cyst
- Ulcerative colitis/primary sclerosing cholangitis)
- Familial adenomatous polyposis (25% of patients with familial adenomatous polyposis have gallbladder dysplasia)
- Peutz-Jeghers syndrome
- Infection with *Salmonella typhi*
- Krabbe disease
- Down syndrome

References

Albores-Saavedra J, Henson DE, Klimstra DS. *Tumors of the Gallbladder, Extrahepatic Bile Ducts, and Ampulla of Vater: Atlas of Tumor Pathology, 3rd Series, Fascicle 27*. Washington DC: Armed Forces Institute of Pathology, 2000.

Burt AD, Portmann BC, Ferrell, LD (eds). *MacSween's Pathology of the Liver. 5th ed.* New York: Churchill Livingstone, 2007.

Dabbs DJ. *Diagnostic Immunohistochemistry*. New York: Churchill Livingstone, 2002.

Hamilton SR, Aaitonen LA (eds). *World Health Organization Classification of Tumours. Pathology and Genetics of Tumours of the Digestive System.* Lyon: IARC Press, 2000.

Ishak KG, Goodman ZD, Stocker JT. *Tumors of the Liver and Intrahepatic Bile Ducts: Atlas of Tumor Pathology, 3rd Series, Fascicle 31*. Washington DC: Armed Forces Institute of Pathology, 2001.

Lee R. *Diagnostic Liver Pathology. 1st ed.* St. Louis: Mosby-Yearbook Inc, 1994.

Mills S, Carter D, Greenson JK, Oberman HA, Reuter V, Stoler MH (eds). *Sternberg's Diagnostic Surgical Pathology. 4th ed.* Philadelphia: Lippincott Williams & Wilkins, 2004.

Odze RD, Goldblum JR, Crawford, JM. *Surgical Pathology of the GI Tract, Liver, and Pancreas.* Philadelphia: WB Saunders, 2004.

Rosai J. *Rosai and Ackerman's Surgical Pathology. 9th ed.* St. Louis: Mosby, 2004.

Scheuer PJ, Lefkowitch JH. *Liver Biopsy Interpretation. 7th ed.* London: Elsevier Saunders, 2006.

Chapter 9

Pancreas

Intraoperative Consultation

Requests for intraoperative consultation during operations on the pancreas typically involve neoplasms in the head of the gland or periampullary region, solid tumors of the body and tail of the gland, cystic lesions, and islet cell tumors.

Neoplastic disease involving the head of the pancreas and periampullary region is typically evaluated quite extensively before surgery. Despite the variety of localizing and diagnostic tests available to evaluate neoplasms in this region, 20% of all lesions felt to be resectable before surgery will be found to be unresectable at the time of exploration. The role of intraoperative consultation on lesions arising in the head of the pancreas or in the periampullary region typically involves evaluation of tissue outside the limits of potential resection. The presence of metastatic disease usually obviates resection. If metastases are present, a palliative procedure is performed.

If there is no obvious extrapancreatic disease, most surgeons do not require tissue confirmation of malignancy before performing a pancreaticoduodenectomy. Reasons for not obtaining intraoperative consultation in this setting include the following:

- A failure to confirm the presence of malignancy should not deter the operating surgeon from resecting what clinically appears to be a malignancy
- Small, eminently curable lesions may not be technically amenable to sampling and tissue confirmation
- Clinical diagnosis of malignancy based on preoperative evaluation is accurate in over 95% of cases
- The morbidity and mortality of a pancreatico-duodenectomy is low enough to justify an occasional resection for benign disease
- A biopsy may result in seeding malignancy outside the pancreas

When pancreaticoduodenectomy is performed, evaluation of the distal pancreatic margin, the margin at the uncinate process where it abuts the superior mesenteric artery (retroperitoneal margin), and the common bile duct margin is frequently requested. Chronic pancreatitis typically accompanies carcinoma. Well-differentiated pancreatic carcinoma may mimic the atypical architectural and cytologic changes seen in the pancreas in the setting of chronic pancreatitis.

Pancreaticoduodenectomy is rarely performed for a distal bile duct lesion without tissue confirmation. Inflammation and fibrosis resulting from the presence of a calculus or biliary stent often produces architectural and cytologic changes that mimic a carcinoma. Once pancreaticoduodenectomy is performed, a frozen section evaluation of the superior bile duct margin and the transected pancreas margins are almost always requested.

Ampullary lesions can be particularly problematic on frozen section. Adenomas arising in the area of the ampulla with or without invasion are difficult to orient, tend to be large, and are frequently associated with the presence of accessory pancreatic ductal tissue in the ampulla which may mimic well-differentiated adenocarcinoma.

A solid tumor in the body or tail of the pancreas is usually a pancreatic carcinoma, a solid-pseudopapillary tumor, or an islet cell tumor. Carcinomas in this location are rarely resectable (<5%). When a resection is performed, intraoperative consultation on the proximal margin will be requested. A solid-pseudopapillary neoplasm is usually not a difficult intraoperative diagnosis. These neoplasms occur almost exclusively in women under the age of 35 years and are readily recognized on gross inspection. Intraoperative consultation on functioning and nonfunctioning islet cell tumors typically involves confirmation of the presence of neoplasm. Islet cell tumors can occasionally demonstrate distinct gland formation, hence may be confused with a well-differentiated adenocarcinoma. In addition, endocrine cell hyperplasia frequently accompanies chronic pancreatitis and can easily be confused with an endocrine neoplasm or an undifferentiated carcinoma. Duodenal gastrinomas are notoriously small (frequently <2 mm in maximal dimension) and require careful examination of the submitted material. Possible intra-abdominal metastasis resulting from a malignant endocrine cell tumor should be examined by frozen section analysis, because the confirmation of malignancy will typically obviate a radical pancreatic resection. The diagnosis of malignancy in an endocrine neoplasm requires the unequivocal presence of local invasion or metastasis. Cytologic atypia and mitotic activity are not enough to warrant the diagnosis of malignancy. Occasionally a nonfunctioning islet cell tumor will be encountered as an incidental finding at operation. These lesions can mimic an undifferentiated carcinoma; the differential diagnosis is an important one.

Cystic lesions of the pancreas include pseudocyst, serous cystadenoma, cystic mucinous neoplasms, and solid-pseudopapillary tumor. A request for an intraoperative evaluation of the surgical margin may accompany a resected cystic lesion. Differentiating a pseudocyst from a serous or mucinous cystic neoplasm can be problematic if the cells lining the cyst desquamate leaving a cyst wall without an epithelial lining. This problem is particularly likely to occur with mucinous tumors. Surgeons faced with what intraoperatively has been confirmed to be a mucinous neoplasm should perform a complete resection with clear margins if at all possible. These tumors even when frankly malignant often show no obvious evidence of invasion. An invasive component may be quite focal and found only after extensive sampling of the lesion.

Specimen Handling

A pancreaticoduodenectomy specimen should be oriented to preserve all the anatomic relationships, pinned on a styrofoam board to preserve those relationships, and completely fixed before sectioning. The common bile duct surgical margin, pancreatic surgical margin, and the margin where the uncinate process abuts the superior mesenteric artery should be inked. The stomach and jejunum, if included with the specimen, can be removed and do not need to be sectioned unless abnormal on gross examination. The remaining pancreatic head, bile duct, and duodenum are serially sectioned from proximal to distal using the duodenum as a reference point. The sections are taken in a transverse plane perpendicular to the long axis of the pancreas. One section should be taken across the ampulla. Whenever possible, sections should be submitted to demonstrate the relationship of neoplasm to the transected pancreatic margin, intrapancreatic bile duct, the duodenum, and the retroperitoneal in origin.

Tumors of Pancreatic Ducts

Ductal Adenocarcinoma

Clinical Manifestations

- Represent 85% of all pancreatic tumors
- Typically occur in the elderly (60-80 years); rare under age of 40 years (~5%)
- Slight male predominance (1.5 to 1)
- 4th most common cause of death from cancer in the United States
- When carcinoma localized to the head, patients present with progressive jaundice, weight loss, puritis, and pain (50%)
- When localized to the body and tail, may cause back pain or be asymptomatic; usually metastatic at time of diagnosis
- Other manifestations include pancreatitis, hypoglycemia, hypercalcemia, endocarditis, and migratory thrombophlebitis *(Trousseau sign)*
- Diabetes present in 70%

Gross Pathology

- 2/3 located in the head (usually upper half) and 1/3 in the body or tail
- 20% multiple
- Cut surface tends to be ill-defined, hard, and yellow-white; foci of hemorrhage and/or necrosis rare; occasionally microcystic areas
- Tumors in the head of the pancreas often obstruct the distal common bile duct and main pancreatic duct causing marked dilatation of both
- Extrapancreatic extension is common with direct extension into the duodenum in 25% of those that arise in the head and into the retroperitoneum in most that arise in the body and tail

Microscopic Pathology

- Irregularly shaped and distributed glands within a concentric desmoplastic stroma
- Perineural invasion present in 90%
- Lobular pancreatic tissue often destroyed; islet tissue may be preserved, especially in well-differentiated tumors
- Changes of pancreatitis (fibrosis and inflammation) in non-neoplastic gland common
- Carcinoma in situ in adjacent ductal epithelium (pancreatic intraepithelial neoplasia—PanIN-III) frequently present
- Well-differentiated:
    - Irregularly distributed large ductlike structures and medium-sized neoplastic glands in tubular or cribriform patterns in a desmoplastic stroma

- Mucin-producing tumor cells are typically columnar with clear to eosinophilic cytoplasm and large round or oval, pleomorphic nuclei with prominent nucleoli
- Normal lobular architecture lost
- Few mitotic figures

- Moderately differentiated:
  - Variably shaped, medium-sized ductlike and tubular structures replace acini and form an irregular pattern in desmoplastic stroma
  - Incompletely formed glands common
  - Large ductlike structures rare
  - Mucin content of tumor cells decreased
  - Cellular atypia with markedly pleomorphic nuclei and mitotic figures common
- Poorly differentiated:
  - Uncommon
  - Densely packed small irregular glands and solid sheets of tumor cells with marked pleomorphism and mitotic activity completely replace acinar tissue
  - Tumor cells in solid sheets often contain large bizarre nuclei
  - Foci of squamoid differentiation, spindle cells, or anaplasia present in 20%
  - Foci of hemorrhage or necrosis may be present
- Microscopic variants:
  - *Adenosquamous carcinoma*: A variable admixture of solid squamoid (at least 30% of tumor) and ductal structures; metastasis consists of adenocarcinoma component
  - *Clear cell carcinoma*: Characterized by nests and sheets of glycogen-rich cells with some mucin-containing cells
  - *Signet ring cell carcinoma*: Composed exclusively of signet-ring cells infiltrating throughout the gland
  - *Mixed ductal-endocrine carcinoma*: Characterized by an admixture of malignant epithelial cells and endocrine cells; endocrine cells must comprise 35% to 50% of tumor
  - *Mucinous non-cystic carcinoma*: Characterized by large pools of mucin containing aggregates, strands, and single tumor cells; mucin represents more than 50% of tumor; pseudomyxoma peritonei may develop
  - *Undifferentiated (anaplastic) carcinoma*: Tumor cells are large and pleomorphic with bizarre nuclei and/or spindle-shaped cells, often with sarcomatoid features and areas of squamoid differentiation
  - *Undifferentiated carcinoma with osteoclastlike giant cells:* Characterized by pleomorphic to spindle-shaped malignant cells and scattered non-neoplastic osteoclastlike giant cells that contain 20 or more small uniform nuclei; in situ or invasive adenocarcinoma often present; giant cells tend to be located near areas of hemorrhage and contain hemosiderin; osteoid may be present

Special Stains

- Tumor cells positive for sulfated (acid) mucins and focally positive for neutral mucins (periodic acid-Schiff [PAS] with diastase and Alcian blue pH 2.5)

Immunohistochemistry

- Most positive for MUC1 (mucin antibody to mucin produced in gastric foveolar cells), MUC3, and MUC5/6 (but not MUC2)
- Tumor cells almost always positive for carcinoembryonic antigen (CEA; luminal contents, luminal border, and cytoplasm of well-differentiated cells stain strongly; poorly differentiated cells stain weakly)
- CEA is negative in normal pancreas, chronic pancreatitis, serous cystadenoma, acinar carcinoma, pancreatoblastoma, and endocrine tumors
- Tumor cells express cytokeratins 7, 8, 18, and 19

Electron Microscopy

- Tumor cells have mucin granules in apical cytoplasm, irregular microvilli on luminal surface, and a generally polarized arrangement of pleomorphic nuclei
- Poorly differentiated tumor cells lose their polarity, basal lamina, luminal spaces, and mucin granules

Molecular Alterations

- 95% have inactivation of tumor suppressor gene *p16* on chromosome 9p
- 90% have a point mutation of the K-*ras* gene on chromosome 12p
- 55% have inactivation of tumor suppressor gene SMAD4 on chromosome 18q
- 50% to 70% have inactivation of tumor suppressor gene *p53* on chromosome 17p
- Other damaged genetic loci include *AKT* (19q), *MYB* (6q), *AIB1* (20q), *BRCA2* (13q), *LKB1* (19p), *MKK4* (17p), *TGFβ-R2* (9q), *TGFβ-R2* (3p), and *RB1* (13q)
- 3% to 10% familial

Differential Diagnosis

- Chronic pancreatitis
- Ampullary carcinoma (ductal adenocarcinoma of the pancreas is indistinguishable from carcinoma of the ampulla and carcinoma arising from the intrapancreatic portion of the common bile duct using histologic and immunohistochemical criteria; differentiation requires gross and microscopic localization which may not always be possible in advanced lesions)
- Pancreatoblastoma
- Intraductal papillary-mucinous tumor
- Acinar carcinoma
- Neuroendocrine tumor
- Solid-pseudopapillary tumor

Treatment

- Surgical resection (10%-20% are resectable at the time of initial abdominal exploration)
- Unresectable lesions typically treated with biliary and/or gastric bypass
- 10% respond to chemotherapy with 5-flurouracil
- Radiotherapy ineffective

Prognosis

- Less than 5% 5-year survival; median survival for resected cases 12 to 18 months with reported 5-year survival of up to 20%
- Prognosis determined by tumor site, stage, microscopic grade, and size

Associations

- Squamous cell carcinoma (possibly a variant of adenosquamous carcinoma) may be associated with hypercalcemia
- Prior partial gastrectomy, smoking, increased intake of dietary fat and coffee, exposure to chlorinated hydrocarbons, radiation exposure, and diabetes mellitus
- Peutz-Jeghers syndrome
- Hereditary nonpolyposis colon cancer (HNPCC)
- FAMMM (*f*amilial *a*typical *m*ultiple *m*ole-*m*elanoma) syndrome, characterized by increased risk of developing both melanoma and pancreatic carcinoma; associated with germline mutations in p16 tumor suppressor gene on 9p
- Hereditary pancreatitis, characterized by early onset of severe recurrent bouts of acute pancreatitis; germline mutations in cationic trypsinogen gene on chromosome 7q35; lifetime risk of developing pancreatic carcinoma 40%
- *BRCA2*: Second breast cancer suppressor gene on chromosome 13q inactivated in 7%

Serous Cystic Neoplasms

Serous Cystadenocarcinoma

Clinical Manifestations

- Extremely rare
- Usually present with an upper abdominal mass with or without jaundice

Gross Pathology

- Usually large (10-12 cm) with a spongy appearance
- Local invasion into adjacent organs (stomach) and metastatic disease may be present

Microscopic Findings

- Histologic features of both primary tumor and metastatic foci essentially the same as serous microcystic adenoma; focal, mild nuclear pleomorphism may be present

Special Stains

- PAS without diastase stains cells lining cysts confirming presence of intracytoplasmic glycogen
- PAS with diastase and Alcian blue both negative
- Mucin stains negative

Immunohistochemistry

- Cells lining cyst are positive for EMA and cytokeratin 7, 8, 18, and 19
- Cells negative for CEA, neuroendocrine markers, S-100 protein, desmin, and vimentin

Electron Microscopy

- Cells contain glycogen and have short, poorly developed microvilli on apical surface
- Myoepithelial cells lie beneath some epithelial cells
- No zymogen or neurosecretory granules

Molecular Alterations

- Loss of heterozygosity at von Hippel-Lindau gene locus (3p25)

Differential Diagnosis

- All other cystic lesions of the pancreas
- Mucinous cystic neoplasms
- Solid-pseudopapillary epithelial tumor
- Acinar cell cystadenocarcinoma
- Lymphangioma
- Renal cell carcinoma

Treatment

- Resection for cure or palliation

Prognosis

- Very slow growing

Associations

- None

Serous Microcystic Adenoma

Clinical Manifestations

- 1% to 2% of all exocrine pancreatic tumors
- Occurs in the elderly and is more common in women (70%)
- Often asymptomatic
- If located in the head of pancreas, may cause bile duct obstruction with jaundice

Gross Pathology

- May occur anywhere in the pancreas; 50% to 65% in body or tail
- Usually solitary and well demarcated from adjacent normal pancreatic tissue; occasionally pancreas diffusely involved
- Usually partially encapsulated and composed of innumerable small cysts of varying sizes filled with serous (clear water) or blood tinged fluid
- Central stellate scar (may be calcified in tumors >5 cm)
- Foci of hemorrhage common

Microscopic Findings

- Neoplasm is separated from adjacent pancreas by a fibrous capsule that may or may not be complete; composed of small cysts lined by a single layer of small, cuboidal epithelial cells with clear cytoplasm (glycogen) and a round, central nucleus with an inconspicuous nucleolus
- Occasionally tumor cells form tiny papillae without fibrovascular stalks
- No atypia and no mitotic activity
- Thin acellular stroma that may contain islets of Langerhans, acini, ducts, nerves, and lymphocytes, and separates cysts
- Central stellate scar consists of hyalinized tissue with aggregates of tiny cysts

Special Stains

- PAS without diastase stains cells lining cysts confirming presence of intracytoplasmic glycogen
- PAS with diastase and Alcian blue both negative
- Mucin stains negative

Immunohistochemistry

- Cells lining cyst are positive for EMA and cytokeratins 7, 8, 18, and 19
- Cells negative for CEA, neuroendocrine markers, S-100 protein, desmin, and vimentin

Electron Microscopy

- Cells contain glycogen and have short, poorly developed microvilli on apical surface
- Myoepithelial cells lie beneath some epithelial cells
- No zymogen or neurosecretory granules

Molecular Alterations

- Loss of heterozygosity at von Hippel-Lindau gene locus (3p25)

Differential Diagnosis

- All other cystic lesions of the pancreas
- Mucinous cystic neoplasms
- Solid-pseudopapillary epithelial tumor
- Acinar cell cystadenocarcinoma
- Lymphangioma
- Renal cell carcinoma

Treatment

- Resection or bilary bypass if neoplasm is symptomatic

Prognosis

- Excellent; minimal risk of malignant transformation

Associations

- von Hippel-Lindau disease: retinal angiomatosis; cerebellar hemangioblastoma; renal cell carcinoma; pheochromocytoma; and renal, liver, lung, and splenic cysts (polycystic changes in pancreas tend to be diffuse)
- Evan syndrome (autoimmune hemolytic anemia and idiopathic thrombocytopenic purpura)
- Coincidental association with gallstones, diabetes mellitus, and extrapancreatic malignancy

Serous Oligocystic Adenoma

Clinical Manifestations

- Much less common than microcystic adenoma
- Occurs in adults over the age of 60 years and affects both sexes equally
- Symptoms consist of upper abdominal pain and discomfort; bile duct obstruction may result in jaundice

Gross Pathology

- Most located in the head and body
- Cut surface demonstrates a few (occasionally one) irregularly arranged cysts separated by broad fibrous septa and filled with clear watery or blood tinged fluid
- A fibrous stroma; no central stellate scar

Microscopic Findings

- Tumor cells similar to serous microcystic adenoma except lining cells may be more cuboidal and have larger nuclei
- Fibrous stroma usually fairly prominent and hyalinized
- Fibrous capsule sparse and small cysts may extend into adjacent pancreas

Special Stains

- PAS without diastase stains cells lining cysts confirming presence of intracytoplasmic glycogen
- PAS with diastase and Alcian blue both negative
- Mucin stains negative

Immunohistochemistry

- Cells lining cyst are positive for EMA and cytokeratin 7, 8, 18, and 19
- Cells negative for CEA, neuroendocrine markers, S-100 protein, desmin, and vimentin

Electron Microscopy

- Cells contain glycogen and have short, poorly developed microvilli on apical surface
- Myoepithelial cells lie beneath some epithelial cells
- No zymogen or neurosecretory granules

Molecular Alterations

- Loss of heterozygosity at von Hippel-Lindau gene locus (3p25)

Differential Diagnosis

- All other cystic lesions of the pancreas
- Mucinous cystic neoplasms
- Solid-pseudopapillary epithelial tumor
- Acinar cell cystadenocarcinoma
- Lymphangioma
- Renal cell carcinoma

Treatment

- Resection or bilary bypass if neoplasm is symptomatic

Prognosis

- Excellent; minimal risk of malignant transformation

Associations

- None

Mucinous Cystic Neoplasms

Classification

- A spectrum of tumors: *mucinous cystadenoma*, *mucinous cystic tumor of borderline malignant potential*, and *mucinous cystadenocarcinoma* (same classification as mucinous tumors of the ovary that they closely resemble)

Clinical Manifestations

- Represents 2% to 2.5% of all exocrine pancreatic neoplasms
- Occurs almost exclusively in young to middle-aged women (40 to 60 years)
- Often presents with vague intermittent or continuous abdominal pain
- Upper abdominal mass frequently palpable
- Presentation may be similar to that of pancreatic cancer with gradual onset of weakness, anorexia, and weight loss, usually without jaundice

Gross Pathology

- Majority (80%) occur in the body and tail of the pancreas; occasionally attached to the pancreas by a narrow tissue stalk
- External surface lobulated and glistening
- Cut surface reveals a single cyst or multiple cysts filled with thick gelatinous (occasionally hemorrhagic) material enclosed in a well-defined dense fibrous capsule (very similar in appearance to a pseudocyst)
- Lining of unilocular tumors usually smooth; multilocular tumors often contain papillary excrescences, solid nodules, and protuberances
- Cyst(s) typically do not communicate with duct system
- Malignant tumors may or may not show obvious evidence of invasion into adjacent pancreas or adjacent organs and/or tissue

Microscopic Pathology

- Cysts lined by a single flat row of tall columnar epithelium with basally oriented nuclei and abundant, predominantly acidic mucin (occasionally papillary or polypoid projections present)
- Cells reminiscent of goblet cells are typically admixed with the columnar cells; endocrine cells are present in 70% to 90%; absorptive-type cells and rare Paneth cells also present
- Various degrees of dysplasia may be present in different areas of epithelium

Mucinous Cystadenoma

- Cells have little evidence of dysplasia (slight increase in size of basal nuclei) and no mitotic activity

Mucinous Cystic Tumor of Borderline Malignant Potential

- Cells of a *borderline mucinous tumor* have moderate dysplasia (cellular pseudostratification with crowded atypical, enlarged nuclei with 1 or more prominent nucleoli) and mitoses; papillary projections or cryptlike invaginations typically present
- Subepithelial stroma consists of an inner layer of moderately dense, plump spindle cells with round nuclei (reminiscent of ovarian stroma often with some degree of luteinization) and an outer layer of collagenous connective tissue; stroma may contain ducts, islets, aggregates of lymphocytes, large blood vessels, foci of hemorrhage and calcification, and chronic inflammatory changes to include a foreign body-type giant cell reaction to extravasated mucin
- Fibrous atrophy may be present in adjacent pancreas

Mucinous Cystadenocarcinoma

- Cells have high-grade dysplasia, carcinoma in situ features that may be very focal (nuclear stratification, marked nuclear atypia, and many mitotic figures; cellular mucin is much reduced); cells form papillae with irregular branching or complex architecture; may be noninvasive or invasive; invasive tumors are characterized by obvious invasion of stroma by atypical glands

Special Stains

- Tumor cells stain with PAS with diastase and Alcian blue
- Endocrine cells can be easily identified with argyrophil and argentaffin stains

Immunochemistry

- Tumor cells positive for EMA, CA19-9, and cytokeratins 7, 8, 18, and 19
- Well-differentiated columnar cells stain in a linear fashion at their apical surface for CEA; highly dysplastic cells demonstrate cytoplasmic staining for CEA
- Endocrine cells are chromogranin A and NSE positive
- Stromal cells positive for vimentin, α smooth muscle actin, and usually estrogen and progesterone receptors

Electron Microscopy

- Columnar epithelial cells lie on a basement membrane and have well-developed microvilli at their apices and mucin granules in apical cytoplasm

Molecular Alterations

- None

Differential Diagnosis

- Pseudocyst
- Intraductal papillary-mucinous tumor
- Serous microcystic adenoma
- Solid-pseudopapillary tumor
- Acinar cell cystadenocarcinoma
- Mucinous noncystic adenocarcinoma
- Cystic endocrine tumors
- Lymphoepithelial cyst

Treatment

- Complete resection
- Internal or external drainage of a mucinous cystic tumor or incomplete excision may result in recurrence as an invasive cystadenocarcinoma

Prognosis

- Excellent if neoplasm completely excised
- Good prognosis if invasive component of mucinous cystadenocarcinoma is limited to stroma
- Unresectable mucinous cystadenocarcinoma has same prognosis as invasive ductal carcinoma

Associations

- Malignant fibrous histiocytoma, mesenchymal giant cell tumor, sarcoma, pseudosarcomatous carcinoma, and anaplastic carcinoma may occur in a mucinous cystic neoplasm
- Presence of endocrine cells may result in production of serotonin, somatostatin, gastrin, and pancreatic polypeptide with the appropriate symptoms
- Diabetes mellitus (replacement of pancreas by tumor)

Intraductal Papillary-Mucinous Tumor (IPMN)

Clinical Manifestations

- 5% to 10% of all exocrine pancreatic tumors
- Twice as common in men as in women; peak age 6th decade
- Presenting symptoms frequently those of acute or chronic pancreatitis as a result of temporary or permanent obstruction of the main pancreatic duct by viscous mucin; 50% develop diabetes mellitus, steatorrhea, or both; tumor involving the ampulla may result in jaundice
- Most reported cases have come from Japan

Gross Pathology

- 80% occur in the head
- Cut surface reveals dilated pancreatic duct (1 to 8 cm) that contains a single or multiple sessile tumors and thick mucinous material; occasionally the entire duct is studded with tumor; mucin may extrude through the ampulla of Vater

- Tumors tend to be soft and friable and gray to tan
- Tumor may involve predominately major ducts or may be limited to the secondary ducts; most occur in the main pancreatic duct and its branches in the head of the gland
- Surrounding pancreatic tissue typically hard, nodular and severely fibrotic
- Invasive tumor usually not readily apparent

Microscopic Findings

- Dilated pancreatic duct(s) lined with tall columnar mucin-producing epithelial cells that form papillary projections of various sizes; intraluminal mucin deposition typically responsible for the ductal dilatation
- Gobletlike cells, argyrophilic cells, and cells with oncocytic differentiation may be admixed with columnar cells
- 2 distinct papillary patterns: intestinal type (85%) and pancreaticobiliary type (15%)
- Degree of differentiation of neoplastic cells ranges from normal to very dysplastic, often in the same tumor
- Pancreatic parenchyma surrounding dilated ducts has the atrophic and fibrotic changes of chronic pancreatitis and lacks any ovarian-type stroma
- No calcifications
- Tumors are graded or classified according to degree of dysplasia and presence or absence of invasion; invasive carcinoma present in about 35%

Adenoma

- Mild dysplasia; well-formed papillae with fibrovascular cores; cells tall and columnar and have apical mucin and basal nuclei; nuclei round or oval and slightly enlarged; no mitotic figures

Tumor of Borderline Malignant Potential

- Mild to moderate dysplasia; irregular elongated papillae with small fibrovascular cores; mucin content of individual cells variable; nuclei tend to be crowded, stratified, irregular, hyperchromatic, elongated, and contain a prominent nucleolus; mitoses frequent

Intraductal Carcinoma (Non-Invasive)

- Severe focal or diffuse dysplasia; papillae are crowded with irregular branching and budding; cribriform pattern may be evident; no fibrovascular cores; cells contain little or no mucin and have large, pleomorphic, very stratified nuclei with a prominent nucleolus; mitoses common

Papillary-Mucinous Carcinoma

- Focal or diffuse invasion of adjacent pancreatic parenchyma; associated findings include intraductal papillary-mucinous borderline tumor or intraductal carcinoma; invasive component usually has features of a mucinous noncystic carcinoma with pools of mucin containing free-floating atypical glandular structures and tumor cells, but may consist of atypical ductal structures

Special Stains

- PAS with diastase stains the columnar tumor cells
- If stained with Alcian blue (pH 2.5 and 1.0) the mucin proves to consist of a combination of sulfomucins, sialomucins, and neutral mucins

Immunohistochemistry

- Most tumor cells positive for EMA, CEA, M1 (a gastric type mucin marker), several keratins, and are frequently positive for CA19-9 and B72.3
- C-*erb*-B-2 product usually overexpressed
- MUC1 (mammary-type mucin) commonly expressed in pancreaticobiliary type; MUC2 more commonly expressed in intestinal type
- Normal duct cells typically secrete sulfated mucins, adenomas characteristically secrete neutral mucin, and dysplastic lesions secrete mostly sialomucin

Electron Microscopy

- Microvilli on apical surface and mucin granules
- Occasional nuclei are cleaved and have pseudoinclusions

Molecular Alterations

- Increased incidence of point mutations at codon 12 in K-*ras* gene
- p53 protein expression in tumors with moderate or severe dysplasia

Differential Diagnosis

- Mucinous cystic tumor (almost always affects women; median age fifth decade; thick wall with "ovarianlike" stroma; no communication with duct system)
- Ductal adenocarcinoma
- Ductal papillary hyperplasia
- Chronic pancreatitis

Treatment

- Complete resection

Prognosis

- Only 10% to 20% are invasive
- Prognosis generally good (overall 5-year survival rate for a composite series 80%-85%), but depends on presence and extent of invasion at the time of surgery

Associations

- May fistulize to duodenum
- 1 case reported in association with a choledochal cyst
- No association with other types of pancreatic neoplasms

Other Rare Exocrine Tumors

Acinar Cell Carcinoma

Clinical Manifestations

- Represents 1% to 2% of all exocrine pancreatic tumors
- Affects males twice as frequently as females
- Mean age at presentation 55 to 60 years; has been reported in children and adolescents (mean age, 8 years)
- Patients typically present with abdominal pain, anorexia, weight loss, and nausea and vomiting; jaundice is unusual; metastases present in 50% at time of diagnosis
- Peripheral eosinophilia may be present

Gross Pathology

- Typically a well-circumscribed, nodular, soft mass evenly distributed throughout the pancreas
- External surface bosselated
- Cut surface reveals a lobular, pale yellow to brown to red neoplasm with fine fibrous strands and focal areas of hemorrhage and necrosis; cystic change may be present especially in the variants; very little stroma

Microscopic Pathology

- Tumor cells typically arranged in large lobules separated by fibrous strands; within the nodule acinar areas frequently alternate with solid areas; occasionally acini are dilated creating "microglandular" structures
- Tumor cells in the acinar areas form small lumina and tend to be uniform in size with abundant finely granular eosinophilic cytoplasm and uniform round basal nuclei, frequently with prominent nucleoli; clumped chromatin may lie next to the inner surface of the nuclear membrane
- Tumor cells arranged in a solid pattern tend to be small, have little cytoplasm and irregular, vesicular nuclei with prominent (often eosinophilic) nucleoli (easily mistaken for being poorly differentiated)
- Trabecular and glandular patterns may be admixed with the more common acinar and solid patterns
- Delicate vessels lie within the fine fibrous bands that course through the tumor
- Mitotic activity in the acinar areas usually <1 mitosis per 10 high power fields (hpf); smaller cells in the solid pattern may have a higher mitotic rate (up to 5 mitoses per 10 hpf)
- A minor component of endocrine cells may be present (as single cells or aggregates)

Special Stains

- PAS with diastase will stain the apical finely granular cytoplasm (zymogen granules) of tumor cells

Immunohistochemistry

- 75% to 100% stain with cytokeratins AE1/AE3 and CAM 5.2 (the latter stains more intensely than the former)
- 90% stain with trypsin and α_1-antichymotrypsin
- 10% to 30% stain focally and weakly with chromogranin
- Tumor cells typically negative for vimentin, α-fetoprotein (AFP), and epithelial membrane antigen (EMA)

Electron Microscopy

- Apical portion of tumor cells contains dense zymogen granules of various sizes
- Cytoplasm also contains abundant rough endoplasmic reticulum, mitochondria, and well-developed Golgi complexes
- Small microvilli present at the apical surface

Molecular Alterations

- p53 and K-*ras* rarely expressed

Differential Diagnosis

- Endocrine tumors (acinar cell carcinomas with a solid and trabecular pattern may mimic low-grade endocrine tumors)
- Solid-pseudopapillary tumors
- Pancreaticoblastoma
- Ductal adenocarcinoma
- Acinar cell adenoma
- Focal acinar cell transformation (a non-neoplastic change in the pancreas characterized by irregular and sharply outlined acinar cell clusters)

Treatment and Prognosis

- Surgical resection with or without radiation and chemotherapy
- 3-year and 5-year survival rates 25% and 5% to 10%, respectively
- Only pathologic parameter of significance is tumor stage

Associations

- May have an endocrine cell component
- 10% to 15% have a *lipase hypersecretion syndrome* characterized by polyarthralgia; extrapancreatic, disseminated fat necrosis; and nonbacterial thrombotic endocarditis

Solid-Pseudopapillary Tumor (Gruber-Frantz Tumor)

Clinical Manifestations

- 1% to 2% of all exocrine pancreatic tumors
- Predominately occurs in adolescent girls and young women; rarely encountered in childhood, older women, or men
- Most frequently diagnosed on routine abdominal examination or because of vague discomfort or pain
- Occasionally the neoplasm is diagnosed after abdominal trauma results in intratumoral hemorrhage
- Jaundice rare even if the tumor is in the head of the gland

Gross Pathology

- May occur anywhere in the pancreas or be parapancreatic; occasionally attached to the surface of the pancreas or located in an extrapancreatic site
- Typically large, round, solitary, and well-demarcated from surrounding normal pancreas
- Cut surface typically lobulated, light brown, and soft with foci of cystic change, hemorrhage, and necrosis; may resemble a pseudocyst
- Calcifications may be present both in the surrounding capsule and in the neoplasm itself
- Rarely invades adjacent organs

Microscopic Pathology

- Tumor is typically well demarcated from normal pancreas, with or without a separating layer of connective tissue; occasional invasion into surrounding pancreas may be present
- Basically 2 architectural patterns: Solid and pseudopapillary
- Small tumors typically have a solid growth pattern characterized by a monotonous population of tumor cells supported by very delicate hyalinized fibrovascular stalks

- Large tumors have a central, pseudopapillary pattern surrounded by a solid pattern (as the neoplasm grows, the cells furthest from the fibrovascular stalks degenerate and lose contact with each other while the cells adjacent to the blood vessels remain viable and attached to the stroma and to each other)
- Amount of preserved or viable tissue in any given tumor depends on its overall size; small tumors are typically well-preserved whereas large tumors only have preserved tissue near the periphery
- Tumor cells tend to be uniform, polygonal to elongated and have eosinophilic to clear cytoplasm and a round to oval, grooved or indented, nucleus with finely dispersed chromatin and an inconspicuous nucleolus
- Solid areas may contain aggregates of tumor cells with foamy cytoplasm and foci of cholesterol crystals surrounded by foreign body giant cells
- Tumor cells lack both mucin and glycogen; large numbers of variably sized intracellular and extracellular eosinophilic globules may be present
- Mitotic figures typically rare (occasionally prominent)
- Hyalinized connective tissue stroma may contain foci of calcification and ossification
- Unequivocal perineural invasion or angioinvasion indicates malignancy (other features indicative of malignant behavior include marked nuclear atypia, increased mitotic rate, and aggregates of necrotic cells)

Special Stains

- Eosinophilic globules within and between tumor cells are PAS-positive; tumor cells themselves do not stain with either PAS or Alcian blue (pH 2.5)

Immunohistochemistry

- Occasional single cells and small clusters of cells stain intensely for both α_1-antitrypsin and α_1-antichymotrypsin
- α_1-antitrypsin will also stain the PAS-positive eosinophilic globules
- Tumor cells typically diffusely positive for both NSE and vimentin
- Tumor cells typically negative for synaptophysin, chromogranin A, CEA, and AFP
- Tumor cells usually estrogen receptor negative; may be progesterone receptor positive
- Cytokeratin positivity present in 30% to 50% (usually focal and faint)

Electron Microscopy

- Tumor cells characterized by an indented nucleus that may contain a small nucleolus and a narrow rim of marginated chromatin; cytoplasm contains numerous mitochondria and may be vacuolated
- Tumor cells contain large zymogenlike granules that may represent deposits of α_1-antrypsin

Molecular Alterations

- None

Differential Diagnosis

- Endocrine tumor
- Acinar cell carcinoma (lack pseudopapillary structures and have a predominantly acinar or trabecular pattern)
- Pancreatoblastoma (tumor cells usually arranged in an acinar pattern and the delicate fibrovascular tissue stalks that characterize a solid-pseudopapillary epithelial tumor are absent)
- Ductal adenocarcinoma
- Cystic tumors

Treatment and Prognosis

- Surgical resection cures 95%
- Vast majority are benign; scattered reports of recurrence or metastases after resection
- Even in the presence of local invasion, recurrence, or metastatic disease, long-term disease-free survival common

Associations

- No associated endocrine syndrome

Pancreatoblastoma

Clinical Manifestations

- Extremely rare, but the most common pancreatic neoplasm in children (30%-50% of pancreatic neoplasms in children)
- Slightly more common in males than females
- Mean age at presentation 4 years; may occur in adults
- More common in Asians than in Caucasians
- Patients frequently have no symptoms and present with an abdominal mass
- Jaundice occurs in fewer than 15%

Gross Pathology

- Neoplasm typically solitary, large, and may be located anywhere in the pancreas
- Tumors may completely replace the pancreas or be attached to it
- Typically a soft, solid mass with a fibrous capsule
- Cut section reveals a well-demarcated mass with lobulation and yellow-tan areas with small pseudocystic, hemorrhagic, and/or necrotic foci
- Neoplasm may invade beyond the pancreas into retroperitoneal tissue and adjacent organs
- Metastases occur in regional lymph nodes, liver, and lung

Microscopic Pathology

- Characterized by relatively uniform, polygonal, epithelial cells arranged in irregular lobules and nests separated by a dense fibrous stroma
- Cells tend to grow in acinar, glandular, trabecular, or solid patterns all of which blend with scattered squamoid cell nests *(squamoid corpuscles)*
- Cells arranged as acinar structures tend to be columnar or cuboidal, have a moderate amphophilic or eosinophilic, finely granular cytoplasm and a round to oval nucleus situated at the basal end of the cell
- Foci of squamoid cell nests and cords are usually present and consist of tumor cells that are polygonal with variably eosinophilic cytoplasm; central keratinization may be present (keratin pearls) as well as foci of necrosis
- Mitotic figures are typically rare
- Dense fibrous stroma separating epithelial areas may contain tubular structures
- Foci of chondroid and osteoid differentiation may be present
- Surrounding fibrous capsule may be infiltrated by tumor cells and frank invasion into the duodenal wall, stomach, and/or peritoneum may be present
- Vascular invasion unusual

Special Stains

- PAS with diastase stains the finely granular eosinophilic cytoplasm of both the cells that make up the acinar areas as well as the cells that make up the squamoid nests
- Alcian blue stain is negative

Immunohistochemistry

- Tumor cells arranged in acinar and solid patterns stain positively for keratin CAM 5.2; they also typically stain positively for lipase, trypsin, chymotrypsin, and α_1-antitrypsin
- Squamoid cells do not stain for CAM 5.2 nor do they stain for pancreatic enzymes or endocrine markers
- Endocrine cells are occasionally scattered throughout the tumor and will stain positively for NSE, synaptophysin, and chromogranin A

Electron Microscopy

- Tumor cells arranged in an acinar pattern have microvilli and are connected to each other by desmosomes; cytoplasm contains large electron-dense zymogenlike granules, well-developed Golgi complexes, and abundant rough endoplasmic reticulum

Molecular Alterations

- Genetic locus for Beckwith-Wiedemann syndrome (see associations below) located on chromosome 11p15.5

Differential Diagnosis

- Acinar cell carcinoma (acinar cell carcinomas do not have squamoid nests)
- Endocrine tumor

- Solid-pseudopapillary tumor (tend to occur in females over the age of 10 years and have a distinct histologic pattern consisting of solid areas alternating with pseudopapillary structures and degenerative pseudocystic lesions)

Treatment and Prognosis

- Surgical excision with adjuvant chemotherapy
- Tumors are malignant and metastasize to lymph nodes and liver (35%)
- 25% of patients alive and disease-free at 5 years if diagnosis made before the development of metastasis

Associations

- Beckwith-Wiedemann syndrome (characterized by exophthalmos, macroglossia, giantism, hemihypertrophy, pancreatic islet cell hyperplasia, pancreatoblastoma, enlarged adrenal glands with cortical cytomegaly, adrenal cortical carcinoma, neuroblastoma, renal medullary cysts, and a predisposition to develop Wilms tumor)

Endocrine Tumors

Clinical Manifestations

- May occur at any age (mean age at diagnosis 58 years)
- Affects males and females equally
- Presents as an incidental finding in approximately 1% of autopsies
- Symptoms typically related to the excessive production of normal pancreatic hormones (insulin, glucagon, somatostatin, and pancreatic polypeptide [PP]), the production of "gut" hormones (gastrin, vasoactive intestinal peptide, and neurotensin), or the production of "ectopic" hormones (adrenocorticotrophic hormone, vasopressin, or parathyroid hormone)
- General signs and symptoms include the presence of abdominal mass and/or abdominal or back pain
- Presence or absence of endocrine symptoms unrelated to tumor size
- Tumors that produce hormones normally produced by the pancreas have a lower malignancy rate (10%-20%) than those producing "gut" hormones (60%-80%) or those producing "ectopic" hormones (90%-100%)

Gross Pathology

- Most are solitary
- Multiple tumors are common in patients with multiple endocrine neoplasia, type 1 (MEN-1)
- Tumors typically well-demarcated and often, at least partly, encapsulated
- Cut surface may be pale gray, tan, pink, red, or yellow depending on amount of stroma, vascularity, and lipid present
- Fibrosis may be quite extensive; foci of hemorrhage may be present; cystic degeneration rare
- Tumors generally evenly distributed throughout the pancreas (gastrin-producing tumors may be found in the duodenum, gastric antrum, along the bile duct, and in parapancreatic soft tissue)

Microscopic Pathology

- 3 characteristic microscopic patterns occur singly or in any combination:
    - Ribbonlike, trabecular or gyriform: Characterized by ribbons and festoons of tumor cells composed of monolayers or bilayers separated by a highly vascular stroma (classic pattern of glucagonoma, pancreatic polypeptide-cell tumor, and insulinoma)
    - Glandular or ductlike: Characterized by tubules and acini with true lumina that often contain secretory material (classic pattern of a gastrinoma and a vasoactive intestinal peptide [VIPoma] secreting tumor)
    - Medullary, solid, or diffuse: Characterized by nodular to diffuse cellular growth with scant intervening stroma that courses through and partially separates large sheets of cells
- Trabecular pattern more common in benign tumors; glandular or solid pattern more common in malignant tumors
- Endocrine cells are typically round or polygonal and relatively uniform in size and shape; nuclei tend to be round with tiny clumps of dense heterochromatin scattered throughout; nucleoli vary from inconspicuous to prominent; cytoplasm varies from pale to moderately eosinophilic
- Occasional tumor cells are elongated (especially in the trabecular pattern)

- Rare cells may be large and pleomorphic and have large or giant nucleoli
- Mitotic activity rare
- Eosinophilic globules may be present in the cytoplasm and in extracellular locations
- Amount of stroma may be quite variable and at times very dense; amyloid may or may not be present; foci of calcification may be present as either irregular masses of calcium or as tiny calcospherites (psammoma bodies)
- Unequivocal evidence of malignancy requires either gross invasion of adjacent organs, metastasis to regional lymph nodes, liver or other distant sites, or blood vessel invasion; histologic features alone correlate poorly with malignant potential, with the exception of vascular invasion

Special Stains

- PAS confirms the relative absence of glycogen in tumor cells
- Argyrophilic stains will highlight cytoplasmic granules in most tumor cells

Immunohistochemistry

- Eosinophilic intracellular and extracellular globules can be highlighted with α_1-antitrypsin
- Tumor cells typically positive for synaptophysin, neuron-specific enolase (NSE), chromogranin, and specific pancreatic and gastroenteric hormones
- Large numbers of cells expressing Ki-67 antigen are associated with malignancy

Electron Microscopy

- Tumor cells characterized by the presence of small dense core secretory granules with or without a crystalline or other kind of regular substructure, enveloped by a thin membrane with or without an intervening space (halo)

Molecular Alterations

- Aneuploid tumors tend to be more aggressive

Differential Diagnosis

- Small cell carcinoma
- Islet cell aggregation in the presence of chronic pancreatitis
- Solid ductal adenocarcinoma
- Solid-pseudopapillary tumor
- Acinar cell carcinoma
- Pancreaticoblastoma

Treatment and Prognosis

- Insulin-producing tumors tend to be benign and can be cured with surgical resection; all other endocrine neoplasms to include nonfunctioning tumors frequently have metastatic foci and the chance for surgical cure is less
- Chance of cure depends on presence and absence of local invasion and metastasis

Associations

- MEN-1
- Functioning pancreatic and parapancreatic endocrine neoplasms present in 80% of patients with MEN-1
- Hyperfunctional syndromes of pancreatic origin seen in patients with MEN-1 include gastrinoma (Zollinger-Ellison syndrome), insulinoma (Whipple triad), VIPoma (watery diarrhea, hypokalemia achlorhydria [WDHA] syndrome), and glucagonoma (glucagonoma syndrome)

Well-Differentiated Endocrine Tumors

Insulinoma

- B-cell differentiation and produce insulin
- Most common functioning pancreatic endocrine tumor
- 90% to 95% benign
- Patients experience symptoms of hypoglycemia
- Tend to occur uniformly throughout the pancreas and are usually single; multiple in 10% (usually in the setting of MEN-1)
- Most significant microscopic feature is the presence of amyloid in fibrovascular stroma adjacent to tumor cells; any growth pattern

Endocrine Tumors: Well-Differentiated>Glucagonoma; Somatostatinoma; Gastrinoma; VIPoma; Enterochromaffin Cell Tumor

Glucagonoma

- A-cell differentiation and produce glucagon
- Typically malignant
- Clinical syndrome of skin rash (necrolytic migratory erythema), stomatitis, diabetes mellitus, weight loss, normocytic normochromic anemia, depression, and tendency to develop deep venous thrombosis
- 8% of all functioning endocrine tumors
- Slightly more common in women
- May be part of the MEN-1 syndrome
- Most located in the distal portion of the pancreas
- Usually have both a trabecular and diffuse pattern of growth
- Nonresectable tumors may respond to streptozotocin, and long-acting somatostatin analogues may reduce glucagon secretion

Somatostatinoma

- D-cell differentiation
- Typically malignant
- More common in the upper small intestine than in the pancreas; when in pancreas, 55% to 60% occur in the region of the head
- Less than 1% of functioning endocrine tumors
- Clinical symptoms include diabetes mellitus, cholestasis, diarrhea (with or without steatorrhea), hypochlorhydria, weight loss, and anemia; symptoms result from the inhibitory action of somatostatin on endocrine cells that produce insulin, secretin, cholecystokinin, and gastrin, as well as on gastric parietal cells, pancreatic acinar cells, intestinal absorptive cells, and gallbladder muscle cells
- Somatostatin-producing tumors frequently contain psammoma bodies
- Strong association with von Recklinghausen disease (neurofibromatosis type I); no association with MEN-1

Gastrinoma

- Predominately malignant
- 30% of all functioning endocrine tumors
- May occur in the pancreas, duodenum, upper jejunum, or stomach; 70% are extrapancreatic; pancreatic tumors are more likely to be functional and malignant than duodenal tumors; duodenal tumors may be quite small and are frequently (50%) associated with metastases
- Produce unregulated hypergastrinemia and the Zollinger-Ellison syndrome (massive gastric acid-hypersecretion, elevated basal serum gastrin levels [above 200 pmol/L], and peptic ulceration; ulcers frequently multiple and unusual in site)
- Tumor cells most frequently arranged in a trabecular pattern with areas of solid sheets or nests
- Most patients survive long-term (10-year survival better for patients with MEN-1 than for patients with sporadic lesions)

VIPoma

- Approximately 10% of all endocrine tumors
- Neoplasm typically solitary; 50% located in the tail of the pancreas
- Most have malignant potential
- Secrete VIP, which produces the Verner-Morrison or WDHA syndrome
- Occasionally seen in patients with MEN-1
- Patients frequently experience a secretory diarrhea up to 6 L per day, hypokalemia, hypochlorhydria, alkalosis, flushing, hypercalcemia, abnormal glucose tolerance test, tetany and a dilated gallbladder (VIP stimulates intestinal secretion, inhibits gastric acid secretion, dilates the gallbladder, and promotes glycogenolysis with consequent hyperglycemia and dilatation of peripheral blood vessels leading to hypotension and flushing)
- Microscopically all 3 patterns may be present
- Streptozotocin and interferon may produce remission in tumors that cannot be resected for cure

Enterochromaffin Cell Tumor

- Usually malignant
- Enterochromaffin cell differentiation
- Produce carcinoid syndrome (diarrhea, cutaneous flushing, hypotension, bronchospasm, right heart endocardial fibrosis, and mesenteric and retroperitoneal fibrosis)

- Tumors secrete a variety of factors to include serotonin, kallikreins (which in turn release bradykinin), substance P, and other tachykinins and prostaglandin
- Most endocrine tumors associated with a carcinoid syndrome have metastases in the liver and regional lymph nodes at diagnosis

Nonfunctioning Tumors

- Tumors with endocrine differentiation that do not produce a clinical syndrome of hormone hyperfunction
- Typically composed of islet A and pancreatic polypeptide cells
- Usually malignant and present with symptoms of expanding mass, pain, jaundice, ascites, steatorrhea, intestinal bleeding, and/or metastatic disease
- Streptozotocin and fluorouracil will produce a response in 60% of those that cannot be resected for cure

Poorly Differentiated Endocrine Tumors

Poorly Differentiated Small Cell Carcinoma

- 1% of all pancreatic tumors; 2% to 3% of all pancreatic endocrine tumors
- More common in men than in women; typically occur after the age of 40 years
- Patients typically present with symptoms of advanced malignant disease (weight loss, jaundice, and metastases)
- Paraneoplastic hormonal syndromes (common in pulmonary small cell carcinoma) tend to be rare
- Tumors typically quite large at the time of diagnosis; cut surface gray to white with areas of necrosis and hemorrhage; invasion into adjacent organs and widespread metastasis are common
- Microscopic appearance indistinguishable from that of small cell carcinoma of the lung; tumor cells arranged in nests and sheets and are characterized by markedly hyperchromatic round to oval nuclei, inconspicuous nucleoli, and poorly defined cell borders; mitoses and foci of necrosis frequent
- Typically unresectable
- Treatment consists of chemotherapy (etoposide and cisplatin) which may produce significant remission

References

Dabbs DJ. *Diagnostic Immunohistochemistry.* New York: Churchill Livingstone, 2002.

Hamilton SR, Aaltonen, LA (eds). *World Health Organization Classification of Tumours: Pathology and Genetics of Tumours of the Digestive System.* Lyon: IARC Press, 2000.

Odze RD, Goldblum JR, Crawford JM. *Surgical Pathology of the GI Tract, Liver, and Pancreas.* Philadelphia: WB Saunders, 2004.

Mills S, Carter D, Greenson JK, Oberman HA, Reuter V, Stoler MH (eds). *Sternberg's Diagnostic Surgical Pathology. 4th ed.* Philadelphia: Lippincott Williams & Wilkins, 2004.

Rosai J. *Rosai and Ackerman's Surgical Pathology. 9th ed.* St. Louis: Mosby, 2004.

Solcia E, Capella C, Kloppel G. *Tumors of the Pancreas: Atlas of Tumor Pathology, 3rd Series, Fascicle 20.* Washington DC: Armed Forces Institute of Pathology, 1997.

Chapter 10

Upper Aerodigestive Tract

Intraoperative Consultation

In keeping with the World Health Organization classification of tumors the upper aerodigestive tract is divided into four distinct anatomic regions—oral cavity and oropharynx, nasal cavity and paranasal cavities, nasopharynx, and hypopharynx, larynx and trachea. Salivary gland lesions, odontogenic lesions, and paraganglionic lesions are discussed in separate chapters.

The ***oral cavity*** extends from the lips to the palatoglossal folds. The outer vestibule is enclosed by the cheeks and lips and forms a groove or slit-like space that separates it from the gingivae and teeth. The superior and inferior limits are the mucosal reflections from the lips and cheeks. The oral cavity proper is bordered by the teeth and gingivae, the floor of the mouth and tongue, and the hard palate.

The ***oropharynx*** lies behind the oral cavity and is bounded by the soft palate, a hypothetical horizonal line level with the tip of the epiglottis. The anterior border is the posterior third of the tongue; the lateral borders consist of the palatopharyngeal arches and palatine tonsils; the posterior border is the pharyngeal tonsils.

The ***nasal cavity and paranasal sinuses*** are separated in the midline by the nasal septum. Superiorly the nasal cavity is bordered by the cribiform plate; the floor is the hard palate. The lateral nasal wall contains the maxillary and ethmoid ostia and the turbinates.

The ***nasopharynx*** is the narrow tubular passage behind the nasal cavity. Its roof and posterior wall consist of the basi-sphenoid, basi-occiput, and the first cervical vertebra. It communicates with the nasal cavity by way of the choanae. The lateral walls contain the orifices of the Eustachian tubes. Behind the Eustachian tubes is a recess called the fossa of Rosenmüller. Inferiorly the nasopharynx tapers into the oropharynx at the level of the soft palate.

The ***hypopharynx*** is the inferior third of the pharynx (the other two thirds are the nasopharynx and oropharynx). The hypopharynx lies behind the larynx and partially surrounds it on either side. The superior border is at the level of the hyoid bone (floor of the vallecula); the inferior border is the cricoid cartilage.

The ***larynx*** extends from the tip of the epiglottis to the inferior border of the cricoid cartilage. Posteriorly the larynx consists of posterior commissure, the arytenoids and the interarytenoid space. Anteriorily the larynx is bounded by the lingual epiglottis, the thyrohyoid membrane, the anterior commissure, thyroid cartilage, the cricothyroid membrane, and the anterior arch of the cricoid cartilage. The larynx is divided into three compartments; supraglottis (epiglottis, aryepiglottic folds, false vocal cords, ventricles, and saccules), glottis (true vocal cords and anterior and posterior commisures), and subglottis (extends one centimeter below the true vocal cords to the inferior margin of the cricoid cartilage.

The ***trachea*** extends from the lower border of the cricoid cartilage to the carina and is about 10 to 11 cm in length. The posterior, noncartilaginous membranous portion contains smooth muscle.

Indications for intraoperative diagnosis during surgery on the upper aerodigestive tract typically involve evaluation of surgical margins during resection of a neoplasm and the determination of resectability. Surgical margins are submitted in one of two ways. When a major resection specimen is received, the pathologist selects the tissue for frozen section based on an inspection of the specimen. Some difficulties can be avoided if the selection of appropriate margins is done in collaboration with the operating surgeon, thus avoiding the sampling of areas not of concern to the operating surgeon. Even the placement of orienting sutures by the surgeon does not necessarily mean that the closest surgical margins will always be obtained. Sectioning and examination of the specimen by both the surgeon and the pathologist may reveal evidence of tumor near surgical margins that represent an unexpected finding. Typically the pathologist will obtain parallel ("shave") sections because these types of sections sample a much larger area and often an entire margin can be easily evaluated. The disadvantage to this technique is that the actual distance from the neoplasm to the surgical margin cannot be determined (an issue that may be of more importance to the pathologist than it is to the surgeon). When parallel sections are made, the true surgical margin should be placed deepest in the block to preserve this margin in case deeper sections are required. A second approach to the evaluation of surgical margins involves having the surgeon submit biopsies from areas of concern during the course of the operation or after the resection is completed. This approach is obviously easier for the pathologist and may be superior for the surgeon as well, in that the risk of sampling error is essentially eliminated.

Biopsies will be submitted for intraoperative consultation whenever a neoplasm that was thought on preoperative evaluation to be resectable appears to be unresectable as the surgical dissection proceeds. In addition, carcinomas that approach the mandible typically require intraoperative microscopic evaluation of adjacent mandibular periosteum to determine whether or not the mandible is involved and can be spared.

Squamous cell carcinoma is the most common malignancy in the upper aerodigestive tract and is frequently treated with radiation. The changes that radiation can induce represent a diagnostic pitfall to the pathologist. Prior to the evaluation of a biopsy from a patient with squamous cell carcinoma, the pathologist should know whether or not the patient has received radiation to that site. In addition, the pathologist should compare the frozen section findings to the original biopsy material. Radiation can result in squamous metaplasia with reactive atypia in mucous glands and minor salivary glands that mimics foci of invasive squamous cell carcinoma.

Poorly differentiated squamous cell carcinoma often has a highly infiltrative growth pattern that at the periphery of the tumor may appear as small nests of cells that seem to be growing in a discontinuous pattern. These small foci of carcinoma may appear quite banal. Occasionally, the only clue on frozen section will be foci of fibrosis.

Biopsies from the area of the retromolar trigone may include a portion of the juxtaoral organ of Chievitz. This structure is composed of nests of squamoid or basaloid cells typically in close relationship to nerve fibers. Microscopically, the findings are reminiscent of invasive squamous cell carcinoma with perineural involvement.

Specimen Handling

Some of the most difficult specimens from the upper aerodigestive tract for the pathologist are those involving partial or total laryngectomy. The pathologist should accurately localize the site of the primary neoplasm, its maximal dimension, depth of invasion and its relationship to the glottis. All the surgical margins (lingual, pharyngeal, and tracheal) should be inked. Occasionally a diagram or photograph of the specimen can be helpful in describing the location of the sections that are taken for microscopic examination.

Sections for microscopic examination should be taken from the following locations:

1) sections of tumor in relationship to its lateral, anterior, inferior, and superior extent
2) sections of larynx to include epiglottis and true and false vocal cords (to include the opposite cord)
3) lateral pharyngeal wall on the side of the neoplasm
4) tracheal cartilage at the inferior margin of resection
5) any cartilage and/or bone near the neoplasm,
6) any associated lymph nodes (preferably by anatomic level)
7) one section of thyroid or parathyroid if included

Oral Cavity and Oropharynx

Squamous Cell Carcinoma

Clinical Manifestations

- Represent more than 90% of all intraoral malignancies
- More common in men than women
- Typically occurs between the 5th and 8th decades
- Tobacco most significant etiologic factor; alcohol abuse appears to act synergistically with tobacco to further increase risk or decrease the time for neoplastic transformation to develop
- Carcinoma can arise in patients who do not use tobacco or alcohol; these patients tend to be elderly women and the lesions rarely involve the floor of the mouth
- 75% of intraoral squamous cell carcinomas arise in a semicircular area of the mouth defined by the floor of the mouth, the lateral-ventral tongue, and the soft palate-retromolar trigone-anterior tonsillar pillar region

Gross Pathology

- First lesion to appear when squamous mucosa is injured or stimulated by carcinogens is leukoplakia (white patch that cannot be scraped off)
- Leukoplakia will disappear with removal of the stimulating agent

- Leukoplakia typically seen in the buccal mucosa, mandibular and maxillary alveolar ridges and sulci, palate, and lip
- A mixed red and white patch (speckled leukoplakia) or erythroleukoplakia represents a more significant risk for the development of squamous cell carcinoma
- Red patches (erythroplakia) represent the most significant risk for the development of squamous cell carcinoma
- Erythroplakia is most frequently seen in the floor of the mouth, retromolar trigone, mandibular gingiva and sulcus, ventral and/or lateral tongue, and palate
- Most squamous cell carcinomas appear as a raised, partially ulcerated hyperkeratotic mass

Microscopic Pathology

- Leukoplakia (white patch):
  - Characterized by varying degrees of epithelial thickening with acanthosis and hyperkeratosis without dysplasia
  - Low incidence of dysplasia and malignant transformation
- Erythroleukoplakia (mixed red/white patch):
  - Characterized by areas of epithelial hyperplasia, hyperkeratosis, epithelial atrophy, and submucosal inflammation
  - Up to 50% represent dysplasia or carcinoma
- Erythroplakia (red patch):
  - Characterized by a thin, atrophic epithelium with prominent subepithelial vascular telangiectasia and inflammation
  - Most demonstrate high grade dysplasia or carcinoma in situ
- Squamous dysplasia and carcinoma in situ:
  - Characterized by a proliferation of basal cells characterized by loss of polarity, irregular epithelial stratification, increased numbers of mitotic figures (especially in the superficial half of the epithelium), cellular and nuclear pleomorphism, enlarged nucleoli, decreased cellular cohesion, increased nuclear cytoplasmic ratio, and keratinization of single cells or groups of cells in the spinous cell layer
- Invasive squamous cell carcinoma:
  - May be well differentiated (nests of closely apposed large squamous cells with keratinization), moderately differentiated (small nests of more pleomorphic, mitotically active squamous cells), and poorly differentiated (single and small nests of poorly developed, very mitotically active squamous cells with a ragged or diffuse margin of infiltration)
  - Characterized by squamous cells invading into underlying tissue from dysplastic epithelium; the presence of single cell keratinization and/or the formation of keratin pearls below the epithelium considered hallmarks of invasive carcinoma
  - Architecturally, invasive tumor may be composed of well-defined, blunt, pushing borders of thick, rounded cords of neoplastic cells (the architectural pattern with the most favorable prognosis), or the tumor may invade as non-cohesive, irregular, jagged small cords and single cells (histologic pattern with the worst prognosis)

Special Stains

- Not helpful

Immunohistochemistry

- Tumor cells cytokeratin positive

Electron Microscopy

- Confirms the epithelial nature of squamous cell carcinoma even when it is poorly differentiated or spindled

Molecular Alterations

- 30% over-express the p53 oncogene
- 65% express *ras*21
- HPV 16 and 18 found in some oral SCCs and in as many as 40% of oropharyngeal cancers
- 70% show loss of heterozygosity of p53 by PCR

Differential Diagnosis

- Undifferentiated solid tumors may resemble malignant lymphoma
- Squamous cell carcinoma of the gingiva may be clinically misdiagnosed as pyogenic granuloma, periodontitis, papilloma, or fibroid epulis (inflammatory hyperplasia)

Oral Cavity and Oropharynx>Squamous Cell Carcinoma: Buccal Mucosa, Floor of Mouth, Gingiva, Lip

Treatment

- Early stage lesions can be treated with equal effectiveness by either surgery or irradiation; treatment decisions based on factors such as functional and cosmetic results and the patient's general state of health
- More advanced lesions are typically treated by a combination of radiation and chemotherapy

Prognosis

- Loss of expression of blood group H antigen associated with increased invasiveness and distant metastasis
- Presence or absence of regional lymph node metastasis is most important predictor of survival
  - 75% 5-year survival with negative regional lymph nodes
  - 50% 5-year survival with 1 positive lymph node
  - 30% 5-year survival with 2 positive lymph nodes
  - 10%-15% 5-year survival with ≥3 positive lymph nodes
- Extracapsular spread of cancer in lymph nodes associated with a 5-year survival of 10%; intact lymph node capsules associated with a 5-year survival of 30%-35%
- Poorly differentiated tumors that invade as single cells or irregular small cords and nests of cells have a higher rate of lymph node metastasis than tumors that invade with blunt pushing borders
- Depth of invasion correlates with metastasis:
- Metastases present in 10% of lesions <4 mm in depth; in 35% of lesions between 4-8 mm in depth; in 85% for lesions >8 mm in depth
- Angiolymphatic invasion and perineural invasion both associated with an increased likelihood of lymph node metastasis

Associations

- Organ transplant recipients appear to be at an increased risk
- Prolonged exposure to sunlight and fair complexion are associated with carcinoma of the lip
- Oropharyngeal lesions are seen with increased frequency in patients with syphilis, oral sepsis, iron deficiency anemia, oral candidiasis, and Fanconi anemia

Buccal Mucosa

- Represents 2% of all intraoral carcinomas
- Metastases usually limited to submandibular lymph nodes
- Five-year survival is 44% for tumors located anteriorly, 15%-20% for tumors in the middle 1/3 and 10% for tumors in the posterior third

Floor of Mouth

- Represents ~15% of intraoral SCCs
- Most common intraoral SCC in the black population
- Usually affects the anterior region of the caruncles of the submaxillary gland and the lingual frenulum
- High likelihood of invasion of contiguous structures at the time of diagnosis
- Most typically metastasizes to submandibular triangle and subdigastric lymph nodes (submental nodes rarely involved)
- Incidence of nodal metastasis dependent upon depth of invasion:
  - 2% for tumors <1.5 mm
  - 33% for tumors 1.6-3.5 mm
  - 60% for tumors thicker than 3.6 mm

Gingiva

- Represents ~5% of all intraoral SCCs
- Typically occurs in the mandibular bicuspid and molar areas
- Tends to invade adjacent bone
- Metastasizes to submandibular lymph nodes

Lip

- Most common (40%)
- 90% arise in the lower lip along the mucocutaneous junction or vermilion border lateral to midline
- Typically metastasize to ipsilateral submandibular and submental lymph nodes
- Mid-line lesions can metastasize to lymph nodes on either side of the neck
- Lesions of the upper lip tend to metastasize to preauricular and periparotid lymph nodes

- Incidence of metastasis directly related to size:
  - 5% in lesions <2 cm
  - 50% in lesions 2-4 cm
  - 75% in lesions >4 cm
- 5-year survival 75%

Oropharynx

- Oropharynx consists of palatine arch and oropharynx proper
- Palatine arch is superior wall of oropharynx and consists of soft palate, uvula, anterior tonsillar pillars, and retromolar trigone
- Oropharynx proper has an *anterior* wall consisting of the posterior 1/3 (base) of the tongue, the intervening vallecula and the lingual surface of the epiglottis; a *lateral* wall consisting of the palatine tonsils, posterior tonsillar pillars (pharyngopalatine folds), and glossotonsillar sulcus; and a *posterior* wall consisting of the posterior and lateral oropharyngeal walls from the soft palate to the level of the hyoid bone including the pharyngoepiglottic fold
- Tumors arising in the palatine arch tend to be less aggressive than tumors arising in the oropharynx proper
- Oropharyngeal SCC tends to be more poorly differentiated than tumors arising more proximally
- Lymphatic drainage to the jugulodigastric, retropharyngeal, and parapharyngeal lymph nodes
- High incidence of contralateral and bilateral cervical lymph node metastases

Palate

- Represents ~5% of all intraoral SCCs
- Soft palate more frequently involved than hard palate
- Most common malignant neoplasm of the palate
- Lymphatic drainage of both the hard and soft palate is through the retromolar triangle to lymph nodes in the internal jugular chain, submandibular, and retropharyngeal regions
- Bilateral cervical lymph node metastases uncommon

Tongue

- Represents 20 to 25% of intraoral SCCs
- Usually occurs only at lateral aspect of the middle 1/3 of the tongue
- Typically first appears as an area of leukoplakia or erythroplakia
- 70% of patients have unilateral or bilateral metastasis at the time of diagnosis
- Primary sites of metastasis ipsilateral subdigastric, submandibular, and mid-jugular lymph nodes
- Tumors in the midline or in the base of the tongue tend to metastasize to lymph nodes in both sides of the neck
- Lesions in the posterior aspect of the tongue usually more poorly differentiated than those arising more anteriorly

Tonsil

- Most common site for primary SCC in the oropharynx (base of tongue second most common)
- Associated with a high rate of lymph node metastasis
- Usually metastasizes to ipsilateral subdigastric lymph nodes; may metastasize to middle and lower jugular lymph nodes and posterior cervical triangle lymph nodes
- Undifferentiated carcinomas may also arise in tonsils

Squamous Cell Carcinoma—Variants

Verrucous Carcinoma

- 75% occur in oral cavity

Basaloid Squamous Cell Carcinoma

- Uncommon in oral cavity; slightly more common in oropharynx
- see Hypopharynx, Larynx, and Trachea

Papillary Squamous Cell Carcinoma

- Rare in oral cavity
- see Hypopharynx, Larynx, and Trachea

Spindle Cell Carcinoma

- More common in larynx than in oral cavity and oropharynx
- see Hypopharynx, Larynx, and Trachea

Acantholytic Squamous Cell Carcinoma

- Lip most frequent site

Adenosquamous Carcinoma

- SCC with obvious areas of adenocarcinoma
- see Hypopharynx, Larynx, and Trachea

Lymphoepithelial Carcinoma

- A poorly differentiated SCC or undifferentiated carcinoma
- Indistinguishable from nasopharyngeal nonkeratinizing carcinoma with lymphocytic infiltrate

Verrucous Carcinoma

Clinical Manifestations

- Represents ~1% of squamous neoplasms of head and neck
- Most commonly found in the buccal mucosa (also seen, in decreasing order of frequency: gingiva, tongue, palate, and tonsillar pillar)
- More common in men than in women and typically diagnosed during the seventh decade of life
- Patients often complain of a mass that interferes with chewing and/or pain and tenderness in what appears grossly as an ulcerated lesion

Gross Pathology

- Typically presents as a circumscribed, elevated, or nodular mass that may have a papillary, "cobblestone", or smooth red to white surface depending upon the amount of surface keratinization
- Cut surface tan to gray; margin of invasion sharp and pushing

Microscopic Pathology

- An extremely well-differentiated squamous epithelium with hyperplastic growth with both superficial and deep orderly maturation
- Surface is typically composed of papillae ("church spires") covered by abundant orthokeratotic and parakeratotic squamous cells; this surface keratin extends into and fills the crevices that give the lesion the papillary appearance
- Downward growth at the base characterized by sharply demarcated broad, bulbous, ridges and nests of well-differentiated, banal squamous cells; cytologic atypia unusual unless the lesion is inflamed
- Lamina propria at advancing edge typically contains a lymphoplasmacytic inflammatory cell infiltrate
- Ragged invasion by small, irregular nests, vascular invasion, and perineural invasion never present
- *Verrucous carcinoma typically is locally invasive and incapable of metastasis*, but if areas of less well-differentiated infiltrating squamous cell carcinoma are present at the deep margin (20%), the diagnosis of a pure verrucous carcinoma is excluded and the lesion is better called a verrucous carcinoma with coexisting foci of squamous cell carcinoma and has the potential to metastasize

Electron Microscopy

- Squamous cells have abundant intracytoplasmic tonofilaments and well-formed desmosomes

Molecular Alterations

- All are diploid

Differential Diagnosis

- Conventional squamous cell carcinoma
- Benign squamous proliferations:
  - Complex squamous papilloma
  - Keratoacanthoma
  - Pseudoepitheliomatous hyperplasia
  - Hyperkeratosis with an exophytic surface (verrucous leukoplakia and verrucous hyperplasia)
- Malignant proliferations
  - Well-differentiated hyperkeratotic dysplasia
  - Squamous cell carcinoma with a papillary or verrucoid surface architecture

Treatment

- Surgical excision
- Advanced disease or disease in patients who are not acceptable surgical candidates can be treated with radiation
- No role for chemotherapy

Prognosis

- A locally invasive neoplasm that does not metastasize unless there is more conventional invasive squamous cell carcinoma at the infiltrating margin (see above)
- Tumor control approaches 85% in patients treated with complete surgical excision and 95% with surgical treatment of recurrences
- Lesions treated with radiation alone may undergo anaplastic transformation within months

Associations

- Tobacco abuse, especially involving chewing tobacco or snuff
- Alcohol not a major etiologic agent
- 30% have HPV DNA (types 6, 11, 16)

Nasal Cavity and Paranasal Sinuses

Olfactory Neuroblastoma (Esthesioneuroblastoma)

Clinical Manifestations

- Arise in cells of neuroendocrine origin scattered in olfactory mucosa
- Bimodal age distribution: small peak during adolescence (15 years) and a second larger peak in adulthood (median age 55 years)
- Typically present as a polypoid mass causing either nasal obstruction or bleeding
- Located in the *roof* of nasal fossa (involves the cribriform plate)
- Reports of catecholamine production without symptoms or vasopressin production with hypertension and hyponatremia

Gross Pathology

- Soft, red to gray, and polypoid with smooth intact surface (occasionally ulcerated)
- Very vascular

Microscopic Pathology

- Usually well-circumscribed nests of uniform small cells with scant cytoplasm and round nuclei, "salt and pepper" chromatin pattern, inconspicuous nucleoli, and indistinct nuclear membranes; slight nuclear pleomorphism; nests separated by stroma
- May grow as diffuse sheets with a prominent vascular background and little stroma
- 85% to 90% have a fibrillary cytoplasmic background
- Mitotic activity very variable
- Usually a suggestion of rosettes, but well-formed Homer-Wright rosettes fairly unusual (25% to 30%); Flexner-Wintersteiner rosettes rare (<5%)
- Ganglion cell differentiation unusual
- Necrosis uncommon
- Rarely focal areas of divergent differentiation (eg, adenocarcinoma-like, rhabdomyoblastic) present

Special Stains

- Not helpful

Immunohistochemistry

- Tumor cells stain positively for NSE (75% to 100%), synaptophysin (65% to 100%), neurofilament protein (75%), microtubular-associated protein, and class III beta-tubulin isotype
- Chromogranin reactivity not particularly reliable
- Cells at the edge of cell nests stain positively for S-100 protein (sustentacular cells); scattered S-100 positive cells may also be present within nests of tumor cells
- Some (up to 30%) may be positive for cytokeratin, particularly those with olfactory rosettes

Electron Microscopy

- Cell processes contain membrane-bound dense core granules, microtubules, and rare intermediate filaments

- Junctional complexes between cells infrequent
- Sustentacular cells covered by basal lamina surround neoplastic cells

Molecular Alterations

- Some with trisomy 8q

Differential Diagnosis

- Sinonasal undifferentiated carcinoma (SNUC)
- Melanoma
- Anterior extension of pituitary adenoma
- Lymphoma
- Peripheral neuroectodermal tumor (PNET) (see Comment below)
- Embryonal rhabdomyosarcoma
- Neuroendocrine carcinoma

Treatment

- Gross total excision with radiation and chemotherapy offers best chance of cure (75%)

Prognosis

- Disease tends to be slowly progressive
- Recurrence may occur late (>10 years)
- Metastasis to lymph nodes and bone (20%)

Associations

- None

Ewing Sarcoma (EWS) / Primitive Neuroectodermal Tumor (PNET)

Clinical Manifestations

- Very rare
- Typically a tumor of children and young adults
- Slight male predominance
- 20% of all EWS/PNET occurs in head; 20% occurs in sinonasal tract (most in maxillary sinus)
- Most present with pain, mass and obstruction

Gross Pathology

- Usually gray-white and glistening with foci of hemorrhage and ulceration

Microscopic Pathology

- Characterized by densely distributed, uniform (occasionally pleomorphic), small to medium sized round cells with little cytoplasm and fine chromatin (occasionally chromatin clumped)
- Mitotic figures easily found
- Foci of necrosis common
- Homer-Wright rosettes rare

Special Stains

- PAS with and without diastase will confirm presence of glycogen in tumor cells

Immunohistochemistry

- Tumor cells reactive for CD99 (MIC2, O13, p30/32, and 12E7) and vimentin and variably positive for S-100 protein, neurofilament protein, NSE, Leu-7 (CD57), synaptophysin and chromogranin

Electron Microscopy

- Interdigiting neuritic processes, neurofilaments, microtubules, neurosecretory granules and glycogen variably seen

Molecular Alterations

- Most have characteristic t(11;22)

Differential Diagnosis

- Malignant melanoma
- Melanotic neuroectodermal tumor
- Rhabdomyosarcoma
- Sinonasal undifferentiated carcinoma
- Pituitary adenoma

Treatment

- Multimodality

Prognosis

- 5-year survival 60% to 70%
- Head and neck tumors have better prognosis than tumors in other anatomic sites

Associations

- Retinoblastoma

Melanotic Neuroectodermal Tumor of Infancy

Clinical Manifestations

- 85% have mass involving craniofacial sites: maxilla (70%), mandible (10%), skull (10%), dura or brain (1%)
- Also reported in epididymis, skin, uterus, and mediastinum
- Patients present with rapidly enlarging pigmented mass in anterior alveolar ridge of maxilla
- Serum levels of vanilmandelic acid may be elevated

Gross Pathology

- Tend to be smooth, hard and grey to blue-black
- Mean 3.5 cm
- May invade adjacent bone

Microscopic Pathology

- Nonencapsulated
- A dual population of small neuroblastic cells and larger melanin-containing epithelial cells in a vascularized dense fibrous stroma
- Epithelial cells usually arranged in an alveolar or tubular pattern and often surround nests of the smaller neuroblastic cells; larger than neuroblastic cells with abundant cytoplasm with melanin granules
- Neuroblastic cells characterized small, round hyperchromatic nuclei, little cytoplasm
- Mitoses and necrosis very rare or absent

Special Stains

- Not helpful

Immunohistochemistry

- Epithelial component reactive for cytokeratin, HMB-45, vimentin, and occasionally EMA
- Both small neuroblastic cells and larger epithelial cell frequently positive for NSE, CD57 (Leu-7)
- Small cells may express synaptophysin, and focally express GFAP and desmin

Electron Microscopy

- Small cells have neurosectetory granules and neuritic processes
- Large cells contain melanosomes and premelanosomes

Differential Diagnosis

- Alveolar rhabdomyosarcoma
- Lymphoma
- EWS/PNET
- Immature teratoma
- Melanoma

Treatment

- Complete local excision

Prognosis

- Usually a benign clinical course (even in presence of bony invasion)
- Metastases occur in 7% (lymph nodes, liver, bone, adrenal glands, or soft tissue)

Associations

- None

Schneiderian Papilloma

Variants

- Fungiform papilloma
- Inverted papilloma
- Oncocytic papilloma (cylindrical cell papilloma)

Clinical Manifestations

- *Fungiform papilloma*
  - Represent 50% of all Schneiderian papillomas
  - Patients typically between ages of 20 and 40 years
- *Inverted papilloma*
  - Represent ~45% of all Schneiderian papillomas
  - Most commonly seen in adult males between the ages of 30 and 50
  - Chief complaints include unilateral nasal obstruction, epistaxis, and facial pain; occasionally proptosis
  - Often multifocal; rarely bilateral
- *Oncocytic papilloma (cylindrical cell papilloma)*
  - Represent ~5% of all Schneiderian papillomas

Gross Pathology

- *Fungiform papilloma*
  - Usually tan to gray, firm, polypoid, exophytic, and lesion on nasal septum
  - Rarely bilateral
- *Inverted papilloma*
  - Usually firm, polypoid lesion arising almost exclusively on lateral nasal wall and in paranasal sinuses
  - Overlying mucosa usually intact
- *Oncocytic papilloma (cylindrical cell papilloma)*
  - Typically a single or multifocal polypoid lesion involving lateral nasal wall or paranasal sinuses
  - Usually soft to moderately firm with granular or finely grooved surface

Microscopic Pathology

- *Fungiform papilloma*
  - An exophytic architecture consisting of thin, branching, fibrovascular stalks covered by 5 to 30 layers of epithelium consisting of squamous, ciliated columnar, and intermediate cells
  - Mucus-secreting cells present
  - Nuclear pleomorphism and mitotic activity rare (latter restricted to basal layer)
- *Inverted papilloma*
  - Characterized by deeply invaginated nests and/or cords of benign, predominantly squamous, epithelium that project into underlying stroma; papillomas lined by 5 to 30 layers of squamous, ciliated columnar, and intermediate epithelium with interspersed mucus-secreting cells; surface usually lined by single layer of ciliated cells regardless of the type of underlying epithelium
  - Fibrous stroma often contains scattered inflammatory cells or lymphoid follicles
  - Occasionally the lesion will have an exophytic surface in addition to the invaginated component
    - Dilated duct-like structures, also lined by multiple layers of epithelium, often present
    - Small mucin-filled microcysts typically present throughout the neoplasm
    - Nuclear pleomorphism may be present (~10%)
    - Mitotic figures rare and limited to basal layers
- *Oncocytic papilloma (cylindrical cell papilloma)*
  - Most have both an inverted and exophytic pattern of growth; exophytic pattern characterized by thin, fibrovascular cores covered by 3 to 8 layers of epithelium; inverted pattern characterized by cords and nests of epithelial cells
  - Epithelial cells are polygonal to columnar oncocytes with abundant granular, eosinophilic cytoplasm and round to oval, dark, uniform nuclei with inconspicuous nucleoli
  - Ciliated cells may cover epithelium
  - Mucous-filled microcysts often present throughout

Special Stains

- Not helpful

Immunohistochemistry

- Epithelial cells of oncocytic papilloma are cytokeratin positive

Electron Microscopy

- Cells of oncocytic papilloma contain many intracytoplasmic mitochondria and have short microvilli and well-formed desmosomes

Molecular Alterations

- None

Differential Diagnosis

- *Fungiform papilloma*
  - Nonkeratinizing squamous cell carcinoma
  - Papillary squamous cell carcinoma
- *Inverted papilloma*
  - Squamous cell carcinoma
- *Oncocytic papilloma (cylindrical cell papilloma)*
  - Rhinosporidiosis (fungus *Rhinosporidium seeberi*)
  - Adenocarcinoma
  - Inflammatory polyp

Treatment

- Complete surgical excision

Prognosis

- *Fungiform papilloma*
  - Lowest recurrence rate (~20%)
- *Inverted papilloma*
  - Recurrence rate ~45%
  - Recurrence rate can be as high as 50%-70% within 1-2 years if the neoplasm is treated by simple local excision
- *Oncocytic papilloma (cylindrical cell papilloma)*
  - Recurrence rate 45%

Associations

- Fungiform papilloma not associated with carcinoma
- Inverted papillomas and oncocytic papillomas occur in association with squamous cell carcinoma which may be present in the papilloma, adjacent to it, or develop later at the same site; other associated carcinomas include spindle cell, transitional cell, clear cell, and high-grade mucoepidermoid carcinoma; all associated carcinomas are aggressive
- Metachronous carcinoma will occur sometime after excision of a papilloma in 3% of patients with or without a recurrence of the papilloma in the interim (hence may or may not be associated with the papilloma); this event is associated with a 25% overall survival
- Human papilloma virus present in many sinonasal papillomas (HPV 6, 11, 16, and 18 most frequent); incidence of HPV positivity is higher for fungiform than inverted papillomas; oncocytic papillomas negative for HPV

Sinonasal Carcinoma

Variants

- Sinonasal squamous cell carcinoma
- Sinonasal intestinal-type adenocarcinoma
- Sinonasal low-grade adenocarcinoma
- Sinonasal undifferentiated carcinoma (SNUC)

Clinical Manifestations

- *Squamous cell carcinoma*
  - Represent 3% of all head and neck neoplasms
  - More common in males than females (both squamous cell carcinoma of the nasal cavity and squamous cell carcinoma of the paranasal sinuses)
  - Most patients are in their 6th or 7th decade
  - Typically present with obstruction, rhinorrhea, epistaxis, or pain
- *Intestinal-type adenocarcinoma*
  - 80% occur in men, usually in ethmoid sinuses
  - Most present with unilateral nasal obstruction, epistaxis, rhinorrhea, mass in cheek, or exophthalmos
  - Tumors that arise sporadically (unassociated with a known exposure to a carcinogen) are more frequently seen in women and involve the maxillary antrum (20%-50%)

- *Low-grade adenocarcinoma*
  - Occur with equal frequency in men and women and in both children and the elderly
  - Most frequent in the nasal cavity, nasal septum, ethmoid, or multiple sinuses
  - No association with tobacco, alcohol, or other carcinogens
- *Sinonasal undifferentiated carcinoma (SNUC)*
  - Slightly more common in females; median age 55 years
  - Multiple sinonasal structures frequently affected; nasal cavity, maxillary antrum, and ethmoid sinuses most commonly involved
  - Usually present with nasal obstruction, proptosis, cranial nerve defects, and periorbital swelling

Gross Pathology

- *Squamous cell carcinoma*
  - Usually papillary, polypoid, or sessile
  - Mucosal surface may be ulcerated and friable
  - Extensive bone destruction usually present at time of diagnosis
  - Intranasal lesions usually occur in the vestibule and lateral wall and can invade into the medial wall of the antrum, ethmoid sinuses, orbit, anterior skull and upper lip; rarely originate in the septum
  - Most paranasal tumors (75%) occur in ethmoid sinus, 15% in sphenoid sinus, and 2% in frontal sinus
- *Intestinal-type adenocarcinoma*
  - Fungating, polypoid, hemorrhagic, pink to white mass
  - Mucosal ulceration typical
  - Cut section often mucoid or gelatinous
- *Low-grade adenocarcinoma*
  - Often a cauliflower or papillary appearance
  - Typically soft; may be gritty on sectioning (calcifications)
- *Sinonasal undifferentiated carcinoma (SNUC)*
  - Large fungating mass obstructing nasal cavity with extensive local invasion

Microscopic Pathology

- *Squamous cell carcinoma*
  - Most are well or moderately differentiated lesions with varying degrees of keratinization
  - Cellular pleomorphism is generally fairly mild and mitotic figures are usually present
  - Rare tumors are completely non-keratinizing; non-keratinizing lesions tend to grow in large cell nests and broad anastomosing cords and have mitotic figures and some nuclear pleomorphism
- *Intestinal-type adenocarcinoma*
  - Cells mimic normal, adenomatous, or carcinomatous intestinal mucosa
  - Well-differentiated tumors closely resemble normal intestinal mucosa and mimic conventional gland-forming colonic adenocarcinoma
  - More poorly differentiated tumors grow in solid sheets and have rare glandular lumina
  - Occasionally neoplasms are more mucinous and closely resemble signet-ring intestinal carcinoma
- *Low-grade adenocarcinoma*
  - Typically characterized by papillary formations with small glands lined by a single layer of cuboidal or columnar cells with basally oriented, non-stratified nuclei and abundant mucin without stroma
  - Occasionally glands are cystically dilated or contain papillary infoldings with overlapping vesicular nuclei and psammoma bodies (reminiscent of papillary carcinoma of thyroid)
  - Nuclear pleomorphism and mitotic figures are unusual
- *Sinonasal undifferentiated carcinoma (SNUC)*
  - Characterized by nests, trabeculae and sheets of medium sized, polygonal, mitotically active cells; round to oval nuclei , slightly pleomorphic and hyperchromatic with diffuse to coarsely granular chromatin; nucleoli typically prominent, but may be inconspicuous

- □ Tumor cells have moderate amounts of eosinophilic cytoplasm and distinct cell borders
- □ Prominent vascular invasion and extensive necrosis typical
- □ No features of squamous or glandular differentiation

Special Stains

- Not helpful

Immunohistochemistry

- Intestinal-type adenocarcinoma positive for epithelial markers (cytokeratin, EMA, B72.3, and Leu M1); rarely positive for carcinoembryonic antigen (CEA)
- Low-grade adenocarcinoma positive for cytokeratin and EMA and focally positive for CEA
- Sinonasal undifferentiated carcinomas positive for cytokeratin and epithelial membrane antigen; 50% positive for neuron-specific enolase (NSE)

Electron Microscopy

- Intestinal-type adenocarcinoma:

Goblet cells, resorptive cells, Paneth cells, and argentaffin cells all present as well as muscularis mucosae-like smooth muscle

- Sinonasal undifferentiated carcinoma (SNUC):

Tumor cells have poorly formed desmosomes and lack cytoplasmic processes and tonofilaments

Molecular Alterations

- None

Differential Diagnosis

- *Non-keratinizing squamous cell carcinoma*
  - □ Fungiform or inverted nasal Schneiderian papillomas
- *Intestinal type adenocarcinoma*
  - □ Metastatic adenocarcinoma from the gastrointestinal tract
  - □ Mucoepidermoid carcinoma
  - □ Low-grade adenocarcinoma of sinonasal or nasopharyngeal region
- *Low-grade adenocarcinoma*
  - □ Intestinal type adenocarcinoma
  - □ Oncocytic Schneiderian papilloma
  - □ Metastatic papillary carcinoma of thyroid
- *Sinonasal undifferentiated carcinoma (SNUC)*
  - □ Nasopharyngeal undifferentiated carcinoma (lymphoepithelioma)
  - □ Lymphoepithelioma-type undifferentiated carcinoma never grows in a trabecular or organoid pattern, typically lacks a prominent lymphoplasmacytic infiltrate and is composed of cells with more prominent cytoplasm, nuclei that are chromatically uniform, vesicular, and usually have small, inconspicuous nucleoli
  - □ Small cell undifferentiated carcinoma
  - □ Olfactory neuroblastoma
  - □ Lymphoma

Treatment

- Combination of surgery and radiation therapy for squamous cell carcinoma and intestinal-type adenocarcinoma
- Low-grade carcinoma treated with surgical excision
- Undifferentiated carcinoma treated with radiation or chemotherapy

Prognosis

- Squamous cell carcinomas usually recur within 2 years; prognosis better for lesions involving nasal cavity than for lesions involving sinuses
- Intestinal-type adenocarcinoma recurs in 50%, but metastases are fairly infrequent
- Intestinal-type adenocarcinoma arising in woodworkers has a 50% 5-year survival
- Sporadic intestinal-type adenocarcinoma has a 20-40% 5-year survival
- Long-term survival typical for completely excised low-grade adenocarcinoma
- Median survival 4 months for SNUC

Associations

- Sinonasal squamous cell carcinoma of the nasal cavity is related to smoking, industrial exposure to nickel ore, chromium, isopropyl alcohol, and radium
- Squamous cell carcinoma of the maxilla is associated with Thorotrast and chronic sinusitis
- Squamous cell carcinoma in the nasal cavity is associated with a 25% incidence of a second primary neoplasm (40% involve the head and neck; 60% develop at more distant sites such as lung, breast and gastrointestinal tract)
- Squamous cell carcinoma arising in the maxillary antrum carries a 5% incidence of bilateral involvement and no increased risk for the development of carcinoma at another site
- Intestinal-type adenocarcinoma is associated with long-term exposure to fine hardwood dust and leather dust
- Sinonasal undifferentiated carcinoma (SNUC) not associated with EBV

Nasopharynx

Nasopharyngeal Carcinoma

Variants

- Keratinizing squamous cell carcinoma
- Nonkeratinizing squamous cell carcinoma
  - Differentiated
  - Undifferentiated carcinoma (lymphoepithelioma)

Clinical Manifestations

- Squamous cell carcinomas more common in men than women and typically occur after age 40
- Undifferentiated carcinomas occur more frequently in children (a bimodal age distribution [2nd and 6th decades])
- Typically arise near the eustachian tube opening in the fossa of Rosenmüller
- Patients often present with complaints referable to a middle ear obstruction (otitis or hearing loss) or local invasion (headache, cranial nerve deficit, epistaxis)
- 50%-80% will present with cervical lymphadenopathy (usually a metastasis from an occult primary of nonkeratinizing or undifferentiated carcinoma); involved cervical lymph nodes may be bilateral and are typically at the level of the jaw and posterior to the sternocleidomastoid muscle
- Nasopharynx may appear normal, have a slight surface granularity, or contain an obvious carcinoma
- Positive serology against Epstein-Barr virus (EBV) is found in almost 100% of nonkeratinizing squamous cell carcinomas (less common in keratinizing carcinomas)

Gross and Microscopic Pathology

- Keratinizing squamous cell carcinoma has obvious squamous differentiation in the form of intercellular bridges and/or cytoplasmic or extracellular keratinization
- Nonkeratinizing squamous cell carcinoma
  - *Differentiated subtype* characterized by solid sheets, irregular islands, discohesive sheets and trabeculae of carcinoma intimately intermingled with variable numbers of lymphocytes and plasma cells; tumor cells often show various levels of maturation and may lack obvious evidence of squamous differentiation; nuclei tend to be pleomorphic and have variable chromatin patterns; tumor cells usually have well-defined cell borders and interdigitate in a "pavement stone" pattern; no evidence of mucin production or glandular differentiation; in comparison to the undifferentiated subtype, the cells may show some stratification, have well-defined cell borders and occasionally intracellular bridges, a lower nuclear-cytoplasmic ratio, less vesicular chromatin, and less prominent nucleoli
  - *Undifferentiated squamous cell carcinoma subtype* characterized by syncytial-appearing large tumor cells with amphophilic or eosinophilic cytoplasm indistinct cell borders, round to oval vesicular nuclei and large central nucleoli (nuclei appear to float in syncytium of cytoplasm); mitotic figures numerous; spindle cells and apoptotic cells may be present, keratinization and no glandular differentiation; rare

desmoplastic stroma; areas of coagulative necrosis may be present; inflammatory infiltrate consisting primarily of lymphocytes and plasma cells and occasionally eosinophils usually present; the density and distribution of lymphocytes and plasma cells may be quite variable; lymphocytes and plasma cells may be very few or so abundant they infiltrate tumor islands, breaking them into tiny aggregates or single cells to the point the epithelial nature of the neoplasm is obscured *(lymphoepithelial carcinoma)*; two patterns (may be admixed) of lymphocyte distribution: *Regaud pattern*: neoplastic cells arranged in well defined, cohesive nests and trabeculae separated by inflammatory cells; *Schmincke pattern*: an admixture of neoplastic cells and inflammatory cells resulting in individual carcinoma cells dispersed throughout an inflammatory (predominantly lymphoid) background

Special Stains

- Not helpful

Immunohistochemistry

- Neoplastic cells of lymphoepithelioma stain positively for keratin; inflammatory (lymphocytic) component stains positively for leukocyte common antigen (LCA)

Electron Microscopy

- Will confirm the epithelial nature of cells in both nonkeratinizing squamous cell carcinoma and undifferentiated carcinoma
- Tumor cells of lymphoepithelioma often contain tonofilaments and complex desmosomes; syncytial appearance the result of complex interdigitations of cell membranes

Molecular Alterations

- Presence of EBV confirmed by in situ hybridization for EBV encoded early RNA (EBER); all infected cells will show nuclear labeling

Differential Diagnosis

- Lymphoepithelioma may resemble nonkeratinizing squamous cell carcinoma and sinonasal undifferentiated carcinoma (SNUC)
- Metastatic lymphoepithelioma with the Schmincke pattern may be impossible to distinguish from non-Hodgkin lymphoma and Hodgkin disease without immunohistochemical stains
- Metastatic lymphoepithelioma with Regaud pattern may resemble sinus histiocytosis

Treatment

- Almost never surgically resectable; primary radiation therapy treatment of choice
- Keratinizing squamous cell carcinoma the least radiosensitive

Prognosis

- Keratinizing squamous cell carcinomas have a greater propensity for locally advanced growth and a lower propensity for lymph node metastasis than nonkeratinizing carcinomas
- Nonkeratinizing squamous cell carcinomas, both differentiated and undifferentiated, metastasize to regional nodes and distant sites
- 5-year disease-specific survival in patients without metastases 80% with an overall survival of 75%
- Survival rate for undifferentiated carcinoma varies according to stage:
  - Stage I (confined to nasopharynx): 98%
  - Stage II A-B (cervical node involvement): 95%
  - Stage III (invasion of surrounding structures): 85%
  - Stage IV-B: 75%

Associations

- Incidence lower in patients with blood group A
- Nonkeratinizing tumors and undifferentiated tumors associated with EBV infection
- Radiation-induced nasopharyngeal carcinoma not associated with EBV
- Chinese patients living in Singapore have significant higher rates of histocompatibility antigens HLA-A2 and HLA-BW46

Nasopharyngeal Angiofibroma

Clinical Manifestations

- Typically seen in adolescent males between the ages of 10 and 17 years (occasionally seen in adults)
- Classically presents as bilateral nasal obstruction (90 to 95%) and repeated episodes of epistaxis (70%)
- Usually presents as a protruding red or red-blue lobulated or polypoid mass arising exclusively in lateral nasopharynx and posterior nasal cavity
- Inflammatory changes may occur adjacent to the neoplasm causing symptoms of mastoiditis, sinusitis, and otitis media

Gross Pathology

- Mass may extend into the anterior portion of the nasal cavity, pterygomaxillary fossa, cheek, maxillary antrum, or orbit
- External surface usually smooth and red or red-blue, but may be ulcerated; cut surface tends to be smooth and fibrous; deceptively avascular
- Peripheral margin typically pushing rather than infiltrative

Microscopic Pathology

- Classic appearance is one of dense partially collagenized fibrous tissue with many interspersed slit-like or wide-open vascular channels that tend to be particularly prominent at the periphery of the lesion
- Vessels tend to be variable in number and configuration and are usually thin-walled, lined by single layer of endothelium, and lack an elastic membrane; an incomplete rim of smooth muscle may or may not be present
- Fibrous component can be quite variable in cellularity and amount of collagen and contain areas of hyalinization and myxoid change
- Stromal elements predominate in center of lesion; periphery characterized by increased vascularity (small, uniform, and closely packed vessels with little intervening stroma)
- Stromal cells often appear spindled or stellate and have nuclei that vary from pyknotic to large and vesicular; occasionally multinucleated or ganglion-like in appearance
- Mitotic figures very rare
- Collagen fibers often have a haphazard arrangement
- Mast cells frequently present
- Focal areas of squamous metaplasia may be seen in association with ulceration

Special Stains

- Not helpful

Immunohistochemistry

- Endothelial cells positive for vascular markers (eg, factor-VIII-related antigen, CD31, and CD34)
- Stromal cells positive for vimentin and testosterone receptors

Electron Microscopy

- Stromal cells are myofibroblasts with both fibroblast and myofibroblast features; tend to have lobulated nuclei with nucleoli and marginal chromatin; electron-dense intranuclear inclusions surrounded by clear halos are usually present
- Vascular channels lined by large endothelial cells, a distinct basal lamina, and variable numbers of smooth muscle cells

Molecular Alterations

- None

Differential Diagnosis

- Lobular capillary hemangioma
- Aggressive fibromatosis
- Fibroma
- Solitary fibrous tumor

Treatment

- Complete surgical excision following oral administration of estrogen
- Radiotherapy can produce rapid regression of tumor and permanent control of symptoms in up to 80%; sarcomatous transformation and development of squamous cell carcinoma and thyroid carcinoma have all been reported following radiotherapy

- Chemotherapy for aggressive unresectable lesions
- Treatment with androgen or testosterone is not particularly effective

Prognosis

- 35 to 60% recur; entirely dependent upon the completeness of excision
- Tumor related mortality results from intracranial extension or exsanguination

Associations

- None

Hypopharynx, Larynx and Trachea

Squamous Cell Carcinoma

Variants

- Glottic carcinoma
- Transglottic carcinoma
- Supraglottic carcinoma
- Infraglottic (subglottic) carcinoma
- Pyriform sinus carcinoma

Clinical Manifestations

- Much more common in men than in women and typically seen in the 5th decade or later
- Tumor typically occurs in one of four regions: glottic, transglottic, supraglottic, and infraglottic
- Glottic carcinoma
    - Most frequent form of laryngeal cancer in the United States; represents 65% of all laryngeal carcinomas
    - Originates from the anterior mobile portion of true vocal cord; tends to produce hoarseness early
    - Staging:
        - T1: tumor confined to free edge of vocal cord with normal mobility
        - T2: tumor extends above or below the vocal cord impaired mobility
        - T3: tumor confined to larynx with complete fixation of vocal cord
        - T4: tumor invades through thyroid cartilage and/or beyond larynx

50% of patients have a T1 tumor at time of diagnosis

- Transglottic carcinoma
    - Typically a glottic carcinoma with supraglottic extension
    - Neoplasm crosses laryngeal ventricle vertically and involves both the vocal cord and supraglottic structures
- Supraglottic carcinoma
    - Represent 30 to 35% of laryngeal carcinomas
    - Often associated with referred pain to the ear, change in quality of voice, dysphagia, or sensation of a mass
    - Neoplasm may involve one or more anatomic areas: epiglottis, ventricular band, angle between the epiglottis and ventricular band, and the aryepiglottic fold or arytenoid body
    - Carcinoma tends to grow upward with involvement of pyriform sinus and base of tongue; downward growth into glottis unusual
    - Staging:
        - T1: tumor confined to one supraglottic site with normal cord mobility
        - T2: tumor invades mucosa of more than one supraglottic site or extends beyond supraglottis; larynx not fixed
        - T3: tumor confined to larynx with fixation of cord or extends into pre-epiglottic soft tissue
        - T4: tumor invades through thyroid cartilage and/or beyond larynx
- Infraglottic (subglottic)
    - Represents ~5% of all laryngeal carcinomas
    - Includes cancers involving the true cord with subglottic extension of more than 1 cm and tumors entirely confined to the subglottic area

- Neoplasms typically extend to the cricoid cartilage and invade the prelaryngeal wall and thyroid gland
- Staging:
  - T1: tumor confined to subglottis
  - T2: tumor extends to vocal cord with or without normal mobility
  - T3: tumor limited to larynx with cord fixation
  - T4: tumor extends through cricoid or thyroid cartilage and/or extends beyond larynx
- Pyriform sinus carcinoma arises below the level of the vocal cords and frequently invades the larynx under an intact mucous membrane; invasion of the larynx usually begins in the posterior edge of the thyroid cartilage or in the upper posterior cricoid

Gross and Microscopic Pathology

- Most tumors appear as an exophytic, fungating, tan, and focally ulcerated mass on mucosal surface; edges may be elevated as a result of submucosal extension
- May be well-differentiated, moderately differentiated, or poorly differentiated depending upon the amount of keratinization, squamous pearl formation, or presence of intracellular bridges between tumor cells
- Microscopically similar to squamous cell carcinomas arising elsewhere
- Well-differentiated tumors demonstrate extensive keratinization of nodules of cells that tend to be located in the center of cords of less well-differentiated invasive cells that frequently have a basaloid appearance
- Poorly-differentiated cancers show only focal evidence of individual cell keratinization
- Microscopic features that have a bearing on clinical behavior include nuclear characteristics, mitotic count, nature of the borders of the neoplasm, and the presence or absence of vascular invasion
- Variants:
  - *Verrucous carcinoma*
    - Represents 1 to 5% of all laryngeal carcinomas
    - Cytologic and architectural features reminiscent of a reactive process; can invade underlying normal tissue; invasion usually limited and metastasis rare
    - Invasion usually limited and metastases very rare
  - *Squamous cell carcinoma with spindle cell features*
    - Typically polypoid
    - Characterized by a squamous cell carcinoma component admixed with a spindle cell component
    - Spindled component may be so bland it resembles granulation tissue or so malignant it resembles malignant fibrous histiocytoma, malignant giant cell tumor of soft parts, or osteosarcoma
    - Lymph node metastasis may be composed of a squamous cell component and/or a spindle cell component
  - *Basaloid squamous cell carcinoma*
    - Tend to involve supraglottic region
    - Characterized by typical invasive squamous carcinoma or squamous cell carcinoma in situ in association with nests and cords of small crowded moderately pleomorphic basaloid cells with scant cytoplasm, small cystic spaces, necrosis, prominent stromal hyalinization, and peripheral palisading; basaloid cell nuclei typically hyperchromatic (occasionally vesicular) and mitotically active
    - Interface between squamous cell components and basaloid components very abrupt
    - Overall architecture of the small nests of cells may appear somewhat adnexal (glandular) as a result of a cribriform growth pattern with nests of cells surrounding mucoid material
    - A very malignant and extremely aggressive neoplasm
  - *Adenosquamous carcinoma*
    - Usually large, exophytic, and ulcerated
    - 3 distinct histologic components, each of which may have varying degrees of differentiation:

- Squamous cell carcinoma (usually predominant)
- Adenocarcinoma
- A mixed pattern of glandular mucous cells and cells with squamous differentiation reminiscent of mucoepidermoid carcinoma

- Tumor cells typically infiltrate the ductal-glandular framework of the minor salivary glands and invade adjacent submucosal soft tissue; perineural invasion frequently present

Special Stains

- Mucicarmine, PAS with diastase, and Alcian blue (pH 2.5 and 1.0) will confirm the presence of intracellular mucin (mucin may be neutral glycoprotein, acidic sialomucin, and sulfomucin) in adenosquamous carcinomas

Immunohistochemistry

- Well-differentiated tumors are immunoreactive for AE1/3
- Poorly-differentiated tumors are typically diffusely positive for CAM5.2 and only focally positive for AE1/3
- Basaloid component of basaloid squamous cell carcinomas weakly positive for cytokeratin
- Glandular cells of adenosquamous carcinoma positive for low molecular weight cytokeratins and CEA; high molecular weight cytokeratin present in both squamous and glandular components

Electron Microscopy

- May be of use in determining if the spindle cell component of a squamous cell carcinoma with spindle cell features is malignant
- Basaloid cells have well-formed desmosomes and few tonofilaments; no neurosecretory granules
- Dense core secretory granules may be present in small cell (oat cell) carcinoma

Molecular Alterations

- Overexpression of p53 present in approximately 60%

Differential Diagnosis

- Verrucous carcinoma may be difficult to differentiate from a benign squamous papilloma and a well-differentiated squamous cell carcinoma
- Basaloid squamous cell carcinoma may resemble small cell undifferentiated carcinoma and adenoid cystic carcinoma
- Adenosquamous carcinoma must be distinguished from high-grade mucoepidermoid carcinoma, basaloid squamous carcinoma, and necrotizing sialometaplasia of minor salivary glands

Treatment

- Glottic cancer
    - 90% of lesions on the free edge of a completely mobile vocal cord can be cured by radiation or limited surgical resection
    - Lesions that extend below the vocal cord but do not cause immobility of the cord treated with partial laryngectomy (radiation therapy is not particularly useful)
    - Lesions causing vocal cord fixation treated with total laryngectomy
- Transglottic cancer is usually treated with total laryngectomy and neoadjuvant chemotherapy and/or postoperative radiation plus elective lymph node dissection
- Supraglottic cancer treated with a horizontal, supraglottic partial laryngectomy (a procedure that preserves the voice)
- Infraglottic (subglottic) tumors treated with laryngectomy and distal resection of trachea with radical lymph node dissection to include removal of paratracheal nodes
- Pyriform sinus carcinoma treated with total laryngectomy with neoadjuvant chemotherapy or adjuvant radiotherapy

Prognosis

- *Glottic carcinoma*
    - Lymph node metastasis present in <10% of patients with T1 and T2 tumors
    - Overall five-year survival 80% (T1 90%, T2 85%, T3 55%, T4 25%)
    - Increased risk of local recurrence if treated with radiation

- *Transglottic carcinoma*
  - 50% of tumors that cross the laryngeal ventricle have lymph node metastases
  - 50% five-year survival
- *Supraglottic carcinoma*
  - Glottis involved in <1%
  - Lymph node metastases present in ~ 40%
  - 65% three-year survival (T1 85%, T2 75%, T3 70%, T4 65%)
  - Neoplasms arising in the aryepiglottic folds have a worse prognosis
- *Subglottic carcinoma*
  - 40% five-year survival
  - Neoplasm frequently extends into the trachea
  - Cervical lymph node metastases present in 15 to 20%; paratracheal node metastasis in 50%
- *Pyriform sinus carcinoma*
  - 65% mortality
- A single positive lymph node decreases 5-year survival by at least 50%

Associations

- Smoking is a major risk factor, increased by concurrent heavy alcohol consumption (excluding glottic carcinoma)
- Patients have increased risk (~10%) for development of a second tumor in upper aerodigestive tract or lung

Adenosquamous Carcinoma

Clinical Manifestations

- Aggressive malignant neoplasm that arises from minor salivary glands and ducts or surface mucosa; may occur in the tongue, floor of the mouth, nasal cavity, and larynx (does not involve major salivary glands)
- Much more common in men than in women; average age at diagnosis 60

Gross Pathology

- Usually presents as a small erythroplakic ulcer or indurated submucosal nodule
- Laryngeal tumors usually large, exophytic, and ulcerated

Microscopic Pathology

- Three distinct histologic components, each of which may have varying degrees of differentiation:
  - Squamous cell carcinoma (usually predominant)
  - Adenocarcinoma
  - A mixed pattern of glandular mucous cells and cells with squamous differentiation reminiscent of mucoepidermoid carcinoma
- Metastases usually contain all three components
- Tumor cells typically infiltrate the ductal-glandular framework of the minor salivary glands and invade adjacent submucosal soft tissue; perineural invasion frequently present
- Multifocal carcinoma in situ involving the salivary gland ducts, extension of intraductal carcinoma upward to involve overlying mucosal epithelium in the form of carcinoma in situ, and the presence of glassy squamous cells may all be present

Special Stains

- Mucicarmine, PAS with diastase, and Alcian blue (pH 2.5 and 1.0) will confirm the presence of intracellular mucin (mucin may be neutral glycoprotein, acidic sialomucin, and sulfomucin)

Immunohistochemistry

- Glandular cells positive for low molecular weight cytokeratins and CEA
- High molecular weight cytokeratin present in both squamous and glandular components

Electron Microscopy

- Can confirm the presence of glandular features

Molecular Alterations

- None

Differential Diagnosis

- High-grade mucoepidermoid carcinoma of salivary type
- Basaloid squamous cell carcinoma
- Necrotizing sialometaplasia of minor salivary glands

Treatment

- Surgical excision with radical neck dissection with or without cervical radiotherapy

Prognosis

- Distant metastatic disease develops in 80% of patients with tumors >1 cm in size
- 10 year survival 25%; no survivors at 15 years

Associations

- None

Basaloid Squamous Cell Carcinoma

Clinical Manifestations

- 90% occur in men with history of smoking and heavy alcohol consumption
- Median age at diagnosis approximately 60 years
- An aggressive variant of squamous cell carcinoma that tends to occur in the oral cavity (base of tongue, pyriform sinus, and palatine tonsil), nasopharynx, and larynx (also reported in the lung, anal canal, thymus, and esophagus)

Gross Pathology

- Rarely exophytic
- Often ulcerated with extensive induration in surrounding mucosa (tumor spreads peripherally under intact mucosa)
- Cut section firm, pale, and infiltrating

Microscopic Pathology

- Characterized by variably sized nests and cords of crowded basaloid cells and foci of conventional squamous cell carcinoma
- Single cell necrosis usually present in smaller nests; areas of comedonecrosis often present in center of larger nests
- Periphery of the basaloid component usually demonstrates nuclear palisading
- Nests of basaloid cells occasionally arranged in a cribriform pattern (appear as small pseudoglandular structures filled with eosinophilic hyalinized or mucoid material)
- Stroma between nests often has a dense, refractile, hyalinized appearance; may be myxoid
- Basaloid cells are moderately pleomorphic and have little cytoplasm; nuclei are usually hyperchromatic but may be vesicular; mitotic figures usually abundant and often atypical
- Areas of typical squamous cell differentiation consisting of cells with abundant eosinophilic cytoplasm, intercellular bridges, and/or keratin pearl formation always present in combination with or separate from the aggregates of basaloid cells
- Interface between basaloid nests and foci of squamous cell carcinoma usually very abrupt
- If surface mucosa intact over the neoplasm, it may be normal, hyperplastic, or dysplastic; regardless strands of basaloid cells often appear to drop off from the mucosal basal layer

Special Stains

- PAS and Alcian blue will highlight material within pseudoglandular spaces formed by basaloid cells

Immunohistochemistry

- Basaloid cells typically weakly positive for cytokeratin
- Majority stain diffusely and weakly for neuron-specific enolase and focally for S-100 protein
- Conventional squamous cells are strongly cytokeratin positive

Electron Microscopy

- Basaloid cells contain well-formed desmosomes and rare bundles of tonofilaments; no neurosecretory granules, myofilaments, or evidence of glandular secretory differentiation
- Prominent basal lamina material lines cyst-like spaces

Molecular Alterations

- None

Differential Diagnosis

- Adenoid cystic carcinoma
- Small-cell undifferentiated carcinoma
- Adenosquamous carcinoma
- Collision tumors with squamous cell carcinoma and adenoid cystic carcinoma or small cell carcinoma

Treatment

- Radical surgical excision with adjuvant radiation or chemotherapy

Prognosis

- Basaloid squamous cell carcinoma and high-grade conventional squamous cell carcinoma have about the same prognosis stage for stage; basaloid squamous cell carcinoma presents at a more advanced stage

Associations

- Tumors in nasopharynx associated with EBV

Spindle Cell Carcinoma

Clinical Manifestations

- Typically arise in the vermillion portion of the lower lip, tongue, alveolar ridge, and gingiva
- Common sites outside the oral cavity include larynx, hypopharynx, and nasal cavity
- Patients usually complain of pain, swelling, and a non-healing ulcer
- Seen more commonly in men than women and usually diagnosed during sixth decade
- Patients typically have a history of alcohol and tobacco use, poor oral hygiene, and occasionally history of previous irradiation to the site

Gross Pathology

- Tumor typically protrudes from the mucosal surface as an exophytic, fungating, polypoid mass; may be attached by a broad base or a narrow stalk giving the erroneous impression that it can be easily amputated
- Surface intact or ulcerated
- Cut section firm and tan to white

Microscopic Pathology

- Diagnosis requires the presence of biphasic population of cells consisting of squamous cell carcinoma and malignant spindle cells
- Two histologic variants:
  - Superficially invasive squamous cell carcinoma (occasionally an in situ squamous cell carcinoma) overlying what appears to be a separate atypical spindle-cell proliferation
  - An invasive squamous cell carcinoma admixed with a malignant spindle cell component (a carcinosarcoma pattern)
- Squamous cell carcinoma component may have all histologic grades of differentiation with an overlying epithelium that can have areas of typical carcinoma in situ, atypical squamous hyperplasia, or verrucous carcinoma
- Spindle cell component can have a variety of histologic patterns:
  - Edematous myxoid stroma with atypical bipolar spindled-cells or plump epithelioid cells mixed with inflammatory cells and blood vessels
  - Densely cellular proliferation that resembles fibrosarcoma, hemangiopericytoma, or MFH
  - Occasional cells that resemble rhabdomyoblasts
  - Numerous osteoclast-like giant cells with features reminiscent of a malignant giant-cell tumor of soft tissue
  - Foci of neoplastic chondroid, cartilage, osteoid, and osseous bony metaplasia
- Metastatic lesions may be purely squamous cell carcinoma, purely spindle cell, or a mixture of both

Special Stains

- Not helpful

Immunohistochemistry

- 50% of lesions will be positive for cytokeratin in the spindle-cell component
- Spindle-cell component may show positivity for muscle-specific actin; desmin rarely positive

Electron Microscopy

- May confirm epithelial nature of the spindle-cell component

Molecular Alterations

- None

Differential Diagnosis

- True sarcoma (usually rhabdomyosarcoma)
- Bizarre granulation tissue and ulcerated irradiated reactions
- Mucosal melanoma

Treatment

- Complete surgical excision
- Primary radiation therapy is ineffective and is associated with an 80% failure rate

Prognosis

- Mortality rate 60% to 65%; mean survival 10 months to slightly <2 years
- Survival rates unaffected by tumor size, gross appearance, grade, histologic features of sarcoma, depth of invasion, and history of prior irradiation
- Most important prognostic factors include the presence or absence of metastasis in cervical lymph nodes

Associations

- Almost 20% have multiple synchronous and metachronous primary carcinomas of the upper respiratory and digestive tracts, a reflection of a common field cancerization to local carcinogen

Papillary Squamous Cell Carcinoma

Clinical Manifestations

- Male predominance
- Most present in 6th or 7th decades
- Smoking and alcohol abuse major etiologic factors
- Role of HPV currently unknown
- Most common in hypopharynx and larynex; in larynx usually foud in supraglottis; rare in subglottis
- Most present with hoarseness or airway obstruction; other symptoms dysphagia, sore throat, cough, and hemoptysis

Gross Pathology

- Soft, friable, polypoid, exophytic papillary mass
- May have a stalk or be broad-based

Microscopic Pathology

- Papillary growth pattern with thin fibrovascular cores that are covered with neoplastic, basaloid cells or pleomorphic cells
- Frequently there is some keratosis, and foci of necrosis and hemorrhage
- May be multiple
- Invasion characterized by single or multiple nests of tumor cells with dense lymphoplasmacytic inflammation at tumor-stromal interface
- If no invasion lesion called atypical papillary hypertplasia or papillary squamous cell carcinoma in situ

Special Stains

- Not helpful

Immunohistochemistry

- Tumor cells stain with cytokeratins and p53

Electron Microscopy

- Not helpful

Differential Diagnosis

- Squamous papilloma

- Verrucous carcinoma
- Exophytic squamous cell carcinoma (papillary stalks better defined in papillary SCC)
- Surgical excision with or without radiation

Prognosis

- Better than squamous cell carcinoma

Lymphoepithelial Carcinoma

Clinical Manifestations

- Male predominance (4:1)
- Mean age at presentation 60 years
- Smoking and alcohol abuse major etiologic factors
- Epstein-Barr virus (EBV) uncommon
- Very rare in hypopharynx, larynx, and trachea (in larynx 65% supraglottic)
- Most present with hoarseness, neck mass, sore throat, cough, otalgia, dysphagia, or hemoptysis

Gross Pathology

- Mass with deep or superficial ulcerations

Microscopic Pathology

- Morphologically indistinguishable from undifferentiated nasopharyngeal carcinoma
- 50% have a squamous cell component (10% to 75% of entire tumor)
- Overlying epithelium may show carcinoma in situ
- Inflammatory infiltrate consisting primarily of lymphocytes and plasma cells and occasionally eosinophils present; lymphocytes and plasma cells infiltrate tumor islands, breaking them into tiny aggregates or single cells sometimes to the point the epithelial nature of the neoplasm is obscured; two patterns (may be admixed) of lymphocyte and plasma cell distribution: *Regaud pattern*: neoplastic cells arranged in well defined, cohesive nests and trabeculae separated by inflammatory cells; *Schmincke pattern*: an admixture of neoplastic cells and inflammatory cells resulting in individual carcinoma cells dispersed throughout an inflammatory (predominantly lymphoid) background

Special Stains

- Not helpful

Immunohistochemistry

- Neoplastic cells of lymphoepithelioma stain positively for keratin; inflammatory (lymphocytic) component stains positively for leukocyte common antigen (LCA)

Electron Microscopy

- Not helpful

Differential Diagnosis

- May resemble nonkeratinizing squamous cell carcinoma and sinonasal undifferentiated carcinoma (SNUC)
- Metastatic lymphoepithelioma with the Schmincke pattern may be impossible to distinguish from non-Hodgkin lymphoma and Hodgkin disease without immunohistochemical stains
- Metastatic lymphoepithelioma with Regaud pattern may resemble sinus histiocytosis

Treatment

- Radiation

Prognosis

- Survival rate varies according to stage:
    - Stage I (confined to nasopharynx): 98%
    - Stage II A-B (cervical node involvement): 95%
    - Stage III (invasion of surrounding structures): 85%
    - Stage IV-B: 75%

Associations

- Presence of EBV rarely demonstrated

References

Mills S, Carter D, Greenson JK, Oberman HA, Reuter V, and Stoler, MH (eds). *Sternberg's Diagnostic Surgical Pathology, 4th ed.* Philadelphia: Lippincott Williams & Wilkins, 2004.

Rosai J. *Rosai and Ackerman's Surgical Pathology, 9th edition.* St. Louis: Mosby, 2004.

Dabbs DJ. *Diagnostic Immunohistochemistry.* New York, Churchill Livingstone, 2002.

Rice DH and Batsakis JG. *Surgical Pathology of the Head and Neck.* Philadelphia, Lippincott Williams & Wilkins, 2000.

Batsakis JG. *Tumors of the Head and Neck. Clinical and Pathological Considerations, 2nd ed.* Baltimore: Williams & Wilkins, 1979.

Kumar V, Abbas AK, Fausto N (eds.) *Robbins and Cotran Pathologic Basis of Disease, 7th ed.* Philadelphia: Elsevier Saunders, 2005.

Barns L, Everson, JW Reichert, P and Sidransky D (eds.). *World Health Organization Classification of Tumours. Pathology & Genetics Head and Neck Tumours.* IARC Press: Lyon 2005.

Chapter 11

Lung

Intraoperative Consultation

Indications for intraoperative consultation involving diseases that affect the lung occur in 1 of 3 clinical settings:

- To ensure that representative tissue has been obtained, particularly in patients undergoing video-assisted thoracoscopic surgery, to obtain pleural, lung, and mediastinal biopsy specimens or for resection for a pulmonary nodule
- To determine that bronchial margins are negative when resection is performed for malignancy
- To determine if unanticipated metastatic disease is present in regional lymph nodes

Surgical specimens of lung tissue obtained in the presence of diffuse interstitial disease or localized infiltrates are often submitted for an intraoperative consultation to ensure that representative (diagnostic) tissue has been submitted. The identification of fungal elements or bacterial organisms will have an obvious immediate effect on patient management. Both the surgeon and pathologist must be aware that several neoplastic processes such as lymphoma, lymphangitic carcinoma, and bronchioloalveolar carcinoma can all produce pulmonary infiltrates that can mimic either acute or chronic inflammatory disease.

Several diagnostic problems are associated with frozen sections on pulmonary nodules. Diagnosis of a lymphoproliferative lesion will typically be deferred to permanent section. The pathologist's role intraoperatively is to ensure that an adequate tissue specimen has been obtained and that an appropriate lymphoma workup can be performed if necessary. Both bronchioloalveolar carcinoma and well-differentiated adenocarcinoma may be difficult to differentiate from papillary adenoma of type 2 pneumocytes, alveolar adenoma, sclerosing hemangioma, and bronchioloalveolar hyperplasia and metaplasia (the latter 3 are usually well-circumscribed and lack the cytologic atypia and mitotic activity that characterize a carcinoma).

Neuroendocrine tumors are important to classify intraoperatively as typical carcinoid, atypical carcinoid, or small cell carcinoma. Typical carcinoids can be problematic for the pathologist if they contain papillary, clear cell, oncocytic, or spindle cell patterns. All of these patterns may mimic various metastatic neoplasms. Atypical carcinoids must be differentiated from typical carcinoids because the latter are treated with simple wedge excision and the former with a lobectomy or pneumonectomy. Atypical carcinoids typically have readily identifiable mitotic figures, small foci of necrosis, and/or nuclear pleomorphism. Differentiating an atypical carcinoid from a small cell undifferentiated carcinoma on frozen section may be all but impossible; in this setting the diagnosis should be deferred. When diagnostic guidance is required in this situation, it is prudent for the pathologist to err on the side of recommending surgical excision. Morphologic features that favor small cell undifferentiated carcinoma include a sheetlike growth pattern, extensive necrosis, abundant mitotic activity, nuclear molding, and deposits of DNA in vessel walls (the Azzopardi phenomenon). Benign and malignant papillary and spindle cell neoplasms involving the lung may appear quite similar and often necessitate a deferred diagnosis. When the diagnosis is to be deferred, a conservative excision with 1 to 2 cm grossly negative margins should be recommended.

Mediastinal staging for lung cancer requires the pathologist to determine if the excised lymph nodes are positive or negative for metastatic carcinoma and if the carcinoma is of the small cell type or non-small cell type. The presence or absence of positive lymph nodes in the mediastinum may determine whether the surgeon abandons the procedure or proceeds to pulmonary resection. One significant pitfall in the evaluation of mediastinal samples is the presence of involuted thymic tissue that may appear on frozen section as a metastatic squamous cell carcinoma. Even the classic Hassall corpuscles of a thymoma may mimic the keratinized pearls of squamous cell carcinoma.

The evaluation of bronchial margins in lobectomy and pneumonectomy specimens probably represent the most common indication for a frozen section on a lung specimen. Microscopic involvement of the surgical margin by carcinoma can be seen as:

1) carcinoma in situ
2) invasive carcinoma in the submucosa
3) invasive carcinoma in the peribronchial soft tissue
4) lymphatic space involvement

When the pathologist is asked to perform a frozen section on a bronchial margin, a complete ring of tissue to include the peribronchial soft tissue should be submitted. The ring of tissue should be embedded so that the true margin is placed deepest in the block.

Occasionally the presence of diagnostic tissue needs to be confirmed by frozen section when the tissue comes from pleura. The differentiation between granulomatous and neoplastic disease can have obvious intraoperative implications. Suspicious visceral and parietal pleural lesions are almost always submitted for frozen section, because positive biopsy findings usually indicate unresectable neoplasms. Benign mesothelial proliferations may mimic metastatic carcinoma. If the lesion is not clearly invasive, the diagnosis is usually best deferred even in the presence of significant cytologic atypia and mitotic activity. The differentiation of atypical mesothelial hyperplasia and mesothelioma can be quite difficult on permanent sections, much less frozen section.

Specimen Handling

Wedge biopsies, lobectomies, and pneumonectomies are best fixed by insufflating the lung parenchyma with formalin before immersing the specimen in formalin. Specimens obtained for neoplasm should be extensively sampled at the interface between the neoplasm and adjacent lung parenchyma as well as at the pleural surface and at the bronchial margin. All peribronchial lymph nodes are also submitted.

Specimens obtained for the evaluation of diffuse interstitial lung disease or localized infiltrate should involve the obtaining of cultures and other diagnostic tests for infectious disease. These studies require that the tissue be handled in a sterile manner until the frozen section has been examined to determine the appropriateness of cultures.

Lymphoproliferative lesions should be fixed in B5 as well as formalin and a sample of tissue should be placed in RPMI medium for flow cytometry. In addition a sample should be frozen so that immunologic studies can be performed if required. If immune-complex-mediated disease is suspected, a representative portion of fresh tissue should be frozen and placed in the appropriate fixative.

Non-Neoplastic Lesions

Bronchogenic Cyst

Clinical Manifestations

- Usually presents in children or young adults
- Males and females affected equally
- Children present with respiratory distress; adults usually present with symptoms secondary to infection involving the cyst
- 15% are asymptomatic
- Chest x-ray demonstrates a sharply defined smooth mass with a dense center located beneath the carina or in the mid-mediastinum; may occur in supraclavicular or subdiaphragmatic location

Gross Pathology

- Typically unilocular and filled with mucus
- Contents may be purulent if infected
- Wall varies in thickness

Microscopic Pathology

- Cyst wall consists of a lining of ciliated cuboidal to columnar respiratory epithelium surrounded by a fibromuscular wall, which contains islands of cartilage and nests of bronchial glands
- Squamous metaplasia may be present in the cyst lining if it has been infected; other signs of infection include a purulent exudate and inflammatory changes
- Cartilage must be present for definitive diagnosis
- If no cartilage or bronchial glands present then lesion is more likely an *undifferentiated foregut cyst*

Special Stains, Immunohistochemistry, and Electron Microscopy

- Not helpful

Molecular Alterations

- None

Differential Diagnosis

- Abscess (often multiple, intrapulmonary, and communicate with a bronchus)

- Enteric cyst (usually located in the posterior mediastinum and lined by gastric epithelium; occasionally associated with vertebral malformations)
- Esophageal cyst (squamous lining and muscular wall reminiscent of esophageal wall)
- Pericardial cyst (typically located in right or left cardiophrenic angle; unilocular with a mesothelial lining)
- Cystic teratoma (usually multiloculated and located in anterior mediastinum; consists of endodermal and ectodermal derivatives, bronchial type epithelium, cartilage, and bronchial type glands)
- Congenital cystic adenomatoid malformation

Treatment and Prognosis

- Surgical resection
- No reports of a malignant transformation

Associations

- None

Congenital Pulmonary Airway Malformation (CPAM; Congenital Cystic Adenomatoid Malformation)

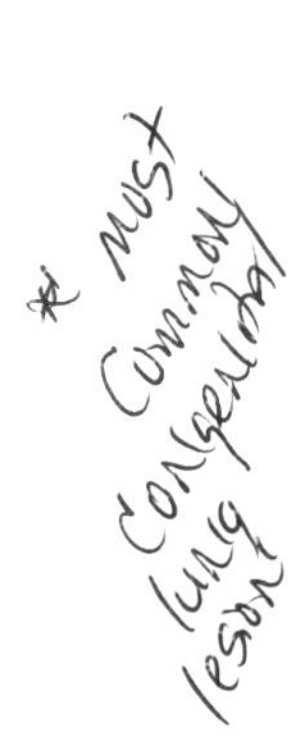

Clinical Manifestations

- Usually seen in stillborn infants or newborn infants with respiratory distress
- Occasionally older children or adults present with an expansile cystic mass
- Slightly more common in boys than in girls
- Occur with equal frequency in either lung; usually unilateral and involve one lobe

Gross Pathology

- Type 0 CPAM:
  - ☐ A malformation of the most proximal tracheobronchial tree
- Type 1 CPAM:

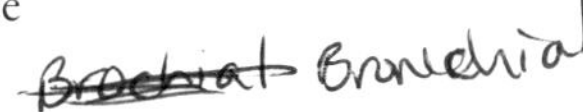

  - ☐ 65% of cases
  - ☐ Characterized by multilocular cysts with broad septa
  - ☐ Cysts typically large (up to 10 cm)
- Type 2 CPAM:
  - ☐ 10% to 15% of cases
  - ☐ Typically small cysts (up to 2.5 cm)
- Type 3 CPAM:
  - ☐ 5% of cases
  - ☐ Usually a large bulky mass that causes a shift of the mediastinum
  - ☐ Essentially solid with cysts <0.5 cm
- Type 4 CPAM:
  - ☐ 10% to 15%
  - ☐ Composed of thin-walled structures suggesting a malformation of distal acinal components

Microscopic Pathology

- Usually communicate with bronchial tree and merge imperceptibly with adjacent normal lung
- Large cysts lined by cuboidal or columnar ciliated respiratory epithelium
- Small spaces lined by type 1 or type 2 alveolar cells
- Type 0 CPAM (acinar dysplasia or agenesis)
  - ☐ Composed of bronchuslike structures with muscle, glands, and numerous cartilage plates
- Type 1 CPAM (large or predominant cyst type)
  - ☐ Composed of bronchuslike and proximal bronchiolelike structures lined with ciliated, pseudostratified columnar epithelium
  - ☐ Mucinous cells present in 30% (usually arranged in small clusters or tufts of well-differentiated goblet cells)
  - ☐ Cyst walls characterized by an increase in elastic tissue and smooth muscle
  - ☐ Fibrous septa tend to be broad
  - ☐ Cartilage present in 5% to 10%
- Type 2 CPAM (medium cyst type)
  - ☐ Composed of bronchiolelike structures and resembles bronchiolar segment of acinus
  - ☐ Some increase in elastic tissue and smooth muscle in cyst walls (not as marked as in type I)
  - ☐ Skeletal muscle present in 5%
  - ☐ Mucinous cells and cartilage plates are rarely present
- Type 3 CPAM (small cystic or solid type)
  - ☐ Composed of bronchiolelike structures and alveolar ducts and saccules lined by cuboidal epithelium (an "adenomatoid" appearance)

Pulmonary sequestration = a benign mass of non-functioning lung tissue that appears during early lung development. The lesion has NO connection c̄ the airway and receives its blood supply from the systemic circulation (Abd or thoracic aorta).

- Resembles early canalicular stage of lung development (16 to 28 weeks)
- Slight increase in elastic tissue and smooth muscle in fibrous septa

■ Type 4 CPAM (peripheral cyst type)

- Cysts lined by flattened epithelial cells type I and II alveolar lining cells)

Special Stains, Immunohistochemistry, and Electron Microscopy

■ Not helpful

Molecular Alterations

■ None

Differential Diagnosis

■ Other congenital and acquired cystic changes

Treatment and Prognosis

■ Surgical resection

■ Recurrent infections likely if not removed

■ Type 0 CPAM incompatible with life

■ Type 1 CPAM can be cured with resection

■ Type 2 and 3 CPAM are associated with a poor prognosis

■ Type 4 CPAM survival excellent with resection

Associations

■ May be complicated by the development of carcinoma (usually a mucinous bronchioloalveolar carcinoma)

■ Type 0, 1, 3, and 4 CPAM

- Other anomalies rare

■ Type 2 CPAM

- Other anomalies present in 50% (eg, bilateral renal atresia/dysgenesis, extralobar pulmonary sequestration, cardiovascular malformations, jejunal atresia, pulmonary hypoplasia, skeletal malformations, and others)

Pulmonary Sequestration (Extralobar and Intralobar)

Clinical Manifestations

■ *Extralobar sequestration*

- 60% diagnosed under the age of 6 months
- 10% asymptomatic
- Boys affected 4 times more frequently than girls
- 65% occur on left
- Most infants present with dyspnea, cyanosis, and problems feeding

■ *Intralobar sequestration*

- 50% present in adults over the age of 20 years
- 15% are asymptomatic
- Affect men and women equally
- 55% occur on the left

Gross Pathology

■ All sequestrations are defined as pulmonary parenchyma that is not in continuity with the normal tracheobronchial tree

■ *Extralobar sequestration*

- A true congenital anomaly consisting of accessory lung tissue with its own pleural covering located in the thorax, diaphragm, or abdomen
- 65% occur between the lower lobe and the diaphragm; fewer than 15% occur within or below the diaphragm
- Usually single with a pyramidal or oval shape
- Fragments of cartilaginous bronchi are present in 50%
- Secondary infection produces fibrosis of the pleural covering with or without an exudate
- Cut section reveals either normal lung parenchyma or cystic change
- Arterial supply almost always systemic (rarely pulmonary)
- Venous drainage may be systemic or portal (only 25% drain completely or partly into pulmonary venous system)

■ *Intralobular sequestration*

- Found in normal pleural investment of the lung
- Tends to occur in the medial aspect of the lower lobes
- Cut surface reveals pleural thickening, adhesions, and a fibrotic parenchyma with variable sized cysts (some up to 5 cm)
- Cysts frequently contain mucinous or purulent material
- Large feeder arteries may be readily apparent and always have a systemic origin
- Venous drainage almost always into pulmonary venous system (very rarely systemic)

Microscopic Pathology

- *Extralobar sequestration*
  - Uninfected cases characterized by dilated airways lined by a bronchiolar epithelium and dilated airspaces that are lined by type 1 and type 2 pneumocytes and contain intraalveolar macrophages
  - Well-formed bronchi may be present
  - Foci of extramedullary hematopoiesis may be present (especially in premature infants)
  - Subpleural lymphatics usually dilated and arteries have thick walls (systemic origin)
  - Infected cases characterized by nonspecific acute and chronic inflammatory changes, fibrosis, and purulent exudate
  - Foci indistinguishable from congenital cystic adenomatoid malformation may be present
- *Intralobar sequestration*
  - Pulmonary parenchyma fibrotic
  - Bronchial remnants dilated and contain mucus or purulent material
  - Alveoli typically filled with foamy alveolar macrophages
  - Epithelial metaplasia typically present
  - Border between sequestered tissue and normal lung parenchyma may be abrupt or indistinct

Special Stains

- Systemic vessels can be highlighted with elastic tissue stains

Immunohistochemistry and Electron Microscopy

- Not helpful

Molecular Alterations

- None

Differential Diagnosis

- Extralobar sequestration:
  - Congenital cystic adenomatoid malformation
  - Abscess

Treatment and Prognosis

- Surgical excision

Associations

- *Extralobar sequestration*
  - Associated anomalies common (60%) and include pectus excavatum and diaphragmatic defects
- *Intralobar sequestration*
  - Associated anomalies uncommon (5%-10%)
  - Squamous cell carcinoma has been reported to occur

Alveolar Hemorrhage Syndromes

Etiologies

- Goodpasture syndrome
- Idiopathic pulmonary hemosiderosis (IPH)
- Wegener granulomatosis and other vasculitides
- Acute lupus pneumonitis
- Underlying diseases, eg, rheumatoid arthritis, polymyositis, mixed connective tissue disease, cryoglobulinemia, Henoch-Schönlein purpura
- Drug reactions, eg, penicillamine, nitrofurantoin, L-tryptophan
- Inhalants, eg, cocaine
- Bone marrow transplantation
- Rapidly progressive glomerulonephritis

Clinical Manifestations

- *Goodpasture syndrome*
  - Antibodies to glomerular basement membrane (type IV collagen), which cross-react with pulmonary basement membrane, in patient's serum
  - Most present with sudden onset of hemoptysis, anemia, azotemia, and diffuse pulmonary infiltrates
  - Men affected twice as often as women; usually young adult cigarette smokers
- *IPH*
  - Clinical picture identical to Goodpasture but without the renal failure; most present with hemoptysis, chest infiltrates on x-ray, and iron-deficiency anemia
  - Affects children under age of 16 years
  - Men and women affected equally
  - 50% have elevated serum IgA; antibodies to basement membrane absent
  - Clinical course characterized by spontaneous remissions and exacerbations

- *Wegener granulomatosis and other vasculitides*
  - See Wegener granulomatosis (p 397)
- *Acute lupus pneumonitis*
  - Patients present with fever, tachypnea, severe hypoxemia, and diffuse infiltrates
- *Underlying diseases (all are rare causes of pulmonary hemorrhage)*
  - Rheumatoid arthritis: Patients present with pleurisy and pleural effusion
  - Polymyositis: Patients may present with bronchopneumonia secondary to a depressed cough reflex and aspiration as a result of respiratory muscle weakness
  - Mixed connective tissue disease: Patients have clinical features of systemic lupus erythematosus, progressive systemic sclerosis, and polymyositis
  - Cryoglobulinemia
  - Henoch-Schönlein purpura
- *Drug reactions*, eg, penicillamine, nitrofurantoin, L-tryptophan, amphotericin B, anticoagulants, cyclophosphamide, haloperidol, hydralazine, mitomycin, propylthiouracil, streptokinase, sulfonamides, and urokinase
- *Inhalants*, eg, cocaine
  - Crack lung syndrome: Acute respiratory distress with non-cardiogenic pulmonary edema and pulmonary hemorrhage
- *Bone marrow transplantation*
  - Pulmonary complications in approximately 50%
  - Rapidly progressive glomerulonephritis

Microscopic Pathology

- *Goodpasture syndrome*
  - Extensive intra-alveolar hemorrhage characterized by both fresh blood and hemosiderin within alveolar macrophages in airspaces
  - Alveolar septa thickened by pneumocyte hyperplasia; occasionally a mild capillaritis with neutrophils may be present
  - Extensive inflammation, vasculitis involving larger vessels, and necrosis are not present
- *Idiopathic pulmonary hemosiderosis*
  - Microscopic findings identical to those of Goodpasture syndrome
  - Vascular elastic tissue often disrupted and covered with iron and calcium; fragments may be present in foreign body giant cells as refractile fragments (*endogenous pneumoconiosis*)
- *Wegener granulomatosis and other vasculitides*
  - See Wegener granulomatosis
- *Acute lupus pneumonitis*
  - Typically a picture of diffuse alveolar damage with interstitial edema, inflammation, and hyaline membranes
  - Occasionally airspaces filled with blood and hemosiderin-laden macrophages (findings almost identical to those of Goodpasture syndrome)
  - Acute necrotizing capillaritis characterized by expansion and destruction of alveolar septa by necrotic neutrophils typically present (not features of Goodpasture)
  - Other vascular changes include intimal thickening, medial hypertrophy, and periadventitial fibrosis; acute changes of fibrinoid necrosis and vasculitis rarely occur outside the setting of pulmonary hemorrhage
- *Underlying diseases rarely reported to cause hemorrhage*
  - Rheumatoid arthritis characterized by pleural lesions of nonspecific pleuritis and necrobiotic nodules; parenchymal lesions consist of an interstitial pneumonia of either the usual type or the nonspecific type; bronchiolitis obliterans with organizing pneumonia (BOOP) or constrictive bronchiolitis obliterans or follicular bronchiolitis; necrobiotic nodules (Caplan syndrome): vasculitis, pulmonary hypertension, and secondary amyloidosis
  - Polymyositis characterized by interstitial pneumonia and interstitial fibrosis, most often of the usual interstitial pneumonia (UIP)-type, but occasionally diffuse alveolar damage (DAD) or rarely nonspecific interstitial pneumonia (NSIP); BOOP may be present in association with the interstitial pneumonia; capillaritis and hemorrhage rare
  - Mixed connective tissue disease characterized by interstitial pneumonia with vascular changes of primary pulmonary hypertension include plexiform lesions, fibrinoid necrosis, and arteritis; hemorrhage rare
  - Cryoglobulinemia
  - Henoch-Schönlein purpura

- *Pulmonary reactions to drugs that can cause hemorrhage*
  - Penicillamine: Obliterative and follicular bronchiolitis, hemorrhage, DAD
  - Nitrofurantoin: DAD, hemorrhage, HP, desquamative interstitial pneumonia (DIP), EP (eosinophilic pneumonia), UIP (usual interstitial pneumonia), CIP (nonspecific chronic interstitial pneumonia) and BOOP
  - L-tryptophan: CIP, hemorrhage
  - Amphotericin B: Hemorrhage
  - Anticoagulants: Hemorrhage
  - Cyclophosphamide: DAD, CIP, UIP, BOOP, hemorrhage
  - Haloperidol: Edema, hemorrhage
  - Hydralazine: Hemorrhage
  - Mitomycin: DAD, BOOP, edema, hemorrhage, hypertension, pleuritis
  - Propylthiouracil: Hemorrhage
  - Streptokinase and urokinase: Hemorrhage, DAD
- *Inhalants*, eg, cocaine
  - Acute crack lung syndrome: Typical changes are those of diffuse alveolar damage; diffuse alveolar hemorrhage may occur
  - Chronic cocaine abuse characterized by evidence of chronic alveolar hemorrhage, interstitial edema, NSIP, and medial hypertrophy of small muscular arteries
- *Bone marrow transplantation*
  - Infectious pneumonia most frequent, with cytomegalovirus being the most common cause
  - Interstitial pneumonia may occur, usually within 3 weeks; may appear as diffuse alveolar damage with intraalveolar fibrin (hyalin membranes), pneumocyte hyperplasia, and fibroblast proliferation or as a nonspecific interstitial pneumonia
  - Diffuse alveolar hemorrhage occurs in approximately 25%; usually within 2 weeks
  - Constrictive bronchiolitis obliterans (obliterative bronchiolitis) occurs in approximately 10% (probably a manifestation of graft-versus-host disease)

Special Stains

- *Goodpasture syndrome:* Linear staining with immunoglobulin (usually IgG) and complement (C3) present along alveolar septa by immunofluorescence
- *IPH:* No immunofluorescent evidence of immunoglobulin or complement deposition
- *Acute lupus pneumonitis:* Capillary basement membranes and alveolar cell and mesothelial cell nuclei stain for immunoglobulin and complement in a granular pattern by immunofluorescence

Electron Microscopy

- *Goodpasture syndrome:* Wide gaps between endothelial cells, fragmented capillary basement membranes, and deposits of ferritin along basement membranes
- *IPH:* Abnormalities in alveolar and capillary basement membranes and damaged alveolar epithelial and capillary endothelial cells
- *Acute lupus pneumonitis:* Electron-dense deposits often present within alveolar capillary basement membranes

Differential Diagnosis

- Causes of alveolar hemorrhage can almost always be determined by a combination of clinical history and laboratory studies and rarely require a biopsy
- Goodpasture, Wegener granulomatosis, and acute lupus pneumonitis represent the most common causes of alveolar hemorrhage to result in a lung biopsy

Treatment and Prognosis

- *Goodpasture syndrome*
  - Plasmapheresis and immunosuppression
  - Prognosis most closely related to severity of renal disease at time of initial diagnosis
  - May recur after apparent successful treatment
- *Idiopathic pulmonary hemosiderosis*
  - Spontaneous remissions and exacerbations common
  - Some benefit from corticosteroids and plasmapheresis

Associations

- Idiopathic pulmonary hemosiderosis
- Celiac disease

Wegener Granulomatosis

Clinical Manifestations

- Characterized by:
  - Necrotizing granulomas of the upper respiratory tract (ear, nose, sinuses, throat), the lower respiratory tract (lung), or both (biopsies from the region of the head and neck often demonstrate nonspecific inflammatory changes)
  - Focal necrotizing or granulomatous vasculitis affecting small to medium-sized vessels (capillaries, venules, arterioles, and arteries) usually in the lungs and upper respiratory tract
  - Focal or necrotizing, usually crescentic, glomerulonephritis
- Occasionally involvement limited to respiratory tract
- Sites of involvement in addition to lungs and kidneys include peripheral nerves, central nervous system, orbit, skin, and breast
- Typically affects adults during middle age (average age 40 years) but all ages may be affected
- Men affected more frequently than women
- Patients with the pulmonary form typically have fever, cough, chest pain, and hemoptysis
- Radiologically, the lungs have nodular masses, occasionally with cavitation, usually involving the lower lobes; occasionally ill-defined infiltrates are present; typically the involvement is bilateral; one reliable radiographic clue that a patient is suffering from Wegener granulomatosis involving the lung is the appearance of infiltrates that wax and wane over a period or nodules that enlarge in one area while resolving in another area
- Serum antineutrophilic cytoplasmic antibody test (ANCA)
  - c-ANCA shows diffuse cytoplasmic staining of neutrophil or monocyte cytoplasm; antibodies are directed against neutrophil serine proteinase 3; positive in 90% of patients with active generalized Wegener granulomatosis and in 60% of patients with limited active Wegener granulomatosis; may be positive in patients with inflammatory bowel disease, pulmonary embolus, and collagen vascular disease
  - p-ANCA stains the cytoplasm of neutrophils and monocytes in a perinuclear distribution; antibody directed against myeloperoxidase and is present in few cases of Wegener; more frequently present in cases of microscopic polyarteritis, inflammatory bowel disease, and crescentic glomerulonephritis (p-ANCA appears as c-ANCA if cells formalin-fixed; cells must be fixed in ethanol)

Gross Pathology

- Typically the lungs are diffusely involved with multiple nodules in various stages of cavitation
- Occasionally a solitary nodule with or without cavitation

Microscopic Pathology

- Characteristic lesion is an irregularly shaped ("geographic") zone of necrotic granulomatous inflammation with a central area of liquefaction necrosis that replaces portions of pulmonary parenchyma; necrotic areas consist of amorphous pink material, nuclear débris and inflammatory cells typically surrounded by a palisade of histiocytes and giant cells often characterized by multiple hyperchromatic nuclei
- Small microscopic microabscesslike foci with a central suppurative exudate surrounded by lymphocytes, plasma cells, neutrophils, and scattered eosinophils are usually present as well as small suppurative granulomas characterized by necrotic collagen surrounded by palisading histiocytes arranged with their long axes perpendicular to the necrotic center
- Necrotic granulomas have a distinct, irregular, "geographic" shape resulting from an overall contour that appears somewhat angulated and the presence of residual islands of viable tissue within the areas of necrosis; many multinucleated giant cells are frequently present in the inflammatory infiltrate
- Foci of inflammatory, necrotizing vasculitis are typically present outside the necrotic granuloma and should be present to establish the diagnosis with certainty
- Vasculitis of Wegener involves both arteries and veins and is characterized by transmural, occasionally eccentric edema in the vessel wall, and infiltration by neutrophils, eosinophils, and plasma cells; necrosis of the vessel or in the infiltrating inflammatory cells is necessary to diagnose necrotizing vasculitis
- Small vessel vasculitis involving alveolar septal capillaries (capillaritis) and venules commonly present; capillaritis characterized by acute inflammation that expands and ultimately destroys alveolar septa
- Histologic variants:
  - *Alveolar hemorrhage and capillaritis*: Acute inflammation of alveolar septal capillaries (capillaritis) rather than large arteries and veins; neutrophils fill capillary lumens, infiltrate alveolar septa, and spill into alveolar spaces; these changes are associated with fresh intraalveolar hemorrhage

- *BOOP-like*: Extensive organizing pneumonia with multinucleated giant cells, small microabscesslike necrotizing granulomas, and necrotizing vasculitis; focal areas of intraalveolar organization may be indications that hemorrhage has occurred in the past
- *Bronchocentric*: Necrotizing granulomatous inflammation primarily affects bronchioles
- *Eosinophilic:* Typical features of Wagener granulomatosis but with prominent eosinophils
- *Interstitial fibrosis with patchy vasculitis*: Necrotizing vasculitis in a background of interstitial fibrosis

Special Stains

- Granulomas in the lung should be stained for acid-fast organisms and fungal elements

Immunohistochemistry and Electron Microscopy

- Not helpful

Molecular Alterations

- None

Differential Diagnosis

- Lymphomatoid granulomatosis (characterized by multiple nodules of atypical lymphoid and plasmacytoid cells; necrotizing and nonnecrotizing granulomas, multinucleated giant cells, neutrophils, eosinophils, and necrotizing vasculitis all absent)
- Allergic angiitis and granulomatosis (Churg-Strauss syndrome) (characterized by necrotizing granulomas, multinucleated giant cells, eosinophilic pneumonia, and a necrotizing vasculitis)
- Bronchocentric granulomatosis (characterized by eosinophilia and necrotizing granulomas centered on the lumens of bronchioles without other features of Wegener granulomatosis; no necrotizing vasculitis)
- Necrotizing sarcoid granulomatosis (characterized by both necrotizing and nonnecrotizing granulomas; acute and chronic inflammatory cells and necrotizing vasculitis very rare)
- Infectious granuloma, eg, tuberculosis and fungal infections (vasculitis may be present but is never necrotizing)
- Rheumatoid nodule
- Infection with *Dirofilaria immitis*

Treatment and Prognosis

- Cytotoxic drugs (particularly cyclophosphamide) in combination with corticosteroids usually produce a dramatic response
- Without treatment Wegener runs an accelerated malignant clinical course; 80% dead within 1 year

Associations

- None

Interstitial Lung Disease

Variants

- Diffuse alveolar damage (DAD)
- Usual interstitial pneumonia (UIP)
- Desquamative interstitial pneumonia (DIP)
- Respiratory bronchiolitis-associated interstitial lung disease
- Acute interstitial pneumonia (Hamman-Rich disease)
- Nonspecific interstitial pneumonia/fibrosis (NSIP)
- Giant cell interstitial pneumonia
- Lymphoid interstitial pneumonia
- Bronchiolitis obliterans-organizing pneumonia (BOOP)
- Constrictive obliterative bronchiolitis
- Sarcoidosis
- Hypersensitivity pneumonitis
- Eosinophilic pneumonia
    - Simple eosinophilic pneumonia (Loeffler syndrome)
    - Tropical eosinophilic pneumonia
    - Chronic eosinophilic pneumonia
    - Acute eosinophilic pneumonia
    - Pulmonary alveolar proteinosis

Diffuse Alveolar Damage (DAD)

Clinical Manifestations

- Clinical correlate is acute respiratory distress syndrome
- Many associated conditions: Infections, toxic inhalation, drugs, ingested toxins, systemic shock, sepsis, radiation, cardiopulmonary bypass, collagen vascular disease, severe burns, and severe physical trauma

- Early manifestations characterized by hypoxemia (defined as a ratio of partial pressure of arterial oxygen to the fraction of inspired oxygen of 200 or less)
- Initially chest x-rays appear normal, but within 24 hours, a diffuse bilateral fluffy infiltrate appears
- Disease passes through several stages: Preclinical stage, exudative phase, proliferative phase, and healing/fibrosis phase
- Biopsies occasionally performed during phase of acute exacerbation ("accelerated IPF")

Gross Pathology

- In the acute, preclinical, and exudative phases, the lungs are heavy, firm, red, and boggy primarily as the result of congestion, interstitial and alveolar edema, and inflammation

Microscopic Pathology

- Early in the course of disease (exudative phase) the histologic appearance is dominated by the presence of edema and hyaline membranes that line the alveolar spaces; interstitial edema with variable numbers of acute and chronic inflammatory cells; and hyaline membranes accompanied by fibrin in the alveolar spaces
- Proliferative (fibroblastic) phase is characterized by the replication and migration of fibroblasts from the interstitium into the alveolar space through damaged epithelial basement membrane; aggregates of fibroblastlike cells give the lung the appearance of BOOP; in addition to the fibroblastic proliferation, type II pneumocytes proliferate in an attempt to repair the damaged alveolar lining; squamous metaplasia of bronchiolar epithelium and fibrin thrombi common
- Complete resolution rarely occurs; the latter phases of disease are characterized by organization of the fibrin exudate with resulting intraalveolar fibrosis; alveolar septa become markedly thickened as a result of the proliferating interstitial cells and the deposition of collagen

Special Stains

- Elastic stains can be useful in identifying bronchioles and alveolar ducts involved with BOOP

Immunohistochemistry

- Immunohistochemical stains for CD20, CD3, and immunoglobulin light chains will confirm the presence of peribronchiolar lymphoid aggregates in which B-cell lymphocytes predominate and CD3-positive T lymphocytes are seen in alveolar septa with polyclonal plasma cells

Electron Microscopy

- The intraalveolar lipoprotein precipitate in pulmonary alveolar proteinosis consists of necrotic alveolar macrophages, type II pneumonocytes, amorphous precipitate, and numerous lamellar osmiophilic bodies that morphologically resemble surfactant material

Differential Diagnosis

- Later stage disease may resemble BOOP
- Acute interstitial pneumonia ("idiopathic" DAD)

Treatment and Prognosis

- Respiratory support
- Mortality approximately 35% to 50%

Usual Interstitial Pneumonia (UIP)

Clinical Manifestations

- Also referred to as fibrosing alveolitis, diffuse interstitial fibrosis, or idiopathic pulmonary fibrosis
- Typically presents between the ages of 40 and 70 years (average age at onset 60 years) with the insidious onset of dyspnea and follows a slowly progressive downhill course

Gross Pathology

- Typically the basilar and subpleural zones are involved and characterized by a honeycomb fibrosis

Microscopic Pathology

- Histologic appearance typically quite heterogeneous with admixture of normal areas, inflamed areas, fibrotic areas, and honeycomb change (best appreciated at low power)
- Inflamed areas tend to consist of interstitial inflammatory cells (small lymphocytes and occasional plasma cells); lymphocytes may form small nodular aggregates

with or without germinal centers; inflammatory cells may be present without associated fibrosis or admixed with variable amounts of collagen; neither epithelioid histiocytes nor granulomas present

- Fibrosis often quite extensive and generally characterized by densely eosinophilic, acellular bundles of collagen; randomly distributed throughout are fibroblast foci, characterized by discrete aggregates of closely associated spindle-shaped cells (myofibroblasts) arranged in lamellae with their long axes parallel to the long axis of the interstitium; these foci have a myxoid-appearing stroma and little collagen
- Hyaline membranes are not present except in occasional patients with superimposed DAD ("accelerated IPF")
- Macrophages frequently accumulate in alveolar spaces, especially in smokers
- Prominent hobnail-shaped or low cuboidal epithelial cells line most of the fibrotic interstitium
- End-stage fibrotic changes include fibrous obliteration of normal architecture and macrocystic enlargement of restructured air spaces (honeycombing), fibrotic thickening of alveolar septa, thickening of pulmonary vascular intima and media, and distortion of bronchioles by peribronchiolar fibrosis (traction bronchiolectasis)

Special Stains

- Elastic stains can be useful in identifying bronchioles and alveolar ducts involved with BOOP

Immunohistochemistry

- Immunohistochemical stains for CD20, CD3, and immunoglobulin light chains will confirm the presence of peribronchiolar lymphoid aggregates in which B-cell lymphocytes predominate and CD3-positive T lymphocytes are seen in alveolar septa with polyclonal plasma cells

Electron Microscopy

- The intraalveolar lipoprotein precipitate in pulmonary alveolar proteinosis consists of necrotic alveolar macrophages and type II pneumonocytes, amorphous precipitate, and numerous lamellar osmiophilic bodies that morphologically resemble surfactant material

Differential Diagnosis

- Lung involvement by collagen vascular diseases
- "Fibrotic" NSIP
- Drug reaction to nitrofurantoin
- Asbestosis
- DIP
- Hypersensitivity pneumonitis
- Chronic eosinophilic pneumonia
- Cases with extensive granulation tissue may be difficult to differentiate from BOOP
- Endstage honeycomb fibrosis (UIP and virtually all chronic infiltrative lung diseases can result in honeycombing)

Treatment and Prognosis

- Death usually occurs within 3 to 6 years of diagnosis
- No effective treatment currently exists other than transplantation
- Mortality secondary to lung disease 65% to 70%

Desquamative Interstitial Pneumonia (DIP)

Clinical Manifestations

- Typically diagnosed in patients in their early 40s (in contrast to patients with UIP who are diagnosed a decade later); most are smokers
- In most cases, patients are symptomatic for <1 year

Gross Pathology

- Gross distribution of disease is similar to that of UIP with subpleural disease characterized by fluffy infiltrates with fibrosis but without honycomb change (the fibrosis is much less extensive than in UIP)

Microscopic Pathology

- Pulmonary involvement tends to be quite uniform from field to field; the alternating patterns of inflammation, fibrosis, fibroblastic foci, honeycomb change, and normal lung parenchyma characteristic of UIP are not present
- Most conspicuous histologic abnormality is the presence of numerous large slightly pigmented macrophages in the alveolar spaces; these macrophages contain iron as finely pigmented cytoplasmic granules

- Variable degrees of interstitial fibrosis typically present; inflammation minimal
- Fibrotic alveolar septa covered by prominent, proliferating alveolar pneumocytes

Special Stains

- The eosinophilic cytoplasmic granules in the alveolar macrophages of DIP are PAS positive

Immunohistochemistry

- Immunohistochemical stains for CD20, CD3, and immunoglobulin light chains will confirm the presence of peribronchiolar lymphoid aggregates in which B-cell lymphocytes predominate and CD3-positive T lymphocytes are seen in alveolar septa with polyclonal plasma cells

Electron Microscopy

- The intraalveolar lipoprotein precipitate in pulmonary alveolar proteinosis consists of necrotic alveolar macrophages and type II pneumonocytes, amorphous precipitate, and numerous lamellar osmiophilic bodies that morphologically resemble surfactant material

Differential Diagnosis

- Usual interstitial pneumonia
- A DIP-like type reaction can occur as a secondary finding in a variety of other conditions: Langerhans cell histiocytosis, rheumatoid nodule, intraparenchymal lymph nodes, infection, localized neoplasia including cancer, UIP, and other forms of chronic interstitial pneumonia
- May be a component of *Pneumocystis jiroveci* (formerly *P. carinii*) infection
- DIP type findings are seen in some cases of pneumonoconiosis and occasionally in cases of drug reaction: eg, nitrofurantoin

Treatment and Prognosis

- 75% will experience improvement or at least stabilization of their disease with smoking cessation and/or steroid therapy
- Average survival after diagnosis is 12 years and mortality from lung disease is approximately 25%

Respiratory Bronchiolitis-Associated Interstitial Lung Disease

Microscopic Pathology

- Typically resembles DIP with collections of intraalveolar macrophages in association with mild interstitial thickening; macrophages tend to aggregate in lumens of respiratory bronchioles and alveolar ducts, but may occur in adjacent peribronchiolar alveolar spaces
- Disease process localized to peribronchiolar parenchyma and is distinctly patchy rather than diffuse (unlike DIP)
  - Large areas of normal lung parenchyma are present throughout

Acute Interstitial Pneumonia (Hamman-Rich Disease)

Clinical Manifestations

- A diagnosis of exclusion (diffuse alveolar damage secondary to an identifiable cause and infection must be excluded)
- Typically previously healthy patients experience the rapid onset of respiratory failure following a nonspecific flulike illness

Gross Pathology

- Lung tissue typically resembles that of diffuse alveolar damage in the proliferative and fibrosing stages

Microscopic Pathology

- Classic picture includes uniform interstitial fibroblast proliferation with little collagen and variable amounts of inflammation; alveolar septa are markedly widened by oval to spindle-shaped fibroblasts admixed with lymphocytes and occasional plasma cells; the residual air spaces are quite variable in size
- Early in the course of the disease edema and hyaline membranes are dominant features
- As the disease progresses, remnants of hyaline membranes are incorporated into the thickened intestinum and become fairly inconspicuous
- Bronchioles may contain focal areas of squamous metaplasia; bronchiolitis and bronchiolar changes are relatively minor compared with the changes in the alveolar septa

- Small pulmonary arteries often contain thrombi in various stages of organization
- In the late stages of disease irreversible fibrosis distorts the underlying lung architecture

Differential Diagnosis

- DAD associated with other causes, especially infection
- Chronic infiltrative lung disease
- Organizing pneumonia (BOOP) (does not have the hyaline membrane material within the alveolar spaces that is typical of AIP)

Treatment and Prognosis

- Typically follows a rapidly fatal course (mortality rates approach 70%)

Nonspecific Interstitial Pneumonia/Fibrosis (NSIP)

Clinical Manifestations

- Etiologic factors include collagen vascular disease (especially lupus, polymyositis, dermatomyositis, scleroderma, Sjögren syndrome, and rheumatoid arthritis), drug reactions (especially nitrofurantoin and amiodarone), inhalation of organic dust (hypersensitivity pneumonia), slowly resolving acute lung injury, inadequate biopsy specimens with UIP or BOOP, and idiopathic
- Patients typically present at an average age of 45 years with dyspnea and cough

Microscopic Pathology

- Characterized by a uniform, occasionally bronchiolocentric, inflammatory and fibrosing process; typically there is interstitial inflammation consisting of small lymphocytes and occasional plasma cells or a combination of interstitial inflammation and fibrosis; interstitial fibrosis without inflammation is rare
- Areas of fibrosis characterized by mature collagen rather than fibroblasts
- Fibroblast foci uncommon
- Alveolar pneumocyte hyperplasia present
- Process may be patchy with intervening areas of normal alveolar parenchyma but areas of abnormality are temporally homogenous
- Foci may have alveolar spaces that contain increased numbers of macrophages with abundant foamy cytoplasm

Differential Diagnosis

- UIP and DIP
- Lung involvement by collagen vascular disease
- Chronic hypersensitivity pneumonia
- Drug-induced lung disease

Treatment and Prognosis

- Prognosis good; majority recover with corticosteroid therapy; the presence of fibrosis does not necessarily prevent recovery
- Approximately 20% die of progressive disease

Giant Cell Interstitial Pneumonia

Clinical Manifestations

- A pneumoconiosis that results from the inhalation of hard metal (a mixture of tungsten carbide and cobalt with or without other metals such as titanium, chromium, tantalum, and/or nickel)
- Typical clinical course consists of progressive respiratory insufficiency secondary to interstitial fibrosis; a restrictive disease by pulmonary function tests

Microscopic Pathology

- Characterized by patchy interstitial and intraalveolar mononuclear inflammatory cell infiltrates with variable degrees of alveolar fibrosis centered around bronchioles
- The most significant diagnostic feature is the presence of alveolar macrophages (a DIP-like reaction); many of these macrophages are multinucleated and appear to engulf smaller inflammatory cells
- Eosinophils may be admixed with the macrophages
- Alveolar pneumocytes are typically hyperplastic and may be multinucleated

Differential Diagnosis

- Other forms of chronic infiltrative lung disease (especially UIP and DIP)
- Granulomatous diseases (sarcoidosis, hypersensitivity pneumonitis, and infections)
- Viral infections (respiratory syncytial virus, parainfluenza virus, and measles virus)

Treatment and Prognosis

- Most patients experience progressive interstitial fibrosis and respiratory insufficiency

Lymphoid Interstitial Pneumonia

Clinical Manifestations

- Patients present with progressive cough or dyspnea
- May represent a prelymphomatous lymphoproliferative disorder
- Typically occurs in the setting of immunologic abnormality: Dysproteinemia, Sjögren syndrome, chronic active hepatitis, and human immunodeficiency virus (HIV) infection (especially in children)
- Lymphoma may develop as a complication

Microscopic Pathology

- Characterized by a diffuse alveolar septal infiltrate of small lymphocytes and plasma cells
- Lymphoid follicles, often with germinal centers, frequently present in peribronchiolar parenchyma
- Lymphoid infiltrates tend to be predominantly of the T-cell type; peribronchiolar lymphoid follicles consist primarily of B cells
- Intraalveolar infiltrates tend to be sparse especially in comparison with the interstitial component
- Alveolar spaces may contain an eosinophilic proteinaceous exudate
- Poorly formed granulomas, some with giant cells, and loose aggregates of histiocytes present in about 40% to 50% of cases

Differential Diagnosis

- Follicular bronchiolitis (lymphoid interstitial pneumonia requires the presence of diffuse involvement of alveolar septal walls beyond the interstitium immediately surrounding bronchioles)
- Hypersensitivity pneumonia
- Pseudolymphoma
- NSIP
- Lymphoma

Treatment and Prognosis

- A lymphoproliferative disorder that may rarely evolve into malignancy
- Mortality approximately 30% and primarily depends on underlying disorder

Bronchiolitis Obliterans-Organizing Pneumonia (BOOP)

Clinical Manifestations

- May be present as the primary cause of respiratory illness:
- Organization of prior viral or bacterial infection
- Drug toxicity, eg, gold, amiodarone, sulfasalazine
- Toxic inhalants, eg, silo-filler disease
- Collagen vascular diseases (10%)
- Bronchial obstruction of almost any cause
- Chronic aspiration

Gross Pathology

- Several patterns are possible on gross examination of the lungs:
  - Few well-defined nodules that resemble neoplasm
  - Multiple patchy areas of consolidation
  - Diffuse interstitial infiltrate reminiscent of some of the other chronic infiltrative lung disease

Microscopic Pathology

- Characterized by the presence of polypoid tufts of proliferating fibroblasts and myofibroblasts arranged in parallel and admixed with variable numbers of lymphocytes, macrophages, and plasma cells in a lightly staining myxoid stroma (rich in acid mucopolysaccharides); very little collagen deposition; these tufts occlude distal bronchioles, alveolar ducts, and nearby alveolar spaces
- Fibroblastic tufts usually covered with bronchiolar or alveolar epithelial cells
- Lesions are typically all of the same age and consist of proliferating fibroblasts; extracellular collagen and well-established interstitial fibrosis are not characteristic features
- The submucosa of involved airways usually contains a mononuclear inflammatory cell infiltrate; neutrophils are rare
- Concentric fibrous narrowing of airways is typically not present, and airway caliber is almost always normal (the lumens are occupied by polypoid tufts of fibroblastic myxoid tissue)
- Alveolar duct involvement is characterized by a branching pattern to the fibroblastic polypoid plugs

- In addition to the fibroblastic plugs, an interstitial mononuclear cell infiltrate accompanied by type 2 pneumocyte hyperplasia and intraalveolar foamy macrophages are usually present

Special Stains

- Elastic stains can be useful in identifying bronchioles and alveolar ducts involved with BOOP

Constrictive Obliterative Bronchiolitis

Clinical Manifestations

- Typically a finding in patients who have undergone lung, heart-lung, or bone marrow transplantation (probably a manifestation of chronic rejection or graft-verus-host disease)
- Patients typically present with progressive dyspnea and cough

Microscopic Pathology

- Characterized by concentric narrowing of bronchioles by fibrous tissue
- Fibrous tissue does not extend into adjacent alveolar ducts and air spaces and a peribronchiolar interstitial pneumonia is not present
- Lumen may be obliterated, leaving a contracted hyalinized scar
- Changes often very focal with large areas of normal-appearing lung parenchyma

Treatment and Prognosis

- Prognosis worse than BOOP and corticosteroids less helpful

Sarcoidosis

Clinical Manifestations

- A systemic disease that affects both thoracic and extrathoracic organs
- Thoracic involvement is seen in 90% and is typically the most common site of disease
- Seen more frequently in blacks than in whites and blacks tend to have more serious disease
- A familial incidence has been postulated
- Symptomatic patients usually present with mild dyspnea and cough; many are asymptomatic
- Longstanding pulmonary disease is characterized by pulmonary insufficiency

Gross Pathology

- 3 types of disease based on anatomic distribution (radiographic staging):
  - Type I: Hilar lymphadenopathy without lung involvement
  - Type II: Both hilar lymphadenopathy and pulmonary infiltrates
  - Type III: Infiltrates in the lung without lymph node involvement

Microscopic Pathology

- Characterized by the presence of well-circumscribed, noncaseating granulomas composed of tight aggregates of epithelioid histiocytes, occasional multinucleated giant cells, and few lymphocytes in a background of partial hyalinization; small foci of central necrosis may be present
- Granulomas often surrounded by a rim of fibroblasts with scattered inflammatory cells and tend to be located along the course of lymphatics and in interlobular septa and lymph nodes; may be scattered throughout the interstitium, causing little distortion or may form confluent masses that replace areas of lung parenchyma resulting in macroscopic nodules
- Active disease is characterized by the presence of lymphocytes of the helper T-cell type in the granulomas; more chronic disease is characterized by the presence of suppressor T cells and B lymphocytes in the granulomas
- Different cytoplasmic inclusions may be found in multinucleated macrophages to include asteroid bodies, Schaumann bodies, and polarizable foreign-looking material (all are nonspecific histologic findings)
- Alveoli between granulomas are typically normal and do not show any evidence of alveolitis (chronic interstitial pneumonia does not extend beyond the granulomatous foci)
- Frequently the juxtalymphatic granulomas lie adjacent to the pleural surface
- Granulomatous and mononuclear cell vasculitis is a common finding, especially in cases with extensive parenchymal involvement

Molecular Alterations

- Some evidence that sarcoidosis has a familial incidence

Differential Diagnosis

- Mycobacterial infections, hypersensitivity pneumonitis
- Berylliosis
- Talc granulomatosis
- Hypersensitivity pneumonia
- Sarcoidlike lesions can be found in the lung, lymph nodes, and various extrathoracic organs in patients with lymphoreticular and solid organ malignant neoplasms, either synchronously with viable tumor or after chemotherapy

Treatment and Prognosis

- Complete resolution is seen in approximately 50% of patients with disease confined to hilar lymph nodes without lung involvement and in patients with both hilar lymph node involvement and lung involvement
- Only 25% of patients will undergo complete resolution if their disease is confined to the lungs without hilar involvement
- The sudden appearance of systemic symptoms of fever, malaise, and erythema nodosum are predictors of a good prognosis
- Chronic disease or patients with evidence of pulmonary insufficiency tend to have a poor prognosis

Hypersensitivity Pneumonitis

Clinical Manifestations

- Typically results from exposure to organic dusts (more than 50 associated substances)
- 2 most well-known entities are farmer's lung (caused by thermophilic *Actinomyces* antigen) and pigeon breeder's lung (caused by avian protein antigen)
- Other associated occupations include sugarcane workers, mushroom farmers, and wood product workers
- Cell-mediated immune mechanisms probably a major etiologic contributor
- Most patients present with a history of respiratory symptoms temporally related to exposure to the appropriate antigen
- Clinical presentation can be quite variable:
    - Acute illness characterized by marked respiratory distress and systemic symptoms of fever, chills, and malaise
    - Subacute and chronic disease characterized by an insidious onset with less severe systemic symptoms

Gross Pathology

- Disease tends to localize to the upper and mid zones of the lung; the bases are usually spared
- Within the zones of involvement the infiltrates tend to be random with neither a subpleural nor juxtalymphatic distribution
- Acute disease characterized by heavy, focally consolidated lung parenchyma
- More chronic disease may produce fibrosis with honeycombing at the periphery of the upper lobes

Microscopic Pathology

- Characterized by the triad of patchy, predominantly peribronchiolar, nonspecific interstitial pneumonia; non-necrotizing granulomas and/or epithelioid histiocytes; and chronic bronchiolitis frequently associated with bronchiolitis obliterans
- Early in the course of the disease infiltrating lymphocytes with variable numbers of plasma cells and enlarged histiocytes surround respiratory bronchioles and extend for variable distances into surrounding alveolar parenchyma
- Small, non-necrotizing, loosely formed granulomas often present in peribronchiolar interstitium
- Foci of bronchiolitis obliterans or BOOP present in over 50%
- Eosinophils and neutrophils not prominent and fibrosis typically minimal
- Distal bronchioles and surrounding alveolar ducts and alveolar spaces usually filled with fibroblasts and chronic inflammatory cells in a light stroma; lipid-laden macrophages may be present in nearby alveolar spaces
- Vasculitis is not a component of the disease
- Extent of alveolar fibrosis a reflection of duration of disease; foci of honeycomb-type fibrosis often present in end-stage disease

Differential Diagnosis

- UIP
- NSIP
- Lymphoid interstitial pneumonia
- Sarcoidosis
- Granulomatous infections

Treatment and Prognosis

- In general the prognosis is good, especially if the offending antigen can be removed
- Corticosteroid therapy may be of benefit in aiding recovery in acute disease; less benefit in chronic disease; overall mortality rate for chronic disease approximately 40%

Eosinophilic Pneumonia

Clinical Manifestations

- 4 diseases:
  - Simple eosinophilic pneumonia (Loeffler syndrome): Mild, self-limited asymptomatic disease characterized by transient pulmonary infiltrates and peripheral eosinophilia that spontaneously resolves, usually within 30 days
  - Tropical eosinophilia: Infection by one of several parasites (usually filarial infections)
  - Chronic disease is more common in women then men and presents insidiously with cough, fever, dyspnea, and weight loss; frequently occurs in asthmatics (50%); numerous etiologic agents, to include drug toxicity (bleomycin, nitrofurantoin, penicillin, and sulfonamides), fungal hypersensitivity (*Aspergillus* and *Candida*), parasites (filaria, *Strongyloides*), and inhalants (cocaine)
  - Acute disease typically seen in nonasthmatics and presents with fever of short duration and respiratory failure; blood eosinophilia usually absent
- Cigarette smoking an initiating factor in some first-time smokers

Microscopic Pathology

- Chronic disease is indistinguishable from acute disease unless there is fibrosis (acute disease usually resolves without fibrosis)
- Characterized by the presence of an alveolar exudate of eosinophils and variable numbers of macrophages filling alveolar spaces; macrophages tend to have eosinophilic cytoplasm and may be multinucleated
- Adjacent alveolar septa are expanded by an admixture of eosinophils, lymphocytes, and plasma cells and are lined by hyperplastic pneumocytes
- The intraalveolar eosinophilic component may be quite pronounced and partially necrotic (eosinophilic microabscess); necrosis does not occur in the interstitium
- A mild, non-necrotizing eosinophilic vasculitis may be present
- Air space organization (BOOP) is frequently present

Differential Diagnosis

- Churg-Strauss disease with tissue eosinophilia and asthma (necrotizing granulomatous inflammation and granulomatous vasculitis are not components of typical eosinophilic pneumonia)
- Langerhans cell histiocytosis (infiltrate primarily interstitial rather than intraalveolar)
- DIP
- Infection with *Coccidioides immitis*
- Wegner granulomatosis, eosinophilic variant

Treatment and Prognosis

- Simple eosinophilic pneumonia: Spontaneously resolves
- Tropical eosinophilic pneumonia: Antifilarial drugs
- Chronic eosinophilic pneumonia: Identify and eliminate etiologic agent if possible; most respond to corticosteroid therapy
- Acute eosinophilic pneumonia: Dramatic response to corticosteroids

Pulmonary Alveolar Proteinosis

Clinical Manifestations

- Patients typically present with slowly progressive shortness of breath, a dry cough, and low-grade fever
- Adults typically affected, but may occur in children in a congenital form
- Chest x-ray shows extensive bilateral infiltrates that radiate out from the hila into the lung parenchyma
- Seen in association with 2 etiologic factors:
  - Exposure to mineral dust (crystalline silica and aluminum)
  - Patients who have been immunocompromised (typically patients with a hematologic malignancy treated with cytotoxic chemotherapy); also seen in patients with AIDS
- Appears to be the result of an acquired defect of alveolar macrophages to clear surfactant related to autoantibodies directed against granulocyte-macrophage colony stimulating factor (GM-CSF); the resulting accumulation of lipoprotein exerts toxic effects on the macrophages

Gross Pathology

- Lungs are large and heavy, and on sectioning, typically have focal to confluent areas of firm, yellow-tan consolidation; turbid fluid extrudes from these congested areas

Microscopic Pathology

- Alveolar spaces are filled by a brightly eosinophilic, granular, almost acellular material that is typically PAS positive and diastase resistant; foamy macrophages and cholesterol crystals often present
- Alveolar septa typically normal except for being lined by hyperplastic alveolar type II pneumocytes; interstitial fibrosis, necrosis, and inflammation rare (presence should suggest an associated infection)
- Secondary superinfection (typically seen in immunocompromised patients) may be present; organisms include *Nocardia* (most common), mycobacteria, fungi, *Pneumocystis*, and cytomegalovirus

Special Stains

- The intraalveolar lipoprotein precipitate in pulmonary alveolar proteinosis is strongly PAS positive and diastase resistant
- Elastic stains can be useful in identifying bronchioles and alveolar ducts involved with BOOP

Immunohistochemistry

- Immunohistochemical stains for CD20, CD3, and immunoglobulin light chains will confirm the presence of peribronchiolar lymphoid aggregates in which B-cell lymphocytes predominate and CD3-positive T lymphocytes are seen in alveolar septa with polyclonal plasma cells

Electron Microscopy

- The intraalveolar lipoprotein precipitate in pulmonary alveolar proteinosis consists of necrotic alveolar macrophages and type II pneumonocytes, amorphous precipitate, and numerous lamellar osmiophilic bodies that morphologically resemble surfactant material

Molecular Alterations

- Some patients with pulmonary alveolar proteinosis have autoantibodies directed against specific defect in GM-CSF

Differential Diagnosis

- Pulmonary edema
- *Pneumocystis jiroveci* (formerly *P. carinii*) pneumonia
- Changes in lung parenchyma distal to bronchial obstruction

Treatment and Prognosis

- Spontaneous resolution often occurs in asymptomatic patients
- Prognosis is good with whole lung lavage or GM-CSF therapy
- Progression to chronic fibrosis unusual

Idiopathic (Cryptogenic Organizing Pneumonia)

Clinical Manifestations

- Often a nonspecific reaction near an unrelated pathologic process, eg, neoplasm, vasculitis, area of infarction, infection, or a minor component of another disease, eg, eosinophilic pneumonia, hypersensitivity pneumonia, NSID
- Most patients are diagnosed between the ages of 40 and 60 years
- 2 clinical pictures:
  - Patients with no prior medical history and no associated disease
  - Patients with some preexisting condition that is associated with lung infiltrates of a pattern similar to that seen in BOOP
- Frequently the onset of disease is characterized by the subacute appearance of dyspnea, cough, fever, and a flulike illness
- Pulmonary function abnormalities indicate restrictive (not obstructive) disease

Differential Diagnosis

- UIP (fibroblastic foci of UIP may be difficult to distinguish from cryptogenic organizing pneumonia; the random interstitial distribution, small size, and presence of collagen coupled with the presence of honeycomb changes elsewhere indicate UIP)
- Organizing stage of DAD and acute interstitial pneumonia

Treatment and Prognosis

- Most patients respond to corticosteroids; some spontaneous regression may occur without treatment
- Mortality typically <15%
- Prognosis better for patients with nodules or patchy consolidation than for patients with diffuse interstitial infiltrates

Malignant Epithelial Tumors

Squamous Cell Carcinoma

Clinical Manifestations

- History of cigarette smoking in almost 100%
- More commonly affects men than women
- Human papillomavirus is found in approximately 20%
- Tumor may be clinically occult
- Generalized symptoms include weakness, anorexia, cachexia, malaise, fever, and orthostatic hypotension
- Local direct effects usually result from endobronchial growth and/or invasion of adjacent structures: cough, dyspnea, wheeze, stridor, and hemoptysis; other symptoms include chest pain or back pain, obstructive pneumonia, and pleural effusion

Gross Pathology

- 65% located centrally; 35% peripherally
- Tumors vary from small endobronchial obstructive lesions to large cavitated neoplasms that replace an entire lung
- Central tumors arise in a major bronchus and demonstrate both endobronchial and invasive growth into peribronchial soft tissue, lung parenchyma, and adjacent lymph nodes; frequently compress pulmonary artery and vein
- Peripheral tumors usually have a nodular growth pattern with circumscribed borders and areas of necrosis and cavitation
- Cut section tends to be gray-white or yellow with a dry, flaky appearance (keratinization); necrosis and hemorrhage are common and cavitation is present in 30%; stromal desmoplasia can result in a hard white tumor mass
- Changes secondary to bronchial obstruction may be seen in parenchyma distal to the tumor: Atelectasis, mycostasis, organization, secondary infection, and/or abscess

Microscopic Pathology

- Well-differentiated lesions characterized by the presence of intercellular bridges and keratinization; some tumor cells may resemble oncocytes; extremely well-differentiated tumors lack cytologic evidence of malignancy; diagnosis based entirely on invasion of surrounding lung parenchyma (this subset typically characterized by large amounts of keratin)
- Moderately-differentiated tumors have less prominent cellular bridges and rare foci of keratinization
- Poorly-differentiated tumors resemble large cell carcinoma and are occasionally very dyscohesive and extensively infiltrated by inflammatory cells
- Tumor cells usually grow in nests with a desmoplastic stroma that may be infiltrated by both acute and chronic inflammatory cells
- Tumor cell nests usually demonstrate some zonation: Cells in the center of the nests have more cytoplasm; 'keratinization and intercellular bridges are both more prominent; central cavitation often seen
- At the periphery of a tumor nodule, cells often grow within intact air spaces
- Occasional mucin vacuoles may be present
- Tumor cell nuclei are hyperchromatic and pleomorphic and often have prominent nucleoli; chromatin tends to be condensed along the inner surface of the nuclear membrane
- Histologic variants:
  - *Small cell variant squamous cell carcinoma*: Tumor cells are small with high nuclear-cytoplasmic ratios and nuclei that show prominent molding (reminiscent of a small cell carcinoma); squamous differentiation may be focal; nuclei tend to be vesicular and have a prominent nucleolus; cellular nests are more clearly defined with less necrosis and a more mature fibrous stroma than in small cell carcinoma
  - *Clear cell variant squamous cell carcinoma*: Composed primarily or almost entirely of tumor cells with a clear cytoplasm; occasionally clear cells represent the majority of the neoplasm, but will still have foci of obvious squamous differentiation
  - *Papillary variant squamous cell carcinoma*: Present as intraepithelial (in situ) and endobronchial; tend to be well differentiated without foci of necrosis; little or no pleomorphism or stromal invasion; tend to occur in older individuals and have a favorable prognosis (5-year survival rate >60%)

  - *Basaloid variant SCC*: May resemble basal cell carcinoma of the skin or basaloid carcinoma of the upper respiratory tract; prominent peripheral palisading of nuclei; associated with a poor prognosis

Special Stains

- PAS may confirm the presence of mucin production in a moderately differentiated squamous cell carcinoma (small foci of mucin production are not unusual)

Immunohistochemistry

- Tumor cells typically immunoreactive for both high- and low-molecular-weight keratins (staining for high-molecular-weight keratins tends to occur in areas of keratinization)
- Tumor cells may also stain positively for vimentin, synaptophysin, and desmin as well as EMA, S-100 protein, Leu-M1, and CEA

Electron Microscopy

- Most useful to confirm squamous differentiation in spindle cell lesions
- Squamous cell carcinoma cells have true desmosomal attachments with tonofilaments that extend into the cytoplasm
- Both mucin and neurosecretory granules may be present
- Tumor cell nests are frequently surrounded by an intact basement membrane
- Oncocytic appearing cells have increased numbers of cytoplasmic mitochondria

Molecular Alterations

- Loss of the p53 gene on the short arm of chromosome 17; most common mutation is a guanine-cytosine (G:C) to thymine-adenine (T:A) transversion (often associated with cigarette smoking)

Differential Diagnosis

- Florid squamous metaplasia (changes that may occur around an organizing infarct or an area of diffuse alveolar damage)
- Squamous metaplasia in the bronchial mucosa overlying another neoplasm (primary or metastatic)
- Postinflammatory squamous metaplasia (infection, radiation)
- Pseudoepitheliomatous hyperplasia seen in association with other tumors (granular cell tumor) or inflammatory process (blastomycosis)
- Other primary neoplasms with a squamous component (eg, mucoepidermoid carcinoma and adenosquamous carcinoma)
- Primary lung tumors with a squamoid or epithelioid appearance
- Metastatic squamous cell carcinoma and metastatic melanoma
- Small cell variant versus small cell carcinoma
- Clear cell variant versus metastatic clear cell carcinoma (eg, renal cell carcinoma)
- Well-differentiated papillary squamous cell carcinoma versus papillomatosis and solitary papilloma

Treatment

- Only chance of cure involves complete surgical excision
- Radiotherapy can provide long-term local control for unresectable tumors, particularly those in the superior sulcus
- Some reports of prolonged survival with combination chemotherapy and radiation therapy

Prognosis

- Overall 5-year survival rate approximately 15%
- 5-year survival rate 50% for stage I, 30% for stage II, and 10% for stage III and higher
- Extent of disease at the time of diagnosis is the most significant prognostic factor

Associations

- Patients may present with hypercalcemia as a result of parathyroid hormone-related protein produced by the tumor (bone metastasis more likely to cause hypercalcemia)

Small Cell Carcinoma

Clinical Manifestations

- Represents 15% to 20% of all lung cancers
- Men affected more commonly than women
- Most patients have a history of heavy cigarette smoking
- Median age at presentation is 60 years
- Most tumors are located proximally and as a result cause symptoms of cough, dyspnea, wheezing, hemoptysis, chest pain, or postobstructive pneumonitis
- Involvement of structures in the mediastinum can result in superior vena cava syndrome (10%), recurrent laryngeal nerve paralysis, and dysphagia
- Other clinical manifestations include:
    - Syndrome of inappropriate secretion of anti-diuretic hormone
    - Ectopic Cushing syndrome
    - Eaton-Lambert (myasthenialike) syndrome
- 30% of patients have limited disease at the time of presentation; remainder have extensive disease
- 70% present with perihilar disease secondary to lymph node metastasis

Gross Pathology

- Cut surface of tumor typically tan-white, soft and friable, and has extensive areas of necrosis
- Neoplasm typically situated in a peribronchial location and may infiltrate submucosally and circumferentially along the bronchial wall

Microscopic Pathology

- 2 histologic types:
    - *Small cell carcinoma*
        - Tumor cells tend to be round or fusiform and have scant cytoplasm, finely granular nuclear chromatin, and either absent or inconspicuous nucleoli
        - Nuclear molding may be readily apparent (less evident in histologic sections than in cytologic preparations)
        - Mitotic figures are typically numerous (9 to 20 per 10 hpfs)
        - Extensive areas of necrosis typically present; within necrotic areas, hematoxyphilic encrustation of vessel walls by DNA from necrotic tumor cells (*Azzopardi effect*)
        - Tumor cells do not always grow with a specific pattern but occasionally they will form nests (with peripheral palisading of cells), ribbons, tubules or ductules, and rosettes
        - There may be marked variation in the size of individual tumor cells with some cells approaching the size of the cells seen in a large cell carcinoma; small cell carcinoma tumor cells are typically 2 to 3 times the size of small resting lymphocytes
    - *Small cell carcinoma with a component of a squamous cell carcinoma or adenocarcinoma*
        - These neoplasms have a greater likelihood of being located in a peripheral location
        - Treatment frequently results in a different morphology; a pure small cell carcinoma may develop morphology of a small cell carcinoma with squamous cell carcinoma or adenocarcinoma

Special Stains

- Not helpful

Immunohistochemistry

- Neuroendocrine markers, chromogranin A, synaptophysin, Leu-7 (CD57), and CD56 positive in 50% to 60% of patients
- NSE is not specific for neuroendocrine differentiation; up to 60% of non-small cell carcinomas will stain positively
- A significant number of small cell carcinoma tumor cells will stain positively for gastrin-related peptide (bombesin)
- Close to 100% of tumors will stain with keratin cocktail of AE1/AE3 and CAM 5.2 and EMA; approximately 90% are positive for TTF-1
- Majority of tumors will stain with CEA

Electron Microscopy

- Tumor cells have scant cytoplasm with few organelles
- Nuclei have moderately and uniformly dense chromatin and small or absent nucleoli
- Cytoplasmic dense core granules are usually few and small (absent in 10% to 35%)

Molecular Alterations

- Retinoblastoma gene (*Rb*) mutated in 80%, and p53 gene, located on the short arm of chromosome 17, also mutated in 80%

Differential Diagnosis

- Non-small cell carcinoma
- Malignant lymphoma
- Chronic inflammation
- Other neuroendocrine tumors: Atypical carcinoids and large cell neuroendocrine carcinoma
- Metastatic carcinoma of the breast or prostate
- Metastatic neuroendocrine carcinoma from other sites

Treatment

- Chemotherapy or radiation therapy
- Role of surgical resection controversial even in patients with limited stage disease
- Surgical resection may be indicated in combined small cell carcinoma

Prognosis

- 5% to 15% of patients survive 2 or more years
- 5% survive 10 years
- Long-term survival is correlated with limited disease, female sex, and the occurrence of herpes zoster

Associations

- Inappropriate secretion of antidiuretic hormone, ectopic Cushing syndrome, and Eaton-Lambert syndrome (see above)

Adenocarcinoma

Clinical Manifestations

- Most common form of lung carcinoma
- More common in women than in men
- Relationship to smoking not as strong as squamous cell carcinoma, small cell carcinoma, or large cell carcinoma

Gross Pathology

- Typically located peripherally in lung as a well-circumscribed mass that may produce some overlying pleural fibrosis; may be located centrally and/or in a bronchus
- Vary in size from <1 cm to lesions that replace an entire lung
- Cut surface usually gray-white, occasionally lobulated, and often has a central scar, which may contain anthracotic pigment; foci of necrosis and hemorrhage common
- Extensive mucus production may be evident
- May be single or multiple, and if associated with a dense desmoplasia, quite firm
- Neoplasms close to the pleura may actually invade the pleura and seed it producing a gross appearance reminiscent of malignant mesothelioma

Microscopic Pathology

- Tubular, papillary, or acinar growth patterns may be present singularly or in combination
- Major individual histologic patterns/subtypes are acinar, papillary, bronchioloalveolar, and solid adenocarcinoma with mucin production; tumors usually have a mixure of histologic subtypes
- All adenocarcinomas produce mucin and/or demonstrate a glandular growth pattern; the demonstration of mucin production is required for diagnostic confirmation in those cases that lack a glandular growth pattern; mucin production varies from rare positive cells in anaplastic tumors to large pools containing nests of malignant cells
- Tumor cells typically form glands but may not contain obvious cytoplasmic mucin vacuoles; these cells tend to be eosinophilic, large, cuboidal, columnar, or polygonal and have large vesicular nuclei with prominent nucleoli
- Nuclear atypia varies with degree of differentiation
- Occasionally, tumors will have large dyscohesive zones with large numbers of single cells that either infiltrate the interstitium or occupy intact airspaces
- Focal or widespread clear cell change may be present
- Intracytoplasmic eosinophilic globules may be present (type 2 cell differentiation)
- Stroma varies from delicate fibrous septa to dense desmoplastic zones

Malignant Epithelial Tumors>Adenocarcinoma

- Dense lymphoid infiltrates may be present as well as secondary granulomatous reactions
- Unusual histologic patterns may be present: signet ring cells, spindle cells, giant cells, and hepatoid cells
- Foci of enteric differentiation may be present: Characterized by cells with features of columnar absorptive, goblet, Paneth, and neuroendocrine cell differentiation
- Grading depends on degree of differentiation (acinar, papillary, bronchioloalveolar, and solid adenocarcinoma with mucin production), proportion of solid foci, architectural regularity, degree of cytologic atypia, and extent of necrosis (well-differentiated neoplasms show architectural regularity, little cytologic atypia, little solid growth, and little necrosis)
- Histologic variants:
    - *Fetal adenocarcinoma*
        - Affects men and women equally; 80% of patients have a history of smoking; mean age at presentation in the 4th decade; 50% to 60% of patients are asymptomatic; most frequent symptoms are fever, cough, chest pain, and hemoptysis; tend to present as a solitary, peripheral or midlung mass and slightly more common in the upper lobes; lymphadenopathy and pleural effusion rarely present
        - Typically solitary, well-circumscribed but not encapsulated; mean 4.5 cm; may be multiple (1 dominant mass with satellite nodules); cut surface bulges and is white to tan to brown with areas of cystic degeneration and hemorrhage; 85% are subpleural
        - Neoplasm resembles fetal lung and is composed of a mass of branching tubules lined by pseudostratified, nonciliated columnar cells with clear or slightly eosinophilic cytoplasm and round to oval nuclei with little or no hyperchromasia or pleomorphism; tumor cells frequently have subnuclear and supranuclear cytoplasmic vacuoles reminiscent of endometrial cells; cytologic atypia rare; morules, consisting of solid nests of cells with abundant eosinophilic cytoplasm almost always present; 50% of morules have optically clear nuclei; glandular lumens may contain small amounts of mucin (intracellular mucin is almost never present); mitotic figures and foci of necrosis frequently present; stroma typically scant and consists of benign spindled myofibroblasts
    - *Mucinous ("colloid") adenocarcinoma*
        - Identical to their counterparts in the gastrointestinal tract; dissecting pools of mucin with islands of neoplastic epithelium; epithelium may be very well differentiated
    - *Mucinous cystadenocarcinoma*
        - Circumscribed with fibrous capsule; cystic change with mucin pooling; mucinous epithelium grows along alveolar walls
    - *Signet ring adenocarcinoma*
        - Usually a focal change seen as part of another histologic variant
    - *Clear cell adenocarcinoma*
        - Usually a focal change in another histologic variant, but may be the major component of the tumor
- Cytologic variants:
    - Adenocarcinoma cells can differentiate into any of the epithelial cells normally present in the bronchus, bronchioles and alveoli and combinations often present
    - *Bronchial surface cell with little or no mucus production*: 8%; a papillary or tubular arrangement of columnar cells that lack cilia
    - *Goblet cell*: A bronchioloalveolar arrangement of cells that resemble goblet cells of normal bronchial epithelium; cytoplasm filled with mucus, which displaces nucleus to the base of the cell
    - *Bronchial gland cell*: 5%; neoplastic tubules, acini, or ductular structures composed of cuboidal cells filled with mucus; solid nests may contain cells that have a signet-ring morphology
    - *Clara cell*: Most common (50%-85%); a papillary arrangement of peg-shaped or low columnar, eosinophilic cells with knoblike protrusions at the apical surface
    - *Type 2 alveolar epithelial cell*: A papillary or bronchioloalveolar arrangement of cuboidal cells that replace the alveolar lining and are characterized by a dome-shaped apical surface and finely vacuolated cytoplasm (lamellar inclusion bodies); alveolar spaces usually filled with exfoliated tumor cells

Special Stains

- Mucin stains (mucicarmine, periodic acid-Schiff [PAS] with diastase and Alcian blue) confirm the presence of mucin
- Phosphotungstic acid hematoxylin (PTAH) and PAS with diastase will reveal apical staining of granules in tumors with Clara cell differentiation
- Eosinophilic inclusions characteristic of type 2 cell differentiation will stain with PAS, Luxol-fast blue, and Sudan black
- PAS confirms the presence of glycogen in clear cells of fetal adenocarcinoma

Immunohistochemistry

- Most tumor cells have a CK7-positive and CK20-negative phenotype and express both high- and low-molecular-weight cytokeratins, epithelial membrane antigen (EMA), carcinoembryonic antigen (CEA), Leu-M1 (CD15), and B72.3
- 75% positive for thyroid transcription factor (TTF-1); metastatic adenocarcinoma and bronchioloalveolar carcinomas typically negative for TTF-1
- 50% positive for neuron specific enolase (NSE)
- 30% positive for Leu-7 (CD57), 10% to 20% for chromogranin or synaptophysin
- 25% positive for vimentin
- 40% positive for peripheral airway markers (surfactant-associated protein and Clara cell protein)
- Cells with hepatoid differentiation typically positive for alpha-fetoprotein
- Morular cells and some epithelial cells of a fetal adenocarcinoma stain positively for chromogranin A, NSE, and synaptophysin; malignant epithelial cells stain positively for cytokeratin, CEA, and EMA

Electron Microscopy

- Acinar structures are generally easily recognized and consist of microvilli that project into an acinar space and have an associated glycocalyx
- Cells contain numerous organelles and mucin and are joined by junctional complexes
- Adenocarcinoma cells typically do not have tonofilaments and have fewer desmosomes than malignant squamous cells
- Malignant epithelial glands of a fetal adenocarcinoma have a distinct basal lamina and microvilli on cell apices; neuroendocrine cells with dense core granules may be present
- 3 basic cell types can be identified by the electron microscope
  - Type 2 alveolar epithelial cell: Osmiophilic whorls resembling myelin figures and intranuclear microtubular arrays that correspond to eosinophilic intranuclear inclusions
  - Clara cell (nonciliated bronchiolar cell): Knoblike projections of cytoplasm with osmiophilic Clara cell granules
  - Mucinous or goblet cells: Both goblet cells and mucin cells

Molecular Alterations

- Point mutations of dominant oncogenes, such as the K-*ras* gene, and tumor suppressor genes such as *p53* and *p16Ink4*
- *p53* mutations not seen in well-differentiated fetal adenocarcinoma

Differential Diagnosis

- Reactive and metaplastic epithelial changes:
  - Organizing diffuse alveolar damage
  - Chemotherapy or radiation effect
  - Reactive atypia associated with inflammatory process
- Benign lesions with glandular features:
  - Sclerosing hemangioma
  - Alveolar adenoma
  - Papillary adenoma of type II cells
  - Atypical adenomatous hyperplasia
  - Bronchiolar adenoma
- Primary lung malignancy with glandular features
- Carcinoid and atypical carcinoid
  - Large cell neuroendocrine carcinoma
- Metastatic adenocarcinoma from extrapulmonary sites (eg, gastrointestinal tract, kidney, breast, prostate)
- Mesothelioma with epithelioid differentiation
- Fetal adenocarcinoma easily confused with clear cell adenocarcinoma

Treatment

- Complete surgical resection provides the only chance for cure
- Fetal adenocarcinoma treated with surgical excision with or without adjuvant chemotherapy; tumor-related mortality rate 10% to 15% at 8 years; prognosis significantly better than for biphasic blastomas

Prognosis

- Resection for cure is associated with a 5-year survival rate of 50% to 80%
- Overall 5-year survival rate is 20%
- Micropapillary pattern (papillary tufts lack a central fibrovascular core) may have a worse prognosis

Associations

- Pulmonary lesions predisposed to develop adenocarcinoma include scarring, atypical adenomatous hyperplasia, and bronchioloalveolar cell adenoma

Bronchioloalveolar Carcinoma

Clinical Manifestations

- 50% asymptomatic at the time of presentation and usually first discovered as solitary peripheral nodules on routine chest x-ray
- Patients with symptoms typically complain of cough, sputum production, dyspnea, chest pain, and weight loss
- Average age at presentation 6th decade
- Unusual for patient to present with symptoms related to metastasis, paraneoplastic syndromes, or hormone production

Gross Pathology

- Typically peripheral nodules or foci of consolidation without destructive or invasive features
- *Nonmucinous tumors* are gray-white with foci of parenchymal consolidation and occasionally have a central scar and anthracotic pigment; foci of hemorrhage and necrosis are typically absent and underlying pulmonary architecture usually preserved
- *Mucinous tumors* tend to be larger and more multifocal than nonmucinous tumors; often replace an entire lobe by glistening mucinous consolidation; underlying lung architecture preserved
- Satellite nodules are common with both forms of neoplasm
- *Mucinous cystic tumors* (colloid carcinomas), are variants of bronchioloalveolar carcinoma, resemble mucinous carcinomas in other sites; characterized by a well-demarcated pools of glistening clear, cloudy, or hemorrhagic mucus; *mucinous cystic tumors of borderline malignancy* and *mucinous cystadenomas* are characterized by mucin pools surrounded by partial or complete fibrous walls

Microscopic Pathology

- 2 main cell types: mucinous and nonmucinous (nonmucinous is more common; up to 75%)
- Typically cuboidal or columnar tumor cells grow along preexisting, intact alveolar walls either as a single layer or occasionally as papillae that protrude into alveolar spaces
- Characteristically single cells, acinar clusters, and papillary groups of tumor cells lie free in alveolar spaces; these cells may spread aerogenously resulting in satellite nodules
- 10% contain psammoma bodies (more common in nonmucinous type)
- *Nonmucinous bronchioloalveolar carcinoma*
    - Tumor cells usually fairly uniform and have Clara cell differentiation (most common; 90%), type 2 cell differentiation, or both; they are typically more cuboidal than tall columnar and have bright eosinophilic cytoplasm
    - Nuclei tend to be large, hyperchromatic, and atypical and have prominent nucleoli
    - Clara cell differentiation characterized by apical snouting of tumor cells (nucleus may protrude into the snout in a hobnail fashion)
    - Cilia rarely present
    - Foci of central scarring usually present
    - Tumor cells become less columnar and less atypical toward the periphery of a tumor nodule and nonmucinous satellite lesions are often lined by cells that are markedly less atypical than those in the main lesion
    - Most have mild interstitial thickening and fibrosis with an interstitial infiltrate of lymphocytes (T cells) and plasma cells
    - A *sclerosing variant of nonmucinous bronchioloalveolar carcinoma* is characterized by extensive interstitial fibrosis that distorts, but does not destroy, lung architecture

- *Mucinous bronchioloalveolar carcinoma*
  - Composed of goblet cells and mucin-producing cells that are usually uniform, tall, columnar, well-differentiated, and lack cilia; cytoplasm clear, foamy, or grey
  - Nuclei tend to be uniform, lack significant hyperchromasia, and are not as atypical in appearance as those of nonmucinous carcinoma; may have clefts or grooves
  - A large amount of mucus is typically produced which fills alveoli both in the tumor and at the periphery
  - Pulmonary interstitium typically normal without any significant inflammatory infiltrate
  - Mucinous tumor cells growing along alveolar septa typically stop abruptly
- *Mucinous cystic tumors* (*mucinous cystadenoma, mucinous tumor of borderline malignancy*, and *mucinous adenocarcinoma*)
  - Characterized by massive pools of mucin and relatively little mucinous epithelium
  - Mucinous cystadenomas and mucinous tumors with borderline malignancy have partial or complete fibrous walls lined by well-differentiated mucinous cells surrounding the pools of mucus

Special Stains

- PAS stain may reveal the presence of cells with PAS-positive intranuclear inclusions (indicative of type 2 cell differentiation)
- PAS stain will reveal the presence of apical PAS-positive granules (an indication of Clara cell differentiation)
- PAS will confirm the presence of both luminal and intracytoplasmic mucin

Immunohistochemistry

- Tumor cells with type 2 cell differentiation stain with antisurfactant antibodies
- Tumor cells with Clara cell differentiation stain with Clara cell antigens
- Non-mucinous tumors reactive for TTF-1 and CK7
- Mucinous tumors may be negative for TTF-1 and CK7 and may stain for CK20

Electron Microscopy

- Clara cell differentiation (present in 90% of nonmucinous tumors) characterized by apical, electron dense granules and few microvilli
- Tumor cells with type 2 cell differentiation have cytoplasmic lamellar granules that resemble surfactant and nuclear inclusions of branching microtubules

Molecular Alterations

- Point mutations of dominant oncogenes, such as the K-ras gene, and tumor suppressor genes such as p53 and p16Ink4

Differential Diagnosis

- Reactive and metaplastic epithelial proliferations (honeycombing)
- Bronchioloalveolar cell adenoma/atypical adenomatous hyperplasia
- Ordinary lung adenocarcinoma with extensive bronchioloalveolar cell growth pattern
- Papillary adenocarcinoma
- Metastatic adenocarcinoma
- Metastatic mucin-producing carcinomas of the ovary and gastrointestinal tract
- Sclerosing hemangioma

Treatment

- Surgical resection for cure can be performed in 50% to 65% of cases

Prognosis

- Overall 5-year survival approximately 90% for stage I disease
- Patients with solitary peripheral tumors have a better prognosis than those with multicentric disease and patients with nonmucinous tumors have a better prognosis than those with mucinous tumors

Associations

- None

Large Cell Carcinoma

Clinical Manifestations

- Diagnosis of exclusion: A malignant epithelial tumor without the characteristics of squamous cell carcinoma, small cell carcinoma, or adenocarcinoma
- Represent 10% to 20% of lung carcinomas
- Almost all patients have a smoking history
- Median age at presentation approximately 60 years
- Most patients present with symptoms due to local effects of the neoplasm
- 10% to 25% of patients have a paraneoplastic syndrome; fewer than 10% have an endocrine syndrome

Gross Pathology

- Often spherical with well-circumscribed borders
- Cut surface bulges and has a fleshy, homogenous, and somewhat sarcomatous texture and appearance; no anthracotic pigment
- Frequently arises in the periphery and may invade overlying pleura and adjacent structures

Microscopic Pathology

- Typically sheets and nests of large polygonal cells with abundant eosinophilic, clear or foamy cytoplasm, prominent cell borders, and large (occasionally multiple) vesicular nuclei with prominent (occasionally multiple) eosinophilic nucleoli (cells may have a distinctly squamoid appearance)
- Stroma varies from almost none to extensive; invasive growth usually associated with desmoplastic stroma
- Foci of hemorrhage and necrosis are usually prominent
- Acute or chronic inflammatory infiltrate may be present as well as giant cells
- Focal areas of cellular dyscohesion may be present; neoplastic cells may be floating in pools of inflammatory cells (usually neutrophils); emperipolesis of inflammatory cells (lymphocytes, plasma cells or neutrophils) into neoplastic cells may be seen in giant cell variants
- Tumor cells may grow along interstitial planes and/or fill alveolar spaces
- Histologic variants:
    - *Large cell carcinoma*: A diagnosis of exclusion requiring that foci of squamous cell carcinoma, adenocarcinoma, or small cell carcinoma are not present; characterized by sheets and nests of large polygonal cells with moderate amounts of cytoplasm, vesicular nuclei, and prominent nucleoli;
    - *Large cell neuroendocrine carcinoma*: Characterized by organoid nesting, trabecular growth, rosettes, and perilobular palisading patterns; tumor cells usually large with moderate to abundant cytoplasm and are typically 2 to 3 times the size of an ordinary non-small cell carcinoma cell; nuclear chromatin usually vesicular with a prominent nucleolus; numerous mitotic figures (30 to 100 per 10 hpfs)
    - *Combined large cell neuroendocrine carcinoma*: Contains components of adenocarcinoma, squamous cell carcinoma, giant cell carcinoma, and/or spindle cell carcinoma
    - *Basaloid carcinoma*: Characterized by a solid or anastomotic trabecular invasive growth pattern; rosettes in 30% to 35%; tumor cells small and monomorphic, and have dense finely granular chromatin and inconspicuous nucleoli; cytoplasm scant; no nuclear molding; high mitotic rate; stroma hyalinized or mucoid; comedo-type necrosis common; no squamous differentiation
    - *Lympholike carcinoma*: Identical to nasopharyngeal counterpart; nests of undifferentiated neoplastic cells growing in a syncytial pattern surrounded by and infiltrated by a dense lymphoplasmacytic cell population; malignant tumor cells have moderate amounts of cytoplasm, prominent vesicular nuclei, and prominent eosinophilic nucleoli; cells tend to lack both squamous and glandular differentiation; surrounding stroma may contain epithelioid granulomas and rare giant cells
    - *Clear cell carcinoma*: Neoplasm is composed entirely of large polygonal clear cells with prominent cell borders, large nuclei and prominent nucleoli; clear cell change more common in large cell carcinomas than in any other type; cells may or may not contain glycogen
    - *Large cell carcinoma with rhabdoid phenotype:* To qualify, at least 10% of the tumor cell population must consist of rhabdoid cells characterized by eosinophilic globules

Special Stains

- Mucin stains should be negative

Immunohistochemistry

- Large cell neuroendocrine carcinoma typically positive for chromogranin, synaptophysin, and CD56; 50% positive for TTF-1
- Basaloid tumor cells generally negative for neuroendocrine markers and TTF-1; cytokeratin 1, 5, 10, and 14 positive
- Lymphoepitheliomalike carcinoma: Epstein-Barr virus-encoded RNA expressed in nuclei of large undifferentiated neoplastic cells but not in the lymphocytic infiltrate
- Large cell carcinoma with rhabdoid phenotype may be positive for vimentin and cytokeratin

Electron Microscopy

- May demonstrate evidence of squamous differentiation (desmosomes and tonofilaments), adenocarcinomatous differentiation (lumina, microvilli, tight junctions, and secretory granules), or neuroendocrine differentiation (neurosecretory-type granules)
- Some neoplastic cells show no evidence of differentiation (anaplastic tumor cells)
- Giant cell tumors have abundant mitochondria, whorls of fibrils, numerous pairs of centrioles, and demonstrate emperipolesis of inflammatory cells

Molecular Alterations

- Share same genetic alterations seen in non-small cell lung cancer

Differential Diagnosis

- Large cell neuroendocrine carcinoma:
  - Squamous cell carcinoma
  - Atypical carcinoid
  - Large cell carcinoma
  - Combined small cell/large cell carcinoma
- Large cell carcinomas with spindled foci and cellular discohesion:
  - Sarcoma
  - Lymphoma
- Clear cell carcinoma:
  - Clear cell tumor
  - Metastatic renal cell carcinoma
- Spindle cell carcinoma:
  - Metastatic fibrosarcoma, leiomyosarcoma and MFH
  - Carcinosarcoma
  - Fibroblastic reaction seen in abscess, focal organizing pneumonia, or inflammatory pseudotumor

Treatment

- Same as for other non-small cell lung cancers (squamous cell carcinoma and adenocarcinoma)

Prognosis

- Large cell neuroendocrine carcinoma has a survival rate similar to those of other non-small cell lung carcinomas
- Conflicting results, with some suggestion that large cell carcinoma may do slightly better (certainly no worse) than other non-small cell carcinomas
- 5-year survival rate for resectable lesions approaches 40%
- Tumors with a cohesive or compact growth pattern all seem to do better than those with a loose or dyscohesive pattern of growth

Associations

- Lymphoepitheliomalike carcinomas may be associated with the Epstein-Barr virus

Adenosquamous Carcinoma

Clinical Manifestations

- A carcinoma that contains both squamous carcinomatous and adenocarcinomatous components (a minimum of 5% of each component required for the diagnosis)
- Most patients are smokers
- Clinical features similar to those of other non-small cell carcinomas
- Represents 3% to 5% of surgically resected lung cancers

Gross Pathology

- Typically peripheral in location, but may arise in the hilar region (major bronchi)
- Cut surface frequently has a central scar

Microscopic Pathology

- Adenocarcinoma elements grow in acinar, papillary, and tubular patterns
- The 2 components (squamous cell carcinoma and adenocarcinoma) may be separate and discrete or admixed; either component can be dominant or they may be equally represented
- Degree of differentiation can vary independently in each component
- A component of large cell carcinoma may be present
- Stromal inflammation and secondary changes in lung parenchyma are similar to those seen in squamous cell carcinoma and adenocarcinoma
- Rarely an amyloidlike stroma present
- Adenocarcinomatous component more likely to metastasize than squamous cell carcinoma component unless the latter is predominant in the primary

Special Stains

- Mucin stains will demonstrate the presence of mucin

Immunohistochemistry

- Tumor cells of both components stain positively for keratin, EMA, and CEA

Electron Microscopy

- Confirms the presence of the features characteristic of squamous cell carcinoma and adenocarcinoma
- Amyloidlike stroma is basement membrane-like material and collagen

Molecular Alterations

- None

Differential Diagnosis

- Squamous cell carcinoma or adenocarcinoma with metaplastic epithelial changes
- High-grade mucoepidermoid carcinoma

Treatment

- Surgical resection

Prognosis

- 5-year survival rate 60% to 65% for patients with localized disease treated with surgical resection
- Overall 5-year survival rate approximately 20%

Associations

- None

Sarcomatoid Carcinoma

Clinical Manifestations

- Represents 0.5% to 1.5% of lung carcinomas
- 90% patients have a smoking history
- Median age at presentation approximately 60 years
- Male-to-female ratio 4 to 1 (except pulmonary blastoma which affects both sexes equally and presents at age 40 years)
- Most patients present with symptoms due to local effects of the neoplasm; central tumors present with cough, hemoptysis, and progressive dyspnea; peripheral tumors may be quite large and present with chest pain or chest wall invasion
- 5 subgroups
  - Pleomorphic carcinoma
  - Spindle cell carcinoma
  - Giant cell carcinoma
  - Carcinosarcoma
  - Pulmonary blastoma

Gross Pathology

- Peripheral tumors usually >5 cm, well circumscribed, and have a grey, yellow or tan, gritty cut surface; mucoid and/or hemorrhagic areas may be present as well as foci of necrosis
- Central tumors often present as a sessile or pedunculated endobronchial mass that infiltrates underlying pulmonary parenchyma
- Biphasic pulmonary blastoma are typically larger than fetal adenocarcinomas, otherwise almost indistinguishable; mean 10 cm

Microscopic Pathology

- Poorly differentiated non-small cell tumors that contain a component of sarcoma or sarcomalike (spindle and/or giant cell) differentiation
- 5 histologic variants represent a morphologic continium:
  - *Pleomorphic carcinoma*: A conventional non-small cell carcinoma (adenocarcinoma, squamous cell carcinoma or any of the types of large cell carcinoma) associated with at least 10% malignant spindle cells and/or giant cells; spindle cells arranged in fascicular or storiform pattern and may resemble epithelioid to mesenchymal cells; numerous mitotic figures; stroma myxoid or fibrous; malignant giant cells polygonal with 1 or more pleomorphic nuclei and densely eosinophilic cytoplasm; emperipolesis often present
  - *Spindle cell carcinoma*: A non-small cell carcinoma consisting of only spindle cells; malignant spindle cells arranged in cohesive nests and irregular fascicles; cells have hyperchromatic nuclei and prominent nucleoli; specific patterns of adenocarcinoma, squamous cell carcinoma, or any of the types of large cell carcinoma not present; lymphoplasmacytic infiltrate permeates tumor
  - *Giant cell carcinoma*: A non-small cell carcinoma composed exclusively of very large pleomorphic, bizarre multi- and/or mononucleated tumor giant cells; specific patterns of adenocarcinoma, squamous cell carcinoma, or any of the types of large cell carcinoma not present; tumor cells are dyscohesive; a dense neutrophilic infiltrate frequently invades the giant tumor cells (emperipolesis)
  - *Carcinosarcoma*: A malignant biphasic tumor with a mixture of conventional non-small cell carcinoma (45%-70% squamous, 20%-30% adenocarcinoma, and 10% large cell carcinoma) and sarcoma containing differentiated sarcomatous elements (osteosarcoma, chondrosarcoma, or rhabdomyosarcoma); malignant stroma often constitutes the bulk of the tumor
  - *Pulmonary blastoma*: A biphasic tumor with a primitive epithelial component (may resemble a well-differentiated fetal adenocarcinoma) and a primitive mesenchymal stroma; epithelial component consists of malignant glands and tubules resembling fetal bronchioles, embedded in an embryonic sarcomatous mesenchyme; tubules resemble well-differentiated fetal adenocarcinoma; glands often have subnuclear or paranuclear vacuoles (endometroid appearance); morular structures consisting of squamoid nests may be present; sarcomatous elements may be focally differentiated

Special Stains

- Not helpful

Immunohistochemistry

- Pleomorphic, spindle cell and giant cell tumors will express epithelial markers if a component of squamous cell carcinoma, adenocarcinoma, or large cell carcinoma present; tumor cells often coexpress cytokeratin, vimentin, CEA, and smooth muscle actins; giant cell tumors may be positive for TTF-1
- Carcinosarcoma: Epithelial component positive for keratins; chondrosarcoma positive for S-100; rhabdomyosarcoma positive for muscle markers
- Pulmonary blastoma: Fetal adenocarcinoma component positive for keratin, EMA, and CEA; may be positive for neuroendocrine markers, Clara cell antigen, and surfactant apoprotein

Electron Microscopy

- Pleomorphic carcinoma may demonstrate evidence of squamous differentiation (desmosomes and tonofilaments), adenocarcinomatous differentiation (lumina, microvilli, tight junctions, and secretory granules), or neuroendocrine differentiation (neurosecretory-type granules)
- Giant cell tumors and spindle cell tumors have aggregates of paranuclear filaments and tonofibrils of fibrils and demonstrate emperipolesis of inflammatory cells

Molecular Alterations

- Pleomorphic carcinoma shares same genetic alterations seen in other non-small cell lung cancer
- p53 mutations present in almost half of biphasic pulmonary blastomas

Differential Diagnosis

- Pleomorphic carcinoma
  - Reactive processes
  - Squamous cell carcinoma
  - Atypical carcinoid
  - Large cell carcinoma
  - Combined small cell/large cell carcinoma
- Spindle cell carcinoma
  - Synovial sarcoma
  - Metastatic fibrosarcoma
  - Inflammatory myofibroblastic tumor
- Giant cell carcinoma:
  - Primary and metastatic sarcomas (eg, pleomorphic rhabdomyosarcoma, metastatic adrenocortical carcinoma, metastatic choriocarcinoma)
- Carcinosarcoma
  - Metastatic teratomas (female or male)
- Pulmonary blastoma
  - Fetal adenocarcinoma
  - Pleuropulmonary blastoma

Treatment

- Treatment same as other non-small cell lung cancers (squamous cell carcinoma and adenosarcoma)
- Adjuvant chemotherapy and radiotherapy not typically helpful

Prognosis

- Outcome stage dependent, but in general sarcomatoid tumors have a worse prognosis than other non-small cell carcinomas
- 5-year survival rate for stage I disease 20%
- Biphasic pulmonary blastomas tend to recur and survival is similar to that of common lung carcinoma; 65% are dead within 2 years; 15% survive 5 years, and <10% survive 10 years

Associations

- None

Carcinoid Tumor, Typical and Atypical

Clinical Manifestations

- Represent 1% to 2% of all lung tumors
- Low-grade indolent malignant neoplasms of neuroendocrine cells
- 50% are asymptomatic
- Most common manifestations include hemoptysis, postobstructive pneumonitis, and dyspnea
- Occur with equal frequency in men and women
- Mean age at clinical presentation 55 years
- Most common lung tumor of childhood
- May present with a variety of paraneoplastic syndromes (see associations later in this section)
- 10% to 25% are atypical

Gross Pathology

- Approximately 1/3 are located centrally, 1/3 in the midportion, and 1/3 in the periphery of the lung; more occur in the periphery of the right middle lobe than in any other lobe
- Central carcinoids usually have a large endobronchial component consisting of a fleshy, smooth, polypoid mass
- Peripheral carcinoids tend to lie in a subpleural location and are not anatomically related to a bronchus; usually circumscribed but not encapsulated; may be multiple
- Central and atypical carcinoids tend to be larger than peripheral and typical carcinoids
- Endobronchial growth is more commonly a feature of typical carcinoid than atypical carcinoid
- Cut surface tends to be tan, yellow, or red (color depends on amount of vascularity)
- Atypical tumors often have areas of necrosis and extensive hemorrhage

Microscopic Pathology

- Both typical and atypical lesions are characterized by an organoid growth pattern consisting of uniform cells with moderate amounts of eosinophilic, finely granular cytoplasm, and nuclei that have a finely granular ("salt and pepper") chromatin pattern (chromatin pattern in an atypical carcinoid may be slightly more coarse)

- Nucleoli tend to be inconspicuous in typical carcinoids and slightly more prominent in atypical carcinoids
- A variety of histologic patterns and combinations of patterns may be present to include trabecular, palisading, glandular, follicular, rosettelike, papillary, and sclerosing papillary
- Peripheral tumors often have spindle cell cytology
- Occasionally tumor cells may appear oncocytic, acinic cell-like, signet ring, mucin-producing, or melanocytic
- Stroma may contain deposits of amyloid and/or bone
- Criteria for separating atypical from typical carcinoid include:
    - Increased mitotic activity (2 to 10 mitotic figures per 10 high-powered fields)
    - Necrosis
- Occasionally prominent cytologic pleomorphism (usually in the absence of necrosis and mitotic activity) can be seen in a typical carcinoid
- Both typical and atypical tumors may demonstrate lymphatic invasion

Special Stains

- Pigment deposits in tumor cells with melanocytic features stain with Fontana-Masson stain
- Argentaffin reaction usually negative; argyrophilia almost always present

Immunohistochemistry

- Tumor cells typically strongly positive for chromogranin (most useful), synaptophysin, and Leu-7 (CD57); this staining pattern is stronger in typical carcinoids than for atypical carcinoids
- TTF-1 positive in most, but not all
- Ectopic hormone production can be confirmed with immunohistochemical stains (corticotropin and gonadotropin-releasing hormone may be seen even in the absence of clinical evidence of Cushing syndrome or acromegaly)

Electron Microscopy

- Tumor cells contain numerous neuroendocrine granules and stacks of rough endoplasmic reticulum
- Cells of atypical carcinoid have fewer and smaller dense core granules
- Cells with oncocytic features have numerous mitochondria in addition to neuroendocrine dense core granules

Molecular Alterations

- Aneuploidy is more common in atypical carcinoids than typical carcinoids

Differential Diagnosis

- Typical versus atypical carcinoid
- Small cell carcinoma
- Metastatic carcinoma (especially from the breast and prostate)
- Spindle cell carcinoid:
    - Smooth muscle tumors
    - Chemodectoma
    - Schwannoma
    - Fibrous mesothelioma
    - Spindle cell carcinoma
    - Metastatic sarcoma
    - Metastatic melanoma
- Carcinoid tumors with oncocytic features:
    - Oncocytoma
- Carcinoid tumors with a papillary growth pattern:
    - Sclerosing hemangioma
- Carcinoid tumors with a glandular growth pattern:
    - Adenoid cystic carcinoma
    - Adenocarcinoma
- Carcinoid tumors with melanocytic features:
    - Melanoma

Treatment

- Central lesions are typically treated with lobectomy
- Small peripheral lesions can be treated with segmentectomy or wedge excision
- Proximal bronchial lesions can occasionally be treated with sleeve resection, but may require pneumonectomy
- Lymph node sampling should always be performed (all carcinoids, both typical and atypical, have some potential to metastasize)
- Tumors relatively resistant to both chemotherapy and radiation

Prognosis

- 5-year survival for typical carcinoids almost 100%; 10-year survival rate 85% to 90%
- 5-year survival for atypical carcinoids 70%; 10-year survival rate 50% to 55%
- Presence or absence of metastasis should not be used to differentiate between typical and atypical carcinoids (see diagnostic criteria above)

Associations

- Paraneoplastic syndromes:
  - Carcinoid syndrome secondary to ectopic ACTH production
  - Seen in 2% to 7% of patients with bronchial carcinoids and in 85% of patients with metastatic carcinoid in the liver
- Cushing syndrome
- Acromegaly
- MEN, type I syndrome
- Central nervous system symptoms, paraneoplastic encephalomyelitis, and subacute dysautonomia (latter characterized by defective lacrimation, skin blotching, emotional instability, motor incoordination, and hyporeflexia)

Salivary Gland Type Tumors

Acinic Cell Carcinoma

Clinical Manifestations

- Extremely rare
- Typically occurs in adults
- May present as a polypoid endobronchial lesion or as a parenchymal lesion (latter usually asymptomatic)

Gross Pathology

- Endobronchial tumors are usually polypoid
- Almost always well-circumscribed but not encapsulated
- Cut surface tan to yellow

Microscopic Pathology

- Characterized by uniform, round to polygonal cells that contain abundant, granular, eosinophilic or basophilic cytoplasm; nuclei usually small round to oval and located centrally
- Tumor cells usually arranged in sheets, nests, acini, small glands, or as tubulopapillary structures
- Bands of fibrous connective tissue sometimes with lymphoid or lymphoplasmacytic infiltrate or vascular stroma separate nests of tumor cells

Special Stains

- Cytoplasmic granules of tumor cells are PAS positive and diastase resistant

Immunohistochemistry

- Focal staining of cytoplasmic granules with amylase and α_1-antichymotrypsin

Electron Microscopy

- Tumor cells contain characteristic zymogenlike granules

Molecular Alterations

- None

Differential Diagnosis

- Metastatic acinic cell carcinoma from the salivary gland
- Oncocytic carcinoid tumor
- Granular cell tumor

Treatment and Prognosis

- Surgical resection
- Recurrence and/or metastasis both extremely rare

Associations

- None

Adenoid Cystic Carcinoma

Clinical Manifestations

- Most common salivary glandlike tumor in lower respiratory tract; represents <0.2% of all primary pulmonary tumors
- Usually arise in the lower trachea, mainstem bronchus, or lobar bronchi
- Symptoms typical of chronic bronchial obstruction or irritation

Gross Pathology

- Typically arise in large cartilage-bearing bronchi
- Tumor usually extends into bronchial lumen as a white to gray to tan soft, sessile, polypoid, annular, or diffusely infiltrative mass
- Usually appear to be well circumscribed, but often extend through the bronchial wall and proximally and distally within the bronchial submucosa

Microscopic Pathology

- Typically a submucosal mass that spreads proximally and distally and circumferentially; usually penetrates the bronchial wall between cartilage plates
- Overlying bronchial epithelium is usually intact, but may undergo squamous metaplasia
- Tumor cells are small and have hyperchromatic angulated nuclei; most often arranged in a cribriform (cylindromatous) pattern; occasionally arranged in trabeculae, glands, tubules, or solid sheets
- Spaces in cribriform pattern represent pseudocysts rather than glands and result from compression of cords of cells coursing through a sclerotic and myxoid stroma; spaces may contain mucinous or eosinophilic, hyaline basal laminalike material
- Solid areas lack luminal structures and may have peripheral cell palisades reminiscent of a basaloid pattern
- Foci of necrosis, cytologic atypia, and mitotic activity are unusual
- True mucin-containing glands lined by a luminal layer of ductal epithelium and 1 or more layers of myoepithelial cells may be present
- Perineural invasion is present in majority; surrounding lung parenchyma and regional lymph node involvement both common

Special Stains

- Eosinophilic, hyaline basal laminalike material seen within pseudocysts and in the surrounding stroma stain strongly with Alcian blue and weakly with PAS
- True glands and tubules contain mucinous material that will stain with both PAS and mucicarmine

Immunohistochemistry

- Tumor cells are strongly reactive for low-molecular-weight cytokeratins, vimentin, and muscle-specific actin
- Focal staining for S-100 protein may be present

Electron Microscopy

- Cords of infiltrating tumor cells surround and entrap matrix pseudocysts
- Cells occasionally lined by replicated basal lamina
- True glands may be present and are characterized by microvilli, junctional complexes, and desmosomes; myoepithelial cells contain cytoplasmic filaments
- Stroma consists of basal lamina and fibrillar material

Molecular Alterations

- None

Differential Diagnosis

- Pleomorphic adenoma
- Mucoepidermoid tumors
- Adenocarcinoma (with cribriform pattern)
- Small cell carcinoma (especially problematic with small crushed biopsies)
- Metastasis from extrapulmonary adenoid cystic carcinoma

Treatment and Prognosis

- Surgical excision is treatment of choice
- Tendency of the neoplasm to extend along airways makes complete excision difficult; recurrences frequent
- 10-year survival rate for patients resected for cure is approximately 50% to 60%

Associations

- None

Mucoepidermoid Carcinoma

Clinical Manifestations

- Represent <0.2% of primary lung cancers
- 50% of patients are younger than the age of 30 years
- Presenting symptoms typically those of large airway irritation or obstruction (cough, hemoptysis, fever); approximately 30% asymptomatic

Gross Pathology

- Usually tan to gray to pink endobronchial nodule in a main or lobar bronchus; rarely peripheral
- Cut surface glistening and mucoid, occasionally cystic
- Low-grade tumors typically confined to the airway; high-grade tumors frequently extend into surrounding lung
- Distal pulmonary parenchyma often demonstrates features of obstructive pneumonia or atelectasis

Microscopic Pathology

- Consists of an admixture of mucin-secreting cells, squamous cells, and intermediate cells in various proportions
- Mucin-secreting cells (glandular component) are typically the dominant cell type; columnar mucinous cells, goblet cells, and cuboidal, clear, or oncocytic cells line glands or dilated cysts
- Intermediate cells are polygonal and have amphophilic or pale eosinophilic cytoplasm and centrally located nuclei; usually appear as solid islands and sheets admixed with the glandular component
- Squamous cells are arranged in a typical pavementlike fashion and usually have abundant eosinophilic or clear cytoplasm; intracellular bridges are present; keratin whorls and pearls are absent
- Occasionally tumors will have prominent foci of oxyphilic or clear cells
- Stroma is usually hyalinized and may be reminiscent of amyloid; foci of calcification may be present
- Low-grade tumors (75%-80%) tend to be endobronchial and polypoid and have little mitotic activity, nuclear pleomorphism or cellular necrosis; glandular component dominant feature in 60%
- High-grade tumors consist primarily of sheets or nests of intermediate and squamoid cells admixed with a smaller population of glandular cells; mitotic figures average 4/10 hpfs; nuclear pleomorphism, hyperchromasia, and cellular necrosis are readily apparent; 50% invade adjacent pulmonary parenchyma

Special Stains

- Mucin stains will highlight the mucin-secreting cells that constitute the glandular component

Immunohistochemistry

- Most tumor cells are positive for EMA
- Intermediate and squamoid cells positive for cytokeratin; well-developed mucous cells usually negative for cytokeratin

Electron Microscopy

- Confirms the presence of undifferentiated cells, glandular cells, and squamous cells with prominent desmosomes and cytoplasmic tonofibrils
- Intermediate cells have few desmosomes and rare cytoplasmic tonofibrils
- Oncocytic cells have abundant cytoplasmic mitochondria

Molecular Alterations

- None

Differential Diagnosis

- Mucous gland adenoma
- Adenocarcinoma
- Carcinosarcoma
- Metastasis to a bronchus
- Adenosquamous cell carcinoma (may be very difficult to differentiate from high-grade mucoepidermoid carcinoma)

Treatment and Prognosis

- Low-grade tumors generally treated with lung sparing (sleeve resection) if clear margins can be obtained; prognosis excellent
- High-grade tumors require surgical resection with or without adjuvant radiation therapy

Associations

- None

Mucous Gland Adenoma

Clinical Manifestations

- Affects both children and adults
- Females 2 to 3 times more commonly affected than males
- Symptoms usually secondary to airway obstruction and/or hemoptysis

Gross Pathology

- Typically soft, round, polypoid endobronchial mass arising in lobar or segmental bronchi of the lower or middle lobes
- Typically well-circumscribed and noninvasive with intact overlying mucosa
- Distal lung may contain dilated bronchi filled with inspissated mucus or pneumonia

Microscopic Pathology

- Characterized by cystic, mucus-filled glands that protrude into a bronchial lumen
- Glands lined by bland, columnar, cuboidal, or flattened mucin-secreting cells that may form small papillae
- Focal areas of oncocytic metaplasia and clear cell change may be present
- Stroma may be fibrous or inflamed

Special Stains

- Tumor cells stain for neutral and acid mucins

Immunohistochemistry

- Typically positive for CEA, keratin, and EMA

Electron Microscopy

- Not helpful

Molecular Alterations

- None

Differential Diagnosis

- Low-grade mucoepidermoid carcinoma
- Adenocarcinoma

Treatment and Prognosis

- Conservative, lung-sparing surgical excision
- Benign neoplasm; no reports of malignant transformation

Associations

- None

Pleomorphic Adenoma

Clinical Manifestations

- Affects adults between the ages of 35 and 75 years
- Sometimes asymptomatic but may cause signs of chronic bronchial obstruction
- May appear adjacent to or actually within a bronchus; also occur in lung periphery without involvement of a bronchus

Gross Pathology

- Usually found in a major or secondary bronchus as a polypoid, occluding intraluminal tumor; 30% to 45% located peripherally
- Cut surface is gray to white, soft, rubbery, or myxoid
- Usually well circumscribed, but not encapsulated

Microscopic Pathology

- Characterized by a biphasic cell population consisting of round to oval epithelial cells with vesicular nuclei and a pale rim of eosinophilic cytoplasm arranged in sheets, anastomosing cords, trabeculae, or small islands that merge with stellate and spindle cells distributed in a myxoid, myxochondroid, chondroid, or hyaline stroma
- Ductal structures are rarely present, characterized by a double layer of epithelial and a myoepithelial cells

Special Stains

- Ductular lumens contain PAS-positive mucinous material

Immunohistochemistry

- Epithelial component stains strongly for low molecular weight keratins
- Basal layer of ductal cells (when present) as well as many spindled and stellate cells stain positively with vimentin, muscle specific actin, S-100 protein, and GFAP

Electron Microscopy

- Epithelioid cells have basal lamina, small microvilli, and well-developed desmosomes
- Stromal cells have tonofilaments, pinocytotic vesicles, and fragments of basement membrane

Molecular Alterations

- None

Differential Diagnosis

- Biphasic pulmonary blastoma (malignant stroma)
- Carcinosarcoma

Treatment and Prognosis

- Conservative surgical resection
- Regional nodes usually free of metastasis at the time of surgery
- May recur and/or metastasize

Associations

- None

Lymphoid/Histiocytic Tumors

Langerhans Cell Histiocytosis (Pulmonary Eosinophilic Granuloma; Langerhans Cell Granuloma; Histiocytosis X)

Clinical Manifestations

- Disease typically limited to lung; extrapulmonary disease unusual
- Typically affects adults who smoke
- Peak incidence 3rd and 4th decades
- Patients present with constitutional symptoms of fever and weight loss accompanied by dyspnea, cough, chest pain, and hemoptysis

Gross Pathology

- Cut surface of lung characterized by discrete and irregular nodules often with associated cystic change
- End-stage disease characterized by diffuse fibrosis and cystic change

Microscopic Pathology

- Low-power appearance one of discrete, peribronchiolar, interstitial nodules separated by large areas of normal lung; nodules often stellate with extensions into adjacent alveolar septa
- Nodules consist of a mixed population of Langerhans cells and variable numbers of eosinophils, plasma cells, and lymphocytes (eosinophils may be absent); central areas of bronchiolectasis may be present in cellular nodules
- Langerhans cells are large and eosinophilic, and have bland, folded, or grooved nuclei with inconspicuous nucleoli; cytoplasmic membranes are indistinct
- A DIP-like reaction, characterized by the accumulation of alveolar macrophages in alveolar spaces surrounding the peribronchiolar fibrous nodules, often present
- Pigmented macrophages tend to accumulate in distal bronchioles and nearby air spaces (respiratory or smoker's bronchiolitis)
- Pulmonary arteries may have a reactive intimal hyperplasia and a transmural infiltrate of eosinophils and other chronic inflammatory cells
- 3 phases of disease
    - *Cellular phase* characterized by presence of Langerhans cells (arranged in clusters and sheets), eosinophils, lymphocytes, plasma cells, and neutrophils
    - *Proliferative phase* characterized by presence of interstitial and intraalveolar fibrosis with chronic inflammation, pneumocyte hypertrophy and hyperplasia, increased numbers of alveolar macrophages, and decreased numbers of Langerhans cells
    - *Healed or fibrotic phase* characterized by presence of stellate scars, and interstitial fibrosis with paracicatrical airspace enlargement ("scar emphysema"); occasionally healing can occur with minimal fibrosis

Special Stains

- Not helpful

Immunohistochemistry

- Langerhans cells positive for S-100 protein and CD1a

Electron Microscopy

- Langerhans cells contain pentalaminar Birbeck granules

Molecular Alterations

- None

Differential Diagnosis

- Eosinophilic pneumonia
- DIP
- Reactive eosinophilic pleuritis
- UIP (healed or fibrotic phase)

Treatment

- Cessation of smoking and steroid therapy for the symptomatic
- Efficacy of treatment uncertain because many cases spontaneously resolve

Prognosis

- Favorable prognosis; 20% progress to fibrosis and end-stage lung disease

Associations

- 10% have extrapulmonary involvement, especially bone and posterior pituitary (with diabetes insipidus)
- Reported in patients treated for Hodgkin disease with combination chemotherapy
- Carcinomas of lung and extrapulmonary sites

Mesenchymal Tumors

Epithelioid Hemangioendothelioma (Intravascular Bronchioloalveolar Tumor [IVBAT])

Clinical Manifestations

- Usually presents as multiple bilateral nodules <2 cm in diameter; occasionally a solitary mass
- 80% in women
- 50% diagnosed before age of 40 years
- Often asymptomatic; occasionally presents with cough or dyspnea

Gross Pathology

- Typically well-circumscribed, firm, and round with a cartilaginous consistency
- Cut surface has a gray to white translucent (chondroid) rim with a somewhat opaque center that may be partially calcified or necrotic
- Unusual growth patterns include diffuse pleural involvement resembling mesothelioma and solitary fibrous nodules

Microscopic Pathology

- Viable tumor best seen at periphery of nodule where nodules of myxochondroid cells fill alveoli; nodules lobulated and grow into alveolar spaces, bronchioles, lymphatics, and blood vessels
- Viable cells arranged in clusters, cords, and as single cells and tend to be polygonal with round nuclei and uniform small nucleoli; cytoplasm eosinophilic and may contain a vacuole (vascular lumen differentiation)
- Rarely tumor cells have some cytologic atypia and mitotic activity
- Tumor cells growing in septa or pleura may have a spindled morphology
- Center characterized as myxochondroid, necrotic, hyalinized, and acellular with scattered polygonal cells with vesicular nuclei

Special Stains

- Not helpful

Immunohistochemistry

- Tumor cells typically positive for vimentin, factor VIII, CD31, and CD34 and negative for cytokeratin

Electron Microscopy

- Tumor cells contain abundant intermediate filaments and Weibel-Palade bodies
- Single large cytoplasmic vacuoles may present in scattered cells

Molecular Alterations

- 2 cases reported with chromosomal translocation involving chromosome 1 and 3 [t(1;3)(p36.3;q25)]

Differential Diagnosis

- Epithelioid angiosarcoma
- Hamartoma
- Fibrous histiocytoma
- Mesothelioma
- Leiomyosarcoma
- Chemodectoma
- Mesothelioma
- Adenocarcinoma
- Metastatic neoplasm
- Chondro (myxo) sarcoma
- Nonneoplastic diseases, eg, granulomatous disease, organizing infarct, amyloid nodules

Treatment

- None

Prognosis

- Patients may have a prolonged indolent or a rapidly fatal course

Associations

- Liver, bone, and soft tissue may be concurrently involved

Pleuropulmonary Blastoma

Clinical Manifestations

- Cystic tumors occur in children under age of 9 years and tend to present with fever, cough, pneumonia, and dyspnea
- Tend to be large, solid, lobulated masses in the mediastinum or pleura of children under the age of 12 years who present with short history of cough, fever, and/ or chest pain

Gross Pathology

- Cystic tumors single or multiloculated with thick walls
- Typically large, multilobulated, and solid with a red to grey to yellow cut surface

Microscopic Pathology

- Characterized by malignant, embryonic-appearing mesenchyme without a malignant epithelial component; foci of anaplasia and pleomorphic cells with numerous mitoses frequently present; malignant mesenchyme may have features of chondrosarcoma, leiomyosarcoma, rhabdomyosarcoma, liposarcoma, undifferentiated sarcoma; various mixtures of these tumors usually present

Special Stains

- Not helpful

Immunohistochemistry

- Malignant mesenchymal cells of cystic and pleuropulmonary blastoma frequently positive for vimentin, α_1-antitrypsin, and α_1-antichymotrypsin; rhabdomyoblasts are positive for desmin and myoglobin; chondroid elements positive for S-100 protein

Electron Microscopy

- Malignant mesenchymal cells of a cystic or pleuropulmonary blastoma have numerous cytoplasmic polysomes and large oval nuclei with prominent reticulated nucleoli

Differential Diagnosis

- May be difficult to differentiate from Askin tumor involving the lung or mediastinum or congenital cystic adenomatoid malformations

Treatment and Prognosis

- Long-term survival 25% to 50% in children with solid lesions and over 50% with thin-walled cystic lesions

Associations

- None

Lymphangioleiomyomatosis

Clinical Manifestations

- A proliferation of modified smooth muscle cells in the lymphatics and lymph nodes of the mediastinum, retroperitoneum, and pulmonary interstitium
- Seen almost exclusively in women and usually diagnosed between the ages of 20 and 50 years (women in their reproductive years); occasionally seen in postmenopausal women, most of whom have a history of taking exogenous hormones

- A manifestation of lung involvement in women (less so with men), with tuberous sclerosis complex
- Patients usually present with dyspnea, often accompanied by recurring pneumothorax
- Chest x-ray reveals the presence of progressively worsening interstitial infiltrates; pulmonary function studies reveal obstructive, restrictive or mixed patterns with paradoxically preserved lung volumes with marked decrease in diffusing capacity; computed tomographic scan reveals the presence of marked cystic change throughout the lung parenchyma which worsens with time

Gross Pathology

- Cut surface of the lung suggests emphysema early in the course of the disease; more advanced disease is characterized by diffusely distributed cystic changes with large cystic spaces resembling a honeycomb change
- Thoracic duct and lymph nodes replaced by a red to gray spongy mass

Microscopic Pathology

- Characteristic findings are a random, multifocal proliferation of immature-appearing smooth muscle cells throughout the interstitium, usually associated with cystic spaces
- Cystic spaces tend to be localized along bronchovascular bundles
- Smooth muscle proliferation consists of a focal fusiform thickening in the walls of cystic spaces with no associated scarring; the smooth muscle proliferation tends to be more disorganized and immature in appearance than that of normal smooth muscle; occasionally the proliferation of smooth muscle will appear almost polypoid and actually protrude into the adjacent cystic lumens
- Pulmonary parenchyma surrounding the lesions frequently contains hemosiderin-laden macrophages
- Proliferating smooth muscle cells may appear spindled or polyclonal and have oval nuclei and distinct nucleoli; cytoplasm tends to be pale
- Lymph node involvement is characterized by replacement by smooth muscle that is identical to that seen in the lung; lymphatics adjacent to lymph nodes show similar smooth muscle proliferation

Special Stains

- Trichrome stain highlights the fuchsinophilia of proliferating smooth muscle cells

Immunohistochemistry

- Proliferating smooth muscle cells are variably immunoreactive for desmin and positive for smooth muscle actin and HMB-45 positive (normal smooth muscle is HMB-45 negative);

Electron Microscopy

- Confirms the immature smooth muscle nature of the proliferating cells which appear shorter and have less cytoplasm than fully developed smooth muscle cells

Molecular Alterations

- Germline mutations in both *TSC1* and *TSC2*

Differential Diagnosis

- Benign metastasizing leiomyoma (lymphangioleiomyomatosis is characterized by cystic spaces with bundles of smooth muscles in the wall without the formation of gross nodules; benign metastasizing leiomyoma consist of nodules, often with entrapped alveolar epithelium, occasionally associated with cystic spaces)
- Cystic lesions of Langerhans cell histiocytosis
- Smooth muscle hyperplasia in late-stage interstitial fibrosis (honeycomb lung)
- Emphysema

Treatment

- Some evidence that the condition is at least partially hormone-dependent thus warranting consideration of oophorectomy with or without medroxyprogesterone in cases of progressive disease
- Obliteration of pleural cavity (chemical pleurodesis) will prevent reaccumulation of pleural effusion
- Transplantation

Prognosis

- Progressive pulmonary insufficiency common, but the survival rate is quite variable (approximately 70% at 10 years)

Associations

- Related to several mesenchymal neoplasms: Angiomyolipoma, clear-cell tumor of lung ("sugar tumor"), pancreas, and uterus (PEComa family of tumors: perivascular epithelial cell tumors that are immunoreactive for HMB-45)
- Multifocal pneumocyte hyperplasia in some patients with either sporadic or tuberous sclerosis-associated lymphangioleiomyomatosis

Inflammatory Myofibroblastic Tumor

Clinical Manifestations

- Most present with asymptomatic mass
- Symptoms include cough, fever, chest pain, hemoptysis, and shortness of breath
- Affects males and females equally
- Most present under age of 40 years
- Many (especially children) have an antecedent history of respiratory infection
- Chest x-ray typically reveals a solitary mass

Gross Pathology

- Typically a solitary, well-circumscribed intrapulmonary mass; occasionally a polypoid endobronchial mass
- Rarely lesions penetrate pleura and involve mediastinal structures
- Cut surface may be yellow, tan, or white depending on the number of xanthoma cells, chronic inflammatory cells, or amount of fibrous tissue present, respectively
- Focal areas of hemorrhage frequently present; calcification and foci of necrosis present in 10%

Microscopic Pathology

- Tend to be well circumscribed, solitary, and peripheral with a pushing rather than invasive margin
- Endobronchial lesions are typically polypoid or sessile
- Tumor destroys underlying pulmonary parenchyma
- Abscess formation rare
- Spindled fibroblasts and myofibroblasts, arranged in long columns and/or short fascicles, admixed with lymphocytes and numerous plasma cells (some with Mott or Russell bodies)
- Spindled cells typically have oval nuclei, small inconspicuous nucleoli, and eosinophilic cytoplasm
- Clusters or linear arrangements of plasma cells follow the course of the fascicles of fibroblasts and myofibroblasts
- Xanthoma cells (foamy macrophages), neutrophils, eosinophils, and numerous mast cells may be present; epithelioid cells, multinucleated giant cells, and granulomas are not present
- Lymphoid follicles may be present at periphery
- Lymphocytes and plasma cells may infiltrate small peripheral veins causing thrombosis and subsequent recanalization; invasion of pleura and mediastinum may also be present (as long as the spindled cells are banal the diagnosis of plasma cell granuloma is warranted; if cytologic atypia is present the diagnosis of inflammatory fibrosarcoma should be considered)

Special Stains

- Not helpful

Immunohistochemistry

- Spindle cells stain with vimentin, muscle-specific actin, and desmin
- Occasional cells are cytokeratin positive (probably represent entrapped pneumocytes)
- Myogenin, CD117 (c-Kit), and S100 protein negative
- Plasma cells are polyclonal
- Xanthoma cells stain for lysozyme and α_1-antichymotrypsin
- Expression of *ALK1* and p80 in 40%

Electron Microscopy

- Confirms presence of fibroblasts and myofibroblasts with variable numbers of lymphocytes, plasma cells, macrophages, and pneumocytes

Molecular Alterations

- Clonal changes in 65% involving chromosome 2 at 2p23 location of the *ALK* gene

Differential Diagnosis

- Sarcomatoid carcinoma
- Inflammatory fibrosarcoma (characterized by atypical fibroblastic cells)
- Extramedullary plasmacytoma
- Metastatic low grade sarcoma (eg, endometrial stromal sarcoma)

Treatment

- Conservative surgical excision with tumor-free margins
- Residual tumor after surgery may be treated with corticosteroids

Prognosis

- Complete surgical excision is essentially curative
- Recurrence typically <5%
- Lesions that invade the mediastinum and/or are unresectable may lead to death

Associations

- None

Miscellaneous Tumors

Hamartoma

Clinical Manifestations

- Lung mass consisting of cartilage, connective tissue, fat, smooth muscle, and respiratory epithelium derived from entrapped lung epithelium in various proportions
- Occur 2 to 4 times more frequently in men than women; rare in children
- Typically discovered in the 6th decade and increase in size after discovery
- Represent 5% to 15% of all pulmonary coin lesions
- 30% have a popcorn pattern of calcification on x-ray
- 2 types:
    - Parenchymal: More frequent; typically measures <4 cm; usually discovered on routine chest x-ray as an asymptomatic round nodule in the periphery of the lung
    - Central (endobronchial): 10% to 20%; symptoms result from airway obstruction

Gross Pathology

- Parenchymal lesions are typically solitary, well circumscribed, bulging, white, or gray
- Cut section has a cartilaginous appearance and consistency
- Flecks of calcium and bone may be present
- No obvious connection to a bronchus and usually easily separated from surrounding lung
- Central (endobronchial) hamartomas usually broad based, lobulated, and lie within the lumen of a large bronchus; may cause a distal obstructive pneumonia or atelectasis

Microscopic Pathology

- Parenchymal hamartoma:
    - Well-circumscribed and consist primarily of lobules of cartilage
    - Foci of fibromyxoid connective tissue, fat, bone, and smooth muscle may be present
    - Cartilage is usually located in the center and comprised of irregular, broad masses surrounded by the other mesenchymal elements (eg, fat and smooth muscle with a rim of fibromyxoid stroma)
    - At the periphery there are typically cleft-like spaces lined by ciliated, non-ciliated and mucus-producing epithelium
    - Occasionally cartilage is completely absent and the dominant component is fat or smooth muscle
- Central (endobronchial) hamartoma:
    - A mixture of mesenchymal tissues with more abundant fat and an association with a bronchial wall
    - Occasionally the cartilaginous element will have areas of atypia and increased cellularity and hyperchromasia

Special Stains

- Not helpful

Immunohistochemistry

- Fibromyxoid tissue stains for S-100 protein and glial fibrillary acidic protein (GFAP)

Electron Microscopy

- Cartilaginous cells have the typical features of cartilage
- Stromal spindle cells are primitive mesenchymal cells
- Epithelial component is a mixture of airway cell types (mucin-secreting cells, Clara cells, type II pneumocytes, and ciliated respiratory cells)

Molecular Alterations

- None

Differential Diagnosis

- Chondroma (tend to occur in young women with Carney triad)
- Leiomyomatous hamartoma (benign metastasizing leiomyoma); characterized by circumscribed nodules of smooth muscle that contain spaces lined by respiratory epithelium
- Lipoma
- Central hamartoma may resemble a chondrosarcoma

Treatment and Prognosis

- Conservative surgery: Wedge resection or enucleation of peripheral lesions
- Sleeve excision of endobronchial lesions
- Large lesions, particularly those producing obstructive pneumonia, may require lobectomy

Associations

- Rare reports of adenocarcinomas and sarcomas arising within or adjacent to hamartoma (possible malignant transformation)

Sclerosing Hemangioma

Clinical Manifestations

- 80% occur in women; average age approximately 45 years
- Most are asymptomatic but occasionally patients complain of cough, chest pain, recurrent upper respiratory tract infections, and hemoptysis
- Typically discovered on routine chest x-ray as a solitary, circumscribed, calcified mass in the periphery of the lung (coin lesion)

Gross Pathology

- Typically a round to oval, well-defined, but not encapsulated, mass within the lung parenchyma
- Occasionally lesions extend into the inner lobar fissure or are found adherent to the pericardium
- 50% occur in the lower lobes
- Rarely multiple
- Cut surface is bulging, gray to tan to yellow with focal areas of hemorrhage

Microscopic Pathology

- Typically characterized by a combination of 4 histologic patterns: solid, papillary, sclerotic, and hemorrhagic; 90% of cases contain 3 of 4 patterns; more than 1 pattern is always present
- Tumor cells tend to be arranged in sheets and are polygonal, round, and uniform with abundant clear cytoplasm (appear as bland epithelioid cells); nuclei are round to oval with finely dispersed chromatin and an inconspicuous nucleolus; cytoplasmic borders tend to be quite distinct;
- Papillary architecture usually present at the periphery of the neoplasm; cells lining papillary structures are large and cuboidal with abundant eosinophilic cytoplasm and prominent nuclei that may contain intranuclear cytoplasmic inclusions and represent non-neoplastic respiratory epithelium
- Other histologic features commonly present include cholesterol clefts, chronic inflammation, foamy macrophages, hemosiderin, mature fat, foci of necrosis, calcification, laminated (scroll-like) whorls, and mast cells

Special Stains

- Not helpful

Immunohistochemistry

- Round, pale staining neoplastic cells that stain for EMA and TTF-1; usually negative for cytokeratin, Clara cell antigen, and surfactant apoprotein
- The cells lining papillary structures stain with antibodies to keratin, surfactant proteins, and TTF-1

Electron Microscopy

- Confirms the epithelial nature of the tumor cells

Molecular Alterations

- None

Differential Diagnosis

- Inflammatory pseudotumor
- Benign clear cell tumor ("sugar" tumor)
- Carcinoid
- Papillary carcinoma (eg, bronchioloalveolar carcinoma or metastatic thyroid or renal cell carcinoma)

Treatment and Prognosis

- Cured by surgical excision
- Rare reports of regional lymph node metastases; no reports of distant metastases or tumor-associated death

Associations

- None

Clear Cell Tumor ("Sugar Tumor")

Clinical Manifestations

- Slightly more common in women than men; median age at diagnosis 50 years
- Typically discovered in an asymptomatic patient as an incidental finding on routine chest x-ray

Gross Pathology

- Usually small (approximately 2.0 cm), circumscribed mass that is easily separated from surrounding lung
- Cut surface tends to be solid and uniform yellow to tan without areas of necrosis or hemorrhage

Microscopic Pathology

- Circumscribed (not encapsulated) nodule that compresses adjacent lung parenchyma
- Tumor cells tend to be large, round to oval with abundant clear cytoplasm (glycogen) and distinct cell membranes; occasionally some are spindle-shaped; nuclei may be small with dense chromatin or large with vesicular chromatin; nuclear membranes and nucleoli are both prominent
- Some large tumor cells have granules radiating from the nucleus in a linear fashion giving them the appearance of "spider cells"; other round or polygonal cells have homogeneous eosinophilic cytoplasm
- Typically there is little in the way of connective tissue stroma but occasionally a dense eosinophilic stroma, associated with psammomatous calcification, may be present between tumor cells
- Tumor cells often contain lipochrome pigment
- Multinucleated cells are usually present, but rarely prominent
- Mitotic figures are usually absent
- Necrosis absent

Special Stains

- Tumor cells are diastase-sensitive and stain with PAS

Immunohistochemistry

- Tumor cells typically stain positively for HMB-45, HMB-50, and cathepsin B
- Focal reactivity for S-100 protein, NSE, synaptophysin, and CD57 (Leu-7)
- Tumor cells negative for keratin

Electron Microscopy

- Confirms the presence of abundant free and membrane-bound cytoplasmic glycogen
- Basement membrane material usually surrounds tumor cells
- Intracytoplasmic filaments may be present
- Cell membranes may have pinocytotic vesicles
- Occasionally neurosecretory granules are present (may represent melanosomes)

Molecular Alterations

- None

Differential Diagnosis

- Clear cell carcinoma (primary or metastatic)
- Carcinoid tumor
- Granular cell tumor
- Oncocytoma
- Metastatic clear cell sarcoma

Treatment and Prognosis

- Surgical excision almost always curative
- 1 report of metastatic disease that eventually resulted in death

Associations

- Clear cell tumors may originate from Kulchitsky cells, nonciliated bronchiolar (Clara) cells, smooth muscle, or pericytic cells and seem to have some melanocytic differentiation (premelanosomes in cytoplasm). These tumors may be related to other perivascular epithelial cell tumors (perivascular epithelioid cell sarcoma [PEComas]) such as angiomyolipoma, clear cell tumor in other organs (uterus and pancreas) and lymphangioleiomyomatosis, all of which have similar immunostaining profiles (HMB-45 positivity)

Granular Cell Tumor

Clinical Manifestations

- Also referred to as granular cell myeloblastoma or Abrikossoff tumor
- 6% of all granular cell tumors occur in the lung
- Affect men and women equally
- Median age at presentation 40 years
- 50% discovered as incidental findings on chest x-ray
- Most common symptoms include cough, recurrent obstructive pneumonitis, chest pain, fever, excessive sputum production, hemoptysis, dyspnea, and weight loss

Gross Pathology

- Tumors usually small (approximately 1 cm in diameter) and circumscribed with a tan-yellow cut surface
- May have a papillary or smooth surface
- Occur with equal frequency in both lungs
- 90% are located within a bronchus, usually near a bifurcation; 10% occur as peripheral lesions without any obvious relationship to a bronchus
- 4% to 10% are multicentric

Microscopic Pathology

- Tumor cells tend to be round or oval (occasionally spindle-shaped) with abundant eosinophilic, granular cytoplasm (granules may be finely dispersed or coarsely clumped)
- Nuclei are small, tend to be positioned somewhat centrally, and have finely granular chromatin and small nucleoli
- Neoplasm tends to infiltrate the submucosa of the bronchus and may extend around the bronchial cartilage rings into peribronchial tissue
- Squamous metaplasia of the overlying mucosa is typically present and may be hyperplastic (pseudoepitheliomatous hyperplasia)
- Subepithelial basement membrane tends to demonstrate hyaline thickening
- Malignancy suggested by >2 mitoses/10 hpfs, >5 cm, increased cellularity, and more elongated cells

Special Stains

- PAS will highlight the eosinophilic granular cytoplasm

Immunohistochemistry

- Tumor cells stain positively for S-100 protein, cathepsin B, myelin-associated protein, myelin basic protein, and NSE
- Tumor cells negative for keratin

Electron Microscopy

- Cytoplasm contains numerous osmiophilic membrane-bound granules of varying sizes and shapes (secondary lysosomes)
- Larger granules tend to be lamellated; smaller granules are granular
- Tumor cells have smooth cytoplasmic borders with a few short projections and desmosomal attachments

Molecular Alterations

- None

Differential Diagnosis

- Oncocytic carcinoid tumor
- Oncocytoma
- Acinic cell carcinoma
- Metastatic renal cell carcinoma (granular cell variant)
- Malakoplakia
- Squamous cell carcinoma (tumors with a prominent pseudoepitheliomatous hyperplastic component)

Treatment

- Lobectomy or pneumonectomy, depending on the amount of obstruction of distal lung parenchyma
- In the absence of lung destruction local excision can be performed
- Occasionally small asymptomatic lesions (especially if multiple) can be followed with careful observation

Prognosis

- No reports of malignant granular cell tumor arising as a primary neoplasm within the lung (malignant granular cell tumors in other sites can metastasize to lungs)

Associations

- 10% of patients will have a granular cell tumor in another organ such as skin, tongue, or esophagus
- 10% to 15% of patients will have another neoplasm of lung, kidney, or esophagus

Meningothelial-like Nodules (Pulmonary Chemodectomas)

Clinical Manifestations

- Typically discovered microscopically as incidental findings in a surgical or autopsy lung specimen
- Asymptomatic except in rare patients with multiple nodules causing diffuse disease ("chemodectomatosis")
- 5 to 6 times more frequent in women than in men

Gross Pathology

- Multiple, 0.1 to 0.3 cm nodules that are often not readily apparent on gross examination
- When visible, appear as ill-defined gray to white nodules bulging above the pleural surface; often found at septal insertions into the pleura
- More common in the upper lobes

Microscopic Pathology

- Typically situated adjacent to a vein and consist of a cellular expansion of alveolar septal interstitium
- Small lesions are generally little more than a cellular nest; larger lesions are frequently associated with fibrotic thickening of the interstitium with fibrosis surrounding individual nests of cells
- Neoplastic cells tend to be round, spindled, or oval and are arranged in nests with a delicate surrounding network of capillaries that may resemble the zellballen pattern characteristic of a paraganglioma
- Tumor cell cytoplasm is usually eosinophilic (may be vacuolated or clear); nuclei are uniform and round with a vesicular or granular chromatin pattern; intranuclear cytoplasmic inclusions may be present; mitoses are absent
- Adjacent lung may show thromboembolic or hyaline vascular change

Special Stains

- Tumor cells do not stain with argyrophil or argentaffin stains

Immunohistochemistry

- Most tumor nodules stain positively with EMA and vimentin
- Tumor cells are typically negative for cytokeratin, NSE, S-100 protein, and actin

Electron Microscopy

- Confirms tumor cell resemblance to cells of a meningioma: cells have prominent interdigitating cytoplasmic processes with a whorling pattern, numerous interconnecting desmosomes, and indented nuclei
- No neuroendocrine granules

Molecular Alterations

- None

Differential Diagnosis

- Carcinoid tumorlets (usually associated with bronchioles rather than venules and have a nesting organoid pattern rather than a zellballen pattern; nuclei have salt and pepper rather than granular or vesicular chromatin)
- Angiomatoid lesions of pulmonary hypertension
- Granulomas
- Interstitial fibrosis
- Metastatic carcinoma

Treatment and Prognosis

- No clinical significance; no treatment required

Associations

- Seen in association with thromboembolism in approximately 50% of cases

References

Chang AM, Myers JL, Trazelaar AD, Wright JL. *Thurlbeck's Pathology of the Lung. 3rd ed.* New York: Thieme, 2005.

Colby TV, Koss MN, Travis WD. *Tumors of the Lower Respiratory Tract: Atlas of Tumor Pathology, 3rd series, Fascicle 13.* Washington DC: Armed Forces Institute of Pathology, 1999.

Colby TV, Lombard C, Yousem SA, Kitaichi M. *Atlas of Pulmonary Surgical Pathology*. Philadelphia: WB Saunders Co, 1991.

Dabbs DJ. *Diagnostic Immunohistochemistry.* New York: Churchill Livingstone, 2002.

Dail DH, Hammer SP (eds). *Pulmonary Pathology*. 2nd ed. New York: Springer-Verlag, 1994.

Dail DH, Hammer SP, Colby TV. *Pulmonary Pathology: Tumors.* New York: Springer-Verlag, 1995.

Katzenstein AA. *Katzenstein and Askin's Surgical Pathology of Non-Neoplastic Lung Disease. 3rd ed.* Philadelphia: WB Saunders Co, 1995.

Mills S, Carter D, Greenson JK, Oberman HA, Reuter V, Stoler MH (eds). *Sternberg's Diagnostic Surgical Pathology. 4th ed.* Philadelphia: Lippincott Williams & Wilkins, 2004.

Rosai J. *Rosai and Ackerman's Surgical Pathology. 9th ed.* St. Louis: Mosby, 2004.

Shimosato Y, Miller R. *Biopsy Interpretation of the Lung.* New York: Raven Press, 1995.

Stocker JT, Dedner LP (eds). *Pediatric Pathology. 2nd ed.* Philadelphia: Lippincott Williams & Wilkins, 2001.

Travis WD, Brambililla E, Muller-Hermelink HK, Harris CC (eds). *World Health Organization Classification of Tumours. Pathology and Genetics Tumours of the Lung: Pleura, Thymus and Heart.* Lyon: IARC Press, 2004.

Travis WD, Colby TV, Koss MN, Rosado-de-Christenson ML, Muller NL, King TE. *Non-neoplastic Disorders of the Lower Respiratory Tract: Atlas of Nontumor Pathology, 1st series, Fascicle 2.* Washington DC: Armed Forces Institute of Pathology, 2002.

Chapter 12

Pleura and Peritoneum

Diffuse Lesions

Malignant Mesothelioma

Clinical Manifestations

- A tumor derived from the cells that line a serous cavity (mesothelium)
- Most develop between the ages of 50 and 70 years and 75% occur in men
- Typically a diffuse lesion that initially involves serous membranes in a multifocal fashion; as disease progresses eventually viscera become completely encased
- An epidemiologic link exists between asbestos and mesothelioma; chrysotile, amosite, and crocidolite forms of asbestos have all been linked to malignant mesothelioma; the greatest risk is associated with crocidolite exposure; x-ray evidence of asbestos exposure found in 50% of patients with peritoneal lesions and in 10% of patients with pleural lesions; no epidemiologic link to smoking
- The interval from first exposure to asbestos to the development of mesothelioma averages 35 years
- Mesothelioma may involve pleura (65%-75%), peritoneum (25%), pericardium (2%), and tunica vaginalis of testis
- With advanced disease the neoplasm can extend into other serosa cavities (peritoneal, pericardial, opposite pleural cavity) and into the mediastinum
- Rarely patients will be hypoglycemic and/or have symptoms of inappropriate secretion of antidiuretic and gonotrophic hormones
- Tumors may produce large amounts of interleukin 6
- Intestinal obstruction frequently develops when peritoneum involved
- Thrombocytosis and thromboembolic episodes are not uncommon
- Initial symptoms of pleural-based lesions include chest pain and dyspnea with subsequent development of cough, weight loss, and generalized muscular weakness; with advanced disease, pain becomes the dominant symptom and is characterized as aching (nonpleuritic) and may be noted in either the abdomen or shoulder; pleural effusion frequently present (only 10% have radiographic evidence of neoplasm without effusion)
- Peritoneal-based lesions cause constant burning abdominal or epigastric pain aggravated by meals and accompanied by constipation, anorexia, nausea, and vomiting; ascites usually present
- Lesions involving the tunica vaginalis associated with hydrocele or scrotal mass
- Pericardial lesions associated with effusion, arrhythmia, and/or cardiac failure

Gross Pathology

- *Pleura*
    - ☐ Initially small foci of tumor that gradually merge into a plaquelike accumulation with eventual encasement of lung
    - ☐ May be several centimeters in thickness
    - ☐ With advanced disease there is extension into soft tissues of the chest wall
    - ☐ Mediastinal involvement is characterized by invasion of the pericardial sac and occasionally the heart
    - ☐ Infiltration into the diaphragm often present with subsequent involvement of the peritoneum
    - ☐ Frequently the neoplasm spreads across the mediastinum to the opposite pleural cavity
    - ☐ Bloodborne metastasis may be seen in the lung, liver, kidney, adrenal gland, and bone (more likely with sarcomatous mesothelial lesions than nonsarcomatous lesions)
- *Peritoneum*
    - ☐ Clinical findings usually indistinguishable from those of carcinomatosis peritonei
    - ☐ Large confluent plaques or masses of tumor typically develop in the omentum and lower abdominal cavity and pelvis
    - ☐ With time abdominal viscera become completely encased and the peritoneal cavity is obliterated
    - ☐ Neoplasm rarely invades the abdominal wall except at site of surgical scars
    - ☐ 50% will have metastasis at the time of diagnosis (usually abdominal lymph nodes)
- *Tunica vaginalis testis*
    - ☐ Multiple nodules or papillary lesions on the serosal surface of the tunica, which eventually encase the scrotal contents
    - ☐ Cystic spaces may be present
    - ☐ Neoplasm can extend into the peritoneum to involve peritoneal surfaces and retroperitoneal lymph nodes
- *Pericardium*
    - ☐ Focal invasion of myocardium often present but the neoplasm does not involve the endocardium or enter a heart chamber
    - ☐ Typically mediastinum and adjacent pleura are involved

Microscopic Pathology

- Marked variation in both cytologic and architectural appearance
- 4 major histologic types of diffuse mesothelioma:
  - *Epithelial (tubulopapillary and epithelioid)*
    - Epithelial tumors are usually tubulopapillary; tumor cells tend to be cuboidal or flattened with acidophilic cytoplasm and uniform vesicular nuclei with prominent nucleoli; a microcystic pattern may be present; focal areas may resemble an adenocarcinoma
    - A nonglandular or solid form of epithelial mesothelioma consists of aggregates or sheets of plump, round, or polyhedral cells with abundant acidophilic cytoplasm; these cells resemble hyperplastic mesothelium; cells may show a fair degree of nuclear pleomorphism and occasionally giant cells are present; large cytoplasmic vacuoles may be present (periodic acid–Schiff [PAS] negative)
    - Stroma of epithelial tumors can be quite variable; may be dense or loosely formed and edematous or myxoid; if cellular, the stroma may be quite difficult to differentiate from the sarcomatous component of a biphasic or mixed tumor
  - *Sarcomatous (including desmoplastic)*
    - Neoplastic cells are spindle shaped or oval and may be arranged in a variety of architectural patterns that overlap the patterns characteristic of malignant fibrous histiocytoma, malignant schwannoma, fibrosarcoma, and rhabdomyosarcoma; classic fascicular patterns are rare
    - Sarcomatous areas may contain foci of malignant osteoid or cartilage
    - Desmoplastic form may appear histologically almost identical to reactive pleural fibrosis; diagnosis hinges on identifying foci of more obviously malignant features, invasion of the chest wall, necrosis, or a combination of these findings
    - Sarcomatous tumors that invade lung often fill alveolar spaces without invading alveolar septa
  - *Biphasic (mixed)*
    - Characterized by malignant epithelial as well as mesenchymal cells (very reminiscent of synovial sarcoma)
  - *Poorly differentiated (or undifferentiated)*
    - Poorly differentiated tumor cells typically arranged in sheets and tend to be polygonal with marked nuclear pleomorphism; occasionally cells will be clear and resemble a clear cell carcinoma originating from other sites such as the kidney or female genital tract
    - 50% of pleural tumors are epithelial, 25% biphasic, 15% sarcomatous, and 10% poorly differentiated
    - 75% of peritoneal tumors are epithelial; the sarcomatous variant is rare in the peritoneum
  - Additional variants:
    - *Lymphohistiocytoid mesothelioma:* Characterized by large histiocytelike tumor cells and a diffuse lymphocytic infiltrate; plasma cells and eosinophils may be present; tubulopapillary differentiation is never present, but sarcomatoid elements may be seen
    - *Small cell mesothelioma:* Tumor cells are small and uniform and have high nuclear-cytoplasmic ratios; superficially resemble small cell carcinoma
    - *Mesothelioma in situ*: Typically seen as a small noninvasive aggregate of mesothelial cells with cytologic features of malignancy arranged in 1 or more layers; can only be reliably identified in patients who have invasive disease elsewhere
    - *Well-differentiated papillary mesothelioma*: A tumor of intermediate malignancy; usually seen in the peritoneum; more common in women often during the 3rd and 4th decades; usually presents as multiple peritoneal nodules; typically a well-developed papillary or tubulopapillary pattern; tubules and papillae lined by a single layer of uniform, cuboidal or flattened mesothelial cells with rather banal nuclear features; psammoma bodies may be present
    - *Malignant mesothelioma of tunica vaginalis testis:* Usually of the papillary type; tumor cells tend to have abundant acidophilic cytoplasm and may have cytoplasmic vacuoles
    - *Localized malignant mesothelioma:* Very rare; typically identical to epithelial and biphasic forms; tends to be quite aggressive, but long-term survival possible with complete excision

- *Deciduoid peritoneal mesothelioma*: Very rare; affects young women; resembles ectopic decidual change in the peritoneum; no relationship with asbestos exposure or endocrine abnormality

Special Stains

- Mucicarmine can be used to help differentiate epithelial mesothelioma from adenocarcinoma (mesothelioma is negative; adenocarcinoma is typically positive)

Immunohistochemistry

- Mesotheliomas stain with low-molecular-weight and high-molecular-weight cytokeratins (the latter feature may be of help in differentiating a mesothelioma from adenocarcinoma; adenocarcinomas do not as frequently express high-molecular-weight cytokeratin)
- Both the normal and neoplastic cells of mesothelioma will express vimentin
- Mesotheliomas rarely express carcinoembryonic antigen (CEA); 70% to 100% of adenocarcinomas will express CEA
- Mesotheliomas are rarely positive for Leu-M1 (CD15); Leu-M1 positivity is seen in 60% to 100% of adenocarcinomas
- Mesotheliomas rarely stain positively for *Ber*-EP4; 85% of adenocarcinomas will stain for *Ber*-EP4
- Fewer than 15% of mesotheliomas will show weak immunoreactivity for B72.3; adenocarcinomas are typically positive for B72.3
- Mesotheliomas often show positivity for the tumor suppressor gene protein p53 (benign mesothelial proliferations are typically negative)
- 75% to 95% of mesotheliomas are positive for calretinin; 5% to 15% of adenocarcinomas are positive for calretinin

Electron Microscopy

- Malignant mesothelial cells typically possess long, thin, "bushy," and sinuous surface microvilli (normal mesothelial cells have similar microvilli; poorly differentiated mesothelial cells lack these distinctive villi)

Molecular Alterations

- Loss of chromosomes 4 and 22 and chromosome arms 9p and 3p
- Gain of chromosomes 5, 7 and 20 with deletion or rearrangement of 3p in occasional hyperdiploid cases

Differential Diagnosis

- Epithelial mesothelioma (well-differentiated)
  - Solid or papillary mesothelial hyperplasia
- Epithelial mesothelioma (moderate to poorly differentiated)
  - Tubulopapillary or tubular adenoma
  - Epithelioid hemangioendothelioma
- Epithelial mesothelioma (undifferentiated)
  - Poorly differentiated tumor, ie, large and small cell carcinoma
- Biphasic (mixed) mesothelioma
  - Synovial sarcoma
  - Carcinosarcoma
  - Epithelioid hemangioendothelioma
  - Carcinoma with cellular stromal reaction
  - Mesothelial hyperplasia
- Sarcomatous mesothelioma
  - Sarcoma
  - Spindle cell carcinoma
  - Metastatic sarcoma
  - Cellular serosal fibrosis
- Desmoplastic mesothelioma
  - Reactive serosal fibrosis

Treatment and Prognosis

- Surgical resection may prolong survival and improve the quality of life
- Radical extrapleural pneumonectomy results in a 3-year survival rate of 15% to 35%
- Radiotherapy for palliation only
- Chemotherapy consisting of adriamycin in multiple drug combinations may result in a significant remission (chemotherapy appears to produce best results in stage I peritoneal disease)

Associations

- Asbestos exposure (especially crocidolite)

Discrete Lesions

Solitary Fibrous Tumor (Localized Fibrous Mesothelioma)

Clinical Manifestations

- May present at any age to include childhood, usually diagnosed between 4th and 7th decades (mean 50 years)
- Slightly more common in women than men
- Most located in thoracic cavity and asymptomatic; typically an incidental finding on a routine chest x-ray that appears as a solitary, round, sharply circumscribed, homogenous mass
- Most common clinical symptoms include chest pain, cough, dyspnea, digital clubbing (osteoarthropathy), and fever
- Large tumors may be associated with ipsilateral pleural effusion and/or hypoglycemia (5%)
- Reported cases associated with galactorrhea
- Also reported in sites unrelated to serosal surfaces (ie, liver, orbit, nasal passages, thyroid, lung, meninges, skin, soft tissue, and breast)

Gross Pathology

- 65% attached visceral pleura, occasionally by a broad-based pedicle
- 35% arise from the parietal, diaphragmatic, or mediastinal pleura
- Tumors have a smooth capsule and average 5 to 6 cm in diameter
- A minority project into lung substance and occasionally are entirely intrapulmonary
- Neoplasms are typically round with a bosselated surface with prominent superficial vasculature
- Interface between the neoplasm and adjacent lung is usually well-defined
- On cut section, the lesion is nodular, firm, and gray-white and may have a whorled pattern; cystic or myxoid areas and foci of hemorrhage and/or necrosis may be present

Microscopic Pathology

- Bland spindle-shaped cells with a variable arrangement from area to area within the same tumor; may be loosely arranged in short, interlacing fascicles or randomly arranged in a "patternless pattern"
- Prominent areas of hyalinization typically present; cells in these hyalinized areas usually arranged singly or in small parallel clusters next to dense collagen; artifactual "cracks" may be present between cells and adjacent collagen; other areas characterized by parallel bands or "wires" of collagen that form complex anastomosing patterns
- More cellular areas often present and typically composed of tightly packed spindled or oval cells arranged in interdigitating fascicles; cells may be pleomorphic and have little intervening stroma; pattern very reminiscent of a hemangiopericytoma
- Vascularity varies from narrow clefts to wide-open, branching channels identical to those of a hemangiopericytoma
- Focal areas of myxoid or cystic change as well as areas of recent necrosis may be present
- Overlying pleura is generally fibrous and thickened with inconspicuous mesothelium (mesothelium may actually be denuded)
- Malignant lesions are more cellular and pleomorphic, have more than 4 mitotic figures per 10 high power fields (hpf), and have areas of hemorrhage and/or necrosis; malignant tumors often have a prominent fascicular pattern (similar to that of a fibrosarcoma)

Special Stains

- Not helpful

Immunohistochemistry

- Tumor cells express CD34 (90% to 95%) and CD99 (70%)
- 20% to 30% express epithelial membrane antigen, *bcl*-2, and smooth muscle actin
- Neoplastic cells typically negative for cytokeratin, desmin, and S-100 protein

Electron Microscopy

- Tumor cells are fibroblastic and myofibroblastic
- No evidence of mesothelial differentiation

Molecular Alterations

- None

Differential Diagnosis

- Hemangiopericytoma (see comment later in this section)
- Desmoplastic mesothelioma
- Fibromatosis
- Fibrosarcoma
- Sclerosing fibrous histiocytoma
- Malignant fibrous histiocytoma
- Malignant peripheral nerve sheath tumor

Treatment

- Complete surgical excision
- Neoplasms that are partly or mainly intraparenchymal should be treated with wide surgical resection
- No evidence that radiation therapy is of benefit
- Nonpedunculated malignant lesions require radical therapy (treated same as diffuse malignant mesothelioma)

Prognosis

- Most are benign (incidence of malignancy quite variable)

Associations

- Hypoglycemia (occurs in approximately 5% and is more common in women than men; hypoglycemia also seen in mesothelioma, fibrosarcoma, hemangiopericytoma, and other nonpancreatic mesenchymal and epithelial neoplasms)

Comment

Extrapleural solitary fibrous tumor and hemangiopericytoma share similar histopathologic features with lipomatous hemangiopericytoma and giant cell angiofibroma. The distinction between these 4 lesions is becoming increasingly indistinct, especially between solitary fibrous tumor and hemangiopericytoma. These 2 tumors occupy the ends of a spectrum of perivascular tumors. At 1 end of the spectrum, the tumor has clinicopathologic features of a "classic" hemangiopericytoma (usually located in an extremity, a marked pericytic vascular pattern, nonspindled cells, and variable to focal zones of hyalinization); at the other end of the spectrum, the tumor has clinicopathologic features of a classic solitary fibrous tumor (usually located in a body cavity, a focal perivascular pattern, spindled cells, and broad zones of hyalinization). Tumors with intermediate features or equal areas of both classic solitary fibrous tumor and classic hemangiopericytoma represent "hemangiopericytoma-solitary fibrous tumor."

References

Battifora H, McCaughey WTE. *Tumors of the Serosal Membranes: Atlas of Tumor Pathology, 3rd Series, Fascicle 15.* Washington DC: Armed Forces Institute of Pathology, 1995.

Churg A, Cagle PT, Roggli VL. *Tumors of the Serosal Membranes: Atlas of Tumor Pathology, Series 4. Fascicle 3.* Washington DC; Armed Forces Institute of Pathology, 2006.

Dabbs DJ. *Diagnostic Immunohistochemistry.* New York: Churchill Livingstone, 2002.

Mills S, Carter D, Greenson JK, Oberman HA, Reuter V, Stoler MH (eds). *Sternberg's Diagnostic Surgical Pathology. 4th ed.* Philadelphia: Lippincott Williams & Wilkins, 2004.

Rosai J. *Rosai and Ackerman's Surgical Pathology. 9th ed.* St. Louis: Mosby, 2004.

Travis WD, Brambililla E, Muller-Hermelink HK, Harris CC (eds). *World Health Organization Classification of Tumours. Pathology and Genetics—Tumours of the Lung, Pleura, Thymus and Heart.* Lyon: IARC Press, 2004.

Weiss SW, Goldblum JR. *Enzinger and Weiss's Soft Tissue Tumors. 4th ed.* St. Louis: Mosby Inc, 2001.

Chapter 13

Mediastinum

Intraoperative Consultation

Intraoperative diagnosis may be requested on specimens taken from the mediastinum for several reasons. The most common indication is to determine if diagnostic material has been obtained from a lesion that is either unresectable or should not be resected because it is best treated by a modality other than surgery. Frozen section diagnosis is also indicated to evaluate surgical margins of lesions that are resected for cure and occasionally to confirm the diagnosis in such a lesion. In the latter instance it is important to realize that a specific diagnosis is not always possible and a differential diagnosis must be offered when there is uncertainty. Finally, intraoperative consultation may be necessary to appropriately triage tissue for ancillary studies such as cultures for microorganisms, electron microscopy, cytogenetics, flow cytometry, immunoperoxidase, and gene rearrangement studies.

The pathologist faces several pitfalls when trying to render a frozen section diagnosis on a specimen from the mediastinum. The presence of Hodgkin disease or non-Hodgkin lymphoma in the mediastinum can be particularly problematic. Superficial biopsies of a lymph node containing Hodgkin disease may reveal a nonspecific cellular infiltrate and fibrosis. Tissue that appears adequate on frozen section may prove to be nondiagnostic on permanent section. The pathologist must ensure that deep representative biopsy specimens are taken in cases of suspected Hodgkin disease. In addition, Hodgkin disease involving the thymus may induce cystic changes that on frozen section resemble a benign cyst. A non-Hodgkin lymphoma, particularly the large cell type (a common lesion in the mediastinum) may induce a diffuse sclerosis that results in the isolation of small aggregates of cells that may mimic a poorly differentiated carcinoma or chronic inflammation.

Thymomas that are completely excised generally do not require an intraoperative diagnosis, but surgical margins around an infiltrating thymoma may require microscopic examination to confirm that they are free of neoplasm. Thymomas, particularly lymphocyte-rich thymomas, are easily confused with low-grade lymphoma, and spindle cell thymoma can mimic a mesenchymal tumor. The differential between a cystic thymoma and a multilocular cyst of the thymus is often not possible on a frozen section.

Among the germ cell neoplasms that involve the mediastinum, only seminomas present a problem for the pathologist. Teratomas are generally easily excised and the diagnosis is usually established preoperatively. The same is true for nonseminomatous malignant germ cell tumors in which serum α-fetoprotein and human chorionic gonadotropin (hCG) levels are elevated in more than 70% of cases. Intraoperative consultation on a seminoma can be problematic if the granulomatous inflammatory reaction is extensive enough to obscure the neoplasm, resulting in a mistaken diagnosis of an infectious process. If the seminoma involves the thymus it may induce cystic change that could be confused with a benign thymic cyst.

Sclerosing mediastinitis represents a potential problem on frozen section. The histologic features of chronic inflammation and sclerosis are quite similar to the secondary inflammatory changes that occur around a number of different neoplasms. If there is no clinical suspicion of sclerosing mediastinitis, the pathologist should request additional deeper biopsy specimens to ensure that diagnostic tissue is obtained.

Specimen Handling

Biopsy specimens from the mediastinum are handled differently depending on the clinical situation. If the patient is undergoing a staging mediastinoscopy for lung cancer the entire biopsy specimen is usually submitted for frozen section so that the intraoperative diagnosis can be as sensitive and specific as possible.

If a biopsy specimen is taken from a primary mediastinal tumor, nonfrozen tissue should be retained. Cultures (fungal and mycobacterial) are indicated in cases of granulomatous inflammation or suspected sclerosing mediastinitis. Tissue specimens of suspected lymphoproliferative disorders should be snap-frozen for immunohistochemical and gene rearrangement studies. Occasionally it is appropriate to fix a portion of tissue in glutaraldehyde for electron microscopy, RPMI medium for flow cytometry, and cytogenetic medium for cytogenetics. Finally, if sufficient tissue is obtained, a portion should be fixed in a mercury-based fixative such as B5 because it provides superior nuclear detail and better antigen preservation for immunohistochemistry.

Specimens intended to represent complete resections are, of course, inked before sectioning.

Germ Cell Tumors

Classification

- Benign teratoma
  - Mature teratoma
  - Immature teratoma, benign
- Malignant teratoma
  - Malignant teratoma with areas of germ cell tumor (germinoma, embryonal carcinoma, choriocarcinoma, yolk sac tumor, and mixed)
  - Malignant teratoma with non-germinal malignant tumor (carcinoma, sarcoma, malignant embryonal tumor, and mixed)
  - Immature teratoma, malignant (a teratoma that can metastasize)
- Germinoma (seminoma and dysgerminoma)
- Embryonal carcinoma
- Yolk sac tumor (endodermal sinus tumor)
- Choriocarcinoma
- Mixed germ cell tumor

Choriocarcinoma

Clinical Manifestations

- Choriocarcinoma occurs in both sexes; elevated serum levels of β-hCG strongly support the diagnosis; men may present with gynecomastia

Gross Pathology

- Cut surface very hemorrhagic
- May be seen in the pure form or in combination with immature teratoma or other germ cell tumors

Microscopic Pathology

- Germinoma, embryonal carcinoma, yolk sac tumor, and choriocarcinoma can all occur in the mediastinum in a pure form, in combination with each other, or in combination with an immature teratoma (microscopic foci of malignant germ cell tumor are frequently present in an immature teratoma and represent malignant transformation)
- An admixture of mononuclear cytotrophoblastic cells and giant syncytiotrophoblastic cells that border areas of hemorrhage

Special Stains

- Not helpful

Immunohistochemistry

- Syncytiotrophoblastic cells and some cytotrophoblastic cells in choriocarcinoma positive for β-hCG; cytokeratin always positive; PLAP and EMA positive in 50%

Electron Microscopy

- Not helpful

Molecular Alterations

- Klinefelter syndrome (47,XXY karyotype)

Differential Diagnosis

- Metastasis from ovarian or testicular primary
- Carcinoma or sarcoma remaining after chemotherapy for a germ cell neoplasm versus primary or metastatic cancer

Treatment and Prognosis

- Nonseminomatous germ cell tumors treated with intensive chemotherapy (cisplatin, vinblastine, etoposide, and bleomycin)
- Poor risk patients with nonseminomatous germ cell tumors usually treated with high-dose etoposide and carboplatin followed by autologous bone marrow transplantation

Associations

- Patients with Klinefelter syndrome at substantial risk for developing all kinds of extragonadal germ cell tumors
- Incidence of Klinefelter syndrome among patients with a mediastinal germ cell tumor is 30 to 40 times the incidence of Klinefelter syndrome in the general population
- Synchronous hematologic malignancies include malignant histiocytosis, anaplastic large cell lymphoma, and acute myelomonocytic leukemia
- Hematologic malignancies reported after chemotherapy for germ cell tumor include acute myelogenous leukemia, acute megakaryocytic leukemia, and acute myelomonocytic leukemia

Embryonal Carcinoma

Clinical Manifestations

- Embryonal carcinoma almost always unresectable; elevated serum levels of α-fetoprotein diagnostic

Gross Pathology

- Usually extensively invasive at the time of diagnosis
- Cut surface necrotic and hemorrhagic

Microscopic Pathology

- Germinoma, embryonal carcinoma, yolk sac tumor, and choriocarcinoma can all occur in the mediastinum in a pure form, in combination with each other, or in combination with an immature teratoma (microscopic foci of malignant germ cell tumor are frequently present in an immature teratoma and represent malignant transformation)
- Characterized by sheets, tubules and papillary structures of large polygonal cells that have round to oval nuclei with prominent nucleoli, pale staining cytoplasm, and indistinct cell borders
- Mitotic figures are frequent
- Multinucleated giant cells reminiscent of syncytiotrophoblastic cells may be present

Special Stains

- Not helpful

Immunohistochemistry

- Syncytiotrophoblasts in both germinomas and embryonal carcinomas are positive for β-hCG
- Tumor cells of embryonal carcinoma usually reactive for PLAP, cytokeratin, and CD30; 30% to 35% positive for α-fetoprotein

Electron Microscopy

- Not helpful

Molecular Alterations

- Klinefelter syndrome (47,XXY karyotype)

Differential Diagnosis

- Metastasis from ovarian or testicular primary
- Germinoma
- Yolk sac tumor (endodermal sinus tumor)

Treatment and Prognosis

- Poor risk patients with nonseminomatous germ cell tumors usually treated with high-dose etoposide and carboplatin followed by autologous bone marrow transplantation

Associations

- Patients with Klinefelter syndrome at substantial risk for developing all kinds of extragonadal germ cell tumors
- Incidence of Klinefelter syndrome among patients with a mediastinal germ cell tumor is 30 to 40 times the incidence of Klinefelter syndrome in the general population
- Synchronous hematologic malignancies include malignant histiocytosis, anaplastic large cell lymphoma, and acute myelomonocytic leukemia
- Hematologic malignancies reported after chemotherapy for germ cell tumor include acute myelogenous leukemia, acute megakaryocytic leukemia, and acute myelomonocytic leukemia

Germinoma (Seminoma and Dysgerminoma)

Clinical Manifestations

- Germinomas typically occur in men between 2nd and 4th decades; rare in women

Gross Pathology

- Tends to be large and soft and well circumscribed
- Cut surface usually homogeneous with foci of hemorrhage and necrosis

Microscopic Pathology

- Germinoma, embryonal carcinoma, yolk sac tumor, and choriocarcinoma can all occur in the mediastinum in a pure form, in combination with each other, or in combination with an immature teratoma (microscopic foci of malignant germ cell tumor are frequently present in an immature teratoma and represent malignant transformation)

- Characterized by sheets of large polygonal cells with distinct cell membranes, clear (glycogen) or finely granular cytoplasm, and a round, partially flattened nucleus with one or more prominent nucleoli
- A loose stroma infiltrated by lymphocytes courses between aggregates of tumor cells: 50% to 60% actually develop a granulomatous reaction that varies from scattered epithelioid histiocytes to ill-defined clusters of histiocytes to discrete, well-formed, noncaseating granulomas with Langerhans-type giant cells
- Isolated multinucleated syncytiotrophoblasts may be present
- Foci of coagulation necrosis may stimulate a granulomatous reaction

Special Stains

- Not helpful

Immunohistochemistry

- Syncytiotrophoblasts in both germinomas and embryonal carcinomas are positive for β-hCG
- Nonseminomatous germ cell tumors are generally positive for cytokeratin
- Germinoma cells tend to be negative for cytokeratin and epithelial membrane antigen (EMA) and positive for placental alkaline phosphatase (PLAP) and CD117 (c-*kit*)

Electron Microscopy

- Not helpful

Molecular Alterations

- Klinefelter syndrome (47,XXY karyotype)

Differential Diagnosis

- Metastasis from ovarian or testicular primary
- Lymphoepitheliomalike carcinoma of the thymus
- Diffuse large cell lymphoma
- Carcinoma or sarcoma remaining after chemotherapy for a germ cell neoplasm versus primary or metastatic cancer

Treatment and Prognosis

- Germinomas are readily curable when treated with surgical excision with adjuvant radiotherapy for mediastinal disease and cisplatin-based chemotherapy for metastatic disease; long-term survival approximately 80%

Associations

- Patients with Klinefelter syndrome at substantial risk for developing all kinds of extragonadal germ cell tumors
- Incidence of Klinefelter syndrome among patients with a mediastinal germ cell tumor is 30 to 40 times the incidence of Klinefelter syndrome in the general population
- Synchronous hematologic malignancies include malignant histiocytosis, anaplastic large cell lymphoma, and acute myelomonocytic leukemia
- Hematologic malignancies reported after chemotherapy for germ cell tumor include acute myelogenous leukemia, acute megakaryocytic leukemia, and acute myelomonocytic leukemia

Benign Teratoma

Clinical Manifestations

- Anterior mediastinum most frequent site; most occur within or adjacent to the thymus gland
  - Mature teratoma most common (75% of the total) and most frequently seen in adolescents; usually asymptomatic, although some patients complain of cough, dyspnea, and/or chest pain; in women, all germ cell tumors are mature teratomas (most of these are cystic)
  - Immature teratomas (both pure form and mixed form) are more frequent in children and adolescents

Gross Pathology

- Mature teratomas are usually cystic (rarely solid), encapsulated, and tend to adhere to surrounding structures; may be unilocular or multilocular; sectioning reveals a variegated surface; cystic areas contain brown, oily fluid, and grumous material with or without hair
- Immature teratomas and malignant germ cell tumors are usually large and solid and either adhere to or invade adjacent structures; sectioning typically reveals extensive areas of hemorrhage and necrosis

Microscopic Pathology

- Germinoma, embryonal carcinoma, yolk sac tumor, and choriocarcinoma can all occur in the mediastinum in a pure form, in combination with each other, or in combination with an immature teratoma (microscopic foci of malignant germ cell tumor are frequently present in an immature teratoma and represent malignant transformation)
- *Mature teratoma*
    - Composed of abnormal mixture of tissues derived from two or all three embryonic layers (ectoderm, endoderm, and mesoderm)
    - Most frequent tissue encountered is skin and its appendages, followed in order of frequency by bronchial tissue, gastrointestinal mucosa, smooth muscle and fat; in addition, bone, cartilage, exocrine and endocrine pancreas (not seen in teratomas of the gonads), salivary gland, central nervous system tissue (including ependymoma), prostate gland, and hepatocytes may be present
- *Immature teratoma*
    - Contains tissue derived from all three germinal layers in various stages of maturation from embryonic to fetal
    - Immature tissue includes epithelium of both ectodermal and endodermal derivation, bone, cartilage, and muscle
    - Many contain large areas of immature neural tissue (eg, glial elements, neuroepithelium with tubules, rosettes, and retinal anlage)
    - Malignant transformation in a mature cystic teratoma (dermoid) in the mediastinum may have features of squamous cell carcinoma, adenocarcinoma, or poorly differentiated carcinoma

Special Stains

- Alcian blue-PAS stain will confirm the presence of cytoplasmic mucus in mature glandular tissue in a mature teratoma

Immunohistochemistry

- Nonseminomatous germ cell tumors are generally positive for cytokeratin

Electron Microscopy

- Not helpful

Molecular Alterations

- Klinefelter syndrome (47,XXY karyotype)

Differential Diagnosis

- Mature versus immature
- Benign versus malignant
- Malignant teratoma with nongerminal malignant tumor

Treatment and Prognosis

- Mature teratoma: Benign neoplasm best treated with surgical removal
- Immature teratoma with a malignant germ cell component usually treated with surgical debulking and adjuvant radiotherapy and chemotherapy; some cases cured

Associations

- Patients with Klinefelter syndrome at substantial risk for developing all kinds of extragonadal germ cell tumors
- Incidence of Klinefelter syndrome among patients with a mediastinal germ cell tumor is 30 to 40 times the incidence of Klinefelter syndrome in the general population
- Synchronous hematologic malignancies include malignant histiocytosis, anaplastic large cell lymphoma, and acute myelomonocytic leukemia
- Hematologic malignancies reported after chemotherapy for germ cell tumor include acute myelogenous leukemia, acute megakaryocytic leukemia, and acute myelomonocytic leukemia

Malignant Teratoma

Clinical Manifestations

- Malignant teratoma and other malignant germ cell tumors are seen exclusively in males and usually present with cough, dyspnea, chest pain, fatigue and weight loss

Gross Pathology

- Malignant component probably arises within teratomatous foci; occurrence of carcinoma in a teratoma is much less frequent than occurrence of a mesenchymal tumor in a teratoma

Microscopic Pathology

- Non-germ cell malignant neoplasm may be found in an immature teratoma
- Malignant tumors include embryonal rhabdomyosarcoma, angiosarcoma, myxoid liposarcoma, chondrosarcoma, leiomyosarcoma, glioblastoma multiforme, neuroblastoma, nephroblastoma, and adenosquamous carcinoma
- Occasionally carcinoma or malignant mesenchymal components may remain after complete disappearance of the germ cell tumor after intensive chemotherapy (may be the result of the selective action of chemotherapy on the germ cell component while sparing the carcinoma or sarcoma component)

Immunohistochemistry

- Nonseminomatous germ cell tumors are generally positive for cytokeratin

Electron Microscopy

- Not helpful

Molecular Alterations

- Klinefelter syndrome (47,XXY karyotype)

Differential Diagnosis

- Mature versus immature
- Benign versus malignant
- Malignant teratoma with nongerminal malignant tumor
- Carcinoma or sarcoma remaining after chemotherapy for a germ cell neoplasm versus primary or metastatic cancer

Treatment and Prognosis

- Immature teratoma with a malignant germ cell component usually treated with surgical debulking and adjuvant radiotherapy and chemotherapy; some cases cured
- Poor risk patients with nonseminomatous germ cell tumors usually treated with high-dose etoposide and carboplatin followed by autologous bone marrow transplantation

Associations

- Patients with Klinefelter syndrome at substantial risk for developing all kinds of extragonadal germ cell tumors
- Incidence of Klinefelter syndrome among patients with a mediastinal germ cell tumor is 30 to 40 times the incidence of Klinefelter syndrome in the general population
- Synchronous hematologic malignancies include malignant histiocytosis, anaplastic large cell lymphoma, and acute myelomonocytic leukemia
- Hematologic malignancies reported after chemotherapy for germ cell tumor include acute myelogenous leukemia, acute megakaryocytic leukemia, and acute myelomonocytic leukemia

Yolk Sac Tumor (Endodermal Sinus Tumor)

Clinical Manifestations

- Yolk sac tumor (endodermal sinus tumor) usually occurs in men in their 20s; highly malignant; elevated serum levels of α-fetoprotein diagnostic

Gross Pathology

- Usually large and invasive at the time of diagnosis
- May be seen in the pure form or in combination with immature teratoma or other malignant germ cell tumors

Microscopic Pathology

- Germinoma, embryonal carcinoma, yolk sac tumor, and choriocarcinoma can all occur in the mediastinum in a pure form, in combination with each other, or in combination with an immature teratoma (microscopic foci of malignant germ cell tumor are frequently present in an immature teratoma and represent malignant transformation)
- Characterized by a diffuse arrangement of tumor cells that form tubular and papillary structures
- Classically the neoplasm has a reticular pattern with various sized spaces lined by flattened cells and Schiller-Duval bodies (papillae composed of a central vessel covered by columnar tumor cells)
- Foci of hepatocytelike cells, entericlike glands, and parietal yolk sac structures present in 20%, 35%, and 90%, respectively
- Eosinophilic hyaline droplets often present in and between cells

Special Stains

- PAS will highlight intracellular and extracellular eosinophilic droplets characteristic of yolk sac tumor

Immunohistochemistry

- Nonseminomatous germ cell tumors are generally positive for cytokeratin
- Yolk sac tumors are immunoreactive for α-fetoprotein, α-1-antitrypsin, and cytokeratin; 50% are positive for PLAP, and 10% are positive for carcinoembryonic antigen (CEA)

Electron Microscopy

- Not helpful

Molecular Alterations

- Klinefelter syndrome (47,XXY karyotype)

Differential Diagnosis

- Metastasis from ovarian or testicular primary
- Embryonal carcinoma
- Carcinoma or sarcoma remaining after chemotherapy for a germ cell neoplasm versus primary or metastatic cancer

Treatment and Prognosis

- Nonseminomatous germ cell tumors treated with intensive chemotherapy (cisplatin, vinblastine, etoposide, and bleomycin)
- Poor risk patients with nonseminomatous germ cell tumors usually treated with high-dose etoposide and carboplatin followed by autologous bone marrow transplantation

Associations

- Patients with Klinefelter syndrome at substantial risk for developing all kinds of extragonadal germ cell tumors
- Incidence of Klinefelter syndrome among patients with a mediastinal germ cell tumor is 30 to 40 times the incidence of Klinefelter syndrome in the general population
- Synchronous hematologic malignancies include malignant histiocytosis, anaplastic large cell lymphoma, and acute myelomonocytic leukemia
- Hematologic malignancies reported after chemotherapy for germ cell tumor include acute myelogenous leukemia, acute megakaryocytic leukemia, and acute myelomonocytic leukemia

Mixed Germ Cell Tumor

Clinical Manifestations

- Can arise not only in gonat but also in the midline of the body

Microscopic Pathology

- Germinoma, embryonal carcinoma, yolk sac tumor, and choriocarcinoma can all occur in the mediastinum in a pure form, in combination with each other, or in combination with an immature teratoma (microscopic foci of malignant germ cell tumor are frequently present in an immature teratoma and represent malignant transformation)

Immunohistochemistry

- Nonseminomatous germ cell tumors are generally positive for cytokeratin

Electron Microscopy

- Not helpful

Molecular Alterations

- Klinefelter syndrome (47,XXY karyotype)

Differential Diagnosis

- Metastasis from ovarian or testicular primary
- Carcinoma or sarcoma remaining after chemotherapy for a germ cell neoplasm versus primary or metastatic cancer

Treatment and Prognosis

- Nonseminomatous germ cell tumors treated with intensive chemotherapy (cisplatin, vinblastine, etoposide, and bleomycin)

- Poor risk patients with nonseminomatous germ cell tumors usually treated with high-dose etoposide and carboplatin followed by autologous bone marrow transplantation

Associations

- Patients with Klinefelter syndrome at substantial risk for developing all kinds of extragonadal germ cell tumors
- Incidence of Klinefelter syndrome among patients with a mediastinal germ cell tumor is 30 to 40 times the incidence of Klinefelter syndrome in the general population
- Synchronous hematologic malignancies include malignant histiocytosis, anaplastic large cell lymphoma, and acute myelomonocytic leukemia
- Hematologic malignancies reported after chemotherapy for germ cell tumor include acute myelogenous leukemia, acute megakaryocytic leukemia, and acute myelomonocytic leukemia

Neurogenic Tumors and Tumors of Paraganglia

Clinical Manifestations

- Represent 20% to 40% of all mediastinal neoplasms
- Occur most frequently in the posterior mediastinum and arise from sympathetic ganglia, paraganglia, and peripheral nerves

Ganglioneuroma

Gross Pathology

- Tends to occur both in the retroperitoneum and the posterior mediastinum of children and young adults
- Usually the result of maturation of a neuroblastoma
- Tends to be large and encapsulated with a cut surface that bulges and has a pale tan and vaguely trabeculated appearance

Microscopic Pathology

- Characterized by mature ganglion cells with Nissl granules, Schwann cells, and nerve fibers
- Scattered granular calcified material often present

Special Stains

- Not helpful

Immunohistochemistry

- Neurogenic tumors are universally positive for S-100 protein

Electron Microscopy

- Not helpful

Treatment

- All neurogenic tumors and tumors of paraganglia that occur in the mediastinum are treated surgically with complete excision when possible

Malignant Peripheral Nerve Sheath Tumor

Gross Pathology

- Rarely occurs in the mediastinum but when present tends to be located posteriorly
- Frequently large and symptomatic as a result of compression, displacement, or invasion of intrathoracic organs and thoracic wall

Special Stains

- Not helpful

Immunohistochemistry

- Neurogenic tumors are universally positive for S-100 protein

Electron Microscopy

- Not helpful

Treatment

- All neurogenic tumors and tumors of paraganglia that occur in the mediastinum are treated surgically with complete excision when possible

Prognosis

- Malignant peripheral nerve sheath tumor carries a worse prognosis when it arises in the setting of neurofibromatosis than when it is solitary

Mediastinal Ependymoma

Gross Pathology

- Has been reported to occur in the paravertebral region with no connection to the spinal canal
- Pigmented neuroectodermal tumor of infancy (melanotic progonoma or retinal anlage tumor)
- Typically occurs in the jaw of an infant, but may occur in the mediastinum

Special Stains

- Not helpful

Immunohistochemistry

- Neurogenic tumors are universally positive for S-100 protein

Electron Microscopy

- Not helpful

Treatment

- All neurogenic tumors and tumors of paraganglia that occur in the mediastinum are treated surgically with complete excision when possible

Neuroblastoma and Ganglioneuroblastoma

Gross Pathology

- Usually occurs in the adrenal medulla, but may arise in extra-adrenal sympathetic ganglia of both the retroperitoneum and posterior mediastinum
- Most patients under the age of 2 years and typically present with symptoms due to compression of neighboring structures by the tumor and Horner syndrome secondary to sympathetic nerve involvement
- Neoplasm tends to be large, encapsulated and soft with focal areas of hemorrhage

Microscopic Pathology

- Neuroblastoma
  - Well-differentiated lesions are characterized by small "neuroblasts," frequent Homer-Wright rosettes, and neurofibrillary material
  - Large and multinucleated cells without ganglion differentiation may be present
  - Poorly differentiated lesions lack rosettes and neurofibrillary material
- Ganglioneuroblastoma
  - Characterized by neuroblasts, ganglion cells and intermediate cells in varying proportions
  - Well-differentiated versus poorly differentiated tumors are diagnosed on the basis of amount of neuroblasts and the degree of maturation toward ganglion cells

Special Stains

- Not helpful

Immunohistochemistry

- Neurogenic tumors are universally positive for S-100 protein
- Neuroblastoma and ganglioneuroblastomas are typically positive for NSE, chromogranin A, PGP9.5, synaptophysin, and neurofilament proteins; tumor cells are always positive for norepinephrine and always negative for epinephrine; cells in fibrovascular septa that separate masses of tumor cells stain positively for S-100 protein

Electron Microscopy

- Not helpful

Molecular Alterations

- Neuroblastoma associated with a loss of heterozygosity for chromosome 1p and amplification of oncogene N-*myc*

Differential Diagnosis

- PNET must be differentiated from poorly differentiated neuroblastoma

Treatment

- All neurogenic tumors and tumors of paraganglia that occur in the mediastinum are treated surgically with complete excision when possible

Prognosis

- Overall 2-year survival rate for neuroblastomas approximately 60%
- Favorable prognostic factors for neuroblastoma include young age (<2 years), a favorable histologic type, no N-*myc* amplification, low serum ferritin, hyperdiploidy, and high expression of *TRK* gene; mediastinal neuroblastomas have a better prognosis than those that occur in the retroperitoneum (perhaps a result of earlier diagnosis)
- 5-year survival for ganglioneuroblastoma almost 90%

Associations

- See neurofibroma, neurofibromatosis, and von Recklinghausen disease (see chapter 20 on Soft Tissue)

Neurofibroma

Gross Pathology

- 2nd most common neurogenic tumor of the mediastinum
- Typically presents as a solitary lesion (multiple in von Recklinghausen disease)
- Grows within a nerve giving the nerve a fusiform shape
- Usually not encapsulated
- No cystic areas on sectioning

Microscopic Pathology

- Wavy elongated cells dispersed through an edematous and partially collagenized stroma

Special Stains

- Not helpful

Immunohistochemistry

- Neurogenic tumors are universally positive for S-100 protein

Electron Microscopy

- Not helpful

Molecular Alterations

- Neurofibromatosis, type I (von Recklinghausen disease)
- An autosomal dominant disease with an abnormality localized to chromosome 17q11.2 (NF1 tumor suppressor gene)
- Neuroblastoma associated with a loss of heterozygosity for chromosome 1p and amplification of oncogene N-*myc*

Treatment

- All neurogenic tumors and tumors of paraganglia that occur in the mediastinum are treated surgically with complete excision when possible

Associations

- See neurofibroma, neurofibromatosis, and von Recklinghausen disease (see chapter 20 on Soft Tissue)

Neurofibromatosis

Gross Pathology

- Plexiform lesion of the vagus nerve and sympathetic chains
- Lesions in the mediastinum are considered peripheral (neurofibromatosis type 1) and are frequently associated with café-au-lait spots and may be associated with various other neoplasms including schwannoma, ganglioneuroma, pheochromocytoma, medullary carcinoma of the thyroid, nephroblastoma, and rarely central nervous system tumors

Microscopic Pathology

Special Stains

- Not helpful

Immunohistochemistry

- Neurogenic tumors are universally positive for S-100 protein
- Neuroblastoma and ganglioneuroblastomas are typically positive for NSE, chromogranin A, PGP9.5, synaptophysin, and neurofilament proteins; tumor cells are always positive for norepinephrine and always negative for epinephrine; cells in fibrovascular septa that separate masses of tumor cells stain positively for S-100 protein

Electron Microscopy

- Not helpful

Molecular Alterations

- Neurofibromatosis, type I (von Recklinghausen disease)
- An autosomal dominant disease with an abnormality localized to chromosome 17q11.2 (NF1 tumor suppressor gene)

Treatment

- All neurogenic tumors and tumors of paraganglia that occur in the mediastinum are treated surgically with complete excision when possible

Prognosis

- Malignant peripheral nerve sheath tumor carries a worse prognosis when it arises in the setting of neurofibromatosis than when it is solitary

Associations

- See neurofibroma, neurofibromatosis, and von Recklinghausen disease (see chapter on Soft Tissue)

Paraganglioma

Gross Pathology

- Arise from the paraganglia present in the aortopulmonary region (superior and middle mediastinum) and from aortic sympathetic paraganglia in the posterior mediastinum

Microscopic Pathology

- Characterized by polygonal tumor cells, frequently with granular cytoplasm, arranged in zellballen nests bordered by capillaries
- Neoplasms may have areas of stromal hyalinization and a prominent spindle cell component

Special Stains

- Not helpful

Immunohistochemistry

- Neurogenic tumors are universally positive for S-100 protein
- Paragangliomas are always positive for neuron-specific enolase (NSE); chromogranin, and synaptophysin are usually positive; sustentacular cells at the periphery of the zellballen nests positive for S-100

Electron Microscopy

- Not helpful

Treatment

- All neurogenic tumors and tumors of paraganglia that occur in the mediastinum are treated surgically with complete excision when possible

Prognosis

- Mediastinal paragangliomas may metastasize

Pigmented Neuroectodermal Tumor of Infancy

Microscopic Pathology

- Characterized by nonpigmented, neuroblastomalike cells with an associated neuropil-like stroma in cystic or alveolar spaces lined by primitive, cuboidal, pigmented cells
- Ganglioneuromalike foci may be present

Special Stains

- Not helpful

Primitive Neuroectodermal Tumor (PNET)

- Very rare; may occur in both the anterior and posterior mediastinum

Microscopic Pathology

- Characterized by sheets of uniform, monotonous, round cells with scant cytoplasm arranged in a vaguely lobular pattern (resembles poorly differentiated neuroblastoma)

Special Stains

- Not helpful

Immunohistochemistry

- Neurogenic tumors are universally positive for S-100 protein
- PNET positive for CD99

Electron Microscopy

- Not helpful

Differential Diagnosis

- PNET must be differentiated from poorly differentiated neuroblastoma

Treatment

- All neurogenic tumors and tumors of paraganglia that occur in the mediastinum are treated surgically with complete excision when possible

Schwannoma (Neurilemmoma, Neurinoma)

- Most frequent neurogenic tumor in the mediastinum
- Typically connected to a peripheral nerve and almost always solitary
- Multiple lesions are associated with von Recklinghausen disease
- Most patients asymptomatic; neoplasm found on routine chest x-ray; large lesions can cause symptoms by compression of nearby organs
- Tends to be spherical or oval and encapsulated
- Cut surface milky white or pale yellow and homogenous with myxoid or cystic areas
- A rare pigmented variant (melanocytic schwannoma) tends to be dumbbell-shaped and extend from the posterior mediastinum into the spinal canal (melanocytes have a common origin from the neural crest)

Microscopic Pathology

- Unless extensive degenerative changes present, characteristic Antoni type A and Antoni type B areas are readily apparent
- Blood vessels tend to be dilated and have a hyalinized wall

Special Stains

- Not helpful

Immunohistochemistry

- Neurogenic tumors are universally positive for S-100 protein

Electron Microscopy

- Not helpful

Treatment

- All neurogenic tumors and tumors of paraganglia that occur in the mediastinum are treated surgically with complete excision when possible

Associations

- Melanocytic schwannoma is a component of Carney syndrome (see chapter on Soft Tissue)

Thymus

Thymoma

Clinical Manifestations

- A benign or low-grade malignant neoplasm of thymic epithelial cell origin
- Most common neoplasm of the mediastinum
- Occurs equally in males and females
- May be seen in children, but most frequent in adults between the 5th and 6th decades
- Most are located in the anterior mediastinum with occasional extension into the superior compartment
- Ectopic locations include upper neck and middle or inferior mediastinum (the result of failure of the thymus to descend or from excessive descent during embryologic development); rarely thymic tissue can be found in the posterior mediastinum, parietal or visceral pleura, and lung
- 40% diagnosed as an incidental finding on routine chest x-ray
- Most common symptoms include cough, chest pain, dyspnea, weight loss, unexplained fever, dysphagia, hoarseness, swollen neck lymph nodes, superior vena cava syndrome, and pleural effusion
- Calcifications may be seen on x-ray

Gross Pathology

- Neoplasms divided into noninvasive (65%) and invasive (35%)
- Noninvasive tumor is encapsulated and/or circumscribed; invasive tumor has clusters of tumor cells that extend beyond its capsule (usually referred to as *malignant thymoma*)

- Neoplasm may be smooth, round or oval, or irregularly nodular; cut surface tan to pink to gray and almost always lobulated
- Calcification may be seen in fibrous capsule or septa that course through the neoplasm
- Occasionally a plaquelike tumor may extend directly from the thymus inferiorly along the anterior thoracic wall
- Cystic changes are frequently present
- Foci of coagulation necrosis are infrequent (more frequent in thymic carcinoma than in thymoma)
- Foci of hemorrhage may be present
- Multifocal involvement of the gland may be present
- Implants of neoplasm on pleura, pericardium, and diaphragm appear similar to the primary tumor as do metastatic foci in lymph nodes and distant organs

Staging

- Stage I: Encapsulated
- Stage II: Microscopic invasion through capsule
- Stage III: Macroscopic and/or microscopic direct invasion of lung, great vessels or pericardium
- Stage IV: "Drop" metastasis to pleura or pericardium or spread outside the chest

Microscopic Pathology

- A cytologically banal epithelial tumor with variable numbers of associated immature T cells
- Typically composed of a mixture of neoplastic epithelial cells and non-neoplastic lymphocytes in varying proportions
- Most are partially or completely encapsulated by a fibrous capsule that may contain flecks of calcium; tumor is divided into lobules by fibrous septa that connect to the fibrous capsule
- 65% have *perivascular spaces* that are formed and bordered by palisading epithelial cells with a basement membrane; these spaces vary in size and typically contain both mature B- and T-type lymphocytes, plasma cells, mast cells, and plasma fluid; near the center there is a small capillary or venule; spaces may contain foamy macrophages and may be hyalinized; perivascular spaces not lined by endothelial cells; occur more frequently in the polygonal cell type than in the spindle cell type
- Epithelial cells may be predominantly polygonal (round or oval), spindled, or a mixture of the 2 (the separation into 1 of these 3 categories may be difficult secondary to the presence of intermediate categories)
- In general, 50% of thymomas will be of the polygonal cell type, 30% the mixed cell type, and 15% the spindle cell type
- Spindle cell thymomas tend to remain localized to the anterior mediastinum; polygonal or mixed cell types are more likely to invade neighboring structures or metastasize
- Mitotic figures may be seen in the polygonal cell type but are rare in the spindle cell type; their numbers increase with the aggressiveness of the lesion
- Lymphocyte population is always non-neoplastic
- Histologic subtypes:
  - *Lymphocytic predominant*
    - Appears to decrease in frequency with advanced stage disease
    - May be misdiagnosed as lymphoma
    - Characterized by the presence of scattered large cells with lightly stained, large, vesicular, round or indented nuclei with distinct nucleoli and clear cytoplasm
    - May have foci of medullary differentiation (superficially resemble germinal centers but with fewer lymphocytes)
  - *Mixed epithelial and lymphocytic*
    - An intimate admixture of epithelial cells and lymphocytes with some variability in their proportions from lobule to lobule
  - *Epithelial predominant*
    - Frequently consists of lobules of polygonal cells with moderately large hyperchromatic vesicular or granular nuclei with small nucleoli and little to moderate amounts of cytoplasm
    - Spindle cells may be arranged haphazardly (an architectural arrangement similar to that of benign localized fibrous tumor of the pleura) or have a storiform pattern that resembles a benign fibrous histiocytoma
    - Lymphocytes are typically inconspicuous
  - Less common cytologic and histologic variations involving the epithelial cells of thymoma include:
    - Marked squamous differentiation with frequent Hassall corpuscles

- *Clear cell thymoma:* Epithelial cells that are predominantly clear (resemble renal cell carcinoma)
- *Rosette-forming cell type:* Characterized by epithelial cells with small basal nuclei arranged in rosettes but without a central lumen
- *Hemangiopericytoma-like*: Small nests and trabeculae of short spindled or oval epithelial cells with a fine vasculature
- *Thymoma with a papillary pattern, glands, and glandlike spaces*
- *Thymoma with myoid cells:* Characterized by large polygonal or round cells with abundant eosinophilic fibrillar cytoplasm scattered throughout the tumor; nuclei tend to be vesicular and have prominent nucleoli

Special Stains

- PAS may highlight the glandular nature of the rare thymoma with glands

Immunohistochemistry

- Epithelial cells are universally positive for both high- and low-molecular-weight cytokeratins (cytokeratins cannot distinguish between nonneoplastic thymic epithelial cells and neoplastic cells)
- Epithelial cells are frequently positive for CD57 (Leu-7) and sometimes for CD3
- Epithelial cells from thymomas associated with myasthenia gravis are much more likely to be positive for acetylcholine receptor-related antigen than the epithelial cells from thymomas unassociated with myasthenia gravis
- Thymomas with metastasis and thymic carcinomas typically express β_2-microglobulin and the α-chain of HLA-DR
- Thymic lymphocytes are typically positive for CD3, CD4, and CD8; immature (cortical) lymphocytes are positive for CD1a; mature (medullary lymphocytes) are typically negative for CD1a
- Areas of medullary differentiation contain CD20-positive B lymphocytes
- Myoid cells, when present in a thymoma, stain positively for desmin, myoglobin, and muscle specific actin

Electron Microscopy

- Epithelial cells are characterized by bundles of intracytoplasmic tonofilaments and large numbers of desmosomes
- Keratinization can be seen in areas of Hassall corpuscles
- Epithelial cell nuclei tend to be oval or irregularly indented and have condensed heterochromatin
- Myoid cells are characterized by numerous sarcomeres and Z bands

Molecular Alterations

- Deletions of chromosome 6p

Differential Diagnosis

- Lymphocyte predominant thymoma
- Lymphoma
- Mixed lymphocytic and epithelial thymoma
- Lymphoepitheliomalike undifferentiated carcinoma or poorly differentiated squamous cell carcinoma
- Thymoma with squamous cell differentiation
- Squamous cell carcinoma
- Thymoma with clear cell differentiation
- Renal cell carcinoma
- Thymoma with glands or glandlike spaces
- Mesothelioma or carcinoma
- Thymoma composed of aggregates of polyclonal epithelial cells and bundles of spindle-shaped epithelial cells
- Sarcomatoid carcinoma
- Thymomas composed primarily of polygonal epithelial cells or haphazardly arranged short spindled epithelial cells
- Thymic carcinoma, localized fibrous tumor of the pleura and other benign mesenchymal tumors

Treatment

- Surgical excision (thymectomy)
- 20% to 40% of patients with pure red cell aplasia can be effectively treated with thymectomy
- Postoperative radiotherapy indicated if tumor incompletely resected or if tumor invades or is adherent to nearby structures

Prognosis

- Benign encapsulated lesions may recur (15%)
- Factors associated with poor prognosis include:
  - Age >60 years
  - Presence of mediastinal or constitutional symptoms
  - Incomplete surgical excision
  - Presence of invasive or metastatic disease at the time of diagnosis
  - Tumor >15 cm
  - Tumors of the predominantly epithelial subtype
- Extrathoracic spread is relatively uncommon
- Spindle cell lesions have a better prognosis than those with polygonal epithelial cells

Associations

- Myasthenia gravis affects 30% to 50% of patients with thymoma (usually lymphocytic predominant lesions)
- Hypogammaglobulinemia, pure red cell aplasia, and aplastic anemia
- Spindle cell thymoma is the most common histologic type
- Pure red cell aplasia is seen in 5% of thymoma patients; 50% of patients with pure red cell aplasia have a thymoma
- Collagen vascular diseases: systemic lupus erythematosus and rheumatoid arthritis
- No association with Epstein-Barr virus
- Single case of thymoma associated with a pedigree of Li-Fraumeni syndrome (other tumors reported in this family were carcinoma of the adrenal cortex, astrocytoma, hepatoblastoma, and carcinoma of the pancreas)

Comment

Since Ewing's classification of thymic tumors in 1916, more than 20 classification schemes have been proposed, most of which represent modifications of those presented previously. The Muller-Hermelink classification is 1 of the more frequently used classifications of thymomas (not any of the other thymic tumors) and is as follows:

- *Medullary thymoma (spindle cell thymoma)*
  - Characterized by medullary-type epithelial cells (usually a spindle cell morphology) with limited numbers of lymphocytes
  - Epithelial tumor cells have dispersed chromatin and no nucleoli
  - May have a storiform, hemangiopericytomalike, rosettelike, or a glandular/adenomalike pattern
- *Cortical thymoma*
  - Epithelial tumor cells have vesicular chromatin and small nucleoli
  - Characterized by sheets of cortical epithelial cells (usually have a polygonal, round, or oval cell morphology) in a well-organized lobular architecture
  - Perivascular spaces tend to be narrow
  - Foci of medullary differentiation are less obvious than in the predominantly cortical thymoma
- *Mixed medullary and cortical thymoma*
  - 3 major patterns:
    1. lobules of medullary-type epithelial cells mixed with lobules of lymphocytes and cortical-type epithelial cells;
    2. nests of medullary-type epithelial cells surrounded by sheets of lymphocytes and cortical-type epithelial cells; and
    3. an admixture of both components
- *Predominantly cortical (organoid) thymoma*
  - Characterized by lobules of lymphocytes bordered by thin delicate fibrous tissue
  - Fewer epithelial cells than seen in cortical type
  - Areas of medullary differentiation with Hassall corpuscles may be present
  - Perivascular spaces may be present and quite dilated

Thymic Carcinoid

Clinical Manifestations

- Usually diagnosed in adults during early 40s
- 30% to 35% asymptomatic and discovered incidentally on chest x-ray
- Symptomatic tumors cause chest pain, cough, and dyspnea
- Carcinoid syndrome rare in the absence of distant metastasis
- Nonfunctional tumors tend to be quite large and easily detected on routine chest x-ray; functional tumors may be quite small and require a computed tomographic scan for diagnosis
- Cushing syndrome most frequent paraneoplastic syndrome seen in patients with a thymic carcinoid

Gross Pathology

- Typically encapsulated or circumscribed
- Cut surface is pale tan to gray and solid and may have scattered areas of necrosis or hemorrhage
- Tumor usually adherent to surrounding organs and occasionally invades adjacent pleura, pericardium, lung, and adventitia of major vessels
- Fibrous bands (so characteristic of thymoma) rarely present
- Occasional reports of multicentricity (may represent metastatic disease to the thymus)

Microscopic Pathology

- Tumor cells are small to medium-sized, uniform, and polygonal (occasionally spindled), and have centrally located round to oval nuclei with stippled chromatin (salt and pepper), thin nuclear membranes, and inconspicuous or small nucleoli; cytoplasm scant, lightly eosinophilic, and finely granular
- Scant, delicately vascular stroma
- Mitotic activity variable, ranging from 2 to 20 per 10 high-power fields (hpf)
- Central areas of coagulation necrosis often present
- Tumor cells classically arranged in solid sheets, rosettes, and trabeculae; solid tumor cell nests usually surrounded by elongated, sustentacular cells
- Unusual histologic patterns include:
    - A sclerotic fibrous stroma that compresses tumor cell clusters occasionally producing an "Indian file" architectural appearance
    - A cribriform pattern
    - Sheetlike masses of tumor cells with little vascular stroma and a vaguely organoid cellular arrangement
    - Focal collections of intercellular brown-gray granular pigment (lipofuscin) scattered throughout a classic carcinoid architectural pattern (presence of a sclerotic stroma and lipofuscin-like pigment probably a manifestation of longstanding tumor)
- Neoplasm may consist primarily of spindle-shaped cells (resembles peripheral carcinoid tumor of lung)
- Occasionally glandular structures may be present (mucin-producing cells not present)
- Very rarely mucin may be found in extracellular stroma, giving the lesion the appearance of a mucinous carcinoid tumor, but there is no cytoplasmic mucin

Special Stains

- Argentaffin reaction negative (also negative in bronchial carcinoid tumor)
- Argyrophil reaction variably positive
- Intracellular lipofuscin can be highlighted with PAS

Immunohistochemistry

- Tumor cells stain positively for NSE, chromogranin A, synaptophysin, and neural cell adhesion molecule
- Both serotonin and somatostatin may be detected
- Evidence of a paraneoplastic syndrome can be confirmed with immunostains: corticotropin (ACTH), calcitonin, human chorionic gonadotropin (hCG), and parathyroid hormone
- Tumor cells are typically immunoreactive for low-molecular-weight cytokeratin (paranuclear distribution)
- Sustentacular cells are typically immunoreactive for S-100 protein (sustentacular cells usually absent in metastatic tumors)

Electron Microscopy

- Tumor cells typically contain abundant membrane-bound dense-core granules (150 to 500 nm in diameter)
- Nuclei tend to be located centrally and have dispersed chromatin and inconspicuous nucleoli
- Cytoplasm contains variable numbers of mitochondria, Golgi apparatuses, rough and smooth endoplasmic reticulum
- Desmosomal-type cellular attachments may be present, but usually poorly developed
- A scanty basal lamina may be present

Molecular Alterations

- None

Differential Diagnosis

- Non-small cell or large cell neuroendocrine carcinoma
- Poorly differentiated carcinoma
- Malignant lymphoma
- Epithelial cell predominant thymoma, especially when rosettelike structures or small spindle cells with finely granular cytoplasm are present

Treatment

- Surgical excision
- Advanced stage disease typically warrants adjuvant radiotherapy with or without chemotherapy

Prognosis

- Tumors producing paraneoplastic syndromes have a poor prognosis
- Local and/or distant recurrence may occur years after primary surgery
- Metastatic disease typically occurs in mediastinal lymph nodes, cervical lymph nodes, lung, and bone (bone metastasis are often osteoblastic)

Associations

- Cushing syndrome: Ectopic production of ACTH
- Multiple endocrine neoplasia (MEN) type 1
- Islet cell carcinoma
- Parathyroid adenoma and hyperplasia (functional and nonfunctional)
- Parathyroid hyperplasia, medullary carcinoma of the thyroid, and adrenal neuroma (a single case representing incomplete Sipple syndrome (MEN type 2))

Thymic Carcinoma

Clinical Manifestations

- Most commonly encountered in middle-aged adults; occasionally seen before age of 40 years; very rare in patients younger than 30 years
- Women slightly more commonly affected than men
- Multiplicity is rare
- Most frequent symptoms are chest pain, fatigue, fever, anorexia, and weight loss
- Occasionally patients present with superior vena cava syndrome
- No reports of accompanying paraneoplastic syndromes or pure red cell aplasia (occasionally a thymoma associated with myasthenia gravis will progress to thymic carcinoma)

Gross Pathology

- Both low-grade and high-grade neoplasms tend to have focal areas of hemorrhage and/or necrosis
- Low-grade tumors (squamous cell carcinoma with keratinization) tend to be firm and have a false capsule at the point where the neoplasm reaches the capsule of the thymus, pleura, or pericardium
- Cut surface of a low-grade neoplasm tends to be ivory-colored with a scalloped border and a granular texture; central areas often sclerotic; areas of necrosis and cystic degeneration relatively unusual

Microscopic Pathology

- A thymic epithelial tumor with marked cytologic anaplasia and atypia with numerous mitotic figures and unassociated with immature T cells; closely resembles carcinomas seen in other organs
- Histologic subtypes:
  - *Squamous cell carcinoma*
    - Characterized by solid nests of polygonal cells that typically have vesicular nuclei, moderately prominent nucleoli, and moderate amounts of eosinophilic cytoplasm
    - Cells have well-defined borders, demonstrate keratinization, and have intercellular bridges
    - Areas of keratinization may resemble Hassall corpuscles
    - Tumor cells almost never palisade in a radial fashion at the borders of nests of tumor (as is typically seen in squamous cell carcinoma of the lung and esophagus)
    - Tumor cell nests are surrounded by broad zones of fibrous stroma, which may be hyalinized, particularly in the center of the neoplasm
    - Rare coagulation necrosis
    - Focal areas in the tumor may have a lobular arrangement of cell nests with intermixed epithelial cells and lymphocytes closely associated with fine blood vessels reminiscent of mixed epithelial and lymphocytic thymoma
    - More poorly-differentiated squamous cell carcinomas have architecture similar to that of well-differentiated tumors but the amount of necrosis is increased and foci of keratinization are much less prominent

Thymus>Thymic Carcinoma

- *Basaloid carcinoma*
  - A very rare low-grade malignancy
  - Neoplasms tend to be solid with areas of hemorrhage and cyst formation
  - Tumor cells usually arranged in trabeculae and anastomosing cords and tend to be small, uniform, spindled to polygonal, with little cytoplasm and a round to oval nucleus with an inconspicuous nucleolus
  - Tumor cells at the periphery of trabeculae show a palisading arrangement similar to that seen in basal cell carcinoma of the skin
  - Small areas of differentiation toward squamous cells may be present
  - Mitotic figures frequent
- *Mucoepidermoid carcinoma*
  - Neoplasm may be solid or cystic and encapsulated
  - Cut surface tends to be granular or mucoid
  - Tumor cells are arranged in nests separated by bands of fibrous stroma and are a mixture of 3 cell types: Most common is the *"intermediate cell"* which is polygonal or spindlelike with a moderate amount of eosinophilic cytoplasm and a finely granular nucleus with an inconspicuous nucleolus; 2nd cell type is larger and has basophilic intracytoplasmic mucin that displaces the nucleus to the periphery giving the cell a *goblet cell* appearance; 3rd cell type is *squamous cells* that have a tendency to keratinize
  - Mitotic figures are rarely evident in any of the cell types
- *Adenosquamous carcinoma*
  - Characterized by combinations of squamous and glandular epithelium
  - Small cystic spaces or tubular structures may be seen in the squamous cell component and may contain mucinous material
  - Mucin-containing cells are relatively rare
- *Adenocarcinoma*
  - Almost inevitably associated with a germ cell tumor
- *Lymphoepithelioma-like carcinoma*
  - Neoplasm resembles the carcinoma with the same name that arises in the nasopharynx
  - Characterized by nests of large polygonal cells with large vesicular nuclei with a single prominent, round, eosinophilic nucleolus
  - Tumor cells have little cytoplasm and ill-defined cell borders and are admixed to various degrees with lymphocytes and plasma cells
- *Large cell carcinoma*
  - Characterized by large tumor cells arranged diffusely or in solid nests; demonstrate no differentiation toward any specific cell type
  - Most are probably poorly-differentiated squamous cell carcinomas
- *Small cell/neuroendocrine carcinoma*
  - Characterized by small polygonal, oval to spindle cells with finely granular nuclei, inconspicuous nucleoli, and little cytoplasm (very similar morphologically to small cell carcinoma of the lung)
  - Cells tend to have ill-defined cell borders and grow diffusely or in large solid nests
  - Occasionally well-differentiated tumors will have a carcinoid histology
  - Not all of the features generally accepted as consistent with neuroendocrine neoplasms are necessarily present in these tumors
- *Clear cell carcinoma*
  - Characterized by lobules or sheets of polygonal, clear (glycogen) cells with small nuclei and inconspicuous nucleoli
  - Little fibrovascular stroma present
  - Generally considered a high-grade neoplasm
- *Sarcomatoid carcinoma*
  - Characterized by a diffuse growth of spindle cells with oval, coarsely granular nuclei and inconspicuous nucleoli
  - Tumor cells may be arranged in bundles, have a storiform pattern, or be haphazard
  - Mitotic figures are frequent
  - Cells displaying some squamous differentiation may be intermixed with the spindle cells
  - Considered a high-grade neoplasm; grows rapidly and is widely metastatic

Special Stains

- PAS will highlight the cytoplasmic mucin present in some of the cells of mucoepidermoid carcinoma and will also highlight the tubular structures or cystic spaces found in squamous cell nests of an adenosquamous carcinoma

Immunohistochemistry

- Epithelioid cells react with cytokeratin and EMA
- Occasional cells of non-small cell carcinoma will be reactive for CEA, B72.3, Leu-7 (CD57), and CD3
- Squamous cell carcinoma is always negative for Leu-7 (CD57)
- Small cell carcinoma ("neuroendocrine") has a lower frequency of positivity for chromogranin A, CD57, and NSE than small cell carcinoma of the lung
- Immature T cells of a thymoma are positive for CD1a, CD3, CD4, CD8, and for terminal deoxynucleotidyl transferase (TdT); lymphocytes in thymic carcinoma are mature and are immunohistologically negative for CD1a, but positive for CD3, CD4, and CD8
- CD1a will also stain Langerhans cells or interdigitating reticulum cells in both thymoma and thymic carcinoma (these cells will also stain for S-100 protein)

Electron Microscopy

- Tumor cells of a small cell thymic carcinoma have relatively few neurosecretory granules (part of the evidence that raises the question as to whether these tumors are truly neuroendocrine)
- Confirms presence of abundant glycogen in the clear cell variant

Molecular Alterations

- Aneuploid cell lines are common

Differential Diagnosis

- Encapsulated and invasive (malignant) thymoma
- Atypical carcinoid
- Germ cell tumors:
  - Dysgerminoma
  - Embryonal carcinoma
  - Choriocarcinoma
- Diffuse large cell lymphoma with sclerosis
- Metastatic carcinoma from lung or malignant mesothelium

Treatment

- Low-grade resectable tumors are treated with surgical resection with or without adjuvant radiotherapy
- Advanced low-grade and high-grade neoplasms are treated with a combination of surgery, radiation, and chemotherapy

Prognosis

- Factors associated with a poor prognosis:
  - Poorly-differentiated neoplasms
  - Neoplasms with infiltrating margins
  - High degrees of mitotic activity
- Metastases tend to occur in lymph nodes, bone, lung, liver, and brain

Associations

- Lymphoepitheliomalike subtype of thymic carcinoma (lesion almost identical histologically to the lymphoepithelioma tumor of the nasopharynx) may possibly be associated with the Epstein-Barr virus

Tumors with Thymic or Branchial Pouch Differentiation

Carcinoma Showing Thymus-Like Elements (CASTLE)

Clinical Manifestations

- Seen in adults; mean age 49 years
- Patients present with a thyroid (usually lower pole) or neck mass

Gross Pathology

- Tends to be well-defined, hard, and lobulated with a gray to pink cut surface
- Predominantly involves the lower pole of the thyroid and frequently extend into adjacent soft tissue

Microscopic Pathology

- Architecturally tumor has pushing margins and is divided into variably sized and shaped lobules by cords of thin and thick fibrous septa that are infiltrated by small lymphocytes and plasma cells
- Lesions typically resemble thymic carcinoma of either the squamous cell type or the lymphoepithelioma type
- Occasional perivascular spaces may be present
- Tumor cells tend to have indistinct borders, vesicular nuclei, and prominent nucleoli
- Residual foci of thyroid tissue may be present
- Focal areas of squamous differentiation (occasionally reminiscent of Hassall corpuscles) may be present
- Mitotic activity can be quite variable

Special Stains

- Reticulin stains will highlight variable amounts of reticulin

Immunohistochemistry

- Tumor cells stain positively for cytokeratin

Electron Microscopy

- Confirms the epithelial nature of both the spindle cells and epithelial cells

Molecular Alterations

- None

Differential Diagnosis

- Primary undifferentiated or squamous cell thyroid carcinoma
- Metastatic carcinoma from an unknown source (aerodigestive tract, lung, and mediastinum)

Treatment

- Local excision or radical excision depending on degree of local tumor infiltration. Carcinoma showing thymus-like differentiation is treated with surgical excision with or without adjuvant therapy

Prognosis

- Spindle epithelial tumor with thymuslike differentiation and carcinoma showing thymuslike differentiation are considered relatively indolent tumors but have a tendency to recur and/or metastasize

Associations

- None

Ectopic Cervical Thymoma

Clinical Manifestations

- Occurs much more commonly in women than men (ratio of 7:1); mean age 42 years
- Patients typically present with a mass in the neck that may be clinically confused with a thyroid nodule
- Neoplasm usually located in the anterior lateral part of neck, deep to the sternocleidomastoid muscle, or adjacent to or inside the lower pole of thyroid gland

Gross Pathology

- Most are encapsulated or circumscribed, but occasionally invasion beyond the main tumor is present
- Cut surface tends to be homogeneous, lobulated, firm, and gray-white-tan

Microscopic Pathology

- Histologic features typically identical to those of mediastinal thymoma
- Encapsulated or invasive with jigsaw puzzle-like lobules
- Epithelial cells are plump or spindled, have indistinct cell borders, pale or dark oval nuclei, and little or no pleomorphism; mixed with lymphocytes
- Perivascular spaces are usually present but rarely prominent
- Mitotic figures are infrequent

Special Stains

- Reticulin stains will highlight variable amounts of reticulin

Immunohistochemistry

- Plump and spindled epithelial cells stain positively for cytokeratin
- Immature T cells stain positively for CD1a (same staining pattern as seen with mediastinal thymomas)

Electron Microscopy

- Confirms the epithelial nature of both the spindle cells and epithelial cells

Molecular Alterations

- None

Differential Diagnosis

- Undifferentiated carcinoma (either primary in the thyroid or metastatic)
- Malignant lymphoma of mixed cell type

Treatment

- Local excision or radical excision depending on degree of local tumor infiltration

Prognosis

- Ectopic cervical thymoma appears to be benign and behaves much like mediastinal thymoma; circumscribed/encapsulated lesions are curable by surgical excision; invasive lesions have the potential to recur and even metastasize although both events are infrequent

Associations

- None

Ectopic Hamartomatous Thymoma

Clinical Manifestations

- Typically found in the supraclavicular or suprasternal region unattached to skin or bone
- Much more common in men than women; mean age at diagnosis 50 years
- Appears to arise from thymic anlage associated with branchial pouches (tumors with morphologic features of ectopic hamartomatous thymoma have never been reported in normally located mediastinal thymus)

Gross Pathology

- Tends to be oval and well-circumscribed and may be as large as 20 cm
- Cut surface solid, gray to white, and may have a fasciculated appearance; foci of adipose tissue or cysts may be visible

Microscopic Pathology

- Typically composed of a haphazard admixture of several elements to include spindled-shaped cells, fat cells, squamous cell nests, and/or glandular epithelial cell nests
- 1st major element usually consists of spindle-shaped, fibroblastlike cells that tend to be arranged in interlacing bundles in a storiform pattern; nuclei tend to be regular, oval to elongated, and have finely distributed chromatin and indistinct nucleoli; no mitotic figures and no necrosis
- 2nd major component consists of epithelial islands, cords, tubules, and branching glands and cysts that are frequently well-demarcated by a rim of fibrous stroma; occasionally epithelial islands merge into spindle cell component; most common type of epithelium is nonkeratinizing stratified squamous, but glandular cells frequently present
- 3rd major component consists of mature fat cells, which may represent 1%-75% of the tumor
- Occasional myoid cells (resemble fetal-type skeletal muscle) may be present

Special Stains

- Reticulin stains will highlight variable amounts of reticulin

Immunohistochemistry

- Both spindle cells and epithelial cells stain positively for cytokeratin

Electron Microscopy

- Confirms the epithelial nature of both the spindle cells and epithelial cells

Molecular Alterations

- None

Differential Diagnosis

- Mixed tumor of salivary or sweat gland
- Peripheral nerve sheath tumor
- Spindle cell carcinoma
- Synovial sarcoma

Treatment

- Local excision or radical excision depending on degree of local tumor infiltration

Prognosis

- Ectopic hamartomatous thymoma does not recur or metastasize

Associations

- None

Spindle Epithelial Tumor With Thymus-Like Elements (SETTLE)

Clinical Manifestations

- Tends to occur in children and young adults; mean age 15 years
- Frequently presents as a thyroid nodule and may cause symptoms related to tracheal compression

Gross Pathology

- May be circumscribed or non-circumscribed, encapsulated or infiltrative
- Most commonly found in or near a lower pole of the thyroid

Microscopic Pathology

- Typically a densely cellular tumor that is traversed by irregular, variably sized sclerotic bands that result in the formation of incomplete nodules
- Tumor cells are spindled (epithelial) and glandular, cytologically bland, and mitotically inactive
- Spindle cells (typically represent 40%-90% of the neoplasm) form short intersecting or streaming fascicles and usually assume a reticulated appearance that is the result of the accumulation of intercellular fluid or mucoid material; nuclei tend to be long and pale with delicate chromatin, inconspicuous nucleoli, and little or no pleomorphism
- Epithelial cells tend to form complex narrow tubules, small papillae, trabeculae, islands, and solid sheets and blend imperceptibly with the spindle-cell component; nuclei tend to be round or oval, pale and bland
- Presence of reticulin fibers can be quite variable
- No lymphocyte component

Special Stains

- Reticulin stains will highlight variable amounts of reticulin

Immunohistochemistry

- Both the spindle cells and epithelial cells stain positively for cytokeratin (the epithelial cells stain more intensively for cytokeratin than the spindle cells)

Electron Microscopy

- Confirms the epithelial nature of both the spindle cells and epithelial cells

Molecular Alterations

- None

Differential Diagnosis

- Malignant (immature) teratoma of soft tissues of neck and thyroid
- Undifferentiated thyroid carcinoma
- Spindle cell variant of medullary thyroid carcinoma
- Columnar cell thyroid carcinoma
- Synovial sarcoma

Treatment

- Local excision or radical excision depending on degree of local tumor infiltration
- Spindled epithelial tumors with thymuslike differentiation and carcinoma showing thymuslike differentiation are treated with surgical excision with or without adjuvant therapy

Prognosis

- Spindle epithelial tumor with thymuslike differentiation is considered a relatively indolent tumor but has a tendency to recur and/or metastasize

Associations

- None

Mediastinal Fibrosis

Sclerosing (Fibrosing) Mediastinitis

Clinical Manifestations

- May occur at any age
- Almost always occurs in anterior-superior mediastinum and appears on chest x-ray as an asymmetric widening of the mediastinum, mass usually projects into an upper lung field
- Patients may present clinically with superior vena cava syndrome or with symptoms of respiratory or cardiac compromise

Gross Pathology

- Firm white fibrous tissue with a distinct interface with adjacent adipose tissue

Microscopic Pathology

- Dense, paucicellular or acellular fibrohyaline, relatively avascular tissue with variably sized collections of entrapped mature lymphocytes
- Caseating or noncaseating granulomas may be present (most cases represent an idiosyncratic response to infection within mediastinal lymph nodes or lungs)
- Approximately 50% of cases result from fungal infection; most common organism is *Histoplasma capsulatum*; additional organisms include *Aspergillus, Cryptococcus*, and *Mucor* (other associations include sarcoidosis, *Nocardia*, *Actinomyces*, syphilis, methysergide therapy, and chest trauma)
- 50% of cases have no obvious etiology and are thought to be a form of delayed cell-mediated hypersensitivity reaction

Special Stains

- Silver stains may help detect causative organisms

Immunohistochemistry and Electron Microscopy

- Not helpful

Molecular Alterations

- None

Differential Diagnosis

- Solitary fibrous tumor
- Desmoid-type fibromatosis
- Nodular sclerosing Hodgkin disease and non-Hodgkin lymphoma
- Metastatic carcinoma
- Malignant desmoplastic mesothelioma

Treatment and Prognosis

- Steroid therapy and surgical excision when symptomatic

Associations

- Sclerosing mediastinitis may occur in association with other sclerosing inflammatory conditions: retroperitoneal fibrosis (most common), sclerosing cholangitis, Riedel struma, and inflammatory pseudotumor of the orbit

References

Dabbs DJ. *Diagnostic Immunohistochemistry.* New York: Churchill Livingstone, 2002.

Kumar V, Abbas AK, Fausto N (eds.) *Robbins and Cotran Pathologic Basis of Disease. 7th ed.* Philadelphia: Elsevier Saunders, 2005.

Mills S, Carter D, Greenson JK, Oberman HA, Reuter V, Stoler MH (eds). *Sternberg's Diagnostic Surgical Pathology. 4th ed.* Philadelphia: Lippincott Williams & Wilkins, 2004.

Rosai J. *Rosai and Ackerman's Surgical Pathology. 9th ed.* St. Louis: Mosby, 2004.

Shimosato Y, Mukai K. *Tumors of the Mediastinum: Atlas of Tumor Pathology, 3rd Series. Fascicle 21.* Washington DC: Armed Forces Institute of Pathology, 1997.

Travis WD, Brambililla E, Muller-Hermelink HK, Harris CC (eds). *World Health Organization Classification of Tumours: Pathology and Genetics—Tumours of the Lung, Pleura, Thymus and Heart.* Lyon, France: IARC Press, 2004.

Chapter 14

Lymph Nodes

Intraoperative Consultation

Intraoperative diagnosis of lymphoid lesions involving lymph nodes is rarely required, but at times may be quite appropriate:

1. ***To ensure that diagnostic tissue has been obtained*** and that there is a sufficient amount of tissue to perform all necessary ancillary studies.
2. ***To ensure proper processing of the specimen***. Lymph node tissue is quite susceptible to artifacts of suboptimal handling. When tissue can be processed immediately, fixation is typically optimized. In addition, fresh tissue may be required for microbial culture, cytogenetics, flow cytometry analysis, frozen section immunohistochemistry or other studies.
3. ***To render an intraoperative diagnosis*** on lymph node tissue obtained from the chest or abdominal cavity. The diagnosis of the presence of metastatic disease has obvious surgical implications, as does even the tentative or suspected diagnosis of lymphoma.

Lymph node tissue that is frozen is irrevocably altered and is consequently rendered sub-optimal for routine histologic examination. When a lymph node is to be frozen for an intraoperative consultation, both surgeon and pathologist must insure that there is additional fresh tissue for routine processing and for ancillary studies.

Often intraoperative consultation can be rendered without performing a frozen section. Cytologic preparations (touch imprints or cytoscrapes) can frequently definitively demonstrate the presence of a lymphoproliferative process or the presence of metastatic carcinoma. When a lymphoproliferative process is suspected, all of the submitted tissue can be submitted for permanent section and ancillary studies. In the case of suspected metastatic carcinoma on cytologic preparation, frozen section can be prepared when the issue is in doubt.

Specimen Handling

Lymph node tissue should be submitted to the pathology laboratory immediately upon removal from the patient and in a fresh state. Once cytologic preparations have been examined with or without subsequent frozen section the tissue is processed in such a way as to insure that all ancillary studies can be performed. Often it is prudent to obtain some tissue for culture even when infection is not a part of the clinical differential diagnosis. Tissue saved for culture can always be retrieved if there is no evidence of infection.

Tissue felt to be representative of a lymphoproliferative disorder is almost always submitted for additional studies. A portion should be fixed in a mercury-based fixative such as B5 (provides superior cytological detail) and in neutral buffered formalin.

Ancillary studies performed on lymph nodes harboring a lymphoproliferative disorder include:

1. ***Flow cytometry***. A portion of tissue is minced, placed in RPMI (Sigma Diagnostics, St. Louis, MO), and refrigerated.
2. ***Molecular genetic studies*** using either the Southern blot technique or polymerase chain reaction (PCR). Tissue is submitted fresh in tissue culture medium or snap frozen.
3. ***DNA PCR-based analysis***. Tissue is fixed in formalin and embedded in paraffin.

Routine sectioning of large lymph nodes involves cutting 0.2 to 0.3 cm serial cross sections of the entire node.

Histiocytic and Dendritic Cell Neoplasms

Follicular Dendritic Cell Sarcoma/Tumor (Reticulum Cell Sarcoma/Tumor; Dendritic Reticulum Cell Sarcoma/Tumor)

Clinical Manifestations

- Typically an indolent clinical course
- Patients typically present with a slowly enlarging, painless mass
- 50 to 65% present in lymph nodes (cervical most common)
- Reported extranodal sites of involvement include tonsils, spleen, oral cavity, gastrointestinal tract, liver, soft tissue, skin, and breast

Histiocytic and Dendritic Cell Neoplasms>Follicular Dendritic Cell Sarcoma/Tumor (Reticulum Cell Sarcoma/Tumor; Dendritic Reticulum Cell Sarcoma/Tumor)

Gross Pathology

- Tend to be well-circumscribed
- Cut surface solid and tan-gray resembling a sarcoma
- Median size about 5 cm

Microscopic Pathology

- Spindled to ovoid cells with elongated nuclei with delicate nuclear membranes, vesicular or finely granular chromatin, and a small but distinct nucleolus
- Individual tumor cells are plump with eosinophilic cytoplasm and indistinct cell borders
- Cells tend to be bland, but may show significant cytologic atypia; mitotic rate varies with degree of atypia (0 to 10 per 10 hpfs to greater than 30 per 10 hpfs)
- Multinucleated cells, reminiscent of Warthin-Finkeldy cells, may be present
- Tumor cells arranged in fascicles, storiform patterns, and whorls
- Proliferating cells often sharply separated from adjacent lymphoid tissue and are typically located between the follicles
- Foci of necrosis may be present
- Uninvolved residual lymphoid tissue often present; may be germinal centers, on clusters of small lymphocytes

Special Stains

- Non-contributory

Immunohistochemistry

- Tumor cells positive for CD21, CD35, CD23, and EMA
- Variably positive for S-100 protein, CD68, CD45, and CD20
- CD1a, CD34, CD3, CD79a, CD30, HMB-45 and cytokeratins consistently negative

Electron Microscopy

- Tumor cells have well-developed, long, numerous cytoplasmic processes joined by desmosomes
- No Birbeck granules

Molecular Alterations

- A germline configuration for the immunoglobulin heavy chain gene and the T-cell receptor genes

Differential Diagnosis

- Lesions in the liver and spleen resemble inflammatory pseudotumors
- Dendritic reticulum cells with a similar morphology may be seen in lymph nodes involved by Castleman disease
- Interdigitating dendritic cell sarcoma/tumor (see Comment below)

Treatment

- Complete surgical excision with or without adjuvant radiotherapy or chemotherapy

Prognosis

- Tends to recur locally (40 to 50%)
- Metastasizes (25%) to distant sites such as lung and liver
- Intra-abdominal tumors tend to be very aggressive
- 10 to 20% of patients die of their disease

Associations

- Castleman disease in 10 to 20% of cases; the Castleman disease either precedes the dendritic cell tumor or the two lesions occur simultaneously

Comment

- Follicular dendritic cells are associated with B zones in a lymph node (specifically germinal centers)
- *Interdigitating dendritic cell sarcoma/tumor* most often involves a single node, but may involve skin (also reported in GI tract, soft tissue, liver, spleen, bone marrow, kidney, and lung); etiology unknown; a neoplastic proliferation of spindled to ovoid cells in a paracortical distribution; cells arranged in fascicles, a storiform pattern and whorls; cells have vesicular nuclei, distinct small or large nucleoli, eosinophilic cytoplasm and indistinct cell borders; cytologic atypia quite variable; usually no necrosis; lymphocytes and occasionally plasma cells admixed with tumor cells; tumor cells consistently express S-100 protein and vimentin; CD1a is negative; *markers for follicular dendritic cells, CD21 and CD23 negative* (see above); clinical course ranges from benign and localized to widespread and lethal

Inflammatory/Hyperplastic Diseases

Acute Nonspecific Lymphadenitis

- Rarely biopsied
- Microscopically the earliest changes consist of sinus dilatation with an accumulation of neutrophils followed by vascular dilatation and edema of the capsule
- Suppurative lymphadenitis is a feature of staphylococcal infections, mesenteric lymphadenitis, lymphogranuloma venereum, and cat-scratch diseases
- Necrotizing features can be seen in bubonic plague, tularemia, anthrax, and typhoid fever

Histiocytic Necrotizing Lymphadenitis (Kikuchi-Fujimoto Disease)

Clinical Manifestations

- Seen in young Asian women and men in all parts of the world
- More common in women then men
- Patients typically present with signs of fever and painless cervical lymphadenopathy that is frequently accompanied by leukopenia
- Fever may or may not be present

Gross and Microscopic Pathology

- The lymph node architecture is usually effaced by large discrete areas of eosinophilic necrosis with abundant nuclear debris surrounded by transformed lymphocytes, histiocytes, and plasmacytoid monocytes
- Granulocytes are essentially always absent
- Follicular centers are usually not hyperplastic
- Occasionally foamy histiocytes
- The necrotic lesions tend to be paracortical and contain abundant karyorrhectic debris, scattered fibrin deposits and collections of large mononuclear cells
- Plasmacytoid monocytes are two to three times the size of small lymphocytes and have small nuclei with open chromatin and small nucleoli and variable amounts of cytoplasm

Special Stains

- Not helpful

Immunohistochemistry

- Plasmacytoid monocytes are CD4 positive
- The transformed lymphocytes are predominately CD8 positive T-cells

Electron Microscopy

- Tubuloreticular structures and intracytoplasmic rods similar to those see in lupus erythematosus are frequently found

Molecular Alterations

- None

Differential Diagnosis

- Malignant lymphoma with secondary necrosis
- When plasmacytoid monocytes grow in a diffuse fashion, they may simulate a malignant lymphoma
- The presence of foamy histiocytes may mimic signet ring adenocarcinoma
- The absence of granulocytes in the areas of necrosis and the absence of follicular hyperplasia differentiate these cases from cat-scratch disease and other bacterial infections

Treatment and Prognosis

- Evolution is generally benign and self limited
- Some cases have been described with recurrent lymphadenopathy or a concurrent association with skin lesions

Associations

- Necrotizing lymphadenitis has been seen following diffuse large B-cell lymphoma
- Necrotizing lymphadenitis has also been reported in cases of stroma-rich Castleman disease and in cases of lupus errythematous

Sarcoidosis

Clinical Manifestations

- World-wide distribution with Scandinavian countries particularly affected
- In the United States, the disease is 10-15 times more common in African Americans (especially women) than in whites
- Practically every organ in the body can be involved (the most commonly involved organs are the lung, lymph nodes, eyes, skin, and liver)
- Characterized by bilateral hilar lymphadenopathy, pulmonary infiltrates and ocular and skin lesions
- Peripheral lymphadenopathy present in most patients
- Functional hypothyroidism is typically present

Gross and Microscopic Pathology

- Typical lymph node appearance is one of total effacement of nodal architecture by epithelioid granulomas that are compact and sharply demarcated from intervening small lymphocytes
- Typically a small granuloma mainly composed of epithelioid cells with scattered Langhans' giant cells and lymphocytes
- Necrosis is either absent or limited to a small central fibrinoid focus
- Schaumann bodies, asteroid bodies, and calcium oxyalate crystals are sometimes found in the cytoplasm of giant cells; Schaumann bodies tend to be round and have concentric laminations and contain iron and calcium
- Follicular centers are absent or rare when lymph nodes are involved with sarcoidosis

Special Stains

- Not helpful

Immunohistochemistry

- Lymphocytes at the site of injury in the lung or lymph node are typically CD4 positive

Electron Microscopy

- Asteroid bodies are composed of radiating filaments enveloped by "myeloid" membranes

Differential Diagnosis

- Fungal infections (special stains and cultures required)
- Mycobacterial infection such as tuberculosis and atypical mycobacteriosis (including swimming pool granuloma)
- Leprosy, syphilis, leishmaniasis, brucellosis, tularemia, chalazion, zirconium granuloma
- Berylliosis
- Crohn disease
- Hodgkin lymphoma
- *When all of these possibilities have been excluded and the clinical picture fits, the diagnosis of sarcoidosis is justified*

Treatment and Prognosis

- Systemic corticosteroids, but such therapy has no affect on long-term prognosis
- One third experience spontaneous remission, one third remain stable, and one third progress (10% progress to severe pulmonary fibrosis)

Associations

- Erythema nodosum often precedes or accompanies the diseases
- Sarcoid type granulomas may coexist in both involved and uninvolved lymph nodes of patients with Hodgkin lymphoma and non-Hodgkin lymphoma and in patients with nonhematologic malignancy

Toxoplasmosis

Clinical Manifestations

- One of the most common parasitic infections of man
- Caused by the protozoan parasite *Toxoplasma gondii* which is acquired by ingesting oocytes in contaminated meat and other foods or by exposure to cat feces
- The lymphadenitis associated with this disease typically involves the posterior cervical nodes
- On palpation the nodes are firm and moderately enlarged
- Diagnosis of lymphadenitis secondary to toxoplasmosis is suspected from the microscopic pattern and must be confirmed serologically

Gross and Microscopic Pathology

- Nodal architecture is typically preserved
- The typical triad (not present in all cases) consists of:
  1. Marked follicular hyperplasia with intense mitotic activity and phagocytosis of nuclear debris
  2. Irregular clusters of epithelioid histiocytes, which may invade follicular centers *(a very specific feature of toxoplasmosis)*
  3. Distention of marginal and cortical sinuses by parafollicular monocytoid B-cells that distort or encroach the subcapsular peritrabecular architecture
- The medullary cords frequently contain immunoblasts and plasma cells

Special Stains

- The parasite will stain with H&E, but rarely seen except in overwhelming infection

Immunohistochemistry, Electron Microscopy, and Molecular Alterations

- Not necessary (accuracy of histologic findings has been confirmed by both molecular genetic and serologic studies)

Differential Diagnosis

- Other infectious diseases
- Areas of resolving toxoplasmosis may resemble Kaposi sarcoma
- Monocytoid B cells commonly found in the lymphadenopathy seen in AIDS

Treatment and Prognosis

- Generally self-limited in immunocompetent host and does not require treatment

Associations

- Immunocompromised individuals are at particular risk for overwhelming infection

Cat-Scratch Disease

Clinical Manifestations

- Zoonotic infection caused by a small, pleomorphic, gram-negative bacterium, *Bartonella henselae*
- Primary skin lesion appears as a red papule at the site of inoculation in 7 to 12 days
- Regional lymphadenopathy (usually axillary or cervical) typically appears 2-3 weeks after primary exposure
- Serologic testing is available to help confirm diagnosis

Gross Pathology

- Lymph nodes are typically enlarged and on sectioning may have obvious suppurative foci

Microscopic Pathology

- Typically, nodes show capsulitis with subcapsular granulomas
- Focal areas of necrosis usually present just beneath the capsule
- Reactive hyperplasia of secondary follicular centers results in some architectural distortion
- Small aggregates of epithelioid histiocytes, primarily in the interfollicular areas, fuse and become stellate areas of necrosis, characterized by neutrophils surrounded by a palisade of histiocytes
- Giant cells often present
- Occasionally suppurative foci drain through the capsule of the node into perinodal soft tissue
- Monocytoid B-cells may fill the sinuses
- Skin lesion typically consists of a focus of necrosis in the dermis that is surrounded by histiocytes, multinucleated giant cells, lymphocytes and eosinophils

Special Stains

- Warthin-Starry silver stains may demonstrate the pleomorphic, small, gram-negative bacterium

Immunohistochemistry

- Not helpful

Electron Microscopy

- May be helpful

Molecular Alterations

- PCR identification of the organism is possible

Differential Diagnosis

- Lymphogranuloma venereum
- Tularemia (results from handling rabbits and usually involves axillary lymph nodes)
- *Yersinia* infections

Treatment

- Antibiotics; but usually is self-limited and resolves spontaneously without antibiotics

Prognosis

- Rare complications include granulomatous conjunctivitis ("oculoglandular syndrome of Parinaud"), thrombotic thrombocytopenic purpura, and central nervous system symptoms

Associations

- None

Lymphogranuloma Venereum

Clinical Manifestations

- Sexually transmitted disease caused by *Chlamydia trachomatis* organisms
- Initial cutaneous lesion a small, painless genital vesicle or ulcer, which heals within a few days followed by inguinal (occasionally axillary or supraclavicular) adenopathy, which may be quite prominent
- Diagnosis can be confirmed with serologic or nucleic acid amplification tests

Gross Pathology

- Lymph nodes are enlarged and may have obvious areas of suppurative inflammation or necrosis

Microscopic Pathology

- Early lesions are characterized by tiny foci of necrosis filled with neutrophils
- Later changes consist of areas that represent coalescence of small suppurative foci into larger stellate abscesses
- Eventually epithelioid cells, Langhans giant cells, and fibroblasts line the walls of these abscesses
- Occasionally abscesses can rupture through the capsule of the lymph node and extend into perinodal soft tissue and skin resulting in a cutaneous sinus tract
- After the disease has run its course, extensive fibrosis may be the only finding in an involved lymph node
- Primary genital lesion typically consists of a flat base of granulation tissue with a bordering zone of necrosis and leukocyte reaction; adjacent skin often shows pseudoepitheliomatous hyperplasia; the inflammatory infiltrate consists of plasma cells and lymphocytes; necrotizing granulomas with giant cells surrounded by plasma cells may be present

Special Stains, Immunohistochemistry, and Electron Microscopy

- Brown-Hopps, Warthin-Starry, or electron microscopy may help

Molecular Alterations

- None

Differential Diagnosis

- Cat-scratch disease
- Atypical mycobacteriosis
- Tularemia

Treatment and Prognosis

- Involves management of the *Chlamydia* infection

Associations

- None

AIDS-Related Lymphadenopathy

Clinical Manifestations

- Patients with HIV infection may have persistent generalized lymphadenopathy in the setting of a stable clinical course before progressing to symptoms of AIDS
- Up to 25% of patients who develop AIDS on follow-up experience cachexia and weight loss

Gross and Microscopic Pathology

- Early in the course of HIV infection, the most common change in the enlarged lymph nodes is *florid hyperplasia* of the follicular centers that may have a dumbbell, serpentine or serrated configuration; follicles contain numerous tingible-body macrophages and plasma cells
- Mantle zones are frequently scant or absent ("naked" germinal centers); mantle zone lymphocytes often invaginate into germinal centers giving them a "moth-eaten" appearance
- Other areas of the same lymph node may take on the appearance of the plasma cell variant of angiofollicular hyperplasia
- Any combination of follicular changes may be seen and none is particularly pathognomonic for AIDS
- Some lymph nodes may show advanced lymphocyte depletion with or without abnormal germinal centers
- Interfollicular areas may contain an easily identified vascular proliferation (resembles Castleman disease)

Special Stains

- Warthin-Starry, AFB, and fungal stains may all be helpful

Immunohistochemistry and Electron Microscopy

- Large numbers of follicular dendritic cells with altered processes
- Fascin stain confirms that the AIDS virus tends to infect these dendritic cells
- HIV core protein P24 positive in abnormal germinal centers

Molecular Alterations

- PCR techniques may be useful in identifying opportunistic organisms

Differential Diagnosis

- Mycobacterial and other opportunistic infections
- Kaposi sarcoma
- Hodgkin lymphoma
- non-Hodgkin lymphoma

Treatment and Prognosis

- Antiretroviral therapy guided by CD4 counts and plasma viral load (PVL) assay results
- Most patients, even without antiviral therapy, survive relatively asymptomatically for 10 to 12 years

Associations

- Lymph node abnormalities in patients with AIDS can include mycobacterial and other opportunistic infections, Kaposi sarcoma, malignant lymphoma of either Hodgkin or non-Hodgkin type and florid reactive hyperplasia (florid reactive hyperplasia is the most common change)
- With progression of HIV infection, lymph nodes begin to involute and lose their follicular centers, with intrafollicular hyalinized vessels resembling those seen in hyaline-vascular type of angiofollicular hyperplasia (Castleman disease)

Comment

- The term *chronic lymphadenopathy syndrome* has been used to describe unexplained enlargement of lymph nodes in two or more extra-inguinal sites for at least three months duration in a patient at risk for AIDS

Infectious Mononucleosis

Clinical Manifestations

- The typical patient presents with a fever, sore throat or splenomegaly and occasionally with lymphadenopathy
- Etiologic agent is EBV which infects B lymphocytes, making them proliferate and differentiate into plasma cells

Gross and Microscopic Pathology

- Typically a marked distortion of the lymph node architecture by a polymorphic lymphoid infiltrate of a variety of different types of immunoblasts, small lymphocytes, and a few plasma cells; capsule and perinodal fat are both infiltrated
- Often there is paracortical expansion with a mottled appearance due to proliferation of immunoblasts; these mmunoblasts may be binucleated and resemble Reed-Sternberg cells
- Various degrees of follicular hyperplasia typical; follicles have a ragged or irregular perimeter
- Necrosis may be present but is usually only focal unless the patient is an immunodeficient child

Special Stains

- Reticulin stains may demonstrate that the sinusoidal pattern is intact and even focally enhanced in the face of what appears to be effacement of the nodal architecture
- One characteristic feature appears to be the presence of clusters of sinusoidal lymphocytes of various sizes

Immunohistochemistry

- The atypical lymphocytes in the blood are CD8 positive cytotoxic T-cells

Electron Microscopy

- Not helpful

Molecular Alterations

- The diagnosis of an infectious mononucleosis can be confirmed by in-situ hybridization techniques

Differential Diagnosis

- Monospot rapid diagnostic test sensitive and specific
- To distinguish a mononucleosis from a lymphoma requires noting the predominately paracortical distribution of the large lymphoid cells, follicular hyperplasia with marked mitotic activity and phagocytosis (these follicles are usually small), an increase in number of plasma cells, and vascular proliferation
- Hodgkin disease
- Hypersensitivity reactions

Treatment and Prognosis

- Typically a benign course treated according to symptoms
- Ampicillin should be avoided (will cause a rash in patients infected with EBV infection)

Associations

- EBV

Castleman Disease

Clinical Manifestations

- The mediastinum is the most frequent site of involvement, but may occur in many other locations, including cervical and axillary regions, within skeletal muscle, pulmonary parenchyma, abdomen and retroperitoneum
- Both sexes affected equally
- May occur anytime between the ages of 10 and 70 years
- May be localized or multicentric (multicentric lesions have been described in multiple lymph node sites and the spleen)
- Patients with hyaline-vascular and transitional types usually asymptomatic; 50% patients with plasma cell type have hematologic abnormalities to include IL-6 syndrome characterized by fever, anemia, and hypergammaglobulinemia (symptoms disappear with removal of the lesion)

- Patients with the multicentric form tend to be older than those with the localized form; men are more commonly affected than women; multiple areas of lymphadenopathy with hepatosplenomegaly

Gross and Microscopic Pathology

- Three types:
  1. Hyaline-vascular
  2. Plasma cell
  3. Transitional or intermediate (features of both hyaline vascular and plasma cell types)
- *Hyaline-vascular type*
  - More common than plasma cell type
  - Usually a single mass
  - Characterized by abnormal follicles and interfollicular vascularity; dysplastic dendritic cells are a key morphologic feature
  - Follicles tend to be small and numerous; frequently contain small blood vessels that radially penetrate the germinal center from vascular perifollicular tissue
  - Penetrating capillaries typically have a thickened, hyalinized wall that results in the presence of hyalin within the follicular center
  - Other follicles have concentric layering (onion skin) of small lymphocytes around a compact germinal center (reminiscent of a Hassall corpuscle of the thymus); when concentrically arranged small lymphocytes are particularly prominent, often obscuring the germinal center, the condition is referred to as *lymphoid variant*
  - More than one germinal center may be present in a single follicle
  - Interfollicular areas contain an extensive network of capillaries intermixed with small lymphocytes, plasma cells, and rare immunoblasts and eosinophils
  - Occasionally large fibrotic masses surround the blood vessels in the interfollicular areas
- *Plasma cell type:*
  - Represents 10% to 20%
  - Usually multiple discrete lymph nodes, more frequently in the retroperitoneum than in the mediastinum
  - Typically solid sheets of plasma cells surround follicles
  - Follicular centers tend to be large and hyperplastic with many mitotic figures and tingible body macrophages
  - The prominent capillary network characteristic of the hyaline-vascular type is typically absent
- *Transitional or intermediate type:*
  - Least common
  - Most of the lesions are predominantly of the hyaline-vascular type with focal areas of plasmacytosis

Immunohistochemistry

- Helpful in assessing plasma cell clonality for discrimination from entities in the differential diagnosis
- Plasma cell type has distinctive features in HIV+ patients co-infected with HHV8; immunoglobulin heavy and light chains, and HHV8 immunohistochemistry may be helpful and is recommended on all systemic and plasma cell types

Molecular Alterations

- Current literature suggests that hyaline-vascular type is a clonal disorder of dendritic cells; cytogenetics of these cells can be quite helpful; may explain the development of dendritic cell neoplasm in some cases (see Associations below)
- PCR or immunohistochemistry to identify HHV8 recommended on all systemic and plasma cell types

Differential Diagnosis

- Localized hyaline-vascular type and multicentric type:
  - Lymphoid depletion histology of lymph nodes in advanced HIV; mantle cell lymphoma; both of these lack the interfollicular vascularity of hyaline-vascular type Castleman
  - Angioimmunoblastic lymphadenopathy
  - Nonspecific reactive lymph nodes
- Plasma cell type:
  - Lymphadenopathy of rheumatoid arthritis, systemic lupus erythematosus, syphilis; all are associated with prominent interfollicular plasmacytosis

Treatment

- Surgical excision

Prognosis

- Patients with multicentric disease may remain stable, have a relapsing or aggressive course, or develop lymphoma

Associations

- 30% of patients with multicentric disease develop malignancy to include a non-Hodgkin lymphoma, Kaposi sarcoma, and carcinoma
- *POEMS syndrome*: ***p***olyneuropathy (peripheral neuropathy, papilledema), ***o***rganomegaly (hepatosplenomegaly, lymphadenopathy), ***e***ndocrinopathy (amenorrhea, gynecomastia, impotence, adrenal insufficiency, hypothyroidism, glucose intolerance), ***m***onoclonal gammopathy (plasmacytosis, paraproteinemia, bone lesions), and ***s***kin lesions (hyperpigmentation, hypertrichosis, glomeruloid hemangiomas); may be associated with multicentric Castleman
- Follicular dendritic cell sarcoma/tumor may occur in association with Castleman disease in about 10% to 20% of cases, usually the hyaline-vascular type; either Castleman disease precedes the follicular dendritic cell sarcoma/tumor or the two occur simultaneously

Dermatopathic Lymphadenitis (Lipomelanosis Reticularis of Pautrier)

Clinical Manifestations

- Lymphadenopathy in patients with a variety of reactive and neoplastic skin disorders; occasionally occurs in patients without significant skin disease
- Represents a T-cell response to skin antigens processed and presented by interdigitating dendritic cells and Langerhans cells

Gross Pathology

- Lymph nodes are enlarged and firm
- Cut surface bulges and is pale yellow; in florid cases, pigmentation may be visible as black linear areas at the periphery

Microscopic Pathology

- Basic nodal architecture is preserved, but at low power, a proliferation of large, pale-staining cells that result in an expansion of the subcapsular paracortical regions with compression of follicles beneath the capsule (occasionally the follicles completely disappear)
- Pale staining cells consist of a mixture of macrophages with abundant pale cytoplasm, Langerhans cells with grooved elongated nuclei and small nucleoli, and interdigitating dendritic cells, characterized by complex nuclei with folded nuclear membranes, delicate chromatin, and inconspicuous nucleoli
- Melanin and/or hemosiderin usually present in cytoplasm of macrophages and in extracellular deposits
- Lymphocytes (some of which have folded or cerebriform nuclei), plasma cells, and eosinophils are admixed with the macrophages and Langerhans cells

Special Stains

- Not helpful

Immunohistochemistry

- Langerhans cells: CD1a positive, S-100 protein positive
- Interdigitating dendritic cells: CD1a negative, S-100 positive
- Lymphocytes in nodules are predominantly T-cells

Electron Microscopy

- Not practical

Molecular Alterations

- Gene rearrangement analysis may be used to document lymphomatous involvement in cases associated with mycosis fungoides

Differential Diagnosis

- Focal involvement of lymph node by T-cell lymphoma, especially mycosis fungoides
- Hodgkin lymphoma
- Langerhans cell histiocytosis
- Monocytic leukemia
- Nodular paracortical T-cell hyperplasia

Treatment and Prognosis

- Lymphadenopathy is typically of no clinical significance; the only treatment involves the associated cutaneous disease

Associations

- Dermatitis, cutaneous lymphoma

Sinus Histiocytosis with Massive Lymphadenopathy (Rosai-Dorfman Disease)

Clinical Manifestations

- Typically presents in children and young adults with fever and bilateral painless cervical lymphadenopathy, leukocytosis, anemia, and polyclonal hypergammaglobulinemia; 10% present with soft tissue involvement with or without associated lymphadenopathy

- Patients with extranodal disease tend to be older than patients with lymph node based disease and may have involvement of the orbit, head and neck, upper respiratory tract, breast, skeleton, skin and subcutaneous tissue, and CNS
- Males and females affected equally

Gross Pathology

- Lymph nodes tend to be matted together by prominent perinodal fibrosis
- Sectioning reveals grey-yellow surface

Microscopic Pathology

- Lymph node involvement characterized by capsular fibrosis and marked distortion of nodal architecture; the nodal sinuses are expanded by histiocytes that characteristically have abundant, granular, occasionally vacuolated eosinophilic cytoplasm which often contains well-preserved lymphocytes (*emperipolesis*), plasma cells, and occasionally erythrocytes and neutrophils; ingested lymphocytes usually distributed around periphery of cytoplasm
- Histiocyte nuclei tend to be round and large and sometimes multinuclear; may be pleomorphic, but not particularly hyperchromatic nor grooved; nucleoli are prominent
- Mitotic figures rare
- Connective tissue between sinuses populated with numerous plasma cells; residual germinal centers vary from hyperplastic to rare or absent
- Extranodal disease is characterized by sheets and irregular aggregates of large, pale, somewhat atypical histiocytes with large, round, vesicular nuclei; mitotic figures are rare or absent; the cytoplasm of these histiocytes contains lymphocytes but not to the extent seen in involved lymph nodes; extensive fibrosis often distorts the sheet-like growth pattern resulting in a storiform pattern

Special Stains

- Not helpful

Immunohistochemistry

- Histiocytes express S-100 protein, CD68, and CD14 and are negative for CD1a

Electron Microscopy

- Helpful in differentiating the condition from a Langerhans cell histiocytosis (the histiocytes of the latter contain Birbeck granules)
- Histiocytes have extensive pseudopodia

Molecular Alterations

- None

Differential Diagnosis

- Langerhans cell histiocytosis
- Extranodal disease:
  - Histiocytic proliferation of infectious etiology
  - Malignant fibrous histiocytoma
- Metastatic melanoma or carcinoma
- Sinus histiocytosis

Treatment

- Surgical excision

Prognosis

- Patients with localized nodal disease usually have a chronic indolent course
- Benign condition with no evidence of malignant transformation
- Occasionally persistent or recurrent disease follows surgical excision
- May spontaneously resolve
- May be fatal in cases of extensive nodal and/or extranodal (renal, liver and/or lung) involvement or in patients who are immunocompromized

Associations

- 25% have an immune disorder such as autoimmune hemolytic anemia, mild joint pain, severe arthritis, and/or glomerulonephritis

Progressive Transformation of Germinal Centers

Clinical Manifestations

- Usually an inciental finding of atypical follicular hyperplasia with irregular expansion of secondary follicles
- May be seen in association with Hodgkin disease, particularly Hodgkin disease of the nodular lymphocyte predominant type; findings may be present prior to, during, or following lymph node involvement with Hodgkin disease

Gross and Microscopic Pathology

- At low power, germinal centers are 2 to 3 times larger than adjacent follicles, which may be hyperplastic

- Large germinal centers result from both an outward as well as an inward expansion of small mantle zone lymphocytes, a process that progressively dilutes and replaces germinal center cells with small lymphocytes
- When the condition is fully developed, the transformed germinal center is composed predominantly of small lymphocytes, residual germinal center cells, and dendritic reticulum cells; tingible body macrophages may be present; the expanded germinal center merges imperceptibly with the surrounding mantle zone (hence, the resemblance to nodules of lymphocyte predominant Hodgkin disease)
- Residual large germinal center cells frequently mimic the L&H (lymphohistiocytic) variant of Reed-Sternberg cells that are characteristic of lymphocyte predominant Hodgkin disease

Special Stains

- Not helpful

Immunohistochemistry

- Not very helpful because both L&H variant Reed-Sternberg cells and residual germinal center cells stain with B-cell antibodies and are negative for CD15 and often for CD30; the small lymphocytes that surround the nodules are polyclonal B-cells in both Hodgkin disease and progressive transformation of germinal centers

Electron Microscopy

- Not helpful

Molecular Alterations

- None

Differential Diagnosis

- Nodular lymphocyte predominant Hodgkin lymphoma
- Follicular lymphoma

Treatment

- None, unless associated with Hodgkin disease

Prognosis

- Entirely dependent upon the presence or absence of Hodgkin disease

Associations

- Nodular lymphocyte predominant Hodgkin disease

Vascular Tumors

Bacillary Angiomatosis

Clinical Manifestations

- Caused by *Bartonella quintana* and *Rochalimaea henselae* infection in immunocompromised patients (usually an AIDS patient)
- Usually appears as violaceous skin lesion that clinically mimics Kaposi sarcoma
- May involve lymph nodes, spleen, liver, and other organs

Gross Pathology

- Lymph nodes often enlarged, and pale brown to red-brown

Microscopic Pathology

- Lymph node architecture focally effaced by large pale nodules composed of exuberant proliferation of small blood vessels lined by plump, somewhat epithelioid, endothelial cells
- Endothelial cells have pale, finely vacuolated cytoplasm
- A deeply eosinophilic, amphophilic, amorphous, or granular material is seen between the blood vessels (aggregates of bacillary organisms)
- Neutrophils, some forming microabscesses, always present

Special Stains

- Warthin-Starry demonstrates bacillary organisms (indistinguishable from those of cat-scratch disease)

Immunohistochemistry

- Not helpful

Electron Microscopy

- Available but not widely used

Molecular Alterations

- PCR identification is possible

Differential Diagnosis

- Kaposi sarcoma;
- Epithelioid hemangioma
- Angiosarcoma

Treatment and Prognosis

- Curable with antibiotics

Associations

- Some cases associated with Epstein-Barr virusin AIDS

Kaposi Sarcoma

Clinical Manifestations

- Lymphoid involvement may or may not be associated with the typical skin lesions
- Nodal involvement without skin lesions mainly seen in African children, but may be seen in adults with HIV-infection

Gross and Microscopic Pathology

- Involved nodes show a proliferation of spindle cells separated by slit-like spaces containing red blood cells
- The spindle cell lesion in the lymph node is often accompanied by lymphoid proliferation with numerous plasma cells and immunoblasts
- The earliest changes are typically seen in the trabecular and subcapsular sinuses but eventually the entire node will be involved with extension into perinodal soft tissue
- Cytoplasmic and extracellular hyaline globules are almost always present

Special Stains

- Hyaline globules positive for PAS and PTAH

Immunohistochemistry

- Spindle cells of nodular lesions strongly immunoreactive for CD34 and CD31 and weakly or focally positive for VWF and *Ulex europaeus*; always negative for factor VIII
- Nuclei of tumor cells stain positively for human herpesvirus 8 (HHV 8)
- Nuclear immunoreactivity for FLI1 always present

Electron Microscopy

- Morphology of most spindle cells closely resembles endothelial differentiation

Molecular Alterations

- Polyclonal; no consistent chromosomal abnormality

Differential Diagnosis

- Spindle cell angiosarcoma
- Spindle cell hemangioendothelioma
- Bacillary angiomatosis
- Nodal angiomatosis
- Castleman disease
- Hemangioma

Treatment and Prognosis

- Patients with AIDS-related Kaposi (usually stage III or IV) treated with chemotherapy

Associations

- Kaposi sarcoma may coexist with malignant lymphoma or leukemia

Malignant Lymphoma

Hodgkin Lymphoma

WHO Histological Classification

- Nodular lymphocyte predominant Hodgkin lymphoma
- Classical Hodgkin lymphoma
- Lymphocyte-rich classical Hodgkin lymphoma
- Nodular sclerosis Hodgkin lymphoma
- Mixed cellularity Hodgkin lymphoma
- Lymphocyte-depleted Hodgkin lymphoma

Clinical Manifestations

- *Nodular lymphocyte predominant Hodgkin lymphoma*
  - 5% of all cases of Hodgkin lymphoma
  - Affects young males between 30 and 50 years
  - 80% to 95% present with localized peripheral lymphadenopathy (stage I or II); 5% to 20% have advanced disease (stage III or IV)
- *Lymphocyte-rich classical Hodgkin lymphoma*
  - 5% of all cases of Hodgkin lymphoma
  - Primarily affects males (70%)
  - Most are asymptomatic
  - Peripheral lymph nodes typically involved; presence of mediastinal disease and bulky disease at time of diagnosis uncommon
  - Patients usually present with clinical stage I or II disease and lack B symptoms
- *Nodular sclerosis Hodgkin lymphoma*
  - 65% to 70% of all cases of classical Hodgkin lymphoma (most common)
  - Tends to affect young adults in their late 20s or early 30s (rare over age of 50)
  - Females and males affected equally
  - Frequently presents with mediastinal involvement (80%); 10% have spleen or lung involvement; 3% have bone marrow involvement; bulky disease in 50% to 55%
  - Most present with clinical stage II disease, and B-symptoms present in 40%

- *Mixed cellularity Hodgkin lymphoma*
  - 20 to 25% of all cases of classical Hodgkin lymphoma
  - 70% males usually between the ages of 30 and 40 years
  - Most present with clinical stage III or IV disease and B-symptoms
  - Peripheral lymph nodes frequently involved; mediastinum less frequently involved than in nodular sclerosis Hodgkin lymphoma; spleen involved in 30%
- *Lymphocyte-depleted Hodgkin lymphoma*
  - Very rare (less than 5%), so there is a lack of reliable epidemiologic and clinical data
  - Primarily involves abdominal organs, retroperitoneal nodes and bone marrow; peripheral nodes often not involved
  - Most present with advanced disease and B symptoms

Clinical Staging (Cotswold revision of Ann Arbor) Classification

- Stage I: involvement of a single lymph node region or lymphoid structure (eg, spleen, thymus, Waldeyer ring)
- Stage II: involvement of two or more lymph node regions on the same side of the diaphragm (the mediastinum is a single site; hilar nodes are lateralized); the number of anatomic sites should be indicated by suffix (eg, II3)
- Stage III: involvement of lymph regions on both sides of the diaphragm
- Stage III1: with or without splenic, hilar, celiac, or portal nodes
- Stage III2; with paraortic, iliac or mesenteric nodes
- Stage IV: involvement of extranodal site(s) beyond those designated E
- All stages further divided on the basis of the absence (A) or presence (B) of systemic symptoms: significant fever, drenching sweats, or unexplained weight loss of greater than 10% normal body weight), the presence of bulky disease (X): defined as >1/3 width of mediastinum and/or > 10 cm maximum dimension of nodal mass, and (E) the presence of involvement of a single extranodal site, or contiguous or proximal to a known nodal site of disease

Gross and Microscopic Pathology

- *Hodgkin and Reed-Sternberg cell (HRS cell):*
  - A large binucleate cell with a huge, round, inclusion-like nucleolus; may have an "owl's eye" appearance
  - Prominent parachromatin clearing produces a paranucleolar halo with a thickened nuclear membrane
  - Cytoplasm is usually acidophilic and abundant
  - *Hodgkin cells* are mononuclear variants of Reed-Sternberg cells
- *Lacunar cell:*
  - A delicate, folded or multilobulated nucleus surrounded by pale cytoplasm
  - Nucleoli smaller than in classic HRS cells
  - By artifact of fixation, the cytoplasm may retract making it appear that the cell is in a lacuna
- *L&H (lymphohistiocytic) cell:*
  - Polypoid nucleus with small, usually multiple nucleoli and moderately abundant cytoplasm (nucleus resembles popcorn kernels, hence "popcorn" cells)
  - Typically found in lymphocyte predominant Hodgkin lymphoma
- Nodular lymphocyte predominant Hodgkin lymphoma
  - Lymph node architecture completely or partially effaced by a nodular infiltrate of small lymphocytes, histiocytes, epithelioid histiocytes, and intermixed L&H cells
- *Lymphocyte-rich classical Hodgkin lymphoma*
  - Characterized by lymph node effacement by a vaguely nodular infiltrate of small lymphocytes admixed with variable numbers of benign histiocytes
  - Some of the Hodgkin and Reed-Sternberg cells may resemble L&H cells
  - Plasma cells, eosinophils, neutrophils, fibrosis, and necrosis are all characteristically absent
  - Two subtypes:
    - Diffuse: characterized by complete lymph node effacement by a lymphocytic/histiocytic proliferation; this subtype is rare
    - Nodular: the lymph node effacement is usually "vague" or "pseudonodular"; HRS cells are generally found in expanded mantle zones
- *Nodular sclerosis Hodgkin lymphoma:*
  - Characterized by the presence of a variant of the Reed-Sternberg cell in lacunar spaces (lacunar cells) and thick, birefringent, bands of collagen that divide the lymph node into circumscribed nodules
  - Lacunar cells and atypical mononuclear cells sometimes present in sheets (syncytial variant) and are usually seen in a polymorphous background of small T lymphocytes, eosinophils, plasma cells, and macrophages
  - Classic Reed-Sternberg cells are less frequent than in mixed cellularity and lymphocyte depleted types

- Necrosis frequent
- Variants of nodular sclerosis:
  - Obliterative total sclerosis: characterized by an admixture of collagen and fibrosis with few or no lacunar cells, lymphocytes, or Reed-Sternberg cells
  - Obliterative "syncytial variant": characterized by lacunar cells and other Reed-Sternberg-like cells that occur in sheets and cohesive clusters reminiscent of metastatic carcinoma, sarcoma, non-Hodgkin lymphoma, thymoma, or germ cell tumor

- *Mixed cellularity Hodgkin lymphoma*
  - Characterized by diffuse effacement of lymph nodes by a heterogeneous cellular infiltrate that consists of small lymphocytes, eosinophils, plasma cells and benign macrophages admixed with HRS cells
  - Classic Reed-Sternberg cells and their mononuclear variants are readily apparent
- *Lymphocyte-depleted Hodgkin lymphoma*
  - Characterized by a predominance of diagnostic Hodgkin and Reed-Sternberg cells accompanied by decreased numbers of lymphocytes
  - Reed-Sternberg cells tend to be very pleomorphic and may appear sarcomatous
  - Represents a final, aggressive, sarcomatous phase of disease in which neoplastic transformation predominates over lymphoid reactivity

Special Stains

- Non-contributory

Immunohistochemistry

- L&H cells (lymphohistiocytic) typically express CD20 and CD45, do not express CD15 and CD30, and may express EMA (50%)
- Hodgkin and Reed-Sternberg cells are positive for CD30 and express CD15 in 75 to 85%; CD45 typically not expressed; however, CD20 may be weak/variable in a subset of HRS cells in up to 40% of cases
- PAX5, Oct2, BOB1, fascin, and in situ staining for EBV are also useful

Electron Microscopy

- Not helpful

Molecular Alterations

- No distinctive or diagnostically specific cytogenetic abnormalities have been found so far
- Possible pathogenetic role for Epstein-Barr virus (EBV) may be present in up to 60% of patients with Hodgkin lymphoma
  - EBV-specific RNA transcripts can be found in 40% of Reed-Sternberg cells in cases of nodular sclerosis and in 60 to 70% of Reed-Sternberg cells in cases of mixed cellularity

Differential Diagnosis

- *Nodular lymphocyte predominant Hodgkin lymphoma*
  - Lymphocyte-rich classical Hodgkin lymphoma
  - Progressive transformation of germinal centers
  - T-cell/histiocyte rich large B cell lymphoma
- *Lymphocyte-rich classical Hodgkin lymphoma*
  - Nodular lymphocyte predominant Hodgkin lymphoma
  - Progressive transformation of germinal centers
  - Small lymphocytic lymphoma
  - Non-Hodgkin follicular lymphoma
- *Nodular sclerosis Hodgkin lymphoma:*
  - Peripheral T-cell non-Hodgkin lymphoma
  - T-cell/histiocyte rich large B cell lymphoma
- Anaplastic large cell lymphoma
  - Mediastinal (thymic) large B-cell lymphoma
  - Necrotizing granulomatous lymphadenitis
  - Mediastinal seminoma
  - Nasopharyngeal carcinoma
  - Metastatic carcinoma, melanoma
- *Mixed cellularity Hodgkin lymphoma*
  - Peripheral T-cell lymphoma
  - Infectious mononucleosis
  - Anaplastic large cell lymphoma
  - Angioimmunoblastic lymphadenopathy
- *Lymphocyte-depleted Hodgkin lymphoma*
  - Anaplastic large cell lymphoma
  - Nodular sclerosis Hodgkin lymphoma
  - Mixed cellularity Hodgkin lymphoma
  - Sarcoma

Treatment and Prognosis

- Combination chemotherapy, tailored to individual patient and stage with or without radiation
- Relapsed disease treated with autologous peripheral blood stem cell transplant
- Five-year survival for patients with stage I and IIA >90%
- Five-year disease-free survival 60 to 70% in patients with advanced disease (stage IVA and IVB)
- Adverse prognostic factors: stage III and IV disease, old age, presence of B symptoms, presence of bulky disease, extensive splenic involvement, and multiple extranodal sites of involvement
- *Nodular lymphocyte predominant Hodgkin lymphoma*
  - 10 year survival 80% for stage I and II disease
  - 3 to 5% of cases progress to B-cell lymphoma (if localized, prognosis generally good)
  - In some centers, stage I disease is not treated after excision of the affected node
- *Classical Hodgkin lymphoma*
  - Histologic subtype not an important predictor of prognosis

Stage and presence of systemic symptoms coupled with clinical and laboratory parameters used to predict outcome Associations

- EBV may play a role in the pathogenesis of classical Hodgkin disease
- Immunosuppressed patients, ie, those with HIV, may be predisposed to development of EBV-associated Hodgkin lymphoma that can present at unusual sites, eg, bone marrow
- Nodular lymphocyte predominant Hodgkin lymphoma is seen before, concurrently, or following progressive transformation of germinal centers

Lymphoid Neoplasms

World Health organization (WHO) Classification of Lymphoid Neoplasms

- Precursor B-cell and T-cell neoplasms (neoplasms of immature B-and T-cells)
  - Precursor B-lymphoblastic leukemia/lymphoma
  - Precursor T-lymphoblastic leukemia/lymphoma
- Mature B-cell neoplasms
  - Chronic lymphocytic leukemia/small lymphocytic lymphoma
  - Lymphoplasmacytic lymphoma (LPL) / Waldenstrom macroglobulinemia
  - Hairy cell leukemia
  - Plasma cell neoplasms
    - Plasmacytoma
    - Plasma cell myeloma
    - Monoclonal immunoglobulin deposition diseases (MIDD)
    - Heavy chain disease
  - Extranodal marginal zone B-cell lymphoma (MALT lymphoma)
  - Nodal marginal zone B-cell lymphoma
  - Splenic marginal zone lymphoma
  - Follicular lymphoma
  - Mantle cell lymphoma
  - Diffuse large B-cell lymphoma
  - Mediastinal (thymic) large B-cell lymphoma
  - Burkitt lymphoma / leukemia
- Mature T-cell and natural killer (NK) cell neoplasms
  - Adult T-cell leukemia/lymphoma
  - Extranodal NK/T-cell lymphoma, nasal type (lethal midline granuloma)
  - Enteropathy-type T-cell lymphoma (refractory sprue)
  - Mycosis fungoides and Sézary syndrome
  - Angioimmunoblastic T-cell lymphoma
  - Peripheral T-cell lymphoma, unspecified
  - Anaplastic large cell lymphoma

Precursor B-Cell and T-Cell Neoplasms (Neoplasms of Immature B Cells and T Cells)

Precursor B-Lymphoblastic Leukemia/Lymphoma

Clinical Manifestations

- Occurs primarily in children
- Symptoms are related to pancytopenia secondary to involvement of bone marrow

Gross and Microscopic Pathology

- Composed of immature, precursor B (pre-B) or T (pre-T) lymphocytes (lymphoblasts)

- Malignant pre-B and pre-T lymphoblasts are morphologically indistinguishable
- Lymph node involvement is characterized by complete effacement by lymphoblasts that are small to intermediate in size and have nuclei that are somewhat larger than the nuclei of small lymphocytes; nuclear chromatin is delicate and finely stippled; nuclear membrane may be indented or grooved giving it a convoluted (lobulated) appearance; nucleoli are either absent or inconspicuous; cytoplasm is agranular and scant
- Presence of multiple benign macrophages throughout the neoplasm give it a "starry sky" appearance
- Mitotic figures are frequent

Special Stains

- Not contributory

Immunohistochemistry

- Pre-B cells express TdT and lack surface Ig
- Most are positive for CD19 and CD22; CD45 may be negative
- Variable expression of CD10, CD20 and CD34

Electron Microscopy

- Not helpful

Molecular Alterations

- Most common rearrangement is t(12;21)(p13;q22) involving TEL1 and AML1 genes
- May have prognostic implications
  - t(9;22)(q34;q11.2) BCR/ABL, unfavorable
  - t(4;11)(q21;q23) AF4/MLL, unfavorable
  - t(1;19)(q23;p13.3) PBX/E2A, favorable
  - t(12;21)(p13;q22), favorable
  - Hyperdiploidy (>50), favorable
  - Hypodiploidy, unfavorable

Differential Diagnosis

- With rare exceptions specific diagnoses can be made with the combination of histologic examination, immunotyping and genotyping

Treatment and Prognosis

- 90% of children with ALL will obtain complete remission with aggressive chemotherapy; 65% will be cured
- Children between the ages of 2 and 10 with a pre-B phenotype have an especially good prognosis
- Factors associated with a worse prognosis include: age under two, high white blood cell count, presentation in adolescence or adulthood, and presence of t(9;22) (Philadelphia chromosome) or t(4;11)(q21;q23)

Associations

- None

Precursor T-Lymphoblastic Leukemia/Lymphoma

Clinical Manifestations

- Male predominance; more common in adolescents than in younger children
- Often present with a mediastinal mass (thymic involvement)
- Splenic, liver, and bone marrow involvement variable

Gross and Microscopic Pathology

- Composed of immature, precursor B (pre-B) or T (pre-T) lymphocytes (lymphoblasts)
- Malignant pre-B and pre-T lymphoblasts are morphologically indistinguishable
- Lymph node involvement is characterized by complete effacement by lymphoblasts that are small to intermediate in size and have nuclei that are somewhat larger than the nuclei of small lymphocytes; nuclear chromatin is delicate and finely stippled; nuclear membrane may be indented or grooved giving it a convoluted (lobulated) appearance; nucleoli are either absent or inconspicuous; cytoplasm is agranular and scant
- Presence of multiple benign macrophages throughout the neoplasm give it a "starry sky" appearance
- Mitotic figures are frequent

Special Stains

- Not contributory

Immunohistochemistry

- Pre-T cells express CD1a and TdT
- Variable expression of other pan T-cell markers CD2, CD3, CD4, CD5, CD7 and CD8

Electron Microscopy

- Not helpful

Molecular Alterations

- One third of translocations involve the T-cell receptor genes
- *TAL1* gene locus dysregulation by microdeletion
- Deletion of 9p (30% or more)

Differential Diagnosis

- With rare exceptions specific diagnoses can be made with the combination of histologic examination, immunotyping and genotyping

Treatment and Prognosis

- 90% of children with ALL will obtain complete remission with aggressive chemotherapy; 65% will be cured
- Children between the ages of 2 and 10 with a pre-B phenotype have an especially good prognosis
- Factors associated with a worse prognosis include: age under two, high white blood cell count, presentation in adolescence or adulthood, and presence of t(9;22) (Philadelphia chromosome) or t(4;11)(q21;q23)

Associations

- None

Mature B-Cell Neoplasms

Chronic Lymphocytic Leukemia (CLL)/ Small Lymphocytic Lymphoma (SLL)

Clinical Manifestations

- CLL is most common leukemia of adults in Western world
- SLL represents 6.7% of all non-Hodgkin lymphomas
- Usually presents in older patients (> 50 y) with bone marrow, lymph node, spleen and liver involvement
- Often asymptomatic, but may present with fatigue, weight loss and anorexia
- Males more commonly affected than females (2:1)
- A minority will have autoimmune hemolysis and thrombocytopenia

Gross and Microscopic Pathology

- The neoplastic cells of CLL and SLL are morphologically indistinguishable
- Involved lymph nodes are diffusely effaced by a population of small lymphocytes with little cytoplasm and round to slightly irregular nuclei with condensed chromatin
- Variable numbers of mitotically active larger cells (prolymphocytes and paraimmunoblasts) may be present in aggregates (proliferation centers); these larger cells are considered to be pathognomonic for CLL and SLL
- Smears of peripheral blood (CLL) reveal increased numbers of small round lymphocytes that are quite fragile and are often disrupted in the process of making the smear (smudge cells)
- Bone marrow is always involved in CLL and consists of interstitial infiltrates or non-paratrabecular aggregates of small lymphocytes
- Splenic white and red pulp and hepatic portal tracts usually infiltrated by tumor cells

Special Stains

- Not contributory

Immunohistochemistry

- B-cells are CD5, CD19, CD23 and CD43 positive and CD10 negative
- Express low levels of surface IgM

Electron Microscopy

- Not helpful

Molecular Alterations

- Trisomy 12 (20%)
- Deletion of 13q14 (up to 50%)
- Deletions of 11q22-23 (20%)
- Deletions of 6q21 (5%) or 17p13 (p53 locus; 10%)

Differential Diagnosis

- With rare exceptions specific diagnoses can be made with the combination of histologic examination, immunotyping and genotyping

Treatment and Prognosis

- Incurable; 5-year survival 50% to 55%
- Presence of trisomy 12 and deletions of 11q associated with higher stage disease and worse prognosis
- CLL and SLL may transform into more aggressive lymph node neoplasms, resembling Hodgkin lymphoma (0.5%) or diffuse large B-cell lymphoma (3.0%); with either of these transformations patients typically survive less than one year

Associations

- Hypogammaglobulinemia is associated with CLL and SLL

Lymphoplasmacytic Lymphoma/ Waldenström Macroglobulinemia

Clinical Manifestations

- Typically occurs in older patients (sixth or seventh decade) with bone marrow, lymph node, spleen and liver involvement
- Neoplastic cells may secrete sufficient IgM (>3 g/dL, Waldenström macroglobinemia) to cause a hyperviscosity syndrome characterized by visual impairment, neurologic symptoms, bleeding, and cryoglobulinemia
- Presenting symptoms weakness, fatigue, and weight loss; 50% have lymphadenopathy, hepatomegaly, and splenomegaly
- Anemia secondary to marrow infiltration common; 10% have autoimmune hemolysis that exacerbates the anemia

Gross and Microscopic Pathology

- Characterized by a diffuse, variably dense, infiltrate of lymphocytes, plasma cells, and plasmacytoid lymphocytes in bone marrow
- Infiltrate typically accompanied by a reactive hyperplasia of mast cells
- PAS-positive inclusions containing immunoglobulin may be present in cytoplasm (Russell bodies) or as nuclear pseudo-inclusions (Dutcher bodies) of tumor cells
- Masses of tumor causing bony erosions (a feature of multiple myeloma) are not present
- An infiltrate similar to that seen in bone marrow may be present in lymph nodes, spleen or liver as well as in nerve roots, meninges, and occasionally the brain

Special Stains

- Not contributory

Immunohistochemistry

- Tumor cells express surface IgM and cytoplasmic immunoglobulin
- Tumor cells positive for CD19 and CD22 and are negative for CD10 and CD23

Electron Microscopy

- Not helpful

Molecular Alterations

- 50% have t(9;14) (p13;q32)
- Aberrant expression of PAX5, a transcription factor essential for normal B-cell differentiation, independent of the translocation

Differential Diagnosis

- With rare exceptions specific diagnoses can be made with the combination of histologic examination, immunotyping and genotyping

Treatment and Prognosis

- An incurable progressive disease, but long-term survival possible with splenectomy
- Hyperviscosity can be alleviated by plasmapheresis
- Transformation to large cell lymphoma may occur but rare

Associations

- None

Hairy Cell Leukemia

Clinical Manifestations

- Typically seen in middle-aged males (male to female ratio 4:1)
- Usually presents with pancytopenia, splenomegaly, and minimal lymphadenopathy

Gross and Microscopic Pathology

- Leukemic cells are larger than small lymphocytes, have round, oval, or reniform nuclei with ground glass chromatin and an inconspicuous nucleolus, modest amounts of pale blue cytoplasm, and poorly defined borders or fine hair-like projections
- The number of circulating cells may be quite variable
- Bone marrow is always involved with a diffuse or interstitial infiltrate entrapped within a reticulin fibrosis
- When the spleen is involved the red pulp is preferentially involved, giving the spleen a beefy-red appearance
- Hepatic infiltration is predominantly sinusoidal

Special Stains

- Not contributory

Immunohistochemistry

- B-cells positive for CD11c, CD19, CD20, CD22, CD25, CD79a and CD103 and are negative for CD5, CD10, CD23, and CD79b

Electron Microscopy

- Not helpful

Molecular Alterations

- No specific chromosomal rearrangements

Differential Diagnosis

- With rare exceptions specific diagnoses can be made with the combination of histologic examination, immunotyping and genotyping

Treatment and Prognosis

- Typically follows a progressive indolent course
- Long-lasting remissions can be achieved with purine analog 2-chlorodeoxyadenosine (2-CdA) in most patients

Associations

- None

Plasma Cell Neoplasms

Clinical Manifestations

- *Plasmacytoma*: an isolated plasma cell mass in bone or soft tissue (eg, oropharynx, lung or nasal sinuses)
- *Plasma cell myeloma*: usually seen in older patients who present with multiple lytic bone lesions and pathologic fractures; may have hypercalcemia, renal failure and primary amyloidosis
- *Monoclonal immunoglobulin deposition disease* (MIDD): characterized by visceral and soft tissue Ig deposition, resulting in compromised organ function; present in 1% of persons over age of 50 and 3% over the age of 70; two major categories are primary amyloidosis and light chain deposition disease
- *Heavy chain disease*: Rare B-cell neoplasms that exclusively produce monoclonal heavy chains and no light chains. There are three of them: *γ heavy chain disease*, *μ heavy chain disease*, and *α heavy chain disease*; the unifying features of all three are the presence of abnormal serum immunoglobulin component and systemic symptoms of anorexia, weakness, fever, weight loss and recurrent bacterial infections and autoimmune manifestations such as hemolytic anemia, and autoimmune thrombocytopenia
- The pathological monoclonal immunoglobulin component is composed of either IgG (γ heavy chain disease), IgA (α heavy chain disease) or IgM (μ heavy chain disease). γ heavy chain disease involves lymph nodes (it also involves Waldeyer ring, bone marrow, liver, spleen and peripheral blood. α heavy chain disease may involve mesenteric lymph nodes as well as the GI tract (usually the small intestine). μ heavy chain disease does not involve lymph nodes.

Gross and Microscopic Pathology

- Bony lesions of both multiple myeloma and plasmacytoma consist of soft red neoplasm with a gelatinous consistency
- More than 30% of the cells in the bone marrow will be plasma cells, which may interstitially infiltrate the marrow or be present in diffuse, sheet-like masses that completely replace normal marrow elements; some cases may have 10-30% plasma cells in conjunction with other criteria
- Well differentiated tumor cells may be indistinguishable from normal plasma cells (an eccentrically placed nucleus with a perinuclear hof); usually they are atypical
- A variety of cytologic variants may be present and dominate the lesion:
- Plasmablasts (less condensed nuclear chromatin and prominent single nucleolus)
- Bizarre multinucleated cells
- Flame cells (fringe of fiery red cytoplasm)
- Mott cells (multiple grape-like cytoplasmic droplets)
- Cells with a variety of cytoplasmic inclusions to include fibrils, crystalline rods, Russell bodies and Dutcher bodies
- Lymph nodes typically contain monomorphic sheets of plasma cells

Special Stains

- Not contributory

Immunohistochemistry

- Terminally differentiated B-cells express CD38 and CD 138 and are usually negative for CD19, CD20, and CD45
- γ heavy chain disease: monoclonal cytoplasmic γ chain without light chain, pan B-cell antigen positive, CD5 negative, and CD10 negative

Electron Microscopy

- Not helpful

Molecular Alterations

- t(4;14) (p16.3; q32); leads to increased expression of FGFR3
- Deletion 13q
- t(14;16)
- t(11;14)

Differential Diagnosis

- With rare exceptions specific diagnoses can be made with the combination of histologic examination, immunotyping and genotyping

Treatment and Prognosis

- Decreased production of immunoglobulins predisposes patients to recurrent infection, the most common cause of death
- Renal failure is the second most common cause of death (most important contributing factor is the presence of Bence Jones proteinuria; excreted light chains are toxic to renal tubular epithelial cells)
- Plasmacytomas involving bone typically progress to classic multiple myeloma
- Plasmacytoma involving soft tissue rarely disseminate
- Solitary plasmacytoma can be cured by surgical excision
- Patients with untreated plasma cell myeloma die within 6 to 12 months
- Chemotherapy with alkylating agents induces remission in 50 to 70% of patients with plasma cell myeloma; median survival is three years
- 20% of patients with monoclonal Ig deposition disease (MIDD) will develop an overt plasma cell dyscrasia (usually plasma cell myeloma, within a period of 10 to 15 years); newer therapeutic options may be used in various combinations with older agents
- Clinical outcome variable ranging from indolent to rapidly progressive with median survival of 12 months

Associations

- None

Extranodal Marginal Zone B-Cell Lymphoma (MALT Lymphoma)

Clinical Manifestations

- GI tract most common site (50%); other common sites include lung (15%), head and neck (15%), ocular adnexa (12%), skin (11%), thyroid (4%), and breast (4%)
- Extranodal disease characterized by tendency to arise in chronic inflammatory disorders of autoimmune type (eg, salivary gland in Sjögren disease and thyroid gland in Hashimoto disease) or infected tissue (eg, stomach in *Helicobacter pylori* gastritis) and a tendency to stay localized for prolonged periods at sites of origin

Gross and Microscopic Pathology

- Neoplasm is composed of cells at various stages of B-lymphoid differentiation frequently found at mucosal sites (***m***ucosa-***a***ssociated ***l***ymphoid ***t***issues—MALT)
- Cells resemble small, cleaved follicle center cells, except they have more cytoplasm
- Marginal zone cells, monocytoid B cells, small lymphocytes, immunoblasts, and plasma cells present in variable numbers

Special Stains

- Not contributory

Immunohistochemistry

- B-cells positive for CD19, CD20 and CD22 and negative for CD5, CD10 and CD23
- Plasma cell component may express cytoplasmic immunoglobulin

Electron Microscopy

- Not helpful

Molecular Alterations

- Trisomy 3; t(11;18)

Differential Diagnosis

- With rare exceptions specific diagnoses can be made with the combination of histologic examination, immunotyping and genotyping

Treatment and Prognosis

- Localized disease can be cured with local treatment (radiation, or antibiotics in gastric MALToma)
- Disseminated disease is indolent and incurable
- Tumors tend to remain localized at site of origin for prolonged periods; some may transform to diffuse large B-cell lymphoma

Associations

- None

Nodal Marginal Zone B-Cell Lymphoma

Clinical Manifestations

- Comprises approximately 0.5% to 2% of lymphoid neoplasms
- Evidence of extranodal lymphoma is seen in approximately 30% of cases
- Peripheral lymph nodes are most typically involved
- Most patients present with either generalized or localized peripheral lymphedema

Gross and Microscopic Pathology

- Marginal zone (centrocyte-like) B-cells, monocytoid B-cells, or small B-lymphocytes, and scattered centroblast and immunoblast-like cells infiltrate the marginal zone and interfollicular areas of lymph nodes
- Some cases demonstrate plasma cell differentiation

Special Stains

- Not contributory

Immunohistochemistry

- Most cases are similar to extranodal marginal zone (MALT) lymphoma
- Some are reported to be IgD positive and CD43 negative, similar to splenic marginal zone lymphoma

Electron Microscopy

- Not helpful

Molecular Alterations

- Very little in the way of genetic studies has been done on these tumors
- t(11;18) (q21;q21) and trisomy 3 characteristic of extranodal marginal zone lymphoma are not often present

Differential Diagnosis

- With rare exceptions specific diagnoses can be made with the combination of histologic examination, immunotyping and genotyping

Treatment and Prognosis

- Majority of patients respond to chemotherapy
- High relapse rate
- Median survival approximately 5 years (consistent with indolent lymphoma)

Associations

- None

Splenic Marginal Zone Lymphoma

Clinical Manifestations

- Less than 1% of lymphoid neoplasms
- Splenic hilar lymph nodes, bone marrow, and peripheral blood involved
- Patients present with splenomegaly with or without autoimmune thrombocytopenia

Gross and Microscopic Pathology

- Both the red pulp and white pulp are infiltrated with small round lymphocytes
- The hilar nodes of the spleen contain tumor cells that surround and replace the germinal centers

Special Stains/Electron Microscopy

- Not contributory or helpful

Immunohistochemistry

- IgM and IgD on surface of tumor cells
- Tumor cells positive for CD20, CD79a, and have surface IgM and IgD
- Tumor cells negative for CD5, CD10, CD23, and CD43

Molecular Alterations

- Heavy and light chain immunoglobulin typically rearranged

Differential Diagnosis

- With rare exceptions specific diagnoses can be made with the combination of histologic examination, immunotyping and genotyping

Treatment and Prognosis

- Indolent
- Splenectomy may result in long-term survival

Associations

- None

Follicular Lymphoma

Clinical Manifestations

- Represents 35% of all adult lymphomas (most common non-Hodgkin lymphoma in the United States)
- Seen in middle-aged men and women with equal frequency
- Presents with generalized lymphadenopathy and bone marrow involvement

Gross and Microscopic Pathology

- Tumor cells closely resemble normal germinal center B-cells
- Lymph node involvement characterized by a predominantly nodular or nodular/diffuse growth pattern
- 2 cell types are typically seen:
  1) small cells with irregular or cleaved nuclear membranes and scant cytoplasm (centrocytes or small cleaved cells)
  2) larger cells with open nuclear chromatin, several nucleoli and modest amounts of cytoplasm (centroblasts)
- 3 grades, dependent on the number of centroblasts in 10 neoplastic follicles at 40× (Grade 1: 0-5; Grade 2: 6-15; and Grade 3: >15)

- 10% will have an involvement of the peripheral blood sufficient to produce a lymphocytosis in the range of 20,000/mm^3
- Bone marrow involved in 85%; characterized by paratrabecular aggregates of tumor cells
- Splenic involvement characterized by expansion of white pulp
- Liver portal tracts frequently involved

Special Stains

- Not contributory

Immunohistochemistry

- B-cells positive for CD10, bcl-6, CD19 and CD20 and negative for CD5
- Express bcl-2 protein, providing helpful distinction from follicular hyperplasia

Electron Microscopy

- Not helpful

Molecular Alterations

- t(14;18) involving bcl-2 gene

Differential Diagnosis

- With rare exceptions specific diagnoses can be made with the combination of histologic examination, immunotyping and genotyping

Treatment and Prognosis

- Median survival 7 to 9 years; no improvement with aggressive chemotherapy
- Symptomatic disease can be palliated with low dose chemotherapy or radiation
- Transformation occurs in 25 to 35%, most commonly to diffuse large B-cell lymphoma; median survival after transformation is one year

Associations

- None

Mantle Cell Lymphoma

Clinical Manifestations

- Occurs in males more commonly than females (median age 60)
- Typically presents with lymphadenopathy and bone marrow involvement
- 35% have peripheral blood lymphocytosis at time of diagnosis
- May arise at extranodal sites or present as splenomegaly (50%)

Gross and Microscopic Pathology

- Tumor cells resemble the normal mantle zone cells that surround follicular centers
- Three patterns of lymph node involvement: 1) a mantle zone pattern in which tumor cells surround or partially efface B-cell follicles, 2) a diffuse pattern, or 3) a vaguely nodular pattern
- Tumor cells are slightly larger than normal lymphocytes and have nuclei that are round to irregular to occasionally deeply clefted (cleaved), condensed chromatin, and inconspicuous nucleoli; scant cytoplasm
- Proliferation centers are typically absent
- Bone marrow involvement is characterized by both non-paratrabecular and paratrabecular lymphoid aggregates
- Spleen is frequently involved and characterized by expansion of the white pulp
- Periportal infiltration may be present in the liver
- Extranodal disease is relatively common and may be seen as lymphomatoid polyposis of small bowel and colon (most common non-Hodgkin lymphoma to spread in this fashion)

Special Stains

- Not contributory

Immunohistochemistry

- Tumor cells are positive for CD5, cyclin-D1, CD19, CD20, CD22, an CD43 and negative for CD10, bcl-6, and CD23
- Express surface IgM and IgD

Electron Microscopy

- Not helpful

Molecular Alterations

- Reciprocal translocation t(11;14)(q13;q32) involving the bcl-1 gene

Differential Diagnosis

- With rare exceptions specific diagnoses can be made with the combination of histologic examination, immunotyping and genotyping

Treatment and Prognosis

- Median survival 3 to 5 years (not curable with conventional chemotherapy)
- Transformation occurs less frequently than in CLL, SLL and follicular lymphoma
- Blastoid variant may have a worse prognosis

Associations

- None

Diffuse Large B-Cell Lymphoma

Clinical Manifestations

- Seen in all ages but most common in adults
- Often presents as a single rapidly enlarging mass: nodal (60%) or extranodal (40%)
- Most common extranodal site is gastrointestinal tract (stomach, ileocecal region)
- Also may present with Waldeyer ring, urinary tract, skin, bone, or brain involvement, or as a large destructive lesion in liver or spleen

Gross and Microscopic Pathology

- Tumor cells are large (2 or 3 times the size of a small lymphocyte; about the size of a histiocyte) and have a diffuse pattern of growth
- Nuclei round or oval with chromatin that tends to aggregate along the inner surface of the nuclear membrane, giving it a vesicular appearance
- Large multilobulated or cleaved nuclei may be present with multiple (2 or 3) nucleoli
- Cytoplasm is typically moderate and pale or basophilic
- Occasionally anaplastic neoplasms contain multinucleated cells with large nucleoli that closely resemble Reed-Sternberg cells

Special Stains

- Not contributory

Immunohistochemistry

- B-cells positive for CD19, CD20, CD22, bcl-6 and variably express CD5 and CD10
- Tumor cells usually positive for surface immunoglobulin and negative for TdT

Electron Microscopy

- Not helpful

Molecular Alterations

- t(14;18) (30%)
- Rearrangements of bcl-6 gene on chromosome 3 in 20 to 30%

Differential Diagnosis

- With rare exceptions specific diagnoses can be made with the combination of histologic examination, immunotyping and genotyping

Treatment and Prognosis

- Rapidly fatal if untreated
- Complete remission can be achieved in 60 to 80% with aggressive chemotherapy; 50% may be cured
- Patients with bcl6 rearrangements have a better prognosis
- Patients with p53 mutations have a worse prognosis

Associations

- None

Mediastinal (Thymic) Large B-Cell Lymphoma

Clinical Manifestations

- A subtype of diffuse large B-cell lymphoma arising in the mediastinum and originating from thymic B-cells
- Most patients in their third to fifth decade, females more commonly affected than males
- Patients with localized disease and signs and symptoms related to large anterior mediastinal mass sometimes with impending superior vena cava syndrome
- When disseminated, extranodal sites often involved (kidney, adrenal, liver, skin and brain)

Gross and Microscopic Pathology

- Massive diffuse proliferation associated with variably dense compartmentalized fibrosis
- Residual remants of thymus may be organized in lobules and mimic carcinoma
- Neoplastic cells vary in size and shape
- Usually the cells have abundant pale pink cytoplasm, small numbers of interspersed benign lymphocytes and eosinophils may be present

Special Stains

- Not contributory

Immunohistochemistry

- Tumor cells express CD19 and CD20
- CD10 and CD5 are not expressed
- Expression of CD30 is usually present but tends to be weak (staining may be focal or extensive)
- Tumor cells express leukocyte common antigen (CD45)

Electron Microscopy

- Not helpful

Molecular Alterations

- Gains in chromosome 9p and amplification of the REL gene
- Overexpression of the *MAL* gene is frequently present
- Cells lack *BCL2, BCL6* and *myc* rearrangements

Differential Diagnosis

- With rare exceptions specific diagnoses can be made with the combination of histologic examination, immunotyping and genotyping
- Hodgkin lymphoma (cells of classical Hodgkin lymphoma are typically negative for CD45)

Treatment and Prognosis

- Response to intensive chemotherapy with or without radiotherapy is usually good
- The chance for a longterm remission correlates with the initial stage of disease; patients with disease extending into adjacent thoracic viscera have a worse prognosis than those with disease confined to the mediastinum
- Spread into infra-diaphagmatic organs predicts an unfavorable outcome

Associations

- None

Burkitt Lymphoma/Leukemia

Clinical Manifestations

- Seen in adolescents and young adults; 30-50% of childhood lymphomas
- Endemic disease occurs in equatorial Africa and presents as a mass in jaw/other facial bones, gastrointestinal tract, ovary, kidney, or breast
- Sporadic disease often presents as a mass involving ileocecal area, ovary, kidney or breast
- Immunodeficiency associated diseases were all seen in association with HIV infection; EBV present in 20%-40%
- Uncommonly presents purely as a leukemia

Gross and Microscopic Pathology

- Tumor cells are intermediate-sized lymphoid cells with round to oval nuclei with coarse chromatin, several nucleoli and a moderate amount of faintly basophilic or amphophilic cytoplasm
- Mitotic figures, apoptotic cells, and macrophages present
- Macrophages tend to be evenly distributed throughout the tumor and are surrounded by a clear space that give the neoplasm a characteristic "starry sky" pattern
- Tumor cells that involve bone marrow have clumped nuclear chromatin, two to five distinct nucleoli and royal blue cytoplasm that contains multiple, clear cytoplasmic vacuoles

Special Stains

- Not contributory

Immunohistochemistry

- B-cells positive for CD10, CD19, CD20, CD22, bcl-6, and Ki-67 (high proliferative fraction nearly 100%), and negative for CD5, CD23 bcl-2, and TdT

Electron Microscopy

- Not helpful

Molecular Alterations

- Translocation of c-myc from chromosome 8 to IgH region on chromosome 14
- t(8;14), or to light chain gene on chromosome 2 or 22 t(2;8), and t(8;22)

Differential Diagnosis

- With rare exceptions specific diagnoses can be made with the combination of histologic examination, immunotyping and genotyping

Treatment and Prognosis

- Cured in 60-90% with intensive, combination chemotherapy

Associations

- Epstein-Barr virus present in a variable portion of cases, especially in entemic disease

Mature T-Cell and Natural Killer (NK) Cell Neoplasms

Adult T-Cell Leukemia/Lymphoma

Clinical Manifestations

- Occurs in areas where HTLV-1 is endemic (Japan, Caribbean, and central America)
- May be transmitted by exposure to blood and in breast milk
- Most have widespread lymph node and peripheral blood involvement along with involvement of the spleen, skin, lung, liver, GI tract and CNS
- Four variants:
  1. Acute variant: characterized by systemic disease (leukemic phase) with a very elevated WBC count, skin rash and generalized lymphadenopathy; hypercalcemia common (with or without bone involvement) opportunistic infections frequent; LDH elevated
  2. Lymphomatous variant: prominent lymphadenopathy without blood involvement; hypercalcemia rare
  3. Chronic variant; skin lesions (exfoliative rash); no hypercalcemia
  4. Smoldering variant: WBC count normal (<55 circulating neoplastic cells); skin and pulmonary lesions frequent; no hypercalcemia
- Progression of chronic and smoldering to acute seen in 25%

Gross and Microscopic Pathology

- Tumor cells typically medium to large with marked nuclear pleomorphism; nuclei often polylobulated (cloverleaf or flower cells); chromatin usually clumped with easily visualized nucleoli
- Some patients with early or smoldering disease have a Hodgkin-like morphology complete with Reed-Sternberg-cells

Special Stains

- Not contributory

Immunohistochemistry

- Tumor cells T-cell antigens (CD2, CD3, CD5); most positive for CD4 and CD25.
- RSB-like cells positive for CD30 and CD15

Electron Microscopy

- Not helpful

Molecular Alterations

- HTLV-1 provirus present in tumor cells

Differential Diagnosis

- With rare exceptions specific diagnoses can be made with the combination of histologic examination, immunotyping and genotyping

Treatment and Prognosis

- Most significant prognostic prognostic factors are serum and LDH levels
- Patients with acute and lymphomatous disease live two week to a year
- Patients with chronic and smoldering disease may have protracted survival unless they transform into acute disease

Associations

- None

Extranodal NK/T-Cell Lymphoma, Nasal Type (Lethal Midline Granuloma)

Clinical Manifestations

- More prevalent in Asia, Mexico and Central and South America
- Typically occurs in adults; more common in males than females
- May occur in immunosuppressed patients
- Tends to occur in the nasal cavity, nasopharynx, palate, skin, soft tissue, gastrointestinal tract and testis
- Some cases are accompanied by secondary lymph node involvement
- Patients with nasal involvement often present with nasal obstruction or epistaxis
- Occasionally patients will present with extensive midfacial destructive lesions (formally called lethal midline granuloma)
- Dissemination to skin, gastrointestinal tract, testis or cervical lymph nodes may be quite rapid
- Involvement of the skin usually presents with nodules, often with ulceration
- Intestinal lesions frequently perforate

Gross and Microscopic Pathology

- A diffuse infiltrate of lymphocytes that frequently demonstrate an angiocentric and angiodestructive (fibrinoid changes in blood vessel walls) pattern
- Tumor cells may vary greatly in size; some may be small with irregular nuclei and be almost indistinguishable from normal small lymphocytes; others may be of medium size with pale cytoplasm; still others may be large and anaplastic and associated with numerous apoptotic bodies
- Tumors comprised predominately of small and mixed cells may be admixed with inflammatory cells: small lymphocytes, plasma cells, eosinophils, and histiocytes
- Nuclei often elongated with irregular nuclear membranes and granular chromatin; nucleoli usually small of inconspicious
- Overlying epithelium may show changes of pseudoepitheliomatous hyperplasia

Special Stains

- Not contributory

Immunohistochemistry

- Typically tumor cells are CD2 positive, CD56 positive, and surface CD3 negative
- Occasional cases are positive for CD7 and CD30

Electron Microscopy

- Not helpful

Molecular Alterations

- EBV can be demonstrated in the tumor cells in most cases
- Most common cytogenetic abnormality is deletion 6 (q21 q25) or i(6)(p10)

Differential Diagnosis

- Inflammatory process
- Overlying pseudoepitheliomatous hyperplasia may minic squamous cell carcinoma

Treatment and Prognosis

- Some patients respond well to therapy while others die of disseminated disease regardless of the type of therapy employed
- There is no clear evidence that the cytologic grade of the tumor has any significance in terms of prognosis
- This type of lymphoma occurring outside of the nasal cavity is highly aggressive, with a survival time that is quite short; response to therapy is limited

Associations

- Most consistently associated with Epstein-Barr virus

Enteropathy-Type T-Cell Lymphoma (Refractory Sprue)

Clinical Manifestations

- Occurs most commonly in the jejunum and ileum, but presentation in the duodenum, stomach, or outside the gastrointestinal tract has been reported
- A few patients have a history of childhood onset of celiac disease, but most have adult onset celiac disease
- Most patients present with abdominal pain often associated with intestinal perforation
- The tumor typically presents as multiple ulcerated, raised, mucosal masses but also may present as one or more ulcers or as one large exophytic mass
- Typically the tumor cells are relatively monomorphic and are of medium to large size; nuclei tend to be angulated and vesicular; nucleoli are prominent; cytoplasm is moderate to abundant and pale staining
- Less commonly the tumor shows marked pleomorphism and takes on the resemblance of an anaplastic large cell lymphoma
- Most tumors are diffusely infiltrated by inflammatory cells to include large numbers of histiocytes and eosinophils; the inflammatory infiltrate may obscure the actual tumor cells
- Adjacent intestinal mucosa usually shows the changes of villous atrophy, crypt hyperplasia, increased lamina propria lymphocytes and plasma cells, and intraepithelial lymphocytosis

Gross and Microscopic Pathology

- Tumor cells within the mucosal mass tend to be monomorphic, round or angulated nuclei; nucleoli prominent; cytoplasm pale staining and may be moderate or abundant
- Typically there is an infiltrate of inflammatory cells consisting of eosinophils and histiocytes

Special Stains

- Not contributory

Immunohistochemistry

- Tumor cells are CD3 positive, CD5 negative, CD7 positive, CD8 may or may not be positive, CD4 negative, CD103 positive
- A variable number of tumor cells may express CD30
- When the tumor is composed predominantly of small to medium sized cells, those cells will frequently be positive for CD8 and express CD56
- The intraepithelial lymphocytes in refractory celiac disease are usually CD8 negative

Electron Microscopy

- Not helpful

Molecular Alterations

- Most patients have the same genotype that characterize celiac disease
- Patients with refractory celiac disease typically have T-cells that are CD3 positive and CD8 negative; celiac disease that responds to dietary therapy typically has CD3 and CD8 positive T-cells

Differential Diagnosis

- With rare exceptions specific diagnoses can be made with the combination of histologic examination, immunotyping and genotyping

Treatment and Prognosis

- Prognosis is typically poor with death secondary to abdominal complications (usually perforation)

Associations

- Seen with increasing frequency in areas with a high prevalence of celiac disease

Mycosis Fungoides/Sézary Syndrome

Clinical Manifestations

- Affects adults; Sézary syndrome usually affects men
- Patients with mycosis fungoides present with cutaneous patches, plaques, nodules, or generalized erythema; often misdiagnosed as psoriasis
- Patients with Sézary syndrome present with generalized exfoliative erythroderma

Gross and Microscopic Pathology

- Mycosis fungoides is characterized by an infiltration of the epidermis and upper dermis by neoplastic T-cells that have markedly cerebriform nuclei (nuclear membrane with marked infolding)
- Tumor cells of Sézary syndrome are identical to those of mycosis fungoides but are found in peripheral blood

Special Stains

- Not contributory

Immunohistochemistry

- T-cells positive for CD2, CD3, CD4, and CD5 and negative for CD8

Electron Microscopy

- Not helpful

Molecular Alterations

- TCR genes clonally rearranged

Differential Diagnosis

- With rare exceptions specific diagnoses can be made with the combination of histologic examination, immunotyping and genotyping

Treatment and Prognosis

- Most are indolent and associated with a mean survival of 8 to 9 years
- Occasionally will transform to a large cell lymphoma of the T-cell type (usually a terminal event)

Associations

- None

Angioimmunoblastic T-Cell Lymphoma

Clinical Manifestations

- One of the more common specific subtypes of peripheral T-cell neoplasms accounting for 15-20% of cases; represents 1-2% of all non-Hodgkin lymphomas
- Typically occurs in middle-aged and the elderly; males and females affected equally
- Patients present with advanced disease with systemic symptoms , a generalized peripheral lymphadenopathy, hepatomegaly, splenomegaly, skin rash, and polyclonal hypergammaglobulinemia
- Other common symptoms include edema, pleural effusion, arthritis and ascites
- The bone marrow is commonly involved

Gross and Microscopic Pathology

- Lymph nodes partially effaced with small follicles
- There is a diffuse infiltrate of polymorphous small to medium-sized lymphocytes in the paracortex; these cells typically have a clear to pale cytoplasm and distinct cell membranes; there is little cytologic atypia
- Tumor cells are typically admixed with small, reactive lymphocytes, eosinophils, plasma cells, histiocytes, and increased numbers of follicular dendritic cells
- Large basophilic blasts of B-cell phenotype may be present; Reed-Sternberg-like cells may also be seen
- Arborizing blood vessels usually very prominent

Special Stains

- Not contributory

Immunohistochemistry

- Tumor cells are typically mature T-cells and represent a mixture of CD4 and CD8 positive cells; CD4 positive cells usually outnumber the CD8 positive cells; may coexpress CD10
- Follicular dendritic cells surrounding venules can be highlighted by CD21

Electron Microscopy

- Not helpful

Molecular Alterations

- Most of the EBV-positive cells are B-cells
- T-cell receptor genes are rearranged in 75%
- Gene rearrangement of immunoglobulin is seen in 10%
- The most frequent cytogenetic abnormalities are trisomy 3, trisomy 5, and an additional X chromosome
- EBV sequences are frequently present in scattered cells (usually B-cells but also T-cells)

Differential Diagnosis

- Atypical T-zone hyperplasia

Treatment and Prognosis

- Clinical course typically aggressive with median survival of less than 3 years
- Patients often succumb to infectious complications

Associations

- None

Peripheral T-Cell Lymphoma, Unspecified

Clinical Manifestations

- Most present with generalized lymphadenopathy
- Occasionally patients will have eosinophilia, pruritus, fever and weight loss,
- Lymphocytosis, and hypercalcemia

Gross and Microscopic Pathology

- Neoplasm diffusely effaces the architecture of involved lymph nodes
- Tumor cells are a pleomorphic mixture of small, intermediate and large malignant T-cells
- A prominent infiltrate of reactive cells such as eosinophils and macrophages typically present
- Prominent angiogenesis occasionally present

Special Stains

- Not contributory

Immunohistochemistry

- Mature T-cells express pan T-cell markers
- Most nodal cases are CD4 positive and CD8 negative
- T-cells do not express TdT and CD1a

Electron Microscopy

- Not helpful

Molecular Alterations

- Often complex karyotypes; no consistent characteristic abnormality

Differential Diagnosis

- With rare exceptions specific diagnoses can be made with the combination of histologic examination, immunotyping and genotyping

Treatment and Prognosis

- Some reports of cure, but incidence of relapse appears to be higher than in diffuse large B-cell lymphoma
- Recurrences are most common in the small intestine

Associations

- None

Anaplastic Large Cell Lymphoma

Clinical Manifestations

- Represents 3% of all adult non-Hodgkin lymphomas and 10-30% of childhood lymphomas
- Most frequently occurs during the first three decades of life
- More common in males than females (especially in the second and third decades)
- Most patients (70%) present with advanced stage disease with peripheral and/or abdominal lymphadenopathy
- Typically lymph nodes and extranodal sites involved; extranodal sites include skin (20%), bone (17%); soft tissue (17%), lung (10%), and liver (8%)
- The GI tract and central nervous system are rarely involved
- Mediastinal disease is less frequent than in Hodgkin lymphoma; bone marrow may be involved (involvement may be very subtle with very few scattered single cells or small clusters of cells)

Gross and Microscopic Pathology

- All cases contain a variable number of large cells with eccentric kidney-shaped nuclei; frequently there is an eosinophilic cuff around the nucleus (these cells are referred to as "hallmark" cells)

- Tumor cells typically have more cytoplasm than the cells of other lymphomas; the cytoplasm may be clear, basophilic or eosinophilic
- Occasionally cells have multiple nuclei and may resemble Reed-Sternberg cells
- Nuclear chromatin is typically finely clumped with multiple small, basophilic nucleoli
- Three variants:
    - ***Common variant*** (70%): typically composed of pleomorphic large cells with hallmark features; tumor cells may be more monomorphic and have rounded nuclei; either cell type may predominate or they may be admixed
    - ***Lymphohistocytic variant*** (10%): tumor cells admixed with large numbers of histiocytes; histiocytes may obcsure the malignant cells
    - ***Small cell variant*** (5%-10%): consists predominately of small to medium-sized neoplastic cells with irregular nuclei; hallmark cells are always present but tend to be concentrated around blood vessels

Special Stains

- Not contributory

Immunohistochemistry

- Tumor cells are positive for CD30 on the cell membrane and in the Golgi region
- Smaller tumor cells may be weakly positive for CD30 or even negative
- ALK expression is seen in 60%-85%; the staining may be cytoplasmic and/or nuclear; *ALK expression is virtually diagnostic for anaplastic large cell lymphoma*
- The majority of tumor cells are positive for EMA with a staining pattern is similar to that of CD30
- The majority of tumor cells express one or more of the T-cell antigens; CD2 and CD4 are also positive in the majority of cases
- CD8 is usually negative
- CD43 is expressed in 65%
- CD15 expression is rare
- Tumor cells are always negative for EBV

Electron Microscopy

- Not helpful

Molecular Alterations

- 90% show clonal rearrangement of the T-cell receptor genes
- ALK expression results from genetic alteration of the ALK locus on chromosome 2
- The most frequent genetic alteration is a translocation, t (2;5) (p23;35), between the *ALK* gene on chromosome 2 and the nucleophosmin (*NPM)* gene on chromosome 5

Differential Diagnosis

- A small cell variant of anaplastic large cell lymphoma may be confused with peripheral T-cell lymphoma
- Hodgkin lymphoma

Treatment and Prognosis

- The most important prognostic factor is the presence of ALK positivity, which is associated with a favorable prognosis
- Overall 5-year survival rate in ALK-positive disease is close to 80%; 5-year survival is 40% in ALK-negative cases
- Relapses are not uncommon (30%) but tend to remain sensitive to chemotherapy

Associations

- No causative agent or predisposing factors have ever been demonstrated

References

Mills S, Carter D, Greenson JK, Oberman HA, Reuter V, Stoler MH (eds). *Sternberg's Diagnostic Surgical Pathology, 4th edition*. Philadelphia: Lippincott Williams & Wilkins, 2004.

Rosai J. *Rosai and Ackerman's Surgical Pathology, 9th edition.* St. Louis: Mosby, 2004.

Dabbs, DJ. *Diagnostic Immunohistochemistry.* Philadelphia: Churchill Livingstone, 2002.

Cotran RS, Kumar V, Collins T. *Robbins Pathologic Basis of Disease, 7th edition*. Philadelphia: W.B. Saunders Company, 2004.

Kjeldsberg CR (ed). *Practical Diagnosis of Hematologic Disorders, 4th edition*. Chicago: ASCP Press, 2006.

Jaffe ES. *Surgical Pathology of the Lymph Nodes and Related Organs, Volume 16. Major Problems in Pathology, 2nd edition.* Philadelphia: WB Saunders Company, 1995.

Warnke RA, Weiss LM, Chan JKC, Cleary ML, Dorfman RF. *Tumors of the Lymph Nodes and Spleen; Atlas of Tumor Pathology, 3rd series. Fascicle 14.* Washington DC: Armed Forces Institute of Pathology, 1995.

Jaffe ES, Harris NL, Stein H, Vardiman JW (eds). *World Health Organization Classification of Tumours. Pathology and Genetics Tumours of Haematopoietic and Lymphoid Tissues*. IARC Press: Lyon, 2001.

Chapter 15

Male Reproductive System

Intraoperative Consultation

Testicular neoplasms, with rare exceptions, are treated by inguinal orchectomy. Prior biopsy confirmation is generally not obtained unless there is a high likelihood the testicular mass is benign or there is a need to preserve the testis. With this definitive surgical procedure, the intraoperative consultation should be limited to gross examination only.

Rarely, an incisional biopsy of the testis is performed and the pathologist will be required to make the distinction between a malignant neoplasm that will lead to an immediate inguinal orchectomy or a benign process that will not require such a resection. There are 2 major pitfalls. The 1st is that granulomatous inflammation in the testis that spares the epididymis might well reflect the presence of a seminoma. The 2nd is that adenomatoid tumors of the testis that arise in the tunica albuginea (rather than in the more common inferior pole of the epididymis) can easily be misdiagnosed as yolk sac tumor. Careful clinical correlation is required by both surgeon and pathologist in these unique situations.

Specimen Handling

The testicle should be weighed and cut longitudinally while in a fresh state. After it has been fixed in formalin it is cut in serial sections 3-mm-thick perpendicular to the original longitudinal line of section. The epididymis is cut longitudinally throughout its length.

At least 3 sections of the neoplasm are submitted or 1 section for each 1 cm of tumor, whichever is greater. One or more of the sections should include some uninvolved testicle, the interface between the tumor and tunica vaginalis, and the epididymis. Sections should always be submitted from areas that appear hemorrhagic or necrotic as well as areas that are solid or fleshy. One section should be taken through the rete testis. The spermatic cord and surrounding soft tissue should be sectioned in 2 places: 1 cross-section taken 1 cm from the testicle, and a 2nd cross-section taken at the surgical margin.

Germ Cell Tumors

Intratubular Germ Cell Neoplasia

- Characterized by the presence of malignant germ cells within seminiferous tubules
- Variants of intratubular germ cell neoplasia show specific forms of differentiation:
  - Intratubular seminoma
  - Intratubular spermatocytic seminoma
  - Intratubular embryonal carcinoma
  - Intratubular yolk sac tumor (rare)
- 5% incidence in contralateral testis in patients with prior germ cell tumor
- More frequently seen in association with nonseminomatous tumors than seminomas
- No association with spermatocytic seminoma
- Infrequent in pediatric cases of yolk sac tumor and teratoma
- In the absence of invasive tumor, intratubular germ cell neoplasia is typically asymptomatic
- Testis usually smaller than normal; oligospermia
- In cases of infertility, the incidence of bilaterality is approximately 40%
- Occasionally patients with intratubular germ cell neoplasia will have no evidence of primary testicular tumor, but will have retroperitoneal germ cell tumor (not true in cases with mediastinal germ cell tumors)

Gross Pathology

- Testis typically appears normal or atrophic
- Occasionally the testis may be firm as a result of tubular shrinkage and intertubular fibrosis

Microscopic Pathology

- Tumor cells resemble tumor cells of seminoma, lie along the basal aspect of the seminiferous tubule and are large, polygonal, and have clear cytoplasm; nuclei are round, large, hyperchromatic, and have 1 or more prominent nucleoli; nuclear membranes tend to be irregular and thickened
- Mitoses may be frequent
- Involved seminiferous tubules tend to be smaller than normal, have a thickened peritubular membrane, and have no normal spermatogenic cells; adjacent seminiferous tubules may be completely normal and show normal spermatogenesis
- Sertoli cells are often admixed with tumor cells and tend to be displaced toward the lumen
- Occasionally there is a peritubular lymphoid infiltrate
- Intratubular calcifications are seen in 40%
- There may be increased numbers of Leydig cells
- Tumor cells may extend in a pagetoid fashion from the seminiferous tubules into the ductal system of the testis and into the rete testis, epididymis, and beyond

Special Stains

- Periodic acid-Schiff (PAS) will readily stain the glycogen in tumor cells
- PAS will also stain non-neoplastic spermatogonia

Immunohistochemistry

- Tumor cells are typically positive for PLAP, OCT 3/4, and C-*kit* (CD117); p53 is present in most cases
- Non-neoplastic spermatogenic cells are almost always PLAP negative

Electron Microscopy

- Confirms the nonepithelial nature of the malignant germ cells (no epithelial junctions) and their similarity to seminoma

Molecular Alterations

- Neoplastic cells are aneuploid
- Presence of isochromosome (12p) in the majority of cases

Differential Diagnosis

- Intratubular germ cell neoplasia, unclassified (IGCNU), must be differentiated from the specific forms of intratubular germ cell neoplasia:
  - Seminoma
  - Spermatocytic seminoma
  - Embryonal carcinoma
  - Yolk sac tumor

Treatment

- Orchiectomy for unilateral disease
- Low-dose radiation for bilateral disease (sterility results)
- Treatment with chemotherapy results in a recurrence rate of 20% and 40% at 5 and 10 years, respectively

Prognosis

- Depends on presence of invasive germ cell neoplasm

Associations

- IGCNU is present in 98% of cases of invasive germ cell tumor when residual seminiferous tubules are present
- 50% of patients with IGCNU develop invasive germ cell tumor within 5 years of initial diagnosis
- 2%-8% incidence in patients with cryptorchidism
- Increased incidence in patients who are infertile, patients with gonadal dysgenesis, and patients with androgen insensitivity syndrome (testicular feminization): 46,XY (phenotypic females with testis)

Seminoma

Clinical Manifestations

- Most common pure germ cell tumor of the testis
- Average age at diagnosis is 40 years
- Typically presents as asymmetric testicular swelling often associated with ill-defined aching sensation in the scrotum, inguinal region, or lower abdomen
- Right testis affected slightly more often than the left
- At the time of presentation, 75% of patients have disease limited to the testis, 20% have disease in the retroperitoneum, and 5% have distant metastasis
- Approximately 2% bilateral (almost never synchronously)
- Patients may present with exophthalmos (paraendocrine abnormality) and hypercalcemia (paraneoplastic)
- Serum AFP levels usually not elevated
- Serum hCG levels may be elevated (tends to correlate with amount of disease and number of syncytiotrophoblastic cells present in the tumor)

Gross Pathology

- 90% are confined to the testis; 10% extend through the tunica albuginea into the epididymis
- On cut section a well-circumscribed, solid, yellow-white to tan to light pink, bulging, lobulated or multinodular mass with a soft and fleshy consistency (occasionally firm and fibrous)
- Foci of hemorrhage may be present (indicative of trophoblastic elements)

Microscopic Pathology

- Tumor cells tend to be arranged in sheets through which thin fibrous septa course
- Scattered normal-appearing lymphocytes and occasionally lymphoid follicles are seen in the fibrous septa (20%); most of the lymphocytes are T cells; a granulomatous reaction is present in 50% to 60%
- Foci of necrosis (sometimes extensive) frequently present
- Focal intratubular growth (neoplastic cells fill and distend seminiferous tubules) frequent

- Tumor cells tend to be round to polygonal, have clear to lightly eosinophilic granular cytoplasm (glycogen), and prominent cytoplasmic membranes; nuclei usually large and centrally located with coarse chromatin, and 1 or 2 (occasionally more) prominent nucleoli; nuclear membrane typically irregularly thickened and often has a somewhat flattened edge
- Mitotic activity is variable but tends to be fairly prominent, especially at the periphery of lobules of tumor
- Syncytiotrophoblastic cells are present in 20% to 25% (positive identification may require immunostain for hCG) and tend to aggregate in small groups around blood vessels

Special Stains

- PAS with and without diastase will confirm the presence of glycogen within the tumor cells

Immunohistochemistry

- Most tumor cells are positive for placental alkaline phosphatase (PLAP) and C-*kit* (CD117)
- Syncytiotrophoblastic cells are positive for hCG
- Tumor cells typically positive for vimentin, LDH, ferritin, and NSE
- Tumor cells negative for CD30
- Tumor cells are highly variable in terms of staining with keratin (reports of positivity range from 0% to 75%)
- Stains for AFP, and EMA negative

Electron Microscopy

- Tumor cells are close to one another and contain variable amounts of glycogen
- Nuclei are round and regular with evenly dispersed chromatin
- Nucleoli may be multiple and tend to be large and are made up of complex, meandering strands of fibrillar material

Molecular Alterations

- Most common abnormality is the presence of an isochromosome derived from the short arm of chromosome 12: i(12p)
- DNA content tends to be 1 to almost 2 times normal
- Decreased expression of the retinoblastoma gene
- C-*kit* oncogene may be expressed in up to 80%

Differential Diagnosis

- Embryonal carcinoma with a solid pattern (nuclei of embryonal carcinoma tend to be more crowded together, irregularly shaped, and vesicular than nuclei of seminoma)
- Yolk sac tumor with a solid pattern
- Presence of syncytiotrophoblastic cells places choriocarcinoma in the differential
- Malignant lymphoma
- Granulomatous orchitis

Treatment

- Seminomas very sensitive to both radiation and chemotherapy
- Neoplasms confined to the testis are treated with orchiectomy with adjuvant radiation therapy to ipsilateral inguinal and iliac lymph nodes and paraortic and paracaval lymph nodes to the level of the diaphragm
- Patients with advanced stage disease and limited retroperitoneal disease are treated with radiation
- Patients with advanced disease and extensive retroperitoneal disease are treated with platinum-based chemotherapy
- Surgery beyond orchectomy not indicated

Prognosis

- Cure rate for stage I disease is approximately 95%
- Patients with limited retroperitoneal disease have an overall survival rate of 90% to 95%
- Patients with extensive retroperitoneal involvement have an overall 80% survival

Associations

- Neoplasm more common in very tall men as well as men with cryptorchidism
- Incidence increased in patients with acquired immunodeficiency syndrome (AIDS)
- Increased incidence of human leukocyte antigen (HLA) type DR5 and Bw41

Spermatocytic Seminoma

Clinical Manifestations

- 2% to 5% of seminomas
- 2nd most common testicular tumor in elderly men (most common is lymphoma)

- Average age at presentation mid 50s (rare under the age of 30 years)
- Most present with painless testicular enlargement
- Approximately 10% bilateral (asynchronous)

Gross Pathology

- Tends to be well-circumscribed and nodular or multilobular
- Cut surface often soft, friable, yellow, and either edematous or gelatinous
- Foci of hemorrhage, cyst formation, and necrosis may be present
- If tumor has undergone sarcomatous transformation, the cut surface may have solid gray areas with more extensive hemorrhage or necrosis

Microscopic Pathology

- Typically a diffuse arrangement of polymorphous tumor cells that lack the monotonous uniformity of classic seminoma cells; tend to be arranged in a diffuse pattern
- Fibrous stroma usually scant, but may be quite prominent and when it is, it is usually very edematous, which gives the tumor cells a pseudoglandular (cystic), trabecular, nested, clustered, or single cell pattern
- Little if any lymphoid infiltrate or granulomatous reaction
- 3 types of tumor cells are present:
    - *Small:* Degenerating cells that resemble lymphocytes; characterized by a densely basophilic nucleus with a homogeneous chromatin pattern and little eosinophilic cytoplasm
    - *Medium-sized (intermediate):* Most numerous; characterized by a uniform, perfectly round nucleus with finely granular chromatin and a modest amount of eosinophilic cytoplasm
    - *Giant:* Least numerous; large cells that resemble primary spermatocytes with 2 or more nuclei that may have a filamentous or "spireme" chromatin pattern and prominent nucleoli
- Mitotic activity is usually prominent; atypical mitoses may be present
- Glycogen is not demonstrable in any of the 3 cell types
- All 3 cell types have indistinct cell borders
- Intratubular growth usually present at periphery of the tumor; no IGCNU
- Foci of sarcoma (usually undifferentiated) present in 5% to 10%

Special Stains

- PAS with and without diastase will confirm the absence of glycogen in the tumor cells

Immunohistochemistry

- Tumor cells are typically negative for vimentin, actin, desmin, AFP, hCG, CEA, leukocyte common antigen, and CD30
- Tumor cells usually negative for PLAP (unlike classic seminoma)
- Tumor cells usually negative for cytokeratin

Electron Microscopy

- Nuclei are round with dispersed chromatin and a prominent nucleolus
- Intracellular bridges exist between adjacent cells
- Tumor cells often contain abundant small, round mitochondria

Molecular Alterations

- None

Differential Diagnosis

- Classic seminoma
- Anaplastic variant of spermatocytic seminoma (tumor characterized by a predominance of monomorphic cells with prominent nucleoli) may resemble classic seminoma and embryonal carcinoma
- Lymphoma

Treatment

- Orchiectomy
- No indication for adjuvant therapy

Prognosis

- Excellent (1 case report of metastasis)
- Tumors with sarcomatous transformation have a poor prognosis secondary to a high rate of metastasis (both lymphatic and hematogenous)

Associations

- No association with cryptorchidism
- No association with IGCNU
- Tumor never admixed with classic seminoma or nonseminomatous germ cell tumors

Embryonal Carcinoma

Clinical Manifestations

- 40% of all testicular germ cell neoplasms have an embryonal carcinoma component
- Embryonal carcinoma is a component of approximately 90% of all nonseminomatous germ cell tumors
- Typically occurs between the age of 25 and 35 years
- Extremely rare in infants, prepubertal children and men older than 50 years
- Most present with a testicular swelling that may be associated with pain
- Approximately 10% present with symptoms of metastatic disease
- 10% present with gynecomastia
- 65% of patients with predominately embryonal carcinoma have metastatic disease at time of diagnosis
- Elevated serum levels of hCG present in 60% (a consequence of the presence of syncytiotrophoblastic cells)
- Advanced disease may result in elevated serum levels of lactate dehydrogenase (LDH) and PLAP

Gross Pathology

- Typically an ill-defined soft, yellow-white to gray to tan granular neoplasm that tends to bulge above the cut surface
- Foci of hemorrhage and/or necrosis and cystic change frequent
- Tends to blend imperceptibly with adjacent normal testis
- Evidence of local extension into the rete testis, epididymis, or beyond present in 25%
- Extensive fibrosis may be present

Microscopic Pathology

- Cohesive large cells arranged in various patterns (solid, glandular, tubular, and papillary)
- Most frequent pattern is solid; papillary and tubular next most frequent
- Tumor cells tend to be polygonal with indistinct cytoplasmic borders and abundant granular cytoplasm that varies from amphophilic, to basophilic, to eosinophilic, to clear; nuclei tend to overlap and be large, polygonal, and vesicular with irregular, coarsely clumped chromatin and prominent parachromatin clearing; nuclei tend to have deep clefts and irregular contours; 1 or more large prominent nucleoli often present
- Areas of necrosis and/or hemorrhage common, especially in association with the solid pattern
- Mitotic rate is high
- Syncytiotrophoblastic cells commonly present
- A cellular, undifferentiated, mitotically active stroma with hyperchromatic, oval to spindle cells may be present
- Papillae are frequent; tumor cells cover fibrovascular cores but occasionally stromal core is absent and the papillae consists simply of piled-up carcinomatous epithelium
- At the periphery of groups of tumor cells (particularly in the solid pattern) there may be darkly staining, smudged, degenerated appearing cells that are reminiscent of syncytiotrophoblastic cells (appliqué pattern—gets its name from the tendency of these degenerated cells to "apply" themselves to adjacent cells); may be confused with choriocarcinoma
- At the periphery of the lesion, intratubular embryonal carcinoma (frequently necrotic) usually present
- Vascular invasion is a common finding (characteristically aggregates of tumor cells conform to the shape of the vessel)

Special Stains

- Not helpful

Immunohistochemistry

- 85% to 95% positive for PLAP
- Most stain for pancytokeratin (AE1/AE3 and CAM5.2)
- 80% are positive for CD30 (Ber-H2, Ki-1)
- Tumor cells typically negative for EMA, CEA, vimentin, and c-*kit* (CD117)
- Scattered tumor cells may stain for β-hCG and α-fetoprotein (AFP)

Electron Microscopy

- Tumor cells have short stubby microvilli and tight junctional complexes with well-defined desmosomes; cytoplasm contains numerous ribosomes, glycogen, prominent Golgi apparatus, rough endoplasmic reticulum, and numerous mitochondria
- Nests of cells frequently surrounded by a basement membrane
- Tumor cell nuclei have deep indentations, clumps of heterochromatin, and large complex, "wandering" nucleoli

Molecular Alterations

- Many have the isochromosome (i) 12p

Differential Diagnosis

- Seminoma
- Yolk sac tumor (nuclei of embryonal carcinoma are larger and more pleomorphic than those of yolk sac tumor; also hyaline globules are absent in embryonal carcinoma)
- Large cell lymphoma (immunoblastic phenotype)

Treatment

- Inguinal orchiectomy with or without retroperitoneal lymph node dissection (nerve sparing)
- Chemotherapy (cisplatin-based) is used for relapse or if retroperitoneal lymph nodes are involved
- Patients with advanced disease are treated with initial cisplatin-based, multidrug chemotherapy followed by inguinal orchiectomy

Prognosis

- Tumors confined to the testis or tumors with relatively limited retroperitoneal involvement typically have an overall survival in excess of 95%
- Patients with extensive retroperitoneal disease have survival rates of 70% to 85%
- The presence of viable nonteratomatous tumor in a nonseminomas germ cell tumor after treatment with chemotherapy represents a high risk for a relapse
- Features associated with a poor prognosis in patients with metastatic nonseminomatous germ cell tumors include:
  - Liver, bone or brain metastasis
  - Elevated serum levels of AFP (>1,000 IU/L) or β-hCG (>10,000 IU/L)
  - A mediastinal mass >5 cm in diameter
  - 20 or more lung metastasis
  - Elderly

Associations

- Less often associated with undescended testis or cryptorchidism than classic seminoma

Yolk Sac Tumor (Endodermal Sinus Tumor)

Clinical Manifestations

- Most common testicular tumor in children; represents 80% to 85% of prepubertal germ cell tumors
- 4 times more common than teratoma
- Most childhood cases occur before the age of 2 years
- When the neoplasm occurs in a prepubertal child, it is almost always pure; in postpubertal patients the tumor is usually component of a mixed germ cell tumor
- Present in approximately 45% of all nonseminomatous germ cell tumors
- Prepubertal tumors are not associated with cryptorchidism
- Patients typically present with a painless testicular mass
- Serum AFP levels elevated in more than 90%

Gross Pathology

- Most unencapsulated with a soft, grey to white to tan cut surface that may appear glistening and have microcystic, hemorrhagic, or necrotic foci of hemorrhage and necrosis are more frequent in postpubertal tumors

Microscopic Pathology

- Several patterns:
  - *Reticular* (microcystic, vacuolated, honeycomb): Most common; a sievelike appearance secondary to prominent cytoplasmic vacuoles; thin cords of neoplastic cells with attenuated cytoplasmic processes create a meshwork of microcysts of varying size; tumor cells with compressed nuclei may have a lipoblastic appearance; stroma is usually myxoid
  - *Macrocystic*: Occurs when microcysts coalesce; microcystic and macrocystic patterns may coexist
  - *Endodermal sinus* (perivascular, festoon): Papillary cores of fibrous tissue with a central vessel covered by a layer of malignant-appearing, cuboidal to columnar cells; papillary structure is typically recessed into a small cystic space that is lined by flattened tumor cells (Schiller-Duval bodies)
  - *Papillary*: Small irregular papillae with fibrous or hyalinized cores lined by low-columnar to cuboidal tumor cells (often appear hobnailed); papillae may project into cystic spaces that frequently contain detached clusters of tumor cells
  - *Solid*: Sheets of polygonal cells with eosinophilic to clear cytoplasm, prominent cytoplasmic borders, and uniform nuclei that do not overlap and have inconspicuous or prominent nucleoli; random pleomorphism may be present; often a prominent vascular network; this pattern resembles seminoma
  - *Glandular-alveolar* (intestinal and endometrioid-like): Usually overlaps with polyvesicular vitelline pattern; glands may have enteric features with pseudostratified columnar cells with eosinophilic cytoplasm and an apical brush border; glandular component can be prominent and complex; nuclei are not as atypical as those in other patterns of yolk sac tumor; basal cytoplasmic vacuolization may be present resulting in a pattern similar to secretory phase endometrium
  - *Myxomatous*: Often seen in conjunction with a reticular pattern; epithelial cells with a stellate or spindled shape are scattered throughout a hypocellular myxoid stroma; prominent blood vessels are present throughout

- *Sarcomatoid* (spindle cell): Sarcomatoid foci may develop in continuity with classic yolk sac tumor patterns, usually reticular or myxomatous
- *Polyvesicular vitelline*: Cysts scattered in a variably cellular mesenchyme that may be edematous or fibrous; cysts often have an eccentric constriction (figure-8 shape); cysts are lined by flattened to columnar epithelium; columnar epithelial cells may have cytoplasmic, basal or apical vacuolation or may have an enteric appearance with a brush border; not a frequent pattern in testicular yolk sac tumors (much more frequent in ovarian yolk sac tumors)
- *Hepatoid*: Present in 20%; small clusters of cells reminiscent of liver cells arranged in nests, tubules, or trabeculae; bile canaliculi may be present; hyaline globules common
- *Parietal*: Neoplastic cells are separated by eosinophilic bands of basement membrane material; residual microcysts may be present

- Reticular and solid patterns most common
- Macrocystic, papillary, and endodermal sinus patterns are more common in childhood tumors than in adult tumors
- Tumor cells characteristically appear to have hyaline eosinophilic globules in their cytoplasm; often occur in clusters

Special Stains

- Intracellular hyaline eosinophilic globules in neoplastic cells are PAS positive and diastase resistant

Immunohistochemistry

- Tumor cells are typically strongly positive for cytokeratin and negative for EMA
- 75% to 100% positive for AFP; staining is cytoplasmic and often weak and focal; hepatoid foci are usually intensely positive for AFP
- Cytoplasmic hyaline eosinophilic globules rarely stain for AFP
- 50% positive for PLAP and α_1-antitrypsin
- Occasionally tumor cells positive for CEA (reactivity localized to cells and glands with enteric features)
- Tumor cells with a spindle cell morphology typically positive for vimentin
- Tumor cells usually negative for CD30 (embryonal carcinoma is almost always positive for CD30)

Electron Microscopy

- Epithelial cells joined by tight junctional complexes and desmosomes
- Cells may form extracellular lumens with apical microvilli
- Intracytoplasmic, non-membrane bound, dense round cytoplasmic globules (corresponding to hyaline globules)
- Cells typically contain conspicuous amounts of glycogen

Molecular Alterations

- Prepubertal tumors lack the i(12p) marker chromosome that is typically seen in postpubertal testicular germ cell tumors
- Frequent abnormalities of chromosomes 1p, 6q, and 3q

Differential Diagnosis

- Seminoma (especially if yolk sac tumor has solid pattern)
- Embryonal carcinoma
- Juvenile granulosa cell tumor
- Immature teratoma
- Sarcomatoid patterns may resemble an unclassified sex cord stromal tumor

Treatment

- Postpubertal patients with yolk sac tumor are treated with orchiectomy with or without retroperitoneal lymph node dissection; patients with negative lymph nodes are followed without adjuvant therapy; patients with positive nodes are given adjuvant chemotherapy
- Pediatric patients are typically treated with radical orchiectomy without retroperitoneal lymph node dissection; chemotherapy is used if relapse occurs

Prognosis

- Yolk sac tumors in prepubertal children are less aggressive than nonseminomatous germ cell tumors in adults
- The presence of a yolk sac tumor component in a stage I mixed germ cell tumor is associated with a better prognosis than is seen with a stage I mixed germ cell tumor without a yolk sac tumor component
- Yolk sac tumor has less metastatic potential than embryonal carcinoma
- Yolk sac tumor is less chemosensitive than embryonal carcinoma
- Some evidence that children under the age of 2 years with yolk sac tumors have a lower mortality than those over the age of 2 years (controversial)

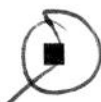

- Stage is the single most important prognostic factor
- 50% of patients with metastatic disease can be cured with chemotherapy
- Relapse typically occurs as a metastasis in the lungs

Associations

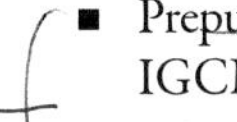

- Prepubertal yolk sac tumors are rarely associated with IGCNU
- Yolk sac tumors in postpubertal patients are almost always associated with IGCNU

Choriocarcinoma

Clinical Manifestations

- Most commonly affects men in their 2nd or 3rd decades (never seen before puberty)
- Rarely seen in pure form (<0.5% of testicular neoplasms)
- Approximately 10% of testicular germ cell neoplasms have foci of choriocarcinoma
- Most patients present with symptoms referable to metastatic disease rather than a testicular mass (tends to disseminate widely before becoming clinically evident at its primary site)
- Presenting symptoms include hemoptysis (pulmonary metastasis), back pain (retroperitoneal spread), gastrointestinal bleeding, or neurologic symptoms (metastasis to the central nervous system)
- 10% present with gynecomastia
- Occasional patients present with symptoms of thyrotoxicosis (similarity of human chorionic gonadotropin [hCG] to thyroid-stimulating hormone)
- Serum levels of hCG higher than 100,000 IU/L typical of pure lesions

Gross Pathology

- On cut section a small, centrally hemorrhagic, necrotic nodule with an ill-defined gray border
- Surrounding testicular parenchyma usually not distorted
- Occasionally entire testis hemorrhagic with or without cystic change
- Cut surface of testis may only reveal a hemosiderin-stained scar

Microscopic Pathology

- Most neoplasms are extensively necrotic and hemorrhagic with relatively small amounts of viable tumor
- Neoplasm is best seen at the periphery where there is typically a mixture of syncytiotrophoblastic and mononuclear cytotrophoblastic cells
- Blood vessel invasion typically prominent
- Cytotrophoblastic cells usually arranged in sheets or small aggregates bordered by multinucleated cells characteristic of syncytiotrophoblastic cells; occasionally the mixture of syncytiotrophoblasts and cytotrophoblasts is random
- Syncytiotrophoblasts are large cells with eosinophilic or amphophilic cytoplasm containing vesicular or deeply chromatic, smudged, irregular nuclei; distinct cytoplasmic vacuoles or lacunae may be present and contain either red blood cells or eosinophilic precipitate; typically not mitotically active
- Cytotrophoblasts tend to be uniform, have a single vesicular nucleus, clear or amphophilic cytoplasm, and well-defined borders (resemble cells of solid variant of yolk sac tumor)

Special Stains

- Not helpful

Immunohistochemistry

- Syncytiotrophoblastic cells always stain positively for hCG; cytotrophoblastic cells generally negative or only weakly positive for hCG
- Syncytiotrophoblastic cells stain positively for inhibin (a marker of sex-cord-stromal tumors) and are frequently positive for EMA (unlike seminoma, embryonal carcinoma, and yolk sac tumor)
- Syncytiotrophoblastic and cytotrophoblastic cells express cytokeratin and CEA
- Approximately 50% of tumors are focally positive for PLAP

Electron Microscopy

- Syncytiotrophoblastic cells have multiple, irregularly shaped nuclei in cytoplasm that contains prominent dilated endoplasmic reticulum that gives the cytoplasm a honeycomblike appearance
- Cytotrophoblastic cells have smooth, round nuclei with cytoplasm that contains short tubular endoplasmic reticulum

Molecular Alterations

- None

Differential Diagnosis

- Hemorrhagic testicular infarction
- Other germ cell neoplasms with syncytiotrophoblastic cells (seminoma and embryonal carcinoma)

Treatment

- Orchiectomy and chemotherapy

Prognosis

- Metastasizes hematogenously (no lymph node involvement); metastatic sites include lungs (most common), liver, gastrointestinal tract, spleen, brain, and adrenal gland
- Worst prognosis of any testicular germ cell tumor
- Chemotherapy can cure some patients

Associations

- None

Teratoma

Clinical Manifestations

- 7% of all germ cell tumors
- 2nd most common germ cell tumor of infancy and childhood (15% to 20% of pediatric GCTs)
- May be seen in postpubertal age group (usually as a component of a mixed germ cell tumor); very rarely occurs in this age group as a pure tumor
- Teratomatous component is present in 50% of all mixed germ cell tumors
- Most present with an enlarged testis
- Presenting symptoms in postpubertal patients may be related to presence of metastatic disease

Gross Pathology

- Pure teratomas are typically nodular
- Extension of neoplasm outside the testis rarely occurs
- Cut surface may have cysts filled with mucus, serous fluid, or keratinous debris admixed with solid areas that may contain obvious areas of cartilage
- Hair is rarely seen except in cases of pure dermoid cyst
- Immature tissues are usually solid with an encephaloid appearance and foci of hemorrhage or necrosis
- Dermoid cysts are rare and are reminiscent of the same lesion that occurs in the ovary (unilocular cyst with keratinous debris and hair with nodules in the inner cyst wall)

Microscopic Pathology

- A germ cell neoplasm consisting of somatic type tissue that is either mature or immature
- *Mature teratoma*
  - Usually contains elements derived from all 3 germ layers
  - Foci of squamous epithelium in a fibrous stroma with or without keratin is common
  - Cysts frequently lined by glandular epithelium (enteric or respiratory)
  - Nests of transitional epithelium may be present
  - Stroma may consist of fibrous tissue or smooth muscle and adipose tissue
  - Foci of neuroglia are common
  - Foci of hyaline cartilage, and occasionally bone, may be present
  - Rarely portions of solid organs may be present (kidney, liver, prostate, pancreas, or thyroid)
  - Mature elements always resemble adult tissue, but usually have increased cellularity, cytologic atypia and occasional mitotic activity
  - Teratomas arising in the prepubertal age group are typically unassociated with other germ cell tumor types and usually have completely mature histologic elements
  - Teratomas arising in the postpubertal age group almost always have some immature elements and are usually associated with other forms of germ cell tumor
  - Intratubular germ cell neoplasm essentially never seen in prepubertal patients with teratoma
  - Intratubular germ cell neoplasm frequently present in postpubertal patients with teratoma
- *Dermoid cyst*
  - Rare in testis, unlike ovary
  - Analogous to the common lesion in the ovary in both gross and microscopic features
  - A lymphogranulomatous reaction usually present
  - Metastases never occur
  - No intratubular germ cell neoplasia or cellular atypia
- *Immature teratoma*
  - Contain elements that resemble normal embryonic tissue of all three germ cell layers
  - Immature elements may be focal, multifocal or diffuse
  - Most common immature elements are neuroepithelium, neuroblastic-type tissue, blastematous tissue (Wilms tumor-like), and rhabdomyoblastic tissue
  - Degree of cellularity and mitotic activity may be quite variable

- *Teratoma with a secondary malignant component*
  - Typically seen in postpubertal patients with immature teratomas
  - Most common secondary malignant neoplasm is a rhabdomyosarcoma (embryonal or alveolar); overgrowth by nephroblastomalike cells may occur
  - Very rarely carcinoma may develop from mature epithelium (adenocarcinoma or squamous cell carcinoma)
  - Development of a carcinoma occurs less frequently in teratomas of the testis than in teratomas of the ovary

Special Stains

- Silver stains may confirm the presence of endocrine cells in enteric glands

Immunohistochemistry

- Focal positivity for AFP may be present in glandular elements
- α_1-antitrypsin may be present in epithelium
- 50% positive for CEA and ferritin

Electron Microscopy

- Not helpful

Molecular Alterations

- i(12p) marker chromosome usually present
- p53 and retinoblastoma gene expression may be present

Differential Diagnosis

- Dermoid and epidermoid cyst (very important in the differential diagnosis because they are both benign) dermoid cysts in postpubertal patients lack immature elements; epidermoid cysts consist of a cyst lined by keratinizing squamous epithelium

Treatment

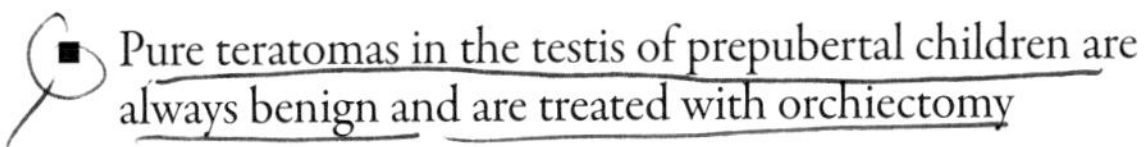

- Pure teratomas in the testis of prepubertal children are always benign and are treated with orchiectomy
- Pure testicular teratomas in postpubertal patients treated with orchiectomy and retroperitoneal lymph node dissection

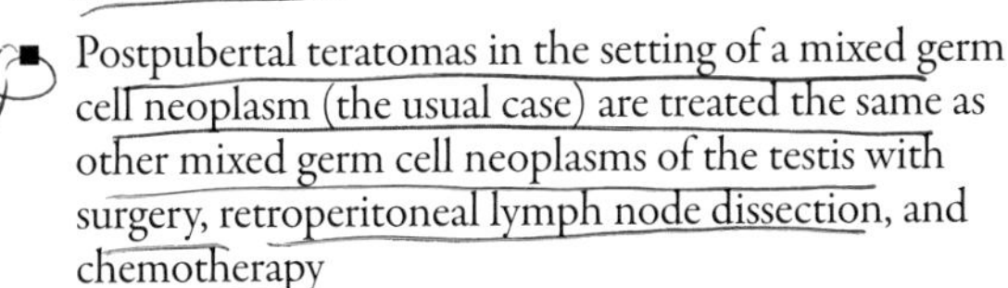

- Postpubertal teratomas in the setting of a mixed germ cell neoplasm (the usual case) are treated the same as other mixed germ cell neoplasms of the testis with surgery, retroperitoneal lymph node dissection, and chemotherapy

Prognosis

- Prepubertal pure teratomas are benign and have an excellent prognosis regardless of the presence of immature elements
- Treatment of a nonseminomatous germ cell tumor with chemotherapy may be followed by the appearance of a metastasis containing pure teratomatous elements
- Teratomatous metastases have a good prognosis after surgical excision

Associations

- Prepubertal teratoma may be associated with inguinal hernia, testicular malformation or maldescent, Down syndrome, Klinefelter syndrome, xeroderma pigmentosa, ataxia, hemihypertrophy, spina bifida, hemophilia, umbilical hernia, and retrocaval ureter

Comment

- Pure teratomas (with or without immature elements) in postpubertal patients have a high incidence of metastasis (unlike a teratoma involving the ovary which can only metastasize if immature elements are present); the histologic features of the metastatic disease may be quite different from the histologic appearance of the teratoma; a pure teratoma can have a metastasis completely free of teratomatous elements and consist of nonteratomatous germ cell elements; conversely a nonteratomatous germ cell tumor can have a metastasis consisting of pure teratoma

Mixed Germ Cell Tumors

Clinical Manifestations

- Represent approximately 30% of all testicular germ cell tumors and 70% to 90% of all nonseminomatous germ cell tumors
- Patients typically present with testicular enlargement with or without pain
- Average age at diagnosis is 30 years (patients with a predominance of embryonal carcinoma present at a slightly younger age than those with the predominance of seminoma)
- Rare before puberty
- 60% have elevated serum levels of AFP
- 55% with metastatic disease have elevated serum hCG levels

Gross Pathology

- Tumors tend to be solid and variegated with gray to white areas that indicate the presence of seminomatous components and areas of necrosis, hemorrhage, and cystic degeneration typically associated with nonseminomatous elements

Microscopic Pathology

- Combination of tumor types including embryonal carcinoma, yolk sac tumor, seminoma, choriocarcinoma, and teratoma
- Embryonal carcinoma is present in almost 95% of all mixed cell germ tumors; teratoma is the next most frequent component (65%); seminoma and yolk sac tumor elements are present in 30% and 25% respectively; choriocarcinoma is present in15%
- Multiple combinations of germ cell types possible: 3 most frequent are embryonal and teratoma, "teratocarcinoma" (~25%); embryonal and seminoma (~15%); and embryonal, teratoma, and yolk sac (~10%)
- Microscopic features of the various components of a mixed germ cell tumor are identical to those seen in the pure germ cell tumors
- Variants:
  - *Polyembryoma*: A mixed germ cell tumor with embryonal carcinoma and yolk sac tumor elements (occasionally with teratomatous elements as well) arranged in a pattern that resembles a presomatic embryo before the 18th day of development; scattered embryolike (embryoid) bodies surrounded by a myxoid mesenchyme; embryolike bodies consist of a central plate of cuboidal to columnar embryonal carcinoma cells of variable thickness, a "dorsal" amnionlike cavity lined by flat epithelium, and a "ventral" yolk sac-like vesicle composed of reticular and myxomatous yolk sac tumor (resembles an embryonic yolk sac)
  - *Diffuse embryoma*: An orderly and intimate admixture of embryonal carcinoma and yolk sac tumor in approximately equal proportions; minor trophoblastic or teratomatous elements may be present

Special Stains, Immunohistochemistry, and Electron Microscopy

- See individual germ cell tumors

Molecular Alterations

- None

Differential Diagnosis

- Adequate sampling ensures that all germ cell elements are represented

Treatment

- The same as for nonseminomatous tumors in general

Prognosis

- Mixed germ cell tumors with a teratomatous component seem to be less aggressive and have a lower rate of metastasis than those without a teratomatous component
- The presence of yolk sac tumor elements in a primary testicular mixed germ cell tumor is associated with a lesser tendency to metastasize
- The higher the percentage of embryonal carcinoma, the worse the prognosis
- Angiolymphatic invasion associated with a worse prognosis

Associations

- None

Sex Cord/Gonadal Stromal Tumors

Leydig Cell Tumor

Clinical Manifestations

- Most common testicular sex-cord stromal tumor
- 2% of all testicular neoplasms
- Occur in all age groups: 20% during 1st decade of life, 25% between the ages of 10 and 30 years, 30% between the ages of 30 and 50 years, and 25% in patients over the age of 50 years
- Patients present with gynecomastia and testicular swelling
- Occasionally patients complain of a decrease in libido or potency
- Children typically present with isosexual pseudoprecocity
- 10% are asymptomatic
- Tumors may produce testosterone (and estrogen)
- 3% bilateral
- 10% to 15% extend beyond the testis at the time of presentation

Gross Pathology

- Usually well-circumscribed, solid, and yellow or tan with a lobulated architecture secondary to the presence of fibrous septa
- 25% have foci of hemorrhage and/or necrosis

Microscopic Pathology

- Diffuse and nodular patterns (determined by the amount of stroma); diffuse pattern has inconspicuous stroma; nodular pattern has prominent, extensively hyalinized stroma
- Stroma may be edematous or myxoid with tumor cells dispersed throughout in irregular clusters and cords
- Tumor cells are typically large and polygonal with abundant, granular, eosinophilic cytoplasm that may be pale, clear, or vacuolated (secondary to the presence of lipid); nuclei tend to be round and have a single prominent nucleolus; nuclear atypia is relatively unusual but may present in up to 30%; mitotic activity tends to be more pronounced when nuclear atypia is present
- Tumor cells may be small with little cytoplasm and grooved nuclei
- Rarely tumor cells are spindle-shaped
- Crystals of Reinke present in cytoplasm of tumor cells in 30% to 35%; 10% to 15% contain lipochrome pigment

Special Stains

- Not helpful

Immunohistochemistry

- Tumor cells are strongly positive for vimentin and inhibin
- Tumor cells show variable immunoreactivity for cytokeratins
- PLAP and EMA negative

Electron Microscopy

- Tumor cells have prominent vesicles of smooth endoplasmic reticulum, mitochondria with tubular cristae, and lipid droplets (all features of a steroid hormone producing cell)
- Reinke crystals may be present (typically geometrically shaped with a striking periodicity)

Molecular Alterations

- None

Differential Diagnosis

- Leydig cell hyperplasia
- Malakoplakia
- Hyperplastic nodules of steroid cells characterized by multifocality, bilaterality, lack of Reinke crystals, and more prominent lipofuscin (typically seen in patients with adrenogenital syndrome and Nelson syndrome the rapid growth of an corticotropin-secreting pituitary adenoma following adrenalectomy for Cushing syndrome)
- Malignant lymphoma
- Plasmacytoma
- Yolk sac tumor
- Tumors with a prominent spindle cell component may be misdiagnosed as sarcoma
- Metastatic carcinoma from the prostate
- Metastatic melanoma

Treatment

- Inguinal orchiectomy
- If malignancy suspected, a retroperitoneal lymph node dissection often performed
- Radiation and chemotherapy usually not effective

Prognosis

- Over 80% are benign
- 10% to 20% behave in a malignant fashion
- Indications that neoplasm may be malignant include:
    - Patient over the age of 60 years
    - Absence of endocrine manifestations
    - Large neoplasms (over 6 cm in diameter)
    - Microscopic features include infiltrative margins, angiolymphatic invasion, foci of necrosis, nuclear atypia, and a high mitotic rate
- Mean survival for patients with malignant tumors 4 years

Associations

- 10% to 15% occur in patients with cryptorchidism
- A rare occurrence in patients with Klinefelter syndrome (Leydig cell hyperplasia is common in Klinefelter syndrome; Leydig cell tumor is quite rare)

Sertoli Cell Tumor (Androblastoma)

Clinical Manifestations

- Fewer than 1% of all testicular neoplasms
- Rarely seen in children under the age of 10 years, but when seen, may present with gynecomastia
- Typically presents as a testicular mass unless associated with another syndrome (see associations later in this section)
- Pure Sertoli cell tumors are rarely associated with endocrine manifestations

Gross Pathology

- Typically a solid, well-circumscribed, tan to yellow to white mass with or without cysts
- Foci of hemorrhage frequent; foci of necrosis rare
- Almost always unilateral and usually confined to the testis

Microscopic Pathology

- Tumor cells form tubules and cords arranged in a diffuse or nested pattern and surrounded by a basement membrane
- Tubules may be hollow and round or solid and elongated and often vary in size and shape (occasionally demonstrate a reticular retiform pattern)
- Neoplastic cells usually have moderate (sometimes abundant) eosinophilic or pale (lipid) cytoplasm; nuclei usually round, oval, or elongated, tend not to be grooved or notched, and usually do not have a particularly prominent nucleolus
- Tumor cells are rarely pleomorphic and/or mitotically active
- Stroma varies from scanty to abundant (when abundant, characterized by dense hyalinized fibrous tissue containing prominent dilated blood vessels)
- Minor calcifications present in 10%
- Occasional tumors are extensively sclerotic with tubules that tend to be small and solid; the sclerotic areas do not have the prominent dilated blood vessels typical of fibrous stroma; these neoplasms are referred to as the *sclerosing variant of Sertoli cell tumor* and represent approximately 15% of all Sertoli cell tumors
- *Large cell calcifying Sertoli cell tumor:* Nests and cords of large polygonal cells with eosinophilic cytoplasm embedded in a myxohyaline stroma with broad areas of calcification; cells have large, vesicular nuclei with prominent nucleoli; 20% malignant; 40% bilateral (see p 511)

Special Stains

- Oil red O stains will highlight the lipid content of tumor cells

Immunohistochemistry

- Sertoli cells are reactive for vimentin (90%), keratin (80%), inhibin (40%), α_1-antitrypsin, and NSE
- Sertoli cells typically negative for EMA

Electron Microscopy

- Sertoli cells have tight junctions, prominent whorls of endoplasmic reticulum, lipid droplets, and interdigitating cell processes
- Charcot-Böttcher filaments, although typical of sertoli cells, rarely present

Molecular Alterations

- None

Differential Diagnosis

- Sertoli cell nodule
- Mixed sex cord tumor
- Stromal tumors
- Adult and juvenile granulosa cell tumor
- Leydig cell tumor
- Seminoma with tubular pattern
- Endometrioid adenocarcinoma
- Adenomatoid tumor
- Metastatic adenocarcinoma

Treatment

- Radical orchiectomy with retroperitoneal lymph node dissection if clinically involved
- Radiation and chemotherapy have not been proven to be of great benefit

Prognosis

- Sclerosing variant of Sertoli cell tumor is inevitably benign as are tumors seen in association with Peutz-Jegher syndrome
- Incidence of malignancy in Sertoli cell tumor, not otherwise specified, is approximately 10% to 15%
- Pathologic features that correlate with a malignant clinical course include large size (>5 cm), necrosis, nuclear atypia, angiolymphatic invasion, and a mitotic rate >5 per 10 high-powered fields

Associations

- Patients with androgen insensitivity syndrome and Peutz-Jeghers syndrome
- Large cell-calcifying variant of Sertoli cell tumor is associated with Carney syndrome

Sertoli-Leydig Cell Tumor

Clinical Manifestations

- Seen in a wide age range (6 months to 7th decade)
- Occasionally associated with gynecomastia

Gross Pathology

- On sectioning, typically solid and yellow with a lobulated appearance

Microscopic Pathology

- Tubules, cords, and trabeculae of Sertoli cells in a background of cellular neoplastic stroma that usually contains foci of Leydig cells
- If the stroma is cellular and neoplastic the presence of Leydig cells is not required to make the diagnosis of Sertoli-Leydig cell tumor
- Retiform pattern and heterologous elements may be present

Special Stains

- Not helpful

Immunohistochemistry

- Both the Leydig cells and Sertoli cells are strongly positive for inhibin

Electron Microscopy

- Sertoli cells have tight junctions, whorls of endoplasmic reticulum, lipid droplets, and interdigitating cell processes
- Leydig cells may contain Reinke crystals

Molecular Alterations

- None

Differential Diagnosis

- Sertoli cell nodule
- Mixed sex cord tumor
- Stromal tumors
- Adult and juvenile granulosa cell tumor
- Leydig cell tumor
- Seminoma with tubular pattern
- Endometrioid adenocarcinoma
- Adenomatoid tumor
- Metastatic adenocarcinoma

Treatment

- Orchiectomy

Prognosis

- 1 reported case of malignancy

Associations

- None

Large Cell Calcifying Sertoli Cell Tumor

Clinical Manifestations

- Mean age at diagnosis 17 years for benign tumor and 39 years for rare malignant tumor
- Most present with mass, gynecomastia, and isosexual pseudoprecocity
- Patients with malignant tumors tend to be older (40 years versus 15 years) and have larger tumors
- Malignant tumors rarely associated with any of the clinical findings of Carney syndrome
- Benign tumors may be bilateral and/or multifocal; malignant tumors almost always unilateral and unifocal

Gross Pathology

- Usually <2 cm in diameter
- May be multifocal and/or bilateral (always in association with Carney syndrome)
- Cut surface reveals a firm, typically well-circumscribed nodule with a yellow to tan, glistening, gritty surface
- Presence of foci of hemorrhage or necrosis may be indicative of malignancy

Microscopic Pathology

- Tumor cells are large and polygonal with abundant eosinophilic, finely granular cytoplasm; tend to be arranged in sheets, nests, trabeculae, cords, and small aggregates
- Nuclei are round or oval with 1 or 2 small nucleoli
- 50% will have areas of intratubular tumor
- Stroma may be loose and myxoid or dense and collagenous
- A prominent neutrophilic infiltrate may be present
- Foci of calcification are usually quite prominent and may be massive with large laminated nodules
- Mitotic activity is relatively rare (unless malignant)

Special Stains

- Not helpful

Immunohistochemistry

- Sertoli cells tend to be reactive for vimentin, keratin, α_1-antitrypsin, neuron-specific enolase (NSE), and inhibin
- Tumor cells are typically negative for EMA

Electron Microscopy

- Confirms the presence of Sertoli cells
- Charcot-Böttcher filament bundles usually seen in the cytoplasm of Sertoli cells

Molecular Alterations

- None

Differential Diagnosis

- Leydig cell tumor
- Sertoli cell nodule (focal, non-neoplastic aggregates of tubules)

Treatment

- Orchiectomy with or without a retroperitoneal lymph node dissection (depending on clinical evidence of retroperitoneal involvement in a neoplasm judged to be malignant)
- Bilateral or multifocal disease tends to be treated more conservatively

Prognosis

- Approximately 15% are clinically malignant

Associations

- 30% to 35% have associated findings of Carney syndrome: Pituitary adenoma (acromegaly and pituitary gigantism), bilateral primary adrenocortical hyperplasia (Cushing syndrome in 20%), testicular Leydig cell tumor and large cell calcifying Sertoli cell tumor (sexual precocity), cardiac myxomas (sudden death), lentigines and blue nevi (spotty mucocutaneous pigmentation), and upper gastrointestinal tract psammomatous melanotic schwannomas; associated large cell calcifying Sertoli cell tumors are usually multifocal and bilateral and almost always benign
- Peutz-Jeghers syndrome (hamartomatous gastrointestinal tract polyps and mucocutaneous pigmentation and predisposition to a wide variety of neoplasms involving the intestine, pancreas, breast, and female genital tract); associated Sertoli cell tumors often have the features of large cell calcifying Sertoli cell tumor but typically lack calcification and tend to more closely resemble sex cord tumor with annular tubules seen in the ovary of females with Peutz-Jeghers syndrome

Tumors Containing Both Germ Cell and Sex Cord/Gonadal Stromal Elements

Gonadoblastoma

Clinical Manifestations

- Almost always occur in patients with dysgenic gonads and intersex syndrome; 80% in phenotypic females, 20% in phenotypic males
- Patients typically have female internal genitalia that result from persistent Müllerian duct-derived structures
- 40% bilateral (frequency of bilaterality in phenotypic males slightly less)
- Gonads typically have the features of mixed gonadal dysgenesis (unilateral streak gonad or streak testis and contralateral testis or bilateral streak testis)
- Phenotypic females typically virilized
- Phenotypic males present under the age of 20 years with feminizing symptoms (gynecomatasia, hypospadias, and cryptorchidism)

Gross Pathology

- 25% are microscopic
- When grossly visible, usually brown to yellow to gray with a soft, fleshly consistency
- Cartilagelike areas and gritty calcifications may be present
- Areas of hemorrhage or necrosis may represent the presence of an invasive germ cell tumor

Microscopic Pathology

- Typically an admixture of germ cells resembling seminoma cells and small, immature Sertolilike cells arranged in round to irregularly shaped nests that contain hyaline deposits of basement membrane that are surrounded by sex cord cells
- Less often the sex cord cells are arranged peripherally around a nest of seminomalike cells or surround individual seminomalike cells within the nest (a pattern reminiscent of a primary ovarian follicle)
- Calcifications in 80%
- Leydiglike cells (without Reinke crystals) in the periphery of 65%
- Typical invasive germ cell tumors (most commonly invasive seminoma) may develop from a gonodoblastoma (the presence of coarse calcifications in an invasive germ cell tumor is an indication that it likely arose from a gonadoblastoma)

Special Stains

- None

Immunohistochemistry

- Seminomalike cells stain for PLAP
- Sertolilike cells stain with cytokeratins and vimentin
- Basement membrane material stains with laminin
- Some of the sex cord cells stain with inhibin

Electron Microscopy

- Immature Sertoli cells may contain Charcot-Böttcher filaments

Molecular Alterations

- Y chromosome almost always present, usually as 45,X/46,XY mosaicism or 46,XY

Differential Diagnosis

- Sertoli cell nodule with IGCNU
- Unclassified germ cell (sex cord) stromal tumor

Treatment and Prognosis

- Bilateral gonadectomy curative unless germ cell neoplasm present

Associations

- Approximately 50% incidence of progression to invasive germinoma (seminoma or dysgerminoma)
- 5% to 10% progress to embryonal carcinoma, yolk sac tumor, or teratoma

Tumors of Paratesticular Structures

Adenomatoid Tumors

- *Epididymis*
    - Most common neoplasm of this organ
    - Most patients are between the 3rd and 4th decade of life
    - Presents clinically as a mass (sometimes associated with pain)
    - On gross examination, a small (usually <2 cm), solid, firm, gray-white nodule, occasionally containing small cysts
    - Microscopically, lesion is unencapsulated and on rare occasions may involve adjacent testis; a proliferation of cells ranging from cuboidal to flattened, which form solid cords with an epithelial appearance alternating with channels having dilated lumina simulating vascular structures; intervening stroma may contain abundant smooth muscle and elastic fibers, may have a reactive desmoplastic quality and be infiltrated by inflammatory cells; tumor cells exhibit prominent cytoplasmic vacuolization
    - Immunohistochemically, strong reactivity for keratin, epithelial membrane antigen (EMA) and calretinin; negative for carcinoembryonic antigen (CEA) and factor VIII-related antigen
    - By electron microscopy, tumor cells have prominent microvilli, desmosomes, and tonofilaments
    - Cell of origin probably mesothelial
    - Generally regarded as benign; frequent coexistence of chronic inflammation and fibrosis suggests that in some cases the lesion may represent a peculiar form of nodular mesothelial hyperplasia
    - Important differential diagnosis includes epithelioid (histiocytoid) hemangioma (the latter lesion is immunoreactive for factor VIII and CD34 and usually negative for keratin)
    - Behavior is invariably benign even when the lesion extends into the testis
- *Urinary bladder/prostatic urethra*
    - Mesonephroid (adenomatoid, nephrogenic) metaplasia
    - Traditionally regarded as a benign neoplasm and designated a nephrogenic adenoma, but most likely represents a localized or diffused metaplastic change of urothelium in response to chronic infection, calculi, or prolonged catheterization
    - Often seen in association with cystitis cystica or glandularis
    - On gross examination, lesions can be papillary, polypoid, or sessile
    - About 20% are multiple
    - Microscopically, small tubular formations lined by cuboidal and hobnail cells having a light microscopic and ultrastructural appearance remarkably similar to mesonephric tubules
    - Main differential diagnosis is with adenocarcinoma of mesonephroid (clear cell) type
- *Adrenal gland*
    - Has been reported in a primary adrenal location
    - Nature most likely mesothelial

- *Fallopian tube*
  - Usually a small lesion within the wall of the tube
  - Gross and microscopic features identical to those of its epididymal counterpart
  - Ill-defined, seemingly infiltrating margins may lead to mistaken diagnosis of carcinoma
  - A marked degree of smooth muscle hyperplasia may be present and obscure the true nature of the lesion
  - Lesion represents a unique variant of benign mesothelioma largely restricted to the genital region
- *Uterus*
  - Identical to those more commonly seen in the fallopian tube
  - Usually small (<2 cm) and lie beneath the serosa close to the cornua
  - Microscopically, adenoid, angiomatoid, solid, and cystic patterns occur singly or in combination; often accompanied by smooth muscle hypertrophy and may be confused with leiomyomas
- *Ovary*
  - Can occur in an intra- or juxta-ovarian location
  - Can simulate the appearance of yolk sac tumor

References

Dabbs DJ. *Diagnostic Immunohistochemistry.* New York: Churchill Livingstone, 2002.

Eble JN, Sauter G, Epstein JI, Sesterhenn IA (eds). *World Health Organization Classification of Tumours. Pathology and Genetics of Tumours of the Urinary System and Male Genital Organs.* Lyon: IARC Press, 2003.

Mills S, Carter D, Greenson JK, Oberman HA, Reuter V, Stoler MH (eds). *Sternberg's Diagnostic Surgical Pathology. 4th ed.* Philadelphia: Lippincott Williams & Wilkins, 2004.

Rosai J. *Rosai and Ackerman's Surgical Pathology. 9th ed.* St. Louis: Mosby, 2004.

Ulbright TM, Amin MB, Young RH. *Tumors of the Testis, Adnexa, Spermatic Cord, and Scrotum; Atlas of Tumor Pathology, 3rd Series. Fascicle 25.* Washington DC: Armed Forces Institute of Pathology, 1999.

Young RH, Scully RE. *Testicular Tumors.* Chicago: ASCP Press, 1990.

Chapter 16

Urinary Tract

Intraoperative Consultation

Most intraoperative consultations rendered on specimens from the urinary tract are requested to determine the presence of appropriate margins of excision and the need for staging. The diagnosis is generally well established in the vast majority of patients undergoing surgery for neoplastic disease of the kidney, bladder, and prostate. Intraoperative consultation to confirm the diagnosis of a renal cell carcinoma can usually be made on gross examination without the need for a frozen section unless the mass is small and found incidentally. Lesions with an atypical gross appearance, such as an oncocytoma, or an extensively cystic lesion may not be amenable to frozen section diagnosis and consequently often result in a deferred diagnosis until permanent sections are available.

Urothelial carcinomas of the upper urinary collecting system are typically treated with a nephroureterectomy with an excision of a cuff of bladder. Occasionally intraoperative consultation to determine the adequacy of the margins of the ureter or bladder cuff are appropriate.

An intraoperative consultation to confirm the presence or absence of metastases in regional lymph nodes does not change the indicated operative procedure of a radical nephrectomy if the lesion is resectable.

Approximately 5% of Wilms tumors are bilateral. This condition is treated with a radical nephrectomy on one side and a partial nephrectomy on the other. Intraoperative consultation on the partial nephrectomy specimen is warranted to evaluate the adequacy of surgical margins (the same issue applies to the surgical margins of a renal cell carcinoma treated by partial nephrectomy).

Radical cystectomy specimens are submitted for frozen section primarily to determine a presence of dysplasia or carcinoma at the ureteral and uretheral margins. If dysplasia is present, additional ureteral tissue is taken until the margins are negative. This is particularly important when a neo-bladder is to be constructed. There is essentially no indication for frozen section diagnosis on a partial cystectomy. The diagnosis is usually well established prior to the procedure, and the presence of dysplasia is generally not an issue because if it is present at the surgical margins the surgeon is most likely to treat the patient with postoperative intravesical chemotherapy rather than extending the partial cystectomy.

Prostate carcinoma is treated with a radical prostatectomy in a majority of cases when the carcinoma is confined to the gland. A more conservative, nerve-sparing procedure may be performed in the setting of a unilateral carcinoma. A radical prostatectomy is generally felt not to be appropriate for carcinomas with obvious extension of cancer beyond the gland or clinically detectable metastatic disease in pelvic lymph nodes. The majority of intraoperative consultations involve the evaluation of the prostatic apex and bladder neck for adequacy of excision. Occasionally, pelvic lymph nodes are submitted to determine the presence of metastatic disease.

Intraoperative consultation on pelvic lymph nodes in patients with prostate cancer are indicated in the following circumstances:

- A large pelvic lymph node is found at surgery. If it contains metastatic cancer, a radical proctectomy will not be performed. If the enlarged node does not contain carcinoma, a pelvic lymph node dissection is performed.
- If it is agreed during the preoperative discussion between patient and surgeon that a radical prostatectomy will not be performed in the presence of nodal metastasis of any size, even grossly involved pelvic lymph nodes will be submitted for frozen section. (Both surgeon and pathologist must realize that the false-negative rate for detecting micrometastasis in a "suspicious" pelvic lymph node is 30%.)

The evaluation of the apical surgical margin and bladder base margin of a prostatectomy specimen by frozen section can be quite difficult if the patient has undergone preoperative treatment with a nonsteroidal antiandrogens and luteinizing hormone-releasing hormone (LHRH) analogues. These modalities of preoperative treatment may reduce the incidence of positive margins in subsequently resected prostate glands. From the pathologist's perspective, the regressive changes that occur in the prostate make recognizing the presence of carcinoma quite difficult and may result in an interpretative error.

Specimen Handling

All surgical margins of both radical nephrectomy specimens and partial nephrectomy specimens should be inked. In partial nephrectomy specimens, the distance between the tumor and the surgical margin should be measured before sections are taken. If the surgical margin is less than 0.5 cm, several sections should be taken at right angles to the margins so that the closest distance to the neoplasm from the margin can be measured under the microscope. These principles apply to both intraoperative consultations as well as to the submission of tissue for permanent sections.

The adequacy of partial cystectomy specimens is generally best determined by taking 2 to 3 mm sections parallel to the margins. Invasive carcinoma anywhere within such a section should be interpreted as a positive margin. Biopsies from sites distant from the main neoplasm are taken to determine the presence of dyplasia.

The significance of ureteral margins in a radical cystectomy specimen has been discussed under the heading of intraoperative consultation.

Prostatectomy specimens are inked in two to three colors with the right lobe, left lobe and base each being colored differently. The bladder base and apex sections are removed separately for margin evaluation. The seminal vesicle sections are also removed separately for staging purposes. The gland is then serially sectioned from the base to the apex and each cassette is labeled with the portion of gland it contains.

Kidney

Pediatric Tumors and Tumorlike Conditions

Nephroblastoma (Wilms Tumor)

Clinical Manifestations

- Affects males and females equally with a mean age at diagnosis of 3 years for males and 3.5 years for females; 90% are diagnosed before the age of 6
- Unusual in neonates and infants
- More common in blacks than whites
- Represents the most common genitourinary cancer in children (80% of GU neoplasms in patients under the age of 15 years)
- Both kidneys are affected equally
- Patients typically present with an abdominal mass and occasionally with pain, hematuria, hypertension, and symptoms related to rupture (usually traumatic)

Gross Pathology

- Tumor is typically solitary and round with a sharply defined border that represents a pseudocapsule
- Cut surface of tumor tends to be soft, friable, gray to tan, and bulges from the surface
- Foci of hemorrhage and necrosis are often present but are rarely a dominant feature
- Tumors consisting primarily of mature stromal elements tend to be firm and have a whorled appearance on cut section
- Tumors frequently distinctly lobulated as a result of prominent fibrous septa
- Cystic spaces may be prominent
- 7% multicentric; 5% bilateral
- Adhesions to adjacent organs often present
- Neoplasm frequently extends into the renal vein and metastases to regional lymph nodes

Microscopic Pathology

- Neoplasm arises from nephrogenic blastemal cells that differentiate along several lines to include *blastemal, epithelial, and stromal*
- Relative proportions of each of the cell types varies from tumor to tumor and the degree of differentiation within each cell type is also quite variable
- Triphasic patterns are most characteristic but biphasic and monophasic lesions are not unusual
- *Blastemal pattern:*
  - Almost always present to some degree
  - Cells are small, densely packed and mitotically active; little evidence of differentiation into recognizable epithelial or stromal structures
  - Blastemal cells may be arranged in diffuse, serpentine, nodular, and/or basaloid patterns
  - Diffuse blastemal pattern: small cells densely packed together with a cohesive appearance; tend to be quite vascular and not particularly aggressive; a vague suggestion of tubular formation may be present; cells tend to be rounded but may be slightly elongated with regular nuclei that are small, round or oval; chromatin may be slightly coarse but is evenly distributed; nucleoli are usually small; mitotic figures are extremely numerous; occasionally sheets of cells show less cohesiveness, are less well circumscribed, and have a more aggressive pattern with invasion into adjacent tissue and blood vessels
  - Serpentine blastemal pattern: a common component; characterized by wavy cords of blastemal cells within a loose, myxoid or fibromyxoid stroma; cells tend to be cohesive and cords of cells are usually sharply defined
  - Nodular blastemal pattern: resembles the serpentine pattern except that the cells are arranged in round islands; well-defined tubules may be present in the central areas of these islands of blastemal cells
  - Basaloid blastemal pattern: blastemal cells in either a serpentine or nodular pattern bordered by a distinctive epithelial layer

- *Epithelial pattern:*
  - Epithelial structures resemble developing collecting ducts, nephrons and glomeruli in the fetal kidney; the degree of differentiation can be quite variable; epithelial differentiation can contain mucinous, squamous, and/or ciliated elements
- *Stromal pattern*:
  - Spindle cells that resemble embryonic mesenchyme within a myxoid background are present in almost all nephroblastomas; smooth muscle, mature fibroblasts, and skeletal muscle (most common) may be present; various types of stromal differentiation may be present to include: adipose, cartilage, bone, osteoid, mature ganglion cells and neuroglial tissue (findings reminiscent of a teratoma)
- Tumors may contain areas of anaplasia defined as extreme nuclear atypia (probably represents the presence of hypertetraploid DNA content); diagnosis of anaplasia requires: 1) presence of multipolar mitotic figures and 2) marked nuclear enlargement with nuclei being at least three times that of non-anaplastic nuclei in other microscopic fields; anaplasia is present in approximately 5% of tumors, but is rare in tumors diagnosed during the first 2 years of life; more common in patients over the age of 6 years

Special Stains

- Not helpful

Immunohistochemistry

- Blastemal cells typically express vimentin and may express NSE; other differentiation markers usually absent

Electron Microscopy

- Nephroblastoma cells resemble cells of the developing metanephros
- Blastemal cells often have well-developed cell junctions and numerous organelles
- A layer of thick, flocculent, electron dense material frequently is found adherent to the blastemal cell surface

Molecular Alterations

- A deletion in chromosome 11p13 found in patients with WAGR syndrome and Denys-Drash syndrome
- 11p15.5 (WT2)
- Other chromosomal abnormalities involve chromosomes 1, 12, and 8
- Abnormalities of 16q (may represent a third nephroblastoma locus)

Differential Diagnosis

- Neuroblastoma (represents most frequent differential diagnosis problem)
- Lymphoma
- Mesoblastic nephroma
- Clear cell sarcoma
- Rhabdoid tumor
- Neurogenic tumors
- Renal carcinoma, oncocytic tumors
- Angiolipoma
- Nephroblastoma with heterologous patterns:
  - Teratoma
  - Mesothelioma
  - Synovial sarcoma
  - Hepatoblastoma
  - Pancreatoblastoma
  - Intra-abdominal desmoplastic small round cell tumor

Treatment

- Stage I and II lesions (tumor confined to the kidney or tumors that can be completely resected) with favorable histology are treated with nephrectomy and adjuvant chemotherapy consisting of dactinomycin and vincristine
- Stage I tumors with unfavorable histology (diffuse anaplasia) are also treated with nephrectomy and adjuvant chemotherapy
- Stage II disease with unfavorable histology and stage III to V disease are treated with nephrectomy if possible, radiotherapy and more toxic chemotherapeutic agents (doxorubicin included)
- Lung metastases typically excised (to confirm diagnosis) followed by radiation
- Actively proliferating and embryonal cell types in blastemal cell populations typically respond well to chemotherapy
- Mature tubular and skeletal muscle cells and anaplastic cells are typically not affected by chemotherapy

Prognosis

- Most signficant factors that contribute to an unfavorable prognosis include age at diagnosis, high stage, and presence of unfavorable histology
- Prognosis not affected by tumor size or weight
- Cells with anaplastic nuclei are more resistant to chemotherapy; presence of anaplasia not a sign of increased aggressiveness
- *Focal anaplasia* is confined to one or more sites in the primary tumor with surrounding cells that have no nuclear or mitotic abnormalities
- *Diffuse anaplasia* characterized by non-localized anaplastic changes, anaplasia in invasive or metastatic sites, and anaplasia at edge of one or more sections

Associations

- Conditions associated with an increased risk for the development of nephroblastoma include:
  - *WAGR syndrome*: increased susceptibility to *W*ilms tumor, *a*niridia, *g*enital anomaly, *r*etardation
  - *Beckwith-Wiedemann syndrome*: enlargement of body organs, hemihypertrophy, renal medullary cysts, and abnormal large cells in adrenal cortex (adrenal cytomegaly)
  - *Denys-Drash syndrome*: glomerulonephritis (renal failure), ambiguous genitalia (male pseudohermaphroditism), streak gonads, and increased susceptibility to Wilms tumor
  - Familial nephroblastoma
- Conditions associated with a *possible* increased risk for the development of nephroblastoma include:
  - Renal malformations
  - Genital malformations
  - Cutaneous nevi, angiomas
  - Trisomy 18
  - Neurofibromatosis
  - Cerebral giantism
  - *Klippel-Trenaunay syndrome:* (port-wine stain, varicose veins, and bony or soft tissue hypertrophy, typically involving one extremity, usually a leg
  - *Bloom syndrome*: (autosomal recessive disorder characterized by hypersensitivity to DNA-damaging agents, such as ionizing radiation; affected individuals typically have short stature, narrow face with prominent nose, skin color changes in face after exposure to sunlight, butterfly-shaped facial rash, high pitched voice, increased susceptibility to infections and respiratory illnesses, increased susceptibility to cancer and leukemia, and occasionally mental retardation

Mesoblastic Nephroma

Clinical Manifestations

- A congenital neoplasm usually diagnosed within three months of birth; rarely diagnosed after a year
- Affects both sexes equally
- Occasionally patients present with hypercalcemia secondary to excessive production of prostaglandin E by the neoplasm
- Entrapped renal elements within the neoplasm may result in hyperreninism

Gross Pathology

- Typically a single, well-demarcated, unilateral mass; may extend beyond renal capsule
- Cut surface may be either soft or firm and typically bulges above the surrounding normal kidney; often resembles a leiomyoma (grossly indistinguishable from nephroblastoma)
- Foci of cystic change, hemorrhage, and necrosis typically present
- Most centered near the hilus and usually involve the renal sinus

Microscopic Pathology

- 2 variants: classic and cellular
- *Classic variant*
  - Characterized by tumor cells that resemble fibroblasts and myofibroblasts and are typically arranged in moderately dense, intersecting fascicles with interspersed thin collagen fibers
  - Mitotic activity variable
  - Margins of the neoplasm are often irregular and bands or tongues of cells extend into the surrounding renal parenchyma entrapping, but not compressing or distorting renal structures

- Neoplasm may extent into adjacent perinephric fat where the advancing edge is typically characterized by angiomatous vascular proliferation
- Small nodules of hyaline cartilage, squamous metaplasia, and foci of extramedullary hematopoiesis often present

- *Cellular variant* (more common than the classic variant)
  - Characterized by densely packed spindled cells with a high mitotic rate; cellular patterns may coexist with classic pattern
  - Tend to be more sharply circumscribed than the classic tumors and usually consist of pleomorphic plump cells with large, vesicular nuclei and abundant eosinophilic cytoplasm
  - A blue cell subtype of the cellular variant resembles infantile fibrosarcoma

Special Stains

- Not helpful

Immunohistochemistry

- Tumor cells of both the classic and the cellular variants are consistently positive for vimentin, often for actin, and rarely for desmin.
- CD34 negative
- Only elements of trapped epithelium are positive for epithelial markers

Electron Microscopy

- Tumor cells are elongated mesenchymal cells with prominent anastomosing, rough endoplasmic reticulum
- Thin cytoplasmic filaments and primitive cell junctions
- Basal lamina is typically absent

Molecular Alterations

- Abnormalities of chromosome 11, 8 and 17 the most frequent finding (a similar genetic abnormality has been reported in congenital fibrosarcoma of the lower extremity); usually increased ploidy
- Cellular mesoblastic nephroma (not classic) demonstrares chromosome translocation t(12;15)(p13;q25)

Differential Diagnosis

- Treated nephroblastoma (especially one with a major component of well-differentiated spindled stroma)
- Rhabdoid tumor

Treatment

- Wide surgical resection with particular attention to the medial aspect of the nephrectomy specimen (mesoblastic nephromas which tend to be centered near the hilus almost always involve the renal sinus and extend into structures medial to the kidney)

Prognosis

- Both recurrence and metastases are uncommon (~5%); occasional reports of metastasis to the lung and brain
- Local recurrence typically occurs within one year of surgery; often confined to the flank and result from incomplete surgical resection
- Patients over the age of 6 months are more likely to have highly cellular lesions and have a higher recurrence rate than younger patients

Associations

- Occasionally seen in patients with Beckwith-Wiedemann syndrome (enlargement of body organs, hemihypertrophy, renal medullary cysts, and abnormally large cells in the adrenal cortex [adrenal cytomegaly]); not seen in other syndromes associated with Wilms tumor
- Hydramnios common during pregnancy

Clear Cell Sarcoma

Clinical Manifestations

- Represent 5% of primary pediatric renal neoplasms
- Peak incidence in the second year of life; rare during the first six months of life and rare in adolescents
- Males affected more frequently than females (1.3:1)
- Not associated with any specific malformations, chromosomal defects, genetic abnormalities, or unusual syndromes

Gross Pathology

- Always unilateral and unicentric
- Rarely involves the renal vein

- Interface between the neoplasm and kidney well-defined and the neoplasm usually confined within the renal capsule
- Typically arises from deep in the medullary regions of the kidney and diffusely infiltrates renal sinus soft tissue
- On sectioning, neoplasm is firm and light brown or gray, homogeneous and gelatinous
- Neoplasms tend to have an irregular surface but are not multinodular
- Cysts may be present and represent a major component of the neoplasm

Microscopic Pathology

- Cell of origin unknown; probably arises from primitive nephrogenic mesenchyme
- Histologic patterns include: classic, epithelioid, spindled, sclerosing, cystic, palisading, sinusoidal (pericytomatous), and pleomorphic (anaplastic)
- *Classic pattern:*
  - Tumor cells tend to be arranged in cords or nests separated by evenly dispersed, arborizing capillary-sized vascular channels (fibrovascular septa); numerous intracytoplasmic and intercellular vesicles are evenly scattered throughout the neoplasm; these *vesicles are a major feature of almost all the variants of this neoplasm* and are either empty or appear filled with a pale-staining or granular, acidophilic mucopolysaccharide
  - Tumor cells are typically uniform, clear, round to polygonal, have indistinct cell borders, and have nuclei that tend to be uniform with finely granular and evenly dispersed chromatin (may appear empty); nucleoli typically small and indistinct; fine nuclear grooves may be present
  - Tumor cells tend to infiltrate short distances into adjacent renal parenchyma (despite the gross appearance of a distinct margin)
  - Mitotic activity is variable
  - Blood vessel invasion is not a prominent feature
  - Individual nephrons or collecting ducts may be entrapped within the neoplasm, especially at periphery (easily mistaken for the tubules of a nephroblastoma)
- *Epithelioid pattern:*
  - May be seen as a component of the classic pattern with discrete hypercellular nodules arranged in cohesive ribbons and occasionally rosettes or tubular structures
  - As condensation of cells increase, distinct ribbons that vary from one to several cells in width develop
- *Spindled pattern:*
  - Results from a combination of spindle cell expansion of the septa of the classic pattern and elongation of the cord cells
  - When spindle cell expansion predominates, the cord cells may disappear; resulting pattern is one of intersecting spindle cell bundles (reminiscent of mesoblastic nephroma or other spindle cell neoplasm)
- *Sclerosing pattern:*
  - Characterized by abundant collagenous sclerosis
  - Sclerosis is usually limited to cord cells with preservation of their original dimensions as well as preservation of the original vascular septa (a "chicken-wire" pattern)
  - Bundles of collagen can be so extensive as to isolate small groups of cells in a dense matrix that may become hyalinized
- *Cystic pattern:*
  - Unlined cysts may result from accumulation of interstitial mucopolysaccharide
  - Cysts lined by renal tubular epithelium result when entrapped nephrons or collecting ducts dilate
  - Cysts lined by pseudoepithelial structures result from the accumulation of mucosubstances within the ribbons of the epithelioid pattern
- *Palisading pattern:*
  - Present in 15%
  - Characterized by focal arrays of parallel spindle cell nuclei alternating with nuclear free zones (resemble the nuclear palisades of neurilemomas)
- *Sinusoidal (pericytomatous) pattern:*
  - Characterized by markedly distended blood vessels giving the neoplasm the appearance of a hemangiopericytoma
- *Pleomorphic (anaplastic) pattern:*
  - Tumor cells are huge with polypoid nuclei and multipolar mitotic figures
  - Occasionally seen in metastatic foci following therapy

Special Stains

- Not helpful

Immunohistochemistry

- Tumor cells frequently positive for vimentin
- Tumor ells negative for epithelial markers, even in epithelioid variants (entrapped renal tubules will be strongly positive for cytokeratin)
- Neural and muscle stains negative

Electron Microscopy

- Tumor cells contain few intermediate filaments and incompletely formed cell junctions
- Vesicles that appear to be intracytoplasmic in usual H&E preparations are actually extracellular

Molecular Alterations

- Most are diploid

Differential Diagnosis

- Nephroblastoma (epithelioid pattern)
- Mesoblastic nephroma (spindled pattern)
- Rhabdoid tumor (sclerosing pattern)
- Schwannoma (palisading pattern)
- Hemangiopericytoma (sinusoidal pattern)

Treatment

- Wide surgical excision with adjuvant chemotherapy that includes doxorubicin

Prognosis

- With appropriate surgery and chemotherapy (most include doxorubicin), survival approximates 70%
- When the neoplasm recurs it tends to do so after a long interval (as long as five years; late recurrence is especially frequent in children treated with doxorubicin); 30% recur after 2 years
- Metastasis to bone in 15% to 20% (especially skull, spine, ribs, and femur); other metastatic sites include regional lymph nodes, brain, lungs, liver, soft tissue (periorbital fat and skeletal muscle of both the trunk and extremities), testis and salivary gland

Associations

- None

Rhabdoid Tumor

Clinical Manifestations

- Represent 2.5% of pediatric renal neoplasms
- Median age at diagnosis approximately one year; 90% are diagnosed under the age of three years
- Males more frequently affected than females (1.5 to 1)
- May be associated with hypercalcemia resulting from secretion of parathormone or prostaglandin E_2 from the neoplasm

Gross Pathology

- Usually soft, pale, tan to yellow with a bulging cut surface
- Tend to be relatively uniform and well-demarcated from adjacent renal parenchyma; no capsule
- Small neoplasms usually arise in the renal medulla
- Typically unicentric and unilateral but multiple satellite nodules representing secondary implants may be present
- Rarely bilateral (synchronous or metastatic)

Microscopic Pathology

- Tumor cells tend to be arranged in loosely cohesive sheets; cells are large and polygonal with abundant acidophilic cytoplasm and distinct cell borders; nuclei tend to be large (occasionally lobulated) and vesicular with very large prominent nucleoli
- Many (but not all) of the tumor cells have eosinophilic cytoplasmic inclusions that have a fibrillary texture; cells with inclusions tend to cluster together rather than be uniformly distributed throughout the tumor
- Growth pattern tends to be infiltrative with invasion of local blood vessels and soft tissue
- Rarely tumor cells are organized into distinctive cords or tubule-like structures (similar to nephroblastoma)
- Areas of necrosis with preservation of cells around blood vessels may be present (giving the neoplasm a superficial resemblance to the serpentine blastemal pattern of nephroblastoma)
- Stroma tends to be densely collagenous and may be hyalinized
- Basophilic ground substance may be present to such a degree that the neoplasm appears to contain chondroid differentiation
- Occasionally infiltrates of eosinophils or multinucleated histiocytes may be present

- Variant patterns include sclerosing (fibrotic, osteosarcomatoid and chondroid), epithelioid (trabecular, mucoid, alveolar, and pseudoglandular), spindled (broad vesicular, myxoid, pericytomatous, storiform, and palisading), and lymphomatoid (solid and histocytoid)

Special Stains

- Not helpful

Immunohistochemistry

- Tumor cells usually positive for vimentin, cytokeratins, and epithelial membrane antigen (EMA)
- Occasionally tumor cells positive for neural markers, desmin, and actin

Electron Microscopy

- Tumor cells contain prominent aggregates of intermediate filaments seen as tightly whorled structures adjacent to the nucleus (represent eosinophilic cytoplasmic inclusions on H&E)
- Primitive cell junctions are usually present

Molecular Alterations

- 80% have loss of heterozygosity on 22q11-12
- Monosomy of chromosome 22 has been reported
- Aberrations of chromosome 11p15.5

Differential Diagnosis

- Desmoplastic small round cell tumor
- Components of nephroblastoma, mesoblastic nephroma, and clear cell sarcoma
- Renal neoplasms:
  - RCC with rhabdoid differentiation
  - Mesoblastic nephroma
  - Rhabdomyosarcoma
- Extrarenal neoplasms:
  - Rhabdomyosarcoma
  - Leiomyosarcoma
  - Neuroendocrine tumor
  - Synovial sarcoma
  - Melanoma
  - Large cell lymphoma

Treatment

- Aggressive surgical excision

Prognosis

- A highly malignant neoplasm with a very aggressive growth pattern and a tendency to disseminate early and metastasize widely; metastasis occur by way of both lymphatics and blood vessels
- 75 to 80% mortality; most within one year of diagnosis

Associations

- Separate primary tumors of primitive neuroepithelial origin that resemble medulloblastomas occur in the midline of the posterior or middle cranial fossa in 15%
- Some cases associated with cutaneous lesions ("neurovascular hamartoma")

Adult Tumors and Tumorlike Conditions

Renal Cell Carcinoma

Clinical Manifestations

- Males affected twice as frequently as females; mean age at presentation 60 years
- Most neoplasms remain clinically occult for most of their lifespan
- When disease is advanced, patients manifest the "classic triad" of hematuria (~ 85%), flank pain (20 to 45%), and a palpable flank mass (up to 50%)
- Occasionally patients will present with a scrotal mass secondary to a varicocele resulting from obstruction of the spermatic vein
- Other nonspecific symptoms include fever, weight loss, fatigue, nausea and vomiting, neuropathy, and muscle tenderness
- 30% present with the signs of metastatic disease
- Polycythemia (typically erythrocytosis) is seen in 6% (2 to 4% of patients with polycythemia have renal cell carcinoma)
- 70% have a normochromic normocytic anemia unrelated to blood loss
- Occasionally patients present with hypercalcemia as a result of the production of parathyroid hormone-like substances by the neoplasm

Variants

- Clear cell (conventional) renal cell carcinoma
- Multilocular cystic renal cell carcinoma
- Papillary renal cell carcinoma (chromophil)
- Chromophobe renal cell carcinoma
- Carcinoma of the collecting ducts of Bellini
- Renal medullary carcinoma
- Renal carcinoma associated with Xp11.2 translocations/*TFE3* gene fusions
- Mucinous tubular and spindle cell carcinoma

Gross Pathology

- *Clear cell (conventional) renal cell carcinoma:*
  - Most common histologic variant (60 to 70%)
  - Most are solitary and randomly distributed in the renal cortex
  - Both kidneys affected equally
  - 4% are multicentric; bilaterality occurs in 0.5 to 3%
  - Multicentricity and bilaterality are associated with von Hippel-Lindau syndrome (see below)
  - Neoplasm typically protrudes from the renal cortex as a rounded, bosselated pushing mass (rarely infiltrative)
  - Cysts are frequently present but separated from the neoplasm
  - On cut section the tumor typically has a golden yellow appearance secondary to the lipid content of the tumor cells (cholesterol, neutral lipids and phospholipids are all present); areas of necrosis, cystic degeneration, hemorrhage and calcification are usually present (calcification may occur in the necrotic zones and is present in 10 to 15%)
- *Multilocular cystic renal cell carcinoma*
  - Well-circumscribed mass of small and large cysts filled with serous or hemorrhagic fluid and separated from the kidney by a fibrous capsule
- *Papillary renal cell carcinoma (chromophil):*
  - Represents 10 to 15%
  - Typically larger than 3 cm and may be multiple
  - Usually well-circumscribed and eccentrically located in the renal cortex; 80% confined to the cortex at the time of surgery
  - Cut surface usually yellow (a function of the number of lipid-laden macrophages in the stroma)
  - 60% have areas of hemorrhage and necrosis
  - A higher association with cortical adenomas than other renal cell carcinomas
- *Chromophobe renal cell carcinoma:*
  - Represents approximately 5%
  - Tumors have a mean diameter of 8 cm
  - Always well-circumscribed and solitary
  - Cut surface tends to be brown and devoid of areas of hemorrhage and necrosis
- *Carcinoma of the collecting ducts of Bellini*
  - <1%
  - Generally located in the medulla but may invade the cortex
  - Typically distorts adjacent calyces
  - Hemorrhage and necrosis not typically present
  - May have a multicystic appearance secondary to dilated tubular structures
- *Renal medullary carcinoma*
  - Tend to be poorly circumscribed and located in the medullary portion of the kidney
  - Usually gray-white with foci of hemorrhage and necrosis
- *Xp11.2 translocation carcinoma*
  - Typically tan-yellow and necrotic
- *Mucinous tubular and spindle cell carcinoma*
  - Well-circumscribed, tan-gray, and uniform

Microscopic Pathology

- *Clear cell (concential) renal cell carcinoma*:
  - Well-differentiated neoplasms tend to have a uniform pattern that is predominantly alveolar or acinar; rounded aggregates of cells are peripherally demarcated by a network of delicate capillaries supported by a network of thin reticulin fibers
  - Poorly differentiated tumors are characterized by solid sheets of neoplastic cells with zones of hemorrhage, necrosis and fibrosis
  - Tumor cells are filled with lipids and cholesterol which dissolve during fixation leaving a clear cytoplasm surrounded by a distinct cell membrane

- Cells with intracytoplasmic globules that resemble Mallory bodies usually present
- Tumor cell nuclei tend to be round and uniform with evenly distributed and finely granular chromatin; nucleoli may be absent, sparse, or large and prominent depending upon the degree of differentiation (see Fuhrman grading system)
- *Sarcomatoid variant:* characterized by interlacing or whorled bundles of spindle cells that may be arranged in a storiform pattern (resemble different types of malignant fibrous histiocytoma); poorly differentiated carcinomatous component may be present and distinctly separate from the spindle cell component (occasionally the transition from the carcinoma to sarcomatoid area quite indistinct)
- *Granular cell variant:* tumor cells have abundant acidophilic or chromophilic cytoplasm and fairly well-defined cell borders and are arranged either in solid sheets or in an alveolar pattern with interspersed focal areas of necrosis; nuclei often high grade, pleomorphic, and have coarsely granular chromatin and prominent nucleoli; mitoses uncommon; lipid and glycogen may be present (usually a minor component)

- *Multilocular cystic renal cell carcinoma:*
  - Cysts lined by a single layer of flat or plump, epithelial cells with clear or pale cytoplasm; cysts may lack an epithelial lining
- *Papillary renal cell carcinoma (chromophil):*
  - Neoplastic cells tend to be arranged as a single layer on fibrovascular stalks
  - Generally the entire tumor is papillary, but tubules may be present
  - Lipid-laden macrophages (foam cells) tend to accumulate in and expand the fibrovascular stalks
  - Areas of tumor necrosis may result in large quantities of lipid and cholesterol crystals
  - Psammoma bodies are often abundant
  - Type 1: Tumor cells tend to be small and cuboidal with darkly acidophilic or slightly basophilic cytoplasm; cells with clear cytoplasm are relatively unusual; cytoplasm of neoplastic cells away from areas of hemorrhage may contain hemosiderin; nuclei tend to be small, regular and low-grade; large, hyperchromatic, and pleomorphic nuclei unusual
  - Type 2: Nuclei of tumor cells tend to be stratified with high nuclear grade and abundant eosinophilic cytoplasm
- *Chromophobe renal cell carcinoma:*
  - Tumor cells tend to be arranged in broad alveoli and have well-defined borders and abundant cytoplasm (actually appear distended with cytoplasm that has numerous microvesicles and a pale acidophilic staining pattern—a plant-like appearance); nuclei tend to be coarsely granular with wrinkled nuclear membranes and perinuclear halos with occasional prominent nucleoli
  - Usually there is an admixture of pale transparent cells and brightly acidophilic cells; the transparent cells tend to be oriented along vascular septa
- *Carcinoma of the collecting ducts of Bellini:*
  - An admixture of tubules and papillae lined by a single layer of cuboidal cells with a high nuclear grade and a hobnail or cobblestone appearance
  - Tubule pattern tends to be dominant and gives the tumor the appearance of a sponge
  - Occasionally tumors composed of anastomosing tubules with pleomorphic and hyperchromatic cells may infiltrate adjacent renal parenchyma and cause a pronounced desmoplastic response
- *Renal medullary carcinoma*
  - Typically tumor consists of poorly differentiated areas of sheets of cells growing in a reticular pattern (yolk-sac like appearance) or in a pattern reminiscent of adenoid cystic carcinoma
  - Cells usually eosinophilic with clear nuclei and a prominent nucleolus
  - Tumor cells may have a squamoid or rhabdoid appearance and neutrophils are often admixed with the tumor; lymphocytes tend to surround the tumor at its advancing edge
  - Between and throughout the tumor there is an edematous or collagenous stroma
  - Most tumors contain droplets of cytoplasmic mucin and sickled red blood cells
- *Xp11.2 translocation carcinoma*
  - Papillary architecture with clear cells; frequently have a nested pattern with eosinophilic cells; tumor cells typically have voluminous clear to eosinophilic cytoplasm, sharp cell borders, vesicular chromatin, and prominent nucleoli; psammoma bodies often extensive

- *Mucinous tubular and spindle cell carcinoma*
  - Tightly packed , small, elongated tubules in a pale mucinous stroma; tumor cells small, spindled and/or cuboidal with low-grade nuclear features (lack obvious cytologic atypia)
- Fuhrman grading system:
  - Grade I: nuclei round, uniform, approximately 10 μm; nucleoli inconspicuous or absent
  - Grade II: nuclei slightly irregular, approximately 15 μm; nucleoli evident
  - Grade III: nuclei very irregular, approximately 20 μm; nucleoli large and prominent
  - Grade IV: nuclei bizarre and multilobulated, 20 μm or greater; nucleoli prominent; chromatin clumped
  - The entire neoplasm is classified by the highest grade of any of its component cells regardless of its prevalence

Special Stains

- *Clear cell (conventional) renal cell carcinoma:*
  - Lipid and cholesterol content of tumor cells can be seen in unfixed material using oil red O and Sudan IV reactions
  - Phospholipid components can be identified with Sudan black B reactions
  - Glycogen can be identified by PAS
- *Papillary renal cell carcinoma:*
  - Areas of necrosis rich in lipid and cholesterol crystals can be highlighted with oil red O and Sudan IV reactions
  - Neoplastic cells with large quantities of hemosiderin can be highlighted with an iron stain
- *Chromophobe renal cell carcinoma:*
  - Microvesicles in the cytoplasm of both types of chromophobe cells (strongly acidophilic and slightly acidophilic) can be stained with Hale colloidal iron (confirming the presence of mucopolysaccharides)

Immunohistochemistry

- *Clear cell (conventional) renal cell carcinoma:*
  - Tumor cells usually react with antibodies to low molecular weight cytokeratins, EMA, vimentin, carbonic anhydrase (G250), CD10, and placental alkaline phosphatase (PLAP)
  - Tumor cells typically negative for high molecular weight cytokeratins, CK 7 and CK 20, CEA, inhibin, and S-100 protein
  - Tumor cells do not react with antibodies to Tamm-Horsfall protein
- *Multilocular cystic renal cell carcinoma*
  - Tumor cells positive for cytokeratins and EMA
- *Papillary renal cell carcinoma:*
  - Staining pattern similar to clear cell type, except CK 7 positive in majority of cases
  - P504S (AMACR) usually positive
- *Chromophobe cell carcinoma*:
  - Tumor cells stain positively with antibodies for CK 7, EMA, and carbonic anhydrase and negatively for vimentin
- *Carcinoma in the collecting ducts of Bellini:*
  - Tumor cells react positively to antibodies for both high and low molecular weight cytokeratins and EMA; CK 5/6 negative
- *Renal medullary carcinoma* Typically positive for keratin AE1/AE3 and EMA; CEA usually positive
- *Xp11.2 translocation carcinoma*
  - Nuclei stain for TFE3 protein, RCC marker and CD10
  - Only 50% express cytokeratin and EMA and labelling is often focal
- *Mucinous tubular and spindle cell carcinoma*
  - Positive for CK7, CK18, CK19, EMA
  - CD10 usually negative

Electron Microscopy

- *Clear cell (conventional) renal cell carcinoma:*
  - Tumor cells have microvilli on the luminal aspect of the cell membrane
  - Abundant cytoplasmic glycogen and lipid droplets are present
  - Cytoplasmic organelles (Golgi and rough endoplasmic reticulum) are usually absent
- *Papillary renal cell carcinoma (chromophil):*
  - Presence of lipid-laden macrophages in the papillary cores and cells with hemosiderin can be confirmed
- *Chromophobe renal cell carcinoma*:
  - Tumor cells are rich in complex cytoplasmic vesicles and mitochondria; vesicles tend to be arranged

around the nucleus; mitochondria tend to be localized to the periphery of the cytoplasm adjacent to the cell membrane

Molecular Alterations

- Clear cell and granular cell renal cell carcinomas have abnormalities of chromosome 3, the most common being a deletion in the short arm beginning at 3p13
- Papillary renal cell carcinoma has abnormalities that consist of trisomy of chromosome 17 and trisomy or tetrasomy of chromosome 7
- von Hippel-Lindau gene located on chromosome 3p25.5
- A BRC/ABL gene rearrangement has been described in renal medullary carcinoma

Differential Diagnosis

- If renal cell carcinoma is small and of papillary type:
  - Renal cortical adenoma
  - Renal cell carcinomas with cells having an oncocytic appearance (granular cell type or chromophobe cell type):
  - Oncocytoma
- Collecting duct carcinomas
  - Papillary type renal cell carcinoma
  - Renal medullary carcinoma
- Sarcomatoid variants of RCC
  - Mesenchymal tumors
  - Melanoma
  - Fibrous renal tumors with chondrosarcomatous or osteosarcomatous elements (designated carcinosarcomas)
- Metastatic sarcomatoid renal cell carcinoma:
  - Primary fibrous histiocytoma
- Metastatic papillary renal cell carcinoma:
  - Primary thyroid carcinoma
- Metastatic clear cell renal cell carcinoma:
  - Primary skin and lung tumors
  - Cerebellar hemangioblastoma
- Medullary carcinoma
  - Collecting duct carcinoma

Treatment

- Radical nephrectomy with removal of any tumor extending into the renal vein and/or vena cava
- Renal medullary carcinoma treated with surgery with or without chemotherapy or radiation (adjuvant therapy of any kind has done little to improve survival)
- A small subset of advanced metastatic RCC benefit from interleukin-2 based immunotherapy

Prognosis

- Factors that adversely affect prognosis include:
  - Large size
  - Infiltrative margin
  - Extension into the renal vein, with or without invasion of the vein wall (has little effect on short-term survival but may decrease survival beyond 10 years)
  - Lymph node metastasis
- Overall survival of 50% for clear cell type with a low Fuhrman grade
- Conventional RCC with granular cytoplasm tend to have a high cytologic grade and are associated with vascular invasion and distant metastasis; prognosis is worse than for clear cell tumors
- Papillary type tumors tend to be well-differentiated; 80% are confined to the kidney at the time of diagnosis; some tendency for late recurrence; type 1 tend to have good prognosis; type 2 usually present with advanced disease
- Chromophobe tumors usually localized to the kidney; survival is better than 80%
- Sarcomatoid variant has the worst prognosis with few survivals beyond one year; high incidence of metastasis to bone and soft tissue of the extremities
- Collecting duct carcinoma: 50% will die from metastasis despite the fact the tumors tend to be localized to the kidney and have only a moderate degree of cellular anaplasia
- Average life span after surgery with medullary carcinoma 15 weeks; metastases occur by way of both lymphatics and blood stream; lung most common metastatic site

Associations

- Other renal diseases, malformations and paraneoplastic syndromes

- Cysts (usually a cortical retention cyst), but also acquired or hereditary polycystic disease
- Acquired polycystic disease in patients on chronic hemodialysis (usually occur after a mean of 3.5 years of dialysis)
- 40% to 55% of patients with von Hippel-Lindau syndrome have RCCA: tumors tend to be bilateral and multicentric and often associated with cysts and angiomyolipomas; 30% of patients with von Hippel-Lindau syndrome die of renal cell carcinoma
- Hepatic disease is seen in 20% and consists of an enlarged liver with chemical studies revealing an elevated alkaline phosphatase, increase indirect bilirubin, increased α-2 globulin and decreased prothrombin time; microscopic changes in the liver include a nonspecific portal infiltrate of chronic inflammatory cells, Kupffer cell hyperplasia and vascular dilatation (peliosis)
- Familial cases have been reported
- Risk factors:
  - Obesity (especially females)
  - Smoking
  - Hypertension
  - Estrogen therapy
  - Prolonged exposure to petroleum products, heavy metals and asbestos
  - Renal medullary carcinoma ssociated almost exclusively with sickle cell trait

Angiomyolipoma

Clinical Manifestations

- A choristoma (a disordered arrangement of mature tissue appearing at a site in which that tissue does not normally occur)
- Represents 0.5% to 2% of all renal tumors
- Women outnumber men (2:1) in sporadic cases; no sex predilection in tuberous sclerosis patients with AML
- Average age at diagnosis approximately 40 years
- Many are asymptomatic; symptomatic patients most typically present with flank pain related to intratumoral or retroperitoneal hemorrhage
- Tumors have been found in the renal capsule (capsulomas), attached to the renal capsule, in the retroperitoneum without attachment to the kidney, and in abdominal organs such as liver, fallopian tubes, spleen, and regional lymph nodes; the presence of this neoplasm in extrarenal sites is probably evidence of multicentricity rather than metastases
- CT scan very sensitive for detection of the fatty component

Gross Pathology

- Typically the lesion resides within the kidney and replaces a portion of the renal parenchyma
- Larger tumors compress surrounding structures
- Neoplasms may rupture into the renal calyces or renal vein and may extend into the renal collecting system, renal vein, or vena cava
- Most are solitary; 20% are multiple
- Most are well circumscribed but not encapsulated
- Occasionally renal tubular elements may be entrapped as the tumor expands; these entrapped tubular elements may dilate and form cysts (a feature associated with tuberous sclerosis)
- On cut surface the lesion is lobular and yellow and may appear slightly oily (fat); tumors composed primarily of smooth muscle may be pale gray and firm
- Small foci of hemorrhage common

Microscopic Pathology

- Neoplasm is composed of a random mixture of blood vessels, interlacing fascicles of smooth muscle, and islands of adipose tissue
- Mature adipose tissue typically makes up the majority of the tumor; fat necrosis, lipid-laden macrophages, and giant cells all frequently present
- Smooth muscle component is usually intimately associated with the outer layers of the muscular walls of blood vessels from which they seem to arise; they tend to be arranged in a radial fashion with their long axis perpendicular to the vessels; smooth muscle cells may have some nuclear enlargement, hyperchromasia and scattered mitoses; occasionally the smooth muscle component will be immature (leiomyoblasts) with rounded nuclei and clear or eosinophilic, granular cytoplasm
- Blood vessels often have very thick, abnormal walls; the muscular wall of the blood vessel may be replaced by dense fibrous connective tissue (the arteries resemble arterialized veins similar to those seen in arteriovenous malformations); the internal elastic lamina is usually either fragmented or absent; vessels tend to be tortuous and have walls that are focally thin and dilated resulting in small cirsoid aneurysms

- *Epithelioid variant*: potentially malignant and characterized by a predominance of large, polygonal, ganglion-like cells with densely eosinophilic cytoplasm (occasionally with focal clearing) and nuclei that often have marked atypia and mitotic activity; extensive necrosis and hemorrhage frequently present *[renal epithelioid oxyphilic neoplasm (REON)]*
- Extrarenal tumors are identical to those that occur in the kidney

Special Stains

- PAS with diastase may reveal presence of granules and rod-shaped crystals in perivascular epithelioid cells

Immunohistochemistry

- Smooth muscle cells positive for actin, desmin, and melanoma associated antigens HMB-45 and Melan-A (MART-1) and C-*kit*
- S-100 and epithelial markers negative

Electron Microscopy

- Cytoplasmic granules and crystals in epithelioid cells morphologically similar to renin granules, but do not stain with antibodies to renin
- Occasionally spherical structures with internal lamellations (reminiscent of abnormal melanosomes) present

Molecular Alterations

- NF-1 gene on chromosome 17
- NF-2 gene on chromosome 22q12
- von Hippel-Lindau gene on chromosome 3p25-26
- Gene for tuberous sclerosis on chromosomes 9q34 and 16p13

Differential Diagnosis

- Grossly resemble renal cell carcinoma
- Epithelioid variant may resemble both oncocytoma and RCCA with granular cytoplasm or rhabdoid differentiation

Treatment

- Total surgical excision

Prognosis

- Benign
- May cause progressive renal failure and/or a massive hemorrhage
- Metachronous lesions may appear in the remaining kidney after nephrectomy
- Epithelioid angiomyolipoma a potentially malignant mesenchymal neoplasm; 30% to 40% metastasize to regional lymph nodes, liver, or lung

Associations

- Tuberous sclerosis (subependymal hamartoma and giant cell astrocytoma, cardiac rhabdomyomas, angiomyolipomas, mental retardation, epilepsy, cutaneous hamartomas primarily involving head and neck, shagreen skin, depigmented spots, and subungual fibromas of the fingers)
  - 80% of patients with tuberous sclerosis will have angiomyolipomas
  - <1/2 of patients with angiomyolipomas will have tuberous sclerosis syndrome
- Tumors tend to be multiple and bilateral
  - von Recklinghausen disease
  - von Hippel-Lindau syndrome
  - Autosomal dominant (adult) polycystic disease
  - Related to several mesenchymal neoplasms: lymphangioleiomyomatosis, clear-cell sugar tumors of lung ("sugar tumor"), pancreas and uterus (PEComa family of tumors—perivascular epithelial cell tumors that are immunoreactive for HMB-45)

Metanephric Adenoma

Clinical Manifestations

- A benign cortical neoplasm
- Seen anywhere between the first decade of life to the ninth
- Females are more commonly affected than males (2:1)
- Polycythemia is seen in 10 to 15%

Gross Pathology

- Well-circumscribed, but not encapsulated, cortical mass usually surrounded by a thin capsule
- Solid with an overall gray-tan appearance

- Focal areas of necrosis, hemorrhage or cystic degeneration may be present
- Calcifications may be seen grossly
- Rarely multifocal and never bilateral

Microscopic Pathology

- Characterized by densely packed, collapsed, small tubules separated by a modest amount of hyalinized stroma
- Tumor cells have small, round or oval, overlapping nuclei with little or no cytoplasm; nucleoli are usually inconspicuous
- Mitotic figures are rare
- Papillary or glomeruloid structures are present in approximately 50% and may be associated with microcalcifications (psammoma bodies)
- Secondary changes of hyalinization, hemorrhage and necrosis commonly present
- *Metanephric adenofibroma* is a biphasic tumor composed of an epithelial component identical to that of a nephrogenic adenoma and a stromal component that consists of interlacing fascicles of bland fibroblast-like cells with focal areas of hyalinization and myxoid change (resembles a mesoblastic nephroma)

Special Stains

- Not helpful

Immunohistochemistry

- Tumor cells are typically pan-cytokeratin and vimentin positive; CK 7 negative
- Tumor cells EMA negative although areas with papillary and/or cystic tubular configurations may be positive

Electron Microscopy

- Tumor cells have varying numbers of microvilli and few cytoplasmic organelles consisting primarily of free ribosomes and mitochondria

Molecular Alterations

- Reports of trisomy of chromosome 7 and 17 and loss of sex chromosomes
- No abnormalities of 11p (argues against any relationship to Wilms tumor)

Differential Diagnosis

- Wilms tumor
- Solid papillary (chromophil) renal cell carcinoma (CK 7 and EMA positive)
- Renal carcinoid

Treatment

- Simple or partial nephrectomy

Prognosis

- A benign neoplasm with no reports of malignant transformation

Associations

- Polycythemia (10%-15%)
- 5% to 10% have a concurrent clear cell renal cell carcinoma either in the ipsilateral or contralateral kidney

Renal Cortical Adenoma (Tubulo-Papillary Adenoma)

Clinical Manifestations

- Usually incidental finding at autopsy (~20%)

Gross Pathology

- <0.5 cm in greatest dimension and located just beneath the capsule of the kidney
- May be multiple
- Unencapsulated, but well-circumscribed

Microscopic Pathology

- Characterized by a tubulo-papillary architecture consisting of densely packed tubules lined by small, cuboidal shaped and round cells with uniform nuclei; no cytologic atypia
- Mitotic figures rare
- Interface between neoplasm and normal renal parenchyma typically devoid of any significant inflammation or stromal reaction
- Occasionally a primarily papillary architecture with psammoma bodies
- Xanthoma cells may be present in the stroma between the tubular or papillary structures

Special Stains, Immunohistochemistry, and Electron Microscopy

- Do not help differentiate this lesion from a renal cell carcinoma

Molecular Alterations

- None

Differential Diagnosis

- Renal cell carcinoma, papillary type

Treatment

- Local excision

Prognosis

- May represent an early renal cell carcinoma, papillary type (the presence of a benign epithelial neoplasm of the kidney that can actually be distinguished from renal cell carcinoma is quite controversial)

Associations

- Associated with kidney scarred from chronic pyelonephritis or renal vascular disease
- Seen in children with von Hippel Lindau syndrome
- May be incidental finding in patients with renal cell carcinoma

Comment

- Caution is advised when an intraoperative consultation is requested. Small lesions are best called "tubulo-papillary" neoplasm of low malignant potential".

Oncocytoma

Clinical Manifestations

- Represent 3% to 7% of all renal tumors
- Occur twice as often in men as in women
- Average age at diagnosis 60 years (approximately 5 years older than the average age of diagnosis of renal cell carcinoma)
- Most patients are asymptomatic
- Symptomatic patients present with flank or abdominal pain (20%) gross hematuria (10% to 15%), flank or abdominal mass (20%) and/or microscopic hematuria (20%)

Gross Pathology

- Typically well-demarcated, homogeneous, and mahogany brown
- Larger tumors usually have a depressed, central zone of scar that may have foci of cystic change
- Usually solitary and unilateral; 3% to 5% multicentric (unilateral or bilateral)
- Occasionally seen coexisting with a renal cell carcinoma or angiomyolipoma
- Areas of hemorrhage and necrosis are not characteristic features

Microscopic Pathology

- Tumor cells typically plump and arranged in alveolar-type nests, trabeculae, or tubules
- Neoplastic cells have granular, acidophilic cytoplasm and small, round, uniform nuclei that measure $<10\mu$ in diameter with finely granular and evenly dispersed chromatin; nucleoli are inconspicuous
- An infiltrative growth pattern with an inflammatory or desmoplastic response never present
- Central scar consists of mature hyalinized fibrous tissue that may entrap nests of tumor cells
- Mitotic figures, clear cells and necrosis extremely rare
- Variants:
  - Scattered aggregates of oncocytic appearing cells that appear incompletely differentiated may be present within the neoplasm; these cells have less cytoplasm and hence appear to have a greater nuclear density; nuclei tend to be slightly larger than the nuclei of typical oncocytes and occasional mitotic figures may be present; typically a gradual transition between these less differentiated appearing oncocytes and more typical oncocytes is apparent
  - Foci of oncocytes with hyperchromatic and frequently bizarre nuclei may be present as single cells or as small groups of cells (oncocytosis); nuclei contain inconspicuous or absent nucleoli and mitotic figures are rarely present (most likely a symplastic or degenerative change)

Special Stains

- Phosphotungstic acid stain (PTAH) or Sudan B black will highlight the lipochrome pigment associated with mitochondria that fill the cytoplasm and give it its densely eosinophilic color

Immunohistochemistry

- Tumor cells express cytokeratin 8, 14 and 18, CD3 and mitochondrial markers (MES-13 and 113-1); cytokeratin 7 usually negative or just focally positive in small clusters of cells, and cytokeratin 20 always negative

Electron Microscopy

- Oncocytes are packed with lipochrome pigment in association with large mitochondria but lack other organelles (oncocytes do not have well-developed endoplasmic reticuli, lipid, glycogen, or abundant Golgi apparatus)

Molecular Alterations

- Deletion of chromosome 1 coupled with loss of Y most common

Differential Diagnosis

- Renal cell carcinoma with oncocytic and/or chromophobic features (a positive reaction to Hale colloidal iron will typically identify a chromophobe cell carcinoma)
- Epithelioid angiomyolipoma
- Eosinophilic variant of chromophobe RCCA (diffusely positive for CK 7)
- RCCA with granular or oncocytic features

Treatment

- Large neoplasms typically treated with simple nephrectomy
- Smaller tumors known to be oncocytomas can be treated expectantly or by percutaneous ablation

Prognosis

- A benign tumor that typically manifests little in the way of progressive disease even when left untreated

Associations

- May coexist with renal cell carcinoma or angiomyolipoma
- No association with von Hippel-Lindau disease, tuberous sclerosis, or chronic dialysis

Medullary Fibroma (Renomedullary Interstitial Cell Tumor)

Clinical Manifestations

- Typically an incidental finding in adults at autopsy (incidence may approach 50%)

Gross Pathology

- A small, pale grey to tan, well-circumscribed spade-shaped lesions located in the center of medullary pyramids
- May be multiple
- Usually <0.3 cm in diameter

Microscopic Pathology

- Tumor cells are typically small, stellate or polygonal and lie within a loose, bland stromal background that may be loosely or densely collagenized and may contain entrapped medullary tubules at the periphery
- Occasionally lesions are extensively hyalinized and almost acellular
- Amyloid may be present

Special Stains

- The presence of neutral fat, phospholipid and acid mucopolysaccharides can be confirmed
- Congo red may confirm presence of amyloid

Immunohistochemistry

- Not helpful

Electron Microscopy

- Tumor cells contain large numbers of electron-dense lipid droplets

Molecular Alterations

- None

Differential Diagnosis

- None

Treatment and Prognosis

- A completely benign tumor of little or no clinical significance

Associations

- Multiple medullary fibromas probably associated with systemic hypertension

Cystic Nephroma

Clinical Manifestations

- Most affected adults are female (8:1)
- Typically asymptomatic; may present as a palpable abdominal mass
- Hematuria a rare presenting symptom

Gross Pathology

- Well circumscribed; typically 5 to 10 cm in greatest dimension
- Consists of several noncommunicating cysts that vary in size and contain clear fluid
- Solid, expansile mural nodules; foci of hemorrhage and necrosis never present

Microscopic Pathology

- Lesion sharply circumscribed from adjacent renal parenchyma
- Cysts lined by flattened, cuboidal, or hobnail cells
- Fibrous septa of varying cellularity course around the cysts; may have the appearance of ovarian-type stroma
- Septa may contain microscopic cysts lined by bland cuboidal cells resembling renal tubules
- Foci of cartilage may be present

Special Stains

- Not helpful

Immunohistochemistry

- Cells lining cysts positive for cytokeratin
- Stroma usually positive for estrogen and progesterone receptors

Electron Microscopy

- Not helpful

Molecular Alterations

- None

Differential Diagnosis

- Polycystic kidney disease
- Multilocular cystic renal cell carcinoma
- Dysplasic kidney
- cystic partially differentiated nephroblastoma

Treatment and Prognosis

- Total resection

Associations

- Cystic nephromas may undergo sarcomatous transformation (rare)

Glomerular Diseases

Acute Proliferative (Poststreptococcal, Postinfectious) Glomerulonephritis

Etiology and Pathogenesis

- An immunologically mediated disease
- Certain strains of group A β-hemolytic streptococci are nephritogenic (90% of cases can be traced to serotypes of group M types 1, 2, 12, 49, 55, 57, and 60)
- One or more of the streptococcal products are elevated in most patients
- Complement levels (CH50, C3) are low
- The streptococcal antigenic component elicits an immune reaction with the formation of immune complexes that are deposited or formed in the glomeruli

Clinical Manifestations

- Patients typically present with the nephritic syndrome characterized by hematuria, red cell casts in urine, azotemia, oliguria, mild to moderate hypertension, proteinuria and edema (less severe than in nephrotic syndrome)
- Typical presentation is that of a young child who suddenly develops malaise, oliguria, hematuria, and rarely nausea and fever one to two weeks after recovering from a sore throat

- Adults are more likely to present with hypertension, edema and an elevation in blood urea nitrogen
- The disease may follow a streptococcal infection (can be confirmed by the presence of elevated titers of antistreptococcal antibody, and/or a decline in serum concentration of C3 in the presence of cryoglobulins in the serum), other bacterial infections (staphylococcal endocarditis, pneumococcal pneumonia, and meningococcemia), viral disease (hepatitis B, hepatitis C, mumps, HIV infection, varicella, and infectious mononucleosis) and parasitic infections (malaria and toxoplasmosis)

Gross and Microscopic Pathology

- Classically the glomeruli are enlarged and hypercellular [hypercellularity is caused by infiltration of leukocytes (neutrophils and monocytes) and to a much lesser degree by proliferation of endothelial cells, mesangial cells and epithelial cells]
- Both the proliferation and leukocyte infiltration are diffuse and involve all lobules of the glomeruli
- Endothelial cells swollen and capillary lumens obliterated (endocapillary proliferation)
- Small deposits of fibrin usually present within capillary lumens and mesangium
- Interstitial edema and inflammation usually present and tubules often contain red blood cell casts

Special Stains

- Trichrome stain may demonstrate subepithelial fuchsinophilic deposits (humps)

Immunofluorescence

- Focal and sparse "lumpy" granular deposits of IgG, IgM and C3 in the mesangium and along the basement membrane

Electron Microscopy

- "Humps" of discrete, amorphous, electron-dense deposits on epithelial side of the basement membrane (represent antigen-antibody complexes at the epithelial cell surface)
- Subendothelial, intramembranous, and mesangial deposits are also present

Molecular Alterations

- None known

Treatment and Prognosis

- 95% of children will recover with conservative therapy designed to maintain normal sodium and water balance
- 1% of children develop rapidly progressive glomerulonephritis
- 1% to 2% progress slowly to chronic glomerulonephritis
- Adults have a worse prognosis than children: 60% quickly recover; the remainder have persistent proteinuria, hematuria and hypertension

Associations

- Infection with group A β-hemolytic streptococci
- Other bacterial infections (staphylococcal endocarditis, pneumococcal, and meningococcemia, viral disease (hepatitis B and C, mumps, HIV infection, varicella, and infectious mononucleosis, and parasitic infections [malaria, toxoplasmosis])

Rapidly Progressive (Crescentic) Glomerulonephritis

Etiology and Pathogenesis

- Most of the glomerular injury is immunologically mediated
- Type I RPGN: an antiglomerular basement membrane disease characterized by antibiodies against the NC1 domain of α3 type IV collagen in the basement membrane and complement activation; antiglomerular basement membrane antibodies cross react with pulmonary alveolar basement membranes to produce pulmonary hemorrhages in association with renal failure (Goodpasture syndrome)
- Type II RPGN: severe immune complex-mediated injury with crescents can complicate any of the immune complex nephritides (postinfectious glomerulonephritis, SLE, IgA nephropathy, and Henoch-Schönlein purpura)
- Type III RPGN: pauci-immune type; characterized by the lack of antiglomerular basement membrane antibodies or immune complexes; most patients have antineutrophil cytoplasmic antibody (ANCA) in their serum which some have suggested causes glomerular injury

Clinical Manifestations

- Characterized by a rapid and progressive loss of renal function with severe oliguria

- Patients present with hematuria, red cell casts in urine, moderate proteinuria [may reach nephrotic range (3.5 gm or more of protein)] and variable hypertension and edema
- Patients with Goodpasture syndrome may present with pulmonary hemorrhage

Gross and Microscopic Pathology

- Kidneys are usually enlarged, pale and have foci of petechial hemorrhage on their cortical surfaces
- Classically glomeruli are collapsed and contain a crescent-shaped mass of proliferating cells and leukocytes internal to Bowman capsule
- Crescents are formed by the migration of monocytes and macrophages into Bowman space and to a lesser extent by the proliferation of parietal cells
- Strands of fibrin are prominent both between the cells of the crescents and in Bowman space

Special Stains

- Trichrome and silver stains may demonstrate deposits in type II rapidly progressive glomerulonephritis

Immunofluorescence

- Type I: Goodpasture syndrome has linear IgG and C3 deposits
- Most cases of type II have granular staining of the glomerular basement membrane with IgG and C3
- Idiopathic cases (type III) have little or no immune deposits (pauci-immune)

Electron Microscopy

- Type I and Type III may have wrinkling of the glomerular basement membrane with focal disruptions in its continuity and lack discrete electron dense deposits
- Type II has granular electron dense deposits in the glomerular basement membrane and/or mesangium

Molecular Alterations

- None

Treatment and Prognosis

- Renal involvement is typically progressive ending with severe oliguria within a matter of weeks
- Recovery may follow intensive plasmapheresis in combination with steroids and cytotoxic agents
- Many patients eventually require chronic hemodialysis or transplantation

Associations

- Type II may represent a complication of postinfectious glomerulonephritis, SLE, IgA nephropathy, or Henoch-Schönlein purpura
- Type III pauci-immune type may represent a component of a systemic vasculitis such as Wegener granulomatosis or microscopic polyarteritis

Membranous Glomerulonephritis (Membranous Glomerulopathy)

Etiology and Pathogenesis

- A chronic antigen-antibody-mediated disease
- Antigen-antibody complexes form "in-situ" in the glomerular capillary wall between the basement membrane and the overlying epithelial cells (podocytes)

Clinical Manifestations

- Most common cause of nephrotic syndrome in adults
- Typically presents with insidious onset of nephrotic syndrome or less frequently with non-nephrotic proteinuria
- 15% to 35% will have hematuria and mild hypertension
- Secondary membranous glomerulonephritis may be associated with:
  - Drugs: penicillamine, captopril and gold
  - Underlying malignant tumor (especially carcinoma of the lung, colon and melanoma)
  - Systemic lupus erythematosus (15% of the glomerulonephritis that results from SLE are of the membranous type)
  - Infectious (chronic hepatitis B, hepatitis C, syphilis, schistosomiasis, malaria)
  - Metabolic disorders (diabetes mellitus and thyroiditis)

Gross and Microscopic Pathology

- Early in the course of disease the glomeruli appear normal or have a uniform, diffuse, thickening of the glomerular capillary wall
- As the disease advances, the membrane thickening encroaches on the capillary lumen; eventually the glomeruli become completely hyalinized
- Epithelial cells of the proximal tubules contain hyaline droplets (result of protein reabsorption)
- Interstitial inflammation consisting of mononuclear cells can be quite extensive

Special Stains

- Silver stains the basement membrane black and will highlight irregular spikes protruding from the glomerular basement membrane
- PAS stain will highlight areas of sclerosis and thickened capillary wall
- Early supepithelial deposits may be stained with trichrome

Immunofluorescence

- Granular deposits of both immunoglobulins and various amounts of complement along the epithelial (subepithelial) side of the glomerular basement membrane

Electron Microscopy

- Electron dense deposits between the basement membrane and the podocytes
- Epithelial cells have effaced foot processes
- Basement membrane material is seen between the deposits and appears as irregular spikes that protrude from the glomerular basement membrane
- Eventually the spikes of basement membrane material envelope the immune deposits and result in intramembranous deposits

Molecular Alterations

- None

Treatment and Prognosis

- Little response to corticosteroid therapy
- 10% die or progress to renal failure within 10 years
- Spontaneous remission occurs more commonly in women than in men, especially women with non-nephrotic proteinuria

Associations

- SLE
- Hepatitis B, *Treponema* antigens, insulin (exogenous antigens) or thyroglobulin (endogenous antigen)
- Some neoplasms; eg, colon carcinoma

Minimal Change Disease (Lipoid Nephrosis)

Etiology and Pathogenesis

- No immune deposits in glomeruli
- May be the result of an immune dysfunction that results in the elaboration of cytokine-like circulating substances that affect podocytes causing cytoskeletal changes and foot process effacement; the end result is proteinuria

Clinical Manifestations

- Most common cause of nephrotic syndrome in children
- Patients typically maintain good renal function despite massive proteinuria (mostly serum albumin; <1 gm/dL can be associated with acute tubular necrosis)
- Hypertension and hematuria rarely encountered
- In adults, the condition may be associated with Hodgkin disease and rarely other lymphomas and leukemias
- Secondary minimal change disease may follow nonsteroidal anti-inflammatory drug therapy in association with acute interstitial nephritis

Gross and Microscopic Pathology

- Glomeruli appear normal
- Cells of proximal tubules are frequently filled with lipid (tubules reabsorb lipoproteins that pass through the diseased glomeruli)

Special Stains

- Trichrome, PAS, and silver stains confirm normal glomerular architecture

Immunofluorescence

- No immunoglobulin or complement deposits

Electron Microscopy

- Basement membrane appears normal and is free of electron-dense material

- The visceral epithelial cells show a uniform and diffuse effacement of foot processes
- The foot processes are replaced by a rim of cytoplasm and show podocyte vacuolization, swelling and villous hyperplasia

Molecular Alterations

- None

Treatment and Prognosis

- 90% of children respond rapidly to corticosteroid therapy
- Long-term prognosis is excellent even in steroid-dependent disease
- Adults are slower to respond than children but long-term prognosis is still excellent

Associations

- NSAIDs
- Respiratory infections and prophylactic immunization
- Eczema and rhinitis (atopic disorders)
- Hodgkin disease and other lymphomas and leukemias

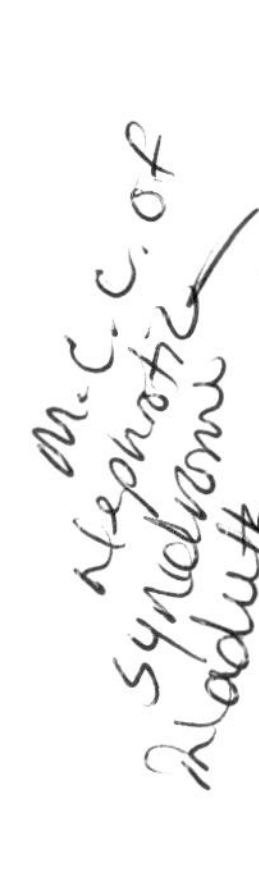

Focal Segmental Glomerulosclerosis

Etiology and Pathogenesis

- Common cause of steroid-resistant nephrotic syndrome in children
- Very rarely represents progression of minimal change disease
- Podocyte injury with detachment may accompany glomerular hyperfiltration with entrapment of plasma proteins and subsequent hyalinosis and sclerosis
- A circulating factor may be the cause of the epithelial damage (recurrence of proteinuria sometimes occurs within 24 hours after renal transplantation)

Clinical Manifestations

- 10% are idiopathic (usually children)
- Most occur in one of the following settings:
  - □ HIV infection with concurrent heroin addiction; sickle cell disease; and massive obesity
  - □ A secondary event as a result of glomerular scarring from another form of glomerulonephritis
  - □ An adaptive response to reduced renal mass (most common in adults)
- Occurs in 5% to 10% of HIV-infected patients (may result from infection of glomerular cells by HIV)

Gross and Microscopic Pathology

- Characterized by segmental sclerosis of selected (frequently a minority of) glomeruli
- Sclerotic lesions initially involve the juxtamedullary glomeruli and gradually become more generalized
- In the sclerotic areas there is collapse of basement membranes, increase in matrix and deposition of hyaline material (hyalinosis) often with lipid droplets and foam cells
- Uninvolved glomeruli appear normal or may show a slight increase in mesangial proliferation and matrix
- Evidence of tubular atrophy often present
- *Collapsing focal segmental glomerulosclerosis* (a variant of focal segmental glomerulosclerosis) is characterized by complete collapse and sclerosis of the entire glomerulus with apparent podocyte hyperplasia (more commonly seen in association with HIV infection)

Special Stains

- PAS stains hyalin accumulation

Immunofluorescence

- Both IgM and C3 present within the masses of hyaline material in the sclerotic areas of the glomeruli

Electron Microscopy

- Both sclerotic and non-sclerotic areas within the glomeruli show diffuse loss of epithelial foot processes
- There is focal detachment of epithelial cells with denudation of the underlying glomerular basement membrane

Molecular Alterations

- Recent advances in elucidating the Mendelian inheritance of familial focal segmental glomerulosclerosis have identified mutations in 4 genes as causing FSGS:
  1) NPHS1 (1q31.1) is mutated in autosomal recessive inherited congenital nephrotic syndrome—Finnish type. This gene encodes "nephrin" a protein associated with the slit diaphragm

2) NPHS2 (1q25-31) is mutated in patients with autosomal recessive inherited steroid-resistant nephrotic syndrome of childhood. This gene encodes a podocin, which may interact with nephrin
3) ACTN4 (19q13) has been identified in autosomal dominant inherited FSGS. It encodes α-actinin-4, a cytoskeletal protein which may be important for maintaining podocyte foot process integrity
4) TRPC6 (11q21-22) has been identified as the causative mutation in some kindreds with autosomal dominant inherited FSGS. It encodes a non-selective cation channel expressed in podocyte foot processes
5) PLCE1 (10q23.32-q24.1) has been identified in kindreds with autosomal recessive nephrosis

Treatment and Prognosis

- Spontaneous remission is rare and response to corticosteroid therapy is variable; angiotensin converting enzyme inhibitors and or angiotensin receptor blockers decrease hyperfiltration and slow progression at the expense of an increase in serum creatinine (resulting from a decrease in glomerular filtration rate)
- Children do better than adults
- 20% of patients follow a rapid course ending in renal failure within two years
- Recurrence is seen in 25% to 50% of patients who receive renal transplantation

Associations

- HIV infection and heroin addiction
- Sickle cell disease
- Massive obesity

Membranoproliferative Glomerulonephritis

Etiology and Pathogenesis

- Type I MPGN results from the deposition of immune complexes in the glomerulus and activation of both the classic and alternative complement pathways; C3 is deposited in the mesangium and occasionally beneath the epithelium
- Type II MPGN (dense deposit disease) results from the activation of the alternative complement pathway; C3 is present on both sides of the basement membrane and in the mesangium; IgG usually absent

Clinical Manifestations

- Most patients are older children or young adults who present with nephrotic syndrome
- Hematuria and mild proteinuria are frequently present
- Secondary membranoproliferative glomerulonephritis may arise in the setting of:
  1) Chronic immune complex disorders (SLE, hepatitis B and C infection, endocarditis, infected ventriculoatrial shunts, chronic visceral abscess, HIV infection, and schistosomiasis)
  2) α_1-antitrypsin deficiency
  3) Malignant diseases (chronic lymphocytic leukemia, lymphoma, melanoma)
  4) Hereditary complement deficiency states
  5) Partial lipodystrophy associated with C3 nephritic factor (C3NeF; type II membranoproliferative glomerulonephritis)

Gross and Microscopic Pathology

- Glomeruli are large and hypercellular (the result of endocapillary inflammatory cells and mononuclear leukocytes infiltrating the mesangium)
- Glomeruli tend to have a "lobular" appearance
- The glomerular basement membrane is thickened (often focally); this thickening is most evident in the peripheral capillary loops

Special Stains

- Silver stains and PAS will highlight the "double-contour" or "tram-track" morphology of the glomerular capillary wall

Immunofluorescence

- Type I is characterized by subendothelial deposits of C3, IgG, and early complement components (C1q and C4) in a granular pattern
- Type II is characterized by irregular linear deposits of C3 on either side of extremely dense material (of unknown composition) distributed in a ribbon-like pattern within the basement membrane; C3 also present in the mesangium in circular aggregates (mesangial rings); IgG and early complement components (C1q and C4) usually absent

Electron Microscopy

- The glomerular capillary wall frequently has a "double-contour" or "tram-track" appearance as a result of duplication of the basement membrane with inclusion of processes of mesangial cells and monocytes (mesangial interposition)
- Type I is characterized by large subendothelial deposits that are incorporated into the basement membrane
- Type II disease is characterized by markedly dense homogeneous deposits within the basement membrane (dense deposit disease)

Molecular Alterations

- None

Treatment and Prognosis

- Spontaneous remissions are rare
- Disease tends to follow a slowly progressive, unremitting course
- 50% develop chronic renal failure within 10 years
- Treatment with steroids, immunosuppressive drugs and antiplatelet drugs has not been particularly effective
- A high incidence of recurrence in patients undergoing renal transplantation (particularly in type II MPGN)

Associations

- Type I may be associated with chronic infections such as infectious endocarditis, ventriculoatrial shunts, malaria, essential cryoglobulinemia, hepatitis B and C infections, SLE, and sickle cell disease; also associated with neoplasms, angiofollicular lymphoid hyperplasia and heroin addiction
- Type II is associated with partial lipodystrophy

IgA Nephropathy (Berger Disease)

Etiology and Pathogenesis

- 50% of patients have elevated levels of serum IgA and circulating IgA immune complexes
- The IgA immune complexes accumulate in the mesangium and activate the alternative complement pathway and initiate glomerular injury
- The increased levels of IgA may be the result of increased synthesis in response to respiratory or gastrointestinal exposure to environmental agents (viruses, bacteria, food proteins)

Clinical Manifestations

- Primarily affects children and young adults
- 50% present with gross hematuria after an infection of the respiratory, gastrointestinal or urinary tract
- Many have only microscopic hematuria and normal renal function for several decades

Gross and Microscopic Pathology

- Glomeruli may have a variety of appearances: normal, mesangial widening and proliferation (mesangioproliferative), segmental proliferation confined to some glomeruli (focal proliferative glomerulonephritis), or rarely full-blown crescentic glomerulonephritis
- When focal proliferative lesions heal, they result in synechiae or segmental sclerosis without hyalinosis
- Occasionally prominent hyaline thickening of arterioles may be present (associated with hypertension and progression to chronic renal failure)

Special Stains

- Not helpful

Immunofluorescence

- Deposits of IgA in the mesangial regions of the glomeruli
- C3, properdin and smaller amounts of IgG and IgM also present
- Early components of complement (C1q and C4) typically absent

Electron Microscopy

- Electron-dense deposits are seen in the mesangium of most cases

Molecular Alterations

- None

Treatment and Prognosis

- 25% to 50% slowly progress to chronic renal failure over a period of 20 years
- Elderly patients and patients with heavy proteinuria and hypertension are at an increased risk of having progressive disease
- Recurrence of IgA deposits in transplanted kidneys occurs in 20% to 60%, but seldom causes graft loss

Associations

- Gluten enteropathy (celiac disease)
- Liver disease that results in defective hepatic reticuloendothelial clearance of IgA complex

Focal Proliferative and Necrotizing Glomerulonephritis (Focal Glomerulonephritis)

Clinical Manifestations

- Patients frequently present with nonspecific complaints (loss of appetite, anemia, vomiting or generalized weakness)
- Occasionally patients present with asymptomatic proteinuria, hypertension or azotemia
- Most patients are hypertensive and may have clinical manifestations of cerebral or cardiovascular disease

Gross and Microscopic Pathology

- Characterized by proliferation and necrosis restricted to segments of individual glomeruli
- Necrotic areas contain neutrophils and fragmented nuclei
- The uninvolved glomerulus appears normal

Special Stains

- Not helpful

Immunofluorescence

- Not helpful

Electron Microscopy

- Not helpful

Molecular Alterations

- None

Treatment and Prognosis

- Prognosis and treatment dependent upon the circumstance under which the disease occurs

Associations

- None

Chronic Glomerulonephritis

Clinical Manifestations

- The percentage of patients with each of the major glomerulonephritides that progress to chronic glomerulonephritis:
    - Acute proliferative glomerulonephritis (poststreptococcal, infectious): 1% to 2%
    - Rapidly progressive (crescentic): 90%
    - Membranous: 50%
    - Focal glomerulosclerosis: 50% to 80%
    - Membranoproliferative: 50%
    - IgA nephropathy: 30% to 50%

Gross and Microscopic Pathology

- Kidneys symmetrically contracted and have a diffusely granular cortical surface
- On sectioning the cortex is thinned and there is an increase in peripelvic adipose tissue
- Endstage disease characterized by hyaline obliteration of glomeruli (appear as acellular eosinophilic masses that represent trapped plasma proteins, increased mesangial matrix, basement membrane-like material and collagen)
- Arteriosclerosis and arteriolosclerosis sclerosis usually prominent
- Marked atrophy of associated tubules, irregular interstitial fibrosis, and lymphocytic infiltration typically present

Special Stains

- Trichrome highlights the collagen that replaces the glomeruli

Immunofluorescence

- Not helpful

Electron Microscopy

- Not helpful

Molecular Alterations

- None

Treatment and Prognosis

- Death is the inevitable result if patients are not maintained on dialysis or do not receive a renal transplant

Tubolointerstitial Nephritis

Xanthogranulomatous Pyelonephritis

Clinical Manifestations

- A form of subacute and chronic renal inflammation that results in a mass that may mimic a renal neoplasm
- More commonly affects women than men
- Typically diagnosed between the 4th and 6th decades
- Patients often present with fever, flank pain and a tender flank mass
- 70% patients will have nephrolithiasis
- The affected kidney is nonfunctioning in 50 to 70% of cases at the time of diagnosis
- Common urinary tract pathogens such as *Proteus mirabilis* and *Escherichia coli* are almost invariably present within the lesion (present in the urine in 30%)

Gross Pathology

- Lesion tends to be unilateral but may involve any part or the entire kidney
- Cut surface of the kidney reveals golden yellow nodules varying in size from a few millimeters to several centimeters that surround renal pelvis and calyces and infiltrate and destroy adjacent renal parenchyma
- Occasionally the inflammatory mass will penetrate Gerota fascia

Microscopic Pathology

- Typical appearance is one of abundant, lipid-laden (foamy) macrophages intermixed with chronic inflammatory cells (lymphocytes and plasma cells)
- Purulent foci with micro-abscesses with many neutrophils may be present
- Multinucleated giant cells and spindled fibroblasts may be present
- The presence of Michaelis-Gutmann bodies in macrophages (not particularly common) warrants the designation of *malakoplakia*

Special Stains

- Macrophages (Hanselman cells) typically PAS positive

Immunohistochemistry and Electron Microscopy

- Epithelial markers negative; CD68 positive

Molecular Alterations

- None

Differential Diagnosis

- Well-differentiated renal cell carcinoma, clear cell type
- The presence of spindled fibroblasts can cause confusion with the spindle cell component of a sarcomatoid renal cell carcinoma

Treatment and Prognosis

- Simple nephrectomy

Associations

- Underlying obstructive chronic pyelonephritis

Ask-Upmark Kidney

Clinical Manifestations

- A form of congenital renal hypoplasia that tends to be unilateral; may mimic a renal neoplasm on radiologic studies
- Typically seen in adolescents who present with hypertension

Gross Pathology

- Typically the surface of the kidney is deformed by grooves that give the kidney the appearance of containing a mass
- Number of medullary pyramids reduced
- Normal areas of renal parenchyma juxtaposed to hypoplastic areas
- Pseudo-diverticular dilatation of the renal pelvis may be present

Microscopic Pathology

- Arcuate and interlobular arteries typically stenotic (likely etiology for the associated hypertension)

Special Stains, Immunohistochemistry, and Electron Microscopy

- Not helpful

Molecular Alterations

- None

Differential Diagnosis

- Most cystic and dysplastic renal lesions (few of which result in an appearance reminiscent of a neoplasm)

Treatment

- Nephrectomy (typically the result of a concern that the clinical appearance of the kidney is that of a neoplasm)

Prognosis

- No particular clinical significance

Associations

- None

Prostate

Adenocarcinoma

Clinical Manifestations

- Affects 20% of all American males; 3% will die from the disease
- Incidence varies by nationality: high incidence in Scandinavian countries and low incidence in Asian countries
- PSA (prostatic specific antigen) used to screen for carcinoma: 50% of organ-confined tumors and a third of extra prostatic extensions are associated with normal PSA levels; elevated PSA level may result from nodular hyperplasia, prostatic biopsy, inflammation, and digital rectal examination
- Diagnosis may be confirmed by a transrectal (or occasionally a transperineal) core biopsy; false negative rate is ~25%
- Occasionally patients present with metastatic disease, usually in the bones but occasionally in the cervical nodes in the left neck, or supradiaphragmatic lymph nodes
- Up to 85% of adenocarcinomas are located in the peripheral portions in the gland and many can be palpated on digital examination of the rectum
- Occasionally lesions will invade rectal mucosa and mimic a primary rectal adenocarcinoma

Gross Pathology

- Small lesions are typically localized to the posterior periphery of the gland and are seen as irregular yellow-white lesions
- More extensive neoplasms appear as an irregularly shaped yellowish mass that may have punctate foci of necrosis

Microscopic Pathology

- At low-power, malignant glands appear pale/amphophilic
- Architecturally glands tend to be small, arranged haphazardly, and infiltrate surrounding stroma at right angles to each other; tend to stand out in marked contrast to surrounding benign glands; may contain intraluminal pink, acellular dense secretions or blue-tinged mucinous secretions (65 to 70%); intraluminal crystalloids are present in 60%
- Malignant glands typically lack a basal cell layer (diagnosis requires more than just a few glands without a basal cell layer because benign glands can show some heterogeneity in the amount of basal cell layer present)
- Tumor cells have abundant cytoplasm and enlarged, hyperchromatic nuclei that are located at the base; most important cytologic feature to separate malignant from benign glands is the increased nuclear enlargement characteristic of carcinoma; other cytologic features include prominent nucleoli and amphophilic cytoplasm (especially as compared to the pale to clear cytoplasm of benign glands)
- Cellular pleomorphism is not a characteristic feature even in poorly differentiated prostatic carcinoma
- Occasional mitotic figures may be present
- Features diagnostic of carcinoma include:
  - Perineural invasion
  - Collagenous nodules (mucinous fibroplasia)
  - Glomerulations: glands that show a cribriform architecture that is not transluminal resulting in an appearance the resembles glomeruli

Grade (Gleason system)

- Based on glandular architectural pattern identified at low magnification
- Cytologic features play no role in grading
  - 2 grades are assigned: a primary (predominant) and a secondary (second most prevalent) architectural pattern; grades are added together for a total score
  - Grades range from 1 to 5; 1 is the most differentiated and 5 is the most undifferentiated
- Gleason grade 1: Tumor consists of a circumscribed nodule of uniform, single, separate, closely packed glands
- Gleason grade 2: Peripheral margin is less sharp than in a Gleason grade 1 (minimal extension of neoplastic glands

into surrounding nonneoplastic prostate); glands are more loosely arranged and not quite as uniform as in Gleason grade 1

- Gleason grade 3: Malignant glands infiltrate in and among non-neoplastic prostate; glands have marked variation in size and shape (many are quite small); circumscribed rounded masses of papillary or loose cribriform tumor of normal gland size may be present
- Gleason grade 4: Tumor glands are fused and nodules of tumor may have a glomeruloid appearance and ragged, infiltrating edges; irregular or large cribriform masses (hypernephroid pattern); clusters of poorly formed glands where tangential sectioning has been ruled out
- Gleason grade 5: Nodule of neoplasm may be circumscribed or ragged; tumor cells show no glandular differentiation and form solid masses of cells or single infiltrating cells; solid areas may have central necrosis (comedocarcinoma)

Variants

- *Mucinous adenocarcinoma*
  - Characterized by the presence of extracellular mucin in sufficient quantities to result in pools of mucin that comprise at least 25% of the resected neoplasm
  - Typically an intermediate grade tumor with a cribriform pattern graded as a Gleason 4+4
- *Carcinoma with neuroendocrine features:*
  - Neuroendocrine cells with argentaffin-argyrophil properties, serotonin, calcitonin, bombesin, and/or somatostatin immunoreactivity are present in 10% to 30% of adenocarcinomas
  - Neuroendocrine cells often resemble Paneth cells (eosinophilic cytoplasmic granules)
  - Architecturally may resemble a typical carcinoid tumor or a small cell carcinoma of the lung
- *Signet-ring carcinoma*
  - Tumor cells grow in solid, acinar, or Indian file fashion and have signet-ring configuration secondary to the presence of intracellular mucin
  - Graded as a Gleason pattern 5
- *Squamous cell carcinoma*
  - Represents 0.5% of prostate tumors
  - Associated with a poor prognosis
  - Not graded
  - Typically do not metastasize to bone, do not respond to hormone therapy and do not develop increased serum levels of PSA when metastatic
  - Squamous differentiation most frequently seen after primary or metastatic deposits of adenocarcinoma have been treated with hormone therapy
- *Adenosquamous carcinoma*
  - Usually occurs after radiation or hormone therapy for ordinary carcinoma, but occasionally seen when there has been no prior therapy
  - Not graded
- *Prostatic duct adenocarcinoma*
  - Represent 0.5% to 1.0% of prostatic carcinomas
  - Typically arises in large primary periurethral prostatic ducts; may grow into the urethra, usually in the region of the verumontanum
  - Characterized by columnar pseudostratified epithelium with abundant, dark (amphophilic) cytoplasm (may be pale or clear)
  - Should be graded as 4+4=8 or 4+5=9 if comedonecrosis present
  - Architectural arrangement of cells frequently papillary but may be cribriform
  - Occasionally the neoplasm will invade as single glands
  - Extensive comedonecrosis and prominent nuclear atypia are typical features
  - Metastasis may be purely ductal, acinar, or a mixture of the two
  - Neoplasm tends to resemble endometrial carcinoma
  - Carcinomas with at least 50% ductal differentiation tend to be large and advanced with extra-prostatic extension, positive margins (50%), seminal vesicle involvement (40%) and metastasis to pelvic lymph nodes (30%)
  - Conventional acinar carcinoma often present
- *Urothelial carcinoma*
  - Typically located within periurethral prostatic ducts
  - Accounts for 1% to 4% of all prostate carcinomas
  - An in situ component is usually present and consists of neoplastic urothelial cells that fill prostatic ducts and frequently have central necrosis
  - Invasive lesions are characterized by small nests of tumor cells that are markedly pleomorphic and mitotically active

- Most have infiltrated the bladder neck and surrounding soft tissue at the time of diagnosis
- 20% have distant metastasis (bone, lung and liver are most common sites; bone metastasis tend to be osteolytic in comparison to the osteoblastic lesions of adenocarcinoma)
- Most commonly urothelial carcinoma involves prostatic ducts and acini in patients with a history of flat carcinoma in situ of the bladder that has been treated with intravesical chemotherapy
- Occasionally prostatic involvement by neoplastic urothelial cells consists of Pagetoid spread characterized by tumor cells that migrate between the secretory and basal cell layers

- *Basaloid carcinoma (adenoid cystic-like tumor)*
  - Resembles adenoid cystic carcinoma of the salivary gland
  - Low malignant potential (no reports of metastasis)
  - May arise from areas of basal cell hyperplasia
  - Nests of tumor cells promote a desmoplastic stromal reaction (an important feature that differentiates a malignant lesion from basal cell hyperplasia)
- *Mesenchymal tumors*
  - Most common benign lesion is a leiomyoma
  - Malignant stromal sarcoma (malignant phyllodes tumor) is characterized by increased stromal cellularity and overgrowth with mitotic figures and necrosis
  - Most frequent malignant tumor in childhood is rhabdomyosarcoma. Most diagnosed during early childhood and are of the embryonal subtype. 15% to 20% die of their tumors
  - Leiomyosarcomas are the second most common malignant mesenchymal tumor involving prostate in adults. Most are diagnosed between the ages of 40 and 70. Average survival 3 to 4 years
  - Other mesenchymal tumors include malignant peripheral nerve sheath tumor, angiosarcoma, hemangiopericytoma, malignant fibrous histiocytoma (MFH) and hemangioma

Special Stains and Electron Microscopy

- Not helpful

Immunohistochemistry

- Malignant cells stain positively for prostate-specific acid phosphatase (PSAP) and prostate-specific antigen (PSA)
- 80% of malignant glands positive for AMACR (P504s); AMACR will also stain high-grade PIN, adenosis, and metaplastic lesions
- Basal cells stain positively for high molecular weight cytokeratin (K903) and p63 (should be negative in well-differentiated adenocarcinoma)

Molecular Alterations

- Expression of *ras* oncogene p21 associated with poorly differentiated tumors
- Expression of p53 tumor suppressor gene is seen in many advanced stage prostatic carcinomas

Differential Diagnosis

- Atrophy: atrophic glands tend to be very basophilic and have open lumina lined by cells with a high nuclear-to-cytoplasmic ratio; the lobular architecture is typically preserved; prominent nucleoli may be present
- Seminal vesicle epithelium: prominent lipofuscin granules within the epithelium; cells may have nuclear pseudoinclusions and show some atypia and hyperchromasia but mitotic activity is absent; PSAP negative
- Squamous metaplasia: may be seen surrounding an infarct, after a transurethral resection, and as a result of estrogen therapy
- Basal cell hyperplasia: usually characterized by small, solid nests of uniform, benign-appearing epithelial cells with somewhat clear cytoplasm and an accompanying area of typical nodular hyperplasia; large stratified nuclei with vesicular chromatin, hyperchromasia, and prominent nucleoli
- Adenosis: consists of numerous crowded, small, pale staining glands that resemble a nodule of low-grade adenocarcinoma; a lobular configuration is usually present; typically there is a gradual transition between small glands that resemble carcinoma into adjacent more easily recognized benign glands; nucleoli, when present, are usually small; only a minority of glands have readily apparent basal cells; blue tinged mucinous secretions are rare; corpora amylacea commonly present; immunostains for high molecular weight cytokeratin should show the presence of basal cells in at least some of the small glands
- Partial atrophy: stellate/undulated gland tumors with pale cytoplasm similar to adjacent benign gland, completely atrophic glands within focus, lack of nuclear enlargement and/or macronuclei. Few cases may show disoranized glandular pattern with poorly formed glands and presence of micronucleoli, which may cause concern at the time of initial evaluation.

- High-grade prostatic intraepithelial neoplasia (PIN): characterized by multilayering of enlarged, pleomorphic and crowded nuclei with prominent nucleoli; infiltrating adenocarcinoma present somewhere in the gland in 30% of cases
- Cowper glands, xanthomas, mucosal gland hyperplasia in the region of the verumontanum, nephrogenic adenoma of the prostatic urethra and mesonephric hyperplasia

Treatment

- Clinical stage T1a (tumor represents an incidental histologic finding in ≤5% of tissue resected by TURP): radical prostatectomy or followup with careful monitoring of PSA levels
- Clinical stage T1b (tumor is an incidental histologic finding in >5% of tissue resected by TURP): radiotherapy or radical prostatectomy
- Clinical stage T1c (tumor identified by needle biopsy usually done for an elevated PSA): generally more significant tumors that warrant definitive therapy that usually consists of radical prostatectomy
- Clinical stage T2 (tumor confined within the prostate, involves one lobe or both lobes): radical prostatectomy
- Clinical stage T3 (tumor extends through prostate capsule and/or involves the seminal vesicles): usually treated with radiotherapy (not a candidate for radical prostatectomy)
- Clinical stage T4 (neoplasm that invades adjacent structures other than seminal vesicles): radiation therapy and/or hormonal therapy
- Metastatic disease: preoperative hormonal therapy followed by radical prostatectomy

Prognosis

- Incidence of lymph node metastasis correlates with overall Gleason score:
  - <1% if Gleason score 2 to 4
  - 2% to 3% if Gleason score 5 to 6
  - 10% if Gleason score 7
  - 20% if Gleason score 8-10
- Serum levels of PSA related to prognosis as an indirect indicator of tumor volume, tumor extension and response to therapy
- Presence of neuroendocrine features is associated with a poor prognosis
- Neoplasms confined to the gland (especially with a low Gleason score) are associated with an excellent prognosis
- Tumors that have extended through the prostatic capsule or involve the seminal vesicles (Stage T3) have an incidence of pelvic lymph node metastasis of 50% to 60%; 50% will develop metastatic disease within 5 years; 75% will die of prostate carcinoma within 10 years
- Patients with distant metastasis have a mortality rate of 15% at 3 years, 80% at 5 years and 90% at 10 years
- Vast majority of patients who relapse after endocrine therapy are dead within a year

Associations

- None

Prostatic Nodular Hyperplasia

Clinical Manifestations

- Urinary obstruction secondary to nodular enlargement of the gland caused by hyperplasia of both glandular and stromal components
- Incidence <10% under the age of 40; 50% in fifth decade, and 75% in the eighth decade
- An androgen-dependent disorder, seen only in men with intact testes

Gross Pathology

- Cut section reveals a multinodular appearance with an admixure of solid and microcystic areas
- Variously sized gray to yellow, granular nodules project above the cut surface
- Typically the nodules first appear in the portion of gland the surrounds the urethra

Microscopic Pathology

- Earliest change typically a stromal proliferation around small sinusoidal spaces in periurethral regions; less proliferation in periductal and intralobular areas
- Stroma contains more smooth muscle and less elastic tissue than normal stroma; occasionally bizarre cells present
- Stromal proliferation followed by hyperplasia of glandular component; nodules contain varying proportions of stroma and glands

- Glands often dilated or even cystic and may contain inspissated secretions of a glycoprotein nature (corpora amylacea) which may consolidate to form calcifications
- Epithelium of glands ranges from flat to columnar with pale cytoplasm and regular, centrally located nuclei; papillary infoldings are common; a continous basal layer is present immediately above a well-developed basement membrane
- Clusters of lymphocytes commonly present
- Several morphologic variations of this basic pattern exist as a result of overgrowth of one component or another (may resemble lesions of the breast such as sclerosing adenosis, fibroadenoma-like and phyllodes tumor-like hyperplasia, leiomyoma, and fibromyxoid-like nodules

Special Stains

- Not helpful

Immunohistochemistry

- p27 (a negative regulator of the cell cycle) is expressed in both the epithelial and stromal cells of a normal prostate but are typically negative in nodular hyperplasia (nodular hyperplasia may result from an initial activation of mesenchymal clones with embryonal functions that stimulate development of the glandular component)
- Basal cells stain positively for high molecular weight cytokeratin (K903) and p63

Electron Microscopy

- Not helpful

Molecular Alterations

- None

Differential Diagnosis

- Adenocarcinoma tends to be a peripheral lesion

Treatment and Prognosis

- Transurethral prostatectomy (TURP) or suprapubic prostatectomy (both these procedures remove the newly formed nodules; the compressed peripheral portion remains and may expand and lead to a recurrence)
- Medical treatment based on blocking the actions of androgens

Associations

- No predisposing or protecting factors have ever been identified
- Infarcts occur and are directly related to the degree of hyperplasia (found in 20% to 25% of prostates removed for nodular hyperplasia); the center of an infarct usually contains epithelial nests with prominent nucleoli, some pleomorphism and occasional atypical mitotic figures; more mature squamous metaplasia is seen at the periphery of the infarct—10% to 25% of prostates with BPH or carcinoma contain vascular amyloid deposits.

Prostatic Infections

- Bacterial prostatitis
  - Acute and chronic prostitis are both typically diagnosed clinically and treated with antibiotics
  - Abscess formation is unusual
- Mycotic prostatitis
  - Blastomycosis, coccidiomycosis, and cryptococcosis most common
  - Almost all occur in setting of systemic hematogenous dissemination in an immunocompromised host
  - Incidence of prostate involvement in systemic Tb ranges from about 5% to 15%.
  - Tuberculous involvement of the prostate seen following bacillus Calmette-Guerin (BCG) immunotherapy for superficial urothelial cell cancer of the bladder (may cause the serum PSA to rise)

Urinary Bladder

Metaplastic Lesions

- Three Types
  - Squamous
  - Intestinal
  - Nephrogenic

Clinical Manifestations

- Typically asymptomatic

- Usually associated with structural defects and chronic irritation
- May coexist with proliferative von Brunn nests

Gross Pathology

- Typically a small reddish nodule on urothelial surface

Microscopic Pathology

- *Squamous metaplasia*
  - Urothelium replaced by stratified squamous epithelium
  - Two types: vaginal and keratinizing
  - Vaginal squamous metaplasia is seen only in females and is so common as to be regarded as normal
  - Keratinizing squamous metaplasia (known as leukoplakia) is more common in males and is usually associated with chronic irritation; basal layers may show considerable atypia
- *Intestinal (cystic) metaplasia*:
  - Urothelium replaced by colonic mucosa; results from chronic inflammation and other causes of mucosal irritation (ureteral reimplantation, neurogenic bladder, or bladder exstrophy); may regress completely if underlying pathogenic factor is removed
  - Trigone area most commonly affected
  - Similar lesions may be present in the ureter and renal pelvis
  - Microscopically, initial change is focal proliferation of the basal layer of transitional epithelium, which produces buds that later become solid nodules (von Brunn nests or islands) located within the lamina propria; some of these nodules developed a central cystic area caused by the accumulation of mucin; when the cells lining the cyst maintain a transitional appearance, the condition is called *cystitis cystica*; when the cells lining the cyst acquire morphologic features analogous to those of colonic epithelium, the process is designated either as *cystitis glandularis* or as *intestinal (glandular, colonic) metaplasia*
  - Extensive intestinal metaplasia is a significant risk factor for the development of adenocarcinoma
- *Nephrogenic metaplasia (nephrogenic adenoma):*
  - Traditionally regarded as a benign neoplasm and designated as nephrogenic adenoma, but probably represents a localized or diffuse metaplastic change of the urothelium in response to chronic infection, calculi, or prolonged catheterization
  - Occasionally seen in association with cystitis cystica or cystitis glandularis
  - Grossly, lesions can be papillary, polypoid, or sessile; 20% are multiple
  - Microscopically, the appearance is that of small tubular formations lined by cuboidal and hobnail cells (remarkably similar to mesonephric tubules)

Special Stains and Electron Microscopy

- Not helpful

Immunohistochemistry

- AMACR (P504s) positive in nephrogenic metaplasia

Molecular Alterations

- None

Differential Diagnosis

- Nephrogenic metaplasia (nephrogenic adenoma) in prostatic urethra may mimic prostatic acinar carcinoma
- Urothelial carcinoma
- Signet ring carcinoma

Treatment

- Excisional biopsy

Prognosis

- Intestinal metaplasia has very low risk for urothelial carcinoma
- Nephrogenic metaplasia tend to recur; no risk for subsequent carcinoma

Associations

- None

Urothelial Carcinoma

Clinical Manifestations

- A disease of the western hemisphere.
- Smoking is a significant risk factor
- In the middle east (Egypt), infestation with *Schistosoma hematobium* causes squamous cell carcinoma
- Men are affected more frequently than women (3:1)

- Whites are affected more frequently than blacks (2:1)
- Majority of urinary bladder neoplasms (neoplastic, nonneoplastic, benign or malignant) occur in the region of the trigone (this anatomic site includes the ureteral orifices and extends into the bladder and bladder neck)
- 60% of all primary neoplasms occur as a single lesion
- Typically seen between the ages of 50 and 70; rare in children and in adults under the age of 40
- Typical symptoms include gross or microscopic hematuria
- Invasive lesions may produce dysuria, frequency, and suprapubic pain
- β-HCG present in the serum of 10 to 30% of patients with high-grade urothelial carcinoma and in 50% of patients with metastatic disease

Variants

- Flat dysplastic urothelial lesions
- Flat urothelial carcinoma in situ
- Papillary urothelial carcinoma, low-grade
- Papillary urothelial carcinoma, high-grade

Gross Pathology

- *Flat dysplastic urothelial lesions:*
  - Usually diagnosed in patients with carcinoma (rarely seen in non-cancer patients)
  - Typically not visible on cystoscopic examination
- *Urothelial carcinoma in situ:*
  - A flat, reddish, non-invasive neoplasm; rarely presents as a primary lesion; usually seen in bladders with an invasive high-grade carcinoma
  - Usually multifocal involving areas of the bladder wall other than the base
  - Patients typically present with hematuria, dysuria, frequency, and suprapubic pain
- *Papillary urothelial carcinoma, low-grade:*
  - Represent 15% to 30% of all transitional neoplasms
  - Usually small papillary lesions on a delicate fibrovascular stalk
- *Papillary urothelial carcinoma, high-grade:*
  - More likely to be multifocal than papillomas or low-grade urothelial carcinoma
  - Represent 50% to 60% of all transitional cell neoplasms and 60% to 80% of all true carcinomas
  - May appear as nodules on the mucosal surface of the bladder

Microscopic Pathology

- *Dysplastic urothelial lesions:*
  - Nuclei tend to be enlarged, disorganized, clustered together, and overlap; nuclear membranes irregular (notches and creases and shallow depressions present but less obvious than in papillomas), chromatin typically finely granular and evenly dispersed
  - Nucleoli are either absent or small
  - Mitoses rare
  - Cytologic atypia less severe than CIS but significantly more than reactive atypia
- *Urothelial carcinoma in situ:*
  - A flat non-invasive lesion with malignant cells that may be present in all layers of the urothelium or present in part of the urothelium (does not need to be full-thickness atypia)
  - Present in almost every bladder with invasive carcinoma
  - Cells tend to resemble the cells of high-grade transitional cell carcinoma but remain confined to an intraepithelial location; tend to lack intracellular cohesion, which often results in extensive denudation
  - Tumor cells have pleomorphic nuclei with chromatin that is coarsely granular and irregularly distributed
  - Nucleoli may be large
  - Mitoses are variably present and may be abnormal
  - Large-cell variant has typical conventional morphology
  - Denuding (clinging) variant characterized by largely denuded urothelium with scattered isolated malignant cells
  - *Small cell variant* resembles other small cell tumors with densely aggregated cells with high nuclear cytoplasmic ratios
  - *Pagetoid variant* characterized by large cells with low nuclear:cytoplasmic ratios, well-defined cell borders and slightly acidophilic cytoplasm; present in 10% of cases
  - All variants are associated with marked inflammation of the underlying lamina propria

- *Papillary urothelial neoplasm of low malignant potential (PUNLMP)*
  - Papillae have an orderly arrangement of cells with minimal architectural abnormality and nuclear atypia
  - The major distinction from papilloma is that the urothelium is much thicker and/or the nuclei are larger
  - Mitotic figures are infrequent and when present are typically limited to the basal layer
- *Urothelial carcinoma, low-grade:*
  - Represent 15% to 30% of all urothelial neoplasms
  - Usually papillary; very rarely has an invasive component
  - Superficial cell layer is usually at least partially preserved
  - Tumor cells tend to be densely packed, uniform and evenly distributed; cell borders usually indistinct with little or no cytoplasmic clearing; nuclei tend to be more rounded and pleomorphic than normal urothelial nuclei; nuclear borders are often irregular (notches and creases); chromatin finely granular and evenly distributed
  - Nucleoli usually small and relatively sparse; occasionally large and prominent
- *Urothelial carcinoma, high-grade:*
  - Represent 50% to 60% of all urothelial neoplasms
  - Tumor cells typically are moderately to poorly differentiated, pleomorphic and usually arranged in nests
  - Often multifocal and associated with separate foci of carcinoma in situ
  - Usually an infiltrating neoplasm with tumor cells arranged in sheets, nests and broad cords
  - Papillary and flat components may be present but are rarely a dominant feature
  - Tumor cells usually have homogeneous cytoplasm but vacuolization is common
  - Nuclei are markedly pleomorphic; chromatin is irregularly dispersed and coarsely granular
  - Large nucleoli may be present
  - Mitotic figures are common and often abnormal
  - Heterologous elements of both epithelioid and stromal origin may be present
- Urothelial carcinoma variants:
  - Urothelial carcinoma with gland-like (pseudoglandular) lumina:
  - Characterized by small clusters of intercellular or intracellular lumina surrounded by neoplastic urothelial or squamous cells
  - Lumina are more commonly seen in high-grade tumors and tend to be small but may appear as empty cysts (occasionally contain acidophilic acid mucins)
  - No prognostic significance
- *Urothelial carcinoma, nested-type:*
  - Urothelial cells arranged in structures that resemble von Brunn nests
  - Tend to be small, multifocal and localized to the ureteral orifices
  - Neoplastic cells are rarely very atypical despite the fact that these tumors can be very aggressive
- *Urothelial carcinoma, sarcomatoid variant:*
  - Tumor cells consist of malignant spindle cells that surround isolated islands of urothelial cell carcinoma
  - Resemble malignant fibrous histiocytoma
- *Urothelial carcinoma with mixed histology:*
  - Urothelium may have very divergent differentiation to include squamous, glandular, micropapillary
- *Small cell neuroendocrine carcinoma:*
  - Very poor prognosis

Special Stains

- Acid mucin present in the gland-like structures of a urothelial carcinoma with "gland-like lumina" can be confirmed with mucicarmine

Immunohistochemistry

- Tumor cells express cytokeratin, CEA, Leu-M1 (CD15), K903, and p63
- CK 7 and CK 20 both usually positive, but may be CK 7 positive and CK 20 negative
- Normal urothelial cells express blood group-related antigens ABH, Lewis a, and Lewis b; neoplastic cells express Lewis X and Lewis T
- Carcinoembryonic antigens can be expressed by both normal and neoplastic urothelial cells
- CK 20 stains umbrella cells in normal urothelium; shows full thickness staining in dysplasia

Electron Microscopy

- Not helpful

Molecular Alterations

- Invasive tumors are associated with loss of heterozygosity of 3p, 5q, and 17p
- Increased expression of c-*erb* B-2 oncogene is seen in 20 to 30% of high-grade tumors
- Most consistent abnormalities are over-expression of the *ras* family and mutations of p53 and Rb

Differential Diagnosis

- *Dysplastic lesions:*
  - Reactive/regenerative epithelium (nuclei tend to be evenly distributed and have prominent nucleoli); CK 20 usually positive in dysplastic epithelium and negative in reactive epithelium
  - Carcinoma in situ
- *Urothelial carcinoma in situ:*
  - Reactive/regenerative epithelium
  - Drug effects on normal urothelium
  - Dysplasia and atypical hyperplasia
- *Urothelial carcinoma, low grade*:
  - Papilloma
  - Urothelial carcinoma, high grade
- *Urothelial carcinoma, high grade:*
  - Urothelial carcinoma, low grade
  - Mixed carcinoma
  - Poorly differentiated prostatic cancer
  - Nonkeratinizing squamous cell carcinoma

Treatment

- Carcinoma in situ: first line of therapy is intravesical BCG; total cystectomy indicated in non-responsive lesions
- Grade I and II lesions without muscle invasion: transurethral resection with or without supplemental intravesical chemotherapy
- Grade III and IV tumors (tumors with muscle invasion irrespective of grade and tumors resistant to conservative therapy): radical cystectomy with or without preoperative chemotherapy
- Urothelial carcinoma, low-grade (without invasion): intravesical immunotherapy with Calmette-Guerin bacillus (BCG) which causes mucosal erosion, submucosal granulomatous inflammation and reactive epithelial atypia
- Radical cystectomy in the male includes removing the bladder, prostate, seminal vesicles and adjacent perivesical tissues with or without en bloc pelvic lymph node resection; in a female, it includes the bladder, uterus, tubes, ovaries, anterior vagina and urethra
- Intravesical triethylene thiophosphoramide (TTP) and mitomycin c (MMC) both cause exfoliation of normal and abnormal urothelial cells with subsequent denudation of the bladder, degeneration, multinucleation and bizarre reactive nuclear changes in superficial umbrella cells

Prognosis

- Presence of dysplasia does not represent a significant risk factor for the development of an invasive cancer
- Prognostic factors:
  - Deeply invasive carcinomas have a five-year survival of 45% to 55%
  - Long-term survival in the presence of lymph node metastasis is essentially zero
  - Local excision of grade I solitary lesions have a 30% to 40% recurrence rate
  - Younger patients are more likely to have well-differentiated and non-invasive lesions
  - Tumors located in the bladder neck tend to have the worst prognosis; tumors in the dome tend to be of a higher grade; tumors at the ureteral surfaces or on the lateral walls tend to be of lower grade
  - Presence of vascular invasion associated with increased recurrence
  - Prominent inflammatory response to the neoplasm is associated with better prognosis
  - Reduced expression of blood group antigens is associated with high-grade lesions
  - Decreased expression of the Rb gene is associated with more aggressive behavior
- Low- and high-grade tumors both have high recurrence rates; low-grade tumors progress slowly; high-grade tumors progress rapidly; PUNLMP has low recurrence rate and rarely progresses

- Carcinoma in situ tends to be an indolent neoplasm that will not spontaneously regress but does not inevitably develop into an invasive lesion; if not treated 35% will develop invasive carcinoma
- Low-grade urothelial carcinomas (predominately papillary) and non-invasive neoplasms have an 80% 10 to 20 year survival rate
- High-grade urothelial carcinomas have a 10 to 20 year survival rate of 40% to 60%

Associations

- Infestation with *S. hematobium*

Urothelial Papilloma

Variants

- Inverted papilloma (Brunnian adenoma)
- Exophytic papilloma

Clinical Manifestations

- Inverted papilloma
  - Represents 1% of urothelial neoplasms
- Exophytic papilloma
  - Represents approximately 25% of urothelial neoplasms

Gross Pathology

- *Inverted papilloma (Brunnian adenoma)*
  - A solitary, raised, pedunculated or polypoid mass with a smooth surface
  - Most larger than 3 cm
- *Exophytic papilloma*
  - Obvious polypoid lesion on the mucosal surface of bladder
- Distinction between inverted papilloma and exophytic papilloma requires microscopic examination

Microscopic Pathology

- *Inverted papilloma (Brunnian adenoma)*
  - Architecturally a "jig-saw" pattern characterized by cords and nests of urothelial cells, in an exophytic lesion that invaginates into the lamina propria
  - Central portion of cords contains maturing urothelial cells and the surrounding tissue is stroma (this is the exact opposite of an exophytic papilloma where the stroma is located centrally and is surrounded by epithelial cells)
  - No true fibrovascular cores
  - Inverted papillomas grow as an expansile mass and do not infiltrate the muscular wall
  - Rarely co-exist with a papillary carcinoma
  - Areas of cystic change and foci of squamous metaplasia common
  - Neuroendocrine differentiation may occur
  - Cellular atypia is common, but true anaplasia is relatively rare; atypical nuclear changes most likely represent compression of cells within tightly packed trabeculae
- *Exophytic papilloma*:
  - Characterized by multiple layers of well-differentiated, essentially normal, urothelial cells (which retain their superficial umbrella cell layer) on delicate fibrovascular stalks
  - Neoplastic cells resemble normal urothelium
  - Tumor cells tend to be evenly distributed on the stalks and have fairly distinct borders and homogeneous, amphophilic to acidophilic cytoplasm
  - Papilloma cells have slightly less cytoplasmic clearing than normal cells from adjacent urothelium
  - Nuclei tend to be round or elongated and maintain their normal perpendicular orientation to the surface and basal lamina; chromatin is evenly dispersed and granular; nucleoli are small or absent
  - Tumor cells often extend onto flat areas of urothelium adjacent to the base of the stalks
  - Fibrovascular stalks contain delicate blood vessels and tend to be edematous; frequently contain foamy macrophages
  - No invasion of the detrusor muscle and no reports of metastasis
  - Mitotic figures are infrequent and when present are typically limited to the basal layer

Special Stains, Immunohistochemistry, and Electron Microscopy

- Not helpful

Molecular Alterations

- None

Differential Diagnosis

- Inverted papilloma
  - Florid proliferation of von Brunn nests
  - Urothelial carcinoma with anastomosing and infiltrating papillae
- Exophytic papilloma
  - Inverted papilloma
  - Polypoid cystitis
  - Nephrogenic metaplasia
  - Low-grade urothelial carcinoma

Treatment

- Cystoscopic removal

Prognosis

- Inverted papillomas recur in <5% of cases
- Progression from a pure inverted papilloma to carcinoma has not been documented

Associations

- Inverted papilloma may be seen with florid proliferation of von Brunn nests

References

Bostwick DG, Eble JN. *Urologic Surgical Pathology*. St. Louis: Mosby-Year Book, 1997.

Dabbs DJ. *Diagnostic Immunohistochemistry*. New York: Churchill Livingstone, 2002.

Mills S, Carter D, Greenson JK, Oberman HA, Reuter V, and Stoler MH (eds). *Sternberg's Diagnostic Surgical Pathology, 4th edition*. Philadelphia: Lippincott Williams & Wilkins, 2004.

Rosai J. *Rosai and Ackerman's Surgical Pathology, 9th edition*. St. Louis: Mosby, 2004.

Murphy WM, Beckwith JB, Farrow GM. *Tumors of the Kidney, Bladder, and Related Urinary Structures: Atlas of Tumor Pathology, 3rd series. Fascicle 11*. Washington DC: Armed Forces Institute of Pathology, 1994.

Murphy WM, Grignon DJ, Perlman EJ . *Tumors of the Kidney, Bladder, and Related Urinary Structures: Atlas of Tumor Pathology, 4th series. Fascicle 1*. Washington DC: Armed Forces Institute of Pathology, 2004

Kumar V, Abbas, AK Fausto, N (eds.) *Robbins and Cotran Pathologic Basis of Disease, 7th edition*. Philadelphia: Elsevier Saunders, 2005.

Eble JN, Sauter G, Epstein JI, Sesterhenn IA (eds). *World Health Organization Classification of Tumours. Pathology & Genetics of Tumours of the Urinary System and Male Genital Organs*. IARC Press: Lyon, 2004.

Chapter 17

Mandible and Maxilla

Odontogenic Tumors

Ameloblastoma

Clinical Manifestations

- Most common odontogenic tumor
- Usually diagnosed in the 3rd and 4th decades (unicystic tumors are more typically diagnosed in the 2nd and 3rd decades)
- Affect men and women equally
- Tend to be associated with unerupted or impacted teeth, especially mandibular third molars
- 80% occur in mandible and 20% in maxilla
- Mandibular lesions usually occur in molar region and ascending ramus (80%)

Radiographic Features

- Usually a well-defined multilocular, radiolucent lesion with a hyperostotic border and displacement of a molar tooth
- Unilocular lesions may occur
- Teeth may be embedded within the neoplasm

Gross and Microscopic Pathology

- A benign but locally invasive lesion consisting of proliferating odontogenic epithelium
- 2 main patterns (multicystic/solid):
  - *Follicular pattern*: Epithelium is architecturally arranged in more or less discrete islands that consist of a central mass of polyhedral cells or loosely connected stellate cells surrounded by a palisaded and polarized layer of cuboidal or columnar cells resembling internal dental epithelium or preameloblasts; cysts frequently form within the islands of epithelium; extensive squamous metaplasia (sometimes with keratin formation) may be present within islands of tumor cells (*acanthomatous variant*); occasionally epithelial cells are large, cuboidal or columnar and have cytoplasm filled with acidophilic granules (*granular cell variant)*
  - *Plexiform pattern*: tumor epithelium arranged in anastomosing strands and cords of cuboidal to columnar cells with hyperchromatic nuclei that are polarized away from surrounding basement membrane (reverse polarity); cyst formation may occur, but usually is the result of stromal degeneration rather than actual cystic change
- *Unicystic ameloblastoma*; three histologic variants:
  - Lining form: cystic space lined by a rather banal epithelium that may have focal areas that are transformed to basal cells with a cuboidal or columnar shape and hyperchromatic nuclei, nuclear palisading with polarization and cytoplasmic vacuolization with intercellular spacing and subepithelial hyalinization
  - Luminal form: lining similar to that described above with localized areas where a nodule of odontogenic epithelium with a plexiform pattern projects into the lumen
  - Mural form: a part of the wall of the cyst is infiltrated by either typical plexiform or follicular ameloblastoma; may infiltrate adjacent bone
- Other variants:
  - Desmoplastic ameloblastoma: Characterized by markedly hyalinized, relatively acellular connective tissue stroma adjacent to the epithelium (usually seen in the follicular type)
  - Basal cell ameloblastoma: Characterized by a predominantly basaloid pattern
  - Peripheral ameloblastoma: Arise directly from surface epithelium or from residual dental lamina lying outside bone; does not invade, and rarely recurs after local excision
  - Keratoameloblastoma: Characterized by extensive keratinization (a feature that is absent or very limited in most ameloblastomas)
  - Papilliferous ameloblastoma: Characterized by microcysts that contain keratin and are lined by parakeratinized epithelium; very rare
  - Malignant ameloblastoma: Characterized by cytologic features of malignancy
  - Sinonasal ameloblastoma: Occur at mean age of 60 years; does not originate from alveolar bone

Special Stains and Immunohistochemistry

- Not helpful

Electron Microscopy

- Eosinophilic granules of the granular cell variant are lysosomes

Molecular Alterations

- None

Differential Diagnosis

- Basal cell ameloblastoma must be distinguished from intraosseous adenoid cystic carcinoma
- Ameloblastomas that have some dystrophic mineralization must be differentiated from calcifying epithelial odontogenic tumor and from adenomatoid odontogenic tumor
- Craniopharyngoma (ameloblastoma lacks wet keratin, "ghost cells")

Treatment

- Complete surgical excision with removal of 1 cm of medullary bone
- If perforation has occurred into overlying alveolar or oral mucosa, the involved tissue should be excised
- Simple unicystic ameloblastomas and plexiform unicystic ameloblastomas can be treated with simple enucleation

Prognosis

- High rate of recurrence (may be late); no tendency to metastasize
- Tend to spread through cancellous bone and cause resorption of compact bone; do not infiltrate Haversian canals
- Unicystic, peripheral, and desmoplastic lesions have lower recurrence rates than the other variants

Associations

- May arise as a result of neoplastic change in the wall of a non-neoplastic odontogenic cyst

Calcifying Epithelial Odontogenic Tumor (Pindborg Tumor)

Clinical Manifestations

- <1% of odontogenic tumors
- Evenly distributed throughout the 20s to 60s
- Men and women affected equally
- 65% occur in the mandible; 35% the maxilla
- 3 times more likely to be in the molar region than in the premolar region
- Most are intraosseous; extraosseous lesions usually located anteriorly
- 50% associated with an unerupted or embedded tooth or teeth
- Most commonly presents as a slowly enlarging painless mass

Radiographic Features

- An irregular radiolucent defect that contains radiopaque masses of varying size and tends to be localized close to the crown of an unerupted tooth
- Periphery of radiolucent zone may or may not be clearly demarcated from adjacent normal bone

Gross and Microscopic Pathology

- Typically tumor cells are polyhedral and have well-defined cell borders with distinct intercellular bridges; cells are typically pleomorphic with large, slightly lobulated nuclei and prominent nucleoli
- Multinucleated cells may be present
- Mitoses rare
- Droplet type calcifications with concentric lamellar appositional rings (Liesegang) commonly present
- Rounded masses of amyloidlike material (which may calcify) lie within sheets of tumor; amyloidlike material may be a degeneration product of epithelial cells or may be actively secreted from epithelial cells
- Intraosseous lesions tend to have more foci of calcification than peripheral or extraosseous lesions

Special Stains

- Thioflavine T and Congo red (polarized light) shows the homogenous material within the sheets of epithelial cells to have a reaction similar to that of amyloid

Immunohistochemistry

- Epithelial cells positive for cytokeratins and *Ulex europaeus*
- Occasional cells positive for S-100

Electron Microscopy

- Cells resemble cells of stratum intermedium of enamel organ

Molecular Alterations

- None

Differential Diagnosis

- Portions of the tumor may closely resemble adenomatoid odontogenic tumor

Treatment

- Wide excision with tumor-free margins

Prognosis

- Locally invasive neoplasm that may recur (up to 15%)
- Generally a less aggressive lesion than an ameloblastoma

Associations

- 6% seen in association with adenomatoid odontogenic tumor

Adenomatoid Odontogenic Tumor

Clinical Manifestations

- Very rare; more common in females than males (2:1)
- Usually seen in the 2nd decade
- Presents as a slowly enlarging painless swelling
- Maxilla involved twice as often as mandible; region of the canines in the anterior maxilla most common site
- Typically associated with an unerupted tooth and may closely mimic a dentigerous cyst both radiographically and at surgery

Gross Pathology

- Usually encapsulated soft tissue mass surrounding the crown of an unerupted tooth
- May be solid or may have extensive cyst formation

Radiographic Features

- Well-defined unilocular or multilocular lesion surrounding the crown of an unerupted or impacted tooth
- Focal or diffuse calcification may be present

Microscopic Pathology

- Well-defined connective tissue capsule surrounding an intracystic, nodular proliferation of epithelial cells
- 2 types of epithelial cells:
  - Spindle-shaped and polyhedral cells arranged in large nodular aggregates with a swirling pattern; nodular aggregates usually solid and have little stroma, but occasionally form small rosettes surrounding eosinophilic, amorphous nodules
  - Cuboidal and columnar cells surrounding microcystic or ductlike spaces resulting in a glandlike pattern; cells lining ductlike spaces have foamy cytoplasm and basally oriented oval nuclei with stippled chromatin
- Amyloidlike material and calcification may be present

Special Stains and Immunohistochemistry

- Acidophilic material that lies between apposing rows of columnar cells is usually periodic acid-Schiff (PAS) positive and immunohistochemical studies confirm this material to be basement membrane-like

Electron Microscopy

- Not helpful

Molecular Alterations

- None

Differential Diagnosis

- Dentigerous cyst
- Ameloblastoma
- Pindborg tumor

Treatment

- Enucleation with preservation of involved tooth if appropriate

Prognosis

- Noninvasive lesion that does not recur once removed

Associations

- None

Odontogenic Myxoma

Clinical Manifestations

- Usually develops in tooth-bearing areas of mandible and maxilla
- 60% occur in the 2nd and 3rd decades
- May be slightly more common in women than men
- Usually asymptomatic, but may grow rapidly
- 65% located in mandible; usually molar regions

Gross Pathology

- Margin may be well-defined or poorly-defined (gelatinous lesions usually less circumscribed)
- Cut section homogenous and slightly translucent

Radiographic Features

- Multiple variably sized radiolucent areas separated by straight or curved bony septa ("soap-bubble" appearance); may expand cortex; rarely perforates into adjacent soft tissue
- Appearance may be indistinguishable from ameloblastoma

Microscopic Pathology

- Stellate or bipolar cells with long, branching cytoplasmic processes scattered throughout an abundant mucoid stroma
- Atypical nuclei may be present
- Collagen uniformly distributed throughout and capillaries may be prominent (if collagen represents a significant component, the lesion is called a *myxofibroma*)
- Occasionally small islands or strands of inactive looking odontogenic epithelium surrounded by a zone of hyalinization may be present

Special Stains

- Stroma rich in acid mucopolysaccharides (chondroitin sulfate and hyaluronic acid) that will stain with Alcian blue

Immunohistochemistry

- Myxoma cells are reactive for vimentin and are negative for S-100 protein and neuron-specific enolase

Electron Microscopy

- Not helpful

Molecular Alterations

- None

Differential Diagnosis

- Myxomatous dental papillae
- Metastatic Wilms tumor with myxoid features

Treatment

- Complete surgical removal

Prognosis

- High recurrence rate if not completely excised
- Do not metastasize

Associations

- None

Odontogenic Fibroma

Clinical Manifestations

- Typically occurs in the maxilla anterior to the molars; when in mandible, tends to occur posterior to first molars
- Much more common in women than in men

Gross Pathology

- Well-defined, smooth, firm, solid white mass
- Cut surface homogeneous and glistening

Radiographic Features

- Usually a unilocular lucency with well-defined thin sclerotic margins

Microscopic Pathology

- Characterized by a wide spectrum of appearances: myxoid and fibroblastic to densely hyalinized; cellular to acellular; calcification and easily recognized odontogenic epithelium may or may not be present

- Often the lesion consists of a well-circumscribed mass of stellate or bipolar fibroblasts arranged in a storiform pattern distributed in a stroma of eosinophilic, finely fibrillar (occasionally coarse) collagen and proteoglycan material; variable numbers of odontogenic epithelial rests
- Occasionally foci of dysplastic cementum or bone may be present
- May occur outside the bone (*peripheral odontogenic fibroma*); a gingival lesion composed of strands and islands of odontogenic epithelium and immature fibrous stroma that is usually <1 cm in size and does not destroy bone

Special Stains, Immunohistochemistry and Electron Microscopy

- Not helpful

Molecular Alterations

- None

Differential Diagnosis

- Odontogenic myxoma
- Myxofibroma

Treatment

- Enucleation and curettage

Prognosis

- Benign
- Recurrence rare

Associations

- Concurrent giant cell granuloma may be present

Cementoblastoma

Clinical Manifestations

- Most arise in the posterior segment of the alveolus of the mandible adjacent to the roots of erupted permanent teeth
- Slightly more common in women than in men
- Typically diagnosed during 3rd decade
- Most present with pain; large lesions may present with localized swelling

Radiographic Features

- An expansile rounded mass of opaque tissue with a thin radiolucent rim in intimate association with the root of a tooth; portions of the tooth root may be resorbed

Gross Pathology

- Typically a round hard mass of cementumlike tissue fused to the root of a tooth

Microscopic Pathology

- Characterized by masses of tissue with prominent basophilic acellular cementumlike lines, irregular lacunae, in a cellular fibrovascular stroma surrounded by a fibrous connective tissue margin; cementum characterized by presence of random and irregular arrays of collagen fibers
- Plump cementoblasts line the nodular masses of cementum
- Cementocytes occupy lacunae, but are smaller than the marginally located cementoblasts
- Periphery characterized by prominent dilated vasculature and radially oriented bony spicules at the interface between the fibrovascular stroma and nodules of cementum
- Foci of resorption of root surface cementum by osteoclast-type giant cells may be present
- Tumor histologically resembles osteoblastoma or osteoid osteoma (the former does not develop in relationship to the root of a tooth)

Special Stains, Immunohistochemistry and Electron Microscopy

- Not helpful

Molecular Alterations

- None

Differential Diagnosis

- Osteoblastoma
- Osteosarcoma

Treatment and Prognosis

- Surgical removal of the affected tooth and the associated mass (occasionally the tooth can be saved)
- Recurrence typical if mass if not completely excised

Associations

- None

Odontoma

Variants

- Complex odontoma
- Compound odontoma

Clinical Manifestations

- Most commonly occur in the premolar or molar region
- Typically diagnosed during the first 2 decades of life
- Small lesions may be incidental findings on x-ray of adults
- May cause expansion of bone
- Affects males and females equally

Radiographic Features

- Lesion typically starts as a well-defined radiolucency in which there is progressive deposition of nodular radiopaque material (impacted, supernumerary teeth may or may not be present)

Gross Pathology

- May contain toothlike structures (compound odontoma tends to contain many toothlike structures that do not resemble the teeth of normal dentition)

Microscopic Pathology

- *Complex odontoma*
  - Consists primarily of a disordered mixture of dental tissues (enamel matrix, tubular dentin, and pulpal tissue)
  - Even if individual tissues are well formed, they tend to have a disordered or haphazard pattern
  - May be difficult to distinguish from ameloblastic fibroma or fibro-odontoma
- *Compound odontoma*
  - Loose myxoid stroma in which dental tissues tend to be arranged in more orderly pattern than complex odontoma and structures that resemble normal teeth are present
  - Components of a tooth—enamel, dentin, cementum, and pulp—are arranged normally

Special Stains, Immunohistochemistry, and Electron Microscopy

- Not helpful

Molecular Alterations

- None

Differential Diagnosis

- Ameloblastic fibroma
- Fibro-odontoma

Treatment

- Conservative local excision

Prognosis

- Tend to be self-limited lesions that may recur if incompletely removed (particularly during their early development)

Associations

- None

Ameloblastic Fibroma

Clinical Manifestations

- 2% of odontogenic tumors
- Typically diagnosed prior to the age of 20
- 80% occur in mandible
- Usually present with local swelling

Radiographic Features

- Usually well-defined unilocular or multilocular cystic lucency in the premolar-molar region of the mandible often associated with an unerupted tooth
- Usually radiologically identical to an ameloblastoma

Gross Pathology

- Well-defined, smooth, tan to white and translucent; usually solid, but may be cystic

Microscopic Pathology

- Characterized by strands, islands, and buds of cuboidal or tall columnar palisaded epithelial cells (reminiscent of early enamel organ development) in a cellular connective tissue stroma
- Centers of epithelial cell islands contain a stellate reticulum; a well-defined basement membrane separates the islands from surrounding cellular stroma
- Cyst formation within the epithelium is rare
- Occasionally stromal cells will contain finely granular cytoplasm (*granular cell ameloblastic fibroma*)
- Hard tooth structures such as enamel and dentin absent

Special Stains, Immunohistochemistry, and Electron Microscopy

- Not helpful

Molecular Alterations

- None

Differential Diagnosis

- Ameloblastoma

Treatment

- Simple excision

Prognosis

- Benign lesion with no evidence of malignant transformation
- Rarely recurs

Associations

- None

Squamous Odontogenic Tumor

Clinical Manifestations

- Most occur during the 3rd decade of life (may be seen from the second decade to the seventh)
- Men and women affected equally
- Affects the maxilla and mandible equally; tends to occur in the anterior maxilla and posterior mandible (lesions in the anterior maxilla are generally more aggressive)
- Most are unilocular, but some are multicentric
- Usually presents as localized loosening of 1 or several teeth

Radiographic Features

- Usually a unilocular radiolucency in alveolar segment of bone directly involving and surrounding a tooth root

Gross and Microscopic Pathology

- Characterized by islands and cords of well-differentiated stratified squamous epithelium with a mature moderately vascularized connective tissue stroma of fibroblasts and collagen
- Islands of epithelium have a peripheral layer of flattened connective tissue cells (the columnar cells typical of an ameloblastoma are not present)
- No atypia within the squamous epithelium and no mitotic activity; individual cell keratinization uncommon; well-developed intercellular bridges prominent
- 50% have microscopic foci of degeneration and/or calcified areas within the islands of squamous epithelium

Special Stains, Immunohistochemistry, and Electron Microscopy

- Not helpful

Molecular Alterations

- None

Differential Diagnosis

- Ameloblastoma with acanthomatous features
- Desmoplastic ameloblastoma

Treatment

- Extraction of involved tooth or teeth and conservative excision of lesion
- Aggressive maxillary lesions require wide local excision

Prognosis

- Recurrence rare

Associations

- None

Odontogenic Cysts

Classification

- *Developmental odontogenic cysts*
  - Gingival cysts of infants (Epstein pearls)
  - Odontogenic keratocyst
  - Dentigerous (follicular) cyst
  - Eruption cyst
  - Lateral periodontal cyst
  - Gingival cyst of adults
  - Glandular odontogenic cyst (sialo-odontogenic cyst)
- *Developmental nonodontogenic cysts*
  - Nasopalatine duct cyst (incisive canal) cyst
  - Nasolabial (nasoalveolar) cyst
- *Inflammatory cysts*
  - Radicular cyst
  - Periapical and lateral cysts
  - Residual radicular cyst
  - Paradental (inflammatory collateral, mandibular infected buccal) cyst

Dentigerous Cyst (Follicular Cyst)

Clinical Manifestations, Gross Pathology and Microscopic Pathology

- Encloses the crown of an tooth and is attached circumferentially to the neck of that tooth
- Fluid accumulates between reduced enamel epithelium and the crown or between layers of the reduced enamel epithelium
- Usually found near mandibular third molars and maxillary cuspids
- Usually diagnosed in the 2nd to 4th decades
- Slightly more common in men than women
- Typically a well-defined lucent area associated with the crown of an unerupted tooth on x-ray
- Cyst wall composed of a thin layer of connective tissue lined by epithelium that is only 1 to 2 cells thick and resembles reduced enamel epithelium; variable numbers of mucus-producing cells, ciliated cells and focal keratinization may be present
- Presence of inflammation causes the epithelium to thicken and appear more squamous; inflammatory cells infiltrate the cyst wall and lie within the cyst lumen (may resemble a radicular cyst with cholesterol and Rushton bodies)

Special Stains, Immunohistochemistry, Electron Microscopy, and Molecular Alterations

- Not helpful

Differential Diagnosis

- Odontogenic keratocyst
- Odontogenic fibroma or myxoma
- Lateral periodontal cyst
- Glandular odontogenic cyst (sialo-odontogenic cyst)
- Collateral odontogenic keratocyst
- Gingival cyst of adults
- Inflammatory cyst lateral to root of tooth

Treatment and Prognosis

- Enucleation of cyst and removal of associated tooth; neoplastic transformation to ameloblastoma, squamous cell carcinoma, and central mucoepidermoid carcinoma reported

Eruption Cyst

Clinical Manifestations, Gross Pathology and Microscopic Pathology

- Surrounds the crown of an erupting tooth and at least partially lies outside the bone (essentially a dentigerous cyst that lies in the soft tissue external to the bone)
- Presents as a bluish swelling in the area where a tooth will erupt

- May impede tooth eruption
- Lined by nonkeratinizing stratified squamous epithelium
- When inflamed, epithelial lining proliferates and thickens

Special Stains, Immunohistochemistry, Electron Microscopy, and Molecular Alterations

- Not helpful

Differential Diagnosis

- Ameloblastoma
- Nasolabial (nasoalveolar) cyst
- Glandular odontogenic cyst

Treatment and Prognosis

- Marsupialization allows tooth to erupt

Gingival Cyst of Adults

Clinical Manifestations, Gross Pathology, and Microscopic Pathology

- Arise from odontogenic epithelial remnants in the gingiva of adults
- Usually present as a well-circumscribed swelling <1 cm in diameter in the canine-premolar region of the mandibular buccal gingiva
- Lining varies from extremely thin epithelium with 1 or 2 cell layers of flat or cuboidal cells to thick stratified squamous epithelium without rete ridges; occasionally epithelial plaques of fusiform or clear cells (similar to those that characterize a lateral periodontal cyst) are present
- Surrounding fibrous connective tissue usually not inflamed

Special Stains, Immunohistochemistry, Electron Microscopy, and Molecular Alterations

- Not helpful

Differential Diagnosis

- Lateral peridontal cyst
- Glandular odontogenic cyst (sialo-odontogenic cyst)

Treatment and Prognosis

- Simple excision; recurrence rare

Gingival Cyst of Infants (Epstein Pearls)

Clinical Manifestations, Gross Pathology and Microscopic Pathology

- Arise from epithelial cell rests in alveolar mucosa
- Usually present at birth; rarely seen after the age of three months
- Present as white or yellow nodules located over the site of a future tooth-bearing area of the alveolar mucosa
- Lined by stratified squamous epithelium with flat basal cells and a parakeratinized surface
- Keratin debris fills the cystic cavity

Special Stains, Immunohistochemistry, Electron Microscopy, and Molecular Alterations

- Not helpful

Differential Diagnosis

- Natal or neonatal teeth
- Lymphangioma

Treatment and Prognosis

- No treatment required; will involute or rupture

Glandular Odontogenic Cyst (Sialo-Odontogenic Cyst)

Clinical Manifestations, Gross Pathology and Microscopic Pathology

- Arise in tooth-bearing areas of jaws
- More common in mandible
- Slightly more common in women
- A multicystic lesion lined by nonkeratinized stratified epithelium with focal plaquelike thickenings (similar to those of lateral periodontal cyst and gingival cyst of adult) partially covered by an epithelial layer that contains eosinophilic cuboidal or columnar cells with cilia that may form irregular papillary projections, mucous cells, and pools of mucin in microcysts

Special Stains, Immunohistochemistry, Electron Microscopy, and Molecular Alterations

- Not helpful

Differential Diagnosis

- Collateral odontogenic keratocyst
- Gingival cyst of adults
- Inflammatory cyst lateral to root of tooth

Treatment and Prognosis

- Marginal resection; locally aggressive and may recur

Lateral Periodontal Cyst

Clinical Manifestations, Gross Pathology and Microscopic Pathology

- Arises from odontogenic epithelial remnants and lies lateral to or between the roots of vital teeth
- Usually located in premolar area of the mandible; anterior maxilla 2nd most common location
- Lined by thin, nonkeratinizing squamous or cuboidal epithelium 1 to 5 cells thick; nuclei tend to be small and pyknotic; localized epithelial plaques that contain fusiform or clear (glycogen) cells frequently present; epithelial lining occasionally separated from underlying connective tissue
- When multiloculated, referred to as *botryoid odontogenic cyst*

Special Stains, Immunohistochemistry, Electron Microscopy, and Molecular Alterations

- Not helpful

Differential Diagnosis

- Gingival cyst of adults
- Nasolabial (nasoalveolar) cyst
- Low-grade cystic central mucoepidermoid carcinoma
- Nasopalatine duct (incisive canal) cyst
- Radicular cyst
- Periapical granuloma

Treatment and Prognosis

- Enucleation of cyst without extraction of adjacent teeth; squamous cell carcinoma has been reported; multicystic variant (botryoid odontogenic cyst) more aggressive and tends to recur

Odontogenic Keratocyst (Primordial Cyst)

Clinical Manifestations, Gross Pathology and Microscopic Pathology

- 5% to 10% of odontogenic cysts
- Mandible more frequently involved than maxilla (2:1); typically arises from dental lamina or its remnants just posterior to the mandibular 3rd molar or the ramus of the mandible
- May be associated with an erupted or unerupted tooth or occur in a non-tooth-bearing region of the jaw
- May present in a dentigerous (associated with crown of impacted tooth), primordial (associated with undeveloped tooth), residual (area where tooth was present), lateral peridontal, globulo-maxillary, or nasopalatine location
- Peak incidence in the 2nd and 3rd decades with a second peak in the 5th decade
- More common in men than women
- May be unilocular or multilocular and wall tends to have a scalloped border on x-ray
- Cyst wall typically thin with a well-defined basal layer composed of palisaded columnar or cuboidal cells under several layers of typical squamous cells that mature to a parakeratotic surface (*parakeratinized odontogenic keratocyst*)
- Basal cell nuclei may have a reversed polarity
- Cyst lining has a corrugated surface and may be focally detached from the fibrous capsule;
- Foci of dysplasia and squamous cell carcinoma may be present in the epithelium
- Occasionally, epithelial islands or daughter cysts may be present in the wall of the main lesion
- *Orthokeratinized odontogenic keratocyst* characterized by presence of orthokeratin overlying granular layer and a well-defined basal layer without palisading
- If the lesion becomes inflamed, the fibrous capsule thickens, the epithelium develops rete processes, and the keratinization may be lost; cholesterol and epithelial hyaline bodies (Rushton bodies) may be present
- Occasionally a tooth will erupt into the cyst cavity
- When multiple, usually a component of the basal cell nevus syndrome (see associations)

Special Stains, Immunohistochemistry, and Electron Microscopy

- Not helpful

Molecular Alterations

- p53 identified in odontogenic keratocysts
- Aberrations of PTCH gene on chromosome 9q in both sporadic and Gorlin syndrome

Differential Diagnosis

- Dentigerous cyst
- Nasopalatine duct cyst (incisive canal) cyst

Treatment and Prognosis

- Treatment controversial: conservative treatment (enucleation, curettage, decompression, marsupialization) associated with a higher recurrence rate than resection
- *Orthokeratinized odontogenic keratocyst* has a lower recurrence rate than a *parakeratinized odontogenic keratocyst*

Associations

- Odontogenic keratocysts (especially when multiple) occur as a component of the autosomal dominant basal cell nevus syndrome (Gorlin-Goltz syndrome) characterized by numerous basal cell carcinomas, cysts of the jaws, skeletal anomalies, a blunted response to parathormone, increased incidence of medulloblastoma, characteristic facies to include frontal and parietal bossing, hypertelorism, and mandibular prognathism, cutaneous epidermoid cysts, pits on the palms and souls, and calcifying ovarian fibromas

Radicular Cyst

Variants, Clinical Manifestations, Gross Pathology and Microscopic Pathology

- *Radicular cyst*
  - Typically arises from epithelial odontogenic remnants (rests of Malassez) in the periodontal ligament secondary to inflammation following necrosis of dental pulp; tends to occur in association with the apical foramen or the lateral root surface of a nonvital tooth; usually the result of dental caries or trauma
- *Periapical and lateral radicular cyst*
  - Most common cyst of jaw
  - May occur in relation to any tooth, but usually seen in the anterior region of the maxilla
  - Tends to occur in the 3rd and 4th decades
  - Men are affected more frequently than women
  - Most are lined by nonkeratinized stratified squamous epithelium; thickness of epithelium varies considerably according to the amount of inflammation present; if inflamed the epithelium will be thickened and have proliferating rete processes; if there is no inflammation the epithelium tends to be thin, lack rete processes, and have extensive juxtaepithelial hyalinization; when hyalinization is extensive the epithelium is usually tenuous and degenerate
  - Epithelium may contain mucous or ciliated cells
  - Intraepithelial hyaline (Rushton) bodies may be present (also seen in dentigerous and odontogenic keratocysts)
  - Foamy macrophages may be present within the cystic cavity and heavy deposits of cholesterol crystals with an associated foreign body cell reaction may be present in the fibrous portion of the cyst wall
  - Cyst wall often has a zone of dense inflammatory cells that lie between the epithelial lining and the outer fibrous wall
- *Residual radicular cyst*
  - A radicular cyst that remains in the jaw after the removal of the associated tooth
- *Paradental (inflammatory collateral, mandibular infected buccal) cyst*
  - Inflammatory process that occurs in a periodontal pocket near the lateral aspect of a root of a vital tooth; may occur on the buccal and distal aspects of erupted mandibular molars (most commonly the third molars) in a patient with a history of pericoronitis; similar lesions occur on the buccal surface of the mandibular first molar in children (*mandibular infected buccal* cyst)

Special Stains, Immunohistochemistry, Electron Microscopy, and Molecular Alterations

- Not helpful

Treatment and Prognosis

- Conservative nonsurgical endodontic therapy; rare cases of carcinoma reported

Fissural Cysts

Nasopalatine Duct Cyst (Incisive Canal Cyst)

Clinical Manifestations, Gross Pathology and Microscopic Pathology

- Arise from remnants of epithelium in the nasopalatine (incisive) canal in the midline of anterior maxilla between and posterior to central incisors
- Most appear in the 4th to 6th decades
- Males are three times more commonly affected than females
- On x-ray, appears as a well-defined round or ovoid lucency in the midline of the maxilla
- Lined by stratified squamous epithelium, pseudostratified ciliated columnar epithelium, or a combination of the two; occasionally transitional types of epithelium may be present; connective tissue in the wall of the cyst usually contains large nerves and vessels as well as mucous glands and adipose tissue; occasionally a small island of cartilage is present

Special Stains, Immunohistochemistry, Electron Microscopy, and Molecular Alterations

- Not helpful

Differential Diagnosis

- Periapical granuloma

Treatment and Prognosis

- Surgical enucleation; carcinoma may occur

Nasolabial Cyst (Nasoalveolar Cyst)

Clinical Manifestations, Gross Pathology and Microscopic Pathology

- Typically located in the soft tissues of the canine fossa beneath the ala of the nose on the maxillary alveolar process
- Peak incidence is 4th and 5th decades
- Much more common in women than in men
- Does not arise within bone but may superficially erode the surface of adjacent bone (maxilla); probably arises from embryonic nasolacrimal duct
- Wall is typically corrugated and the lining may be ciliated or nonciliated, pseudostratified columnar epithelium which may contain numerous mucous cells; foci of squamous epithelium or cuboidal epithelium

Special Stains, Immunohistochemistry, Electron Microscopy, and Molecular Alterations

- Not helpful

Treatment and Prognosis

- Intraoral surgical excision; recurrence very rare

Bone-Related Lesions

Giant Cell Granuloma (Giant Cell Reparative Granuloma, Central Giant Cell Lesion)

Clinical Manifestations

- Usually diagnosed in 3rd decade of life
- More frequent in women than men (3:2)
- Tends to occur in anterior tooth-bearing area of mandible
- Lesion may expand bone, penetrate cortex, and present as a localized gingival swelling

Variants

- Small nonaggressive lesion
- Large aggressive lesion

Radiographic Features

- Small, nonaggressive lesion usually a well-defined lucency unrelated to a tooth
- Large, aggressive lesion characterized by focus of destruction with a smooth or lobulated outline; interior may be traversed by slender bony septa giving the lesion a multilocular appearance (radiologically similar to an ameloblastoma)

Gross and Microscopic Pathology

- Characteristically composed of cellular fibrous tissue containing multiple foci of hemorrhage, aggregates of osteoclastlike giant cells, and spicules of woven bone; endothelial-lined vascular spaces in association with fibroblasts give the lesion an appearance resembling granulation tissue

- Multinucleated giant cells tend to be smaller and have fewer nuclei than giant cells of a typical giant cell tumor
- Foci of fresh hemorrhage and deposits of fibrinoid material often present
- Mitotic figures not uncommon
- Aggressive lesion closely resembles giant cell tumor of bone; some lesions have relatively large vascular spaces and resemble aneurysmal bone cyst

Special Stains

- Not helpful

Immunohistochemistry

- Giant cells stain with monoclonal antibody against osteoclasts (eg, CD68)

Molecular Alterations

- None

Differential Diagnosis

- Cherubism
- Brown tumor of hyperparathyroidism
- Giant cell tumor of bone (giant cells of giant cell tumors tend to be larger and contain more nuclei than the giant cells in giant cell granulomas; true giant cell tumors do not occur in the jaws)
- Solid variant of aneurysmal bone cyst

Treatment

- Simple curettage and complete resection for small non-aggressive lesions and large aggressive lesions respectively

Prognosis

- May recur if incompletely excised (presence or absence of cortical disruption most significant predictor of recurrence)
- Neoplasm is not invasive and does not metastasize

Associations

- None

Cherubism (Familial Multilocular Cystic Disease of the Jaws)

Clinical Manifestations

- Lesions typically occur during early childhood and have a familial tendency
- Tend to affect all four quadrants of the jaw in a symmetric fashion and cause malocclusion
- More common in boys than in girls (2:1)
- Lesions tend to be more active in young patients; activity diminishes after puberty; eventually becomes completely inactive

Radiographic Features

- Lesions appear as multilocular, radiolucent areas that expand bone; trabeculation produces "soap bubble" appearance
- Cortical surface usually intact
- Teeth absent, displaced, or floating in the lesion
- As lesion regresses bone fills the lytic areas

Gross and Microscopic Pathology

- May begin as unilateral involvement
- Essentially indistinguishable from giant cell granuloma, solid variant of aneurysmal bone cyst, and brown tumor of hyperparathyroidism
- A reactive-looking fibrovascular stroma that contains varying numbers of multinucleated giant cells, multiple foci of hemosiderin, and occasional seams of osteoid and woven bone
- A cuff of acidophilic material may surround blood vessels
- As activity diminishes, lesion becomes progressively more fibrotic with diminution of giant cells and simultaneous appearance of new bone

Special Stains

- Eosinophilic cuff that surrounds blood vessels is van Gieson (collagen) positive

Immunohistochemistry and Electron Microscopy

- Not helpful

Molecular Alterations

- Autosomal dominant mode of inheritance mapped to chromosome 4p16.3

Differential Diagnosis

- Central giant cell granuloma
- Solid variant of aneurysmal bone cyst
- Hyperparathyroidism

Treatment

- Surgical intervention (correction of cosmetic deformity) should be performed only after cessation of bone growth since lesion regresses with time
- No role for radiotherapy

Prognosis

- Condition typically completely inactive after the age of 20 years

Associations

- *Noonan syndrome*: multiple giant cell granulomas of jaws in patients with phenotype of Noonan syndrome (body habitus of Turner, hypertelorism, downward slanting palpebral fissures, ptosis, low set ears, cryptorchidism, heart defects, and abnormal oral features, eg, micrognathia, cleft palate, bifid uvula, and dental malocclusion)

Melanotic Neuroectodermal Tumor of Infancy (Melanotic Progonoma)

Clinical Manifestations

- Typically seen before the age of 1 year
- Affects boys and girls equally
- Craniofacial region involved in 70%; usually arises in the anterior part of the maxilla
- Also reported to occur in the mandible, skull, long bones, epididymis, uterus, mediastinum, and soft tissues of extremities
- Usually nonfunctional; catecholamine secretion reported

Radiographic Features

- Expansion and osteolytic destruction of affected bone

Gross Pathology

- Lesion may be completely contained within bone or present as an exophytic gingival mass
- Typically associated with bone destruction; adjacent developing teeth often displaced
- Cut surface reveals varying degrees of pigmentation from focal areas of discoloration to uniform deep black

Microscopic Pathology

- Characterized by alveolar nests and tubules composed of 2 cell types, large peripheral pigmented cells and small neuroblastic-type cells, in a fibrous stroma
- Epithelial-like cells are large and pale staining, contain variable numbers of melanin granules, and are arranged in sheets, cords or ductlike structures which surround groups of small neuroblastic type cells; a fibrillar network is usually present between nuclei of neuroblastic cells
- Neuroblastic cells tend to resemble small lymphocytes with dense round (smudged) nuclei and scant cytoplasm; occasionally these cells have larger nuclei with fine chromatin
- Margin characterized by irregular extension into surrounding bone giving the tumor an invasive appearance

Special Stains

- Not helpful

Immunohistochemistry

- Large pigmented cells are positive for cytokeratin, vimentin, and HMB-45 and are variably positive for epithelial membrane antigen (EMA) and S-100 protein
- Small neuroblastic cells stain for synaptophysin, glial fibrillary acidic protein , and S-100 protein
- Both cell types stain with CD57 (Leu-7)

Electron Microscopy

- Large pigmented cells contain premelanosomes, melanosomes, tonofilament bundles, and desmosomes
- Neuroblastic cells contain neurosecretory type granules, neurotubules, and neurofilaments

Molecular Alterations

- None

Differential Diagnosis

- Melanoma
- Metastatic neuroblastoma
- Rhabdomyosarcoma

Treatment and Prognosis

- Local excision; may recur (10% to 50%); metastasis rare (5%)

Associations

- None

References

Barns L, Everson JW, Reichert P, Sidransky D (eds). *World Health Organization Classification of Tumours: Pathology and Genetics Head and Neck Tumours.* Lyon: IARC Press, 2005.

Kramer IRH, Pindborg JJ, Shear M. *Histologic Typing of Odontogenic Tumours: World Health Organization International Histological Classification of Tumours. 2nd ed.* Berlin: Springer Verlag, 1992.

Mills S, Carter D, Greenson JK, Oberman HA, Reuter V, Stoler MH (eds). *Sternberg's Diagnostic Surgical Pathology. 4th ed.* Philadelphia: Lippincott Williams & Wilkins, 2004.

Rosai J. *Rosai and Ackerman's Surgical Pathology. 9th ed.* St. Louis: Mosby, 2004.

Sciubba JJ, Fantasia JE, Kahn LB. *Tumors and Cysts of the Jaw: Atlas of Tumor Pathology, 3rd series. Fascicle 29.* Washington DC: Armed Forces Institute of Pathology, 2001.

Chapter 18

Salivary Glands

Intraoperative Consultation

There are 3 indications for an intraoperative consultation on a salivary gland neoplasm. The 1st is to establish the diagnosis so that the optimal surgical procedure can be performed. In this regard, it is most important to establish the nature of the neoplasm in terms of its benign or malignant potential. The pathologist must distinguish between benign neoplasms, low-grade carcinomas, and high-grade carcinomas. The pathologist does not necessarily have to diagnose the specific histologic type of neoplasm in each of these categories, although some familiarity with specific features of salivary gland tumors is necessary to determine the correct category.

Tumors that fall into the benign category include pleomorphic adenoma (benign mixed tumor), myoepithelioma, Warthin tumor, canalicular adenoma, basal cell adenoma, and oncocytoma. All of these neoplasms, with the exception of a pleomorphic adenoma, are removed by complete excision with a narrow margin of normal tissue. Pleomorphic adenomas are excised intact with a margin of normal tissue that is wide enough to include the surface protuberances frequently present, and thereby avoid local recurrence. Low-grade carcinomas include low-grade mucoepidermoid, myoepithelial carcinoma, acinic cell, low-grade polymorphous, epithelial-myoepithelial, and basal cell adenocarcinoma. All of these low-grade carcinomas are treated with complete resection. Lymph nodes are removed if clinically positive. Low-grade, but highly aggressive tumors, include adenoid cystic carcinoma, which must be treated with complete resection with clear margins. High-grade carcinomas include high-grade mucoepidermoid adenocarcinoma, lymphoepithelial carcinomas, squamous cell carcinoma, and salivary duct carcinoma. All of these tumors are treated with radical resection to include the removal of involved nerves. Lymph node dissections are performed therapeutically for positive nodes and electively for clinically negative nodes.

The second indication for frozen section is to evaluate the adequacy of surgical margins. Salivary gland neoplasms should be inked, serially sectioned in 1 to 2 mm parallel sections. Frozen section samples should be taken at the interface between tumor and normal salivary gland and at the point(s) where the neoplasm most closely approaches the margin. Sections at the interface between normal and abnormal may demonstrate an infiltrating margin, perineural invasion, and the presence of a chronic inflammatory infiltrate at the periphery of the neoplasm, all features more likely to be seen in carcinomas than in benign lesions.

The final indication for frozen section in salivary gland tumors is the evaluation of regional lymph nodes to determine the appropriateness of lymph node dissection.

The pathologist is faced with a number of pitfalls in performing a frozen section for diagnosis on a salivary gland neoplasm. Salivary glands can produce a wide variety of neoplasms, many of which have similar architectural patterns. A limited sample obtained for frozen section purposes may not reveal the overall diagnostic pattern necessary to make the correct diagnosis. In addition there is often significant histologic overlap between benign and malignant tumors; for example, pleomorphic adenomas frequently have small foci that resemble adenoid cystic carcinoma. Many salivary gland cancers, particularly those of low-grade, have banal cytologic features. With the loss of cytologic morphology as a reliable indicator of carcinoma, the overall architectural pattern (to include the presence or absence of invasion) may be the only reliable criterion to determine malignancy. The site to sample for the frozen section must adequately represent the neoplasm as well as demonstrate the interface between the neoplasm and surrounding tissue.

Specimen Handling

The external surface of all surgical specimens that contain a salivary gland is inked. In the case of the parotid gland it may be advisable to ink the superficial surface a different color from the deep surface. The specimen is then serially sectioned in 2- to 3-mm parallel sections and, when possible, submitted in its entirety. Special care should be taken to ensure that all of the surgical margins as well as the interface between neoplasm and surrounding gland or soft tissue will be well demonstrated on permanent section.

Non-Neoplastic Lesions

Necrotizing Sialometaplasia

Clinical Manifestations

- Twice as common in men as in women
- Average age at diagnosis approximately 45 years
- 75% involve the minor salivary glands of the palate (usually the hard palate or the junction of the hard and soft palate); also reported in the parotid gland and oral cavity (lower lip, retromolar mucosa, tongue, and buccal mucosa)
- Usually unilateral but may be in the midline or bilateral
- Typically presents as a rapidly developing ulcer
- Most patients complain of pain or numbness in the area of the lesion

Gross Pathology

- May be a nonulcerated localized area of swelling or a craterlike ulcer

Microscopic Pathology

- Pathogenesis generally felt to be related to ischemic necrosis or infarction
- Characterized by lobular coagulative necrosis of solitary salivary gland acini, squamous metaplasia of salivary gland ducts, pseudoepitheliomatous hyperplasia of overlying or adjacent mucosal epithelium, and surrounding inflammation
- Typically the lobular architecture of the salivary gland is preserved but numerous acini demonstrate coagulative necrosis
- Necrotic cells leave mucin pools surrounded by necrotic fibrous septa and an inflammatory infiltrate consisting of both neutrophils and lymphocytes
- Squamous metaplastic change in salivary gland ducts and residual acini is always present and may be extensive; ducts retain their lobular pattern despite the metaplastic change
- Nests of cytologically bland squamous epithelium usually have smooth edges and no mitotic figures
- Mucous cells may be present in the metaplastic squamous areas
- Overlying or adjacent surface epithelium is often hyperplastic and thickened with elongated rete pegs (pseudoepitheliomatous hyperplasia)

Special Stains, Immunohistochemistry, and Electron Microscopy

- Not helpful

Molecular Alterations

- None

Differential Diagnosis

- Low-grade mucoepidermoid carcinoma
- Mucosal squamous cell carcinoma
- Distinguishing features of necrotizing sialometaplasia include:
  - A lobular architecture of the involved salivary gland
  - Coagulative necrosis of salivary gland acini and/or lobules
  - Bland cytologic appearance of both the metaplastic ducts and surface epithelium
  - Intense mixed inflammatory reaction; none of these features is characteristic of the malignancies that enter the differential diagnosis

Treatment and Prognosis

- A benign lesion that will eventually heal (usually within 3-12 weeks)

Associations

- Patients may give a history of traumatic injury, dental infection, denture use, adjacent cysts or tumors, surgery for benign or malignant tumors, and upper respiratory tract infection or allergy

Malignant Epithelial Tumors

Acinic Cell Carcinoma

Clinical Manifestations

- 3rd most common epithelial malignancy of salivary glands (mucoepidermoid carcinoma is first and adenocarcinoma, not otherwise specified [NOS], is second)
- Comprises approximately 15% of primary malignant salivary gland tumors and about 5% of all salivary gland tumors
- 85% occur in the parotid gland; 5% in the submandibular gland; most of the remainder occur in intraoral minor salivary glands
- Rarely occurs in the sublingual gland

- 3% are bilateral (most common malignant salivary gland tumor to occur bilaterally)

- More common in women; mean age 45 years
- Typically presents as a solitary enlarging mass of the parotid gland; pain or tenderness in approximately 30%; facial muscle weakness (involvement of the facial nerve) in 5% to 10%

Gross Pathology

- Most are single, firm or soft, and well-circumscribed; may even appear encapsulated
- Cut surface is lobular and tan and may be solid or cystic

Microscopic Pathology

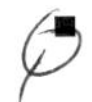

- Growth pattern may be solid, papillary-cystic, microcystic, or follicular
- Tumor cells are typically large and polygonal with granular, basophilic cytoplasm; nuclei are small, uniform, round, and located eccentrically in the cytoplasm (resemble serous cells of the normal parotid gland)
- Tumor cells may be clear (contain variable amounts of glycogen)
- Follicular pattern characterized by numerous cystic structures of various sizes filled with eosinophilic proteinaceous material
- Papillary-cystic lesions have branching papillae that protrude into cystic lumens and are lined by epithelium of variable thickness

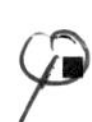

- Lymphoid follicles, some with germinal centers, often seen in the periphery of the neoplasm

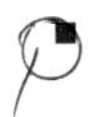

- Psammoma bodies occasionally seen

Special Stains

- PAS with diastase highlights the cytoplasmic secretory granules

Immunohistochemistry

- Tumor cells reactive for cytokeratin, transferrin, α_1-antitrypsin, α_1-antichymotrypsin, IgA, carcinoembryonic antigen (CEA), Leu-M1, and amylase

Electron Microscopy

- Tumor cells contain multiple, round, electron-dense cytoplasmic secretory granules (similar to zymogen secretory granules of normal serous acinar cells)

- Rough endoplasmic reticulum and many mitochondria are typical

Molecular Alterations

- None

Differential Diagnosis

- If minor salivary gland involved:
  - Polymorphous low-grade adenocarcinoma
- If a papillary cystic or follicular pattern predominates:
  - Cystadenocarcinoma
  - Mucoepidermoid carcinoma
  - Metastatic thyroid carcinoma
- If abundant clear cells present:
  - Clear cell adenocarcinoma
  - Clear cell oncocytoma
  - Metastatic renal cell carcinoma
  - Mucoepidermoid carcinoma

Treatment

- Complete surgical excision
- Radiation indicated only if complete excision cannot be accomplished
- Lymph node dissection performed if cervical lymph nodes clinically involved

Prognosis

- Local recurrence in 20%
- Regional lymph node metastasis present in 10% of papillary cystic variant, which has a significantly worse prognosis
- 5-year survival figures are unreliable; most recurrences seen within 5 years but death may not occur for many years
- Mortality approximately 15%

Associations

- None

Mucoepidermoid Carcinoma

Clinical Manifestations

- Most common malignant salivary gland tumor (15% of all salivary gland tumors)
- Most occur in the parotid gland (45%)
- Minor salivary glands of the palate site of origin in approximately 20%
- Approximately 20% occur in the buccal mucosa, lips (more often in the lower lip than the upper lip), retromolar region, and tongue
- More common in women than men
- Most common malignant salivary gland tumor in children (usually between ages of 10 and 20 years)
- Reported in skin, esophageus, thymus, thyroid gland, breast, lacrimal sac, and lung
- Present as asymptomatic swelling (low-grade) or as painful, hard mass with facial nerve involvement (high-grade)

Gross Pathology

- Tend to be poorly circumscribed and unencapsulated
- Cut surface firm, gray or pink, and lobulated with cysts of various size that contain bloody, mucoid material

Microscopic Pathology

- 4 cell types:
  - *Intermediate (basal) cells:* Cells that range in size from that of a lymphocyte to 2 to 3 times the size of a lymphocyte; usually seen in clusters or solid sheets and may be intermixed with other cell types
  - *Mucus-producing cells:* The neoplastic cells of the lesion that contain epithelial mucin, regardless of morphology; may resemble intermediate, epidermoid, clear, and columnar cells; may be found in clusters or as single cells
  - *Epidermoid cells:* Tend to form small solid nests or may partially line a cystic space; foci of epidermoid differentiation may be very difficult to find; keratin pearl formation and individual cell keratinization very rarely seen (more common in inflamed tumors)
  - *Clear cells:* Constitute approximately 10% of the carcinoma; contain glycogen
- Abundant fibrous hyalinized stroma
- Prominent lymphoid proliferation may be present
- Mitotic figures, nuclear atypia, and extensive necrosis all rare
- Low-grade tumors tend to be well circumscribed with a majority of well-differentiated mucous cells that form glandular or microcystic structures (>80% cystic/<20% solid)
- High-grade tumors tend to be more solid with an infiltrating pattern; intermediate, epithelial, and clear cells outnumber mucous cells (>80% solid/<20% cystic)

Special Stains

- PAS confirms presence of glycogen in the clear cells
- Mayer mucicarmine and Alcian blue will confirm the presence of both extracellular and intracellular mucin

Immunohistochemistry

- Intermediate, columnar, and epidermoid cells are positive for cytokeratin
- Clear cells are variably reactive for cytokeratin
- Well-developed mucous cells are usually negative for cytokeratin
- Most tumor cells are positive for EMA
- Tumor cells are variably reactive for muscle-specific actin, vimentin, S-100 protein, CEA, α-fetoprotein, and GFAP

Electron Microscopy

- Luminal cells have goblet cell features, secrete mucus, have microvilli on their apical surfaces, and contain tonofilaments
- Intermediate cells have basal lamina partially lining their surface

Molecular Alterations

- Expression of p53 protein in 25%
- Several known to have t(11;19)(q21;p13)

Differential Diagnosis

- Sialometaplasia
- Inverted papilloma, cystadenoma and cystadenocarcinoma
- If a predominance of epidermoid cells:
  - Primary or metastatic squamous cell carcinoma

- If a predominance of intermediate cells:
  - Pleomorphic adenoma
- If a predominance of clear cells:
  - Clear cell carcinoma
  - Epithelial-myoepithelial carcinoma
- If extensive cystic change:
  - Benign cyst

Treatment

- Stage I and II can be treated by conservative excision if the lesion is in the parotid gland
- Tumors in the submandibular gland require complete surgical excision and radiation therapy
- Tumors in minor salivary glands are treated with wide surgical excision
- Radical neck dissection is appropriate for patients with T3 disease (extraparenchymal extension or >4 cm) or high-grade tumors

Prognosis

- Depends on grade:
  - Intracystic component more than 20%: 2 points
  - Neural invasion: 2 points
  - Necrosis: 3 points
  - 4 mitotic figures per 10 high power fields: 3 points
  - Anaplasia: 4 points
- Low-grade tumors (0 to 4 points):
  - 98% 5-year survival
  - 5% metastasize to regional lymph nodes
- Intermediate-grade tumors (5-6 points):
- High-grade tumors (≥7 points):
  - 56% 5-year mortality
  - 55% metastasize to regional lymph nodes
- Recurrence likely if surgical margin not free of neoplasm

Associations

- Prior exposure to ionizing radiation
- May occur simultaneously with mixed tumor, Warthin tumor, and oncocytoma
- Extravasated mucous may result in an inflammatory response and granulation tissue reaction that may make detection of the underlying neoplasm particularly difficult
- Squamous metaplasia, as seen in necrotizing sialometaplasia and Warthin tumor may mimic mucoepidermoid carcinoma

Adenoid Cystic Carcinoma

Clinical Manifestations

- 7% to 8% of all salivary gland carcinomas; 5% of all benign and malignant epithelial salivary gland neoplasms
- More frequent in women; peak incidence in 4th and 5th decades
- 50% to 60% occur in parotid or submandibular gland
- When intraoral, 50% are in the palate
- Typically presents as a slow-growing mass in the para-auricular or submandibular region
- Intraoral lesions associated with ulcerated mucosa

Gross Pathology

- When small, typically well-circumscribed and rarely encapsulated
- Gross impression often misleading because neoplasm has a tendency to invade along nerve tracts (50% of all tumors)

Microscopic Pathology

- 3 architectural patterns: Solid, tubular, and cribriform (cribriform most common; solid least common)
- Tumor cells generally have a banal basaloid myoepithelial appearance with basophilic or clear cytoplasm and indistinct cell borders; nuclei tend to be either round or angulated and hyperchromatic or occasionally lightly basophilic; small nucleoli may be present; nuclear-cytoplasmic ratio usually 1:1
- Foci of ductal cells are scattered among the basaloid myoepithelial cells; ductal cells are about the same size, have eosinophilic cytoplasm, uniform round nuclei, and small nucleoli
- Neoplastic cells are supported by a collagenous stroma that is continuous with the cystic lumens seen in the tubular and cribriform types, hence the cystic structures are not true ductal or glandular lumens but rather pseudocysts

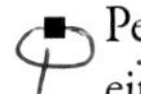

- Peripheral nerve invasion quite common and can be either perineural or intraneural

Special Stains

- Pseudocysts of tubular and cribriform types Alcian blue positive (Alcian blue positivity abolished with heparinase and chondroitinase but not hyaluronidase)

Immunohistochemistry

- Most tumor cells positive for S-100 protein
- Ductal cells lining true lumens are positive for CEA and epithelial membrane antigen (EMA) and negative for muscle-specific actin, vimentin, and α_1-antichymotrypsin
- Nonluminal and pseudocyst lining cells are positive for muscle-specific actin, vimentin, and α_1-antichymotrypsin and negative for CEA and EMA
- Cytokeratin and vimentin coexpressed in cells with myoepithelial differentiation
- Both chondroitin sulfate and heparin sulfate typically present

Electron Microscopy

- Luminal surface of ductal cells covered with microvilli
- Pseudolumens contain basal lamina and proteoglycans

Molecular Alterations

- Abnormalities of the terminal part of 6q and 9p
- Frequent loss of 12q and 19q

Differential Diagnosis

- Polymorphous low-grade adenocarcinoma (tumor cells tend to be uniform with round or oval nuclei with stippled chromatin and indistinct nucleoli)
- Epithelial-myoepithelial carcinoma
- Pleomorphic adenoma
- Basaloid squamous cell carcinoma

Treatment

- Wide to radical surgical excision with postoperative radiation therapy
- Some reports that chemotherapy with cisplatin and high-dose melphalan may be beneficial

Prognosis

- Neoplasm tends to be indolent, persistent, and recurrent
- 5-year survival rate good; 10- to 20-year survival rates poor

- Tumors with solid areas tend to do worse than those with tubular or cribriform patterns

Associations

- None

Comment

- Pleomorphic adenoma, canalicular adenoma, and polymorphous low-grade adenocarcinoma may have foci that are indistinguishable from adenoid cystic carcinoma
- Tubular pattern of adenoid cystic carcinoma frequently resembles a benign neoplasm

Polymorphous Low-Grade Adenocarcinoma (PLGA)

Clinical Manifestations

- Limited to minor salivary glands; 60% in soft or hard palate; 15% in buccal mucosa; 12% in upper lip
- 2nd most common salivary gland carcinoma to involve palate (adenoid cystic most common)
- More common in women than in men
- Typically presents as a small, nontender nodule in the mucosa of the hard or soft palate (frequently at their junction)
- Ulceration and bleeding from mucosa over the tumor may occur
- Bone adjacent to tumor may be infiltrated

Gross Pathology

- Typically circumscribed but not encapsulated
- Cut surface glistening, firm, and tan

Microscopic Pathology

- A large variety of architectural patterns: Solid, trabecular, tubular, and ductular in various combinations; cribriform, cystic, and papillary-cystic foci may be present
- Invasive features typical at periphery and sometimes assume an linear pattern (similar to invasive lobular carcinoma of breast)

- Central portion of tumor typically solid or lobulated; lobules or cords of tumor and individual cells becoming more frequent at the periphery
- Characteristically there is formation of small tubules with distinct lumens lined by cuboidal cells
- Most tumor cells are uniform with round or oval nuclei with stippled chromatin and indistinct nucleoli
- Mitotic figures scarce and atypical mitoses absent
- Focal oncocytic change may be present
- Usually limited collagenous stroma; occasionally abundant hyaline or mucohyaline stroma present

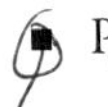

- Perineural invasion almost always present

Special Stains

- Tumor cells PAS positive

Immunohistochemistry

- Tumor cells reactive for cytokeratin, vimentin, muscle-specific actin, EMA, CEA, GFAP, and S100

Electron Microscopy

- Randomly arranged oval and spindled cells with variably dense cytoplasm and prominent junctional complexes

Molecular Alterations

- None

Differential Diagnosis

- Adenoid cystic carcinoma (tumor cells of an adenoid cystic carcinoma generally have a banal basaloid, myoepithelial appearance with basophilic or clear cytoplasm, indistinct cell borders and either round or angulated, hyperchromatic nuclei with small nucleoli)
- Pleomorphic adenoma
- Carcinoma ex pleomorphic adenoma

Treatment

- Wide excision with tumor-free margins (both bone and soft tissue)
- Cervical lymph node dissection only with clinical evidence of lymph node metastasis
- No evidence adjuvant chemotherapy or radiation of benefit

Prognosis

- 15% to 20% recur
- Approximately 10% have regional lymph node metastases

Associations

- None

Epithelial-Myoepithelial Carcinoma

Clinical Manifestations

- 1% of all salivary gland neoplasms
- Primarily involves the major salivary glands (usually the parotid)
- Intraoral minor salivary glands involved in 10% to 15%
- Generally a tumor of adults with peak incidence in the 7th decade
- A slight female predominance
- Typically presents with a localized painless swelling; involvement of the facial nerve may result in pain and/or facial weakness

Gross Pathology

- Neoplasm typically 2 to 3 cm in diameter
- Usually well circumscribed, firm, gray to tan to white, and at least partially encapsulated
- Recurrent neoplasms tend to be multinodular, irregular, hemorrhagic, or focally necrotic

Microscopic Pathology

- A biphasic cell population consisting of epithelial cells (ductal) and myoepithelial cells
- Typically 75% of the cell population will be myoepithelial and 25% ductal, but this ratio can be quite variable
- Epithelial or ductal cells usually border small lumens and tend to be cuboidal with eosinophilic cytoplasm and large round nuclei
- Myoepithelial cells are large and polygonal with clear cytoplasm (glycogen); they tend to surround the ductal cells and are usually the dominant cell type
- Myoepithelial cells tend to have large, irregularly shaped nuclei and indistinct cytoplasmic borders

- Tumor cells tend to be arranged in sheets, have an organoid pattern, or form discrete nests; hyalinized eosinophilic stroma that may be loose, collagenous, or myxoid surrounds aggregates of neoplastic cells
- A cystic or papillary cystic component may be present; the lining of the cysts and papillae maintains the biphasic relationship of myoepithelial cells surrounding ductal cells
- Cytologic atypia tends to be mild or absent
- Some nuclear pleomorphism and mitotic figures may be present
- At the periphery of the neoplasm tumor cells tend to infiltrate adjacent tissue
- Perineural invasion may be present

Special Stains

- Lumens of ductal structures contain PAS positive, mucicarmine negative eosinophilic material
- PAS stains confirm the presence of glycogen in the clear myoepithelial cells and highlights the eosinophilic hyalinized stroma that courses between aggregates of neoplastic cells
- Mucicarmine stains will occasionally demonstrate foci of cells containing mucin

Immunohistochemistry

- Epithelial (ductal) cells are immunoreactive for cytokeratin
- Myoepithelial (clear) cells are immunoreactive for S-100 protein (may be quite variable from tumor to tumor)
- Myoepithelial cells usually stain intensively for muscle specific actin, p63, and occasionally for glial fibrillary acidic protein (GFAP)
- Hyalinized stroma is often positive for type IV collagen

Electron Microscopy

- Epithelial (ductal) cells tend to be electron dense, surround small lumens, have microvilli on their luminal surfaces, and are attached to one another by well-formed junctional complexes and desmosomes; occasionally dense core secretory granules are present
- Myoepithelial cells are electron-lucent and contain glycogen

Molecular Alterations

- None

Differential Diagnosis

- Pleomorphic adenoma
- Adenoid cystic carcinoma
- Polymorphous low-grade adenocarcinoma
- Mucoepidermoid carcinoma
- Acinic cell carcinoma
- Sebaceous carcinoma
- Oncocytoma
- Clear cell adenocarcinoma
- Metastatic renal cell carcinoma

Treatment

- Complete surgical excision with or without adjuvant radiation therapy

Prognosis

- A low-grade malignancy with a tendency to recur and metastasize to periparotid and cervical lymph nodes
- Recurrence occurs in approximately 30% and lymph node metastasis in 20%
- Approximately 8% develop distant metastasis and die

Clear Cell Adenocarcinoma

Clinical Manifestations

- Represents about 1% of epithelial cell salivary gland neoplasms
- 60% involve minor salivary glands
- Involvement of intraoral salivary glands tends to occur in the palate
- Most occur between the 5th and 7th decade
- Men and women are affected equally
- Typically present with painless swelling, occasionally ulceration of the overlying mucosa; pain may be present (intraoral tumors)

Gross Pathology

- Usually <3 cm at the time of initial diagnosis
- Poorly circumscribed with infiltration of adjacent tissues (both mucosal surface and bone)
- Cut surface gray to white

Microscopic Pathology

- Tumor cells uniform, polygonal or round with clear, or occasionally pale, eosinophilic cytoplasm
- Some pleomorphism typical and cells tend to be larger than normal acinar cells
- Nuclei tend to be round, eccentric, and have small nucleoli; some nuclear pleomorphism may be present; mitotic figures rare
- Nuclear-cytoplasmic ratio generally low
- Tumor cells arranged in a variety of architectural patterns to include sheets, nests, and cords with variable amounts of intervening fibrous stroma
- Rarely microcysts present
- Ductal structures almost never present
- Connective tissue stroma may have a variety of patterns:
    - Interconnecting, thin fibrous septa
    - Thick, cellular collagenous bands
    - Sclerotic or hyalinized collagenous tissue
    - Short and fine strands of collagen
- Perineural invasion is usually present

Special Stains

- PAS with and without diastase will confirm the presence of glycogen in many tumor cells
- Mucicarmine or Alcian blue confirm the absence of intracytoplasmic mucin

Immunohistochemistry

- Most tumors focally or diffusely immunoreactive for cytokeratin
- Tumor cells may or may not be immunoreactive for S-100 protein, GFAP, muscle-specific actin, and vimentin

Electron Microscopy

- Tumor cells show features of epithelial and duct cell differentiation
- Features of myoepithelial differentiation (arrays of fine filaments with focal dense bodies and pinocytotic vesicles) absent

Molecular Alterations

- None

Differential Diagnosis

- Clear cells may be a prominent component of several salivary gland neoplasms:
    - Mucoepidermoid carcinoma (the most common clear cell-containing salivary gland neoplasm)
    - Acinic cell carcinoma
    - Epithelial-myoepithelial carcinoma
    - Clear cell oncocytoma
    - Sebaceous adenoma
    - Sebaceous carcinoma
    - Metastatic renal cell carcinoma

Treatment

- Complete surgical excision with or without adjuvant radiotherapy

Prognosis

- A low-grade neoplasm that tends to be locally infiltrative but rarely metastasizes
- No reported deaths

Associations

- None

Oncocytic Carcinoma

Clinical Manifestations

- Approximately 5% of oncocytic salivary gland neoplasms and fewer than 1% of all salivary gland tumors
- Men outnumber women 2:1
- Mean age about 63 years
- 80% involve parotid; 8% submandibular gland; remainder minor salivary glands
- Patients present with painful, rapidly enlarging mass that may be associated with paralysis
- Overlying skin may be discolored or wrinkled

Gross Pathology

- Firm, tan-gray unencapsulated mass; obvious necrosis may be present

Microscopic Pathology

- Tumor cells large, round, or polygonal, arranged in solid sheets islands, cords, or as individual cells
- Cells characterized by fine, granular, eosinophilic cytoplasm and central vesicular nuclei each with a prominent nucleolus
- Multinucleated cells may be present as well as ductlike structures of variable caliber
- Neoplasm is unencapsulated and often invades adjacent muscle, lymphatics, and nerves

Special Stains

- PTAH stains mitochondria-rich cytoplasm dark blue (occasionally PTAH stain will be falsely negative)

Immunohistochemistry

- Ki-67 helpful in differentiating benign from malignant

Electron Microscopy

- Tumor cells contain large numbers of mitochondria that are frequently misshapen

Molecular Alterations

- None

Differential Diagnosis

- Multifocal oncocytosis
- Oncyctoma
- Acinic cell carcinoma
- Salivary duct carcinoma

Treatment

- Aggressive excision
- Radiation not proven to be effective

Prognosis

- Characterized by multiple local recurrences and regional (cervical lymph nodes) or distant metastases (lungs, kidney, liver, thyroid, mediastinum, and bone)

Associations

- None

Salivary Duct Carcinoma

Clinical Manifestations

- An uncommon malignant neoplasm (3%-4% of salivary gland malignancies)
- Vast majority involve parotid gland (85%); may occur in submandibular gland and intraoral minor salivary glands
- More common in men (75%)
- Peak incidence 5th and 6th decades
- Typically presents with rapid onset of parotid swelling; facial nerve dysfunction in 25%; palpable cervical lymph nodes in 30% to 35%

Gross Pathology

- Typically unencapsulated and poorly circumscribed
- Grey-white to yellow multinodular neoplasm
- Cut surface fibrotic with small, variably sized cysts and foci of necrosis

Microscopic Pathology

- Rounded nodules of cuboidal and polygonal tumor cells with moderately abundant eosinophilic cytoplasm; nuclei typically large and round but may be slightly irregular; presence of a nucleolus and the number of mitotic figures is variable
- Small nodules of tumor can be either solid or cystic; larger nodules are almost always cystic
- Cystic nodules have epithelium arranged in bandlike, papillary, and cribriform patterns (all configurations typically present)
- Comedonecrosis a frequent finding
- Small aggregates of neoplastic epithelium frequently seen in the stroma between larger nodules of tumor
- Perineural and lymphatic infiltration frequent
- Dense fibrosis with focal hyalinization of stroma typical
- Typically some areas histologically quite similar to intraductal carcinoma of the breast

Special Stains

- Tumor cells typically unreactive to mucicarmine, Alcian blue, and PTAH

Immunohistochemistry

- Tumor cells reactive for cytokeratin, EMA, CEA, and androgen receptor

Electron Microscopy

- Tumor cells have basal lamina, microvilli, desmosomes, tight junctions, rough endoplasmic reticulum, moderate numbers of mitochondria, and some glycogen (all features of ductal cells)

Molecular Alterations

- Frequent p53 mutations and amplification of HER-2/neu

Differential Diagnosis

- Oncocytic carcinoma
- Mucoepidermoid carcinoma
- Acinic cell carcinoma
- Cystadenocarcinoma
- Polymorphous low-grade adenocarcinoma

Treatment

- Wide surgical excision with radical neck dissection and radiation

Prognosis

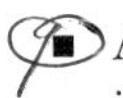

- A very aggressive salivary gland carcinoma with local invasion, angiolymphatic metastasis, and poor prognosis

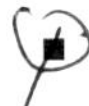

- 60% die of their tumor, often within 5 years of diagnosis

Associations

- None

Adenoarcinoma, NOS

Clinical Manifestations

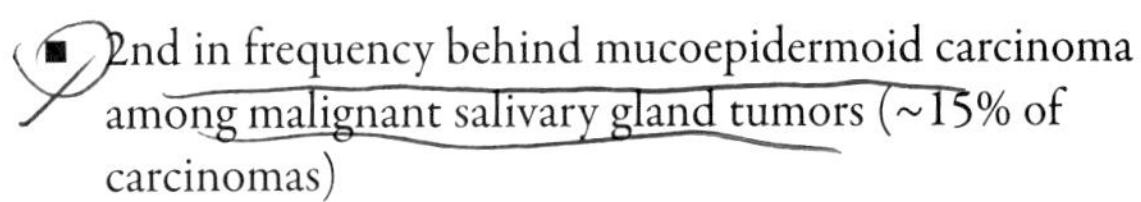

- 2nd in frequency behind mucoepidermoid carcinoma among malignant salivary gland tumors (~15% of carcinomas)
- More common in women than men
- Mean age at diagnosis 58 years; very rare in children
- 60% in major glands usually parotid; 40% in minor glands, usually hard palate, buccal mucosa, and lips
- Most present with solitary, hard asymptomatic mass; 20% have pain or facial weakness; pain more often associated with submandibular tumors
- May be ulcerated.

Gross Pathology

- Often partially circumscribed, but may be irregular
- Cut surface white to yellow and may have areas of hemorrhage or necrosis

Microscopic Pathology

- Ductal or glandular differentiation without morphologic features that characterize other defined types of salivary gland carcinomas
- Infiltrative growth into surrounding glandular parenchyma or adjacent tissue
- A variety of architectural patterns: Small nests or cords, large islands with trabeculae and fibrous stroma, large solid, densely cellular sheets
- Small cysts may be present
- Typical tumor cells oval or cuboidal; scattered clear cells and oncocytic cells may be present
- Small deposits of eosinophilic acellular material and extracellular mucin may be present
- *Low-grade tumors* characterized by distinct ductal differentiation, cells with little pleomorphism, and uniform nuclei with small nucleoli; mitoses rare
- *Intermediate-grade tumors* characterized by more pleomorphism in both size and shape; nucleoli more prominent; scattered mitoses often present
- *High-grade tumors* characterized by large, hyperchromatic, pleomorphic nuclei and numerous mitoses; ductal differentiation harder to recognize

Special Stains

- Mucin stains may help identify presence of extracellular mucin

Immunohistochemistry

- Immunoreactivity with prostate specific antigen possible

Electron Microscopy

- Not particularily useful, but can confirm ductal morphology of tumor cells

Molecular Alterations

- None

Differential Diagnosis

- Metastatic adenocarcinoma
- Polymorphous low-grade carcinoma

Treatment

- Aggressive excision; radiation not proven to be effective

Prognosis

- Mostly determined by site and grade; minor gland tumors have better prognosis than major gland tumors

Associations

- None

Carcinoma Ex Pleomorphic Adenoma

Clinical Manifestations

- Approximately 4% of all salivary gland tumors and approximately 10% of malignant salivary gland tumors
- Most commonly occurs in the parotid gland followed by the submandibular gland and minor salivary glands (very rare in the sublingual gland)
- Incidence of malignant transformation of a pleomorphic adenoma increases with the duration of the latter with an estimated incidence of 2% for tumors present for ≤ 5 to an incidence of 10% for tumors present more than 15 years
- Unusual in patients under the age of 30 years
- 20% of patients present with a history of having ≥ 1 operations for pleomorphic adenoma
- Many patients give a history of the presence of a mass for ≥ 3 years
- Typically presents as a painless mass (occasionally pain or facial nerve palsy may be present)
- On physical examination the mass is usually fixed to underlying soft tissue or bone (especially if recurrent)

Gross Pathology

- Usually poorly circumscribed and infiltrative
- Cut surface tends to be white or tan-gray with foci of hemorrhage, necrosis, and cystic degeneration

Microscopic Pathology

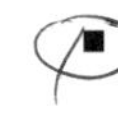

- *A focus of pleomorphic adenoma always a component of the neoplasm*; occasionally the benign element is clearly demarcated from the carcinomatous element, but more typically foci of malignant transformation are scattered within the benign element

- Carcinomatous element *always* arises from the epithelial component of the pleomorphic adenoma
- Carcinomatous cells are usually enlarged and pleomorphic and have hyperchromatic nuclei with prominent nucleoli (resemble high-grade adenocarcinoma, NOS)
- Occasionally carcinomatous element can be classified as ductal, mucoepidermoid carcinoma, epidermoid carcinoma, adenoid cystic carcinoma, clear cell adenocarcinoma, acinic cell carcinoma, or myoepithelial carcinoma
- Mitotic figures readily apparent
- Occasionally tumor confined by a capsule (encapsulated or noninvasive)
- Perineural and vascular invasion typically present
- Prominent hyalinization and foci of hemorrhage and/or necrosis common

Special Stains

- Mucicarmine stain will demonstrate intracytoplasmic mucin in tumors with mucinous cells

Immunohistochemistry

- Epithelial nature of the carcinoma can be demonstrated with stains for EMA, keratin, and CEA
- If carcinomatous cells have a myoepithelial component, they can be demonstrated with stains for muscle-specific actin and S-100 protein

Electron Microscopy

- Not helpful

Molecular Alterations

- Alterations of 5q, 8q, and 12q fairly frequent

Differential Diagnosis

- Pleomorphic adenoma with focally atypical features
- Carcinosarcoma

Treatment

- If neoplasm encapsulated, complete surgical excision with preservation of the facial nerve
- Unencapsulated tumors and large and recurrent tumors best treated with radical parotidectomy (often with sacrifice of at least part of the facial nerve) with or without lymph node dissection
- Some recommend radical neck dissection for major gland involvement with or without clinical evidence of lymph node involvement
- Some evidence adjuvant radiation therapy may be helpful

Prognosis

- Cervical lymph node metastasis occur in 25%
- 40% to 55% recur (appearance of recurrence may be as long as 25 years after primary surgery)
- Recurrence typically signifies a poor prognosis
- 5-year survival 25% to 65%; 10-year survival 25% to 50%; 15-year survival 10% to 35%, and 20-year survival 0% to 40%

Associations

- None

Benign Epithelial Tumors

Benign Mixed Tumor (Pleomorphic Adenoma)

Clinical Manifestations

- Most common neoplasm of the salivary glands
- Parotid gland (75%-85%)
- Submandibular gland (5%-10%)
- Remainder occur in minor salivary glands
  - Palate (60%-65%)
  - Cheek (15%)
  - Tongue and floor of mouth (10%)
- Most common in adults between 3rd and 5th decades
- More frequent in women
- Usually presents as a painless mobile mass

Gross Pathology

- Arises in lower pole of superficial lobe of parotid (50%), in anterior portion of superficial lobe (25%), and in deep lobe (25%)
- Usually solitary
- Other salivary glands may contain metachronous or synchronous tumors
- A well-circumscribed partially encapsulated, solid mass that on cut section is tan to white and shiny with a matrix of delicate fibrous connective tissue

Microscopic Pathology

- A mixture of epithelium and mesenchymal-like tissue
- Epithelial component includes both epithelial and myoepithelial cells and may be spindled, clear, squamous, basaloid, cuboidal, plasmacytoid, oncocytic, mucous, or sebaceous
- Epithelial cells may be arranged in a variety of patterns: solid, broad sheets, cystic structures, anastomosing trabeculae with tubular or ductal structures, and intersecting fascicles
- Stroma contains significant amounts of mucopolysaccharide and is both myxoid and mucoid and is often hyalinized
- Both chondroid and osseous tissue may be found in the stroma
- Excessive proliferation of both the epithelial and myoepithelial cells can result in an extremely cellular (malignant appearing) neoplasm
- 60% to 70% are either predominantly myxoid or have an equal mix of myxoid and epithelial elements; 20% are predominately cellular, and 10% are extremely cellular
- 2 types of mucin: Epithelial (characterized by high content of neutral glycoprotein) and connective tissue (sulfated and nonsulfated glycosaminoglycans)
- A variety of extracellular substances may be found: Tyrosine-rich crystalloids in the myxoid areas, collagenous spherules, calcium oxalate crystals, amyloid, and other birefringent crystalloids

Special Stains

- Collagenous spherules can be highlighted with a trichrome stain

Immunohistochemistry

- Epithelial component positive for keratin, EMA, CEA, lysozyme, lactoferrin, and α_1-antitrypsin
- Amylase usually absent
- Myoepithelial cells immunoreactive for keratin, actin, fibronectin, myosin, S-100 protein, and p63
- Cartilaginous foci are positive for S-100 protein

Electron Microscopy

- Proliferating tumor cells have basal lamina, small microvilli, and well-developed desmosomes
- Stromal (mesenchymal) cells may have tonofilaments and microfilaments, pinocytotic vesicles, and fragments of basement membrane
- Extracellular spaces often contain elastic fibers

Molecular Alterations

- May have a normal karyotype, rearrangement of 8q12 or rearrangement of 12q13-15
- Overexpression of p53 rare

Differential Diagnosis

- If insufficient tissue processed and submitted:
  - Canalicular adenoma
  - Polymorphous low-grade adenocarcinoma
  - Dermal mixed tumor (chondroid syringoma)
- If neoplasm composed almost exclusively of myxoid, chondroid, or osseous tissue:
  - Myxoma
  - Myxoid lipoma
  - Myxoid neurofibroma
  - Osteoma
  - Osteochondroma
- If squamous differentiation and mucous cells present:
  - Mucoepidermoid carcinoma

Treatment

- Superficial parotidectomy or extracapsular dissection with a margin of normal tissue are surgical procedures of choice

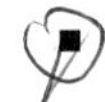

- Frey syndrome (gustatory sweating) and injury to the marginal mandibular branch of facial nerve are significant surgical complications

Prognosis

- If total excision not achieved, recurrence likely (especially in case of parotid gland tumors)
- Mixed tumors in minor salivary glands much less likely to recur

Associations

- None

Comment

- If the section taken for frozen section evaluation is particularly cellular and primarily epithelioid with little or no myxochondroid component, the differential diagnosis includes low-grade adenocarcinoma and polymorphous low-grade carcinoma
- Pleomorphic adenomas that arise in minor salivary glands tend to be quite cellular and frequently lack a prominent myxochondroid component; in addition, they may not have a well-formed capsule (all features of malignancy)
- Carcinoma, NOS, mucoepidermoid carcinoma, and adenoid cystic carcinoma all mimic pleomorphic adenoma on frozen section

Myoepithelioma

Clinical Manifestations

- Represents 1.5% of all salivary gland tumors
- Men and women are affected equally; average age at diagnosis 45 years
- 40% occur in the parotid gland; 20% occur in the hard and soft palates
- Typically presents as an asymptomatic mass

Gross Pathology

- Well circumscribed with a solid, tan to yellow, shiny cut surface
- Most have fibrous capsule, but tumor may extend through the capsule in a pushing nodular fashion and come into direct contact with surrounding salivary gland or soft tissue

Microscopic Pathology

- Tumor cells may have pronounced heterogeneity; the overall growth pattern is largely dependent on the predominant cell type
- Tumors that consist primarily of *spindle cells* have the appearance of a mesenchymal neoplasm rather than an epithelial neoplasm; spindle cells tend to be arranged in compact interlacing fascicles with little or no myxoid or mucoid stroma; spindle cell nuclei are usually vesicular with blunt or tapered ends and inconspicuous nucleoli; cytoplasm eosinophilic and finely granular; cell borders indistinct
- Predominantly spindle cell tumors frequently have foci of polygonal epithelioid cells that have pale eosinophilic or clear cytoplasm
- Large oval or polygonal *epithelioid cells* may predominate and are often associated with small cystic spaces; tumors with this cellular morphology frequently have few spindle cells and few plasmacytoid cells; occasionally epithelioid cells arranged in interconnecting cords surrounded by abundant mucoid stroma (reticular variant)
- Occasionally the predominant cell type is *plasmacytoid cells* (more frequent in palatal lesions than parotid gland lesions); typically small aggregates of plasmacytoid cells lie in a loosely collagenous mucoid stroma; these cells tend to be round or ovoid and have a large amount of eosinophilic cytoplasm, and an eccentrically placed nucleus with a small nucleolus

Special Stains

- Not helpful

Immunohistochemistry

- Myoepithelial cells are immunoreactive for cytokeratin, muscle-specific actin, and p63
- They are negative for desmin
- Spindle cells tend to be less reactive for cytokeratin than the other cell types
- Spindle cells are more reactive for muscle-specific actin than are epithelioid cells; plasmacytoid cells are generally nonreactive for muscle-specific actin

Electron Microscopy

- Spindled myoepithelial cells contain microfilaments, intermediate filaments, tonofilaments, pinocytotic vesicles, basal lamina, and desmosomes
- Epithelioid cells contain limited numbers of filaments and some glycogen

Molecular Alterations

- None

Differential Diagnosis

- Tumors with a variety of cell types are most likely to be misdiagnosed as pleomorphic adenomas
- Solid cellular tumors with clear cells may mimic adenocarcinoma
- Spindle cell myoepitheliomas:
    - Nerve sheath tumor
    - Fibrous histiocytoma
    - Nodular fasciitis
    - Synovial sarcoma
    - Leiomyoma and leiomyosarcoma
    - Hemangiopericytoma

Treatment

- Complete surgical excision

Prognosis

- Recurrence rare (much less common than in pleomorphic adenoma)

Associations

- None

Basal Cell Adenoma

Clinical Manifestations

- Most occur in superficial lateral lobe of parotid gland (70%); 5% arise in submandibular gland
- Occur in adults (mean age 58 years)
- More frequent in women than in men (2:1)
- Usually single and present with swelling

Gross Pathology

- Usually solitary and circumscribed with a distinct fibrous capsule (membranous type may be multifocal and unencapsulated)
- Cut surface homogenous gray to tan to brown and may be cystic

Microscopic Pathology

- Nests of basaloid epithelial cells with peripheral palisading (tumor has a "basaloid" appearance)
- Tumor cells may be light or dark; light cells have pale nuclei and pale cytoplasm and usually predominate in the central areas; dark cells have less cytoplasm and darker nuclei and tend to be located peripherally; both cell types have indistinct cell borders
- Aggregates of tumor cells regardless of pattern separated from vascular stroma by well-defined basement membrane
- Stroma typically fibrous without a myxochondroid matrix
- Cystic change, squamous whorls, frank keratinization, and/or a cribriform pattern may occasionally be present
- Several patterns:
  - *Solid*: Most common pattern; characterized by variably sized aggregates of cells with prominent palisading of nuclei along stromal interface; collagenized stroma
  - *Trabecular*: Interlacing bands of cells; stroma less collagenous than in solid variant
  - *Trabecular-tubular*: Stroma characterized by a subtle spindled cellularity
  - *Tubular*: Small lumens lined by ductal or basaloid cells
  - *Membranous*: Neoplasm histologically very similar to dermal eccrine tumors (eccrine spiradenoma and cylindroma); characterized by nests of cells that fit together like a jigsaw puzzle, contain coalescent membrane droplets, and are surrounded by dense hyaline bands of basal lamina

Special Stains

- Periodic acid–Schiff (PAS) highlights the hyaline basal lamina material surrounding tumor cell nests, especially in membranous type

Immunohistochemistry

- Typically cytokeratin positive, but with variable reactivity
- Immunoreactivity for S-100 protein (focal), muscle-specific actin, and vimentin localized to peripheral tumor cells bordering connective tissue stroma; muscle-specific actin and p63 positivity confirm presence of cells with myoepithelial differentiation
- Luminal cells frequently EMA and CEA positive

Electron Microscopy

- Ductal cells have tight junctions, microvilli, and a few secretory granules
- Basal lamina material is associated with basal and myoepithelial cells

Molecular Alterations

- None

Differential Diagnosis

- Pleomorphic adenoma
- Adenoid cystic carcinoma
- Basal cell adenocarcinoma

Treatment

- Total excision with a rim of normal salivary gland

Prognosis

- Excellent except for membranous type which tends to be multifocal and unencapsulated hence has a high recurrence rate (25%)
- Malignant transformation may occur; more likely with membranous type than other types (25% versus 4%); malignant transformation characterized by infiltration, perineural involvement, angiolymphatic invasion, and cytologic atypia

Associations

- Brooke-Spiegler Syndrome: 25% to 40% of membranous adenomas coexist with skin adnexal tumors (dermal cylindromas, trichoepitheliomas, and spiradenomas)

Canalicular Adenoma

Clinical Manifestations

- Approximately 1% of salivary gland neoplasms
- Slightly more common in women (1.8:1)
- Most occur in the upper lip
- A benign neoplasm that grows slowly in the mucosa and is both mobile and compressible
- Average age 65 years (unusual under age of 50 years)

Gross Pathology

- Overlying mucosa tends to have a bluish discoloration
- Usually well-circumscribed, yellow to tan, and range in size from 0.5 to 2.0 cm
- Usually single and encapsulated, but may be multinodular or multifocal
- Cut surface typically homogeneous and gelatinous with multiple small cysts

Microscopic Pathology

- Double rows of short columnar epithelial cells arranged in branching and interconnecting cords in a background of loose stroma
- In areas the double rows of cells may separate slightly to produce narrow channels (canaliculi, hence the name); in other areas the double rows of epithelium may be more widely separated resulting in small cysts
- Epithelial cells tend to have a short columnar configuration and eosinophilic or amphophilic cytoplasm; nuclei tend to be round or oval with finely stippled chromatin
- Little or no pleomorphism
- Mitotic figures very rare
- Stroma is very loose with scant amounts of collagen, occasional fibroblasts, and scattered small capillaries

Special Stains

- None

Immunohistochemistry

- Tumor cells stain positively for cytokeratin and S-100 protein and negatively for muscle-specific actin (which indicates no myoepithelial differentiation)

Electron Microscopy

- No myoepithelial differentiation
- Luminal surface of cells have few microvilli
- Few secretory granules

Molecular Alterations

- None

Differential Diagnosis

- Basal cell adenoma
- Adenoid cystic carcinoma

Treatment and Prognosis

- Local excision; recurrence uncommon

Associations

- None

Oncocytoma (Oncocytic Metaplasia, Nodular or Diffuse Oncocytosis)

Clinical Manifestations

- About 1% of salivary gland neoplasms
- 85% to 90% occur in parotid gland, rare in minor salivary glands
- Rare under age of 50 years; peak incidence 7th to 9th decades (mean age 58 years)
- Slightly more common in women, especially clear cell variant
- Typically presents as painless mass
- A few have been reported to occur after exposure to radiation

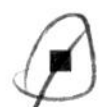

- Bilateral disease (synchronous or metachronous)

Gross Pathology

- Usually single, well-circumscribed, tan to red-brown; typical size from 3 to 4 cm cm
- Occasionally one or more cysts within tumor nodule(s)

Microscopic Pathology

- Oncocytes characterized by abundant, very eosinophilic, and finely granular cytoplasm; intensity of eosinophilic staining variable
- Cells typically large (1 to 2 times the size of a normal acinar cell) and have a single round nucleus with evenly dispersed chromatin and a easily seen nucleolus

- Cell borders usually distinct
- Cells typically arranged in organoid pattern with clusters of cells surrounded by a very thin band of fibrovascular stroma; lumens may be present within clusters
- Some nuclear and cellular pleomorphism; mitotic figures very rare
- Micro- or macrocysts may be present and have an associated lymphoid infiltrate (resemble Warthin tumor)
- Clear cells may dominate lesion (clear cells particularily common in nodular oncocytosis); clear cytoplasm due to accumulation of cytoplasmic glycogen

Special Stains

- PAS with and without diastase confirms presence of glycogen in clear cells
- Phosphotungstic acid-hemotoxylin (PTAH) has an affinity for mitochondria

Immunohistochemistry

- Not helpful

Electron Microscopy

- Tumor cells almost filled with mitochondria are round to oval in shape
- Desmosomal attachments typically present

Molecular Alterations

- None

Differential Diagnosis

- Oncocytic metaplasia and oncocytosis (see comment later in this section)
- Oncocytic carcinoma
- Pleomorphic adenoma and mucoepidermoid carcinoma most common salivary gland neoplasms to have oncocytic metaplasia
- Clear cell neoplasms (clear cell mucoepidermoid carcinoma, clear cell adenoma, epithelial-myoepithelial carcinoma and metastatic renal cell carcinoma)
- Warthin tumor

Treatment and Prognosis

- Local excision; recurrence uncommon, but seen with incomplete excision or multifocal disease

Associations

- None

Comment

- Oncocytic cells most commonly seen in salivary gland, thyroid gland, parathyroid gland, respiratory tract, and kidney
- Oncocytic metaplasia characterized by transformation of ductal and acinar epithelium to oncocytes (uncommon under age of 50 years, but almost universal over age of 70 years)
- Nodular oncocytosis characterized by 2 or more nodules of oncocytes (usually not encapsulated); diffuse oncocytosis consists of the replacement of the entire gland by oncocytes

Warthin Tumor (Cystadenoma Lymphomatosum Papilliferum)

Clinical Manifestations

- 2nd most common benign parotid gland tumor (5% of all parotid tumors and 10% of benign parotid tumors)
- Almost all occur within the parotid gland or in periparotid tissue; most involve tail (10% in deep lobe)
- May be multicentric, synchronous or metachronous, unilateral or bilateral (bilateral in 5%-10%)
- More common in men; unusual in blacks
- Mean age at diagnosis 62 years; rare before age 40 years
- Typically presents as painless (occasionally fluctuant) mass in inferior portion of parotid gland
- May be associated with acute onset of pain with a simultaneous increase in size secondary to leakage of fluid into surrounding tissues and subsequent infection

Gross Pathology

- May be adherent to overlying skin
- Usually round or oval and well-circumscribed
- Cut surface reveals cysts with clear, mucoid, or brown fluid
- Small excrescences line cysts (papillary epithelial proliferations)
- Cystic spaces separated by grey fibrous septa of varying thickness

Microscopic Pathology

- Cystic spaces lined by papillary, double layer of columnar oncocytic epithelial cells with a supporting lymphoid stroma, often with germinal centers
- Luminal epithelial cells have finely granular, eosinophilic cytoplasm, oval nuclei located in the center or apical end of the cell, and distinct cell membranes
- Randomly distributed small basaloid cells lie beneath and between columnar epithelial cells
- Squamous metaplasia within proliferating epithelium may be present
- Lymphoid stroma closely resembles normal lymph node with normal lymphoid follicles; plasma cells may be seen
- Cystic lumens typically contain secretions mixed with cellular debris and structures that resemble corpora amylacea
- Proportion of epithelial and lymphoid elements varies within the same tumor and between different tumors; typically proportion is 50/50; epithelial component can be as much as 70% to 80% or as little as 20% to 30%

Special Stains

- PTAH stain highlights the granular cytoplasm of epithelial cells

Immunohistochemistry

- 50% of B-lymphocytes produce IgA; 30% to 35% produce IgG

Electron Microscopy

- Oncocytic epithelial cells packed with mitochondria

Molecular Alterations

- None

Differential Diagnosis

- Papillary oncocytic cystadenoma
- If squamous metaplasia present:
  - Epidermoid carcinoma
  - Mucoepidermoid carcinoma
- If lymphoid component prominent:
  - Lymphoepithelial cyst
  - Lymphoma
  - Lymphoepithelial carcinoma
  - AIDS-related lymphadenopathy
  - Metastatic carcinoma
- Lymphoid proliferation often associated with mucoepidermoid carcinoma, acinic cell carcinoma, and cystadenocarcinoma

Treatment

- Surgical excision with an awareness of the possibility that these tumors may be multifocal

Prognosis

- Recurrence rate should be <2%

Associations

- Heavy smoking (smokers are at an 8-fold higher risk)
- Metastatic carcinoma or melanoma may be present
- Lymphoma may arise from lymphocytic component
- Adenocarcinoma, squamous cell carcinoma, undifferentiated carcinoma, and oncocytic carcinoma may arise from epithelial component

References

Barns L, Everson JW, Reichert P, Sidransky D (eds). *World Health Organization Classification of Tumours: Pathology and Genetics—Head and Neck Tumours.* Lyon: IARC Press, 2005.

Dabbs DJ. *Diagnostic Immunohistochemistry.* New York: Churchill Livingstone, 2002.

Ellis GL, Auclair PL. *Tumors of the Salivary Glands: Atlas of Tumor Pathology, 3rd Series, Fascicle 17.* Washington, DC: Armed Forces Institute of Pathology, 1995.

Mills S, Carter D, Greenson JK, Oberman HA, Reuter V, Stoler MH (eds). *Sternberg's Diagnostic Surgical Pathology. 4th ed.* Philadelphia: Lippincott Williams & Wilkins, 2004.

Rice DH, Batsakis JG. *Surgical Pathology of the Head and Neck.* Philadelphia: Lippincott Williams & Wilkins, 2000.

Rosai J. *Rosai and Ackerman's Surgical Pathology. 9th ed.* St. Louis: Mosby, 2004.

Chapter 19

Bones and Joints

Intraoperative Consultation

Frozen sections are obtained on bone tumors for 1 of 5 indications:

1. To determine if sufficient, viable tissue has been obtained to ensure accurate diagnosis on permanent sections.
2. In the case of benign lesions and metastatic disease, to render a diagnosis that can lead to the performance of a definitive procedure without the need for reoperation.
3. To obtain tissue specimens for ancillary studies, such as culture for microorganisms, electron microscopy, and flow cytometry.
4. To evaluate surgical margins for completeness of excision in the case of malignant tumors.
5. To confirm the presence of obviously malignant tissue, so long-term venous access can be placed while the patient is under general anesthesia.

Tissue from malignant bone tumors submitted to the pathologist for frozen section should be of sufficient volume to allow representative tissue to be fixed in formalin for permanent sections without having been frozen.

Request for a frozen section diagnosis on malignant bone tumors should be accompanied when possible by either the appropriate x-rays or the report from the radiologist. The impression of the radiologist as well as the surgeon can be of benefit to the pathologist trying to make a frozen section diagnosis or determine the presence of lesional tissue. Evaluation of radiographs by radiologist, surgeon, and pathologist helps narrow the differential diagnosis and, most importantly, helps make the distinction between benign and malignant. Making a diagnosis without knowledge of the radiologic findings increases the likelihood of an error. A classic example is the frozen section evaluation of an enchondroma. Enchondromas taken from the digits are often quite cellular and pleomorphic and can be easily interpreted as being malignant. Similarly, well-differentiated chondrosarcomas from the pelvis can be quite bland and easily interpreted as benign. Both of these errors are easily avoided when radiographs accompany the specimen.

Specimen Handling

Once the pathologist has determined that sufficient tissue has been submitted for histologic diagnosis, consideration should be given to submitting some of the tissue for microbial culture when appropriate, placing a portion of tissue in glutaraldehyde for possible electron microscopy, and finally, in the case of suspected lymphoma, ensuring that a piece of the tissue specimen is frozen for possible immunohistochemistry or gene rearrangement studies.

When fragments of bone are accompanied by attached or unattached fragments of soft tissue, the 2 components should be separated so that only the bony portions are subjected to decalcification. A bone should not be decalcified until it is adequately fixed in formalin. Ideally, bone fragments should be fixed for 24 hours before being decalcified. The decalcification process should be as short as possible; overdecalcification introduces artifacts that can alter the morphologic findings on permanent section.

Large resection specimens that include a segment of bone should be fixed and then divided longitudinally along the long axis of the bone and then fixed again. The cut surfaces of the specimen can then be photographed, copied on a standard copier, or sketched. The diagram or picture allows for visual assessment of the presence and absence of necrosis (especially important in cases of neoadjuvant chemotherapy or irradiation), and allows the pathologist to measure the size of the tumor, the width of the margin of resection, and the distance the neoplasm penetrates into adjacent soft tissue. The specimen should then be mapped so that precise histologic information concerning margins of resection and extent of tumor necrosis can be assessed.

Benign Cartilage Lesions

Chondroblastoma

Clinical Manifestations

- <1% of all bone tumors
- Peak incidence is the 2nd decade of life (50% diagnosed in skeletally immature patients)
- Males more frequently affected than females

- Tend to occur in the epiphysis of major long tubular bones; most frequent location distal femur or proximal tibia (30%); 3rd most common site is proximal humerus
- May involve craniofacial bones (base of the skull and temporal fossa) as well as pelvis, scapula, vertebrae and ribs
- Rarely multifocal
- Patients usually present with pain referred to the nearest joint and mild functional impairment

Radiologic Features

- Typically a centrally located, sharply demarcated, round, lytic epiphyseal defect with a surrounding rim of sclerotic bone; overall shape of bone usually not changed
- Tumor usually abuts articular cartilage

Gross Pathology

- A well-defined, gray mass with foci of calcification, hemorrhage, and/or cystic change
- Curettings typically hemorrhagic and friable with tiny foci of bone

Microscopic Pathology

- Tumor cells are immature, round to polygonal chondroblasts with central or eccentric, round nuclei with longitudinal clefts or grooves and distinct nuclear membranes; cytoplasm eosinophilic and cell borders distinct; individual chondroblasts may be cytologically atypical (not a sign of malignancy)
- Scattered mitotic figures may be present (never atypical)
- Cells tend to be closely packed together with foci of osteoclastlike giant cells scattered throughout
- Focal areas of cartilaginous differentiation vary from immature to mature
- Foci of calcification often present and characteristically appear as fine, linear strands that course between and around the chondroblasts ("chicken wire" pattern); coarse calcifications may be present as well
- Areas of spindle cell change may be present and at times can be the dominant microscopic feature
- Extensive myxoid change may be present
- A secondary aneurysmal bone cyst is present in 15% to 20%
- Occasionally unilocular or multilocular cystic spaces filled with serous fluids represent a major portion of the lesion (*cystic chondroblastoma*)

Special Stains

- Not helpful

Immunohistochemistry

- Tumor cells are positive for S-100 protein and vimentin
- Multinucleated giant cells are typically negative for S-100 protein
- Lesions with extensive cystic change or aneurysmal bone cyst formation are only focally positive for S-100 protein
- Some cytokeratin positive cells may be present

Electron Microscopy

- Nuclei of chondroblasts have deep indentations corresponding to the grooves seen on routine hematoxylin-eosin (H&E) stain; inner surface of the nuclear membrane has a thick lamina (a classic EM finding in chondroblastoma)
- A mineralized stroma ("chicken wire") may be present

Molecular Alterations

- Rearrangements of chromosome band 8q21 seen in aggressive chondroblastoma

Differential Diagnosis

- Chondromyxoid fibroma (usually no calcification)
- Giant cell tumor (usually occurs in the epiphysis of a mature bone)
- Eosinophilic granuloma
- Aneurysmal bone cyst
- Solitary bone cyst
- Clear-cell chondrosarcoma

Treatment

- Curettage and bone grafting (10% recur)
- Soft tissue tumoral nodules can result from surgical implantation

Prognosis

- A benign lesion with the potential to "metastasize" (a benign lung implant not a true metastasis)
- *Aggressive chondroblastoma* can destroy bone and may undergo malignant transformation

Associations

- 15% to 20% develop secondary aneurysmal bone cysts; usually involve the tarsal bones
- Aneurysmal bone cysts may engraft on a chondroblastoma resulting in an almost complete obliteration of the chondroblastoma
- Extensive cystic change with serous-filled cavities may obliterate an underlying chondroblastoma

Chondromyxoid Fibroma

Clinical Manifestations

- Represents <1% of all bone tumors
- More common in males than females with a peak incidence in the 2nd and 3rd decades
- Tends to occur in the metaphysis of major long bones of the lower extremity (proximal tibia most common site); bones of upper extremities rarely affected; 30% occur in the region of the knee (proximal tibia and distal femur); small bones of the feet may be affected; ilium is the flat bone most frequently affected
- Patients usually present with pain and localized swelling in soft tissue overlying the lesion

Radiographic Features

- Typically benign-appearing, lytic, oval lesion in the metaphysis; may extend into diaphysis or epiphysis; attenuates and expands closest adjacent cortex
- Sharply defined sclerotic, scalloped border

Gross Pathology

- An eccentrically located, sharply circumscribed, lobulated, firm, bluish, gray-white mass confined by intact periosteum
- Foci of myxoid change typically present; chondroid foci usually grossly discernible
- No necrosis, cystic change, or liquefaction

Microscopic Pathology

- Rounded and confluent lobules of hypocellular myxomatous and chondroid areas separated by intersecting bands of highly cellular fibroblastlike spindle cells and multinucleated giant cells
- A pseudolobulated pattern with central hyaline cartilage and immature myxoid tissue undergoing cartilaginous differentiation with a highly cellular periphery
- Typical tumor cell is a plump spindled cell that may have a stellate shape with elongated cytoplasmic processes; these cells are chondroblasts but are not present in discrete lacunae
- Tumor cells may be pleomorphic, hyperchromatic, and multinucleated
- Mitotic figures are uncommon and never atypical
- Foci of mature cartilage with calcifications may be present
- An aneurysmal bone cyst may be present (10% of long bone and flat bone lesions)

Special Stains

- Not helpful

Immunohistochemistry

- Cells within the area of mature chondroblastic differentiation are strongly positive for S-100
- Tumor cells in the myxoid areas and in the areas of hypercellular septa are weakly and focally positive for S-100

Electron Microscopy

- Tumor cells are immature stellate mesenchymal cells that have long irregular cytoplasmic processes embedded in a loose myxoid matrix
- Cells have thick lamina on the inner surface of the nuclear membrane and glycogen in the cytoplasm

Molecular Alterations

- Rearrangements of chromosome 6q13 and 6q25 reported

Differential Diagnosis

- Conventional chondrosarcoma
- Dedifferentiated chondrosarcoma
- Chondroblastoma

Treatment

- En bloc resection or aggressive curettage
- Simple curettage usually results in recurrence
- Radiation therapy useful to treat inaccessible lesions

Prognosis

- Benign, with no reports of malignant transformation

Associations

- Aneurysmal bone cyst

Enchondroma

Clinical Manifestations

- 10% to 25% of all benign bone tumors and 5% to 10% of all bone tumors
- Typically asymptomatic and often present as an incidental finding on radiograph
- Fairly evenly distributed throughout life
- Males and females affected equally
- Small bones of the hands and feet most frequently involved (60%); hands more frequently involved than feet
- May occur in long bones: proximal humerus and proximal and distal femur
- Never reported in craniofacial bones and rare in pelvis, ribs, spine, and sternum
- Lesions in the phalanges, metacarpals, and metatarsals may present with a palpable mass or pathologic fracture

Radiologic Findings

- A localized radiolucent lesion with stippled calcifications
- When located in a small bone, lesion tends to be centered in the diaphysis, often with extension into the epiphysis; cortex may be expanded and thinned
- When located in a long tubular bone, lesion tends to be located in the metaphysis

Gross Pathology

- An obviously cartilaginous lesion with a lobular architecture; lobules vary in size
- Ivory-white foci of calcification easily identified

Microscopic Pathology

- A lobular arrangement of mature cartilage
- Lobules partially separated by a thin, fibrovascular stroma and normal marrow elements
- Cellularity is low and chondrocytes appear quite banal (chondrocytes closely resemble those seen in normal hyaline cartilage)
- Chondrocytes typically arranged in loose clusters and have small, hyperchromatic nuclei and finely granular cytoplasm that is often vacuolated; cells sit in sharp-edged lacunar spaces
- Prominent myxoid change is rare; its presence suggests malignancy (except in lesions involving the small bones of the hands and feet)
- Periphery of cartilage lobules usually consists of a rim of lamellar bone
- Tumors of small bones of hands and feet may be more cellular and cytologically atypical than long bone tumors

Special Stains

- Not helpful

Immunohistochemistry

- Staining patterns similar to other cartilage lesions; cells positive for S-100 protein and vimentin

Electron Microscopy

- Cartilage cells have irregular cell contours, centrally located nucleus with condensed chromatin and a convoluted nuclear membrane

Molecular Alterations

- None

Differential Diagnosis

- Low-grade chondrosarcoma (especially when found in the metaphysis of long bones in the middle-aged or elderly)
- Chondroid differentiation in fibrous dysplasia

Treatment

- Asymptomatic lesions require no treatment
- Painful or worrisome lesions are treated with complete curettage with or without bone grafting

Prognosis

- Recurrence can occur after incomplete curettage
- Recurrence is suspicious for malignancy

Associations

- See "Enchondromatosis"

Enchondromatosis: Ollier Disease

Clinical Manifestations

- Multifocal intramedullary proliferation of hypercellular dysplastic cartilage
- Typically a unilateral distribution, but occasionally bilateral
- Males and females affected equally
- Most frequent presentation is that of extensive involvement of a single extremity
- Extent of skeletal involvement varies greatly
- Appendicular skeleton more frequently involved than axial skeleton
- Short tubular bones in the hands are most frequently affected, followed by the bones of the feet, femur, humerus, and bones of forearm
- Craniofacial bones and vertebrae rarely involved
- Typically the onset of symptoms occurs between the ages of 10 and 25 years
- Involvement of long bones of the extremities usually results in length discrepancy
- Patients may present with pathologic fracture (typically occurs late in the course of the disease)

Radiologic Features

- Lesions usually eccentric, multifocal, and located in metaphysis and diaphysis
- Short tubular bones have lytic defects with punctate calcifications oriented perpendicularly to the long axis of the bone
- Long tubular bones have long intramedullary grooves or parallel lucent columns (parallel rows of dysplastic cartilage) that extend from the growth plate toward the diaphysis (fluted-column sign)

Gross Pathology

- Affected bone is typically expanded and shortened
- On sectioning, metaphyseal areas contain longitudinal rows of nodular cartilage or irregular masses of cartilage and extend from the metaphysis into the diaphysis

Microscopic Pathology

- Findings similar to that of a solitary enchondroma with the exception that in general the lesions are more cellular, less calcified, and have more nuclear atypia
- Cartilage cells are typically larger, have a more open chromatin pattern, and are more frequently binucleate than cartilage cells of a solitary enchondroma
- Nuclear atypia and myxoid change are fairly frequent
- In general, the microscopic findings are quite similar to those of a grade I chondrosarcoma

Special Stains

- Not helpful

Immunohistochemistry

- Tumor cells positive for S-100 protein and vimentin

Electron Microscopy

- Cartilaginous nature of cells very evident: centrally located nucleus with condensed chromatin and irregular nuclear membrane

Molecular Alterations

- A nonhereditary skeletal disorder

Differential Diagnosis

- Low-grade chondrosarcoma
- Polyostotic fibrous dysplasia (some overlap radiologically)

Treatment

- Corrective surgery for deformities and length discrepancy
- Osteotomy and lengthening procedures for growth disturbance

Prognosis

- Typically a progressive, slow-growing disease that tends to stabilize at puberty
- Secondary sarcomatous change may occur (estimated incidence as high as 30%) most are low-grade conventional chondrosarcomas, but high-grade sarcomas (osteosarcoma or dedifferentiated chondrosarcoma) can occur

Associations

- Increased incidence of extraskeletal neoplasms, especially ovarian neoplasms (juvenile granulosa cell tumor and Sertoli-Leydig cell tumors) and astrocytoma

Enchondromatosis: Maffucci Syndrome

Clinical Manifestations

- Multiple enchondromas identical to those of Ollier disease with extraskeletal, soft tissue angiomatosis
- Angiomas typically involve the skin but may involve viscera (lungs, liver, and gastrointestinal tract) and tend to be more pronounced in areas of skeletal involvement

Gross and Microscopic Pathology

- Identical to Ollier disease
- Vascular lesions, usually cavernous hemangiomas with frequent thrombosis (thrombi may be calcified)
- Other vascular lesions: arteriovenous aneurysms or fistulae, lymphedema, and lymphangiomas

Prognosis

- Patients at an increased risk for the development of low-grade conventional chondrosarcoma
- Dedifferentiated chondrosarcoma and angiosarcoma have been reported
- Malignant transformation more likely than in Ollier disease

Associations

- Nodular goiter
- Adrenal insufficiency
- Juvenile granulosa cell tumor

Osteochondroma

Clinical Manifestations

- 35% of all benign bone tumors and 8% of all bone tumors
- More common in males than females (2:1)
- Peak incidence between the ages of 15 and 35 years
- Typically present as a hard localized swelling of long duration
- Tend to occur in the appendicular skeleton on the surface of metaphyseal portions of major long bones; region of the knee most frequently affected (35%); distal femur, proximal humerus, and proximal tibia and fibula
- May involve flat bones (ilium and scapula)
- Rare in small bones of the hands and feet, ribs,or vertebral column
- Essentially never occur in craniofacial bones
- 15% of patients have multiple lesions (see "Multiple Hereditary Exostoses" below)

Radiologic Features

- A pedunculated lesion arising from the surface of the bone as a bony stalk continuous with adjacent cortex in the region of the metaphysis; tends to point away from the nearest joint
- End of stalk covered by lobulated cartilaginous cap that may have calcifications
- In flat bones, lesion may be sessile

Gross Pathology

- A lobulated cartilage cap covers the distal end of a pedunculated lesion or the surface of a sessile lesion and is covered with a fibrous membrane that is continuous with the periosteum of the stalk
- Spongiosum of stalk is continuous with cancellous bone of underlying medullary cavity
- All lesions have an area of endochondral ossification

Microscopic Pathology

- Characterized by 3 layers: fibrous perichondrium (continous with periosteum of underlying bone), cartilage cap, and bone
- Cartilage cap consists of hyaline cartilage similar to that seen in the epiphyseal growth plate; cartilage cells may show some individual atypia and may be multinucleated; loss of normal architecture, wide fibrous bands, myxoid change, increased chondrocyte cellularity, mitotic activity, significant chondrocyte atypia, and necrosis may indicate malignant transformation
- At the interface with the cancellous bone, the cartilage cap shows endochondral ossification
- Spongy bone beneath the cartilage cap may contain irregular masses of necrotic, calcified chondroid material

- Bulk of the lesion consists of mature bone trabeculae and normal bone marrow beneath cartilaginous cap
- Older lesions may not have a cartilaginous cap

Special Stains

- Periodic acid-Schiff (PAS) stains may highlight eosinophilic inclusions within the cytoplasm of the cartilaginous cells

Immunohistochemistry and Electron Microscopy

- Not helpful

Molecular Alterations

- See "Multiple Hereditary Exostoses" below

Differential Diagnosis

- Parosteal osteosarcoma
- Juxtacortical myositis ossificans
- Reactive periostitis
- Subungual exostosis
- Bizarre parosteal osteocartilaginous proliferation (Nora lesion)
- Periosteal chondroma

Treatment

- Simple excision for cosmesis, relief of pain, or limitation of motion
- Recurrence may occur if a portion of the cartilage cap or perichondrium is left behind

Prognosis

- Benign, with self-limited growth (no growth once skeleton is mature)
- Low, but definite, risk of malignant transformation (1%-2%); usually a low-grade chondrosarcoma

Associations

- Reported to occur after irradiation for malignant nonosseous tumors of childhood such as Wilms and neuroblastoma
- *Multiple Hereditary Exostoses (Multiple Osteochondromas)*
    - An autosomal dominant hereditary disorder, slightly more common in males than females
    - A genetic defect linked to *EXT1* gene at 8q 22-24.1 and *EXT2* gene at 11p11-12 in some families; other studies have identified abnormal loci on chromosome 19
    - Characterized by multiple osteochondromas associated with bone deformities that consist of growth disturbances with bowing
    - Lesions typically larger, more sessile, and have a more lobulated cartilage cap than is seen in solitary exostoses
    - Region of the knee almost always involved
    - Gross and microscopic features identical to that of the solitary lesion
    - Affected individuals characteristically have a short stature, skeletal deformity, and as many as 30 individual lesions
    - Corrective surgery may be necessary to deal with the growth disturbances, functional impairment, and deformity
    - Risk of malignant transformation ranges from 5% to 25% (most common malignancy is a low-grade conventional chondrosarcoma)

Periosteal Chondroma (Juxtacortical Chondroma)

Clinical Manifestations

- 2% of chondromas
- Typically presents as a palpable mass (a surface lesion on bone)
- Proximity to a tendon insertion site causes pain with movement
- Most present between the 2nd and 3rd decades
- Males slightly more commonly affected than females;
- Typically affect long tubular bones; proximal humerus the most common site (50%); also occur in small tubular bones

Radiologic Features

- A well-circumscribed cartilaginous lesion on the surface of bone with scattered punctate calcifications
- Cortex beneath the lesion typically partially eroded resulting in a craterlike appearance ("saucerization"); cortex almost never completely disrupted

Gross Pathology

- A well-marginated, lobulated mass of cartilage on the surface of bone and covered with fibrous tissue (periosteum)
- On sectioning, calcifications easily identified
- Lesion separated from medullary cavity by rim of indented, sclerotic cortical bone

Microscopic Pathology

- Tend to be more cellular than enchondroma of long bones
- Mild nuclear atypia and occasional binucleate chondrocytes may be present
- Outer cortex usually scalloped and eroded; a margin of lamellar bone always separates the lesion from the underlying medullary cavity

Special Stains

- Not helpful

Immunohistochemistry

- Cartilaginous cells positive for S-100 protein and vimentin

Electron Microscopy

- Cartilage cells have centrally located nuclei with a wrinkled nuclear envelope and condensed chromatin

Molecular Alterations

- None

Differential Diagnosis

- Juxtacortical chondrosarcoma
- Periosteal osteosarcoma

Treatment and Prognosis

- Complete, wide local excision to include underlying cortex (necessitated by radiologic similarity to juxtacortical chondrosarcoma)
- Lesions in "nonessential" bones should be treated with segmental resection
- En bloc excision is almost always preferred over curettage
- Complete excision is always curative

Associations

- None

Benign Osteoblastic Lesions

Osteoblastoma

Clinical Manifestations

- Fewer than 1% of all primary bone tumors
- Occurs between the ages of 5 and 45 years with a peak incidence in the 2nd decade
- Males more commonly affected than females (2:1)
- 40% involve the vertebra (dorsal portion of arch) and sacrum; also seen in the jaw, craniofacial bones, and extremities (lower more often than upper)

Radiologic Findings

- Similar to osteoid osteoma except nidus exceeds 1.5 cm in diameter and sclerotic zone typically less extensive (may even be absent)
- Lesions in jaw usually near root of a tooth
- May expand the bone with thinning and focal destruction of the overlying cortex

Gross Pathology

- Nidus is well demarcated (an important finding that differentiates osteoblastoma from osteosarcoma), granular, very vascular, and easily separated from surrounding bone
- Surrounding bone may be expanded with a thinned and partially destroyed cortex
- Evidence of cystic degeneration and hemorrhage characteristic of a secondary aneurysmal bone cyst may be present

Microscopic Pathology

- Findings similar to those of osteoid osteoma: bony trabeculae evenly distributed in a loose well-vascularized fibroblastic stroma
- Prominent osteoblastic rimming may be present
- Some osteoclastlike giant cells often found along border of trabeculae and in areas of hemorrhage
- Mitotic figures may be present, but are never atypical
- Microscopic evidence of aneurysmal bone cyst with cystic spaces filled with blood may be present, especially in larger lesions

Special Stains, Immunohistochemistry, and Electron Microscopy

- Not helpful

Molecular Alterations

- None

Differential Diagnosis

- Osteoid osteoma (<1.5 cm)
- Osteosarcoma
- Aneurysmal bone cyst (not seen in association with osteoid osteoma)

Treatment

- Complete surgical (en bloc) excision
- Recurrence after surgery approximately 25%
- Lesions that are inaccessible to surgery can be treated with radiotherapy

Prognosis

- Malignant transformation has been reported

Associations

- Osteomalacia (oncogenic osteomalacia syndrome)
- Aneurysmal bone cyst (see above)

Aggressive osteoblastoma

- A neoplasm midway between benign osteoblastoma and osteosarcoma
- Tend to be larger than osteoblastomas (typically >4 cm in diameter)
- Males and females affected equally; most occur between ages of 30 to 50 years
- Anatomic location and radiologic and gross features similar to those of conventional osteoblastoma
- Classic microscopic finding is the presence of *epithelioid osteoblasts* that rim osteoid trabeculae; these epithelioid osteoblasts may form sheets of cells that fill the spaces between the trabeculae
- Trabeculae may be wider and more irregular than those of a benign osteoblastoma
- Epithelioid osteoblasts are twice the size of ordinary osteoblasts, have abundant eosinophilic cytoplasm, a round nucleus with a prominent nucleolus and may have a clear area (Golgi apparatus) that compresses and displaces the nucleus; 1 to 4 mitotic figures per 20 high-power fields; but never atypical)
- Secondary aneurysmal bone cyst formation often present
- No evidence of transformation or progression to osteosarcoma
- Treated with wide surgical excision

Osteoid Osteoma

Clinical Manifestations

- Represent approximately 10% of all benign bone tumors
- Typically occur between the ages of 10 and 30 years
- More common in males than females (3:1)
- 50% occur in long bones of the lower extremity (especially proximal femur)
- May occur in the small bones of the hands and feet; rare in the axial skeleton and craniofacial bones
- Usually (80%) present with pain that typically is worse at night and is relieved by aspirin and other nonsteroidal anti-inflammatory agents
- Pain and reactive sclerosis the result of a prostaglandin E_2 and prostacyclin released from osteoblasts in the center of the lesion

Variants According to Anatomic Site

- Osteoid osteoma: long tubular bone
  - Femoral neck most common site; tibia second
  - Intracortical lesion associated with fusiform cortical thickening with or without periosteal reaction
  - Intramedullary lesions typically produce surrounding sclerosis
  - Rarely can result from localized bone overgrowth
- Osteoid osteoma: small bones of hands and feet
  - More common in the hands than in the feet (2:1)
  - Usually associated with adjacent soft tissue swelling and synovitis in the closest joint
- Osteoid osteoma: vertebral column
  - 10% to 15% of all osteoid osteomas
  - Typically located in the neural arch of the lower thoracic or lumbar vertebra
  - May produce pain and scoliosis
  - Most frequently located in the posterior arch

- Osteoid osteoma: juxta-articular
  - Less painful and less responsive to aspirin
  - Typically little sclerosis or periosteal reaction
  - Intraarticular lesions usually associated with inflammatory changes in the adjacent synovium
- Osteoid osteoma: subperiosteal
  - A lucent defect on the surface of bone with adjacent periosteal reaction
  - Nidus tends to be less sclerotic, have thinner trabeculae and more stromal tissue than the more common intracortical lesion

Radiologic Findings

- A well-demarcated lytic lesion surrounded by distinct rim of sclerotic bone
- Center of the nidus opaque and surrounded by a lucent halo
- May be intracortical or intramedullary

Gross Pathology

- On cut section, soft and/or granular tissue nidus easily separates from surrounding sclerotic bone
- Nidus may be more sclerotic in center than at its periphery and is usually surrounded by a zone of dense sclerotic bone

Microscopic Pathology

- Nidus histiologically similar to osteoblastoma with numerous bony trabeculae of different size, thickness, and degree of mineralization distributed evenly throughout a highly cellular, vascular stroma
- Irregular osteoid trabeculae bordered by prominent osteoblasts and osteoclastlike giant cells
- Central area of nidus more calcified and less cellular than the highly cellular peripheral zone

Special Stains, Immunohistochemistry, and Electron Microscopy

- Not helpful

Molecular Alterations

- None

Differential Diagnosis

- Osteoblastoma (osteoid osteoma <1.5 cm; osteoblastoma >2 cm)
- Intracortical hemangioma
- Bone island
- Stress fracture
- Ewing sarcoma
- Intracortical osteosarcoma

Treatment

- Complete surgical excision of the nidus and some of the surrounding bone
- Curettage with bone graft is also acceptable (in sites where surgical excision not possible)
- If nidus is not completely removed, recurrence likely
- Long term (3-4 years) treatment with nonsteroidal inflammatory agents can lead to a reduction in the size of the nidus and permanent relief of symptoms

Prognosis

- Limited growth
- May spontaneously disappear

Associations

- Transformation of osteoid osteoma to osteoblastoma has been reported

Cystic Lesions

Aneurysmal Bone Cyst

Clinical Manifestations

- Represents 2% to 3% of all primary bone tumors
- Females affected slightly more often than males
- 80% occur in patients under the age of 20 years (skeletally immature); median age 13 years
- Any bone in the body can be affected with a slight increased incidence in craniofacial bones (20%) and the vertebral column (25%)
- When long bones involved, the metaphyseal region is most frequently affected
- Typically present with pain and swelling; symptoms may worsen during pregnancy

- Involvement of the vertebral column results in signs and symptoms related to compression of the spinal cord and nerves

Radiologic Findings

- Classically an ill-defined lucency (blowout) that distends the periosteum and is lined by a thin shell of subperiosteal bone
- Lytic portion of the lesion may have a "soap-bubble" pattern
- Typically eccentrically located in the metaphysis; may extend across a joint and involve adjacent bones

Gross Pathology

- Usually a sharply demarcated, spongy, or multilocular cystic lesion filled with blood
- Portion extending outside the bone is sharply circumscribed and surrounded by periosteum with a thin shell of reactive bone

Microscopic Pathology

- Multilocular cystic spaces bordered by septa of loose, well-vascularized, bland fibrous tissue (resembles granulation tissue) with multinucleated giant cells, inflammatory cells, extravasated red blood cells, trabeculae of osteoid and reactive woven bone rimmed by osteoblasts, and in 30% a peculiar filamentous bluish, chondro-osteoid calcified matrix (*"blue bone"*)
- Partially mineralized osteoid tends to form long strands that are oriented parallel to the long axis of the fibrous septa; vascular channels also tend to parallel the fibrous septa
- Cystic spaces typically have no recognizable lining
- Focal areas of reactive bone formation are typically present
- Clusters of giant osteoclastlike cells often present and tend to aggregate in areas of extravasated blood
- Surrounding bone typically shows features of resorption with prominent osteoclastic activity
- Mitotic figures commonly present, but never atypical
- *Solid variant of aneurysmal bone cyst* has same components as seen in the trabeculae of an ABC and is essentially identical to a giant cell reparative granuloma

Special Stains

- Not helpful

Immunohistochemistry

- Vascular markers will demonstrate focal presence of endothelial cells

Electron Microscopy

- Confirms the absence of endothelial cells lining cystic spaces

Molecular Alterations

- None

Differential Diagnosis

- Telangiectatic osteosarcoma is the most important consideration in the differential diagnosis
- Conventional osteosarcoma with secondary aneurysmal bone cyst
- Giant cell tumor
- Aneurysmal bone cyst engrafted on a preexisting giant cell tumor
- Giant-cell reparative granuloma
- Solitary bone cyst, especially if complicated by a pathologic fracture

Treatment

- Complete extraperiosteal surgical excision when lesion is anatomically accessible; 90% cured
- Inaccessible lesions are treated with curettage and bone grafting; probably >50% recur
- Radiation therapy is occasionally used for inoperable cases in adults
- Selective arterial embolization for lesions in spine, pelvis, and proximal femur

Prognosis

- Spontaneous malignant transformation has been reported
- Osteosarcoma and MFH may develop following radiation therapy

Secondary Aneurysmal Bone Cyst

- 50% of all aneurysmal bone cysts arise from a precursor lesion
- Rare after the age of 30 years

- Most often develop in weight-bearing bones
- Precursor lesions include giant cell tumor, chondroblastoma, osteoblastoma, nonossifying fibroma, fibrous dysplasia, giant cell reparative granuloma, chondromyxoid fibroma, fibrous histiocytoma, solitary bone cyst, eosinophilic granuloma, hemangioendothelioma, myositis ossificans, osteosarcoma, MFH, metastatic carcinoma, and other lesions containing a prominent vascular component (ie, hamartoma)

Solitary Bone Cyst (Unicameral Bone Cyst)

Clinical Manifestations

- More common in males than females (2:1)
- 80% are diagnosed between the ages of 3 and 14 years; rare over the age of 20 years
- Tend to involve the metaphysis of major long bones (proximal humerus and femur) of an immature skeleton; become inactive soon after end of skeletal growth
- Pain is the most common symptom with or without swelling or deformity
- May be complicated by a pathologic fracture

Radiologic Findings

- A lytic lesion with fine trabeculation and a scalloped sclerotic border that arises in the medullary cavity of the metaphysis with extension toward the growth plate and diaphysis
- Overlying cortex is distended and thinned, but never disrupted
- Evidence of a pathologic fracture frequently present

Gross Pathology

- A large intramedullary unilocular cystic cavity filled with clear or yellow, watery fluid
- Typically a single cyst but septations may be present
- A spongy component consisting of multiple small cysts may be present at the periphery or attached to the wall of the cyst
- Wall of cyst consists of thin, tan-yellow fibrous tissue with bony ridges

Microscopic Pathology

- Cyst wall has no lining and consists of a thin layer of fibrous tissue that contains dilated blood vessels, multinucleated giant cells, and occasional inflammatory cells
- Macrophages and hemosiderin typically present
- Focal areas of mineralization may be present in the cyst wall (mineralized fibrin) and resemble cementum
- Bone resorption with osteoclastic activity usually present in surrounding tissue
- Reactive bone formation with prominent osteoblasts may be present and indicate the presence of a fracture

Special Stains, Immunohistochemistry, and Electron Microscopy

- Not helpful

Molecular Alterations

- None

Differential Diagnosis

- Aneurysmal bone cyst
- Fibrous dysplasia (if patient an adult)
- Giant cell lesions

Treatment

- Dual needle aspiration with the instillation of methylprednisolone
- Curettage with bone grafting may be necessary for enlarging cysts in weight-bearing bones

Prognosis

- Recurrence after injection and curettage approximately 20%
- Secondary malignancy may occur (chondrosarcoma)

Associations

- None

Fibrous, Fibro-Osseous, and Fibrohistiocytic Lesions

Fibrosarcoma of Bone

Clinical Manifestations

- Males and females affected with equal frequency
- Typically involves metaphyseal portions of long tubular bones; distal femur most common site (50%), followed by proximal femur (15%), distal humerus (15%), and proximal tibia (10%); rarely multifocal

- Usually diagnosed between the 2nd and 7th decades of life with a peak incidence in the 5th decade
- Most patients present with pain, swelling, and tenderness; pathologic fracture may be the initial manifestation of disease

Radiographic Features

- An ill-defined lytic lesion with a destructive growth pattern
- Destroyed bone may have a moth-eaten appearance
- A Codman triangle (periosteal elevation) may be present
- Usually centered in the metaphysis
- Epiphysis may serve as an early barrier to the spread of the tumor in immature skeletons

Gross Pathology

- Low-grade lesions tend to be firm and fibrous; high-grade lesions tend to be soft and fleshy
- Focal areas of myxoid change, necrosis, and hemorrhage may be present
- Invasion in the bone may be irregular resulting in indistinct margins
- Destruction of the cortex with extension into soft tissue frequently present

Microscopic Pathology

- Uniform fibroblastlike cells arranged in a fasicular or "herringbone" pattern
- Cells tend to be uniform with ovoid, blunt-ended nuclei with single small nucleoli and finely dispersed chromatin; collagen fibers appear to emanate from nuclear poles
- Well-differentiated tumors tend to have abundant collagen
- No evidence of cartilage or bone matrix production
- Focal myxoid areas may be present (*myxofibrosarcoma*)
- Less well-differentiated and most high-grade fibrosarcomas are more cellular with less collagen, have greater nuclear atypia, and a high mitotic count with abnormal mitotic figures (usually classified as malignant fibrous histiocytomas)

Special Stains

- Not helpful

Immunohistochemistry

- Tumor cells strongly positive for vimentin and weakly positive for smooth muscle actin

Electron Microscopy

- Tumor cells demonstrate myofibroblastic differentiation with variable amounts of extracellular collagen

Molecular Alterations

- None

Differential Diagnosis

- Malignant fibrous histiocytoma (differentiation of fibrosarcoma from malignant fibrous histiocytoma can be quite arbitrary)
- Fibroblastic osteosarcoma
- Desmoplastic fibroma
- Metastatic carcinoma with spindle cell features

Treatment

- Low-grade lesions are treated with radical excision (either limb salvage or amputation)
- High-grade lesions are treated the same as malignant fibrous histiocytoma with surgery and adjuvant chemotherapy

Prognosis

- 10-year survival 80% for low-grade lesions
- 5-year survival 35%-45% for high-grade lesions (most classified as MFH)

Associations

- May be seen in association with giant cell tumor, Paget disease, irradiation damage, chronic osteomyelitis, fibrous dysplasia, and bone infarct (most sarcomas that complicate these conditions are currently classified as malignant fibrous histiocytomas)

Fibrous Dysplasia

Variants

- Monostotic (6 times more frequent than polyostotic)
- Polyostotic

Clinical Manifestations

- Typically presents before age of 30 years
- Lesions in long bones may present with pathologic fracture
- *Monostotic*
  - Usually a single focus of involvement
  - Typically asymptomatic and discovered incidentally on an x-ray taken for another reason
  - Most common clinical symptom is mildly painful swelling or deformity
  - Most frequent sites in men are rib, followed by craniofacial bones; most frequent sites in women are proximal femur and tibia; involvement of bones of hands and feet and flat bones (pelvis and scapula) rare
- *Polyostotic*
  - *Monomelic*: Usually exclusive involvement of a single lower extremity and the ipsilateral pelvis or scapula
  - *Polymelic*: Widespread, bilateral skeletal involvement to include both lower extremities, trunk, and craniofacial bones
  - Involvement of the vertebral column is uncommon with both variants

Radiographic Features

- Typically well-defined areas of rarefaction ("ground-glass" appearance) in the medullary cavity with a surrounding narrow rim of sclerotic bone; extension into epiphysis unusual
- Overlying cortex may be thinned and bone contour usually expanded (especially in narrow and flat bones)
- Degree of radiographic density dependent upon the amount of osseous component
- If lesions superimposed on an aneurysmal bone cyst, appearance may be suggestive of sarcoma

Gross Pathology

- Typically a centrally located fibrous or gritty, tan or gray lesion with sharp borders
- Areas of cartilaginous tissue may be seen as well as focal areas of hemorrhage or cystic change
- Lesions may have extensive ossification and resemble an osteoma

Microscopic Pathology

- Small irregularly shaped trabeculae of immature woven bone without rimming osteoblasts dispersed in a background of bland spindle cells arranged in a whorled or storiform pattern
- Most typical bone pattern consists of thin, curved, or branching fragments of woven bone characterized as "Chinese characters" (occasionally trabeculae are few and the lesion consists predominantly of spindle cells and resembles a benign fibrous histiocytoma)
- Under polarized light, the bony trabeculae consist of typical woven bone with disorganized, haphazard deposits
- Foci of cartilaginous differentiation are frequent and may be quite prominent (*fibrous dysplasia with massive cartilaginous differentiation* or *fibrocartilaginous dysplasia*)
- Occasionally there is a dense infiltrate of foamy histiocytes
- Intralesional hemorrhage may promote a giant cell reaction
- Older lesions may have focal or extensive areas of myxoid change
- If the lesion is complicated by a pathologic fracture, reactive bone with prominent osteoblastic rimming may be present
- A secondary aneurysmal bone cyst is a common finding

Special Stains, Immunohistochemistry, and Electron Microscopy

- Not helpful

Molecular Alterations

- Increased levels of *c-fos*
- Clonal structural alterations involving chromosomes 3, 8, 10, 12 and 15
- Mutation in *GNAS1* gene in chromosome 20q13 (seen in McCune-Albright syndrome)

Differential Diagnosis

- Osteofibrous dysplasia (**T2.1**)
- Desmoplastic fibroma
- Polyostotic fibrous dysplasia with large amounts of cartilage may mimic endochondromatosis or conventional chondrosarcoma
- Low-grade central osteosarcoma

Treatment

- Bony deformities treated with corrective surgery (prepubertal age group)
- A lesion prone to pathologic fracture can be treated with curettage and bone grafting, but only after puberty when lesion becomes quiescent; if this lesion must be treated before puberty, osteotomy with internal fixation is usually the procedure of choice
- Smaller lesions in non-weight-bearing bones treated with segmental resection

Prognosis

- 20% recur
- Monostotic variant typically does not progress to polyostotic variant
- Lesions grow slowly and have a tendency to stabilize after puberty
- Pregnancy appears to stimulate growth
- Secondary sarcoma develops in approximately 1% (more likely in patients treated with radiation therapy)
- Malignant transformation more likely in polyostotic variant (a reflection of extent of involvement)
- MFH and high-grade osteosarcoma are the 2 sarcomas most likely to complicate fibrous dysplasia
- Foci of fibrous dysplasia in the craniofacial skeleton and in the femur are the most likely lesions to undergo malignant transformation
- Prognosis following the development of sarcoma extremely poor (mean survival 3 to 4 years)

Associations

- Café-au lait spots (most common extraskeletal association; usually polyostotic variant)
  - Tuberous sclerosis
  - *McCune-Albright Syndrome*
- Occurs sporadically as a result of mutation in *GNAS1* gene located in chromosome band 20q13

T2.1
Differential Diagnosis of Osteofibrous Dysplasia (OFD) and Fibrous Dysplasia (FD)

	OFD	FD
Location	Tibia and fibula	Any bone, often polyostic
Age	0-10 y	Usually >10y
Bowing	Very frequent	No
Imaging	Intracortical	Intramedullary
Spontaneous regression	Possibly	No
Histology	Less cellular	More cellular
	Osteoblastic rimming	No
	Some lamellar bone	No
	Keratin + cells	No
	Zonal architecture	No

- Polyostotic fibrous dysplasia
- Café-au-lait spots
- Multiple endocrinopathies:
  - Sexual precocity (usually females)
  - Pituitary adenoma (acromegaly, Cushings)
  - Hyperthyroidism
  - Hyperparathyroidism
- Other reported abnormalities:
  - GI polyps; hyperplasia of spleen, thymus, and pancreatic islets; hepatobiliary disease; cardiac disease; failure to thrive; metabolic acidosis; abnormalities in serum electrolytes, glucose, or insulin levels; hyperphosphaturic hypophosphatemia; osteosarcoma (4%); developmental delay; microcephaly; sudden or premature death
- Cases of familial association between MEN I and McCune-Albright syndrome have been reported
- *Mazabraud syndrome*
- Polyostotic fibrous dysplasia associated with solitary or multiple intramuscular myxomas (very rare)

Comment

Generally considered a dysplastic abnormality of bone-forming mesenchymal tissue characterized by a solitary or multifocal inability of bone-forming tissue to produce mature lamellar bone; bone formation is arrested at the level of woven bone

Malignant Fibrous Histiocytoma of Bone

Clinical Manifestations

- A rare primary bone tumor (<2%)
- Males more frequently affected that females
- May occur any time between the ages of 20 and 80 years with a peak incidence in the mid-50s; only 10% diagnosed under the age of 20 years
- Most likely to occur in major long tubular bones; 30% arise in the region of knee and involve the metaphysis of the distal femur (30%-45%) or proximal tibia; may extend into epiphysis; diaphysis rarely involved
- Very rarely multifocal

Radiographic Features

- Typically a lytic, ill-defined, intramedullary defect that involves the metaphyseal portions of long tubular bones with occasional extension into adjacent epiphysis; infrequently centered in the diaphysis
- A destructive growth pattern
- Cortical disruption and extension into soft tissue both early findings
- Periosteal new bone formation usually scant
- Pathologic fracture frequent

Gross Pathology

- Neoplasm typically has irregular, ill-defined borders and on cross-section is tan to grey with fleshly yellow foci and areas of necrosis and hemorrhage; overall consistency of the neoplasm varies from soft to fibrous
- Cortical disruption with irregular infiltration of adjacent soft tissue often usually present

Microscopic Pathology

- Tumor typically consists of an admixture of histiocytoid cells, spindled cells arranged in a storiform pattern, and pleomorphic cells
- Broad range may be present resulting in several histologic subtypes more than 1 of which may be present in any given tumor:
  - *Storiform-pleomorphic MFH*: Most common, characterized by spindled cells that resemble fibroblasts arranged in storiform patterns; throughout the storiform areas, less differentiated cells are present and are characterized by nuclear atypia and increased mitotic activity; large mononuclear cells that resemble histiocytes are present and contain very atypical, pleomorphic nuclei (represent undifferentiated mesenchymal components); multiple atypical mitotic figures usually present as both malignant giant cells and osteoclast-type giant cells; focal areas of necrosis and scattered histiocytes with vacuolated cytoplasm (foamy) and inflammatory cells usually present
  - *Giant cell-rich MFH:* Characterized by a pattern that appears to be dominated by numerous multinucleated, osteoclastlike giant cells (easily confused with giant cell tumor of bone or other giant cell containing lesions of bone)
  - *Myxoid MFH* characterized by conventional MFH areas admixed with mucoid areas; mucoid areas must make up >50% of the neoplasm to warrant the diagnosis
  - MFHs that primarily arise in bone frequently have inflammatory cells dispersed throughout but a distinct inflammatory variant (as seen in soft tissue neoplasms) is rarely seen in bone
  - *Angiomatoid MFH* is not considered a variant of MFH in bone; this lesion is currently referred to as angiomatoid fibrous histiocytoma; tends to occur in children and young adults and is composed of solid areas of undifferentiated histiocytoid-appearing mesenchymal cells with telangiectatic spaces throughout (lesion mimics aneurysmal bone cyst or telangiectatic osteosarcoma); rarely metastasizes and has a good prognosis

Special Stains

- Not helpful

Immunohistochemistry

- Tumor cells strongly positive for vimentin and weakly positive for smooth muscle actin
- CD68 (macrophage-monocyte marker) may be positive, not particularly helpful

Electron Microscopy

- Tumor cells have features similar to those found in the soft tissue counterpart

Molecular Alterations

- Some reports of a familial incidence

Differential Diagnosis

- Undifferentiated osteosarcoma (defined as having unequivocal osteoid and/or bone formation)
- Fibrosarcoma
- Desmoplastic fibroma
- Metastatic carcinoma and melanoma with spindle cell features

Treatment

- Combined modality treatment consisting of surgery, chemotherapy, and radiotherapy
- After preoperative chemotherapy, the proportion of necrosis that remains is used as a prognostic factor and to modify subsequent treatment protocol (similar to the management of osteosarcoma)

Prognosis

- A highly aggressive malignancy with a high likelihood of metastasis, especially to the lungs (45%-50%); lymph node metastases unusual
- Localized disease has a 5-year disease-free survival of ~50%
- Tumors that arise from preexisting conditions tend to be more aggressive than those that arise de novo
- In general, the 5- and 10-year survival rates are similar to the soft tissue counterpart

Associations

- May be seen in association with giant cell tumor, Paget disease, irradiation change, chronic osteomyelitis, fibrous dysplasia, and bone infarct

Nonossifying Fibroma (Fibrous Cortical Defect; Histiocytic Fibroma)

Clinical Manifestations

- Most asymptomatic and found incidentally on a radiograph
- Peak incidence in 2nd decade with an age range of 5 to 20 years
- Typically occur in individuals with unfused growth plates
- Most common site is distal femoral metaphysis followed by proximal tibial metaphysis and distal tibial metaphysis
- Occasionally multifocal
- May be symptomatic if large (may present as a pathologic fracture)
- Rapid enlargement with development of a mass indicates presence of a superimposed aneurysmal bone cyst

Radiographic Findings

- Typically an eccentric, sharply circumscribed lytic lesion in the metaphysis that has a scalloped border and a narrow rim of marginal sclerosis
- Matrix mineralization not present
- Overlying cortex may be thinned and slightly expanded

Gross Pathology

- On cut section the lesion is fibrous and fleshy with a tan to brown color
- Cystic change, hemorrhage, and/or necrosis may be present particularly in the setting of a pathologic fracture

Microscopic Pathology

- Typically a highly cellular mass of fibrous tissue with a fibroblastic appearance arranged in a storiform pattern; collagen and hyaline change may be present
- Scattered osteoclasts and focal collections of foamy and hemosiderin-laden macrophages typically present throughout the lesion
- Mitotic figures often found within the fibroblastlike spindle cell areas, but cytologic atypia and atypical mitoses are both absent
- Small numbers of mononuclear inflammatory cells may be present
- Fresh hemorrhage and cystic change similar to that seen in an aneurysmal bone cyst may be present
- Multinucleated giant cells may be the dominant feature, but their distribution tends to be focal and often localized to areas of hemorrhage
- Focal areas of necrosis likely
- Lesion shares many microscopic features with both giant cell tumor of bone and benign fibrous histiocytoma

Special Stains

- Iron stains confirm the presence of hemosiderin in macrophages

Immunohistochemistry and Electron Microscopy

- Not helpful

Molecular Alterations

- None

Differential Diagnosis

- Benign fibrous histiocytoma (BFH is histologically identical to NOF; distinction must be based on clinical and radiographic features; BFH usually occurs in patients over the age of 20 years, may occur in non-long bones, when in a long bone usually centered in the epiphysis or diaphysis, and on x-ray lacks a well defined, sclerotic, scalloped border)
- Giant cell tumor (GCT is similar to nonossifying fibroma except less fibroblastic and giant cells more diffusely distributed)
- Fibrous dysplasia
- Desmoplastic fibroma (the intraosseous counterpart of soft tissue fibromatosis)
- Cortical irregularity syndrome (an avulsion lesion at site of insertion of muscle tendon on posterior-medial aspect of distal femur)

Treatment

- Usually do not require treatment (tend to resolve spontaneously)
- Large lesions that distort bone or develop a secondary aneurysmal bone cyst are treated with curettage and bone grafting
- A pathologic fracture is treated with a cast until healed and then the underlying lesion is curetted with or without bone grafting

Prognosis

- Most stabilize at puberty and spontaneously heal

Associations

- Osteosarcoma has been reported in bones with a nonossifying fibroma
- Reports of malignant transformation exist (but not generally accepted)
- Multiple nonossifying fibromas
- A well-documented familial incidence exists
- Increased incidence in patients with neurofibromatosis (von Recklinghausen disease)
- *Jaffe-Campanacci syndrome*: Congenital disorder characterized by multifocal nonossifying fibromas, café-au-lait pigmentation, hypogonadism, cryptorchidism, ocular anomalies, and cardiovascular malformations (to include mitral insufficiency and aortic stenoses), occasional precocious puberty, and kyphoscoliosis; the skeletal involvement tends to be symmetric; the trunk, axial skeleton and craniofacial bones are often involved; pathologic fractures common

Osteofibrous Dysplasia (Ossifying Fibroma of Long Bones)

Clinical Manifestations

- Occurs almost exclusively in the proximal and middle 3rd of the tibia and occasionally in the proximal ipsilateral fibula (may present as synchronous involvement of both bones on 1 side)
- Represents fewer than 1% of all bone tumors
- May be present at birth but usually occurs before the age of 10 years
- Males and females affected equally

Radiographic Features

- A multiloculated lytic expansion of the anterior lateral cortex of the tibia with a synchronous lytic lesion near the distal or proximal end of the fibula
- Anterior-bowing deformity is usually present

Gross Pathology

- A multilocular intracortical lesion in the anterior lateral cortex
- Surrounding sclerosis usually evident
- On sectioning a gritty, fibrous texture
- Cortical disruption and invasion into soft tissue rare

Microscopic Pathology

- Fibroblastlike spindle cells arranged in loose bundles usually in a storiform pattern
- Scattered throughout the fibroblastic component are small irregular fragments of woven bone rimmed by a lamellar layer of new bone laid down by well-developed osteoblasts

- Lesion tends to have a zonal architecture with progressively larger, more mature, and more numerous trabeculae of mineralized bone at the periphery compared with the center (center of the lesion contains fibrous tissue and immature woven bone; the periphery has more lamellar bone)
- Osteoclasts may be present
- Pathologic fracture with hemorrhage and collections of multinucleated giant cells may be present

Special Stains

- Not helpful

Immunohistochemistry

- Single keratin-positive cells may be present (evidence that osteofibrous dysplasia may represent an indolent form of adamantinoma)

Electron Microscopy

- Confirms the presence of epithelial elements

Molecular Alterations

- Clonal chromosomal abnormalities have been identified suggesting that the underlying lesion may be neoplastic in nature

Differential Diagnosis

- Fibrous dysplasia (see **T2.1**)
- Classic adamantinoma
- Differentiated adamantinoma

Treatment

- Corrective surgery (osteotomy) for deformity

Prognosis

- A self-limited process that progresses until puberty and then stabilizes and spontaneously repairs itself
- Rarely recurs
- Small minority develop adamantinoma

Associations

- See Adamantinoma of Long Bones

Comment

There may be a relationship between adamantinoma and osteofibrous dysplasia of long bones; adamantomas with a microscopic appearance predominantly of osteofibrous dysplasia and an inconspicuous component of epithelial elements may represent a special variant of adamantinoma characterized by exclusive, often multicentric, involvement of the cortex of the tibia with frequent synchronous involvement of the ipsilateral fibula

Adamantinomata may represent a continuum of neoplasms with classic adamantinoma at one end, osteofibrous dysplasia at the other end, and differentiated adamantinoma somewhere in the middle

Giant Cell Lesions

Giant Cell Reparative Granuloma

Clinical Manifestations

- Typically occur between the ages of 15 and 25 years
- Most frequently occurs in the craniofacial bones (mandible and maxilla)
- 2nd most common site is the small bones of the hands and feet
- Very rare in long tubular bones and vertebrae

Radiographic Findings

- In the craniofacial bones, lesion produces a round or oval lucency with fine trabeculations, a distinct border, and minimal reactive sclerosis; cortex is usually intact with little or no periosteal reaction
- In the small bones of the hands and feet, lesion can be either metaphyseal or diaphyseal or both but never crosses an unfused growth plate

Gross Pathology

- Tan or brown, friable, and gritty usually with cystic change or hemorrhage

Microscopic Pathology

- Moderately cellular fibrous stroma consisting of spindle-shaped fibroblasts and collagen
- Multinucleated giant cells are *unevenly* distributed and tend to form obvious clusters separated by bundles of stroma tissue; clusters of giant cells tend to occur in areas of hemorrhage (which are almost always present)

- Extensive reactive bone formation usually present (osteoid and immature bone)
- Changes suggestive of an aneurysmal bone cyst often present

Special Stains and Immunohistochemistry

- Not helpful

Electron Microscopy

- Giant cells are similar to those seen in giant cell tumor
- Stromal spindle cells show myofibroblastic differentiation (macrophagelike differentiation is not present)

Molecular Alterations

- None

Differential Diagnosis

- Brown cell tumor of hyperparathyroidism (microscopically indistinguishable)
- Giant-cell tumor (giant cells evenly distributed, ie, do not cluster and less fibroblastic)
- Aneurysmal bone cyst
- Nonossifying fibroma (usually metaphysis of long bone)
- Pigmented villonodular synovitis

Treatment

- Curettage with or without bone grafting
- Lesions of the maxilla can be treated with steroids
- Lesions involving the small bones of the hands and feet that destroy the majority of the bone may have to be treated with amputation

Prognosis

- Recurrence occurs in a third to a half of patients treated with curettage and bone graft
- Malignant transformation does not occur
- Pulmonary implants (a rare feature of giant cell tumor) never occur

Associations

- A reactive process to the presence of intraosseous hemorrhage either in normal bone or in bone with a preexisting lesion such as fibrous dysplasia, brown tumor of hyperparathyroid disease, or rarely, Paget disease
- Relationship probably based on trauma
- Some evidence of overlap with solid aneurysmal bone cyst

Giant Cell Tumor of Bone

Clinical Manifestations

- 4% of all bone tumors
- Most commonly occurs between the ages of 25 and 45 years; unusual in patients under the age of 20 years or over the age of 55 years
- Usually found in the epiphyseal ends of long tubular bones
- Epiphysis of distal femur, proximal tibia, and distal radius 3 most frequent sites; may occur in the vertebral bodies (especially sacrum), flat bones, ribs, or craniofacial bones
- More common in women than in men and occurs more frequently in Asian than in Western countries
- May be multifocal (rare in absence of Paget disease); typically involve small bones of distal extremities

Radiographic Findings

- Typically centered in the epiphysis and entirely lytic and expansile without peripheral bone sclerosis or periosteal reaction
- Overlying cortex usually expanded and may be focally destroyed
- 5% to 10% have an associated pathologic fracture
- Radiologic diagnosis difficult because there is marked overlap with fibrosarcoma, MFH, multiple myeloma, and other destructive bone lesions

Gross Pathology

- A soft, friable, fleshy lesion in the epiphyseal end of bone with extension into the medullary cavity
- Articular cartilage rarely involved
- Overlying cortex often destroyed with expansion of the contour of bone
- Focal areas of hemorrhage, cyst formation, and necrosis frequently present

Microscopic Pathology

- Two main components:
  - A moderately vascularized stroma consisting of spindle-shaped mononuclear cells with regular round or oval nuclei that have evenly distributed chromatin and a prominent nucleolus
  - Multinucleated giant cells characterized by large size and large numbers of nuclei (50 to 100 or more) that tend to be clustered in the middle of the cell; giant cell nuclei are similar to the nuclei of the spindle cells in that they have regular outlines and are round or oval with evenly distributed chromatin and a prominent nucleolus
- Giant cells resemble osteoclasts; they are not neoplastic and simply represent the fusion of intravascular monocytes that have been recruited to the lesion by various cytokines; *mononuclear stromal cell is the neoplastic cell and is the only proliferating element of the lesion*; stromal cells produce types I and III collagen and have receptors for parathyroid hormone
- Mitotic figures frequently present in stromal cell population; no mitotic activity is seen among the multinucleated giant cells
- Osteoid and bone often present at periphery and may be present in central areas
- Intravascular invasion of neoplasm frequent (approximately 30%)
- Secondary changes within a giant cell tumor include: malignant transformation (dedifferentiation), necrosis, fibrohistiocytic (xanthomatous) change, and secondary aneurysmal bone cyst formation
- Areas of hemorrhage and/or necrosis may be fairly extensive

Special Stains

- Not helpful

Immunohistochemistry

- Mononuclear stromal cells and multinucleated giant cells positive for α_1-antrypsin
- Mononuclear stromal cells express both parathyroid hormone and calcitonin receptors (an indication that these stroma cells are undergoing osteoclastic differentiation)

Electron Microscopy

- Mononuclear stromal cells have similarities with cells of histiocytic and/or macrophage lineage

Molecular Alterations

- Most neoplasms are aneuploid
- Most have a random or clonal chromosomal aberration with telomeric fusion being the most common abnormality

Differential Diagnosis

- If located in a tubular long bone:
  - Chondroblastoma
  - Nonossifying fibroma
  - Chondromyxoid fibroma
  - Aneurysmal bone cyst
  - Pigmented villonodular synovitis
  - Osteogenic sarcoma
- If located in the small bones of the hands and feet:
  - Giant-cell reparative granuloma
  - Pigmented villonodular synovitis
- If located in the vertebral column:
  - Aneurysmal bone cyst
  - Osteoblastoma
  - Giant-cell reparative granuloma
  - Eosinophilic granuloma
- If located in a flat bone:
  - Chondroblastoma
  - Fibrosarcoma
  - Malignant fibrous histiocytoma
- If located in the craniofacial bones:
  - Fibrous dysplasia
  - Brown tumor of hyperparathyroidism
  - Giant-cell reparative granuloma

Treatment

- Curettage with bone grafting or en bloc excision; 25% to 35% recur and are treated the same as primary lesions
- Treatment with radiation may result in malignant transformation

Prognosis

- 25% locally aggressive
- 1% to 2% may metastasize to lung (referred to as a pulmonary implant and hence distinguished from a true metastasis from a malignant giant cell tumor); prognosis good but some will die

- Pulmonary metastases usually occur after removal of the primary bone lesion and may represent mechanical seeding of the bloodstream at the time of surgery

Associations

- May complicate Paget disease (a less frequent complication of Paget disease than the development of a sarcoma); often multifocal
- *Goltz syndrome*: Focal dermal hypoplasia with multiple congenital anomalies of skin, teeth, and bone

Malignant Giant Cell Tumor

Clinical Manifestations

- May occur as a primary lesion (very rare) or as secondary lesion (malignant transformation of a benign giant cell tumor)
- Malignant change usually occurs in the setting of multiple local recurrences or an irradiated lesion (usually 5 years or more after radiation exposure)

Radiographic Features

- Large, lytic, destructive lesion with cortical disruption and invasion of adjacent soft tissue

Gross Pathology

- May be indistinguishable from benign giant cell tumor that has resulted in a cortical disruption and soft tissue invasion

Microscopic Pathology

- Malignant change in secondary lesions resembles fibrosarcoma, malignant fibrous histiocytoma, or osteosarcoma; malignant features are characterized by the presence of atypical mitoses and nuclear pleomorphism in the spindle cell (monocyte) population; a focus of benign giant cell tumor is usually present
- Osteoid is not produced; but reactive bone is almost always present at the periphery
- Primary malignant tumors have high mitotic rates with numerous atypical mitoses involving both stromal cells and giant cells

Special Stains, Immunohistochemistry and Electron Microscopy

- Not helpful

Molecular Alterations

- None

Differential Diagnosis

- Other sarcomas that contain giant cells: Osteosarcoma and malignant fibrous histiocytoma

Treatment

- Complete surgical excision if possible
- Radiation can be used for palliation in surgically inaccessible lesions

Prognosis

- Primary malignant giant cell tumors may have a slightly better prognosis than secondary malignant giant cell tumors

Associations

- Secondary lesions typically follow previous therapy (incomplete surgical excision or curettage and/or radiation)

Malignant Cartilage Lesions

Clear Cell Chondrosarcoma

Clinical Manifestations

- 2% of all chondrosarcomas
- More common in males than females (3:1)
- Proximal femur most frequently affected site (45%) followed by the proximal humerus
- Peak incidence between 25 and 50 years
- Patients typically present with pain in the affected area

Radiographic Findings

- A lytic defect that resembles chondroblastoma in the epiphysis of a long tubular bone
- Sclerotic margins may be present
- Cortical disruption not a typical feature

Gross Pathology

- Usually well-circumscribed and on sectioning soft, gray to tan with focal calcification

- Foci of cystic change and hemorrhage may be present
- Large lesions expand bone, stimulate new bone formation, and may erupt into joint
- Features of cartilage usually absent

Microscopic Pathology

- Tumor cells large and contain abundant clear or granular cytoplasm and are embedded in a loose cartilaginous matrix; they tend to be oval with uniform centrally located nuclei with prominent nucleoli; cellular membranes usually distinct; few mitotic figures
- Typically a lobulated architecture with bands of fibrovascular stroma (typical of conventional chondrosarcomas)
- Foci of coarse calcification and multinucleated osteoclast-like giant cells usually present
- Infiltrative growth pattern
- Areas of aneurysmal bone cyst often present

Special Stains

- PAS with and without diastase confirms presence of glycogen within tumor cells

Immunohistochemistry

- Tumor cells strongly positive for S-100 protein and negative for epithelial markers

Electron Microscopy

- Not helpful

Molecular Alterations

- Unusual karyotypic findings

Differential Diagnosis

- Chondroblastoma
- Osteoblastoma
- Central osteosarcoma
- Conventional chondrosarcoma
- Metastatic clear cell carcinoma

Treatment

- En bloc excision with clear margins with or without joint replacement usually curative
- Chemotherapy may prolong survival

Prognosis

- A low-grade malignant neoplasm with a definite metastatic potential (usually following incomplete excision)

Associations

- None

Chondrosarcoma (Conventional; Intramedullary)

Clinical Manifestations

- 2nd most frequent primary malignant neoplasm of bone (25% of all primary sarcomas of bone)
- Peak incidence between the 5th and 6th decades
- Rare under the age of 40 years and very rare in children
- Affects males and females equally
- Involves the pelvis (usually ilium) and ribs 25% and 20%, respectively; proximal femur (15%) and proximal humerus (10%)
- Rare in the spine (5%), craniofacial bones (2%), and small bones of hands and feet (1%)
- May occur in extraskeletal site (usually a myxoid variant)
- Typically presents as a dull, aching, intermittent pain that seems to be more pronounced at rest and at night; restriction of range of motion may occur if located near a joint

Radiographic Findings

- An area of lucency with variable amounts of evenly distributed punctate or ringlike calcifications
- Typically cortex is thinned with erosions on its inner surface; cortical sclerosis may be seen
- Advanced lesions usually disrupt cortex and extend into adjacent soft tissue

Gross Pathology

- On cut section, lobules of typically normal-appearing cartilage with peripheral mineralization
- Foci of enchondral ossification are readily apparent as ivorylike bony areas
- Focal areas of myxomatous change, hemorrhage, and/or necrosis may be present
- Cortex often eroded or destroyed with extension into adjacent soft tissue (especially when tumor involves flat bones)

Malignant Cartilage Lesions>Chondrosarcoma (Conventional; Intramedullary)

Microscopic Pathology

- Neoplasm uniformly cartilaginous
- Tumor cells are uniformly distributed and look like normal chondrocytes and occupy lacunae in a partially myxoid or calcified hyaline cartilage matrix
- Tumor cells may be vacuolated and appear as clear cells
- Lobulated architecture very evident with irregularly shaped lobules separated by narrow bands of fibrovascular tissue
- At periphery of the lesion, lobules of cartilage may infiltrate cortical and/or medullary bone
- Little or no reactive bone formation at the periphery
- Three grades
  - Grade I: Very similar to benign enchondroma except the cellularity is increased; occasional enlarged, hyperchromatic nuclei or double nuclei; infiltrative growth pattern
  - Grade II: Uniformly increased cellularity; tumor cells have enlarged, hyperchromatic nuclei with open chromatin and prominent nucleoli; binucleate cells are frequent and atypical nuclei often present; foci of myxoid change frequent (the presence of myxoid change denotes at least a grade II lesion)
  - Grade III: High cellularity which tends to gradually increase toward the periphery of the lesion with prominent nuclear atypia and multiple mitoses (>1 mitotic figure per high-powered field denotes a grade III lesion)
- Most are grade I or grade II (~3% are grade III)

Special Stains

- Not helpful

Immunohistochemistry

- Tumor cells positive for S-100 protein and vimentin
- Grade III lesions may be focally negative for S-100

Electron Microscopy

- Tumor cells have abundant rough endoplasmic reticulum and glycogen

Molecular Alterations

- Deletions of numerous chromosomes have been reported
- Non-random rearrangements of chromosome 1p and possibly 4, 5, 9, and 20
- p53 protein overexpression may be present in high-grade lesions

Differential Diagnosis

- Chondroblastic osteosarcoma
- Enchondroma (cytologically almost indistinguishable from low-grade chondrosarcoma; *most significant feature of chondrosarcomas is permeation through cortex and into cancellous bone*)
- Enchondromatosis (Ollier disease)
- Fibrous dysplasia with cartilaginous differentiation
- Fracture callus
- Synovial chondromatosis

Treatment

- Wide surgical excision
- Irradiation and chemotherapy play a limited role in high-grade chondrosarcomas

Prognosis

- Risk of recurrence and metastasis dependent upon grade (most important), tumor necrosis, mitotic count, and myxoid tumor matrix
- 5-year survival 90% for grade I
- 5-year survival 80% for grade II
- 5-year survival 30% for grade III
- Metastasis to lymph nodes more frequent than in other sarcomas, but lung primary metastatic site
- Grade I lesions do not metastasize (death results from local uncontrolled growth)
- Recurrent tumors usually show an increase in grade

Associations

- May represent a malignant transformation of an enchondroma in a patient with enchondromatosis (Ollier disease or Maffucci syndrome)

Variants

- *Periosteal chondrosarcoma* (occurs on surface of bone; metaphysis of distal femur most common site; histologic features similar to conventional chondrosarcoma with nodules of tumor invading adjacent soft tissues)
- *Secondary chondrosarcoma* (arises in benign precursor lesion—osteochondroma or enchondroma)

- *Secondary chondrosarcoma in Ollier disease and Maffucci syndrome* (histologic features characterized by increased cellularity and nuclear atypia in comparison to enchondromas of Ollier disease and Maffucci syndrome; enchondromas of Ollier disease and Maffucci syndrome have increased cellularity and nuclear atypia in comparison to sporadic enchondromas)

Dedifferentiated Chondrosarcoma

Clinical Manifestations

- 10% of all chondrosarcomas
- Average age at presentation 50 to 60 years
- Typically present with a long history of vague discomfort followed by a rapidly enlarging mass
- 30% involve the femur, 20% pelvis, 15% humerus, 5%-10% ribs, and 5%-10% scapula
- 50% present with pathologic fracture

Radiographic Features

- A lytic lesion with punctate opacities in the center and a periphery characterized by complete loss of bony architecture
- Complete cortical disruption and extension into soft tissue usually present

Gross Pathology

- 2 components of the lesion (low-grade cartilaginous and high-grade sarcoma) easily identified; cartilaginous portion is lobulated; dedifferentiated portion has a soft fleshy consistency often with areas of hemorrhage and necrosis
- Cartilaginous component located centrally

Microscopic Pathology

- Low-grade cartilaginous lesion and a high-grade sarcoma with a distinct zone where the 2 components interface
- Dedifferentiated area looks like a high-grade sarcoma; most commonly resembles a pleomorphic malignant fibrous histiocytoma)
- Dedifferentiated component may have features of osteosarcoma, fibrosarcoma, and/or rhabdomyosarcoma

Special Stains

- Not helpful

Immunohistochemistry

- Low-grade cartilaginous regions stain positively for S-100 protein
- Dedifferentiated sarcomatous areas stain negatively for S-100
- Specific features of differentiation can be highlighted with muscle markers and/or epithelial markers

Electron Microscopy

- Dedifferentiated cells are very pleomorphic mesenchymal cells with various features of differentiation (ie, osteoblastic, chondroblastic, smooth muscle, or skeletal muscle)

Molecular Alterations

- See conventional chondrosarcoma
- Precursor cartilage lesion diploid; dedifferentiated component aneuploid

Differential Diagnosis

- High-grade conventional chondrosarcoma
- Mesenchymal chondrosarcoma
- Chondroblastic osteosarcoma
- Malignant fibrous histiocytoma
- Fibrous dysplasia with abundant cartilage
- Metastatic high-grade spindle cell sarcoma

Treatment

- Chemotherapy

Prognosis

- Fewer than 10% survive 1 year

Associations

- None

Comment

Dedifferentiation is defined as the development of high-grade sarcoma in a preexisting locally aggressive low-grade tumor; may be seen in giant cell tumors, low-grade intramedullary and parosteal osteosarcomas, and liposarcomas. Extraskeletal chondrosarcomas can also dedifferentiate.

Mesenchymal Chondrosarcoma

Clinical Manifestations

- 2% of all chondrosarcomas
- Males and females affected equally
- Peak incidence between ages of 10 and 30 years
- Maxilla and mandible most frequently affected; also ribs, ilium, and vertebrae
- Bones of appendicular skeleton rarely involved
- 30% present as extraskeletal soft tissue lesions (meninges one of the most common sites)
- Often present with pain and swelling in the affected area

Radiographic Features

- An eccentrically located radiolucent lesion with variable amounts of stippled calcification
- May have a sclerotic margin
- Bone often expanded or disrupted with extraosseous extension into soft tissue

Gross Pathology

- Typically well-demarcated with a lobular architecture
- Lesional tissue gray to pink; areas of necrosis and hemorrhage may be present
- Disruption of cortex with extension into soft tissue frequent

Microscopic Pathology

- Consists primarily of solid, highly cellular areas of primitive round or spindled mesenchymal cells that may be arranged in a hemangiopericytomalike pattern with multiple vascular spaces (cells resemble cells of Ewing sarcoma)
- Islands of cartilage are scattered throughout and may contain focal areas of calcification
- Proportion of cellular, mesenchymal elements, and cartilaginous elements highly variable between tumors and within the same tumor
- Osteoclastlike giant cells may be present

Special Stains

- PAS with diastase confirms presence of glycogen in cartilaginous areas

Immunohistochemistry

- Areas of cartilaginous differentiation typically positive for S-100 protein
- Cellular areas of primitive mesenchymal cells are negative for S-100 protein
- Primitive mesenchymal cells may be weakly positive for neuron-specific enolase (NSE)
- Muscle markers may confirm the presence of rhabdomyoblastic differentiation

Electron Microscopy

- Confirms the presence of oval, elongated primitive mesenchymal cells

Molecular Alterations

- A reciprocal translocation (11;22) of the Ewing family of tumors is not present

Differential Diagnosis

- Dedifferentiated chondrosarcoma
- Ewing sarcoma of bone
- Primitive neuroectodermal tumor
- Embryonal rhabdomyosarcoma
- Malignant lymphoma
- Small-cell osteosarcoma
- Hemangiopericytoma

Treatment

- Surgical excision

Prognosis

- A highly aggressive neoplasm that frequently recurs and metastasizes, occasionally late (>20 years)
- Tumors of the jaws tend to have a more indolent course
- 30% survive 10 years
- 50% die within 5 years

Associations

- None

Metabolic Conditions

Paget Disease (Osteitis Deformans)

Clinical Manifestations

- Usually an insidious onset with no symptoms for many years
- Slightly more frequent in men than women
- Rarely diagnosed in patients under the age of 40 years; age range 45 to 80 years
- Skeletal deformities include enlarged head, outward bowed femora, forward bowed tibiae, and bowed back
- Long bones appear to be thickened
- Spine, pelvis, skull, and femur are the most frequently involved sites

Radiographic Findings

- Classic findings are areas of irregular increased density with a "cotton wool-like" appearance intermixed with lucent areas
- Areas of sclerosis may be present
- Bones are typically enlarged and have an altered shape secondary to prominent deformity
- Early cranial lesions appear as well-circumscribed lytic areas (*osteoporosis circumscripta*)
- Bowing deformities and pathologic fractures both common in weight-bearing bones

Gross Pathology

- Cortex and trabeculae of medullary bone typically thickened

Microscopic Pathology

- In the early phases of the disease, there is increased osteoclastic (lytic) activity with fibrosis and prominent vascularization of the spaces between the trabeculae
- In the active phase of the disease, there is a mixture of osteoclastic activity and osteoblastic activity; the osteoclasts tend to be enlarged and aggregate in clusters (often in Howship lacunae) producing an irregular scalloped appearance of the trabeculae; the osteoblastic activity may be focal and result in the formation of new osteoid
- The final phase of disease is characterized by bone sclerosis in which there are multiple irregular lines of mineralization; the disorganized nature of lamellar bone leads to the formation of *cement lines* (represent abrupt interruptions and changes in direction of bone lamellae and fibers resulting from reabsorption and regeneration of bone)

Special Stains and Immunohistochemistry

- Not helpful

Electron Microscopy

- Viruslike intranuclear and cytoplasmic inclusions are frequently present in osteoclasts

Molecular Alterations

- A familial incidence exists (<10%); a Mendelian-dominant pattern

Differential Diagnosis

- None

Treatment

- Stabilization of pathologic fracture (fracture may be result of development of a sarcoma)

Prognosis

- Largely dependent upon the development of an associated sarcoma

Associations

- Sarcomatous transformation occurs in <10%; incidence increases with age until the 7th decade
- Most frequent sites are pelvis, humerus, and femur
- Most common type of Paget sarcoma is osteosarcoma; fibrosarcoma, chondrosarcoma, malignant giant cell tumor, and pleomorphic malignant fibrous histiocytoma also occur
- Prognosis for sarcoma arising in the setting of Paget worse than for de novo sarcoma (<10% 5-year survival vs 50% to 65% 5-year survival)
- Paramyxovirus

Tophaceous Gout

Clinical Manifestations

- Hyperuricemia coupled with deposition of monosodium urate crystals in synovium
- Men much more frequently affected than women (9:1)
- Affects adults between the ages of 35 and 65 years, with a peak incidence in 6th decade

- Joints of the foot and ankle most frequently involved; >1 joint may be involved
- 50% of patients with gouty arthritis have deposits of monosodium urate crystals (tophi)

Radiographic Findings

- Usually a periarticular, noncalcified mass that often shows evidence of erosion into adjacent bone
- 20% show calcifications

Gross Pathology

- Cut surface white to yellow with a chalky consistency surrounded by a pseudocapsule of fibrous tissue
- Older lesions tend to be multilobular, fibrotic, and calcified

Microscopic Pathology

- Crystals of monosodium urate are needle-shaped, doubly refractile that are strongly negatively birefringent under polarized light
- Crystals are found both free floating and within leukocytes
- Crystals in tophi elicit a granulomatous response that is dominated by the presence of histiocytes and foreign body giant cells; histiocytes tend to palisade around the nodule (reminiscent of a rheumatoid nodule)
- Urate deposits eventually destroy cartilage and bone

Special Stains

- Tissue should be fixed in alcohol to preserve monosodium urate crystals

Immunohistochemistry and Electron Microscopy

- Not helpful

Molecular Alterations

- None

Differential Diagnosis

- Chondrocalcinosis (tophaceous pseudogout)

Treatment

- Aimed at controlling the hyperuricemia

Associations

- None

Tophaceous Pseudogout (Chondrocalcinosis)

Clinical Manifestations

- Typically affects adults between the ages of 45 and 65 years
- More common in women than in men
- Knee joint most frequent site of involvement; also reported in hip, cervical spine, toe, and temporomandibular joint
- Serum levels of calcium and phosphate tend to be normal

Radiographic Findings

- A variably calcified mass
- Calcification has a granular or fluffy appearance
- No peripheral density (as seen in myositis ossificans)
- Adjacent bone may show evidence of pressure erosion

Gross Pathology

- Typically circumscribed, gray or white with a chalky appearance

Microscopic Pathology

- Deposits of calcium pyrophosphate dihydrate crystals in articular and periarticular tissue
- Variably cellular tissue with small to large islands of basophilic calcified crystalline material
- Crystals tend to be short and rhomboid in shape and are weakly birefringent under compensated polarized light
- Cellular component contains large numbers of histiocytes and foreign body giant cells surrounding foci of calcification
- Metaplastic chondroid tissue with some cellular atypia may be present

Special Stains

- Decalcification will remove the calcium pyrophosphate dihydrate crystals

Immunohistochemistry and Electron Microscopy

- Not helpful

Electron Microscopy

- Not helpful

Molecular Alterations

- None

Differential Diagnosis

- Synovial chondromatosis
- Chondrosarcoma
- Chondroma

Treatment and Prognosis

- A benign condition with no evidence of a malignant transformation
- Surgical excision (high rate of recurrence even after complete excision)

Associations

- None

Neuroectodermal Tumors

Askin Tumor

- (See Ewing Sarcoma and Primitive Neuroectodermal Tumor [PNET] in chapter 20)
- A malignant small, round, blue cell tumor involving the thoracopulmonary region of children
- Most arise in the periosteum of ribs (may arise in soft tissue and within the lung); frequently involves intercostal nerves
- Generally felt to be a variant of Ewing sarcoma and PNET that *occurs exclusively in the thoracopulmonary region*; may demonstrate features of either Ewing sarcoma or features of PNET (by light microscopy, immunohistochemistry, and electron microscopy)
- Probably more closely related to PNET than Ewing sarcoma (tends to express neural markers more frequently than does Ewing sarcoma)
- Glycogen may or may not be present in neoplastic cells
- Frequently positive for neural markers to include NSE, neurofilaments, and chromogranin; also positive for MIC2 gene product; focally positive for low-molecular-weight cytokeratins
- Same t(11; 22)(q24; q12) as seen with Ewing sarcoma and PNET

Ewing Sarcoma

Clinical Manifestations

- Represents 6% to 8% of all primary malignant bone tumors; 3rd most frequent sarcoma of bone (following osteosarcoma and chondrosarcoma)
- Occurs between the ages of 1 and 25 years, with the peak incidence in the 2nd decade
- More common in males than females
- Almost never seen in black patients
- Most commonly involves the shaft of long tubular bones, the pelvis, and the ribs in immature skeletons (essentially any bone can be affected)

Radiographic Findings

- Ill-defined diaphyseal, intramedullary destructive lesion often with an ill-defined adjacent soft tissue mass
- Prominent multilayered periosteal reaction (onion skin) typical
- Most are purely lytic and have a moth-eaten appearance
- Surface of bone may have a concave defect (saucerization)

Gross Pathology

- Gray to white, well-demarcated, intramedullary mass that permeates and penetrates the overlying cortex; often necrotic and hemorrhagic
- Extension to adjacent soft tissue with a large extraosseous mass is typical

Microscopic Pathology

- Solid sheets and nests of small round blue cells (undifferentiated mesenchymal cells) fill intertrabecular spaces
- Tumor cells have scant eosinophilic or clear cytoplasm and centrally located nuclei with fine granular chromatin and 1 to 3 nucleoli
- A biphasic pattern consisting of small, round, blue cells with dark, condensed chromatin and small, round, blue cells with lighter, open chromatin (the dark nuclei represents cells undergoing apoptosis)

- Small foci to large geographic areas of necrosis usually present
- Homer-Wright rosettes may be present (usually <20% of the tumor); if >20% consider PNET
- Little, if any, stroma present

Special Stains

- Presence of cytoplasmic glycogen can be demonstrated by PAS stain with diastase control

Immunohistochemistry

- Tumor cells are positive for MIC2 gene (CD99) product located on the X-Y pairing region (Xp22.32 region of X chromosome); a membranous pattern
- MIC2 positivity also seen in pediatric lymphomas, lymphocytic lymphoma, occasional rhabdomyosarcomas, and rare synovial sarcomas
- Tumor cells also positive for vimentin (80%-90%)
- If neural differentiation present, then NSE will tend to be positive as will other neuromarkers: Leu-7, HNK-1, gliofibrillar acid protein, and S-100 protein
- The presence of neurosecretory granules can be confirmed with chromogranin
- Tumor cells of a Ewing sarcoma positive for TrkB and TrkC receptors; if neural differentiation present (PNET), then tumor cells will express TrkA

Electron Microscopy

- Densely packed, primitive, round to oval mesenchymal cells with fine cytoplasmic processes and little or no stroma
- Abundant glycogen arranged in rosettelike deposits in the cytoplasm
- Biphasic nature of tumor cells with dark cells showing features of apoptosis

Molecular Alterations

- Reciprocal t (11;22)(q24;q12)
- In 10% there is a reciprocal t (21;22)(q22;q12)
- t(7;22); t(17;22); and t(2;22) have all been reported (<1%)

Differential Diagnosis

- Metastatic neuroblastoma
- Small-cell osteosarcoma (no [11;2] translocation)
- Mesenchymal chondrosarcoma
- Rhabdomyosarcoma
- Hematopoietic malignancy

Treatment

- Multidrug chemotherapy and surgery with or without radiation

Prognosis

- 70% survive 5 years with localized, resectable disease treated with chemotherapy and surgery
- 30% survive 5 years with disseminated disease
- Younger patients (<10 years of age) tend to do better than older patients
- Resectable lesions in the appendicular skeleton do better than those with a disease in the axial skeleton
- Patients with a larger tumor volume (>100 mm) do worse than patients with smaller neoplasms
- Extensive necrosis, increased numbers of apoptotic (dark) cells, and increased numbers of mitotic figures are all associated with a poor prognosis
- Prognosis very dependent upon response to chemotherapy:
    - 90% 5-year survival with complete necrosis of tumor
    - 50%-55% 5-year survival with microscopic residual tumor
    - 30%-35% 5-year survival with gross evidence of residual tumor

Associations

- None

Comment

Ewing sarcoma and PNET may represent a single group of bone and soft tissue tumors in which typical undifferentiated Ewing sarcoma and PNET with obvious neural differentiation represent opposite ends of a spectrum

The term Ewing sarcoma is used for tumors that lack evidence of neuroectodermal differentiation by light microscopy, immunohistochemistry, and/or electron microscopy

Primitive Neuroectodermal Tumor (PNET)

Clinical Manifestations

- Occurs less frequently than Ewing sarcoma
- Tend to occur between the ages of 10 and 25 years
- Anatomic distribution same as Ewing sarcoma

Radiographic Features and Gross Pathology

- Same as Ewing sarcoma

Microscopic Pathology

- Tumor cells are small, round, primitive, and mesenchymal and essentially identical to those seen in Ewing sarcoma
- Rosettes of the Homer-Wright type (circular arrangement of cells with fibrillar processes that radiate toward center) should comprise >20% of the neoplasm (*these rosettes are the morphologic evidence of neural differentiation that allow the diagnosis of PNET on microscopic examination*); in actuality the presence of Homer-Wright rosettes making up >20% of the neoplasm is an extremely rare finding

Special Stains

- Glycogen in the cytoplasm can be demonstrated with PAS with diastase (70% of both Ewing sarcomas and PNETs)

Immunohistochemistry

- Tumor cells are positive for MIC2 gene product located on the X-Y pairing region (Xp22.32 region of X chromosome); a membranous pattern
- MIC2 positivity also seen in pediatric lymphomas, lymphocytic lymphoma, occasional rhabdomyosarcomas, and rarely synovial sarcomas
- 80% to 90% of tumor cells positive for vimentin
- If neural differentiation present, then NSE will tend to be positive as will other neuromarkers: Leu-7, HNK-1, gliofibrillar acid protein, and S-100 protein
- The presence of neurosecretory granules can be confirmed with chromogranin
- Tumor cells of a Ewing sarcoma positive for TrkB and TrkC receptors; if neural differentiation present (PNET), tumor cells will express TrkA

Electron Microscopy

- Diagnosis of PNET dependent upon the identification of neural differentiation (may be focal), which is characterized by neurosecretory granules and cytoplasmic projections
- Well-differentiated cells often contain filaments or neurotubules (both features of neuritic differentiation)

Molecular Alterations

- Reciprocal t(11;22)(q24;q12)

Differential Diagnosis

- Metastatic neuroblastoma
- Small cell osteosarcoma (no [11;22] translocation)
- Mesenchymal chondrosarcoma
- Rhabdomyosarcoma
- Hematopoietic malignancy

Treatment

- Multidrug chemotherapy and surgery with or without radiation

Prognosis

- Worse than for Ewing sarcoma (Ewing sarcomas tend to be more localized than PNETs)

Associations

- None

Comment

PNET and Ewing sarcoma are most likely related tumors within a continuous spectrum of prominent (PNET) to minimal (Ewing) neural differentiation

The term *PNET* is used for tumors that demonstrate neuroectodermal features on light microscopy, immunohistochemistry, and/or electron microscopy

Osteosarcoma

Conventional (Intramedullary) Osteosarcoma

Clinical Manifestations

- Most common primary malignant neoplasm of bone
- A bimodal age distribution (10 to 20 years and after 50 years); 60% in patients <25 years
- Males more commonly affected than females
- Metaphysis of the distal femur most common site, followed by proximal tibia; metaphysis and diaphysis of the proximal humerus is the 3rd most frequent site
- In patients over the age of 50 years, the axial skeleton and flat bones are more frequently affected
- Most common presenting symptom is pain followed by swelling and limitation of range of motion
- Overlying skin frequently feels warm and has a prominent vasculature
- Serum levels of alkaline phosphatase and lactic acid dehydrogenase frequently elevated

Radiographic Findings

- Tumor may be either completely sclerotic or lytic or have any combination of these features
- Mineralization of matrix produces cloudy opacities
- A destructive growth pattern with ill-defined borders
- Focal destruction of the cortex is typically present with extension into adjacent soft tissue
- When tumor grows on the surface of the bone, the periosteum may be elevated forming an open triangle on the diaphyseal side of the lesion (*Codman triangle*)

Gross Pathology

- Typically arises in the metaphysis of a long bone
- Cut surface is heterogeneous in terms of color, consistency, and degree of ossification; may be soft or gritty, depending upon amount of osteoid present; 25% have significance amounts of cartilage
- An invasive/destructive pattern of growth with indistinct margins between neoplasm and bone or neoplasm and soft tissue
- Growth plate rarely penetrated by tumor
- Destruction of articular cartilage with extension into joint space infrequent

Microscopic Pathology

- A very heterogeneous neoplasm
- Two basic components: Sarcomatous tumor cells and extracellular matrix
- Direct production of osteoid by sarcomatous tumor cells required for the diagnosis
- 3 major subtypes based upon matrix component: osteoblastic (50%), chondroblastic (25%), and fibroblastic (25%)
- Malignant tumor cells are typically quite pleomorphic and may be spindled, fusiform, oval, small and round, clear, epithelioid, plasmacytoid, or mono- or multinucleated giant; most cases have a complex mixture of 2 or more of these cell types
- Tumor cells produce osteoid which appears as an eosinophilic glassy substance with irregular contours surrounded by osteoblasts; the amount of osteoid varies from almost none to abundant, and is usually fine and lacelike with variable amounts of mineralization
- Areas of osteoid may be mixed with fibroblastic and/or chondroblastic foci
- Tumor cells typically have marked nuclear atypia and numerous mitoses many of which are atypical
- Neoplastic bone frequently merges with preexisting normal lamellar bone forming a large ossified solid area
- Malignant-appearing tumor cells may be entrapped by osteoid; these cells appear less malignant than the cells that lie outside the osteoid
- When infiltrating tumor destroys or entraps preexisting normal bone, the neoplasm is referred to as an *osteoblastomalike variant*
- Cartilaginous differentiation may be present and may be quite extensive, but osteoid production will always be present; cartilage appears malignant with spindling at the periphery of lobules of cartilage (*chondroblastic variant)*
- Fibroblastic differentiation may occur and resemble a fibrosarcoma or malignant fibrous histiocytoma although the spindled tumor cells are quite pleomorphic and mitotically active; the osteoid formation may be quite inconspicuous (*fibroblastic variant*)
- A *small-cell variant* consists of undifferentiated small cells that are easily confused with lymphoma or Ewing sarcoma; osteoid production may be difficult to identify
- Some tumors have large numbers of osteoclastlike giant cells admixed with pleomorphic (but occasionally banal) spindle cells; osteoid formation may be very inconspicuous *(giant cell-rich variant)*

Special Stains

- Not helpful

Immunohistochemistry

- Tumor cells typically positive for vimentin
- Areas of cartilaginous differentiation stain positively for S-100
- Focal areas of positivity for keratin, EMA, smooth muscle actin, and desmin usually present

Electron Microscopy

- Tumor cells are pleomorphic, undifferentiated, and mesenchymal; they have eccentric nuclei, abundant and dilated rough endoplasmic reticulum, and prominent Golgi centers
- Intracytoplasmic lipid may be present
- Osteoid is composed of collagen with deposits of calcium hydroxyapatite crystals

Molecular Alterations

- Chromosomal rearrangements tend to occur in 1p, 1q, 3p, 3q, 11p, 17p, and 22q
- Loss of chromosomes 3, 10, 12, and 15
- Mutations of the retinoblastoma (*Rb*) gene on chromosome 13 frequently present
- Alteration of *p53* is frequent (also a feature of the Li-Fraumeni syndrome); tumors with altered p53 tend to be aggressive and likely to metastasize

Differential Diagnosis

- Fracture callus
- Acute suppurative osteomyelitis
- Osteoblastoma and aggressive osteoblastoma
- Chondrosarcoma
- Fibrosarcoma and malignant fibrous histiocytoma
- Giant cell tumor of bone
- Ewing sarcoma, peripheral neuroectodermal tumor, and lymphoma
- Metastatic carcinoma (osteosarcoma with epithelioid cells arranged in a nesting pattern may mimic renal cell carcinoma)

Treatment

- Neoadjuvant multimodality chemotherapy with or without irradiation (50% of patients have a substantial reduction of tumor mass) followed by limb-sparing surgical excision and postoperative chemotherapy determined by the extent of tumor necrosis. The greater the amount of necrosis the better the prognosis (**T2.2**)

T2.2
Histologic Grading Based on Chemotherapeutic Effect

Grade I	No or minimal tumor response
Grade II	Extensive necrosis with >10% of viable tumor
Grade III	Extensive necrosis with scattered foci of viable tumor (<10%)
Grade IV	Complete necrosis

Prognosis

- 5-year survival 90% if >90% of the tumor is necrotic at the time of surgery
- 5-year survival 15% if <90% of the tumor is necrotic at the time of surgery
- If neoplasm is treated with surgical excision alone, the rate of metastasis will exceed 80% (most common sites lungs and liver)
- Surgical excision of metastasis may prolong life
- Survival better for tumors involving the appendicular skeleton than the axial skeleton

Associations

- May arise in the setting of Paget disease (most common precursor lesion to give rise to osteosarcoma), postradiation, bone infarct, fibrous dysplasia, metallic implant, and chronic osteomyelitis
- May have an inherited familial incidence associated with retinoblastomas (alterations in a specific locus of chromosome 13)
- *Li-Fraumeni syndrome*: Increased incidence of osteosarcoma and other tumors (breast cancer, soft tissue sarcomas, leukemia, brain tumors, and adrenal cortical carcinoma) in kindreds with a germ cell mutation of the tumor suppressor gene *p53*

- *Rothmund-Thompson syndrome* (congenital poikiloderma): Increased incidence of squamous cell carcinoma of the skin and osteosarcoma (may be multicentric) in patients with erythematous and maculopapular skin lesions with areas of hyperpigmentation, cataracts, photosensitivity, hypogonadism, psychomotor retardation, and various skeletal abnormalities
- Multifocal osteosarcoma (synchronous [childhood 5 to 15 years] and metachronous [adults])

Intracortical Osteosarcoma

Clinical Manifestations

- Fewer than 10 cases have been described
- Occurs between the 2nd and 3rd decades of life
- More common in males than females
- Presents with pain, tenderness, and swelling of <1 year duration
- Occur in tibial diaphysis and femoral shaft

Radiographic Features

- An intracortical lytic defect with an irregular margin and surrounding sclerosis
- No evidence of intramedullary or soft tissue involvement
- Little or no periosteal reactive changes

Gross Pathology

- Cortex is expanded and thickened by a well-demarcated neoplasm with irregular borders; cut section gray to tan and gritty

Microscopic Pathology

- A very high-grade osteoblastic lesion with extensive bone formation
- At the periphery invasion characterized by remnants of cortical bone surrounded by anaplastic cells
- Cartilage formation is rare

Differential Diagnosis

- Osteoid osteoma
- Osteoblastoma
- Fibrous dysplasia
- Nonossifying fibroma
- Adamantinoma of long bones

Treatment and Prognosis

- Surgical excision associated with excellent prognosis
- Curettage and/or irradiation likely to result in recurrence

Parosteal (Juxtacortical) Osteosarcoma

Clinical Manifestations

- Represents 4% of all osteosarcomas
- Peak incidence in 3rd and 4th decades
- More commonly affects females than males
- 70% located on the posterior aspect of the distal femur within the region of the superior popliteal space; also occur on proximal tibia and proximal humerus
- Typically presents as a slow growing, painless, firm, fixed mass with inability to flex knee

Radiographic Features

- Neoplasm grows on the surface of bone as an exophytic mass that does not raise the periosteum or stimulate the growth of new periosteal bone; attached by a broad base to the underlying cortex; tends to wrap around involved bone
- Usually lobulated and densely mineralized

Gross Pathology

- A sharply demarcated, exophytic/polypoid bony mass attached by a broad base to the external surface of cortex of a long bone
- Surfaces lobulated with overhanging edges
- Satellite nodules may be found (usually a feature of recurrence)
- Periphery of neoplasm typically softer (may be cartilage) than base, which tends to be heavily ossified
- Cut surface tan to white with foci of soft, fleshly tissue and hyaline cartilage

Microscopic Pathology

- A banal, hypocellular, fibroblastic spindle cell population mixed with well-developed bony trabeculae
- Tumor cells usually lack atypia; mitotic figures rare (no atypical mitotic figures)
- Cartilage may be found both within tumor and at periphery; chondrocytes usually atypical
- At the base, erosion through underlying cortex into the medullary cavity present in 25%

- Foci of high-grade neoplasm may be present (15%) and resemble malignant fibrous histiocytoma (usually a feature of a recurrence)

Electron Microscopy

- Fibroblastlike tumor cells surrounded by dense bundles of collagen

Differential Diagnosis

- Reactive lesions: Posttraumatic periostitis, florid reactive periostitis, juxtacortical myositis ossificans, and postavulsive lesions (ie, cortical irregularity syndrome)
- Periosteal osteosarcoma
- Convential (intramedullary) low-grade osteosarcoma
- Sessile osteocartilaginous exostoses
- Fibromatosis and fasciitis

Treatment and Prognosis

- Radical surgical excision
- High-grade and dedifferentiated lesions are treated with chemotherapy in addition to excisional surgery
- 85%-90% 5-year survival
- Dedifferentiation associated with metastases and a prognosis similar to conventional osteosarcoma

Associations

- Previous radiation exposure

Periosteal Osteosarcoma

Clinical Manifestations

- 2% of all osteosarcomas
- Slightly more common in males than females
- Almost all involve the diaphysis of the femur or tibia; tends to affect anterior, lateral, or medial portion of shaft
- Tend to occur between the ages of 15 and 40 years
- Typically presents with extremity swelling with or without pain

Radiographic Features

- A lucent fusiform lesion on the surface of a long bone with nonhomogeneous, calcified speculations disposed perpendicular to the cortex ("sunburst" appearance)
- Periosteum is elevated with prominent periosteal new bone formation
- Codman triangle frequently present

Gross Pathology

- Neoplasm arises beneath and elevates the periosteum and stimulates prominent periosteal new bone formation
- Advancing margin well delineated by a capsule or pseudocapsule
- On cut section, a lobular architecture with grossly visible cartilage
- Spicules of bone traverse the tumor centrally and run perpendicular to the area where the tumor attaches to the cortex
- A solid ossified mass is usually seen adjacent to and blending in with the underlying cortex

Microscopic Pathology

- Prominent features of cartilage differentiation (predominantly a chondroblastic tumor with the appearance of a moderately differentiated chondroblastic osteosarcoma)
- Poorly demarcated lobules of cartilage separated by bands of primitive sarcomatous tumor cells; cartilaginous component has cytologic atypia and areas of calcification
- Tumor osteoid and immature bone production found in the areas of sarcomatous cells
- Ossified mass of mature bone usually found arising from the cortex, to which it is intimately attached; the periphery tends to be uncalcified or minimally calcified
- Perpendicular spicules of reactive bone with prominent osteoblastic rimming traverse the tumor centrally and become coarser at the base where the neoplasm attaches to the cortex (accounts for the perpendicular spicules seen radiographically)

Differential Diagnosis

- Parosteal osteosarcoma
- High-grade surface osteosarcoma
- Conventional intramedullary osteosarcoma
- Juxtacortical chondrosarcoma
- Periosteal chondroma

Treatment and Prognosis

- Radical surgical excision and amputation

- No data concerning role of chemotherapy
- 25% dead of metastasis within 3 years, but overall prognosis generally favorable

Telangiectatic Osteosarcoma

Clinical Manifestations

- ~ 4% of all osteosarcomas
- Most frequently occurs during 2nd decade
- Slight male predominance
- Typically occur in metaphyseal region of long bones; 50% located in the region of the knee (metaphysis of distal femur most common site)
- Pain, swelling, and limitation of range of motion
- Alkaline phosphatase level elevated in 30%
- 25% have pathologic fracture

Radiographic Features

- Usually a purely lytic lesion with a destructive growth pattern without distinct surrounding bony sclerosis
- Typically does not have the mixture of blastic and lytic areas characteristic of a conventional osteosarcoma
- Expansile growth pattern with sharply demarcated margins; mimics an aneurysmal bone cyst

Gross Pathology

- On cut surface, hemorrhagic without an identifiable sarcomatous component ("bag of blood")
- A mixture of large cystic and spongy areas
- Often well demarcated, but areas of invasive growth can usually be readily identified
- Cortical erosion and/or complete cortical disruption with soft tissue mass occasionally seen

Microscopic Pathology

- Septa consisting of highly atypical sarcomatous cells form hemorrhagic, cystlike spaces
- Tumor cells very pleomorphic with atypical nuclei and numerous atypical mitotic figures
- Tumor cells usually in direct contact with areas of hemorrhage
- Benign and malignant-appearing sarcomatous giant cells may be present
- Osteoid production is typically minimal and focal and may be hard to find without extensive sampling

Special Stains

- Not helpful

Immunohistochemistry

- Tumor cells positive for vimentin

Electron Microscopy

- Undifferentiated pleomorphic sarcomatous cells

Differential Diagnosis

- Aneurysmal bone cyst (distinction based on presence of highly malignant cells in septa)
- Conventional osteosarcoma with telangiectatic features
- Benign or malignant giant cell tumor

Treatment and Prognosis

- Typically has a better response to chemotherapy than conventional osteosarcoma

Well-Differentiated Intramedullary Osteosarcoma

Clinical Manifestations

- Represents 1% of all osteosarcomas
- Typically involves the metaphysis of long bones (distal femur and proximal tibia) in individuals between the ages of 25 and 45 years
- 50% occur in the femur
- Both sexes affected equally
- Presenting complaint usually pain and a palpable mass
- Pathologic fracture rare

Radiographic Features

- Lytic foci intermixed with poorly demarcated patches of "cloudlike" density
- Periosteal new bone formation rare
- Involvement of subarticular bony endplate at a joint may occur
- Typically the bone is expanded rather than invaded; 50% have adjacent soft tissue mass
- Codman triangles rarely seen

Gross Pathology

- Typically located in the center of the medullary cavity of the metaphysis and diaphysis of a long bone
- Cut surface is gray with fibrous and osseous (gritty) features
- Neoplasm tends to fuse with inner surface of the cortex; cortical disruption with or without soft tissue mass may be present

Microscopic Pathology

- Generally hypocellular, fibroblastic stroma with abundant collagen and variable amounts of osteoid
- Spindled tumor cells and their osseous component are well differentiated and have a bland appearance that simulates benign fibrous dysplasia; tend to be plump with elongated nuclei and prominent nucleoli, have little pleomorphism, and are rarely atypical; mitotic figures rare but almost always present
- At the periphery a peritrabecular, invasive growth pattern may be seen
- Occasionally (15% to 20%), dedifferentiation occurs resulting in focal areas of high-grade pleomorphic osteosarcoma within an otherwise low-grade lesion (usually a feature of tumor recurrence)

Differential Diagnosis

- Conventional osteosarcoma
- Fibrous dysplasia
- Fibrosarcoma
- Malignant fibrous histiocytoma
- Leiomyosarcoma

Treatment and Prognosis

- Wide excision or amputation
- Chemotherapy is reserved for neoplasms that have areas of dedifferentiation
- Incomplete excision typically results in recurrence with an increased likelihood that dedifferentiation will occur
- 15% incidence of metastasis (usually lungs)

Synovial Lesions

Pigmented Villonodular Synovitis (Giant Cell Tumor, Diffuse Type)

Clinical Manifestations

- Patients usually present with pain and swelling in a joint with some limited range of motion
- Hemorrhagic joint effusion usually present
- Symptoms may be intermittent but are generally progressive
- Typically affects adults between the ages of 25 and 45 years
- Intraarticular disease usually involves knees (80%), hips (15%), ankles, elbows, and shoulder; extraarticular tumors typically involve the knee region, thigh, and foot and tend to be located in periarticular soft tissues
- Intra- and extraarticular disease may coexist in same patient, with the latter being a soft tissue extension of the former

Radiographic Features

- An ill-defined periarticular soft tissue mass
- Findings of degenerative joint disease (multiple subchondral cysts) typically present
- Bone erosion frequently present

Variants

- *Intraarticular*
  - Diffuse involvement of joint synovium
  - Localized (polypoid or nodular) synovial lesion
- *Extraarticular*
  - Diffuse: Multifocal involvement of extraarticular synovial membrane (tendons)
  - Nodular: Localized extraarticular nodular lesion (aka "giant cell tumor of tendon sheath")

Gross Pathology

- *Diffuse intraarticular variant* characterized by synovium covered with variably sized, tan to brown, papillary or nodular lesions; joint capsule is thick; on sectioning, deposits of hemosiderin and lipid deposits are evident (brown and light yellow); articular cartilage and adjacent bone may be eroded

- *Localized intraarticular variant* characterized by a discrete, frequently necrotic, nodule attached to the synovial membrane by a stalk (resembles a polyp) that protrudes into the joint space
- Extraarticular diffuse and nodular variants similar in appearance to intraarticular form, but usually with a nodular architecture rather than villous

Microscopic Pathology

- An infiltrative lesion growing in expansile sheets with variable cellularity; cleftlike spaces common and appear as artifactual tears or as synovial-lined spaces
- Variable numbers of mononuclear histiocytic cells admixed with larger cells; histiocytelike cells are ovoid or spindle-shaped with pale, eosinophilic cytoplasm, and small ovoid, grooved nuclei; larger cells are rounded with abundant cytoplasm, hemosiderin granules and lobulated nuclei with prominent nuclear membranes
- Hemosiderin deposits prominent
- Foamy histiocytes present individually and in clusters or sheets
- Osteoclastic giant cells less common than in localized form and may be completely absent
- A thickened layer of synovial cells covers the nodules and merges with the underlying cellular infiltrate
- Mitotic figures are frequent but never atypical

Special Stains

- Not helpful

Immunohistochemistry

- Histiocytes and multinucleated cells positive for KP-1 (CD68) and other macrophage markers
- Cellular infiltrates negative for both cytokeratin and epithelial membrane antigen (EMA)

Electron Microscopy

- Confirms histiocytic nature of the mononuclear cells as well as the multinucleated giant cells

Molecular Alterations

- Trisomy 5 and 7

Differential Diagnosis

- Reactive inflammatory conditions:
  - Rheumatoid arthritis
  - Osteoarthritis
  - Posttraumatic reactive synovitis
  - Hemarthrosis associated with hemophilia
- Extraarticular nodular variant may resemble epithelioid sarcoma

Treatment

- Excision of the affected synovium
- Occasionally excision of the synovium and adjacent bone require prosthetic joint replacement
- Aggressive cases can be treated with low-dose radiation

Prognosis

- A locally aggressive disease with frequent recurrences (30%)
- Erosion of adjacent joint often results in compromise of joint function
- Transformation to a spindle cell malignancy has been reported

Associations

- Degenerative joint disease (see above)
- May coexist with synovial chondromatosis

Synovial Chondromatosis

Clinical Manifestations

- Males affected twice as often as females
- Peak incidence 5th decade
- Preferentially involves major weight bearing joints (knee and hip) and elbow
- 70% involve area around knee
- 10% bilateral
- Symptoms include long history of pain, swelling, and limitation of motion
- Rarely presents as painless periarticular soft tissue mass

Variants

- *Primary synovial chondrometaplasia:*
  - De novo formation of cartilage nodules in the synovial membrane; as nodules mature they calcify and detach and eventually fill the joint cavity

- Usually only involve a single joint; knee most frequent
- Chondrocytes in these nodules typically arranged in clones and often show cytologic atypia

- *Secondary synovial chondrometaplasia:*
  - Stimulated by preexisting joint disease
  - Detached portions of subchondral bone or degenerated articular cartilage become embedded in synovial membrane and stimulate cartilage metaplasia
  - Microscopically a nidus of cartilage surrounded by concentric rings of metaplastic cartilage; cartilage is cellular but lacks both atypia and clonal arrangement

Radiographic Features

- Multifocal, articular, and/or periarticular nodules with stippled or ringlike calcifications with a central lucency
- Older lesions are more densely calcified
- Bone erosion may be present (not an indication of aggressive behavior)

Gross Pathology

- Synovium is covered with multiple granular nodules of cartilage varying from <0.1 to 2 cm
- Nodules may be loose within the joint space or attached to synovium
- Involvement of synovium can be diffuse or localized

Microscopic Pathology

- Multiple, well-circumscribed nodules of cartilage with hyaline or myxoid change
- Typically cartilage cells are arranged in loose clusters; nuclei have small nucleoli and may show significant atypia and binucleated forms (the atypia may be comparable to that seen in low-grade chondrosarcoma)
- Enchondral ossification of cartilage nodules usually present, and characterized by a well-developed peripheral ring of lamellar bone (lesions with well-developed enchondral ossification are referred to as *osteochondromatosis*)
- A single cartilaginous nodule within a joint capsule is called a *synovial chondroma* (more common in smaller joints)

Special Stains, Immunohistochemistry, and Electron Microscopy

- Not helpful

Molecular Alterations

- None

Differential Diagnosis

- Chondrosarcoma
- Osteocartilaginous loose bodies of osteoarthritis

Treatment

- Synovectomy with removal of the loose nodules of cartilage

Prognosis

- A local, nonneoplastic, self-limited disease
- Recurrence common especially with diffuse involvement of the joint and incomplete synovectomy

Associations

- Chondrosarcomas may develop in a joint capsule involved by synovial chondromatosis; usually diagnosed after multiple recurrences of apparent chondromatosis
- Occasional PVNS concurrently present

Miscellaneous

Adamantinoma of Long Bones

Variants

- Classic
- Differentiated

Clinical Manifestations

- Classic
  - Typically affects individuals over the age of 20 years; rare under age 10 years
  - Usually involves the tibia, fibula, or both; synchronous involvement of both bones occurs in 50%
  - Usually presents as pain and bowing deformity of the tibia
  - Palpable mass may be present
- Differentiated
  - Typically affects individuals under the age of 20 years
  - Exclusively involves tibia and fibula
  - Presents with pain and bowing deformity

Radiographic Features

- Classic
  - May be intracortical or show evidence of cortical disruption with involvement of the medullary cavity and/or adjacent soft tissue
  - 70% are located in the midshaft of the tibia
  - Anterolateral cortex usually involved
  - Typically the lesion represents a mixture of lytic and sclerotic regions or multiple lucencies with well-defined margins and sclerosis of intervening bone
  - A destructive growth pattern is frequently seen
  - Lesions in the fibula typically expand the bone without causing a bowing deformity
- Differentiated
  - Identical to osteofibrous dysplasia with lytic expansion of anterolateral cortex of tibia with a 2nd lytic lesion in proximal or distal fibula

Gross Pathology

- Classic
  - Typically a fleshy soft mass that may be multifocal and involve a large area of the medullary cavity
  - Frequently there is a gradual transition from soft fleshy areas to gritty fibrous areas
  - Complete cortical disruption and involvement of adjacent soft tissue and/or bone may be present
- Differentiated
  - Cortex expanded anteriorly toward medullary cavity by multiple foci of fibrous tissue delineated by a rim of sclerotic cortical bone
  - Cortex is not disrupted and tumor does not extend into medullary cavity and/or adjacent soft tissue

Microscopic Pathology

- Classic
  - Typically small epithelial islands in a dense fibrous or fibro-ossous stroma
  - 5 basic patterns (any combination of patterns may be present):
    - *Basaloid pattern*: Most common; nests or large masses of epithelial cells with a peripheral layer of cells that palisade at right angles to an inner mass of cells; cystlike spaces usually separate outer layer of cells from inner cells; solid areas consist of cells arranged in sheets with parallel, oval nuclei
    - *Spindled pattern*: Spindle cells with elongated nuclei that resemble a fibrosarcoma; no peripheral palisading of cells
    - *Tubular pattern*: Small, flat, or cuboidal cells line small open spaces embedded in a fibrous stroma; may resemble vascular channels or adenocarcinoma
    - *Squamoid pattern*: Areas with obvious squamoid differentiation embedded in a background of nonsquamoid cells
    - *Osteofibrous dysplasialike pattern*: Loose bundles of fibroblastlike cells usually in a storiform pattern with trabeculae of bone rimmed by osteoblasts; small nests of epithelial cells lie within the fibroblastic stroma and often have squamoid differentiation; immature woven bone in center with mature lamellar bone at periphery; foci of this pattern seen in all classic adamantinomas
- Differentiated
  - Fascicles of spindled cells with a storiform pattern and a fibroblast morphology with trabeculae of bone with prominent osteoblastic rimming; zonal maturation from central woven bone to peripheral lamellar bone present (very similar to osteofibrous dysplasia); small nests of epithelial cells may be present centrally in the fibrous stroma

Special Stains

- Not helpful

Immunohistochemistry

- Tumor cells of the basaloid, spindle, tubular, and squamoid patterns are strongly positive for keratin as are the nests of epithelial cells and tubular structures seen in the osteofibrous dysplasialike pattern
- Tumor cells strongly positive for vimentin
- Negative staining for factor VIII, *Ulex europaeus*, actin, and S-100 protein

Electron Microscopy

- Epithelial nature of tumor cells confirmed by the presence of prominent desmosomes, tubular structures, and features of keratinization

Molecular Alterations

- Translocation involving *13q14* has been reported
- Multiple complex chromosomal abnormalities with multiple translocations and extra chromosomes

Differential Diagnosis

- Epithelial elements in basaloid, tubular, and squamoid variants raise the possibility of metastatic carcinoma or adenocarcinoma
- Spindle cell or small tubular variant may be confused with fibrosarcoma or vascular neoplasm (hemangioendothelioma) respectively
- Fibrous dysplasia
- Osteofibrous dysplasia (ossifying fibroma)

Treatment

- En bloc excision or amputation; lymph nodes removed if clinically positive

Prognosis

- Most have an indolent course
- Cure rate ~90%
- Metastasis typically occur late by either hematogenous or lymphatic routes (20%)
- Recurrence rate as high as 30%; recurrence associated with an increase in epithelial-to-stroma ratio and more aggressive behavior

Associations

- See Osteofibrous Dysplasia

Comment

There may be a relationship between adamantinoma and osteofibrous dysplasia of long bones; adamantinomas with a microscopic appearance predominantly of osteofibrous dysplasia and an inconspicuous component of epithelial elements may represent a special variant of adamantinoma characterized by exclusive, often multicentric, involvement of the cortex of the tibia with frequent synchronous involvement of the ipsilateral fibula

Adamantinomata may represent a continuum of neoplasms with classic adamantinoma at one end, osteofibrous dysplasia at the other end, and differentiated adamantinoma somewhere in the middle

Chordoma

Clinical Manifestations

- Represents 3% to 4% of all primary malignant bone tumors and is 4th most common primary malignant bone tumor (following osteosarcoma, chondrosarcoma, and Ewing sarcoma)
- Most frequently arises in the sacrococcygeal (50%) and sphenooccipital regions (30%); remainder in cervical and lumbar spine (20%)
- Affects males and females equally
- Peak incidence in the 5th to 6th decades
- Occasionally seen in children during the first 2 decades of life (often involves the 2nd cervical vertebra in this age group)
- Almost never seen in black patients
- Pain is a common symptom
- Sacrococcygeal lesions may compress nerves or obstruct the rectum
- Sphenooccipital lesions may produce symptoms from impingement on the optic nerves or pituitary gland
- Cervical lesions may present as a pharyngeal mass

Radiographic Features

- Typically a lytic lesion with scattered intralesional calcifications
- Sphenooccipital lesion may destroy clivus, sella turcica, or both; sacrococcygeal lesions expand native bone

Gross Pathology

- Typically soft, gray or tan and multilobulated with a myxoid or gelatinous texture
- Foci of hemorrhage, necrosis, and cystic change common

Microscopic Pathology

- Resembles normal notochord tissue in different stages of development
- A lobular pattern with lobules surrounded by fibrous septa which contain numerous, thin-walled, and often gaping vessels
- Cells are arranged in anastomosing chords, nests, and/or solid areas separated by variable amounts of mucoid intracellular stroma

- Tumor cells tend to be large with vacuolated cytoplasm and prominent vesicular nuclei (*physaliphorous cells*) with distinct nucleolus; the classic physaliphorous (from Greek "physallis" = bubble) cell has a centrally positioned nucleus that is surrounded by a small rim of cytoplasm, which in turn is surrounded by cytoplasmic vacuole(s)
- Physaliphorous cells are not always present and occasionally completely absent
- Mitotic figures are rare
- Some neoplasms have a sarcomalike appearance with spindled, atypical nuclei; others can be densely cellular and eosinophilic without cytoplasmic vacuoles and resemble epithelial neoplasms
- Cartilaginous differentiation may be present (neoplasms with extensive cartilaginous differentiation are occasionally referred to as *chondroid chordoma*)

Special Stains

- Physaliphorous cells contain a glycoprotein that stains with PAS and is diastase sensitive

Immunohistochemistry

- Tumor cells coexpress S-100 protein and epithelial markers (cytokeratins and EMA)
- Tumor cells may be positive for neurofilaments and carcinoembryonic antigen (CEA)

Electron Microscopy

- Confirms vacuolated nature of the cytoplasm of physaliphorous cells that are connected by desmosome-like junctions
- Patchy areas of glycogen and intermediate filaments usually present

Molecular Alterations

- Frequent abnormalities of chromosome 21, specifically the loss or structural rearrangement of 21q22

Differential Diagnosis

- Chondrosarcoma
- Epithelial neoplasm (especially if tumor has highly cellular areas arranged in sheets with marked nuclear atypia)
- Metastatic adenocarcinoma (some adenocarcinomas [as well as chordoma] coexpress S-100 protein and epithelial markers)

Treatment

- Wide en bloc surgical excision
- Lesions that cannot be removed surgically usually treated with adjuvant irradiation therapy

Prognosis

- A locally aggressive neoplasm with a high incidence of recurrence and a high mortality rate
- Mean survival approximately 4 years
- 5-year survival 50-60%; very few survive 10 years
- Metastatic rate averages 40%, but metastasis tend to occur late in the course of the disease (most common sites are skin, bone, and lungs)

Variants

- Chondroid chordoma
  - □ More frequent in the spheno-occipital region
  - □ Prognosis better than conventional chordoma
  - □ Features in common with both chordoma and chondrosarcoma
  - □ Contains a mixture of chondroid and cartilaginous elements
  - □ The importance of this tumor is the difficulty in differentiating it from a chondrosarcoma
- Dedifferentiated chordoma
  - □ More frequent in the sacrococcygeal region
  - □ A biphasic neoplasm with high-grade sarcoma (usually has MFH-like features) admixed with more histologically typical chordoma; high-grade sarcoma component usually develops after multiple recurrences of a more typical chordoma

Associations

- None

Langerhans Cell Histiocytosis

Clinicopathologic Variants:

- *Unifocal Langerhans cell histiocytosis* (eosinophilic granuloma)
- *Multifocal Langerhans cell histiocytosis* (Hand-Schüller-Christian disease)
- *Acute disseminated Langerhans cell histiocytosis* (Letterer-Siwe disease)

Clinical Manifestations

- *Unifocal Langerhans cell histiocytosis (eosinophilic granuloma)*
  - Most common variety of Langerhans cell histiocytosis
  - Typically affects children and young adults (80% <30 years; 50% <10 years)
  - More common in males than females (2:1)
  - Typically involves a single focus of 1 bone (hands and feet are *never* involved)
  - Most common sites are cranial vault, jaw, humerus, rib (most common site in an adult), and femur; also found in skin, lungs, and stomach
  - X-ray typically reveals a lytic lesion in the metaphyseal region of a long bone
  - With a fracture, the neoplastic process can extend into adjacent soft tissue
  - 5%-10% have fever, malaise, and peripheral eosinophilia
- *Multifocal Langerhans cell histiocytosis (Hand-Schüller-Christian disease)*
  - Primarily affects children <3 years
  - Patients present with fever, diffuse cutaneous eruptions particularly on the scalp and in the ear canals, frequent and recurrent bouts of otitis media, mastoiditis, and upper respiratory tract infections; clinical course long and characterized by alternating episodes of regression and recrudescence
  - Mild lymphadenopathy, hepatomegaly, and splenomegaly not uncommon clinical features
  - 50% of patients have a diabetes insipidus (secondary to involvement of the posterior lobe of the pituitary)
- *Acute disseminated Langerhans cell histiocytosis (Letterer-Siwe syndrome)*
  - Typically affects infants and children <2 years
  - Classically presents with fever and infection (otitis media or mastoiditis) followed by a diffuse micropapular eczematous or purpuric skin rash with splenomegaly, hepatomegaly, and massive lymphadenopathy (both above and below the diaphragm)
  - Most experience severe lung disease characterized by respiratory compromise secondary to fibrosis
  - Laboratory studies typically reveal the presence of anemia, thrombocytopenia, and leukopenia (all secondary to neoplastic replacement of bone marrow); peripheral monocytosis (>20% of differential count)

Radiolographic Features

- Early lesions appear aggressive
- Typically a purely lytic, well-demarcated lesion with thick periosteal bone formation

Staging System for Langerhans Cell Histiocytosis

- Stage I:
  - A single monostotic bone lesion
  - Multiple lesions in 1 bone or multiple bones
- Stage II:
  - Age ≥24 months at diagnosis with ≥1 of the following findings: diabetes insipidus, lymphadenopathy, involvement of the skin, seborrhea at any site, mild lung involvement (infiltrate on chest x-ray without pulmonary symptoms), and/or focal involvement of bone marrow
- Stage III:
  - Age <24 months at diagnosis with any of the symptoms seen in stage II, or
  - Age ≥24 months with involvement of liver and/or spleen, massive nodal involvement (several sites above and below the diaphragm), honeycomb lung (major lung involvement with fibrosis), extensive diffuse bone marrow involvement
- Stage IV:
  - Spleen palpable ≥6 cm below the costal margin and fever for more than a month with or without any or all of the aforementioned sites involved
- Stage V:
  - Monocytosis in peripheral blood (>20% of differential cell count), in combination with stage III or stage IV findings

Gross Pathology

- Affected bone has a sharply demarcated gray to tan lytic focus usually with cortical disruption
- Occasionally foci of tan or yellow tissue with fibrosis may be present indicating that the lesion may be undergoing some regression

Miscellaneous>Langerhans Cell Histiocytosis

Microscopic Pathology

- Eosinophilic granuloma, multifocal Langerhans cell histiocytosis, and acute disseminated Langerhans histiocytosis all have identical microscopic features
- Tumor cells represent proliferating Langerhans cells that are normally present within the epidermis and are related to the mononuclear phagocyte system
- Typical lesion composed of 2 basic cell types; eosinophils and Langerhans cells (proportion of each, especially the eosinophils, may vary greatly from lesion to lesion)
- Langerhans cells typically have oval nuclei and abundant well-demarcated, eosinophilic or clear cytoplasm; most nuclei have prominent nuclear grooves that run parallel to the long axis of the nucleus giving it a "coffee bean shape"
- Occasional nuclei have round or oval nucleoli
- Nuclear atypia and mitotic activity both characteristically low; atypical mitosis never present
- Occasional multinucleated giant cells present and have nuclear features of either Langerhans cells or ordinary osteoclasts
- Ordinary histiocytes may also be present and can be distinguished from Langerhans cells by their high phagocytic activity and the absence of nuclear grooves; may appear as foam cells and contain Charcot-Leyden crystals (fragments of degenerated eosinophils)
- Eosinophils may be quite prevalent throughout the lesion and may actually form aggregates with areas of necrosis (eosinophilic abscess)
- Other inflammatory cells to include lymphocytes and plasma cells may be present
- Lesions that are undergoing regression are typically associated with fibrosis and an increase in foamy histiocytes (may be reminiscent of nonossifying fibroma or chronic osteomyelitis)
- Bone adjacent to the lesion may show prominent resorptive osteoclastic activity

Special Stains

- Not helpful

Immunohistochemistry

- Histiocytes are strongly positive for both S-100 protein and CD1a and negative for CD45

Electron Microscopy

- Langerhans cells have nuclei with prominent indentations, long cytoplasmic processes, few lysosomes and *Birbeck granules* (a pentalaminar, rodlike, tubular structure, with characteristic periodicity and sometimes a dilated terminal end that resembles a tennis-racket)

Molecular Alterations

- None

Differential Diagnosis

- Osteomyelitis
- Granulomatosis inflammation
- Hodgkin disease and non-Hodgkin lymphoma

Treatment

- Both unifocal and multifocal lesions can be cured by curettage of the bony lesions, or low-dose radiation and steroid therapy, or both
- Acute disseminated Langerhans cell histiocytosis requires intensive chemotherapy

Prognosis

- Unifocal Langerhans cell histiocytosis may heal spontaneously
- Both unifocal and multifocal Langerhans cell histiocytosis carry a good prognosis and are essentially curable diseases, but occasionally progress to a systemic disease (a phenomenon that occurs almost exclusively in children during the first 2 years of life)
- Acute disseminated disease is rapidly fatal if not treated; 50% 5-year survival with chemotherapy
- Stage of disease is single most important prognostic factor followed by the number of organs involved and their functional compromise

Associations

- Multifocal Langerhans cell histiocytosis (Hand-Schüller-Christian disease) may have *Christian triad* of lytic skull lesions, exophthalmos, and diabetes insipidus

References

Dabbs DJ. *Diagnostic Immunohistochemistry.* New York: Churchill Livingstone, 2002.

Dorfman D, Czerniak B. *Bone Tumors.* St. Louis: Mosby Inc, 1998.

Fletcher CDM, Unni KK, Mertens F (eds). *World Health Organization Classification of Tumours: Pathology and Genetics of Tumours of Soft Tissue and Bone.* Lyon: IARC Press, 2002.

Helliwell TR. *Pathology of Bone and Joint Neoplasms, Volume 37:Major Problems in Pathology.* Philadelphia: WB Saunders Co, 1999.

McCarthy EF. *Bone and Joint Disorders: Differential Diagnosis in Pathology.* New York: Igaku-Shoin, 1996.

Mills S, Carter D, Greenson JK, Oberman HA, Reuter V, Stoler MH (eds). *Sternberg's Diagnostic Surgical Pathology. 4th ed.* Philadelphia: Lippincott Williams & Wilkins, 2004.

Rosai J. *Rosai and Ackerman's Surgical Pathology. 9th ed.* St. Louis: Mosby, 2004.

Weiss SW, Goldblum JR. *Enzinger and Weiss's Soft Tissue Tumors. 4th ed.* St. Louis: Mosby Inc, 2001.

Chapter 20

Soft Tissue

Intraoperative Consultation

With the exception of some superficial benign lesions, intraoperative frozen section is rarely used to make the primary diagnosis on a soft tissue tumor. Sampling is a major problem. Benign soft tissue tumors frequently have features that overlap with intermediate or frankly malignant tumors, while intermediate and malignant tumors often have focally benign features. In addition, malignant tumors frequently have areas of dedifferentiation that can have a major impact on both the final diagnosis and therapeutic options. Occasionally, however, the operating surgeon needs to know if a lesion is obviously malignant, so long-term venous access for chemotherapy can be placed while the patient is under anesthesia.

There are 3 generally accepted reasons to perform an intraoperative consultation on a soft tissue tumor. The most common is to ensure that sufficient viable, lesional tissue is present for permanent section diagnosis. The second is to evaluate the adequacy of surgical margins. Less frequently, tissue is obtained for ancillary studies such as electron microscopy and chromosomal analysis.

A request for an intraoperative consultation to confirm the presence of viable, lesional tissue can be problematic if the section to be frozen is obtained from the periphery of the neoplasm. Frequently soft tissue tumors are encased in a pseudocapsule or are surrounded by reactive tissue. A section of insufficient depth will indicate the presence of abnormal tissue but not necessarily lesional tissue. The distinction may be all but impossible to make on frozen tissue.

Requests for frozen sections to determine the adequacy of resection are the most frequent indication for intraoperative consultation in soft-tissue cases. The pathologist orients the specimen and inks the surgical margins so that when sections are taken, the exact location is always known. At sites where the tumor appears closest to a margin, the exact location is recorded and perpendicular sections into the tumor are taken, frozen, and stained. Frozen sections to assess the adequacy of margins are ideally obtained in the presence of the operating surgeon who can not only assist in orienting the specimen, but who usually has some sense of where the neoplasm may be closest to the margin.

Frozen sections to assess the adequacy of margins can be easily misinterpreted when the neoplasm is of low enough grade to resemble non-neoplastic tissue. Soft-tissue tumors that are most easily confused with normal or reactive tissue include desmoids, low-grade angiosarcomas, low-grade fibrohistiocytomas, well-differentiated fatty lesions and well-differentiated fibrosarcomas. This problem can be compounded when the margin is taken at a site showing the reactive changes of a previous biopsy or resection.

Soft-tissue tumors subjected to intraoperative injury or extensive electrocauterization can also cause problems in determining the status of the surgical margins. The actual margins of a distorted specimen are difficult to ink and consequently difficult to assess. Likewise, cauterization can distort tissue to the point that margins are essentially impossible to assess by either frozen section or permanent section. A surgeon aware of these diagnostic pitfalls can make more informed intraoperative decisions concerning the conduct of the operation and the extensiveness of resection.

Specimen Handling

As mentioned, under frozen section considerations, excised soft tissue neoplasms are carefully oriented and inked. The specimen is serially sectioned in parallel 3 to 4 mm thick sections. After appropriate frozen section analyses are performed and recorded, the entire specimen is fixed in formalin for the time required to obtain complete fixation. Tissue samples are taken for permanent sections from all areas that show any gross variation in morphology. A minimum of 1 section for every centimeter of neoplasm in maximum dimension is customarily submitted. Sections are taken from necrotic, cystic, or hemorrhagic foci, as well as from solid, viable areas of the neoplasm, which should include sections from the margin, and the interface of the neoplasm with surrounding normal tissue.

Extraskeletal Osseous and Cartilaginous Tumors

Extraskeletal Chondrosarcoma

Variants

- Well-differentiated extraskeletal chondrosarcoma
- Extraskeletal myxoid chondrosarcoma
- Extraskeletal mesenchymal chondrosarcoma

Clinical Manifestations

- *Well-differentiated extraskeletal chondrosarcoma*
  - Too few cases to characterize typical clinical manifestations
- *Extraskeletal myxoid chondrosarcoma*
  - Typically a deep-seated slowly growing mass in the deep musculature of adults
  - Median age at onset 50 years
  - Men affected almost twice as frequently as women
  - Extremities (thigh and popliteal space) and limb girdles involved in 70%, followed by trunk, paraspinal region, foot, and head and neck region
- *Extraskeletal mesenchymal chondrosarcoma*
  - Slightly more common in women than men
  - Soft-tissue lesions arising in head and neck region (meningeal and periorbital) tend to occur at an average age of 25 years and cause symptoms of increased intracranial pressure or changes in vision
  - Soft-tissue tumors that involve the deep musculature (thigh) occur at an average age of 45 years and tend to present as a painless slow-growing deep-seated mass

Gross Pathology

- *Extraskeletal myxoid chondrosarcoma*
  - Tends to be well circumscribed and soft to firm with a lobulated or nodular appearance
  - Cut surface usually gelatinous and gray with areas of hemorrhage (may be so extensive that the lesion grossly resembles a hematoma)
- *Extraskeletal mesenchymal chondrosarcoma*
  - Typically a multilobulated well circumscribed mass
  - Sectioning reveals a gray to white fleshly neoplasm with small foci of cartilage, bone, necrosis, and hemorrhage (hemorrhage much less prominent than in myxoid chondrosarcoma)

Microscopic Pathology

- *Well-differentiated extraskeletal chondrosarcoma*
  - Well-circumscribed mass of hypercellular, well-differentiated hyaline cartilage with mild nuclear atypia
  - Binucleated chondrocytes typically present
  - Mitoses rare
  - Calcification may be present
- *Extraskeletal myxoid chondrosarcoma*
  - Neoplasm has a multilobular appearance (a result of fibrous septae) and is well circumscribed (a result of a fibrous capsule)
  - Chondroblasts have eosinophilic cytoplasm, cytoplasmic glycogen, and hyperchromatic nuclei and are arranged in interanastomosing strands with abundant myxoid matrix
  - Mitotic figures, areas of necrosis, and hyaline cartilage may all be present
  - Calcification is rare
  - Secondary changes of hemorrhage, hemosiderin deposition, and fibrosis may be present
  - A cellular variant is composed of large cells with intensely eosinophilic cytoplasm and vesicular nuclei
- *Extraskeletal mesenchymal chondrosarcoma*
  - Relatively uniform, primitive round to spindled cells with scant cytoplasm arranged in a hemangiopericytomalike pattern around sinusoidal vascular spaces admixed with small nodules of cartilage, dense collagen, or bone

Special Stains

- *Well-differentiated extraskeletal chondrosarcoma:* Tumor cells are positive for periodic acid-Schiff (PAS) and are diastase sensitive (intracellular glycogen)
- *Extraskeletal myxoid chondrosarcoma* (chondroitin 4-sulfate, chondroitin 6-sulfate, and keratin sulfate) stains with colloidal iron, Alcian blue, mucicarmine, and toluidine blue
- *Extraskeletal mesenchymal chondrosarcoma:* Absence of intracellular glycogen confirmed by a negative PAS staining

Immunohistochemistry

- *Extraskeletal myxoid chondrosarcoma*
  - Tumor cells stain strongly for vimentin; approximately 50% stain for S-100 (may be both weak and focal)
- *Extraskeletal mesenchymal chondrosarcoma*
  - Cartilaginous portions and isolated cells within the undifferentiated areas are S-100 positive
  - The undifferentiated cells may be positive for neuron-specific enolase (NSE) and Leu-7
  - Desmin, actin, cytokeratin and epithelial membrane antigen (EMA) negative

Electron Microscopy

- *Extraskeletal myxoid chondrosarcoma*
  - Tumor cells have multiple mitochondria, microtubules, glycogen granules, and grooved nuclei
- *Extraskeletal mesenchymal chondrosarcoma*
  - Cells resemble cells of the Ewing sarcoma but without the intracytoplasmic glycogen

Molecular Alterations

- Extraskeletal myxoid chondrosarcoma characterized by a balanced reciprocal translocation between chromosomes 9 and 22 [t(9;22) (q22;q12)]

Differential Diagnosis

- *Well-differentiated extraskeletal chondrosarcoma*
  - Chondroma of soft parts
  - Osteochondroma
  - Benign or malignant mesenchymoma of cartilage
  - Chondrosarcoma arising in an osteochondroma
  - Well-differentiated chondrosarcoma of bone
  - Periosteal osteosarcoma
  - Malignant peripheral nerve sheath tumor (MPNST) with chondroid metaplasia
- *Extraskeletal myxoid chondrosarcoma*
  - Myxoma
  - Myxochondroma of soft parts
  - Parachordoma
  - Chordoma (myxoid variant)
  - Chondromyxoid fibroma with soft tissue extension
  - Lipoma
  - Myxoid liposarcoma
  - Periosteal osteosarcoma
  - Myxopapillary ependymoma
  - Pleomorphic adenoma
  - Chondroid syringoma
- *Extraskeletal mesenchymal chondrosarcoma*
  - Hemangiopericytoma
  - Synovial sarcoma
  - Localized fibrous tumor of pleura/peritoneum
  - Ewing sarcoma
  - Primitive neuroectodermal tumor (peripheral neuroepithelioma; PNET)

Treatment

- Radical local excision with or without adjuvant chemotherapy or radiotherapy

Prognosis

- *Well-differentiated extraskeletal chondrosarcoma*
  - Too little data
- *Extraskeletal myxoid chondrosarcoma*
  - 75% survive 10 years
  - Local recurrence rate 50% to 55% with metastasis in 40% to 45%
  - Local recurrences frequently multiple
  - Survival may be as long as 5 to 15 years even after development of lung metastasis
  - Poor prognostic factors include tumors >10 cm and advanced age
- *Extraskeletal mesenchymal chondrosarcoma*
  - Neoplasm characterized by a rapid clinical course and high incidence of metastasis
  - 50% survive 5 years; 25% survive 10 years
  - Lymph node metastasis more common than in myxoid chondrosarcoma

Associations

- Reports of extraskeletal mesenchymal chondrosarcoma arising after radiotherapy

Extraskeletal Osteosarcoma

Clinical Manifestations

- Typically occurs in adults at about 50 years; rare under age of 40 years
- Men and women probably affected equally
- May arise after irradiation therapy for other malignant neoplasms (ie, Hodgkin disease, carcinoma of the breast, carcinoma of the female genital tract, and retinoblastoma)
- Reported to occur after administration of radioactive thorium dioxide (Thorotrast)
- Typically presents as a deep-seated, fixed mass in the thigh, retroperitoneum, pelvic and shoulder girdles; 30% are painful

Gross Pathology

- Either well circumscribed with obvious pseudocapsule or infiltrative
- Typically firm or hard
- On sectioning, tends to have a white granular surface with multiple foci of necrosis and hemorrhage
- No attachment to bone, but may secondarily involve bone

Microscopic Pathology

- All major subtypes of osteosarcoma that arise in bone may be seen (osteoblastic, fibroblastic, telangiectatic, small cell, and well-differentiated)
- Malignant cells produce osteoid and bone, often with neoplastic cartilage, that may be arranged in lacelike strands or trabeculae throughout the neoplasm
- Pleomorphic, bizarre spindled or polyhedral cells with mitoses (some atypical) usually present
- Benign or malignant multinucleated giant cells may be present as well as osteoclastlike giant cells
- Neoplasm may contain areas that resemble fibrosarcoma or malignant fibrocytic histiocytoma, pleomorphic malignant fibrous histiocytoma, chondrosarcoma (chondroid variant), or Ewing sarcoma (small cell variant)
- Neoplasm may demonstrate a "reverse zoning pattern": osteoid material in the central portion with atypical spindle cells at the periphery (unlike myositis ossificans where the bony elements are located at the periphery)

Special Stains

- Not helpful

Immunohistochemistry

- Tumor cells stain positively for vimentin
- Antibody to osteocalcin positive in 80% to 85%
- 70% express smooth muscle actin, 50% EMA, 25% desmin, 20% S-100 protein, and approximately 10% keratin

Electron Microscopy

- Features indistinguishable from primary osteosarcoma of bone

Molecular Alterations

- None

Differential Diagnosis

- Myositis ossificans
- Synovial sarcoma, epithelioid sarcoma, pleomorphic malignant fibrous histiocytoma, and melanoma with metaplastic bone
- Malignant mesenchymoma
- Chondrosarcoma of bone with ossification
- Parosteal osteosarcoma

Treatment

- Radical surgery, radiotherapy, and pre- or postoperative chemotherapy

Prognosis

- Most die within 2 to 3 years of diagnosis
- Metastases frequently present at the time of initial diagnosis
- Most common metastatic sites: Lung, regional lymph nodes, bone, and soft tissue
- Most important prognostic factor is size of tumor (>5 cm)

Associations

- Prior radiation therapy and Thorotrast (see clinical manifestations earlier in this section)
- Trauma seems to have an etiologic role

Myositis Ossificans

Clinical Manifestations

- Typically occurs in the musculature of young active men between the 2nd and 3rd decades
- Occurrence in children distinctly uncommon
- Most common locations: Flexor muscles of the upper arm (brachialis muscle), quadriceps femoris, adductor muscles of the thigh, gluteal muscles, and soft tissues of the hand
- Tends to be a self-limited lesion
- History of trauma in most cases
- May occur in subcutis (panniculitis ossificans), fascia (fasciitis ossificans) and periosteum of digits (fibro-osseous pseudotumor of digits)

Gross Pathology

- Tends to be well-circumscribed and solitary
- On cross section, soft, white and gelatinous (sometimes hemorrhagic) in the center with a gritty, granular periphery

Microscopic Pathology

- Most characteristic feature is a zonal pattern of cellular maturation with maturation occurring first at the periphery and proceding centrally
- Interior of lesion typically composed of immature highly vascular fibroblastic tissue that resembles nodular fasciitis or granulation tissue; fibroblasts may be mildly pleomorphic and mitotically active
- An intermediate zone (between the center and periphery) contains fibroblasts, osteoblasts, and osteoid arranged in poorly defined trabeculae and separated by ectatic vessels
- Peripheral zone characterized by presence of cartilage, osteoid, and mature lamellar bone; a 4th zone of loose fibrous tissue, that may have myxoid component, separates peripheral bone from surrounding muscle
- Inflammatory cells, fibrin, and multinucleated giant cells may be present
- Surrounding muscle may be atrophic

Special Stains

- Colloidal iron may highlight areas of endochondral calcification
- Osteoblasts contain alkaline phosphatase
- Osteoclastlike giant cells contain acid phosphatase

Immunohistochemistry

- Centrally located fibroblasts and myofibroblasts express vimentin, smooth muscle actin, and desmin
- Peripheral osteoblasts and osteocytes positive for osteocalcin

Electron Microscopy

- Fibroblasts, myofibroblasts, macrophages, and osteoblasts with numerous mitochondria and prominent rough endoplasmic reticulum

Molecular Alterations

- None

Differential Diagnosis

- Extraskeletal osteosarcoma (usually no zoning, but if present, osteoid/bone will be located in center with spindle cells at the periphery)
- Nodular fasciitis
- Proliferative fasciitis and myositis
- Fracture callus
- Fibrosarcoma
- Posttraumatic periostitis

Treatment

- May spontaneously regress
- No need for treatment if diagnosis confirmed (unless symptomatic)

Prognosis

- Excellent
- No confirmed cases of malignant transformation

Associations

- Trauma (see above)

"Fibrohistiocytic" Tumors

Atypical Fibroxanthoma (AFX) (Superficial Malignant Fibrous Histiocytoma)

Clinical Manifestations

- Considered superficial form of pleomorphic MFH (see differential diagnosis later in this section)
- Tends to occur in the head and neck area (actinic damaged skin) of elderly persons; particularly common on the nose, cheek, and ear
- 25% occur on the limbs and trunk of young patients (probably a variant of fibrous histiocytoma)
- Typically a solitary nodule or ulcer that may bleed but otherwise causes little by way of symptoms

Gross Pathology

- Typically a solitary nodule or ulcer <2 cm in diameter (gross appearance not particularly diagnostic)

Microscopic Pathology

- Typically centered in the dermis; may make contact with the epidermis, resulting in some pressure atrophy or ulceration

- Tumor cells vary in size and are predominantly spindled with pleomorphic, bizarre nuclei with malignant features; typically a haphazard or vaguely fascicular or storiform arrangement, cytoplasm may be vacuolated (small droplets of neutral fat) or glassy and eosinophilic
- Mitotic figures are abundant and may be atypical
- Scattered inflammatory cells may be present as well as small foci of osteoid
- Amount of background collagen or myxoid change may be quite variable
- Areas adjacent to the neoplasm may show actinic damage, vascular dilatation, and capillary proliferation
- Necrosis almost never present

Special Stains

- Droplets of neutral fat within occasional tumor cells are PAS-positive and diastase-resistant

Immunohistochemistry

- Occasional Langerhans histiocytes may be present in the lesion and stain positively for S-100 protein
- 50% positive for CD68 (KP1)

Electron Microscopy

- Tumor cells have characteristics of fibroblasts, myofibroblasts, and histiocytes
- No evidence of epithelial differentiation (prominent intercellular junctions, tonofibrils)

Molecular Alterations

- None

Differential Diagnosis

- Spindled carcinoma and melanoma (most problematic)
- Fibrous histiocytoma
- Pleomorphic malignant fibrous histiocytoma (PFMH; a superficially located lesion will typically extensively involves the subcutis, invades fascia and muscle, and contains foci of necrosis and/or evidence of vascular invasion)
- Leiomyosarcoma of the skin

Treatment and Prognosis

- Conservative surgical excision
- If lesion recurs following excision, it should be considered a pleomorphic malignant fibrous histiocytoma

Associations

- Solar radiation (frequently associated with other actinic-related lesions such as BCCA and SCCA)
- May be associated with either occupational or therapeutic irradiation

Dermatofibrosarcoma Protuberans (DFSP)

Clinical Manifestations

- A nodular cutaneous mass that typically presents in early to midadult life (20 to 40 years); rarely seen in children
- Affects men more frequently than women
- 50% occur on the trunk, 20% on the proximal upper and lower extremities (even distribution and rare on distal extremities), and 15% in the region of the head and neck
- Average size at time of excision 4 to 5 cm
- Early lesions are typically raised, firm, and flat with a surrounding area of red to blue discoloration; eventually the lesion may begin to grow rapidly and result in the appearance of a nodule
- Occasionally multiple, small cutaneous nodules may be the presenting finding (usually a feature of recurrence)

Gross Pathology

- Lesion typically consists of a solitary, bulging, gray-white mass lying in the dermis and subcutis
- Overlying skin may be normal, atrophic, and/or ulcerated
- Extension into underlying skeletal muscle is uncommon (with the exception of recurrent lesions and lesions arising in the head and neck region)
- Cut section may reveal presence of translucent or gelatinous areas (myxoid change)
- Hemorrhagic and cystic areas may be seen; necrosis is distinctly uncommon

Microscopic Pathology

- Tumor typically diffusely infiltrates both dermis and subcutis
- Neoplasm may extend to the overlying epidermis or leave an uninvolved zone of dermis just beneath the epidermis (Grenz zone); the overlying epidermis is not hyperplastic as it usually is over a benign fibrous histiocytoma
- Tumor cells bland, uniform, and monomorphic; nuclei vary from elongate and small with dense chromatin to large, round, and vesicular; no significant nuclear pleomorphism; cytoplasm faintly eosinophilic; cell borders indistinct; low to moderate mitotic activity; no abnormal mitoses

- Peripheral and especially superficial margins of the neoplasm characterized by benign-appearing spindle cells admixed with preexisting collagen (very reminiscent of a cutaneous fibrous histiocytoma); in deeper regions the tumor spreads along connective tissue septa and between adnexa or interdigitates with lobules of subcutaneous fat
- Central portion of the neoplasm consists of a uniform population of bland, slender fibroblasts usually arranged in a very distinct storiform pattern; blood vessels often inconspicuous
- Giant cells, xanthoma cells, and inflammatory cells rare or absent
- Focal myxoid areas may be present; myxoid change may obscure the characteristic storiform pattern resulting in a microscopic appearance that resembles a myxoid liposarcoma
- Occasionally focal areas of transformation to a higher grade of sarcoma such as fibrosarcoma or pleomorphic malignant fibrous histiocytoma may be present
- May contain areas indistinguishable from giant cell fibroblastoma or hemangiopericytoma
- *Bednar tumor* (pigmented dermatofibrosarcoma protuberans)
    - Microscopically identical to DFSP, with the exception of the presence of variable numbers of melanin pigment-containing dendritic cells
    - Melanin-containing cells have a bipolar or multipolar morphology as a result of tentaclelike processes that radiate from a central, nucleus-containing area

Special Stains

- Fontana stain and Warthin-Starry (pH 3.2) stain will confirm the presence of melanin in a Bednar tumor

Immunohistochemistry

- Tumor cells usually CD34 positive and S-100 negative; may be smooth muscle actin positive
- Melanin-containing cells of a Bednar tumor positive for S-100 protein and negative for HMB-45 and EMA

Electron Microscopy

- Fibroblastic cells (fusiform cells with organized lamellae of rough endoplasmic reticulum), cells with neuroendocrine differentiation, and cells that resemble histiocytes (cell of origin yet to be determined)
- Both mature and immature melanosomes are present within the dendritic cells of a Bednar tumor

Molecular Alterations

- 75% have a ring chromosome 17 and 22 (same alteration seen in giant cell fibroblastoma)

Differential Diagnosis

- DFSP (typically a DFSP has a more uniform, distinctly storiform pattern, smaller cells, and fewer giant cells and inflammatory cells than either benign fibrous histiocytoma or pleomorphic malignant fibrous histiocytoma)
- Pleomorphic malignant fibrous histiocytoma

Prognosis and Treatment

- A locally aggressive neoplasm that has a 50% recurrence rate
- Treatment consists of wide local excision (the recurrence rate correlates with the completeness of excision; if margin is ≥3 cm, recurrence rate 20%; if margin is ≤2 cm, recurrence rate 40%)
- Local recurrence usually appears in 3 years
- May recur as a giant cell fibroblastoma
- Metastases rare and are associated with tumors that have transformed to fibrosarcomas or pleomorphic malignant fibrous histiocytoma; tend to occur by way of the blood stream and involve lung; lymphatic spread to regional lymph nodes occurs in 25%; a recurrent lesion is much more likely to metastasize than a primary lesion
- Isolated pulmonary metastasis should be excised
- Little role for radiotherapy

Associations

- May be associated with acanthosis nigricans and chronic arsenic exposure
- May rapidly enlarge during pregnancy
- Some develop at sites of previous trauma, especially scars

Fibrous Histiocytoma

Clinical Manifestations

- Usually occurs in the dermis and superficial subcutis of the extremities; occasionally in deeper subcutaneous tissue, deep soft tissue, and rarely in visceral organs
- Typically affects adults between the ages of 20 and 45 years

- Usually solitary; 30% are multiple and may appear metachronously
- Superficial (cutaneous) lesions usually present as a painless, elevated, or pedunculated nodule measuring between a few millimeters to several centimeters in diameter; overlying skin may be red to red-brown and occasionally blue or black; lateral compression of the lesion often produces a central dimple
- Deep lesions centered in subcutaneous tissue or deep structures are less common, and like their superficial counterparts, tend to occur in the extremities and are usually painless

Gross Pathology

- On cut section, tend to be circumscribed, yellow or white (resulting from the presence of lipid), and have focal areas of hemorrhage

Microscopic Pathology

- *Cutaneous lesions* typically characterized by a nodular proliferation of fibroblastic spindle cells arranged in short intersecting fascicles that form a vague storiform or fascicular pattern
- Peripheral margins typically ill-defined and overlying epidermis usually hyperplastic
- Frequently more rounded "histiocytic" cells are seen admixed with the fibroblastic cells
- Multinucleated giant cells of the foreign body or Touton type are usually present and frequently contain lipid and hemosiderin (Touton giant cells are characterized by a "perfect" wreath of nuclei surrounding foamy cytoplasm)
- Both lymphocytes and xanthoma cells often scattered throughout the lesion
- Background stroma usually consists of delicate collagen fibrils that surround individual cells; occasionally extensive hyalinization may be present
- Focal areas of hemorrhagic cystic change commonly present ("aneurysmal" variant)
- Tumor cells generally not very pleomorphic and have little or no mitotic activity; cellular lesions may have some mitotic activity and completely benign lesions may have foci of degenerative change manifest as markedly atypical and pleomorphic nuclei ("monster cells"); the obvious presence of both mitotic activity and pleomorphism suggests malignancy
- *Deep-seated lesions* tend to be well circumscribed and pseudo-encapsulated with a hemangiopericytomalike vascular pattern;they have a more pronounced storiform pattern, fewer xanthoma cells and giant cells, and less cytologic pleomorphism than their cutaneous counterparts; in addition the background stroma tends to be more myxoid or hyalinized

Variants

- *Cellular fibrous histiocytoma*
    - Tends to occur in extremities and head and neck region of young men
    - Characterized by increased cellularity and more fascicular (less storiform) pattern of growth
    - Spindle cells tend to be plump with prominent eosinophilic cytoplasm
    - Inflammatory cells, giant cells, and xanthoma cells are less conspicuous than in the more typical lesion
    - Usually extends into subcutaneous tissue
    - Necrosis present in 10%
    - 25% recur
- *Epithelioid fibrous histiocytoma*
    - Tends to occur as a polypoid red nodule in the lower extremity of adults
    - 50% of tumor cells have an epithelioid shape with abundant eosinophilic cytoplasm and a round to oval vesicular nucleus with a small red to purple nucleolus
    - Multinucleated giant cells are rare; xanthoma cells usually present as well as bi- and trinucleated cells
- *Aneurysmal fibrous histiocytoma*
    - Present as blue to brown nodule on extremity of middle-aged adult
    - Characterized by scattered blood-filled spaces surrounded by discohesive fragments of tumor
    - Hemosiderin-laden macrophages, xanthoma cells, and inflammatory cells all present

Special Stains

- Not helpful

Immunohistochemistry

- Lysosomal and oxidative enzymes typically present (confirm the histiocytic origin of this tumor)
- α_1-antitrypsin present in up to 75%

- A significant number of cells stain positively for factor XIIIa
- Tumor cells typically negative for CD34 (helpful in distinguishing benign fibrous histiocytoma from DFSP; latter is positive for CD34), epithelial markers, desmin, and S-100 protein

Electron Microscopy

- Various cell types ranging from fibroblasts (contain organized lamellae of rough endoplasmic reticulum) to round cells that resemble histiocytes (numerous cell processes, mitochondria, and phagolysosomes)

Molecular Alterations

- Cellular variant associated with chromosomal translocation t(4;17)

Differential Diagnosis

- Nodular fasciitis
- Neurofibroma
- Leiomyoma (especially sclerotic forms)
- DFSP
- pleomorphic malignant fibrous histiocytoma

Treatment and Prognosis

- Local excision; recurrence usually in <5%
- Deep-seated lesions are more likely to recur than cutaneous lesions (probably related to ease of excision)

Associations

- Synchronous lesions are occasionally seen in the setting of immunosuppression

Giant Cell Fibroblastoma (GCF)

Clinical Manifestations

- Typically presents as a painless nodule or mass in the dermis or subcutis of a male child; 65% of patients are under the age of 5 years
- Most commonly occurs in the posterior thigh, inguinal region, and chest wall
- Almost twice as common in males as in females

Gross Pathology

- Typically a poorly circumscribed mass between 1 and 5 cm with a cut surface that is gray to yellow and mucoid

Microscopic Pathology

- Characterized at low power by pseudovascular or gaping spaces that simulate vascular channels and are often lined by multinucleated giant fibroblastlike cells that appear to contain multiple, large, overlapping, vesicular angulated-nuclei with prominent nucleoli and have eosinophilic cytoplasm; these giant cells also scattered throughout solid areas
- Solid areas contain tumor cells that tend to be elongated, wavy, and fibroblastlike and are often arranged in ill-defined, randomly placed fascicles; these cells infiltrate the deep dermis and subcutis and encircle adnexal structures in a pattern reminiscent of DSFP
- Degree of cellularity quite variable
- Stroma may be fibrous to myxoid
- Occasionally storiform foci are present
- Mast cells and lymphocytes almost always present

Special Stains

- Not helpful

Immunohistochemistry

- Tumor cells express vimentin; some express CD34
- Tumor cells negative for S-100 protein and vascular markers

Electron Microscopy

- Overlapping nuclei of the giant fibroblastlike cells that line the pseudovascular spaces are actually multiple lobulations of a single nucleus
- Tumor cells most closely resemble fibroblasts and primitive mesenchymal cells

Molecular Alterations

- Ring chromosome 17 and 22 (same alteration seen in DFSP)

Differential Diagnosis

- Presence of a myxoid matrix may lead to the erroneous diagnosis of myxoma, myxoid lipoblastoma, myxoid liposarcoma, and myxoid fibrosarcoma
- Presence of a fibrous background can lead to the erroneous diagnosis of fibrous histiocytoma

Treatment

- Wide local excision

Prognosis

- Recurrence rate almost 50%
- May recur as a DFSP
- No reports of metastatic disease

Associations

- Lesion closely linked to DFSP and may represent a juvenile analogue of DFSP

Juvenile Xanthogranuloma

Clinical Manifestations

- Usually diagnosed during infancy
- Presents as ≥1 cutaneous nodules: occasionally (5%) occur in deep soft tissue and/or internal organs
- 20% of patients have the lesion(s) at birth; 65% develop the lesion(s) by the age of 6 months; occasionally lesion(s) develop after the age of 20 years
- 50% occur in the region of the head and neck; most of the remainder involve the trunk and extremities; eye is the most common extracutaneous site (symptoms may result from hemorrhage in the anterior chamber and glaucoma); also seen in lung, epicardium, oral cavity, and testis
- After a variable period , lesions regress leaving a slightly depressed and sometimes hyperpigmented (yellow to brown) area of skin
- Lesions that develop after the age of 20 years tend not to regress

Gross Pathology

- Lesions tend to be red papules when they first appear; older lesions are yellow-brown

Microscopic Pathology

- Lesions involving the skin consist of sheets of histiocytes in the dermis that extend to a flattened epidermis (with thin, elongated rete ridges), infiltrate adnexal structures, and extend into the subcutis
- Lesions involving deep soft tissue may appear circumscribed but tend to have infiltrative margins
- Histiocytes that comprise the lesion show no pleomorphism and mitoses are rare; the amount of cytoplasm varies with the amount of lipid, and the amount of lipid is frequently a function of the age of the lesion
- Giant cells of both the Langerhans and Touton type are typically present
- Inflammatory cells consisting of lymphocytes, plasma cells, and eosinophils usually present
- Inconspicuous vascularity
- Focal areas of fibrosis present in 50%
- Longstanding lesions or lesions that are regressing may have significant interstitial fibrosis with a vague storiform pattern and resemble a benign fibrous histiocytoma

Special Stains

- Not helpful

Immunohistochemistry

- Histiocytes express α_1-antichymotrypsin (100%) and α_1-antitrypsin (100%)
- Staining for S-100 negative (except for occasional dendritic cells)

Electron Microscopy

- Neoplastic cells have numerous pseudopodia, lipid droplets, and lysosomes (all characteristics of histiocytes)

Molecular Alterations

- No evidence of a familial incidence

Differential Diagnosis

- Histiocytosis X (histocytes of histiocytosis X consistently express S-100 protein; the histiocytes of a juvenile xanthogranuloma do not)
- Xanthoma
- Longstanding lesions that have regressed may resemble a fibrous histiocytoma

Treatment and Prognosis

- Surgical excision (no recurrence)
- Cutaneous lesions (in infants and children) typically regress or at least stabilize with time and the prognosis is quite good
- Occasionally deep-seated or parenchymal lesions may need to be removed surgically
- Radiotherapy can be used to treat lesions involving the eye

Associations

- No underlying lipid abnormality
- Associated with neurofibromatosis and urticaria pigmentosa

Malignant Giant Cell Tumor of Tendon Sheath/Pigmented Villonodular Synovitis

Clinical Manifestations

- Occurs in distal extremities
- Extremely rare

Gross Pathology

- Similar to benign counterparts

Microscopic Pathology

- Areas of typical benign giant cell tumor with focal areas of malignancy characterized by large prominent atypical mononuclear cells with abundant cytoplasm and hyperchromatic nuclei with large nucleoli; both typical and atypical mitoses present
- Giant cells are less numerous than in benign lesions
- Mononuclear neoplastic cells grow in sheets or large nodules and may have areas of hemorrhage and necrosis and little stromal collagen

Special Stains, Immunochemistry and Electron Microscopy

- Not helpful

Molecular Alterations

- None

Differential Diagnosis

- Includes all of the items listed in the differential diagnosis of benign tenosynovial giant cell tumor (both localized and diffuse)

Treatment

- Wide excision or amputation

Prognosis

- Locally aggressive with high local recurrence rate
- Metastasis occurs

Associations

- Malignancy may develop in an otherwise typical benign lesion, may appear in a recurrent originally benign lesion, or may develop as a primary lesion

Pleomorphic Malignant Fibrous Histiocytoma (PMFH)

Variants

- *Storiform PMFH/Undifferentiated high-grade pleomorphic sarcoma*
- *Giant cell PMFH/Undifferentiated pleomorphic sarcoma with giant cells*
- *Inflammatory PMFH/Undifferentiated pleomorphic sarcoma with prominent inflammation*

Clinical Manifestations

- *Storiform PMFH*
  - Peak incidence 7th decade
  - Most occur in extremities (especially the legs)
  - May (<3%) develop at site of previous radiation (most common postradiation sarcoma); also appears at sites of infarction, foreign body, or scar
  - Majority involve deep fascia or skeletal muscle; 10% subcutaneous
  - May grow rapidly and if they do, will be associated with pain
- *Giant cell PMFH/Undifferentiated pleomorphic sarcoma with giant cells*
  - Most present as deep-seated, painless mass of extremities or trunk
  - Giant cell tumor of soft tissues presents as a small, mass in the subcutaneous tissue or dermis of the extremities (70%), trunk (20%), and head and neck (7%)
- *Inflammatory MFH/Undifferentiated pleomorphic sarcoma with prominent inflammation*
  - Most patients over age 40 years
  - May present with fever, weight loss, and leukocytosis with neutrophilia or eosinophilia
  - Tends to occur in the abdomen (rarely in an extremity)

Gross Pathology

- *Storiform PMFH and giant cell PMFH*
  - Usually solitary, well circumscribed (pseudoencapsulated) but may infiltrate for considerable distance; gray/white and fleshy; may have foci of necrosis, hemorrhage, or myxoid change)
- *Inflammatory MFH*
  - Usually large and yellow (large collections of xanthoma cells)

Microscopic Pathology

- *Storiform PMFH*
  - Features typically include a storiform or pinwheel pattern surrounding slitlike vessels of an admixture of uniform fibroblastic cells and bizarre, pleomorphic cells arranged in short fascicles with atypical mitoses; inflammatory cells usually mixed with neoplastic cells; metaplastic bone and cartilage may be present; xanthoma cells, giant cells, and areas of hyalinization and necrosis frequently present; collagen fibrils surround individual tumor cells
- *Giant cell MFH/Undifferentiated pleomorphic sarcoma with giant cells*
  - Shares morphologic features with malignant giant cell tumor of soft tissues, malignant giant cell tumor of bone, extraskeletal osteosarcoma, leiomyosarcoma with prominent osteoclastic giant cells, and osteoclast-rich carcinoma
  - Typically a multinodular or plexiform proliferation of ovoid to spindled fibroblastlike cells and histiocytes intermixed with osteoclastlike giant cells; nodules separated by fibrous bands
- *Inflammatory MFH/Undifferentiated pleomorphic sarcoma with prominent inflammation*
  - Characterized by sheets of benign xanthoma cells with intermixed inflammatory cells (neutrophils, eosinophils, and occasional lymphocytes and plasma cells); scattered (sometimes rare) large, xanthomatized atypical cells with ≥1 irregular, hyperchromatic nuclei with prominent nucleoli; tumor cells may contain phagocytosed neutrophils in their cytoplasm; hyalinized collagenous stroma with delicate vasculature

Special Stains

- PAS and reticulin stains highlight the vasculature in storiform-pleomorphic type

Immunohistochemistry

- *Storiform PMFH*
  - Most high-grade, pleomorphic sarcomas show a reproducible line of differentiation (ie, pleomorplic leiomyosarcoma, liposarcoma, rhabdomyosarcoma, and myxofibrosarcoma)
  - Rare cells may show reactivity for epithelial or myogenic antigens *(findings that do not rule out the diagnosis)*
  - Histiocytic markers such as α_1-antitrypsin, α_1-antichymotrypsin, lysozyme, and CD68 of no value
- *Giant cell MFH/Undifferentiated pleomorphic sarcoma with giant cells*
  - Leiomyosarcoma with osteoclastic giant cells positive for smooth muscle actin and desmin
  - Osteoclastlike or giant cell rich MFH always positive for keratin
- *Inflammatory MFH/Undifferentiated pleomorphic sarcoma with prominent inflammation*
  - May be useful in showing epithelial, lymphoid, or smooth muscle lines of differentiation (see differential diagnosis later in this section)
  - Occasional cells positive for CD68
  - Tumor cells negative for CD15, CD20, CD30, CD43, and CD45

Electron Microscopy

- Confirms presence of undifferentiated, nonspecific fibroblasts, histiocytes, and primitive mesenchymal cells

Molecular Alterations

- 30% of storiform/pleomorphic MFHs have mutant p53

Differential Diagnosis

- *Storiform PMFH* (a diagnosis of exclusion)
  - Pleomorphic liposarcoma
  - Pleomorphic rhabdomyosarcoma
  - Metastatic pleomorphic carcinoma
  - Melanoma
  - Hodgkin disease (Leu-M1 staining of Reed-Sternberg cells helpful) and lymphoma
  - DFSP and benign fibrous histiocytoma
- *Giant cell MFH/Undifferentiated pleomorphic sarcoma with giant cells*
  - Giant cell tumor of soft tissue
  - Extraskeletal osteosarcoma (dependent upon amount of osteoid present)
  - Leiomyosarcoma with prominent osteoclastic giant cells
  - Osteoclast-rich carcinoma (pancreas, thyroid, breast, and kidney)
- *Inflammatory MFH/Undifferentiated pleomorphic sarcoma with prominent inflammation*
  - Inflammatory dedifferentiated component of carcinoma, lymphoma, leiomyosarcoma, inflammatory myofibroblastic tumor, and liposarcoma

Treatment

- Complete surgical excision (tumor tends to infiltrate along fascial planes and between muscle fibers)

Prognosis

- *Storiform PMFH*
  - Tend to recur (45%) and metastasize (45%) (lung most common site)
  - 5-year survival rate 50% to 60%
- *Giant cell MFH/Undifferentiated pleomorphic sarcoma with giant cells*
  - Local recurrence 10 to 15%; metastases rare
- *Inflammatory MFH/Undifferentiated pleomorphic sarcoma with prominent inflammation*
  - Prognosis grim secondary to inaccessibility to complete surgical excision

Associations

- Storiform PMFH may be induced by radiation; 10% develop a 2nd neoplasm (may be an age-related phenomenon); reported in patients with Lynch II syndrome (increased risk for colorectal cancer and extraintestinal cancer, especially endometrial carcinoma); patients may be hypoglycemic secondary to the secretion of an insulin-like substance from the tumor

Comment

- 10 years ago a "pleomorphic MFH" was considered to be the most common sarcoma to affect the adult population. Currently a PMFH, also called an "undifferentiated high grade pleomorphic sarcoma," is considered a diagnosis of exclusion and represents a tumor that affects fewer that 5% of adults. Storiform PMFH, giant cell MFH—also called an "undifferentiated pleomorphic sarcoma with giant cells"—and inflammatory MFH—also called undifferentiated pleomorphic sarcoma with prominent inflammation—are all treated in this text as variants of PMFH (undifferentiated high-grade pleomorphic sarcoma).
- Giant cell malignant fibrous histiocytoma shares a morphologic pattern with various tumor types; giant cell tumor of soft tissues (see above), malignant giant cell tumor of bone, extraskelatal osteosarcoma, leiomyosarcoma with giant cells, and osteoclast-rich carcinoma

Tenosynovial Giant Cell Tumor, Diffuse Type (Proliferative Synovitis, Extra-Articular Pigmented Villonodular Synovitis, Pigmented Villonodular Bursitis, and Florid Synovitis)

Clinical Manifestations

- The soft tissue counterpart of pigmented villonodular synovitis
- Intra-articular and extra-articular disease may coexist in the same patient; the latter representing a soft-tissue extension of the former
- Less common than localized type of tenosynovial giant cell tumor and tends to occur in younger patients (often <40 years of age)
- Females more frequently affected than males
- Most commonly involves the knee (80%); also ankle and foot
- Pain and swelling of long duration are characteristic symptoms

Gross Pathology

- Lesions tend to be large, multinodular masses varying in color from yellow to white to brown
- Tends to be unencapsulated with an infiltrative growth pattern at the periphery (no mature collagenous capsule)
- Adjacent joint may be involved

Microscopic Pathology

- Sheets of round or polygonal mononuclear cells with a high nuclear-cytoplasmic ratio and clear to eosinophilic to brown (hemosiderin) cytoplasm admixed with xanthoma cells and spindle cells; overall pattern infiltrative
- Mitotic activity may be vary noticable
- Slitlike or pseudoglandular spaces usually distributed throughout
- Chronic inflammatory cells and multinucleated giant cells tend to be scattered throughout the spindle cell population giving the lesion a very pleomorphic appearance (giant cells tend to be less numerous than in localized type)
- Lesion may destroy adjacent tissue and focal areas of necrosis may be present
- Cellular areas relatively devoid of collagen; hypocellular areas often quite hyalinized

Special Stains

- Iron stains may highlight presence of hemosiderin

Immunohistochemistry

- Mononuclear cells and giant cells reactive for CD68 (KP1) and leukocyte common antigen (LCA)

Electron Microscopy

- Most of the mononuclear cells have histiocytelike features with abundant cytoplasm and lysosomes

Molecular Alterations

- Clonal rearrangements of 1p11-13 and trisomy 5 and 7

Differential Diagnosis

- Intra-articular, pigmented villonodular synovitis
- Localized tenosynovial giant cell tumor
- Villous hypertrophy of synovium as a reactive response to a failed orthopedic prosthetic device
- Chronic hemarthrosis
- Pseudoglandular spaces may be interperated as the glandular spaces of a biphasic synovial sarcoma or the alveolar spaces of an alveolar rhabdomyosarcoma
- Inflammatory or xanthomatous MFH

Treatment

- Wide surgical excision

Prognosis

- Locally aggressive
- Recurrence rate approximately 40% to 50%
- Lesions involving the knee most likely to recur
- 1 report of a recurrent lesion in the foot metastasizing to lung

Associations

- When in soft tissue, probably represents an extra-articular (soft tissue) variant or extension of pigmented villonodular synovitis

Tenosynovial Giant Cell Tumor, Localized Type (Nodular Tenosynovitis)

Clinical Manifestations

- More common in women than in men
- Typically occurs between the ages of 30 and 50 years
- Most commonly (85%) occurs along extensor or flexor surfaces of interphalangeal joints of the hand (less commonly feet, ankles, and knees)
- Tends to develop slowly and remain unchanged in size for years
- Usually adherent to deep structures (usually tendon) and are not attached to overlying skin

Gross Pathology

- A small (<4 cm), smooth, circumscribed lobulated mass that may have grooves on its surface created by adjacent tendons
- Lesions on the feet usually larger than lesions on the hands
- On sectioning, a mottled, white to gray surface with scattered foci of lipid (yellow) and hemosiderin (brown)

Microscopic Pathology

- Sheets of round or polygonal mononuclear cells with fibrous septa and cleftlike spaces that form a vague nodule that is attached to a tendon or tendon sheath and has a mature fibrous capsule
- Cells have small, oval to round, uniform nuclei that frequently have clefts and may have prominent nucleoli
- Multinucleated benign giant cells, xanthoma cells, and hemosiderin (interstitial and within macrophages) typically present in variable numbers and amounts
- Evidence of chronic inflammation usually present (lymphocytes and histiocytes)
- Mitoses present in 50%
- Hyalinization may be present
- A histologic continuum exists between nodular and diffuse tenosynovial giant cell tumors

Special Stains

- None

Immunohistochemistry

- Cells reactive for HLA-A, B, C, and DR
- Mononuclear cells and giant cells reactive for CD68 (KP1) and LCA

Electron Microscopy

- Most of the mononuclear cells have histiocyte-like features with abundant cytoplasm and lysosomes

Molecular Alterations

- Chromosomal abnormalities largely localized to 1p11 and 16q24

Differential Diagnosis

- Tenosynovial giant cell tumor, diffuse type
- Necrobiotic granuloma
- Foreign body granuloma
- Xanthoma of tendon sheath
- Fibroma of tendon sheath

Treatment

- Local excision with small rim of normal tissue

Prognosis

- A benign lesion with capacity for local recurrence
- Local recurrence rate approximately 20% to 30%; usually the result of incomplete excision
- Recurrence more likely in densely cellular lesions with numerous mitoses

Associations

- None

Xanthoma

Clinical Manifestations

- Usually occurs in the skin and subcutis; occasionally involves deep soft tissue (tendon or synovium)
- Typically develops in the clinical setting of either primary hyperlipoproteinemia or secondary hyperlipoproteinemia (primary biliary cirrhosis and diabetes mellitus)
- Occasionally seen in patients who are normolipidemic

Variants

- Eruptive xanthoma
- Tuberous xanthoma
- Tendinous xanthoma
- Xanthelasma
- Plane xanthoma

Gross Pathology

- Eruptive xanthoma
  - Small yellow papules that tend to occur on the buttocks
- Tuberous xanthoma
  - Large plaquelike lesions that involve the subcutis and typically occur on the buttocks, elbows, knees, and fingers
- Tendinous xanthoma
  - Tends to occur on the tendons of the hands and feet and the Achilles tendon
  - Usually painless, slowly enlarging mass
  - May be solitary and well-circumscribed or diffuse or multiple and tend to occur at sites subjected to minor trauma
  - Tends to be firmly attached to tendon but not attached to overlying skin
  - Cut surface has variegated color ranging from white to yellow to brown depending upon the amount of lipid, hemorrhage, and fibrosis present
- Xanthelasma
  - Involves the eyelid
- Plane xanthoma
  - Tends to occur in skin folds (palmar creases)

Microscopic Pathology

- Eruptive xanthoma
  - Sheets of nonfoamy (majority), foamy histiocytes, and occasional inflammatory cells
- Tuberous xanthoma and tendinous xanthoma
  - Sheets of foamy histiocytes with an admixture of inflammatory cells
  - Histiocytes are bland and have small pyknotic nuclei and occasionally contain hemosiderin
  - Aggregates of extracellular cholesterol surrounded by giant cells
  - Varying amounts of fibrosis may be present and tends to be more prominent in longstanding lesions
- Xanthelasma and plane xanthoma
  - Sheets of foamy histiocytes with little fibrosis

Special Stains and Immunohistochemistry

- Not helpful

Electron Microscopy

- Xanthoma cells contain numerous clear vacuoles (cholesterol or its esters)
- Eruptive xanthomas have both fat and tissue macrophages in vessel walls

Molecular Alterations

- Cerebrotendinous xanthomatosis is a rare autosomal recessive inherited disease

Differential Diagnosis

- Tendinous xanthoma may clinically resemble a sarcoma
- Giant cell tumor of tendon sheath
- Diffuse villonodular synovitis
- Lipogranuloma

Treatment and Prognosis

- Xanthelasma and tuberous xanthomas may both regress on medical therapy
- Large and/or symptomatic xanthomas may be treated surgically but have a tendency to slowly recur

Associations

- Eruptive xanthoma
  - Associated with hyperlipidemia types I, III, and V
- Tuberous xanthoma
  - Associated with hyperlipidemia types IIa and III
- Tendinous xanthoma
  - Associated with hyperlipidemia types II and III and occasionally type IV
  - Associated with cerebrotendinous xanthomatosis (an autosomal recessive disease characterized by bilateral xanthomas involving the Achilles tendons, dementia, ataxia, and cataracts that result from abnormal bile acid synthesis with deposition of cholesterol in nerve myelin both centrally and peripherally)
- Xanthelasma
  - May be associated with hyperlipidemic types IIa and III, but usually seen in patients who are normolipidemic
- Plane xanthoma
  - May be associated with hyperlipidemia type II which in turn is associated with primary biliary cirrhosis
  - Also seen in type III hyperlipidemia and in normolipemic patients
  - When seen in normolipemic patients, there is a high association of reticuloendothelial malignancies
  - Minor trauma that results in a localized histamine release will cause an increase in vascular permeability allowing serum lipoproteins to escape the vascular compartment and become engulfed by soft tissue macrophages (xanthoma formation)

Fibroblastic/Myofibroblastic Tumors

Calcifying Aponeurotic Fibroma

Clinical Manifestations

- Tends to occur in children and adolescents (birth to 15+ years); adults rarely affected
- Painless mass involving aponeuroses or tendons of the hands and feet (more common in hands than feet)
- Lesions in the hand tend to occur on the palm or the fingers; lesions in the foot tend to occur in plantar or ankle regions

Gross Pathology

- Typically an ill-defined infiltrating mass or nodule in subcutaneous tissue attached to a tendon or aponeuroses
- On cut section, firm and gray with occasional foci of calcification
- Rarely larger than 3 cm

Microscopic Pathology

- Multiple cellular nodules consisting of fibroblasts surrounding a hyalinized collagenous zone which in turn surrounds a central, punctate zone of calcification and/or cartilage; fibroblasts tend to palisade near these areas of calcification and are plump with oval or round, vesicular nuclei (chromatin that appears condensed along the inner surface of the nuclear membrane), eosinophilic cytoplasm, and indistinct cell borders
- Nodules separated by a fibrous stroma that contains smaller, mature fibroblasts with nuclei with dense, evenly distributed chromatin
- Degree of calcification and cartilage formation largely a function of the age of the tumor and the age of the patient; longstanding lesions in teenagers more likely to be calcified

- At periphery, adjacent fat and muscle may be infiltrated by rays of fibrous tissue that appear to radiate from the main lesion
- Atypical cytologic features and mitoses rare
- Osteoclastlike giant cells frequent in areas of calcification
- Cells inside and adjacent to calcified foci resemble chondrocytes

Special Stains

- Trichrome will highlight collagen

Immunohistochemistry

- Variable expression of vimentin, smooth muscle actin, muscle-specific actin, CD99, and S-100 protein

Electron Microscopy

- A biphasic pattern of fibroblasts and to a lesser extent, myofibroblasts and chondrocytes
- Cells surrounded by intercellular matrix of fibrils and round granules

Molecular Alterations

- None

Differential Diagnosis

- Fibrous hamartoma of infancy
- Infantile digital fibromatosis
- Chondroma of soft parts (calcifying and noncalcifying)

Treatment and Prognosis

- Conservative surgery (even considering likelihood of recurrence)
- 50% recur locally (more likely to recur in infants and children than in adults)
- Malignant transformation may occur (extremely rare)

Associations

- None

Elastofibroma

Clinical Manifestations

- Typically occurs beneath the rhomboid and latissimus dorsi muscles and is adherent to the underlying periosteum, fascia, and ligaments of the chest wall in the region of the 6th, 7th, and 8th ribs; other sites include gastrointestinal tract (stomach, small intestine, and rectum), tracheobronchial tree, omentum, foot, cornea, deltoid region, and greater trochanter
- Usually deep-seated, solitary, painless, and very slow growing
- More common on the right than the left; 10% bilateral
- Typically affects adults over the age of 55 years; much more common in women than men
- Patient often has a history of hard, repetitive manual labor

Gross Pathology

- Typically oval or round with ill-defined margins
- Firm, white shiny surface with foci of cystic degeneration and adipose

Microscopic Pathology

- Tends to consist primarily of a hypocellular, hyalinized collagenous (types I, II, and III) tissue admixed with thickened, serrated, eosinophilic, refractive elastic fibrils that usually contain a central dense core (resemble pipe cleaners), mucoid stroma, and entrapped mature adipose
- Elastic fibers may be fragmented into round, serrated discs or globules (*chenille bodies*) arranged in a linear pattern ("beads on a string")
- Rare fibroblasts may be scattered throughout the lesion

Special Stains

- Elastic fibrils highlighted with both collagen and elastic stains

Immunohistochemistry

- Not helpful

Electron Microscopy

- Elastic fibers consist of granular electron dense material with a central core
- Spindle cells have characteristics of fibroblasts and myofibroblasts

Molecular Alterations

- A possible genetic predisposition

Differential Diagnosis

- Fibrolipoma
- Fibromatosis

Treatment

- Surgical excision or radiation

Prognosis

- A completely benign reactive process; no reports of malignant transformation
- Local recurrence very rare

Associations

- None

Fibroma of Tendon Sheath

Clinical Manifestations

- Typically occurs in adults between the ages of 20 and 50 years
- Men affected twice as often as women
- Typically presents as a slowly enlarging mass involving the fingers, hand, and wrist; may involve the feet
- Thumb, index, and middle fingers most commonly involved
- Typically painless, but may limit range of motion

Gross Pathology

- Well-circumscribed, multilobulated mass attached to a tendon or tendon sheath
- Firm with a uniform gray to gray-white cartilaginous appearance
- Typically ranges between 1 and 2 cm in size

Microscopic Pathology

- An overall multilobular architecture; individual lobules separated by deep, narrow clefts
- Widely separated (hypocellular) fibroblasts and stellate-shaped cells in a densely eosinophilic, hyalinized collagenous stroma
- Fibroblasts tend to have elongated nuclei with finely granular chromatin and small basophilic nucleoli
- Zones of increased cellularity may be present; cells in these areas often arranged in storiform or fascicular pattern (resemble nodular fasciitis)
- Often a gradual transition between densely hyalinized collagenous areas to more cellular areas
- May have a component of pleomorphic tumor cells without mitotic activity
- Foci of myxoid change may be present and quite prominent; stellate cells may be prominent in these areas
- Multinucleated giant cells may be present (rare) as well as bizarre cells and foci of osseous and chondroid metaplasia; xanthoma cells and hemosiderin deposits absent

Special Stains

- None

Immunohistochemistry

- Spindle cells are reactive for vimentin and both muscle specific and smooth muscle actin
- Tumors express both factor XIIIa and CD34

Electron Microscopy

- Spindle cells represent a mixture of myofibroblasts and fibroblasts
- Myofibroblasts more common in cellular areas; fibroblasts more common in collagenous areas

Molecular Alterations

- Translocations involving chromosome 2q31-32

Differential Diagnosis

- More cellular forms may be confused with nodular fasciitis and fibrous histiocytoma
- Pleomorphic lesions may resemble MFH

Treatment

- Local excision and re-excision of recurrences

Prognosis

- Recurrence rate up to 25%

Associations

- Approximately 10% of patients has a history of trauma to the area

Fibromatosis

Clinical Manifestations

- Most commonly occurs in adults
- May be superficial (palmar, planter, and penile) or deep (musculoaponeurotic desmoid tumor)

Gross Pathology

- Ill-defined and nonencapsulated
- Sectioning reveals firm, white irregularly whorled surface
- Usually arise in muscular fascia

Microscopic Pathology

- A proliferation of well-differentiated fibroblasts and myofibroblasts with an infiltrative pattern of growth
- Usually not very cellular, and nuclei tend not to touch one another
- Variable amounts of collagen between proliferating cells
- No cytologic features of malignancy, but mitoses occasionally seen
- A perivascular lymphocytic infiltrate often found at the advancing edge (more characteristic of deep lesions)
- Thin-walled, elongated, and compressed blood vessels tend to be very obvious and stand out from the surrounding tissue
- Dystrophic and metaplastic calcification rarely present

Variants

- *Superficial (fascial) fibromatosis*
  - Penile fibromatosis (Peyronie disease)
    - Most patients between ages of 55 and 75 years
    - Proliferation of myofibroblasts in tissue layer between corpora cavernosa and tunica albuginea
    - Causes penial curvature toward side of lesion
    - Longstanding disease characterized microscopically by hyalinized fibrous tissue that may contain cartilage and/or bone
    - May be a reaction to recurrent episodes of urethritis
    - Treated with radiation, steroids, or excision
  - Palmar fibromatosis (Dupuytren contracture) and plantar fibromatosis (Ledderhose disease)
    - Occurs predominately in adults (55-75 years)
    - Causes contracture of fingers and toes
    - Lesions typically multiple and bilateral
    - Plantar form usually more localized than palmar form
    - Microscopically, nodules of a variably cellular, uniform population of fibroblasts and myofibroblasts with uniform vesicular to dark nuclei arranged in short fascicles in a collagenous stroma; mitotic figures may be present
- *Deep (musculoaponeurotic) fibromatosis*
  - Extra-abdominal fibromatosis (extra-abdominal desmoid):
    - Typically arises from connective tissue of muscle and overlying fascia or aponeurosis in adults between 25 and 35 years
    - Most commonly arise in the musculature of the shoulder; also seen in the chest wall, back, thigh, and neck
    - Patients typically present with relatively painless poorly circumscribed mass
    - May be multicentric but tend to be confined to a single anatomic region
    - Typically a dense, white, trabeculated fibrous mass that infiltrates adjacent skeletal muscle
    - Neoplasm consists of uniform, long, slender spindle-shaped cells (fibrocytes, fibroblasts, and myofibroblasts) surrounded and separated from one another by abundant myxoid to collagenous stroma; nuclei tend to be small, well-defined and pale with 1 to 3 small nucleoli; the cells and collagen tend to be arranged in ill-defined sweeping bundles
    - Most tumors contain thin-walled slitlike vessels and thick-walled arteries
    - At the periphery, the tumor typically infiltrates muscle with fragments of muscle occasionally becoming entrapped within the neoplasm
  - Abdominal fibromatosis (abdominal desmoid):
    - Typically arises from the musculoaponeurotic structures of the abdominal wall and their fascicular coverings and presents as a deep-seated solitary mass that tends to become more prominent when the abdominal muscular is contracted
    - Usually seen in women between the ages of 20 and 30 years during gestation or within the first year after childbirth
    - Also seen in males and in young children, particularly boys
    - Less frequent than extra-abdominal fibromatosis
    - Gross and microscopic features identical to extra-abdominal fibromatosis

- Intra-abdominal fibromatosis (desmoid):
  - *Pelvic fibromatosis*: A variant of abdominal fibromatosis, but located in the iliac fossa or lower portion of the pelvis; arises from muscle or aponeurosis; usually seen in young women between the ages of 20 and 35 years; unlike abdominal desmoids, unrelated to recent pregnancy
  - *Mesenteric fibromatosis*: Occurs in the mesentery of the small bowel and may extend into the retroperitoneum; usually presents as an asymptomatic mass that may be palpable in the lower abdomen; occasionally obstructs the small or large intestine or the ureter; tend to be more myxoid than other desmoids
  - *Mesenteric fibromatosis and Gardner syndrome*: The incidence of fibromatosis in patients with Gardner syndrome ranges from 10% to 15%; slightly more common in women than men; neoplasm tends to arise in the mesentery and retroperitoneum but may occur in the abdominal wall; usually develops after surgery and seen microscopically and is indistinguishable from desmoids in other anatomic sites

Special Stains

- Reticulin and trichrome stains highlight collagen between individual tumor cells

Immunohistochemistry

- Proliferating cells are actin positive and usually focally desmin positive
- β-catenin demonstrates nuclear positivity

Electron Microscopy

- Features of myofibroblasts: cells have long thin cytoplasmic processes; nuclei are round or oval with undulated outline; cytoplasm contains rough endoplasmic reticulum and actin-type microfilaments

Molecular Alterations

- 20% to 25% of patients with deep fibromatosis (desmoid) have trisomy for chromosome 8; 10% have a deletion of 5q

Differential Diagnosis

- Extra-abdominal fibromatosis:
  - Scar
  - Fibrosarcoma
  - Nodular fasciitis
  - Myxoid MFH
- Abdominal fibromatosis:
  - Scar
  - Fibrosarcoma
  - Nodular fasciitis
  - Myxoid MFH
- Mesenteric fibromatosis:
  - GI stromal tumor
  - Myxoid MFH
  - Idiopathic retroperitoneal fibrosis (Ormond disease)

Treatment

- Wide radical excision
- Radiation therapy (local control)
- Tamoxifen

Prognosis

- Recurrence rate for extra-abdominal desmoids 35% to 65%
- Recurrence rate for abdominal desmoids 15% to 30%

Associations

- Mesenteric fibromatosis
- *Gardner syndrome*: Autosomal dominant; intestinal adenomatous polyps identical to those in familial adenomatous polyposis occur in the large and small intestine and stomach in association with multiple osteomas (particularly of mandible, skull, and long bones), epidermal cysts, and fibromatosis (most of the fibromatoses are intra-abdominal and develop after surgical intervention); significant potential for development of large bowel carcinoma and carcinomas of small bowel, particularly in the periampuallary area; other associations include abnormalities of dentition, such as unerupted and supernumerary teeth, benign lymphoid polyposis of the terminal ileum, and congenital hypertrophy of retinal pigment epithelium resulting in solitary or multiple oval pigmented lesions in 1 or both eyes
- Fibromatosis colli
  - Trauma
  - Congenital dislocation of hip (15%)

- Palmar fibromatosis
  - Chronic alcoholism
  - Epilepsy, diabetes, and cirrhosis
- Penile fibromatosis
  - More common in patients with palmar and plantar fibromatosis
- Extra-abdominal fibromatosis
  - Surgical scar (cicatricial fibromatosis)
  - Irradiation (post-irradiation fibromatosis)
- Intra-abdominal fibromatosis
  - Tends to occur after trauma in genetically susceptible patients

Fibrosarcoma

Clinical Manifestations

- 2 major types:
  - *Adult-type fibrosarcoma*
    - Typically occurs between ages of 40 and 55 years
    - Slightly more common in men than women
    - Usually presents as a deep-seated, solitary, palpable, and painless mass
    - Most frequently occurs in the extremities, trunk, and head and neck
  - *Juvenile/infantile-type fibrosarcoma*
    - By definition patient must be under the age of 10 years
    - 90% develop during 1st year of life; often present at birth
    - Most occur in extremities (usually distal), but also trunk and head and neck
    - Tends to grow rapidly
    - Overlying skin tense, erythematous, and ulcerated

Gross Pathology

- *Adult-type fibrosarcoma*
  - Arises from superficial and deep connective tissue (fascia, tendon, periosteum and scar)
  - Often well-circumscribed or lobulated and soft (may contain areas of necrosis); a "fish flesh" consistency
  - Rarely involves subcutaneous tissue unless there is a pre-existing dermatofibrosarcoma protuberans, scar, burn, or history of irradiation
- *Juvenile/infantile-type fibrosarcoma*
  - Poorly circumscribed, lobulated, and infiltrarive into adjacent soft tissue
  - Cut surface fleshy and gray to tan with myxoid or mucinous change, cystic degeneration, necrosis, and hemorrhage

Microscopic Pathology

- *Adult-type fibrosarcoma*
  - Uniform dense population of fusiform or spindle cells arranged in fascicles that intersect at acute angles resulting in a "herringbone pattern"
  - Individual cells resemble fibroblasts with tapered, hyperchromatic nuclei; delicate collagen fibers separate and parallel the cells (occasionally collagen "keloidlike")
  - Mitoses (some of which may be atypical) usually present but significant pleomorphism unusual
  - Occasionally a myxoid matrix, necrosis, and/or osseous or chondroid metaplasia may be present
  - Typically more cellular than fibromatosis, but fibromatosis areas may be present
- *Juvenile/infantile-type fibrosarcoma*
  - Typically densely cellular consisting of intersecting fascicles of oval or spindled cells with a "herringbone" pattern
  - Zonal necrosis and hemorrhage frequent with or without dystrophic calcifications
  - Pleomorphism rare, collagen formation variable
  - Scattered inflammatory cells usually present
  - Various findings include hemangiopericytomalike pattern, dilated vessels with fibrin thrombi, and areas of myxoid change

Special Stains

- Reticulin stain demonstrates collagen fibers wrapped around each spindle cell

Immunohistochemistry

- *Adult-type fibrosarcoma:* Reactive for vimentin and very focally for smooth muscle actin
- *Infantile-type fibrosarcoma:* Tumor cells always reactive for vimentin; rarely positive for S-100, CD34, CD57, CD68, and cytokeratin

Electron Microscopy

- *Adult-type fibrosarcoma:* Tumor cells are fibroblasts with prominent rough endoplasmic reticulum and no myofilaments

Molecular Alterations

- *Adult-type fibrosarcoma*
  - No characteristic chromosomal anomalies
- *Infantile fibrosarcoma*
  - Contains chromosomal translocation t(12;15)(p13;q26)
  - Shares the same molecular alterations associated with cellular mesoblastic nephroma

Differential Diagnosis

- Nodular fasciitis
- Fibrous histiocytoma
- Fibromatosis
- Monophasic synovial sarcoma (fibrous type)
- Pleomorphic malignant fibrous histiocytoma
- Malignant peripheral nerve sheet tumor
- Malignant fibrous mesothelioma
- Spindle cell desmoplastic melanoma

Treatment

- Radical excision with postoperative radiation for residual disease or positive margins

Prognosis

- *Adult-type fibrosarcoma*
  - Survival rate related to histologic grade, cellularity, amount of collagen, number of mitotic figures (>20 per 10 high power fields [hpf]), and necrosis
  - 5-year survival rate for adult type ranges from 60% for grade 1 or 2 to 20% for grade 4
  - Recurrence rate depends on extent (adequacy) of primary surgical excision
  - Metastasis occurs via blood stream (lung most common site)
- *Infantile fibrosarcoma*
  - Excellent prognosis (much better than adult fibrosarcoma) with a mortality rate of <25%
  - Metastases rare

Associations

- Adult-type may be associated with hypoglycemia (neoplasms may produce insulinlike substances resulting in increased utilization of glycogen) and may arise in irradiated tissue and burn scars or result when a DFSP dedifferentiates
- *Adult fibrosarcoma variant: Sclerosing epithelioid fibrosarcoma*
  - Occurs in deep soft tissues of lower upper extremities and limb girdles, trunk, upper exrtremities, and head and neck
  - Most commonly well-circumscribed and lobulated; may have a firm gritty cut surface with myxoid or cystic areas
  - Typically hypocellular; tumor cells predominately epithelioid and arranged in nests, cords, and strands and separated by extensive areas of densely hyalinized collagen; nuclei round to oval and angulated with vesicular chromatin and small nucleoli; cytoplasm scanty and clear or faintly eosinophilic
  - Mitotic figures usually fairly rare
  - Consistently positive for vimentin
  - Recurrence rate 50%; metastases in 40% (usually lungs)

Infantile Digital Fibromatosis (Inclusion Body Fibromatosis)

Clinical Manifestations

- Typically a small, firm, broad-based, nontender nodule in a finger or toe (fingers more common than toes)
- Tend to be located on the sides or dorsum of the distal or middle phalangeal joints and most commonly involve the 3rd, 4th, and 5th digits; overlying skin may be pale or red
- May be single or multiple and may involve more than 1 digit of the same hand or foot
- 30% to 35% present at birth; most diagnosed by 1 year of age

Gross Pathology

- Cut surface solid, white, and fibrous

Microscopic Pathology

- A uniformly circumscribed proliferation of fibroblasts and myofibroblasts surrounded by dense collagenous stroma

- Neoplasm appears to extend from a normal, slightly flattened epidermis into underlying dermis and subcutis; typically surrounds dermal appendages
- Small, round eosinophilic inclusions (resemble intracytoplasmic red blood cells) are present in the cytoplasm of variable numbers of fibroblasts and tend to be near the nucleus
- Normal mitotic figures frequently present

Special Stains

- Eosinophilic cytoplasmic inclusions stain deep red with Masson trichrome stain and purple with phosphotungstic acid hematoxylin (PTAH); they do not stain with PAS nor Alcian Blue

Immunohistochemistry

- Cytoplasm of spindle cells typically stains positively for muscle actins
- Cytoplasmic inclusions stain positively for actin if tissue is fixed in alcohol

Electron Microscopy

- Spindle cells are fibroblasts and myofibroblasts
- Cytoplasmic inclusions appear to arise in endoplasmic reticulum, consist of intermediate filaments, and lack a limiting membrane

Molecular Alterations

- Not familial

Differential Diagnosis

- Calcifying aponeurotic fibroma (early phase)

Treatment and Prognosis

- Surgical excision
- Lesions may spontaneously regress
- 50% will recur locally, typically at the same site within weeks or months of excision
- A 2nd tumor may develop in an adjacent finger or toe
- Tumors may result in a deformity or contracture, even when surgically excised

Associations

- None

Inflammatory Myofibroblastic Tumor (Extrapulmonary Inflammatory Pseudotumor)

Clinical Manifestations

- Typically occur in infants and children under age of 14 years; girls affected slightly more frequently than boys
- Most develop in the abdomen (mesentery and omentum)
- Other locations include urinary bladder, mediastinum, head and neck region, and soft tissue (other sites include GI tract, pancreas, skin, breast, bone, nerve, and central nervous system)
- Intra-abdominal lesions typically cause pain associated with an abdominal mass; systemic manifestations include fever, night sweats, weight loss, and generalized malaise; patients may also have an elevated erythrocyte sedimentation rate, anemia, thrombocytosis, and hypergammaglobulinemia

Gross Pathology

- Lesions typically circumscribed and lobular or multinodular; occasionally have infiltrating margins
- Cut surface hard and white to gray to tan-yellow (occasionally red), often with focal myxoid areas
- Focal calcifications may be present
- Usually a solitary lesion, but multiple lesions in a single anatomic site may be seen in up to 30%

Microscopic Pathology

- 3 histologic patterns that vary from tumor to tumor and within the same tumor:
  - Elongated myofibroblasts with abundant eosinophilic cytoplasm and large vesicular nuclei in a loose myxoid stroma with abundant blood vessels (resemble granulation tissue or nodular fasciitis); inflammatory cells include neutrophils, lymphocytes, and eosinophils (few plasma cells)
  - Spindled fibroblasts and myofibroblasts densely packed together and arranged in nests with a storiform or fascicular pattern surrounded by a myxoid or hyalinized stroma; mitotic figures often present; inflammatory cells include small aggregates of plasma cells (majority) and lymphoid nodules
  - Fibroblasts and myofibroblasts in a densely hyalinized and largely acellular stroma; inflammatory cells consist of a few plasma cells; eosinophils, and lymphocytes scattered throughout the stroma

- The first 2 patterns may have cells with marked cytologic atypia; these cells resemble ganglion cells; they have large vesicular nuclei, prominent eosinophilic nucleoli, and abundant amphophilic cytoplasm
- Mitotic figures may be present, but are never atypical
- Small foci of coarse or psammomatous calcifications and osseous metaplasia may be present

Special Stains

- Not helpful

Immunohistochemistry

- Cells usually positive for smooth muscle actin, muscle-specific actin, and vimentin
- Tumor cells focally positive for cytokeratin in approximately 30% to 35%
- CD68 positivity in approximately 25%
- Tumor cells stain negatively for myogenin, myoglobin, and S-100 protein

Electron Microscopy

- Tumor cells have features of fibroblasts and myofibroblasts

Molecular Alterations

- Clonal abnormalities at 2p23

Differential Diagnosis

- Inflammatory malignant fibrous histiocytoma/Undifferentiated pleomorphic sarcoma with prominent inflammation
- Sclerosing mediastinitis and retroperitoneal fibrosis,

Treatment and Prognosis

- Surgical excision
- Abdominal and retroperitoneal tumors tend to be more aggressive with recurrence rates as high as 35%
- Metastases have been reported (<5%)
- More aggressive tumors are associated with cytologic atypia, the presence of ganglionlike cells, expression of *p53,* and DNA aneuploidy

Associations

- Reported following treatment for Wilms tumor

Low-Grade Fibromyxoid Sarcoma (Adult Fibrosarcoma Variant)

Clinical Manifestations

- Tends to occur as a slowly enlarging painless mass in proximal extremities or trunk of young adults (median age 34 years)
- May also occur in head or retroperitoneum

Gross Pathology

- Cut surface yellow-white and glistening; no hemorrhage or necrosis

Microscopic Pathology

- Classic low-grade fibromyxoid sarcoma
- An admixture of densely collagenized, hypocellular areas and more myxoid nodules; bland spindle cells arranged in short fascicles in a whorling pattern, mitoses rare; 10% have areas of increased cellularity and nuclear atypia
- Low-grade fibromyxoid sarcoma with giant collagen rosettes
- Foci of poorly formed collagen rosettes in an otherwise typical appearing low-grade fibromyxoid sarcoma, rosettes consist of a central core of dense collagen surrounded by a rim of epithelioid fibroblasts (*hyalinizing spindle cell tumor with giant rosettes*)

Special Stains

- Reticulin stain demonstrates collagen fibers wrapped around each spindle cell

Immunohistochemistry

- Typically only express vimentin and rarely focal smooth muscle actin
- Tumor cells negative for desmin, histiocytic markers, cytokeratin, CD34, EMA, and S-100

Electron Microscopy

- Show fibroblastic differentiation

Molecular Alterations

- Chromosomal aberrations rare

Differential Diagnosis

- Nodular fasciitis
- Fibrous histiocytoma
- Fibromatosis
- Monophasic synovial sarcoma (fibrous type)
- Malignant peripheral nerve sheet tumor
- Malignant fibrous mesothelioma
- Spindle cell desmoplastic melanoma

Treatment

- Radical excision with postoperative radiation for residual disease or positive margins

Prognosis

- Recurrence 10%, metastastes 6%, death from disease 2%

Associations

- None

Low-Grade Myofibroblastic Sarcoma

Clinical Manifestations

- Typically occur in adults with slight male predominance
- Typically a painless swelling or soft tissue mass in thigh or head and neck (especially tongue)

Gross Pathology

- Typically a firm, pale, ill-defined mass with a fibrous texture

Microscopic Pathology

- Fascicles of spindle-shaped cells arranged in a storiform pattern that is usually diffusely infiltrative; in deep-seated lesions, tumor cells grow between individual skeletal muscle fibers
- Tumor cells characterized by ill-defined pale, eosinophilic cytoplasm and elongated and wavy nuclei with evenly distributed chromatin; some nuclei may be more oval and indented with vesicular chromatin and small nucleoli
- Focal moderate nuclear atypia, characterized by enlargement, hyperchromatism, and pleomorphism always present
- Chronic inflammatory cells not a prominent feature

Special Stains

- Not helpful

Immunohistochemistry

- May be smooth muscle actin positive or negative and desmin positive or negative
- Tumor cells may focally express CD34 and CD99
- S-100 and epithelial markers negative

Electron Microscopy

- Tumor cells have clefted or indented nuclei and are surrounded by a discontinuous basal lamina

Differential Diagnosis

- Fibromatosis

Treatment

- Wide excision

Prognosis

- Local recurrences common
- Metastases rare

Associations

- None

Myofibroma and Myofibromatosis

Clinical Manifestations

- Typically a solitary mass in the dermis or subcutis (*myofibroma*); may be multiple (*myofibromatosis*)
- Most commonly occur in head and neck region (scalp, forehead, orbit, parotid region, and oral cavity) followed by trunk, lower and upper extremities
- Solitary lesions may occur in bone (usually skull)
- Multicentric disease may involve soft tissue, bone, and viscera (lungs, heart, GI tract, liver, kidney, pancreas, and rarely the central nervous system); if bone involvement, usually a long bone
- Often first diagnosed at birth; may occur in adults
- Males affected twice as often as females

Gross Pathology

- Cutaneous lesions may appear as a purple macule

- Subcutaneous lesions usually painless and mobile; deep lesions often fixed
- Usually firm with a fibrous, white to gray cut surface; center of lesion may be cystic and filled with yellow, necrotic, caseous material or blood

Microscopic Pathology

- Typically a nodular or multinodular growth pattern
- Periphery of nodule(s) characterized by plump myofibroblasts arranged in short fascicles or whorls; cells have pink cytoplasm, elongated, tapering nuclei with a vesicular chromatin pattern and 1 or 2 small nucleoli; extensive hyalinization may be present giving the area a pseudochondroid appearance
- Center of nodules characterized by primitive round to polygonal to spindle-shaped cells that typically have slightly larger, pleomorphic, and hyperchromatic nuclei; these cells have little cytoplasm, vesicular nuclei, indistinct cell borders and are usually arranged around hemangiopericytomalike vessels
- Mitotic figures usually rare but on occasion may be quite numerous
- Foci of hemorrhage, necrosis, and cystic degeneration with calcification may be present
- Chronic inflammatory cells (lymphocytes and plasma cells) may be present at the periphery of the nodule(s)

Special Stains

- Not helpful

Immunohistochemistry

- Peripheral myofibroblasts stain for pan-actin HHF-35
- Central primitive cells stain weakly if at all for actin
- Both cell types negative for S-100, EMA, and keratin

Electron Microscopy

- Predominant cell is fibroblast and myofibroblast with dilated endoplasmic reticulum, cytoplasmic filament bundles, dense bodies, and focal basal lamina

Molecular Alterations

- May have an autosomal dominant inheritance pattern

Differential Diagnosis

- Peripheral areas resemble nodular fasciitis, fibrous histiocytoma, neurofibroma, or infantile fibromatosis
- Central areas may resemble sarcoma such as PNET, mesenchymal chondrosarcoma, malignant hemangiopericytoma, and poorly differentiated synovial sarcoma

Treatment

- Local excision (10% recur)

Prognosis

- May regress spontaneously, even when multiple
- Pulmonary involvement associated with a bad prognosis
- 75% of newborns and infants with multifocal visceral disease die of respiratory disease and/or diarrhea

Associations

- None

Myxoinflammatory Fibroblastic Sarcoma

Clinical Manifestations

- Also referred to as an inflammatory myxohyaline tumor of distal extremities with virocyte or Reed-Sternburg-like cells)
- Typically a slow-growing, poorly defined mass on the hand or wrist (65%) or the feet (35%)
- May cause pain or decreased mobility
- Develop in subcutaneous tissue and are attached to underlying fascia
- Males and females affected equally
- Peak incidence between the 4th and 5th decades

Gross Pathology

- Poorly defined and multinodular with alternating fibrous and myxoid areas

Microscopic Pathology

- Alternating hypocellular or cellular hyaline areas and myxoid areas with a prominent acute and chronic inflammatory infiltrate
- Aggregates of macrophages and uniform mononuclear cells with foci of hemosiderin deposition typically present
- 3 types of cells: Spindle cells with slight to moderate atypia, large polygonal, bizarre ganglionlike cells with huge inclusion-like nucleoli, and variably sized multivacuolated lipoblastlike cells scattered singly or in nodular aggregates

Special Stains

- Stains for bacteria, fungal elements, and mycobacteria negative (help to rule out an infectious process)

Immunohistochemistry

- Tumor cells always positive for vimentin and variably positive for cytokeratin (weak and focal), CD68 (focal and punctate), and CD34; cells do not express leukocyte common antigen, T and B cell markers, or CD30
- Cytomegalovirus and Epstein-Barr virus not present by either immunohistochemistry or polymerase chain reaction (PCR)

Electron Microscopy

- All cell types show features of fibroblasts
- Lipoblastlike cells have cytoplasmic pseudoinclusions of mucinous material

Differential Diagnosis

- Pigmented villonodular synovitis
- Reaction to an infectious agent
- Lymphoma

Treatment

- Wide local excision or amputation

Prognosis

- Local recurrence in 20%
- Regional or distant metastases very rare (<2%)

Associations

- None

Myxofibrosarcoma

Clinical Manifestations

- Very common sarcoma in the elderly (6th to 8th decade)
- Typically occurs in dermal/subcutaneous tissues (65%) or in fascia or skeletal muscle in the extremities (lower more often than upper)
- Still occasionally referred to us as a myxoid malignant fibrous histiocytoma

Gross Pathology

- Superficially located tumors usually multilobulated and solitary
- Deep-seated tumors tend to be single with infiltrating borders
- Gray/white and fleshy; may be myxoid

Microscopic Pathology

- Low-grade lesions typically hypocellular with a multinodular growth pattern and a prominent myxoid matrix of hyaluronic acid; tumor cells are plump, spindled, or stellate with slightly eosinophilic cytoplasm and atypical, enlarged, hyperchromatic nuclei; mitotic figures rare; prominent curvilinear, thin-walled, elongated vessels with a perivascular condensation of tumor cells and inflammatory cells; vacuolated neoplastic fibroblastic cells (pseudolipoblasts) often present
- High-grade lesions typically consist of solid sheets and fascicles of spindled and pleomorphic tumor cells with foci of hemorrhage and necrosis; mitotic figures are numerous and often atypical; bizarre multinucleated giant cells with prominent eosinophilic cytoplasm often present; focal areas of low-grade tumor usually present

Special Stains

- Not helpful

Immunohistochemistry

- Tumor cells positive for vimentin and occasionally for smooth muscle actin and muscle-specific actin (focal myofibroblastic differentiation)
- Histiocytic markers (CD68) negative

Molecular Alterations

- Chromosome numbers in triploid or tetraploid range in most cases
- Ring chromosomes reported

Differential Diagnosis

- Pleomorphic malignant fibrous histiocytoma
- Myxoid chondrosarcoma
- Liposarcoma (myxoid and pleomorphic types)
- Leiomyosarcoma with myxoid stroma
- Metastatic myxoid carcinoma
- Nodular fasciitis

Treatment

- Complete surgical excision (deep tumors tend to infiltrate along fascial planes and between muscle fibers)

Prognosis

- A better prognosis than the more typical storiform/pleomorphic MFH; recurrence rate 65%; metastatic rate 25% (both recurrence rate and mortality higher in high-grade, deep-seated tumors)
- Low-grade lesions may become higher grade in subsequent recurrences

Associations

- None

Comment

- Myxoid MFH (currently called a myxoid fibrosarcoma), once thought to be a specific type of MFH, is now considered to be distinctive and discrete entity

Nodular Fasciitis

Clinical Manifestations

- Typically affects young adults (males and females equally) with a peak incidence at 40 years (20 to 50 years); rare over age of 60 years
- Most commonly occurs on the upper extremities (flexor aspect of forearms), trunk, neck, face, and shoulder
- Tends to be small (2-3 cm) with a history of rapid growth (much more rapid than the usual sarcoma)
- 50% are painful
- Occasional history of trauma to the area

Gross Pathology

- Typically located immediately superficial to muscle layer in what appears to be the fascial layer and usually involves the subcutis, but may be localized to fascia or dermis, or involve underlying skeletal muscle
- Usually round to oval and well-circumscribed, but with an infiltrative margin, giving it a malignant gross appearance
- Cut surface tan to gray and myxoid, mucoid, or fibrous

Microscopic Pathology

- Proliferating cells are bland immature fibroblasts arranged in short S-shaped or C-shaped bundles or fascicles that may intersect (storiform pattern); cells typically have large, uniform, vesicular, and spindled nuclei with prominent nucleoli and abundant, pale eosinophilic or basophilic cytoplasm
- Irregular pools of stromal mucin frequently present and give the tumor the appearance of being "torn" or of having a "feathery" background
- Vessels tend to be small and thin-walled and often have a branching pattern
- Lymphocyte and macrophage infiltration and extravasated red blood cells are all typically present; scattered mast cells, plasma cells, neutrophils, and osteoclast-like giant cells may also be present
- Mitotic figures are common (average one per hpf); no atypical mitotic figures
- Focal areas of metaplastic bone formation may be present
- Longstanding lesions typically have variable amounts of thick hyaline bands between fibroblasts ("keloidlike" collagen)

Variants

- Intravascular fasciitis
  - Involves small or medium sized arteries and/or veins
  - Tends to occur in children and young adults
- Cranial fasciitis
  - Grows rapidly and occurs predominantly in infants during the 1st year of life
  - Involves soft tissue of scalp and underlying skull (may penetrate the skull and involve the leptomeninges)
  - May result from birth trauma
- Ossifying fasciitis
  - Similar to myositis ossificans but without zonal pattern
  - Occurs near periosteum
- Proliferative fasciitis
  - Much less common than nodular fasciitis
  - Proximal extremities most frequently affected
  - Primarily occurs in adults over the age of 50
  - Mainly involves the interlobular fibrous tissue septa of the subcutis (tends to be more well-demarcated than nodular fasciitis)
  - Classic microscopic finding is the presence of large, polygonal, eosinophilic ganglion cell-like myofibroblasts scattered in a variably myxoid or collagenized stroma

Special Stains

- □ Alcian blue stains mucopolysaccharides of myxoid matrix
- □ Spindle cells are fuchsinophilic when stained with trichrome

Immunohistochemistry

- Proliferating spindle cells stain positively for vimentin, smooth muscle actin, and muscle specific actin and stain negatively for desmin and S-100 protein

Electron Microscopy

- Features typical of myofibroblasts (long bipolar cells with abundant rough endoplasmic reticulum and intracytoplasmic microfilaments)
- No evidence of smooth muscle differentiation

Molecular Alterations

- Diploid

Differential Diagnosis

- Nodular fasciitis most frequent benign mesenchymal tumor to be misdiagnosed as sarcoma
- Fibromatosis
- Low-grade fibrosarcoma
- Benign fibrous histiocytoma (subcutaneous and deep)
- Myxoma
- Myxoid MFH

Treatment

- Local excision (recurrence rate 1%-2%)

Prognosis

- Benign; spontaneous regression may occur

Associations

- Not a true neoplasm (considered a "pseudosarcoma")
- A self-limiting, reactive process

Lipomatous Tumors

Hibernoma

Clinical Manifestations

- Tends to occur in subcutis of the scapular region, mediastinum, chest wall, back, thigh, popliteal fossa and axillary and inguinal regions of young adults (median age ~25 years)
- Typically slow growing and painless

Gross Pathology

- Usually well-defined and soft
- Cut surface has yellow to orange to brown color

Microscopic Pathology

- A lobular pattern of variably differentiated round to oval cells with centrally located nuclei and granular to multivacuolated eosinophilic cytoplasm; cell membrane quite distinct
- Typical lipocytes found throughout
- Prominent vascularity (responsible for typical brown color)
- Lipofuscin typically present in cytoplasm
- 6 variants: granular/eosinophilic, pale, mixed, "lipoma-like," myxoid, and spindle cell

Special Stains

- Lipid droplets positive on oil red O stain
- PAS-positive cytoplasm at periphery of neoplasm

Immunohistochemistry

- Cells variably, sometimes strongly, positive for S-100 protein

Electron Microscopy

- Multivacuolated cells filled with mitochondria with parallel cristae, pinocytotic vesicles, and variable numbers of lipid droplets

Molecular Alterations

- Translocation involving 11q13 and 10q22

Differential Diagnosis

- Adult rhabdomyoma
- Granular cell tumor
- Round cell liposarcoma

Treatment and Prognosis

- Local excision curative
- No reports of malignant behavior

Associations

- May be mixed with ordinary lipoma (probably more common than pure hibernoma)
- Pheochromocytoma

Lipoblastoma and Lipoblastomatosis

Clinical Manifestations

- Typically occurs in children under the age of 3 years; may be present at birth
- Boys affected twice as often as girls
- May be localized and subcutaneous (*lipoblastoma*) or diffuse and infiltrating (*lipoblastomatosis*)
- Lipoblastomas typically involve extremities; lipoblastomatosis more likely to be in a deeper location (skeletal muscle, retroperitoneum, or mesentery)
- Painless

Gross Pathology

- Soft and lobulated
- Cut surface pale and myxoid or gelatinous

Microscopic Pathology

- Typically irregular lobules of immature fat composed of stellate spindle cells, vacuolated (single or multiple) lipoblasts in various stages of development, hibernoma-like areas, and mature fat cells in a myxoid intercellular material that contains a plexiform vascular network
- Degree of fat cell maturation quite variable and inversely proportional to amount of myxoid matrix
- Lobular architecture results from variably sized fibrous septa
- Mast cells and extramedullary hematopoiesis may be present

Special Stains

- Not helpful

Immunohistochemistry

- None

Electron Microscopy

- Immature mesenchymal cells to multivacuolated lipoblasts and lipocytes
- Pinocytotic vesicles present along plasma membrane

Molecular Alterations

- Associated with rearrangements of 8q11-13

Differential Diagnosis

- Myxoid liposarcoma-lipoblastoma, lipoblastomatosis, and paucicellular myxoid liposarcoma usually indistinguishable (lipoblastoma and lipoblastomosis typically more cellular than myxoid liposarcoma; myxoid liposarcoma rare before the age of 20 years; lobulation usually more prominent in lipoblastoma and lipoblastomatosis than in myxoid liposarcoma)
- Lipoma
- Lipomatosis
- Spindle cell lipoma

Treatment

- Local excision for lipoblastoma and wide local excision for lipoblastomatosis

Prognosis

- Excellent
- Recurrence more common in patients with lipoblastomatosis than lipoblastoma

Associations

- Sequential biopsies of a lipoblastoma show that in time the lipoblasts will mature into adult-type adipocytes

Lipoma

Clinical Manifestations

- Most common soft tissue tumor
- Slightly more common in men than women
- Can arise in any location where adipose tissue is present
- Most occur in upper half of the body, primarily trunk and neck
- Usually painless
- Most are subcutaneous but may be intramuscular (trunk) and intermuscular (anterior abdominal wall)
- Tends to occur during the 5th or 6th decade; rare before age of 20 years
- May be multiple

Gross Pathology

- When superficial, tends to be encapsulated and occurs in upper back, neck, shoulder and abdominal wall
- When deep, tends to be poorly circumscribed
- Typically lobulated with or without a fibrous capsule
- Usually pale yellow with vaguely lobular pattern

Microscopic Pathology

- Consists of mature adipose tissue without cellular atypia
- Fat cells vary in size and shape and have uniform, band nuclei
- Focal areas of fat necrosis, infarct and calcification may be present
- Thin fibrous septa
- Always well-vascularized, but vascularity very inconspicuous

Variants

- *Fibrolipoma*
  - Prominent bundles of mature fibrous tissue traverse mature fat lobules
  - Lacks the vascular pattern and thick collagen bundles that characterize a spindle cell lipoma which it resembles
- *Myxolipoma*
  - Focally well-developed myxoid changes
  - May be overdiagnosed as myxoid liposarcoma
- *Chondroid lipoma*
  - Usually in subcutis or muscle of extremities
  - Characterized by lobules of nests and cords of eosinophilic, uni- and multivacuolated lipoblasts that contain glycogen and lipid and resemble brown fat cells, embedded in a prominent myxoid to hyalinized chondroid matrix
  - Cells typically immunoreactive for vimentin, S-100 protein, and CD68
  - May have foci of mature metaplastic cartilage
- *Myolipoma*
  - May be in subcutis or deep; also occurs in abdomen and retroperitoneum
  - An admixture of mature adipose tissue and fascicles of well-differentiated smooth muscle
- *Spindle cell lipoma*
  - Typically located in the regions of the shoulder and posterior neck of men older than 40 years
  - On gross examination, resembles a typical lipoma except for the presence of mucoid foci
  - An admixture of mature adipose and uniform spindle cells in a mucinous background and associated with thick "ropelike" collagen bundles
  - Spindle cells resemble cells of a neurofibroma with wavy, streaming nuclei
  - A prominent plexiform vascular pattern may be present
- *Pleomorphic lipoma*
  - Typically located in the regions of the shoulder and posterior neck of men of about 45 years
  - Fibrous septae with abundant collagen traverse neoplasm and contain hyperchromatic, multinucleated "floret-like" cells (pedals of a flower)
  - Occasionally lipoblastlike cells and atypical mitotic figures are present
- *Angiolipoma*
  - Typically located in the subcutis of the trunk or extremities (forearm most common site) and present as multiple painful nodules shortly after puberty
  - Branching, small vessels with hyaline thrombi divide adipose into nodules, vascularity more prominent beneath fibrous capsule
  - Degree of vascularity unrelated to the amount of pain
  - If vascular component predominant, it may be confused with Kaposi sarcoma or angiosarcoma

Special Stains

- Alcian blue stains mucoid component of myxolipoma
- Vacuolated cells of chondroid lipoma stain with PAS

Immunohistochemistry

- Cytoplasmic rim of fat cells positive for S-100 protein
- Smooth muscle of myolipoma positive for smooth muscle actin and desmin
- Both spindle cell lipoma and pleomorphic lipoma are CD34 positive

Electron Microscopy

- Mature lipocytes with central large lipid vacuole and peripheral cytoplasm and nucleus

Molecular Alterations

- 80% of solitary lipomas have chromosomal aberrations affecting 12q (translocation 12q13-15), 6p (rearrangement involving 6p21-23), and 13q (interstitial deletion)
- Multiple lipomas typically have a normal karyotype
- Spindle cell and pleomorphic lipomas have aberrations of chromosome 16q13
- No known chromosomal abnormalities associated with angiolipoma

Differential Diagnosis

- Fibrolipoma
    - Spindle cell lipoma
- Myxolipoma
    - Myxoid liposarcoma
    - Myxoma
- Chondroid lipoma
    - Liposarcoma
    - Myxoid chondrosarcoma
- Myolipoma
    - Angiomyolipoma
    - Leiomyoma
    - Leiomyosarcoma
    - Liposarcoma with smooth muscle differentiation
- Spindle cell lipoma
    - Myxoma and myxolipoma
    - Spindle cell liposarcoma
    - Myxofibrosarcoma
    - Myxoid malignant fibrous histiocytoma
- Pleomorphic lipoma
    - Sclerosing WD liposarcoma
    - Pleomorphic liposarcoma
    - Pleomorphic malignant fibrous histiocytoma
- Angiolipoma
    - Kaposi sarcoma
    - Angiosarcoma
    - Lipoma
    - Spindle cell lipoma

Treatment

- Local excision

Prognosis

- Recurrence rate <5%
- Deep lesions tend to recur more frequently (harder to remove)

Associations

- Solitary lipoma:
    - Obesity
    - Diabetes mellitus and hypercholesterolemia
    - Multiple endocrine neoplasia
    - GI lipomas may cause ulceration and bleeding, intussusception and may be seen in Crohn disease and malignancy
- Multiple lipomas:
    - Bannayan-Zonana syndrome: Multiple lipomas, hemangiomas, and microcephaly
    - Cowden syndrome: Multiple lipomas; hemangiomas; nodular hyperplasia of thyroid (goiter); and lichenoid, papular, and papillomatous lesions of skin and mucosa
    - Fröhlich syndrome: Multiple lipomas, obesity, and sexual infantilism
    - Proteus syndrome: Multiple lipomas, fibroplasia of hands and feet, skeletal hypertrophy, bony exostoses, scoliosis, and linear verrucous epidermal nevi

Liposarcoma

Clinical Manifestations

- Peak incidence between the ages of 40 and 60 years
- More common in men than in women
- 2nd most common soft tissue sarcoma in adults
- Most common retroperitoneal soft tissue tumor (retroperitoneal liposarcoma is more common in women than in men)
- Most commonly occur in the lower extremity (popliteal fossa and anterior thigh); retroperitoneum (second most common site); less frequent in upper extremities, shoulder, and head and neck
- May arise in breast as a primary neoplasm or in cystosarcoma phylloides
- Usually painless, deep-seated mass

Gross Pathology

- Typically well-circumscribed and lobulated

- Often bright yellow with a distinctly lobulated architecture; small lobules may become detached from the main tumor mass to form satellite tumors
- On cut section, a variety of appearances depending on the amount of mucinous material, lipid, fibrosis, necrosis, and cyst formation; vary in color from almost white to pale yellow to orange

Microscopic Pathology

- Pathognomonic feature is the presence of the lipoblast: A mononuclear or multinucleated cell with cytoplasmic vacuoles of fat; the nucleus may be pushed to the periphery giving the cell a signet-ring configuration or it may remain in the center of the cell and be indented by multiple small vacuoles

Variants

- *Atypical lipomatous tumor/Well-differentiated liposarcoma*
  - On gross examination, resembles ordinary lipoma and when located in the subcutaneous tissue or skeletal muscle, these are referred to as *atypical lipoma* or *atypical intramuscular lipoma*
  - Microscopically, tumor cells vary significantly in size and usually demonstrate nuclear atypia and hyperchromasia; multinucleate stromal cells usually present; hyperchromatic stromal cells tend to congregate in fibrous strands that traverse lobules; lipoblasts may be present *(the presence of lipoblasts does not make, nor is required for a diagnosis of liposarcoma);* 4 morphologic subtypes: 1) adipocytic (lipoma-like), 2) sclerosing 3) inflammatory, and 4) spindle cell; more than 1 type often present in same lesion
  - Adipocytic (lipomalike) is most common and resembles an ordinary lipoma; tumor cells with irregularly shaped, hyperchromatic nuclei often found within fibrous bands or septae that surround irregular lobules of fat
  - Sclerosing type (2nd most common) typically seen in the groin and the retroperitoneum; bizarre stromal cells with marked nuclear hyperchromasia and lipoblasts found in a matrix of dense fibrosis with abundant eosinophilic collagen fibrils
  - Inflammatory type (rare) occurs most frequently in the retroperitoneum; tumor cells are associated with chronic inflammatory cells (lymphocytes and plasma cells) in a background of mature adipose; inflammatory infiltrate may predominate
  - Spindle cell type consists of a bland neural-like spindle cell population in a fibrous and/or myxoid background; an atypical lipomatous component with lipoblasts almost always present
- *Myxoid liposarcoma*
  - Most common type (~50%)
  - Most commonly occurs in the lower extremity in the area of the thigh
  - Microscopically consists of proliferating lipoblasts with few or no mitotic figures in a myxoid matrix, often with cystic spaces filled with granular eosinophilic material, and a prominent anastomosing capillary network (this "chicken-wire" vascular network is the most important diagnostic feature)
  - Lipoblasts found in various stages of differentiation (univacuolated or multivacuolated)
- *Round cell liposarcoma (Poorly differentiated myxoid liposarcoma)*
  - A subset of myxoid liposarcoma
  - Microscopically consists of solid sheets of back-to-back small round tumor cells with a high nuclear-cytoplasmic ratio, distinctly acidophilic cytoplasm, and vesicular nuclei with prominent nucleoli; no intervening myxoid stroma
  - Lipoblasts are rare
  - Mitoses are more common than in myxoid liposarcoma
  - Vascular network much less prominent than in myxoid liposarcoma
- *Pleomorphic liposarcoma*
  - 5% of all liposarcomas
  - Tend to occur on the extremities; less frequent in retroperitoneum
  - May be well circumscribed or infiltrative
  - Characterized by pleomorphic spindle-shaped tumor cells, round cells, and multinucleated giant cells (similar to the cells in an undifferentiated high-grade pleomorphic sarcoma/pleomorphic MFH) admixed with pleomorphic, multivacuolated lipoblasts, with bizarre, hyperchromatic, and scalloped nuclei
  - 2 predominant cell types:
    - Large, spindled, bizarre cells with hyperchromatic, indented nuclei and eosinophilic cytoplasm (areas of these cells may resemble high-grade myxofibrosarcoma)
    - Giant, pleomorphic cells with lipid vacuoles and large (may be huge), scalloped, irregularly shaped, hyperchromatic nuclei (bizarre lipoblasts)

- Intra- and extracellular eosinophilic hyaline droplets or globules frequently present
- Rarely a heavy neutrophilic infiltrate; neutrophils may be found within the cytoplasm of the multinucleated giant cells
- Mitotic activity is much more prevalent than in any other variant of liposarcoma
- Necrosis and hemorrhage directly related to the degree of pleomorphism

- An *epithelioid variant* is characterized by solid, cohesive sheets and clusters of atypical epithelioid cells that have round to oval nuclei with prominent nucleoli, eosinophilic cytoplasm, and distinct cell borders
- *Dedifferentiated liposarcoma*
  - Tumor characterized by the presence of both well-differentiated and poorly differentiated areas
  - Poorly differentiated areas often have the appearance of a pleomorphic malignant fibrous histiocytoma (60%-65%); remainder resemble fibrosarcoma, leiomyosarcoma, or rhabdomyosarcoma
  - Most commonly found in the retroperitoneum and groin
  - The presence of dedifferentiation within the liposarcoma is probably a function of the duration that the tumor has been present

Special Stains

- Mucinous matrix will stain with Alcian blue and colloidal iron
- Intracellular glycogen is diastase sensitive and PAS positive
- Lipid stains typically of little value in light of the paucity of lipid in some liposarcomas

Immunohistochemistry

- Both mature and immature fat cells stain positively for vimentin and S-100 protein (tumor cells of a poorly differentiated liposarcoma are negative for both)
- Some tumor cells stain positively for smooth muscle actin

Electron Microscopy

- Tumor cells resemble developing fat with a range of differentiation from primitive mesenchymal cells to mature lipocytes

Molecular Alterations

- 75% of myxoid liposarcomas have a reciprocal translocation t(12;16) (q13;p11.2)
- Tumor progression is usually accompanied by overexpression of p53
- Well-differentiated and dedifferentiated liposarcomas have a ring chromosome 12 (80%)

Differential Diagnosis

- Atypical lipomatous tumor/Well differentiated liposarcoma:
  - Fat necrosis, myxoid change in benign fat, hibernoma, myxoid liposarcoma, dedifferentiated liposarcoma, and pleomorphic liposarcoma
- Myxoid or round cell liposarcoma:
  - Spindle cell lipoma, hibernoma, angiolipoma, lipoblastoma, intramuscular myxoma, angiomyxoma, myxoid DFSP and myxoid fibrosarcoma
- Pleomorphic liposarcoma:
  - Well-differentiated sclerosing liposarcoma, myxoid fibrosarcoma, pleomorphic malignant fibrous histiocytoma, and dedifferentiated liposarcoma
- Dedifferentiated liposarcoma:
  - pleomorphic malignant fibrous histiocytoma, fibrosarcoma, and pleomorphic liposarcoma

Treatment

- Wide/radical excision
- Amputation has no advantage over radical excision
- Adjuvant postoperative radiation especially valuable for myxoid liposarcomas and incompletely excised tumors

Prognosis

- Size and histologic subtype determine prognosis (myxoid and well-differentiated types tend to recur locally and rarely metastasize; round cell and pleomorphic types often exhibit widespread metastasis)
- 5-year survival rate for myxoid and well-differentiated forms >85%
- 5-year survival rate for round cell and pleomorphic types is 50 - 60%
- 5-year survival rate 45% for retroperitoneal tumors and 70% for tumors in the extremities
- Recurrent or metastatic liposarcomas frequently present as dedifferentiated liposarcomas

Associations

- Reports of antecedent trauma

Lymphatic Tumors

Lymphangioma

Clinical Manifestations

- Most appear to be malformations that arise from lymphatics that do not communicate normally with either lymphatic system or venous system
- Presents as soft mass that may periodically change size
- Most appear during childhood and both sexes affected equally
- 50% are congenital and 90% are present by the time the child reaches the age of 2 years
- *Cutaneous lymphangioma (lymphangioma circumscriptum)*
  - Presents as multiple small vesicles or nodules in localized areas of skin
  - Usually involves skin of proximal limbs, thigh, and buttocks
- *Cavernous lymphangioma*
  - Tend to occur in oral cavity, upper trunk, neck, and inguinal region or may be deep and infiltrate muscle and fascia
- *Cystic hygroma* (a dilated form of cavernous lymphangioma) occurs in neck, axilla, or groin

Gross Pathology

- Vary from well-circumscribed to ill-defined lesions
- Well-circumscribed lesions tend to be of the cystic type; infiltrative or poorly circumscribed lesions tend to be of the cavernous type

Microscopic Pathology

- Anastomosing, thin-walled, dilated, irregular lymphatic channels with variably thick vessel walls that contain disorganized smooth muscle fibers and fibrous connective tissue
- Endothelial lining typically flat and banal
- Cystic spaces and lumens contain proteinaceous fluid with lymphocytes, lipid droplets, and red blood cells
- Lymphoid aggregates may be present in stroma
- *Cutaneous lymphangioma*
  - Composed of small, thin-walled, dilated lymphatic channels located immediately beneath epidermis
  - Overlying skin hyperplastic and pushed up into complex folds
  - Endothelium attenuated
- *Cavernous lymphangioma*
  - Consists of larger lymphatic channels with attenuated endothelium
  - Walls of large lymphatic spaces contain collagen, discontinuous bundles of smooth muscle, and lymphoid aggregates
- Some lymphangiomas have both cystic and cavernous components

Special Stains

- Not helpful

Immunohistochemistry

- Lymphatic endothelium usually positive for factor VIII-associated antigen, CD34, CD31, and occasionally *Ulex europaeus*

Electron Microscopy

- Typically few tight junctions between endothelial cells and absent or disrupted basal lamina (also features of hemangiomatous lesions)

Molecular Alterations

- Cystic hygroma associated with cytogenetic abnormalities of Turner syndrome (45,XO or 46,XO/46,XX)

Differential Diagnosis

- *Cavernous lymphangioma*
  - Multicystic mesothelioma
  - Microcystic adenoma of the pancreas
  - Hemangioma (especially cavernous)

Treatment

- Surgery modified by location of the lesion and the importance of achieving an acceptable cosmetic result
- Cystic lymphangiomas are more circumscribed and hence easier to remove than cavernous hemangiomas that tend to be more infiltrative

Prognosis

- A totally benign condition; prognosis primarily determined by site and extent
- Malignant transformation reported after radiation treatment

Associations

- Cystic lymphangioma (cystic hygroma)
  - Turner syndrome
  - Hydrops fetalis
  - Noonan syndrome (heard defects, webbed necl, "trident"hairline, typical facial abnormalities
  - Familial pterygium colli
  - Fetal alcohol syndrome
- Lymphangiomas occur with hemangiomas in Maffucci syndrome

Lymphangiomatosis

Clinical Manifestations

- Visceral form consists of a diffuse or a multifocal involvement of parenchymal organs (especially lung) by lymphangiomas
- Patients with pulmonary or pleural lesions are usually dyspneic secondary to chylothorax
- May involve bone and skin
- When confined to somatic soft tissue tends to affect infants and children (males more frequently than females); patients present with boggy swelling of a portion or all of a limb
- 50% to 75% of patients have multiple, asymptomatic osteolytic bone lesions

Gross Pathology

- A soft cystic or multicystic mass that may or may not be well-circumscribed

Microscopic Pathology

- Anastomosing, thin-walled, bland lymphatic channels with variably thick walls that may contain disorganized smooth muscle fibers and fibrous connective tissue
- Channels lined by attenuated endothelium ramify and dissect throughout skin, subcutis and normal structures leaving islands of normal tissue "hanging in midair"
- Channels tend to be empty or contain small amounts of proteinaceous fluid
- Lymphoid aggregates scattered throughout a delicate collagenous stroma
- Typically an infiltrative appearance (suggestive of malignancy)
- Stromal hemosiderin (without hemorrhage) may be present

Special Stains

- Not helpful

Immunohistochemistry

- Lymphatic cells are positive for factor VIII-associated antigen and CD31, and sometimes *Ulex europaeus;* focally positive for CD34

Electron Microscopy

- Typically few tight junctions between endothelial cells and absent or disrupted basal lamina (also features of hemangiomatous lesions)

Molecular Alterations

- None

Differential Diagnosis

- Angiomatosis (distinction may not be possible)
- Multicystic mesothelioma
- Involvement of the bone may be confused with fibrous dyplasia or bone changes secondary to hyperparathyroidism
- Well-differentiated angiosarcoma

Treatment

- Surgical excision if localized

Prognosis

- Involvement of liver, spleen, lung, or thoracic duct usually results in a poor prognosis as a result of the extent of disease and inability to obtain adequate surgical excision
- Prognosis for skeletal disease is quite excellent; lesions tend to stabilize; involvement of the vertebra may cause cord compression

Associations

- None

Lymphangiomyoma and Lymphangiomyomatosis

Clinical Manifestations

- A localized or diffuse proliferation of smooth muscle in lymphatics of lungs, thoracic duct, and/or mediastinal and retroperitoneal lymph nodes

- 2 forms of the disease: Localized and diffuse (localized form called *lymphangiomyoma*; diffuse form called *lymphangiomyomatosis*)
- Exclusively involves reproductive age (mean 40 years) women many of whom have taken birth control pills
- Patients typically complain of shortness of breath (secondary to chylous pleural effusion or pulmonary involvement); other signs or symptoms include pneumothorax, hemoptysis, ascites, abdominal pain, and chyluria

Gross Pathology

- A gray-white or red spongy mass that may replace the thoracic duct and/or mediastinal lymph nodes
- Chylous effusion typically present
- Lung involvement characterized by a honeycomb appearance with blebs and/or bullae

Microscopic Pathology

- A proliferation of disorganized smooth muscle in lymphatics and lymph nodes of mediastinum, retroperitoneum, and lung
- Muscle cells arranged in short fascicles around a ramifying network of endothelial lined spaces
- Individual cells characterized by abundant eosinophilic cytoplasm and uniform, banal nuclei; no mitotic figures
- Lymphoid aggregates may present between muscle cells
- Eosinophilic proteinaceous fluid with or without lymphocytes and lipid droplets typically present in lymphatic spaces
- Pulmonary involvement characterized by fascicles of disorganized smooth muscle that surround angiolymphatic structures and fill or partially fill alveolar system

Special Stains

- Trichrome stain will highlight the proliferating smooth muscle cells

Immunohistochemistry

- Immunohistochemical staining pattern is similar to that of angiomyolipoma, a neoplasm associated with tuberous sclerosis complex (both are HMB-45 positive)
- Smooth muscle cells positive for smooth muscle actin and usually desmin
- Pulmonary tissue may be both estrogen and progesterone receptor positive

Electron Microscopy

- Smooth muscle cells contain electron dense granules with a lamellar substructure, which may be responsible for the immunoreactivity for HMB-45

Molecular Alterations

- None

Differential Diagnosis

- Lymphangiomatosis
- Benign metastasizing leiomyoma
- Metastatic leiomyosarcoma

Treatment

- Localized disease can be treated surgically
- Good therapeutic results with medroxyprogesterone therapy and/or oophorectomy
- Low-dose irradiation

Prognosis

- Pulmonary involvement typically results in death within 1 to 10 years from progressive pulmonary insufficiency

Associations

- Tuberous sclerosis complex
- Lymphangiomyomatosis is not inherited, is not associated with CNS lesions and is never seen in men (all features of tuberous sclerosis)
  - 15% of patients with lymphangiomyomatosis have renal angiomyolipomas (angiomyolipoma present in 80% of patients with tuberous sclerosis)
  - 1% of patients with tuberous sclerosis have pulmonary changes of lymphangiomyomatosis
- Lymphangiomyomatosis belongs to a family of perivascular epithelioid tumors (PEComas) that coexpress muscle and melanocytic markers. Other tumors in the PEComa family include angiomyolipoma, clear cell "sugar" tumor of lung, clear cell myomelanocytic tumor of the falciform ligament/ligamentum teres, and unusual clear cell tumors of the pancreas, rectum, abdominal serosa, uterus, vulva, proximal lowere extremity, and heart

Lymphangiosarcoma

Clinical Manifestations

- Typically arises in clinical setting of chronic lymphedema (upper and lower extremity); usually affecting the breast or upper extremity following mastectomy and extensive axillary dissection (referred to as *Stewart-Treves syndrome*) and is indistinguishable from angiosarcoma

Gross Pathology

- Typically a blue or purple elevation in edematous skin
- Frequently multiple

Microscopic Pathology

- Histologically almost indistinguishable from angiosarcoma with areas of freely anastomosing capillary-sized vascular channels lined by atypical endothelial cells that infiltrate adjacent soft tissue and skin
- Lumina may be empty or contain proteinaceous fluid, lymphocytes, or red blood cells

Special Stains

- Not helpful

Immunohistochemistry

- Typically tumor cells are positive for CD31 (platelet-endothelial cell adhesion molecule; very specific) and CD34 (human hematopoietic progenitor cell antigen; less specific)
- Angiosarcomas of soft tissue often coexpress cytokeratin and EMA and are more likely to express von Willebrand factor than more conventional lesions

Electron Microscopy

- Ultrastructure study unable to determine if lesion is a lymphangiomatous neoplasm or a hemangiomatous neoplasm

Molecular Alterations

- A variety of nonclonal deletions and translocations

Differential Diagnosis

- Distinction between angiosarcoma and lymphangiosarcoma is often impossible and hence arbitrary. The differential diagnosis for a "lymphangiosarcoma" is the same as for an angiosarcoma

Treatment

- Radical surgery and/or chemotherapy

Prognosis

- Similar to that of angiosarcoma

Associations

- See section on angiosarcoma

Myogenic Tumors

Leiomyoma

Clinical Manifestations

- Relatively common in the genital, urinary, and GI tracts
- Typically a tumor of adults (regardless of location)

Gross Pathology

- Typically sharply circumscribed and firm with a yellow to yellow-pink whorled cut surface

Variants

- *Cutaneous leiomyoma (leiomyoma cutis)*
  - Leiomyoma of pilar erector muscle origin
  - May be solitary or multiple
  - Typically develops as a small brown-red to gray, discrete papule on the extensor surfaces of the extremities during adolescence or early adult life
  - Frequently produces pain on exposure to cold (nitroglycerine used to treat pain)
  - Typically lies within the connective tissue of the dermis; overlying epidermis is atrophic and a *Grenz* zone separates the tumor from the epidermis
  - Tumor cells are spindled, eosinophilic, have longitudinal myofibrils and uniform, oval, blunt-ended nuclei and are arranged in interlacing fascicles; tends to blend with surrounding collagen and pilar muscle
- *Genital leiomyomas*
  - Typically solitary and painless
  - Occur in the nipple, areola, scrotum, labia, and penis
  - More circumscribed, more cellular, and more variation in microscopic appearance than pilar leiomyomas

- *Angiomyoma (vascular leiomyoma)*
  - More frequent in women than in men (unless in the oral cavity)
  - Usually located in the subcutis of the lower extremities
  - Typically painful; pain worse with cold, pregnancy or menses
  - Microscopically consists of well-circumscribed nodule consisting of bundles of smooth muscle which originate from medium-sized blood vessels that lack elastic fibers; thick-walled blood vessels are present throughout
  - Vessel(s) of origin typically have orderly circumferentially arranged inner smooth muscle and a disorderly outer layer of smooth muscle that blend with smooth muscle tissue of the tumor
  - Myxoid change, hyalinization, calcification and fat may be present
  - Morphologically subdivided into capillary (solid), cavernous, and venous subtypes
- *Leiomyoma of deep soft tissue*
  - A rare lesion that occurs in adults
  - Typically involves the deep muscle of the extremities, abdominal cavity and retroperitoneum
  - A gray-white well-circumscribed mass of well-differentiated smooth muscle arranged in interlacing fascicles; mitoses absent
  - Paranuclear glycogen vacuoles may be present (variable); fibrosis, hyalinization, calcification, and myxoid change variably present (represent regressive change)
- *Intravenous leiomyomatosis*
  - An intravascular growth of benign smooth muscle within the uterine or pelvic veins that represent vascular invasion from an uterine leiomyoma or may arise de novo within the a vessel
  - Seen primarily in premenopausal middle-aged women many of whom have been pregnant
  - On gross examination, a coiled mass in the myometrium that occasionally extends into uterine veins and beyond
  - Microscopically consists of an intravascular growth of variably cellular smooth muscle cells with round to oval nuclei that occasionally have clear cytoplasm; mitoses are rare; thick-walled vessels are present in "plugs" of intravascular smooth muscle (a vessel within a vessel)
- *Leiomyomatosis peritonealis disseminata*
  - A subserosal proliferation of smooth muscle nodules disseminated throughout the peritoneal cavity
  - Frequently found as an incidental finding in pregnant black women
  - May arise from fibroblasts and myofibroblasts of the peritoneum that have been induced to differentiate into smooth muscle and decidualized cells by hormones (lesions will regress with estrogen and progesterone suppression, but recur with subsequent pregnancy)
  - Microscopically well-oriented fascicles of mature smooth muscle; rounded decidual cells typically scattered amongst the smooth muscle cells; mitoses rare; no hemorrhage or necrosis; some pleomorphism

Special Stains

- Masson trichrome will stain myofibrils within tumor cells
- PAS will stain basal lamina and small connective tissue fibers surrounding individual smooth muscle cells

Immunohistochemistry

- Smooth muscle actin, desmin, and vimentin positive; S-100 protein negative

Electron Microscopy

- Majority of cells resemble mature smooth muscle and are characterized by the presence of mitochondria, rough endoplasmic reticulum, and ribosomes all located near the nucleus, pinocytotic vesicles and longitudinally oriented myofilaments make up the remainder of the cytoplasm; delicate basal lamina separates cells

Molecular Alterations

- Leiomyoma of pilar erector origin may be inherited as an autosomal dominant trait

Differential Diagnosis

- Cutaneous:
  - Fibrous histiocytoma (dermatofibroma), hamartoma or choristoma, and leiomyosarcoma
- Deep:
  - Fibrous histiocytoma and leiomyosarcoma
  - If palisading present, may resemble schwannoma
- Angiomyoma:
  - Fibroma, fibrous histiocytoma, and leiomyosarcoma

- Intravenous:
  - Benign metastasizing leiomyoma or leiomyosarcoma
- Leiomyomatosis peritonealis disseminata:
  - Decidual reaction, leiomyosarcoma, and mesothelioma

Treatment

- Local excision; cutaneous leiomyoma difficult to treat surgically because they are usually multifocal (recurrence rate ~50%)
- Nitroglycerine, phenoxybenzamine, and hyoscine hydrobromide used to manage pain of cutaneous lesions

Prognosis

- Benign
- Reports of intravenous leiomyomatosis extending into the inferior vena cava, right atrium, and pulmonary veins
- No evidence of malignant transformation

Associations

- Multiple cutaneous leiomyomata of pilar erector origin may be associated with dermatitis herpetiformis and HLA-B8, premature uterine leiomyomas, increased erythropoietin activity, and multiple endocrine neoplasia (MEN) type 1

Leiomyosarcoma

Clinical Manifestations

- Accounts for 5 to 10% of soft tissue sarcomas
- Typically occurs in adults
- More common in women than in men (especially if located in the retroperitoneum or arise from vena cava or large veins of the lower extremity); smooth muscle growth in women stimulated by pregnancy and estrogen
- May arise in nonretroperitoneal soft tissue (usually lower extremity of men)
- Has been associated with the production of β-human chorionic gonadotrophin

Gross Pathology

- Seems to be well-circumscribed and may have a gray-white whorled appearance with areas of necrosis, hemorrhage, and cystic degeneration

Microscopic Pathology

- Spindled tumor cells with blunt-ended nuclei and eosinophilic fibrillary cytoplasm; cytoplasmic vacuoles often located at both ends of the nucleus (sometimes indenting the nucleus)
- Nuclear pleomorphism and hyperchromatism usually prominent, but may be focal, mild, and even absent; mitotic figures usually readily apparent, but may be focal and scarce
- Tumor cells arranged in a fascicular pattern with bundles intersecting each other at right angles
- Tumor cells seem to merge with blood vessel walls
- Myxoid change and osteoclastlike multinucleated giant cells may be present, but uncommon
- Variants:
  - *Epithelioid leiomyosarcoma (malignant leiomyoblastoma)*
    - Occurs most frequently in the mesentery and omentum; less frequently in the retroperitoneum
    - Characterized by prominent round cells with clear cytoplasm that represent primitive smooth muscle cells that do not have intracytoplasmic desmin or collagen
    - Mitotic figures are present in variable numbers
    - Tumor may metastasize to regional lymph nodes and distant sites; survival after metastasis may be prolonged
  - *Myxoid leiomyosarcoma*
    - Spindled smooth muscle cells in a background consisting of pools of mucin (hyaluronic acid)
    - May be quite hypocellular and appear benign
  - *Inflammatory leiomyosarcoma*
    - Characterized by xanthoma cells and a prominent lymphoid infiltrate (easily mistaken for inflammatory pleomorphic malignant fibrous histiocytoma)
  - *Cutaneous and subcutaneous leiomyosarcoma:*
    - Men affected 2×-3× more frequently than women
    - Typically occurs in the 5th to 7th decades
    - 2 types: intradermal and subcutaneous
    - Tends to involve extensor surfaces of extremities, be solitary, and almost always painful

        - Dermal lesions usually have ill-defined borders and merge with adjacent dermal collagen and pilar erector muscle; often resemble retroperitoneal leiomyosarcomas
    - *Retroperitoneal, intra-abdominal, and deep soft tissue leiomyosarcoma:*
        - Retroperitoneum most common site and commonly involves other adjacent structures
        - Deep soft tissue tumors affect the sexes equally and usually present as a mass in the lower extremity
        - A wide variety of patterns seen microscopically; multinucleated giant cells are frequently present; tumor cells elongated with cigar-shaped nuclei and eosinophilic cytoplasm; a vacuole may indent 1 end of nucleus
        - In well-differentiated areas, fascicles of tumor cells tend to intersect at right angles; in other areas a more disorderly pattern reminiscent of a fibrosarcoma may be present
        - Occasionally nuclei will be arranged in palisades similar to the Verocay bodies of a schwannoma
        - Mitotic activity quite variable but always present and usually over 5 per 10 hpfs
    - *Leiomyosarcoma of vascular origin:*
        - More frequent occurrence within large veins than arteries
        - Main vascular sites include inferior vena cava, saphenous, iliac and femoral veins as well as pulmonary artery; very rarely arise in systemic arteries
        - Leiomyosarcomas involving the inferior vena cava usually occur in women and involve the suprahepatic vena cava; leiomyomas arising from other vascular sites affect both sexes equally
        - Tends to be circumscribed, firmly attached to the vessel of origin and have typical leiomyosarcoma features
        - Histologically similar to tumors in the retroperitoneum

Special Stains

- Intracytoplasmic glycogen can be demonstrated with PAS stains; myofibrils with Masson trichrome (deep red) and striations with PTAH (purple)
- Reticulin forms will highlight fine interstitial reticulin fibers in well-differentiated leiomyosarcomas

Immunohistochemistry

- Most are positive for muscle-specific actin and smooth muscle actin
- Reactivity for desmin is variable (50% to 100%)
- Cytokeratin may be positive (as a result of the presence of keratins 8 and 18)
- S-100 protein and EMA sporadically positive

Electron Microscopy

- Tumor cells have many of the same characteristics as normal smooth muscle cells but tend to be less well developed
- Pinocytotic vesicles and basal lamina are both prominent

Molecular Alterations

- Some deep leiomyosarcomas have deletions in the RB1 locus

Differential Diagnosis

- Retroperitoneal, intra-abdominal, and deep leiomyosarcoma:
    - Fibrosarcoma
    - Malignant peripheral nerve sheath tumor
    - Reactive fibroblastic nodules (postoperative spindle cell nodule, pseudotumor, pseudosarcomatous fibromyxoid tumor)
- Cutaneous and subcutaneous leiomyosarcoma
    - Leiomyoma, synovial sarcoma, monophasic type, fibrosarcoma, pleomorphic malignant fibrous histiocytoma
- Leiomyosarcoma of vascular origin:
    - Leiomyoma, malignant peripheral nerve sheath tumor, synovial sarcoma (monophasic type), fibrosarcoma, pleomorphic malignant fibrous histiocytoma, extraskeletal myxoid chondrosarcoma, and postoperative spindle cell nodule

Treatment

- Radical excision if possible (tumor frequently too large for resection if located in other than cutaneous or subcutaneous site)

Prognosis

- Tumors in the deep soft tissue of the extremities have a better prognosis than those arising in the retroperitoneum (the latter tend to be aggressive and are usually unresectable)
- Tumor necrosis may be associated with a poor prognosis
- Leiomyosarcomas of vascular origin tend to metastasize and have a poor prognosis

Associations

- Estrogen receptors have been found in some neoplasms
- Leiomyosarcoma may be a 2nd neoplasm in patients with bilateral (hereditary) retinoblastomas
- Cutaneous leiomyosarcomas may develop at site of previous irradiation

Rhabdomyoma

Clinical Manifestations

- Approximately 2% of all skeletal muscle tumors
- Much less common than the malignant counterpart, rhabdomyosarcoma

Gross and Microscopic Pathology

- *Rhabdomyoma of the heart*
  - A hamartomatous lesion
  - Tends to occur in the pediatric age group
  - Typically a multifocal (rarely diffuse) process involving the myocardium of both ventricles and the intraventricular septum
  - May be asymptomatic or cause of arrhythmias, tachycardia, or sudden death
  - Tumors generally well-demarcated from adjacent cardiac muscle
  - Tumor cells are large and vacuolated with little cytoplasm; vacuolation the result glycogen; cells similar to those of adult rhabdomyoma except more vacuolated and larger
  - Occasional spider cells may be scattered throughout; characterized by a centrally located nucleus and surrounded by a rim of cytoplasm with radial extensions (myofibers) to the periphery
  - Spontaneous regression may occur
- *Adult rhabdomyoma*
  - Typically presents as a solitary mass (20% are multifocal) in the region of the head and neck of an adult over the age of 40 years
  - Men more frequently affected than women
  - 65% arise in mucosa of oropharynx, nasopharynx, or larynx; remainder arise from branchial musculature of 3rd and 4th branchial arches
  - Typically asymptomatic but may partially obstruct the pharynx or larynx
  - Usually round or lobulated with a gray-yellow or red, granular cut surface
  - Microscopically consists of distinct lobules of large, rounded or polygonal cells with pink cytoplasm and variable amounts of lipid and glycogen; some cells have features reminiscent of "spider cells" (cells that contain a small central eosinophilic aggregate of cytoplasm that is connected to a rim of cytoplasm at the cell periphery by thin strands); cross-striations and intracytoplasmic rodlike (jackstraws) crystalline inclusions are frequent; no nuclear atypia; no mitotic figures
- *Fetal rhabdomyoma*
  - Tends to be fairly well circumscribed and superficial
  - 25% congenital, 15% occur before 1 year; 45% occur after age 15 years (mean 19 years)
  - Usually solitary and polypoid; may be multicentric
  - 65% arise in soft tissues of face, preauricular and postauricular regions, neck, and periorbital area; remainder arise in mucosa of nasopharynx, oropharynx, and larynx
  - Microscopic appearance ranges from immature predominantly myxoid tumors *(myxoid type)* to tumors with a high degree of cellular differentiation and very little myxoid matrix (*cellular type*)
  - Myxoid tumors tend to occur in subcutaneous and submucosal areas of the head and neck (particularly pre- and postauricular) in boys under the age of 3 years and consist of oval or spindled cells with indistinct cytoplasm admixed with muscle fibers in a very myxoid stroma
  - Cellular tumors tend to occur in head and neck region (orbit, tongue, nasopharynx, and soft palate) of adults (men more frequently affected than women) and have many differentiated muscle fibers, few spindled cells, and almost no myxoid matrix
  - A special variant is associated with peripheral nerve (*benign Triton tumor*)
  - Mitotic figures are rare
- *Genital rhabdomyoma*
  - Typically present as a slowly growing polypoid mass or cyst in the vagina or vulva of young or middle-aged women
  - Most are asymptomatic, but may cause dyspareunia
  - Microscopically, mature, broad, round or straplike skeletal muscle cells with distinct cross-striations in a fibrous stroma containing dilated vascular channels

Special Stains

- PTAH and trichrome stains will highlight cross-striations and intracellular crystalline structures
- PAS will highlight the presence of intracellular glycogen

Immunohistochemistry

- Tumor cells of adult rhabdomyoma immunoreactive for desmin, myoglobin, muscle-specific actin, and myosin
- Some cells stain for CD56, CD57, S-100 protein, and smooth muscle actin
- 40% of fetal tumors will stain for glial fibrillary protein (GFAP)
- Tumor cells of a genital rhabdomyoma positive for muscle-specific actin, myoglobin, and desmin; negative for smooth muscle actin, cytokeratin, S-100 protein, GFAP, EMA, and CD68

Electron Microscopy

- Adult rhabdomyoma:
    - Cytoplasm with mitochondria, glycogen, myofilaments (both thick and thin) and distinct Z lines (better organized and more prominent in cardiac rhabdomyoma)
- Fetal rhabdomyoma:
    - Differentiated muscle cells have organized bundles of myosin and actin, glycogen, and few mitochondria

Molecular Alterations

- Adult rhabdomyoma
    - Reciprocal translocation of chromosomes 15 and 17
    - Minor abnormality of 10q

Differential Diagnosis

- Adult rhabdomyoma:
    - Granular cell tumor
    - Hibernoma
    - Paraganglioma
    - Rhabdomyosarcoma
    - Reticulohistiocytoma
    - Oncocytoma
- Fetal rhabdomyoma:
    - Embryonal and spindle cell rhabdomyosarcoma
    - Infantile (desmoid-type) fibromatosis
- Genital rhabdomyoma:
    - Benign vaginal polyp
    - Botryoid embryonal rhabdomyosarcoma

Treatment

- Local excision

Prognosis

- Fetal tumors can undergo malignant transformation
- All types have low recurrence rates (recurrence depends on completeness of excision)
- Spontaneous regression may occur in cardiac rhabdomyomas

Associations

- Cardiac rhabdomyomas associated with *tuberous sclerosis*: Subependymal hamartoma and giant cell astrocytoma, cardiac rhabdomyomas, angiomyolipomas, mental retardation, epilepsy, cutaneous hamartomas primarily involving head and neck, shagreen skin, depigmented spots, and subungual fibromas of the fingers
- Multicentric fetal rhabdomyomas may be associated with Gorlin syndrome (*nevoid basal cell carcinoma syndrome*): Development of multiple BCCs early in life, medulloblastoma, hypertelorism, ectopic dural calcification, keratocysts of mandible and maxilla, osseous anomalies, ovarian fibromas, lymphatic mesenteric cysts, and palmar and plantar dyskeratosis (pits)
- No evidence that a fetal rhabdomyoma is a precursor lesion for an adult rhabdomyoma

Rhabdomyosarcoma

Clinical Manifestations

- The most common sarcoma of children and adolescents
- Distinctly unusual in individuals over the age of 45 years
- Anatomic location:
    - Head and neck (45%)
    - Orbit, eyelid, skull (20%)
    - Nasal cavity, nasopharynx, palate, mouth, pharynx (10%-15%)
    - Sinuses, cheek, neck (10%)
    - Ear, mastoid (3%-5%)
    - Trunk (40%)
    - Paratesticular (20%)
    - Retroperitoneum, pelvis (5%-10%)
    - Chest wall, back, flank, abdominal wall (5%-10%)
    - Urinary bladder, prostate (5%)
    - Vagina, vulva (1%)
    - Extremities (15%)
        - Upper (5%-10%)
        - Lower (5%-10%)

Variants

- *Embryonal rhabdomyosarcoma*
  - Most develop during first 2 decades of life
  - Most common malignant soft tissue tumor in childhood
  - 4 subtypes:
  - Embryonal rhabdomyosarcoma, not otherwise specified (NOS):
    - Most common variant (70%-75% of embryonal rhabdomyosarcomas)
    - Typically occurs in children under the age of 15 and usually involves the head and neck region; but may involve the orbit, genitourinary tract, retroperitoneum, and extremities
  - Botryoid rhabdomyosarcoma
    - Approximately 10% of embryonal rhabdomyosarcomas
    - A polypoid grapelike growth pattern
    - Most frequently seen in tumors arising in hollow organs with mucosal surfaces such as the genitourinary tract (80%), head and neck (pharynx, conjunctiva, and auditory canal: 15%), and GI tract
  - Spindle cell rhabdomyosarcoma
    - Approximately 5% of embryonal rhabdomyosarcomas
    - Most (30%-35%) paratesticular; also head and neck (15%) and orbit (12%)
    - Mimics fibrosarcoma and leiomyosarcoma
    - Has the best prognosis of all rhabdomyosarcomas
  - Anaplastic rhabdomyosarcoma
    - 3% to 4% of embryonal rhabdomyosarcomas
    - Most frequently involves lower extremities (25%); also involves paratesticular region, head and neck, retroperitoneum, and pelvis
- *Alveolar rhabdomyosarcoma*
  - 2nd most common type of rhabdomyosarcoma (20%)
  - Tends to occur in individuals between the ages of 2 and 25 years
  - Tends to occur in the same locations as embryonal except for a higher incidence in the extremities
- *Pleomorphic rhabdomyosarcoma*
  - Rarest of all rhabdomyosarcomas (<5%)
  - Typically presents in patients over the age of 40 years
  - Often located deep in lower extremity (especially the thigh)
  - Variant of rhabdomyosarcoma most likely to metastasize (lungs, regional lymph nodes, and bone marrow)

Gross Pathology

- Neoplasms that grow into body cavities tend to be circumscribed, nodular, polypoid, and have a gelatinous cut surface with focal areas of hemorrhage or cyst changes
- Deep-seated tumors that arise in muscle tend to infiltrate adjacent structures and have a firm consistency with a gray to tan, granular, and bulging cut surface with focal areas of necrosis and cystic degeneration

Microscopic Pathology

- *Embryonal rhabdomyosarcoma*:
  - Embryonal rhabdomyosarcoma, NOS, characterized by "small round blue cells" (rhabdomyoblasts) that may be spindled, "strap-shaped," ribbon-shaped, and round with eosinophilic cytoplasm; nuclei may be variable in shape, but are usually hyperchromatic with smooth chromatin and an invisible or small and inconspicuous nucleolus; cells haphazardly arranged in an infiltrative pattern, with alternating hypercellular and myxoid, hypocellular zones; cross-striations seen in 30%; minimal collagen; mitoses vary according to the degree of differentiation; significant pleomorphism rare; approximately 1% contain cells with rhabdoid features
  - Botryoid rhabdomyosarcoma characterized by a polypoid (grapelike) growth pattern with few, scattered, spindled to rounded rhabdomyoblasts in an abundant myxoid matrix; typically there is a subepithelial zone of increased cellularity (cambium layer) separated from the mucosa by a zone of loose stroma (overlying epithelium usually hyperplastic); cross-striations rare
  - Spindle cell rhabdomyosarcoma characterized by elongated, fusiform rhabdomyoblasts with abundant deeply eosinophilic fibrillary cytoplasm and elongated, oval (cigar-shaped) nuclei arranged in a fascicular pattern; few mitoses; abundant interstitial, partly hyalinized collagen separates tumor cells (occasionally there is little interstitial collagen)
  - Anaplastic rhabdomyosarcoma characterized by cells with very hyperchromatic nuclei that are 3 times larger than nuclei of surrounding cells; bizarre mitotic figures and rare cells with skeletal muscle differentiation often present

- *Alveolar rhabdomyosarcoma:*
  - Aggregates of poorly differentiated, small, round or oval tumor cells with deeply eosinophilic cytoplasm separated into discrete nests by fibrous tissue septa; occasional tumors have a clear cell morphology
  - Tumor cells in contact with fibrous septa tend to be well-preserved and firmly attached to septa while cells in the center of the alveolar spaces tend to be less well-preserved (degenerated or necrotic) and "float" as a result of lack of cohesiveness (hence the alveolar or pseudoglandular appearance)
  - Solid variants lack alveolar pattern and resemble round cell areas of an embryonal rhabdomyosarcoma (no fibrosis)
  - Multinucleated giant cells with peripherally placed ("wreathlike") nuclei usually present
- *Pleomorphic rhabdomyosarcoma:*
  - An infiltrative, loose disorderly arrangement of small primitive rhabdomyoblasts and large (sometimes bizarre) pleomorphic cells with hyperchromatic nuclei and intensely eosinophilic cytoplasm
  - Cross-striations extremely rare
  - Very little collagen

Special Stains

- PAS with and without diastase (most rhabdomyosarcomas contain significant amounts of intracellular PAS-positive glycogen)
- Colloid iron and Alcian blue will stain extracellular mucin (which can be removed by hyaluronidase) and will highlight the fibrous septa in alveolar tumors
- Reticulin stains confirm the absence of interstitial collagen
- Differentiated rhabdomyoblasts will stain with Masson trichrome stain, PTAH, and iron hematoxylin

Immunohistochemistry

- Desmin, muscle-specific actin, and myoglobin all positive in proportion to the amount of differentiation in the rhabdomyoblast population
- Myo D1 and myogenin both stain rhabdomyoblasts according to degree of differentiation
- Both undifferentiated and well-differentiated tumors are vimentin positive

Electron Microscopy

- Tumor cells have the appearance of embryonal muscle tissue at various stages of development with a mixture of thick (myosin) and thin (actin) fibrils with distinct Z bands
- Tumor cells have a prominent Golgi apparatus and cytoplasmic glycogen

Molecular Alterations

- Embryonal rhabdomyosarcoma has a loss of heterozygosity for multiple loci at chromosome 11p55 and trisomy 8
- Alveolar rhabdomyosarcoma associated with translocation t(2;13)(q35;q14); this translocation not present in the embryonal variant

Differential Diagnosis

- Embryonal rhabdomyosarcoma, NOS
  - PNET/Ewing sarcoma
  - Lymphoma
  - Desmoplastic small round blue cell tumor
  - Neuroblastoma
- Embryonal rhabdomyosarcoma with rhabdoid features
  - Malignant rhabdoid tumor (cells of a malignant rhabdoid tumor usually have vesicular nuclei and prominent nucleoli; cytoplasm positive for cytokeratin and negative for desmin and muscle-specific actin)
- Botryoid embryonal rhabdomyosarcoma
  - Upper respiratory and genitourinary tract polyps
  - Genital rhabdomyoma
- Spindle cell embryonal rhabdomyosarcoma
  - Leiomyosarcoma
  - Fibrosarcoma
  - Pleomorphic malignant fibrous histiocytoma
  - Myofibroma
  - Infantile fibromatosis
- Anaplastic embryonal rhabdomyosarcoma
  - Pleomorphic rhabdomyosarcoma
- Alveolar rhabdomyosarcoma
  - Alveolar soft part sarcoma (cells of an alveolar soft part sarcoma are larger and the alveoli tend to be more uniform and are separated by delicate fibrous septa with sinusoidal vascular channels)

- Pleomorphic rhabdomyosarcoma:
    - Other rhabdomyosarcoma variants (all of which may have pleomorphic foci, especially anaplastic embryonal)
    - Pleomorphic leiomyosarcoma and pleomorphic malignant fibrous histiocytoma

Treatment

- A combination of surgery, radiation, and chemotherapy

Prognosis

- Tumors with the best prognosis include those that occur in infants and children in the orbital or genitourinary (nonbladder) areas, botryoid or spindle cell types, noninvasive tumors without regional lymph node metastasis, and tumors <5 cm
- Unfavorable prognostic factors include tumors that occur in adults and are located in the head and neck (nonorbital), abdomen, biliary tract, retroperitoneum, or extremities, alveolar and pleomorphic types, size >5 cm, and invasive tumors with regional lymph node involvement
- Metastasizes most frequently to lung (65%), lymph nodes, and bone marrow; metastases present at time of initial diagnosis in approximately 20%

Associations

- None

Neuroectodermal Tumors

Clear Cell Sarcoma (Malignant Melanoma of Soft Parts)

Clinical Manifestations

- Most patients are young adults; peak incidence in the 3rd decade
- Usually deep-seated and arise from tendons and aponeuroses of extremities (especially foot and ankle)
- Women more commonly affected than men
- Patients present with slowly enlarging mass; 50% are painful

Gross Pathology

- Tumor usually firm, circumscribed (unencapsulated), and lobulated or multinodular with a gray-white gritty cut surface and focal areas of hemorrhage, necrosis, or cystic change
- Foci of pigmentation are seen in approximately 20%
- Often attached to tendon or aponeuroses; never attached to skin
- May invade into deep dermis or muscle; rarely involve epidermis

Microscopic Pathology

- Packets or nests of round or spindled cells with clear (glycogen) to eosinophilic cytoplasm arranged in fascicles (reminiscent of a fibrosarcoma) or whorls with delicate or sometimes thick fibrous septa
- Tumor cells are medium-sized to large, round to polygonal to spindled, and have round to oval nuclei with a vesicular chromatin pattern and prominent, basophilic nucleoli; nuclear pleomorphism fairly unusual; cytoplasm clear to lightly eosinophilic to densely eosinophilic
- Multinucleated giant cells with 10 to 15 peripherally oriented nuclei that are similar to the nuclei of other tumor cells are commonly present
- Neoplasm typically contains abundant extracellular and intracellular iron
- Tumor cells may contain melanin (frequently inconspicuous)
- Mitotic figures rare (usually <2 to 3 per 10 hpf)

Special Stains

- PAS stains, with and without diastase, confirm the presence of glycogen in approximately 65% of tumors
- Hemosiderin can be detected with a Fontana stain or Warthin-Starry preparation; helpful in distinguishing hemosiderin from melanin
- Reticulin stains highlight fibrous collagen framework that separates cell packets

Immunohistochemistry

- Tumor cells typically reactive for S-100 protein, HMB-45, and Melan A/MART-1
- NSE and leu-7 may be positive
- Cytokeratin, EMA, desmin, and LCA negative

Electron Microscopy

- Cytoplasm filled with swollen mitochondria, membrane-bound vesicles, ribosomes, and polyribosomes, aggregates of rough endoplasmic reticulum, and melanosomes

Molecular Alterations

- 75% associated with a reciprocal chromosomal translocation t(12;22)(q13;q12)

Differential Diagnosis

- Metastatic melanoma
- Primary desmoplastic or spindle cell melanoma
- Cellular blue nevus
- Synovial sarcoma
- Fibrosarcoma
- MPNST (most problematic)
- Renal cell carcinoma
- Paraganglioma

Treatment

- Radical excision and/or amputation with radiotherapy and multiagent adjuvant chemotherapy
- Regional lymph node dissection if clinically involved

Prognosis

- A highly malignant neoplasm with high likelihood of both multiple local recurrences and distant metastasis (50% metastasize within 5 years)
- Metastasizes to lungs, lymph nodes, and bone (also heart)
- Recurrence or metastasis can occur as long as 10 years after initial therapy
- Size and presence or absence of necrosis most important prognostic features

Associations

- Neoplasm should not be interpreted as a melanoma despite the fact it is often referred to as a *malignant melanoma of soft parts*
- History of trauma at site of tumor in 45% to 50%

Extraskeletal Ewing Sarcoma

Clinical Manifestations

- Men affected slightly more often than women
- Average age 20 years; rarely seen after age 40 years
- Tumor usually presents as a rapidly enlarging, deep-seated mass
- 30% are painful
- Involvement of a peripheral nerve or the spinal column often results in progressive sensory or motor deficits
- Most commonly located in the paravertebral region and chest wall in close association with the vertebra or ribs (50%-65%) and extremities (20%-25%)

Gross Pathology

- Usually multilobulated and soft
- Cut surface tends to be gray to tan with areas of necrosis, cystic degeneration, and/or hemorrhage; calcification unusual

Microscopic Pathology

- Sheets of uniform, monotonous round cells with scant, pale pink, ill-defined cytoplasm arranged in a vaguely nodular pattern with a rich, delicate, inconspicuous vasculature
- Intracytoplasmic glycogen present
- Nuclei are uniform with fine granular chromatin and small nucleoli
- Pleomorphism and pseudorosettes both rare
- Mitotic figures are usually sparse
- Crushed, necrotic cells frequently result in a "filigree" pattern
- Little if any reticulin fibers between tumor cells and essentially no collagen
- Extensive hemorrhage and coagulative necrosis common features

Special Stains

- Reticulin stains confirm the absence of reticulin fibrils between tumor cells while confirming the nodular architecture
- PAS stains with and without diastase confirm the presence of abundant intracellular glycogen

Immunohistochemistry

- A cell membrane protein (p30;32) which is encoded by the MIC2 gene (present on both the X and Y chromosomes) is detected by the antibody HBA71 (CD99)
- Typically positive for vimentin and *bcl*-2
- Tumor cells stain variably for NSE, Leu-7 (CD 57), and synaptophysin
- Tumor cells usually stain negatively for S-100 protein and chromogranin

Electron Microscopy

- Primitive undifferentiated cells with round nuclei and finely granular chromatin
- Cytoplasm typically contains glycogen, small lipid droplets, and neurosecretory granules
- Little or no collagen in the extracellular spaces

Molecular Alterations

- 80% to 90% have reciprocal translocation of the long arm of chromosomes 11 and 22 [t(11;22)(q24;q12)]
- Same chromosomal abnormality is seen in peripheral neuroepithelioma, Askin tumor, and esthesioneuroblastoma
- A similar translocation, t(11;22) (q13;q12), has been seen in intra-abdominal desmoplastic small cell tumor of childhood

Differential Diagnosis

- Ewing sarcoma of bone
- Peripheral neuroepithelioma
- Askin tumor
- Neuroblastoma
- Rhabdomyosarcoma
- Non-Hodgkin lymphoma
- Neuroendocrine carcinoma (Merkel cell tumor and metastatic small cell carcinoma of lung)
- Melanoma
- Granulocytic sarcoma
- Small cell osteosarcoma
- Hemangiopericytoma
- Angiosarcoma
- Hematolymphoid neoplasm

Treatment

- Sequential chemotherapy (doxorubicin hydrochloride, cyclophosphamide, dactinomycin, and vincristine) coupled with limited radical excision with or without adjunctive radiation therapy

Prognosis

- Unfavorable prognostic factors include large size and presence of extensive necrosis
- A second malignant neoplasm may appear after radiotherapy
- Late central nervous system recurrences have been noted after chemotherapy
- 65%-70% survival at 5 years

Associations

- None

Comment

- Ewing sarcoma and PNET may represent a single group of bone and soft tissue tumors within a continuous spectrum of minimal (Ewing) to prominent (PNET) neural differentiation

Granular Cell Tumor

Clinical Manifestations

- Tends to occur in adults in the 4th through 6th decades of life
- Relatively uncommon in children
- More common in women than in men (2:1)
- Several reports indicate African-American patients are more frequently affected than whites
- Typically presents as a solitary painless nodule in the dermis, subcutis, or submucosal tissues; may also be found in smooth muscle or striated muscle
- Classic location is tongue (25%)
- Also seen in breast (5%-15%), larynx (7%), bronchus, esophagus, stomach, appendix, rectum, anus, bile ducts, pancreas, urinary bladder, vulva, uterus, brain, and pituitary gland

Gross Pathology

- Typically solitary, circumscribed, small and hard
- May be multiple (10%-15%)
- Cut surface gray-white to yellow

Microscopic Pathology

- Neoplastic cells are monomorphous, large, and round or polygonal (occasionally spindled) with coarsely granular eosinophilic cytoplasm, distinct cell borders, and a nucleus that tends to be in the center of the cell and is either small and hyperchromatic or large and vesicular; multinucleation, nuclear pleomorphism, prominent nucleoli, and mitotic figures uncommon
- Cells may be arranged in sheets, ribbons, nests, or lobules or may be haphazardly arranged with no particular pattern; marked desmoplasia may be present (especially in older lesions)

- Occasional cells contain ≥1 densely eosinophilic cytoplasmic globules surrounded by a clear halo
- Stromal histiocytes contain refractile eosinophilic lysosomes ("angulate bodies")
- Cells typically closely associated with peripheral nerves
- Aggregates of lymphocytes at periphery of most tumors
- Elastotic change may present in the stroma
- Tumors arising in the dermis or subcutis often associated with acanthosis or pseudoepitheliomatous hyperplasia of the overlying squamous epithelium
- A malignant variant (extremely rare) exists and comprises 1% to 2% of all granular cell tumors (criteria for malignancy include necrosis, spindling, vesicular nuclei with large nucleoli, >2 mitotic figures/10 hpfs, high nuclear-cytoplasmic ratio, and pleomorphism)

Special Stains

- Cytoplasmic granules of tumor cells (phagolysosomes), globules, and angulate bodies strongly positive for PAS with diastase
- Tumor cells have a red-brown color when stained with trichrome
- Tumor cells positive for Luxol fast blue (granules contain large amounts of hydrolytic enzymes, eg, acid phosphatase)
- Silver stains highlight residual remnants of associated peripheral nerve

Immunohistochemistry

- Cells positive for S-100 protein, NSE, laminin, CD68 (Kp1), and some myelin proteins
- Tumor cells negative for neurofilament proteins and GFAP

Electron Microscopy

- Cytoplasmic granules are membrane-bound secondary lysosomes that contain cellular debris; mitochondria, myelin figures, fragmented rough endoplasmic reticulum, and other components of the cell
- Small interstitial histiocytes contain angulated bodies that consist of microtubules, microfilaments and lipid

Molecular Alterations

- None

Differential Diagnosis

- Congenital (gingival) granular cell tumor (congenital epulis); seen exclusively in infants; usually located on labial aspect of dental ridge of upper jaw
- Granular cell leiomyoma
- Malignant granular cell tumor
- Reactive granular cell change in scars or foreign body granulomas
- Rhabdomyoma (adult)
- Hibernoma
- Paraganglioma
- Secondary granular cell change in neoplasms, such as fibrous histiocytoma, leiomyoma, leiomyosarcoma, and angiosarcoma
- Alveolar soft part sarcoma
- Squamous cell carcinoma
- Fibroxanthoma
- Granular cell tumors of breast may be difficult to distinguish from carcinoma

Treatment

- Local excision with tumor free margins

Prognosis

- Benign clinical course
- Local recurrence rare, usually after incomplete excision

Associations

- Cell of origin is probably the Schwann cell
- No association with neurofibromatosis

Malignant Peripheral Nerve Sheath Tumor

Clinical Manifestations

- Most arise from a neurofibroma or de novo in a peripheral nerve; very rarely arise in a schwannoma, ganglioneuroma, ganglioneuroblastoma, or pheochromocytoma
- Incidence of 4% in patients with von Recklinghausen disease; 50% occur in patients with von Recklinghausen disease

- In cases that occur in the setting of von Recklinghausen disease, the average age at diagnosis is 29 years and there is a 4:1 male predominance
- In sporadic cases, the average age at diagnosis is 40 years and women are affected slightly more often than men
- Tend to occur in the trunk (45%), extremities (35%), and head and neck (20%)
- Usually enlarge rapidly and produce pain and/or symptoms of nerve deficit
- Rarely multifocal unless arising in a plexiform neurofibroma

Gross Pathology

- Most arise in association with a major nerve trunk (sciatic nerve, brachial plexus, and sacral plexus)
- A large (>5 cm) fusiform mass within a major nerve; nerve just proximal and distal may be thickened
- On sectioning, a fleshy white or tan surface with focal areas of hemorrhage or necrosis
- Appears well-circumscribed, but often invades adjacent soft tissue and extends intraneurally

Microscopic Pathology

- Histologic pattern most varied of any soft tissue tumor
- Elongated cells with wavy, serpentine, or comma-shaped nuclei arranged in sharply demarcated hypercellular and hypocellular zones
- Cells may be arranged in whorls (rarely), sweeping fascicles, herringbone, storiform, or a patternless pattern
- Common features include geographic palisading necrosis, diffuse necrosis with perivascular sparing of tumor cell cuffs, condensation of tumor cells around vessels, and patchy hyalinization
- Tumor cells have moderate amounts of weakly eosinophilic cytoplasm and hyperchromatic nuclei that are wavy or tapered at 1 end (not blunt)
- 30% contain large, pleomorphic, and multinucleated tumor cells
- Nuclear palisading is very rare
- Tumor may have a hemangiopericytic vascular pattern with staghorn-shaped vessels
- A variety of different heterologous components may be present in 15% to 20%:
  - Rhabdomyoblastic differentiation (*malignant Triton tumor*)
  - Glandular differentiation (benign or malignant glands)
  - Chondroid and/or osseous differentiation (benign or malignant)
  - Malignant epithelioid differentiation (closely resembles carcinoma or melanoma and unless areas of typical MPNST, a nerve trunk, or a neurofibroma are present the diagnosis can be quite difficult)

Special Stains

- Reticulin stains reveal dense pericellular network of reticulin fibers in both spindle cell and pleomorphic lesions

Immunohistochemistry

- No *specific* markers for MPNST, with or without heterologous elements
- 30% to 65% are positive for S-100 protein; S-100 staining pattern tends to be focal and limited to small numbers of cells
- Staining for Leu-7 (CD 57) variable
- Usually negative for GFAP and EMA

Electron Microscopy

- Spindle cells have long branching cytoplasmic processes with microtubules and neurofilaments, interdigitating cell membranes, and a basal lamina
- Matrix contains different types of collagen (long-spacing collagen—Luse bodies)

Molecular Alterations

- Tumors arising in setting of von Recklinghausen disease often have abnormalities involving chromosome 17 (but not the same locus as the NF-1 gene)

Differential Diagnosis

- Cellular schwannoma
- Cellular neurofibroma
- Leiomyosarcoma
- Fibrosarcoma
- Synovial sarcoma (monophasic)
- Hemangiopericytoma
- Clear cell sarcoma (melanoma of soft parts)
- Melanoma, especially spindle cell neurotrophic melanoma

Treatment

- Complete radical surgical excision
- Adjuvant radiation and chemotherapy of questionable value

Prognosis

- Both local recurrence (typically from the cut nerve ends) and distant metastasis (lung most common) are frequent
- Little correlation between microscopic grading and prognosis
- Lesions associated with von Recklinghausen disease (tend to have a higher grade), incomplete excision, and size over 5 cm have a worse prognosis
- Location not a major prognostic factor
- Overall 10-year survival rate approximately 25%

Associations

- von Recklinghausen disease
- Prior irradiation a risk factor (mean latency period of 17 years)
- 15% to 20% have a concurrent or 2nd non-neurogenic tumor

Melanotic Neuroectodermal Tumor of Infancy (Retinal Anlage Tumor, Melanotic Progonoma)

Clinical Manifestations

- Typically occurs in infants <1 year of age
- Classically presents as a mass in upper or lower jaw; also reported in the epididymis, mediastinum, brain, and anterior fontanelle
- Tends to be radiolucent and locally destructive

Gross Pathology

- Cut surface may have various colors from gray to blue-black depending on the amount of melanin present

Microscopic Pathology

- Primitive, nonpigmented neuroblastomalike cells lie within irregular cystic or alveolar spaces lined by primitive, cuboidal, pigmented cells
- A neuropil-like stroma may be associated with the primitive neuroblastomalike cells
- Ganglioneuroma-like foci may be present
- Fibrous stroma between the cysts

Special Stains

- None

Immunohistochemistry

- Cuboidal cells are strongly positive for cytokeratin and melanoma-associated antigen (HMB-45)
- Both the large pigmented cells that line the cystic spaces and the primitive neuroblastoma cells are variably positive for NSE, Leu-7, and synaptophysin

Electron Microscopy

- The large primitive pigmented cells that line the cystic spaces contain both mature and immature melanosomes
- The small primitive neuroblastoma cells contain neurosecretory granules and have cytoplasmic processes

Molecular Alterations

- None

Differential Diagnosis

- Neuroblastoma
- Ganglioneuroblastoma
- PNET
- Melanoma
- Rhabdomyosarcoma

Treatment

- Complete surgical excision

Prognosis

- Generally considered benign, but a 5% to 10% incidence of metastasis
- Recurrence rate may be as high as 50%
- Ability to predict recurrence or metastasis requires flow cytometry

Associations

- Neoplasm may arise from pigmented epithelial cells of neural crest
- Rarely associated with elevated levels of vanillylmandelic acid
- Despite its name there is no reason to compare this tumor to developing retina other than the fact that they both develop from pigmented neuroepithelium

Melanotic Schwannoma

Clinical Manifestations

- Most commonly arise from spinal or autonomic nerves near the midline; also reported to occur in the stomach, bone, and soft tissue
- Almost always seen in adults; usually forth decade
- Typically cause pain and neurologic symptoms involving the affected nerve
- Multiple in 20% (patients with Carney syndrome have a higher incidence of multiplicity)

Gross Pathology

- Typically circumscribed but not encapsulated
- Cut surface usually solid and black-brown to blue-gray

Microscopic Pathology

- Deposits of coarsely clumped or finely granular pigment often obscure cellular detail although focal areas free of pigment are usually present
- Tumor cells are spindled and epithelioid; the former have indistinct cytoplasmic borders giving the neoplasm a syncytial quality similar to that of a typical schwannoma; the latter have well-defined cell borders
- Tumor cell nuclei often have clear intranuclear vacuoles or (pseudo) inclusions (typical of Schwann cells) and are frequently hyperchromatic and have prominent nucleoli
- Scattered multinucleated giant cells often present
- Vague palisading may be present but uncommon
- Ganglion cell differentiation is rarely if ever seen
- Psammoma bodies present in 40% to 50% (*psammomatous melanotic schwannoma*)
- Majority involve alimentary tract
- 50% seen in Carney syndrome and may be multiple (see Associations below)
- 60% have tumor cells with large cytoplasmic inclusions (reminiscent of mature fat)
- Vessels tend to be thin-walled
- Foci of hemorrhage and/or necrosis may be present
- Osseous metaplasia occasionally present at periphery

Special Stains

- Melanin pigment stains positively for Fontana stain and negatively for iron and PAS

Immunohistochemistry

- Tumor cells strongly express S-100 protein, melanoma-associated antigen (HMB-45), and collagen type IV

Electron Microscopy

- Cytoplasm of tumor cells contain a spectrum of melanosomes in different stages of maturation (premelanosomes to melanosomes)
- Tumor cells resemble Schwann cells with elongated, interdigitating cytoplasmic processes

Molecular Alterations

- None

Differential Diagnosis

- Conventional schwannoma
- Pigmented neurofibroma
- Metastatic melanoma

Treatment

- Complete surgical excision

Prognosis

- Generally regarded as a low-grade malignancy (especially after a recurrence) as a result of a tendency for local recurrence as well as an incidence of metastasis of approximately 25%
- Tumors with significant mitotic activity are considered frankly malignant

Associations

- Melanotic schwannoma not seen in association with NF-2
- 50% of psammomatous melanotic schwannomas seen in patients with *Carney syndrome* (other features of Carney syndrome include lentiginous pigmentation [65%], usually involving face; myxoma of the heart [65%] and other sites such as skin [25%] and breast [25%]; endocrine overactivity [10%] that may result in Cushing syndrome [25%] secondary to pigmented multinodular adrenocortical disease; sexual precocity [30%] secondary to large cell calcifying Sertoli cell tumor or steroid cell tumor of testis; blue nevi [10%]; and acromegaly [8%] secondary to pituitary adenoma)

Merkel Cell Carcinoma

Clinical Manifestations

- A neuroendocrine carcinoma of skin
- Occurs primarily in adults and especially the elderly; rare cases reported in children
- Slightly more common in women than men (1.5:1)
- Commonly involves head and neck or the extremities
- Usually presents as a slowly enlarging firm nodule with a pink to purple hue; overlying skin may be ulcerated
- May suddenly and rapidly enlarge

Gross Pathology

- Neoplasm typically located in the dermis; occasionally centered in the subcutaneous tissue
- Overlying epidermis not involved

Microscopic Pathology

- Typically a diffuse arrangement of small, uniform, discohesive, round cells (occasionally ill-defined nodules or trabeculae)
- Tumor cells have scant eosinophilic cytoplasm that appears as a small rim around a round or oval nucleus with fine granular chromatin and a small (occasionally multiple) nucleolus
- Some tumor cells have eccentrically located nuclei and more abundant cytoplasm; round eosinophilic inclusion-like bodies may be present
- Extensive single cell necrosis may be present throughout
- Mitotic figures frequent
- Stroma typically vascular with vascular spaces lined by plump endothelial cells
- Rarely tumors have focal areas of squamous or glandular differentiation or rosette formation

Special Stains

- Tumor cells argyrophilic with the Grimelius reaction (staining is particularly prominent if tissue fixed in Bowen solution)

Immunohistochemistry

- Tumor cells positive for low-molecular-weight keratin (especially cytokeratin 20 which highlights a distinct perinuclear inclusionlike globule), NSE, and neurofilaments (a feature that separates this neoplasm from small cell carcinoma of the lung and other organs, which typically do not contain neurofilaments)
- Tumor cells occasionally positive for chromogranin (<50%) and synaptophysin
- S-100 protein, LCA, and HMB-45 always negative

Electron Microscopy

- Tumor cells are round or dendritic and contain dense-core neurosecretory granules (occasionally arranged beneath the cell membrane), tightly packed perinuclear intermediate filaments (may displace the nucleus), and primitive junctional complexes

Molecular Alterations

- 30% associated with abnormalities of chromosomes 1, 11, and 12

Differential Diagnosis

- Malignant lymphoma
- Metastatic neuroendocrine (oat cell) carcinoma of the lung
- Primary extraskeletal Ewing sarcoma of dermis and subcutis
- Amelanotic melanoma
- Adnexal tumors
- Lymphoepitheliomalike carcinoma

Treatment

- Wide surgical resection (2-3 cm) and regional lymph node dissection with or without adjuvant radiation therapy
- Chemotherapy is appropriate in absence of local control or for metastatic disease
- Irradiation may have a role both prophylactically and as treatment for recurrent or metastatic disease

Prognosis

- Tends to metastasize to regional lymph nodes early
- An aggressive neoplasm that is usually fatal when recurrent or metastatic
- Sites of distant metastatic spread in decreasing frequency: lymph nodes, liver, bone, brain, lung, and skin

Associations

- Occasionally seen in association with both in situ and invasive squamous cell carcinoma, basal cell carcinoma, adnexal carcinoma, and Bowen disease

Neurofibroma

Clinical Manifestations

- Variants:
  - *Localized cutaneous neurofibroma*
    - Most common
    - May be single or multiple and affect dermis and subcutis
    - Painless and quite mobile
    - 90% unassociated with NF-1
  - *Diffuse cutaneous neurofibroma*
    - A superficial variant of neurofibroma that occurs as a solitary mass in children and adolescents
    - 10% associated with NF-1
    - An ill-defined plaquelike thickening of dermis and subcutis in head and neck region
    - Tends to surround dermal adnexal structures and spread along connective tissue septa
  - *Localized intraneural neurofibroma*
    - 2nd most frequent
    - Marked variation in size; <1cm to many centimeters
    - Multiple lesions tend to occur in patients with NF-1
    - May affect any nerve of any size to include autonomic nervous system
  - *Plexiform neurofibroma*
    - Seen almost exclusively in patients with NF-1
    - Involve the same nerves as localized intraneural neurofibroma
  - *Massive soft tissue neurofibroma*
    - Least common
    - Only seen in patients with NF-1
    - Large and diffuse and produce massive enlargement of local soft tissue
    - Tumor widely infiltrates adjacent soft tissue and muscle

Gross Pathology

- Localized cutaneous neurofibroma
  - Appears circumscribed but is not encapsulated
  - Tends to have a soft consistency with a cut surface homogenously gray or tan; no degenerative changes
- Diffuse cutaneous neurofibroma
  - Cut surface yellow-white
- Localized intraneural neurofibroma
  - Causes a fusiform expansion of nerve in which it originates
  - Cut surface translucent and gray to tan
- Plexiform neurofibroma
  - Diffuse enlargement and distortion of involved nerve resulting from haphazard growth both within and occasionally adjacent to a nerve trunk
  - If a plexus of nerves is involved, appearance will be reminiscent of a "bag of worms"; if a medium to large, nonbranching nerve involved, the appearance will be of a ropy cylinder
  - A rubbery consistency and a translucent cut surface

Microscopic Pathology

- Elongated cells consisting of Schwann cells (majority), perineurial-like cells, transitional cells, and fibroblasts with thin wiry acidophilic processes arranged in fascicles, whorls, or a storiform pattern embedded in a mucopolysaccharide-rich matrix
- Neoplastic cells tend to have hyperchromatic serpentine, wavy, or comma-shaped nuclei and are admixed with strands of collagen that has the appearance of "shredded carrots"
- Collagen in localized and diffuse cutaneous neurofibromas and diffuse soft tissue neurofibromas tends to be delicate and wirelike; the collagen of intraneural neurofibromas tends to be coarse and refractile; collagen content of plexiform neurofibromas increases with age (as mucoid content decreases)
- Neoplastic cells diffusely infiltrate nerve and/or soft tissue
- Mast cells frequently present
- Lymphocytes, melanin pigment, and xanthoma cells may be present
- Plexiform neurofibromas have a more prominent mucoid matrix than any of the other types
- Tactoid structures resembling Pacinian corpuscles or Wagner-Meissner bodies frequently present in diffuse cutaneous neurofibromas, massive soft tissue neurofibromas, and plexiform neurofibromas
- Plexiform neurofibromas may contain nodules of Schwann cells with Verocay bodies

- Unusual variants:
  - Epithelioid neurofibroma
    - Characterized by the presence of epithelioid cells arranged in nests and cords
    - May be hard to recognize as being a neoplasm of peripheral nerve unless the peripheral nerve is included with the specimen
  - Pigmented neurofibroma
    - Fewer that 1% of all neurofibromas
    - Characterized by the presence of melanin in the cytoplasm of the neoplastic nerve cells

Special Stains

- Collagen best highlighted with trichrome stain
- Mucoid matrix of neurofibromas (especially plexiform) can be highlighted with Alcian blue

Electron Microscopy

- Schwann cells characterized by thin, arborizing cell processes, intermediate filaments, microtubles, and continuous basement membrane
- Perineurial-like cells characterized by long, straight, thin cytoplasmic processes with numerous pinocytotic vesicles
- Fibroblasts have abundant branching endoplasmic reticulum, a well-developed Golgi apparatus, and no basement membrane

Immunohistochemistry

- All variants have cells positive for S-100 protein (staining not as intense or as uniform as in schwannoma)
- More than 50% positive for Leu-7 (CD57)
- EMA staining seen in residual, compressed normal perineurium
- CD34-positive cells present throughout

Molecular Alterations

- Non-NF-1 related neurofibromas may be associated with abnormalities involving the NF-1 gene on chromosome 17

Differential Diagnosis

- Schwannoma
- Low-grade MPNST (most likely a problem with cellular neurofibromas)
- Ganglioneuroma
- DFSP (neurofibroma with pigment vs Bednar tumor)
- Fibrous histiocytoma
- Plexiform fibrohistiocytic tumor vs. plexiform neurofibroma
- Nerve sheath myxoma and neurothekeoma
- Spindle cell lipoma
- Blue nevus and cellular blue nevus
- Spindle cell or desmoplastic melanoma

Treatment

- Simple excision of localized and diffuse cutaneous neurofibromas
- Resection of localized intraneural and plexiform neurofibromas will result in loss of parent nerve
- Pain and rapid increase in size may herald malignant transformation

Prognosis

- Sporadic neurofibromas may undergo malignant change
- Neurofibromas that arise in the setting of NF-1 (especially plexiform neurofibromas) are most likely to undergo malignant transformation; when malignant transformation occurs, the prognosis is particularly poor

Associations

- Diffuse, plexiform, and massive soft tissue neurofibromas associated with NF-1

Neurofibromatosis

Variants

- Neurofibromatosis, type 1 (NF-1)
  - NF-1 is diagnosed in a patient with ≥2 of the following:
  - ≥6 café-au-lait macules >5 mm in greatest diameter in a prepubertal patient, and >15 mm in greatest diameter in a postpubertal patient
  - ≥2 neurofibromas of any type or 1 plexiform neurofibroma
  - Presence of freckles in the axillary or inguinal region
  - Optic glioma (tumor of optic pathway)
  - ≥2 Lisch nodules (benign pigmented iris hamartomas)

- An osseous lesion such as sphenoid dysplasia or thinning of long bone cortex with or without pseudoarthrosis
- A first-degree relative with NF-1 by the above criteria

- Neurofibromatosis, type 2 (NF-2)
  - NF-2 is diagnosed in a patient who has the following:
  - Bilateral 8th cranial nerve (vestibular branch of acoustic nerve) Schwannomas or a 1st-degree relative with NF-2 plus
  - Unilateral 8th cranial nerve schwannoma and any 2 of the following:
    - Neurofibroma
    - Meningioma
    - Glioma
    - Schwannoma
    - Juvenile posterior subcapsular lenticular opacity/juvenile cortical cataract

Clinical Manifestations

- NF-1 (peripheral form; von Recklinghausen disease)
  - Café-au-lait spots develop early followed by neurofibromas
  - Central nervous system (CNS) tumors (optic nerve glioma, astrocytomas, and heterotopias)
  - 90% develop pigmented hamartomas of iris (Lisch nodules)
  - 40% develop primary (nonossifying fibroma) or secondary (local erosion) skeletal defects
- NF-2 (central form)
  - Bilateral acoustic (vestibular) schwannomas hallmark of disease
  - Onset in late adolescence or early adulthood with tinnitus and hearing loss
  - Café-au-lait spots (tend to be small and few in number)
  - Cutaneous neurofibromas may occur, but are rare; cutaneous schwannomas seen in approximately 70%
  - Meningiomas often coexist with acoustic schwannoma and are often multifocal
  - Spinal cord gliomas (70% are ependymomas) less frequent than schwannomas or meningiomas

Gross Pathology

- 5 distinct variants of neurofibroma in NF-1:
  - Localized and diffuse cutaneous neurofibroma
    - Typically multiple
    - Most common lesion in neurofibromatosis
    - Larger than sporadic neurofibromas
    - Appears circumscribed but is not encapsulated, but often tends to have a soft consistency with a cut surface homogenously gray or tan; no degenerative changes
    - Microscopically identical to sporadic lesions; varies from highly cellular to highly myxoid
  - Localized intraneural neurofibroma of peripheral nerve
    - Usually multiple
    - Causes a fusiform expansion of nerve in which it originates
    - Cut surface translucent and gray to tan
  - Plexiform neurofibroma typically involving major nerve trunk
    - Diffuse enlargement and distortion of involved nerve resulting from haphazard growth both within and occasionally adjacent to a nerve trunk
    - If involvement a plexus of nerves the appearance will be reminiscent of a "bag of worms"; if a medium to large, nonbranching nerve involved the appearance will be of a ropy cylinder
    - A rubbery consistency and a translucent cut surface
  - Massive soft tissue neurofibroma
    - Diagnostic of NF-1
  - Visceral neurofibromas
    - May be the only manifestation of disease
    - GI tract most frequently involved with most lesions occurring in esophagus, stomach, and small intestine
    - Lesions include ganglioneuromatosis, localized and plexiform neurofibromas, GI stromal tumors (GIST) including the frequent variant GI autonomic nerve tumor (GANT), and neuroendocrine tumors

Microscopic Pathology

- Neurofibroma
  - Elongated cells consisting of Schwann cells (majority), perineurial-like cells, transitional cells, and fibroblasts with thin wiry acidophilic processes arranged in fascicles, whorls, or a storiform pattern embedded in a mucopolysaccharide-rich matrix

- Neoplastic cells tend to have hyperchromatic serpentine, wavy, or comma-shaped nuclei and are admixed with strands of collagen that has the appearance of "shredded carrots"
- Collagen in localized and diffuse cutaneous neurofibromas and diffuse soft tissue neurofibromas tends to be delicate and wirelike; the collagen of intraneural neurofibromas tends to be coarse and refractile; collagen content of plexiform neurofibromas increases with age (as mucoid content decreases)
- Neoplastic cells diffusely infiltrate nerve and/or soft tissue
- Mast cells frequently present
- Lymphocytes, melanin pigment, and xanthoma cells may be present
- Plexiform neurofibromas have a more prominent mucoid matrix than any of the other types
- Tactoid structures resembling Pacinian corpuscles or Wagner-Meissner bodies frequently present in diffuse cutaneous neurofibromas, massive soft-tissue neurofibromas, and plexiform neurofibromas
- Plexiform neurofibromas may contain nodules of Schwann cells with Verocay bodies

- Schwannoma
  - Spindle cells with spindled to oval to angulated nuclei with mild nuclear pleomorphism and hyperchromasia arranged in short fascicles or swirls and encapsulated with epineurium
  - Nuclear palisading (*Verocay bodies*), compact cellular zones (*Antoni A areas*), and hypocellular zones (*Antoni B areas*) are typically all present
  - Intranuclear cytoplasmic invaginations or vacuoles often present
  - Myxoid change and large, irregular vessels usually conspicuous in Antoni B areas
  - Cystic spaces lined by round, epithelioid Schwann cells may be present (pseudoglandular schwannoma)
  - Mitoses variably present
  - Melanin pigment may be present

Special Stains

- Collagen best highlighted with trichrome stain
- Mucoid matrix of neurofibromas (especially plexiform) can be highlighted with Alcian blue

Immunohistochemistry

- All variants positive for S-100 protein (staining not as intense as in schwannomas)
- More than 50% positive for Leu-7
- EMA staining seen in residual, compressed normal perineurium
- Tactoid structures of a plexiform neurofibroma stain with S-100 and have a peripheral rim of EMA-positive cells (true Pacinian corpuscles stain predominately with EMA, not S-100; normal Wagner-Meissner corpuscles do not have a rim of EMA-positive cells)

Electron Microscopy

- Schwann cells characterized by thin arborizing cell processes, intermediate filaments, microtubles, and continuous basement membrane
- Perineurial-like cells characterized by long, straight, thin cytoplasmic processes with numerous pinocytotic vesicles
- Fibroblasts have abundant branching endoplasmic reticulum, a well-developed Golgi apparatus, and no basement membrane

Molecular Alterations

- *NF-1* gene located on chromosome 17q11.2 (this gene encodes protein, *neurofibromin*, which is necessary for the correct negative regulation of *ras* proteins)
- *NF-2* gene on chromosome 22q12 (encodes *merlin [schwannomin]* protein)

Differential Diagnosis

- See section on neurofibroma

Treatment

- Typically large number of lesions makes definitive surgery impossible
- Surgery is reserved for symptomatic lesions or lesions that have the potential to cause a complication

Prognosis

- Risk of malignant transformation of neurofibroma in NF-1 approximately 2%; the longer the duration of the disease the greater the likelihood of malignant transformation
- All acoustic schwannomas in NF-2 are benign; no MPNST

- Patients with NF-2 usually die of complications of the acoustic neuromas or the spinal cord ependymomas

Associations

- NF-1 associated tumors:
    - Bilateral pheochromocytoma
    - Rhabdomyosarcoma
    - Duodenal paraganglioma and carcinoid tumor
    - Ganglioneuroma
    - Juvenile chronic myelogenous leukemia (CML)
    - Juvenile xanthogranuloma
    - Non-ossifying fibroma
- NF-1 associated central nervous system tumors:
    - Astrocytomas; to include unilateral and bilateral optic gliomas (15%), pilocytic astrocytoma, and fibrillary astrocytoma
- NF-1 associated central nervous system lesions:
    - Neuroglial and retinal glial hamartomas
    - Macrocephaly and hydrocephaly
    - Learning disabilities and epilepsy
- Other NF-1 associated lesions:
    - Skeletal dysplasias
    - Congenital pseudoarthroses
    - Arterial intimal hyperplasia and fibrosis with aneurysm or stenosis
    - Hypertrophic (obstructive) cardiomyopathy
- NF-2 associated central nervous system lesions:
    - Multiple glial microhamartomas
    - Spinal cord cellular ependymal ectopias
    - Syringomyelia

Neuroma

Variants

- *Traumatic neuroma*
    - Proximal end of a transected or crushed peripheral nerve proliferates into a tangled mass of nerve fibers that do not meet distal end
    - Painful, firm, and tender
    - Circumscribed, gray-white nodule in continuity with proximal end of injured nerve
- *Mucosal neuroma*
    - Involves mucosal surface of mouth, lips, eyelids, and GI tract
    - Occur in setting of MEN-2b
    - Slightly more common in women
- *Pacinian neuroma*
    - Localized hyperplasia of Pacinian corpuscles
    - Typically seen in digits as rice-like, pearl gray ovoid nodules embedded in fibroadipose tissue
    - May lie under perineurium or be attached to nerve by a thin stalk
- *Palisaded encapsulated neuroma*
    - Typically a small, asymptomatic, nonpigmented papule in the skin of the face of middle-aged adults
    - Slightly more common in women
    - Most occur in skin (reticular dermis)
- *Morton neuroma (localized interdigital neuritis)*
    - Typically located in an interdigital plantar nerve between the 3rd and 4th toes
    - Most commonly affects adult women
    - A fusiform enlargement of a plantar digital nerve typically at a point of bifurcation (resemble traumatic neuroma or neurofibroma)

Clinical Manifestations

- All neuromas are painful except mucosal and palisaded encapsulated variants

Gross Pathology

- See variants earlier in this section

Microscopic Pathology

- *Traumatic neuroma*
    - A random proliferation of nerve fascicles that include axons, Schwann cells, and perineural fibroblasts
    - Proliferating fascicles of nerve elements may be surrounded by and embedded in collagen
    - Myxoid areas may be present
- *Mucosal neuroma*
    - Irregular, tortuous nerves with prominent perineurium within submucosal tissue
    - Myxoid change may be prominent
    - In GI tract all elements of plexus (Schwann cells, neurons, and ganglion cells) increased

- *Pacinian neuroma*
  - Mature Pacinian corpuscles that typically have an irregular shape and a thickened capsule in association with small peripheral nerves
  - Capsular and interlamellar collagen deposition (degenerative changes) commonly present
- *Palisaded encapsulated neuroma*
  - A solid proliferation of Schwann cells and axons within a thin capsule of perineurium; cells tend to be aligned and fasciculated and course in various directions
  - Mast cells frequently present
- *Morton neuroma (localized interdigital neuritis)*
  - Ill-defined with extensive perineural fibrosis that may extend into adjacent soft tissue
  - Degenerative changes of edema, fibrosis, hyalinization of endoneurial, and endoneurial mucin accumulation typically present
  - Elastic tissue typically decreased in center and increased at periphery of lesion

Special Stains

- Silver stains will highlight axons in close association with Schwann cells traversing a palisaded encapsulated neuroma

Immunohistochemistry

- *Traumatic neuroma*
  - Schwann cells positive for S-100 and Leu-7 (CD57)
  - Axons positive for neurofilament protein
  - Perineural cells surrounding fascicles positive for EMA
- *Mucosal neuroma*
  - Schwann cells positive for S-100 protein
  - Axons positive for neurofilament protein
  - Ganglion cells positive for NSE, neurofilament protein, and synaptophysin
- *Pacinian neuroma*
  - Perineural cell lamella of outer core EMA positive
  - Schwann cells positive for S-100 protein
  - Axons positive for neurofilament protein
- *Palisaded encapsulated neuroma*
  - Schwann cells positive for S-100
  - Variable numbers of axons positive for neurofilament and Leu-7 (CD57)
  - Perineural cells within thin capsule EMA positive
- *Morton neuroma (localized interdigital neuritis)*
  - Neurofilament stain and S-100 protein will demonstrate reduction in axons and Schwann cells respectively
  - EMA will demonstrate abnormal (fibrotic) perineurium

Electron Microscopy

- *Traumatic neuroma*
  - Schwann cells, axons, and perineurium all present in a tangled mass
- *Pacinian neuroma*
  - Outer lamellae consists of long perineurial processes with pinocytotic vesicles
- *Palisaded encapsulated neuroma*
  - Well-differentiated Schwann cells
- *Morton neuroma (localized interdigital neuritis)*
  - Confirms degenerative changes in nerve fibers and myelin loss

Molecular Alterations

- None

Differential Diagnosis

- *Traumatic neuroma*
  - Schwannoma
  - Morton neuroma
  - Palisaded encapsulated neuroma
  - Neurofibroma
- *Mucosal neuroma*
  - Traumatic neuroma
  - Palisaded encapsulated neuroma
- *Pacinian neuroma*
  - Normal Pacinian body
  - Dermal nerve sheath myxoma (neurothekeoma)
- *Palisaded encapsulated neuroma*
  - Traumatic neuroma
  - Schwannoma
  - Neurofibroma
  - Angioleiomyoma
- *Morton neuroma (localized interdigital neuritis)*
  - None

Treatment

- *Traumatic neuroma*
  - Simple excision with reapproximation of severed ends or embedding of proximal nerve stump in normal adjacent soft tissue
- *Pacinian neuroma*
  - Excision with sparing of parent nerve
- *Palisaded encapsulated neuroma*
  - Simple excision
- *Morton neuroma (localized interdigital neuritis)*
  - Resection (may be followed by development of a traumatic neuroma)

Prognosis

- Benign with no reports of malignant transformation

Associations

- Traumatic neuroma, Morton neuroma, and Pacinian neuroma associated with trauma (transection of a nerve in the case of the first and repeated blunt trauma in the case of the latter two)
- Mucosal neuromas seen in patients with MEN-2b (bilateral pheochromocytoma, C-cell hyperplasia, medullary carcinoma of thyroid, and parathyroid hyperplasia)
- Diffuse intestinal ganglioneuromatosis associated with disorders other than MEN-2b: Cowden syndrome, juvenile polyposis, colonic adenoma, colonic adenocarcinoma, and Hirschsprung disease
- Pacinian neuromas occur in association with traumatic neuromas and glomus tumors
- Palisaded encapsulated neuroma not associated with neurofibromatosis, mucosal neuromatosis, or trauma; some association with acne

Neurothekeoma

Clinical Manifestations

- Typically occurs in children and young adults
- Tends to involve the upper portion of the body especially the head and neck and shoulder regions
- May also involve the fingers especially of young adults
- Tends to be localized to the dermis or subcutis; mucous membranes rarely involved
- Occasionally originates from a nerve

Gross Pathology

- Solitary, circumscribed, and firm; may be multilobular
- Cut surface gray-tan and myxoid

Microscopic Pathology

- Uniform round or plump spindled cells typically arranged in packets with a surrounding thin collagen band containing delicate blood vessels (an overall multilobular architecture); cells within lobules tend to have a whorled arrangement
- Tumor cell nuclei hyperchromatic with little pleomorphism and few mitotic figures
- Cellular tumors are less myxoid, tend to have nuclear atypia and mitoses, and are locally invasive
- Invariably there is a prominent myxoid matrix that consists of either hyaluronic acid or sulfated acid mucins
- Benign giant cells may be present
- No necrosis

Special Stains

- Alcian blue will highlight mucin (rich in hyaluronic acid)

Electron Microscopy

- Schwannian or perineurial cell differentiation usually present (not all investigators agree)
- Cells have features suggestive of fibroblastic differentiation

Immunohistochemistry

- Neoplastic cells typically positive for vimentin and S-100 protein (S-100 positivity more pronounced in highly myxoid tumors than in highly cellular lesions)

Molecular Alterations

- None

Differential Diagnosis

- Nerve sheath myxoma
- Focal mucinosis
- Myxoid neurofibroma and schwannoma
- Myxoid MFH
- Cellular neurothekeoma may resemble Spitz nevus and desmoplastic (neurotrophic) melanoma

Treatment and Prognosis

- Local complete excision
- A benign neoplasm that rarely recurs

Associations

- May be a variant of myxoid nerve sheath tumor

Neurotropic-Desmoplastic Melanoma

Clinical Manifestations

- 75% occur in the head and neck region of adults
- May occur in children
- Occasionally occurs in unusual sites (ie, vulva)
- Lentigo maligna melanoma is the most common precursor lesion; neoplasm may also arise from a superficial spreading or an acral lentiginous melanoma
- Most present as a Clark level IV or V

Gross Pathology

- The neoplasm has a firm fibrous consistency similar to scar

Microscopic Pathology

- Spindled or oval (epithelioid) cells arranged in short fascicles that infiltrate connective tissue
- Collagen fibrils (both fine and dense) typically surround tumor cells
- Tumor cells may focally infiltrate surrounding tissue as single cells
- Typically tumor cells found within the endoneurium and perineurium of normal nerves
- Melanin pigment absent (but present in precursor lesion)

Special Stains

- Not helpful

Immunohistochemistry

- Neoplastic cells positive for S-100 protein (staining may be focal) and typically negative for HMB-45

Electron Microscopy

- No melanosomes or premelanosomes
- Schwann cell features usually evident

Molecular Alterations

- None

Differential Diagnosis

- Reactive fibroblastic proliferation
- Benign or malignant nerve sheath tumor
- Squamous cell carcinoma
- Spitz nevus

Treatment

- Wide local excision with lymph node dissection if lymphadenopathy present

Prognosis

- A malignant lesion with a very high recurrence rate; 50% recur locally (tumors most likely to recur are those excised with <1 cm of margin, in the head and neck region, and more than 4 mm in thickness)
- Metastatic sites include regional lymph nodes and lung

Associations

- None

Perineurioma

Variants

- Intraneural
- Extraneural (soft tissue)

Clinical Manifestations

- Intraneural
  - Usually develops in nerve of upper extremity in young adults
  - Patients usually present with muscle weakness
- Extraneural
  - Usually presents in soft tissue of hand

Gross Pathology

- Intraneural
  - Fusiform expansion of affected nerve
  - Entire nerve expanded by "onion bulbs"
- Extraneural
  - Circumscribed and white on sectioning

Microscopic Pathology

- Intraneural
  - Concentric layers of perineural cells (onion bulbs) surround a central axon and Schwann cell; perineurial cells spin off to join others
- Extraneural
  - Composed of extremely elongated cells that resemble perineurium arranged in parallel bundles of short fascicles that may have a storiform pattern
  - May have an appearance similar to that of a neurofibroma or Pacinian neurofibroma
  - Lesion may be very cellular and mimic a cellular schwannoma or transitional meningioma
  - Frequently has a myxoid background

Special Stains

- Not helpful

Immunohistochemistry

- Intraneural
  - EMA stains perineural cells but not central Schwann cells and axons
  - S-100 protein stains Schwann cells and axons but not perineurial cells
- Extraneural
  - EMA positive and S-100 protein negative

Electron Microscopy

- Cells have nonbranching, long, thin cytoplasmic processes covered with an external basal lamina and joined at their ends by tight junctions; pinocytotic vesicles tend to be surface oriented

Molecular Alterations

- Abnormalities of chromosome 22 have been seen in some cases

Differential Diagnosis

- DFSP
- Benign fibrous histiocytoma
- Neurofibroma
- Meningioma

Treatment

- Local excision

Prognosis

- Always benign
- No evidence of malignant transformation

Associations

- None

PNET/Peripheral Neuroepithelioma

Clinical Manifestations

- Most patients are adolescents or young adults; median age 20 years (reported age range 1 to 80 years)
- Males (55%) are more often affected than females (45%)
- Usual sites of involvement are the paravertebral region (50%-60%) and extremities (20%-25%)
- 30% are associated with major peripheral nerve trunks (no known association with von Recklinghausen disease)
- 30% are painful
- Does not arise from sympathetic nervous system

Gross Pathology

- Typically neoplasm is multilobulated and soft
- Cut surface is gray to tan with large areas of necrosis, hemorrhage, or cystic degeneration
- Grossly detectable calcification is unusual

Microscopic Pathology

- Sheets of uniform, monotonous, round cells with scant or ill-defined cytoplasm arranged in a vaguely lobular pattern (resemble neuroblastoma)
- Nuclei tend to be hyperchromatic with clumped chromatin pattern
- Pleomorphism rare
- Mitotic figures usually present
- Areas of crushed, necrotic cells often give the tissue a "filigree" pattern
- Neoplasm typically has a rich, delicate, and inconspicuous vasculature
- Rosettes with a central neurofibrillary core (Homer-Wright type) and/or a central vesicle or lumen (Flexner-Wintersteiner type) are present in highly variable numbers (the presence of rosettes is considered a prerequisite for the diagnosis)

Special Stains

- Reticulin stains highlight the distinctly lobular arrangement of the tumor and confirm the absence of reticulum fibers between tumor cells (this feature helps distinguish this neoplasm from poorly differentiated fibrosarcoma, chondrosarcoma, and small cell osteosarcoma all of which have reticulin fibers between individual tumor cells)
- PAS with and without diastase confirms the absence of digestible glycogen granules in tumor cells

Immunohistochemistry

- A cell membrane protein (p30/32) which is encoded by the *MIC2* gene located on the short arm of both the X and Y chromosomes is detected by the antibody HBA-71 (CD99)
- Tumor cells typically positive for *bcl*-2
- Tumor cells variably positive for S-100 protein, neurofilament protein, NSE, Leu-7 (CD57), synaptophysin, and chromogranin
- Tumor cells do not express GFAP, desmin, muscle-specific antigen, myoglobin, factor VIII, or LCA

Electron Microscopy

- Tumor cells are primitive and undifferentiated with uniform round or oval nuclei and coarsely granular chromatin
- Cells have elongated or interdigiting cellular processes with filaments and microtubules

Molecular Alterations

- 80% to 90% have a reciprocal translocation of long arm of chromosomes 11 and 22 (t[11;22] [q24;q12]); this chromosomal abnormality is also been detected in Askin tumor and esthesioneuroblastoma
- A similar translocation, t(11;22) (q13;q12) is associated with intraabdominal desmoplastic small cell tumor of childhood
- Tumors overexpress n-*myc* and c-*myb*

Differential Diagnosis

- Extraosseous Ewing sarcoma
  - Neuroblastoma (may be virtually indistinguishable from PNET on light microscopy)
  - Neuroendocrine carcinoma (Merkel cell tumor, metastatic small cell carcinoma of lung)
  - Desmoplastic small round cell tumor
  - Poorly differentiated synovial sarcoma
  - Lymphoblastic lymphoma
  - Extraskeletal mesenchymal chondrosarcoma and small cell osteosarcoma
  - Rhabdomyosarcoma

Treatment

- Combination surgery, chemotherapy, and radiation

Prognosis

- Aggressive neoplasm with frequent metastases to lung, bone, and liver
- Most significant prognostic factors are size and amount of necrosis
- 30% to 50% survival at 3 years

Associations

- None

Variant

- *Askin Tumor*
  - A malignant small round blue cell tumor involving the thoracopulmonary region of children
  - Most arise in the periosteum of ribs (may arise in soft tissue and within the lung) and frequently involves intercostal nerves
  - Generally felt to be a variant of Ewing sarcoma and PNET that *occurs exclusively in the thoracopulmonary region*; may demonstrate features of either Ewing sarcoma or features of PNET (by light microscopy, immunohistochemistry, and electron microscopy)
  - Probably more closely related to PNET than Ewing sarcoma (tends to express neural markers more frequently than does Ewing sarcoma)
  - Glycogen may or may not be present in neoplastic cells
  - Frequently positive for neural markers to include NSE, neurofilaments, and chromogranin; also positive for *MIC2* gene product; focally positive for low-molecular-weight cytokeratins
  - Same t(11; 22)(q24; q12) as seen with Ewing sarcoma and PNET

Comment

- PNET and Ewing sarcoma may represent a single group of bone and soft tissue tumors in which typical undifferentiated Ewing sarcoma and PNET with obvious evidence of neural differentiation lie at opposite ends of a spectrum

Schwannoma (Neurilemoma)

Clinical Manifestations

- Affects adults between the ages of 20 and 50 years
- Men and women affected equally
- Neoplasm tends to occur in the head and neck region and flexor surfaces of extremities
- Also found in the posterior mediastinum, retroperitoneum, posterior spinal roots, and arising from the vestibular branch of cranial nerve VIII (acoustic neuroma) at the cerebellopontine angle
- Almost always solitary, but may be multiple (especially if associated with NF-2)
- May occur in the setting of von Recklinghausen disease
- Typically grows slowly and rarely causes pain
- Patient may report that tumor waxes and wanes in size
- Lesions arising in the posterior mediastinum frequently extend into the vertebral channel (dumbbell tumors); these lesions produce neurologic symptoms

Gross Pathology

- Tumor arises in nerve sheath, peripherally displaces nerve fibers, has a true fibrous capsule, and forms a globoid eccentric mass
- Nerve of origin usually identifiable in the periphery of the neoplasm (flattened along the capsule but not penetrating the substance of the tumor)
- May contain cystic areas (especially when large)
- Cut section reveals a white to pink firm encapsulated nodule
- Larger neoplasms (retroperitoneal or mediastinal) typically have foci of hemorrhage, cystic change, and/or calcification

Microscopic Pathology

- A well-formed fibrous, hyalinized capsule containing displaced nerve
- Schwann cells with spindled to oval to angulated nuclei with mild nuclear pleomorphism and hyperchromasia arranged in short fascicles or swirls
- Nuclear palisading (Verocay bodies), compact cellular zones (Antoni A areas) and hypocellular zones (Antoni B areas) are typically all present if neoplasm extensively sampled
- Antoni B areas often characterized by presence of nuclei with cytoplasmic inclusions, myxoid change (mucopolysaccharide), mast cells, and both thick-walled and ectatic, thin-walled vessels
- Antoni A areas tend to have prominent collagen
- Cystic spaces lined by round, epithelioid Schwann cells may be present (pseudoglandular schwannoma)
- Mitoses variably present
- Melanin pigment may be present
- Degenerative or reactive changes of hemorrhage, organizing thrombi, hemosiderin, xanthoma cells, lymphoid aggregates, cyst formation, necrosis, calcification, extreme hyalinization and vessels with thickened hyalinized walls coupled with bizarre hyperchromatic nuclei are diagnostic of "ancient" schwannoma (see below)

Variants

- *Cellular schwannoma*
  - Consists almost exclusively of Antoni A areas with cells that have very hyperchromatic and pleomorphic nuclei
  - Approximately 4 mitotic figures per 10 hpf
  - Necrosis in 10%
  - Easily confused with malignant peripheral nerve sheath tumor
- *Plexiform schwannoma*
  - Usually occurs in skin
  - Patients may have NF-1 or NF-2 (latter more common)
- *Ancient schwannoma (degenerated schwannoma)*
  - Usually of longstanding duration and located in the retroperitoneum
  - Degenerative changes include cyst formation, hemorrhage, hyalinization, and calcification
  - Marked nuclear atypia characterized by large hyperchromatic multilobed nuclei
  - *No mitotic figures*
- *Epithelioid schwannoma*
  - Superficial encapsulated mass
  - Nests or cords of small epithelioid Schwann cells with distinct cell borders and occasional nuclear inclusions in a collagenous or partially myxoid stroma
  - Cells S-100 positive and type IV collagen outlines both individual cells and nests of cells

Special Stains

- Trichrome will confirm absence of longitudinal striations (when differentiation from leiomyosarcoma problematic) and will highlight collagen
- Reticulin stains highlight intracellular collagen bundles and basement membrane material in Antoni A areas

Immunohistochemistry

- Schwann cells are immunoreactive for S-100 protein and Leu-7 (CD57)
- Neurofilament protein will identify residual nerve fibers
- CD34-positive cells present in Antoni B areas
- Collagen IV demonstrates a distribution of collagen corresponding to reticulin

Electron Microscopy

- Cells have a continuous basal lamina, numerous thin cytoplasmic processes, aggregates of intracytoplasmic microfibrils, intracytoplasmic lamellar bodies, and extracellular long-spacing collagen (Luse body)

Molecular Alterations

- Loss of *NF-2* gene product (Merlin) on chromosome 22

Differential Diagnosis

- Neurofibroma (Antoni B areas of a Schwannoma closely mimic a neurofibroma)
- Leiomyoma (may have areas that closely resemble Verocay bodies) and leiomyosarcoma
- Malignant peripheral nerve sheath tumor
- If melanin pigment present:
  - Metastatic melanoma
  - Melanotic schwannoma

Treatment and Prognosis

- Local excision with sparing of parent nerve
- A benign neoplasm that rarely recurs and probably never undergoes malignant transformation

Associations

- No association with NF-1 (except plexiform variant); occasionally associated with NF-2 (especially tumors that involve cranial or spinal nerve roots)
- Prior irradiation may be a predisposing factor
- 50% of psammomatous melanotic schwannomas occur in Carney syndrome

Tumors of Uncertain Histogenesis

Alveolar Soft Part Sarcoma

Clinical Manifestations

- Typically occurs in adolescents and young adults between the ages of 15 and 35 years
- More common in females than males (particularly if under the age of 25 years)
- Occurs predominately in the lower extremities (anterior portion of the thigh) in adults; also may occur in the cervix and uterus, mediastinum, and lung
- Reported in infants and children in whom it is more commonly located in the region of the head and neck (especially orbit and tongue)
- Typically presents as a slowly enlarging asymptomatic mass that may be pulsatile or have a bruit
- Destruction of adjacent bone may occur

Gross Pathology

- Poorly circumscribed, friable, and soft and often surrounded by large tortuous blood vessels
- On sectioning, typically yellow to white with large areas of necrosis and hemorrhage

Microscopic Pathology

- At low power the tumor is divided by dense fibrous septa into compact irregularly sized aggregates or groups of cells that are further subdivided into fairly uniform nests and islands of cells separated by delicate fibrous septa with a delicate sinusoidal-like vasculature
- Tumor cells are large, polygonal, and uniform with abundant granular eosinophilic or clear cytoplasm, distinct cell borders, and large, round, vesicular nuclei (sometimes more than one) with prominent nucleoli; pleomorphism and mitoses both rare
- Often there is a of loss of cellular cohesion with necrosis in the central portion of the cellular aggregates (a pseudoalveolar pattern)
- Large dilated veins typically at the periphery and vascular invasion invariably present
- Occasionally (especially in children) tumor grows in sheets of large granular cells with few vascular septa (hence no recognizable alveolar pattern)

Special Stains

- PAS-positive, diastase-resistant, rhomboid or rod-shaped crystals present in 80%; PAS will also confirm presence of intracellular glycogen
- Reticulin stain will outline nests of tumor cells and highlight alveolar pattern

Immunohistochemistry

- Tumor cells occasionally express S-100 protein and NSE and are variably positive for desmin, muscle-specific actin, and vimentin
- Tumor cells negative for cytokeratin, EMA, neurofilaments, GFAP, serotonin, and synaptophysin

Electron Microscopy

- Tumor cells contain numerous mitochondria, smooth endoplasmic reticulum, and glycogen
- Rhomboid crystals arranged in a cross-grid pattern are typically present

Molecular Alterations

- Abnormalities of chromosomes 17q25
- Trisomy 8 and gains at 1q, 8q, 12q and 16p (detected with genomic comparative hybridization)

Differential Diagnosis

- Alveolar rhabdomyosarcoma (cells of an alveolar rhabbomyosarcoma are smaller; alveoli tend to be more irregular and elongated and are separated by fibrovascular septa)
- Metastatic renal cell carcinoma, paraganglioma (cells more pleomorphic and not discohesive), adrenal carcinoma, and melanoma
- Granular cell tumor
- Clear cell sarcoma

Treatment

- Radical surgical excision of both primary and metastatic lesions with radiotherapy and/or adjuvant chemotherapy
- Recurrence rate 20% to 35%

Prognosis

- 2-year survival rate approximately 75%; 5-year survival rate 60%; 10-year survival rate 40%; 20-year survival rate 15%
- Metastasis tends to occur early; principal metastatic sites are lungs, brain, and skeleton
- Cerebral metastasis may be first manifestation of disease and is more common with this neoplasm than any other soft-tissue sarcoma
- Lymph node metastases unusual
- Tumors with a sheetlike or solid pattern (usually seen in infants and children) have a better prognosis

Associations

- None

Angiomatoid Fibrous Histiocytoma

Clinical Manifestations

- Still referred to as angiomatoid MFH
- Usually occurs in the extremities of children and young adults; mean age 20 years
- Typically a slow-growing, painless, nodular mass involving the dermis or subcutis; 65% occur in areas in which normal lymph nodes occur
- May cause systemic symptoms such as anemia, fever, and weight loss

Gross Pathology

- Usually solitary, firm, circumscribed, tan-gray and resembles a lymph node
- Cut surface multinodular and fleshy with red-brown cystic spaces

Microscopic Pathology

- A multinodular proliferation of generally uniform, eosinophilic, histiocytoid or myoid cells with ovoid vesicular nuclei; some cellular pleomorphism and mitiotic activity may be present
- Focal areas of hemorrhagic cystlike spaces (pseudoangiomatoid spaces) that are not lined by endothelium but rather are true cystic spaces within the tumor
- Aggregates of chronic inflammatory cells typically arranged at the periphery of the tumor giving it the overall appearance of a lymph node
- A thick fibrous pseudocapsule
- Cannonball-like architectural pattern and myxoid change may be present

Special Stains

- Not helpful

Immunohistochemistry

- Tumor cells often reactive for CD68, desmin (50%), EMA (40%), and CD99 (50%)
- Tumor cells always negative for CD31, CD34, S-100 protein, HMB-45, and cytokeratins

Electron Microscopy

- No consensus on line of differentiation of tumor cells

Molecular Alterations

- Only 1 tumor with chromosomal abnormalities reported

Differential Diagnosis

- Metastatic sarcoma in a lymph node

Treatment

- Wide local surgical excision

Prognosis

- Indolent growth with low (<10%) local recurrence rate and <1% metastases (usually to regional lymph nodes and not fatal)

Associations

- May be related to other hematopoietic tumos that can cause systemic symptoms such as anemia, fever, and weight loss (eg, fibroblastic reticulum cell sarcoma)

Comment

- Angiomatoid MFH (currently called angiomatoid fibrous histiocytoma), once thought to be specific type of malignant fibrous histiocytoma, is now considered to be distinctive and discrete entity.

Desmoplastic Small Round Cell Tumor

Clinical Manifestations

- Typically affects young adult males between the ages of 15 and 35 (mean age 22 years)
- Usually involves abdominal and/or pelvic peritoneum; also rarely reported in the scrotum, ovary, parotid gland, hand, and central nervous system
- Frequently associated with multiple peritoneal implants when first diagnosed; may replace omentum and mesentery and involve retroperitoneum
- Usually painful
- When located in the abdomen, may cause abdominal distension, constipation, and intestinal or ureteral obstruction

Gross Pathology

- Typically large, multinodular, and solid
- Cut section reveals a firm, grey to white surface that may have foci of cystic change, necrosis, and/or hemorrhage

Microscopic Pathology

- Tumor cells typically quite uniform, small, round or oval, have little cytoplasm, and indistinct cell membranes; nuclei tend to be hyperchromatic and granular; nucleoli are usually inconspicuous
- Tumor cells typically arranged in well-demarcated large, solid, round to elongated nests or masses (occasionally cells are arranged in trabeculae or cords of single cells); irregular cystic spaces that contain central foci of necrosis may be present within nests; tumor cells may palisade along periphery of nests
- Aggregates of tumor cells invariably surrounded by vascular fibrous connective tissue that contains widely scattered spindle-shaped fibroblasts and myofibroblasts in a loose, occasionally edematous or myxomatous, extracellular material or collagen; the stromal vessels are hyperplastic and vary in appearance from complex capillary tufts to large vessels with eccentric thickened walls and prominent endothelial cells; *appearance is one in which the islands of tumor cells appear to be trapped within a desmoplastic stroma*
- Mitotic figures are numerous; significant pleomorphism is rare
- Rhabdoidlike cells present in about 50%
- Some tumors (30%) have focal areas of epithelial differentiation, with glands formation or rosettes

Special Stains

- Rhabdoidlike cells may contain glycogen and can be highlighted with PAS stain

Immunohistochemistry

- Tumor cells are usually immunoreactive for keratin (90%), EMA (90%), desmin (90%) (desmin immunoreactivity characterized by a perinuclear dotlike pattern), vimentin (85%), NSE (80%), CD15 (75%), and CD57 (50%)
- Tumor cells are variably reactive for S-100 protein and synaptophysin

- Myogenin always negative
- Stromal cells positive for smooth muscle actin

Electron Microscopy

- Tumor cells contain paranuclear whorls and packets of microfilaments, moderate numbers of mitochondria, and small foci of glycogen
- Dense core granules may be present in the cytoplasm (rare)

Molecular Alterations

- A reciprocal translocation t(11;22)(p13; q12); the breakpoints are located on the *EWS* gene at 22q12 and the Wilms tumor gene at 11p13; this translocation very similar to that seen in Ewing sarcoma/PNET [t(11;22)(q24; q12)]

Differential Diagnosis

- Other small round blue cell tumors: Ewing sarcoma/PNET, neuroblastoma, embryonal rhabdomyosarcoma (none of which have a prominent desmoplastic stroma)
- Malignant mesothelioma
- Neuroendocrine carcinoma
- Malignant extrarenal rhabdoid tumor
- Merkel cell carcinoma
- Lymphoma
- Poorly differentiated carcinoma
- Small cell carcinoma

Treatment

- Intra-abdominal tumors are usually unresectable as a result as their irregular margins and the presence of multiple metastatic implants within the abdomen at the time of initial surgery
- Extensive surgical debulking in combination with adjuvant chemotherapy and radiotherapy to high-risk sites provides modest increased survival

Prognosis

- Highly aggressive neoplasm
- 75% mortality within 2½ years of diagnosis; 5% live beyond 5 years

Comment

- Tumor may arise from subserosal cells of peritoneum or pleura

Epithelioid Sarcoma

Clinical Manifestations

- Typically occurs on the flexor surface of the fingers, hands, wrist, and forearm of young adults between the ages of 10 and 40 years (median 26 years)
- Most common soft tissue neoplasm to involve the hand or wrist; also occurs in pretibial region, ankle, foot, and toes
- Tend to be superficial but may involve deeper tissues; deep-seated lesions are typically attached to tendons, tendon sheaths, or fascial structures
- Men affected more commonly than women
- Typically presents as a painless, firm nodule; may be solitary or multiple
- Superficial lesions may ulcerate overlying skin

Gross Pathology

- Usually multinodular, ill-defined mass with a tan to gray cut surface with focal areas of necrosis or hemorrhage

Microscopic Pathology

- A nodular pattern of uniform rounded or polygonal epithelioid cells with deeply acidophilic cytoplasm and sharp cell borders and plump spindle cells with eosinophilic or clear cytoplasm; both have relatively large, slightly atypical vesicular nuclei with small readily apparent nucleoli
- Extensive intercellular collagen often surround nodules
- Epithelioid and spindled cells are so admixed they merge imperceptibly
- Mitotic figures usually present (may be numerous)
- Typically there are degenerative changes and necrosis in the center of the nodules resulting in a pseudogranulomatous appearance; in addition chronic inflammatory cells (lymphocytes and plasma cells) may surround the tumor nodules and contribute to the relatively circumscribed, granulomatous appearance
- Tumor cells tend to palisade around the central necrotic areas
- Multinucleated giant cells are rare
- Hemorrhage and cystic change may be present
- Calcification or bone present in 10% to 20%

Special Stains

- Intracellular glycogen may be demonstrated; mucin negative
- A dense network of reticulin fibers separates individual tumor cells
- Cytoplasm of tumor cells stains deeply with trichrome

Immunohistochemistry

- Tumor cells express both low- and high-molecular-weight cytokeratin, vimentin, and EMA
- 50% to 60% stain positively for CD34
- CD31 and S-100 protein may be focally positive, but are usually negative
- Tumor cells are typically negative for desmin, factor VIII-related antigen, CEA, and neurofilament protein

Electron Microscopy

- Polygonal cells with paranuclear masses of intermediate filaments

Molecular Alterations

- Loss of heterozygosity of chromosome 22q reported
- Gains at 11q, 1q, 6p, and 9q and abnormalities of 18q and 9q have all been described

Differential Diagnosis

- Infectious or necrobiotic granuloma (necrotizing infectious granuloma, necrobiosis lipoidica, granuloma annulare, and rheumatoid nodule)
- Malignant extrarenal rhabdoid tumor
- Tenosynovial giant cell tumor, localized type
- Sweat gland tumors
- Nodular fasciitis
- Fibrous histiocytoma
- Squamous cell carcinoma
- Synovial sarcoma
- Epithelioid hemangioendothelioma
- Epithelioid angiosarcoma
- Melanoma
- Clear cell sarcoma
- Fibrosarcoma
- Rhabdomyosarcoma
- Epithelial MPNST
- Metastatic carcinoma

Treatment

- Early radical excision to include amputation if lesion located in the fingers or toes
- Amputation often procedure of choice for recurrence
- Regional lymph node dissection at the time of primary excision
- Adjuvant radiotherapy and multi-agent chemotherapy may help with local control and decrease the recurrence rate

Prognosis

- Overall, long-term survival approximately 65% to 70%
- Neoplasm tends to grow insidiously along fascial planes making the extent of tumor hard to determine both clinically and pathologically
- Overall recurrence rate 80% at 10 years
- Metastatic rate approximately 40%
- Most common metastatic sites are lung, regional lymph nodes, scalp, bone, and central nervous system
- Prognosis related to male sex, advanced age at diagnosis, tumor site, large size, deep location, mitotic rate, and presence or absence of necrosis, vascular and/or nerve invasion, and positive regional lymph nodes at time of diagnosis

Associations

- Neoplasm may arise in sites of trauma

Variant

- A "proximal" variant of epithelioid sarcoma that tends to occur in the pelvis, perineum, and genital tract; characterized by a multinodular pattern with epithelioid carcinomalike cells with marked cytological atypia, abundant eosinophilic cytoplasm, and vesicular nuclei with prominent nucleoli; tumor cells may have pronounced rhabdoid features and mimic the cells of a malignant extrarenal rhabdoid tumor

Fibrous Hamartoma of Infancy

Clinical Manifestations

- Typically presents during the first 2 years of life
- 15% to 25% present at birth
- 2 to 3 times more common in boys than girls
- Typically located superficially in the region of the anterior or posterior axillary fold; also seen in the upper arm, thigh, inguinal and pubic regions, shoulders, back, and forearm

- Never occurs in the hands or feet
- Almost always solitary and usually mobile
- May arise at a site of previous trauma

Gross Pathology

- Usually poorly circumscribed and composed of whitish fibrous tissue intermixed with islands of adipose
- Average size at diagnosis 3 to 5 cm

Microscopic Pathology

- 3 different tissue components arranged in a vaguely organoid pattern:
  - Intersecting bundles or trabeculae of fibrous tissue of various sizes and shapes composed of spindle cells (mostly myofibroblasts) and collagen (may resemble a keloid)
  - Loosely cellular areas of small immature rounded or stellate cells in a mucoid matrix (may be centered around small veins)
  - Mature fat (may be a major component of the neoplasm or be present only at the periphery)
- Typically has ill-defined margins
- May have areas of fibrosis that resemble neurofibroma

Special Stains

- Alcian blue will stain the mucoid matrix surrounding the immature cells
- Trichrome and colloidal iron stains will highlight all 3 components of the lesion

Immunohistochemistry

- Cells that make up the bundles of fibrous tissue and cells in the mucoid matrix are both vimentin positive
- Cells in fibrous areas are actin positive and occasionally desmin positive

Electron Microscopy

- A mixture of fibroblasts and myofibroblasts
- Immature cells resemble immature mesenchymal cells (few intracytoplasmic organelles)
- No elastic fibers

Molecular Alterations

- None

Differential Diagnosis

- Infantile fibromatosis
- Infantile myofibromatosis
- Calcifying aponeurotic fibroma

Treatment

- Local excision (~15% recur)

Prognosis

- Completely benign

Associations

- No associated malformations or other neoplasms
- No evidence of a hereditary incidence

Giant Cell Angiofibroma

Clinical Manifestations

- Usually involves orbital region and eyelids of middle-aged adults
- May occur outside the orbital region in the head and neck as well as posterior mediastinum, back, axillary and inguinal regions, retroperitoneum, and vulva
- Men more frequently affected than women

Gross Pathology

- Usually well circumscribed with a hemorrhagic/cystic cut surface

Microscopic Pathology

- A variable admixture of bland round or spindled cells with pale, indistinct cytoplasm and plump nuclei, collagenous to myxoid stroma with foci of sclerosis, small to medium-sized thick-walled vessels, and variable numbers of giant multinucleated stromal cells that tend to line vascular spaces

Special Stains

- Not helpful

Immunohistochemistry

- Mononuclear and multinucleated stromal cells express CD 34 and CD 99

Treatment and Prognosis

- Excision curative

Associations

- May belong to the solitary fibrous tumor/hemangiopericytoma group of tumors

Hemangiopericytoma

- *Pericytes* are cells that lie adjacent to capillaries, have multiple extensions that partially encircle vascular channels and by virtue of their contractile nature function to regulate vascular caliber thereby controlling capillary blood flow and permeability

Clinical Manifestations

- Usually occurs in adults; median age 45 years (rare in infants and children)
- Men and women affected equally
- Often deep-seated; thigh, pelvic retroperitoneum, and the region of the orbit are common locations; also reported to occur in the meninges, nose, and paranasal sinuses
- Typically presents as a slowly enlarging painless mass; overlying skin may appear telangiectatic and have an elevated temperature; auscultation may reveal the presence of a bruit
- Patients with large tumors in the pelvis or retroperitoneum may have hypoglycemia

Gross Pathology

- Typically a solitary circumscribed mass covered with a highly vascularized pseudocapsule
- On cut section neoplasm has a gray-white to brown color, dilated vascular channels, areas of hemorrhage and cystic degeneration
- Necrosis is uncommon

Microscopic Pathology

- Typically a well-circumscribed, vaguely lobulated neoplasm of densely packed cells with a focal storiform arrangement and numerous, thin-walled, branching vessels of variable caliber that are lined by a single layer of flattened endothelium
- Large, collapsed vessels are typically seen at the periphery of the lesion and frequently have a "stag-horn" appearance
- Thick-walled vessels are uncommon
- An intervascular and perivascular proliferation of relatively uniform cells (pericytes) that characteristically have round to oval to slightly angulated, vesicular nuclei and ill-defined cytoplasmic borders (morphologically very similar to endothelial cells, fibroblasts, and histiocytes); cytologic pleomorphism rare; mitotic activity variable
- Hypocellular, myxoid, or hyalinized areas not typical
- Some tumors have an extensive lipomatous component (*lipomatous hemangiopericytoma*)
- Malignant tumors are typically >5 cm, have tumor cell necrosis, have pleomorphic cells with abnormal chromatin patterns, and more than 4 mitoses per 10 hpf (areas of unequivocal hemangiopericytoma or evidence of malignant transformation must be present)

Special Stains

- PAS and reticulin stains will highlight basal lamina surrounding both vessels and tumor cells

Immunohistochemistry

- Tumor cells are invariably positive for vimentin and rarely focally positive actin and desmin
- A subset of tumors comparable to solitary fibrous tumor usually stain positively for CD34 and CD99 (*normal endothelial cells are positive for CD34*)
- Tumor cells do not stain for factor VIII-related antigen, but do stain for factor XIIIa
- Cytokeratin, S-100 protein, and CD31 negative (*normal endothelial cells positive for CD31)*

Electron Microscopy

- Pericytes with large round or oval nuclei with few organelles and numerous long cytoplasmic extensions which contain microfilaments surround vascular spaces lined by normal endothelium
- Pinocytotic vesicles typically prominent

Molecular Alterations

- Abnormality localized to 13-15 region of chromosome 12

Differential Diagnosis

- Tumors most likely to be misinterpreted as hemangiopericytoma:
- Deep fibrous histiocytoma
- Extrapleural solitary fibrous tumor

- Monophasic synovial sarcoma
- Mesenchymal chondrosarcoma
- Metastatic endometrial stromal sarcoma
- Tumors that may have a hemangiopericytomalike vascular pattern:
- Synovial sarcoma
- Fibrous histiocytoma
- Mesenchymal chondrosarcoma
- Extrapleural solitary fibrous tumor
- Myofibroma
- Leiomyosarcoma
- Endometrial stromal sarcoma
- Other tumors in the differential:
  - Cellular hemangioma
  - Glomus tumor
  - Leiomyoma
  - Liposarcoma
  - Angiosarcoma
  - MPNST

Treatment

- Complete excision
- Radical surgery with or without preoperative embolization and with or without adjuvant radiation therapy is required for borderline or malignant neoplasms

Prognosis

- Malignant lesions may metastasize but usually late
- Recurrence usually the forerunner of a distant metastasis

Associations

- Hypoglycemia
- 3 other soft tissue tumors appear to be histogenetically related to hemangiopericytoma:
  - Extrapleural solitary fibrous tumor
  - Giant cell angiofibroma
  - Lipomatous hemangiopericytoma

Comment

- Extrapleural solitary fibrous tumor and hemangiopericytoma share similar histopathological features with lipomatous hemangiopericytoma and giant cell angiofibroma. These 4 lesions are becoming increasingly indistinct, especially solitary fibrous tumor and hemangiopericytoma. These 2 tumors occupy the ends of a spectrum of perivascular tumors. At 1 end of the spectrum, the tumor has clinicopathologic features of a "classic" hemangiopericytoma (usually located in an extremity, a marked pericytic vascular pattern, nonspindled cells, and variable to focal zones of hyalinization); at the other end of the spectrum, the tumor has clinicopathologic features of a "classic" solitary fibrous tumor (usually located in a body cavity, a focal perivascular pattern, spindled cells, and broad zones of hyalinization). Tumors with intermediate features or equal areas of both classic solitary fibrous tumor and classic hemangiopericytoma represent "hemangiopericytoma-solitary fibrous tumor."

Malignant Extrarenal Rhabdoid Tumor

Clinical Manifestations

- Typically occur in infants and children (may affect adolescents and adults); mean age 8 to 9 years
- Usually solitary, rapidly growing, and painful
- Involves deep soft tissue of trunk (30%), proximal extremities (25%), head and neck region (15%), solid organs, other than the kidney (15%), and abdomen, pelvis, and retroperitoneum (20%)
- Has been reported in the prostate, liver, central nervous system, skin, GI tract, and thymus

Gross Pathology

- Usually solid, irregularly shaped, nonencapsulated, nodular, and soft
- May be fairly well circumscribed
- Cut surface soft, gray to tan with foci of necrosis and hemorrhage

Microscopic Pathology

- Tumor cells tend to be round or polygonal or spindle-shaped with eccentric round or bean-shaped, vesicular nuclei with large, prominent, eosinophilic nucleoli; cytoplasm tends to be eosinophilic or amphophilic and abundant and contains a densely eosinophilic, globular intracytoplasmic inclusion (intermediate filaments) located near the nucleus
- Tumor cells usually grow in densely cellular discohesive sheets or trabeculae in an infiltrative and destructive pattern (occasionally other patterns such as alveolar, nesting, and trabecular)

- Mitotic figures (usually 1 or 2 per hpf) and areas of necrosis frequent
- Occasionally non-neoplastic, osteoclastlike giant cells, a myxoid stroma, and increased amounts of collagen may be present

Special Stains

- Intracytoplasmic eosinophilic inclusions tend to stain with PAS

Immunohistochemistry

- Tumor cells positive for keratin (paranuclear), EMA, and vimentin; also frequently positive for CD99, synaptophysin, and NSE
- Expression of muscle-specific actin and focal expression of S-100 protein fairly common
- Tumor cells negative for desmin, myoglobin, and CD34

Electron Microscopy

- Intracytoplasmic hyaline inclusions represent whorls of intermediate filaments and tend to have a paranuclear distribution

Molecular Alterations

- No consistent chromosomal abnormality, but some have abnormalities of chromosome 22q11-12
- Tumors in CNS have monosomy 22

Differential Diagnosis

- Epithelioid sarcoma (distinction may be quite difficult; both epithelioid sarcoma with rhabdoid features and rhabdoid tumors with features of epithelioid sarcoma exist)
- Rhabdomyosarcoma (cytokeratin negative; rhabdoid tumor cytokeratin positive)
- Poorly differentiated carcinoma
- Melanoma
- Desmoplastic small round cell tumor of infancy and childhood
- PNET/Ewing sarcoma

Treatment

- Wide surgical excision with or without lymph node dissection

Prognosis

- A very aggressive neoplasm; fewer than 50% live 5 years

Comment

- There is some feeling that malignant rhabdoid tumor may not be a specific tumor but rather a "rhabdoid" phenotype that may develop during the evolution of many tumors to a higher histologic grade such as occurs in epithelioid sarcoma, intra-abdominal desmoplastic small cell tumor, rhabdomyosarcoma, melanoma, and various types of carcinoma. The diagnosis of malignant rhabdoid tumor requires the exclusion of an underlying alternative line of differentiation

Malignant Mesenchymoma

- Historically the term *malignant mesenchymoma* was used to encompass a group of sarcomas that exhibit ≥2 tissue elements sufficiently differentiated to permit clear recognition of histologic type with light microscopy, immunohistochemistry, or electron microscopy. Most commonly the tumors given this diagnosis were myxoid liposarcomas with cartilaginous metaplasia, well-differentiated liposarcomas with osseous, cartilaginous, smooth muscle, or skeletal muscle elements, and pleomorphic liposarcomas with osteogenic areas.
- Nonfatty tumors included in the definition of malignant mesenchymoma included rare leiomyosarcomas with focal areas of osteosarcoma or rhabdomyosarcoma differentiation and embryonal rhabromyosarcomas with foci of cartilage.
- Sarcomas with ≥2 lines of differentiation are best diagnosed by identifying, quantifying, and grading the various lines of differentiation with appropriate emphasis on the most aggressive component. "Lumping" all these neoplasms together under 1 diagnosis is misleading and should be abandoned.

Myxoma

Variants

- *Intramuscular myxoma*
- *Digital myxoma (digital mucous cyst)*
- *Juxta-articular myxoma*
- *Cutaneous myxoma (superficial angiomyxoma)*

Clinical Manifestations

- *Intramuscular myxoma*
  - Tends to occur in the large skeletal muscles: thigh, buttock, shoulder, and upper arm
  - Typically present in the 5th to 7th decades
  - More common in women than men
  - Most present with a palpable painless mass; may be mobile and fluctuant
  - May be multiple (see associations later in this section)
- *Digital myxoma (digital mucous cyst)*
  - A dome-shaped nodule in the dermis of the distal and dorsal portions of the fingers
  - Typically solitary and painful
  - Twice as common in women as in men
  - Nodule may be covered with verrucous (wartlike) skin or atrophic skin
- *Juxta-articular myxoma*
  - 90% occur in the region of the knee
  - 25% involve a meniscus
  - Usually involve a large joint, ie, shoulder, elbow, hip and ankle; wrist and hand rarely involved
  - More common in men than women
  - Typically present in the 4th through 6th decades
  - May be associated with degenerative joint disease in adjacent joint
- *Cutaneous myxoma (superficial angiomyxoma)*
  - Affects men and women equally; 4th to 6th decades
  - Slow-growing dermal or subcutaneous mass
  - Most common on trunk, genital region, or head and neck region
  - Rarely multiple *(multiple lesions should raise possibility of Carney complex; presence of lesion in external ear essentially pathognomonic for Carney)*

Gross Pathology

- May appear well-circumscribed but often ill-defined
- Cut surface mucoid and gelatinous
- Angiomyxomas usually multilobulated

Microscopic Pathology

- *Intramuscular myxoma*
  - Small numbers of bland spindled to stellate fibroblast-like cells with small, hyperchromatic nuclei and scant, tapering, eosinophilic cytoplasm; a myxoid stroma (mucopolysaccharide composed of hyaluronic acid) may be prominent
  - No nuclear atypia, pleomorphism, mitoses, or multinucleate cells
  - Very few intralesional blood vessels
  - Periphery appears infiltrative; lesion merges with adjacent muscle and fascia with atrophic muscle cells and fat cells in mucoid stroma
  - Macrophages with lipid or mucin may be present
  - Areas of increased cellularity with numerous collagen fibers may be present
- *Digital myxoma (digital mucous cyst)*
  - Morphologically similar to intramuscular myxoma, but more cellular
- *Juxta-articular myxoma*
  - Morphologically indistinguishable from the cellular form of intramuscular myxoma
  - Cystic spaces lined by a delicate layer of fibrin or thicker layer of collagen
  - May have foci of inflammation, hemorrhage, or fibrosis
- *Cutaneous myxoma (superficial angiomyxoma)*
  - Multilobulated dermal or subcutaneous mass
  - Characterized by bland plump, spindle-shaped or stellate-shaped fibroblasts and elongated thin-walled vessels in a myxoid matrix
  - No cytologic atypia or pleomorphism; rare mitoses present
  - Neutrophils and other inflammatory cells present in stroma
  - 30% contain entrapped epithelial elements and adipose (usually epidermoid cyst, strands of squamous cells, or small islands of basaloid cells)

Special Stains

- Reticulin stain will demonstrate loose network of reticulin fibers
- Mucoid stroma stains with Alcian blue, mucicarmine, and colloidal iron

Immunohistochemistry

- Tumor cells stain positively for vimentin and negatively for S-100 protein

Electron Microscopy

- Cells are fibroblast and myofibroblast features
- Macrophagelike cells with small lipid droplets or secretory vacuoles and cytoplasmic processes

Molecular Alterations

- Superficial angiomyxoma may be transmitted as an autosomal dominant trait (see Carney syndrome later in this section)

Differential Diagnosis

- *Intramuscular myxoma*
  - Juxta-articular myxoma
  - Low grade myxofibrosarcoma
  - Myxoid neurofibroma
  - Dermal nerve sheath myxoma (neurothekeoma)
  - Myxoid liposarcoma
  - Myxoid leiomyosarcoma
- *Digital myxoma (digital mucous cyst)*
  - Mucoid neurofibroma
  - Dermal nerve sheath myxoma (neurothekeoma)
  - Dermal mucinosis (tends to occur in head and neck region)
- *Juxta-articular myxoma*
  - Intramuscular myxoma
  - Ganglion cyst
- *Cutaneous myxoma (superficial angiomyxoma)*
  - Dermal nerve sheath myxoma (neurothekeoma)
  - Digital myxoma (usually more cellular and unilocular)

Treatment

- Wide local excision

Prognosis

- Intramuscular myxomas rarely recur (even after incomplete excision)
- Juxta-articular myxomas and superficial angiomyxomas have a 30% local recurrence rate

Associations

- Intramuscular myxoma
  - When multiple may be a component of *Albright syndrome*: Monostotic or polyostotic fibrous dysplasia of bone, melanotic pigmentation of the skin, endocrine abnormalities (precocious puberty), GI polyps, hypophosphatemic osteomalacia, and benign and malignant bone tumors
  - *Mazabraud syndrome*: Intramuscular myxoma(s) and skeletal fibrous dysplasia
  - Cutaneous myxoma (superficial angiomyxoma)
  - *Carney syndrome*: Cardiac, breast myxomas and superficial angiomyxomas, spotty pigmentation, endocrine tumors (adrenal and pituitary), large-cell calcifying Sertoli cell tumor of testis, and psammomatous melanotic schwannoma
- Juxta-articular myxoma is not associated with other syndromes or tumors

Ossifying Fibromyxoid Tumor

Clinical Manifestations

- Typically occurs in the deep subcutaneous tissue of adults (median age of onset 50 years)
- Presents as a slowly enlarging, painless, subcutaneous mass of the extremities (70%), trunk, and head and neck; also mediastinum and retroperitoneum
- May be attached to tendon, fascia, or skeletal muscle
- Usually solitary but may be multiple
- Slightly more common in men than women

Gross Pathology

- Typically well circumscribed and surrounded by a thick fibrous capsule
- Areas of calcification may be seen in subcapsular region
- Cut surface may be bony hard and lobulated

Microscopic Pathology

- Small nests or trabeculae of uniform, round or polygonal cells with small amounts of pale eosinophilic to clear cytoplasm, ill-defined cytoplasmic borders, and uniform round to oval vesicular nuclei, sometimes with a small nucleolus, in an abundant fibromyxoid collagenous matrix
- Pleomorphism and atypia are rare and nuclear features are bland
- Mitoses may be present, but rare
- No necrosis

- Fibromyxoid matrix contains prominent thin-walled vessels, some of which are thrombosed
- Surrounding capsule may be fibrous or consist of an incomplete shell of lamellar bone (80%); fibrous septa may extend from capsule into lesion
- Lobules of tumor may extend beyond capsule
- *Atypical or malignant ossifying fibromyxoid tumor* characterized by:
  - Centrally located foci of osteoid laid down by plump neoplastic cells
  - Increased cellularity with a high mitotic rate
  - Usually a less complete shell of bone than conventional lesions

Special Stains

- Tumor cells negative for PAS (do not contain glycogen)
- Myxoid matrix will stain with Alcian blue

Immunohistochemistry

- Neoplastic cells usually positive for vimentin
- 75% to 80% are positive for S-100 protein; 50% for desmin; 30% to 40% for actin
- Cells typically negative for cytokeratin and EMA

Electron Microscopy

- Tumor cells contain parallel bundles of intermediate filaments and short cytoplasmic processes

Molecular Alterations

- None

Differential Diagnosis

- Epithelial nerve sheath tumors (epithelioid neurofibroma, schwannoma, and MPNST)
- Extraskeletal myxoid chondrosarcoma (typically large and deep-seated)
- Extraskeletal osteosarcoma (only in differential of atypical or malignant ossifying fibromyxoid tumor)

Treatment

- Surgical excision

Prognosis

- Overwhelming majority benign
- 10% will recur locally after surgical treatment; result of incomplete excision
- 2 reports of metastasis

Comment

- Neoplasm may be a neural tumor of Schwann cell origin (based on immunohistochemical features)

Synovial Sarcoma

Clinical Manifestations

- Generally seen in young patients between the ages of 15 and 40 years
- Males affected more commonly than females
- Typically presents as a slowly enlarging, palpable, painful, and tender deep-seated mass
- 80% occur in the area of the knee or ankle
- Also seen in the region of the hip, soft tissues of the neck (particularly retropharyngeal), oral cavity, anterior abdominal wall, retroperitoneum, and mediastinum
- Typically grows close to a joint but rarely involves the synovial membrane

Gross Pathology

- Tends to be well circumscribed and firm with yellow to white cut surface
- Cystic changes common
- Usually adherent to adjacent tendons, tendon sheaths, or exterior surface of joint capsule

Microscopic Pathology

- 2 variants: Biphasic and monophasic (more common)
  - Biphasic pattern consists of uniform round to spindled cells with a high nuclear-cytoplasmic ratio admixed with columnar or cuboidal epithelial cells
- Epithelial cells are large and cuboidal or columnar with prominent cytoplasmic membranes and round vesicular nuclei; usually arranged in cords, nests, glandular structures, or covering papillary structures
- Spindled cells tend to be plump with scant cytoplasm and oval, hyperchromatic nuclei arranged in dense sheets, "herringbone" fascicles resembling a fibrosarcoma; nuclei have finely dispersed chromatin and frequently abut each other or overlap; alternating hypo- and hypercellular areas typical (reminiscent of nerve-sheath tumors)

- Stroma may be collagenous, delicate, and fibrovascular, or myxoid (focal)
- Hemorrhagic or mucinous cysts may be present
- 30% show tumoral calcification with or without ossification
- On low power, tumor tends to have a vaguely multinodular architecture and be well circumscribed with a pseudocapsule or invasive periphery
- Mitotic activity often sparse in both spindle cell and epithelioid cell areas (<2 per hpf)
- Mast cells may be present
- Degree of vascularity variable: May be a dominant feature with multiple dilated, irregularly shaped vessels similar to those of a hemangiopericytoma or may be inconspicuous and few in number
- Vascular invasion may be present
- Some neoplasms do not have obvious epithelial foci (monophasic fibrous type); others do not have spindle cell component (monophasic epithelial type)
- Approximately 20% are poorly differentiated (3 patterns: *large cell or epithelioid* characterized by pleomorphic, rounded nuclei with prominent nucleoli, *small cell* characterized by nuclei similar to those of other small cell tumors, and *high-grade spindle cell* characterized by high grade vesicular nuclei and increased numbers of mitoses)

Special Stains

- Mucin stains confirm presence of acidic mucopolysaccharides (hyaluronic acid, chondroitin sulfate, and heparan sulfate) in spindle cell areas
- Epithelial foci contain PAS-positive, sialic acid-containing glycoproteins
- Stromal mucin is negative for PAS
- Reticulin stains will outline epithelioid cell clusters in tumors where they are indistinct

Immunohistochemistry

- 90% reactive for cytokeratin and/or epithelial membrane antigen in both the epithelial areas and spindle cell areas (staining in epithelial areas usually stronger); cytokeratin staining in monophasic fibrous type may be limited to a few isolated cells
- 60% to 70% of cases are immunoreactive for CD99 (product of *MIC-2* gene), a marker associated with Ewing sarcoma/PNET
- 80% demonstrate strong positivity for *bcl*-2 protein in spindle cell component
- 30% focally positive for S-100 protein
- Tumor cells negative for CD34

Electron Microscopy

- Biphasic tumors have epithelial cells, spindle cells, and transition forms
- Epithelial cells may have microvilli and be arranged in clusters
- Even lesions that appear to be monophasic will have areas of epithelial differentiation characterized by slitlike glandular spaces and microvilli
- Spindle cells resemble fibroblasts with irregular nuclear membranes, marginated chromatin, and small nucleoli

Molecular Alterations

- 90% associated with chromosomal translocation t(X;18)(p11.2;q11.2); translocation results in fusion of *SS18* gene at chromosome 18q11.2 to either of 2 genes, *SSX1* or *SSX2*, at Xp11.2

Differential Diagnosis

- Biphasic variant:
  - Epithelioid sarcoma
  - Malignant mesothelioma
  - Carcinosarcoma
  - Metastatic carcinoma
- Monophasic variant:
  - Solitary fibrous tumor
  - Hemangiopericytoma
  - Fibrosarcoma
  - Leiomyosarcoma
  - MPNST
  - Spindle cell carcinoma

Treatment

- Wide local excision with adjuvant high-dose radiation
- Childhood lesions often very sensitive to chemotherapy

Prognosis

- Prognosis appears to be better for tumors that have osseous metaplasia and/or extensive calcification

- Prognosis better for young patients (<15 years), distal extremity lesions, small tumors (<5 cm), tumors with low mitotic rates, and tumors with little necrosis
- Tumors with extensive necrosis (>50%), rhabdoid cells, high mitotic rates (>10 per hpf) and high-grade nuclei have the worst prognosis
- Late metastasis (up to 20 years) develop in 50%; lung most frequent site
- Low-risk lesions (>50% epithelial or glandular and <15 mitotic figures/10 hpf) have 5-year survival close to 100%
- High-risk lesions (monophasic and high mitotic rate) have 5-year survival of 20%

Associations

- Trauma may or may not be associated antecedent event (most patients do not report a history of trauma; tumors have been documented to arise in areas of previous trauma)

Vascular Tumors

Angiosarcoma

Clinical Manifestations

- Usually seen in adults; men and women affected equally
- 35% arise in the skin and subcutis, 25% in soft tissue, and the remainder in other sites (breast, liver, bone, spleen, heart, and great vessels)
- 50% multicentric
- Rarely arise from major vessels
- May arise in previously irradiated fields, around long-standing foreign bodies, and in arteriovenous fistulas
- May be seen engrafted on mediastinal or retroperitoneal germ cell tumors and may exist within a preexisting benign tumor such as a hemangioma, neurofibroma, intramuscular lipoma, or leiomyoma

Gross Pathology

- *Variants*
  - Cutaneous without associated lymphedema
    - Usually occurs in scalp and upper forehead and appear as an ill-defined bruise with an indurated border
    - 50% are multifocal
    - Advanced lesions nodular and may ulcerate
  - Cutaneous in setting of long-standing lymphedema
    - 90% occur after mastectomy (Stewart-Treves syndrome)
  - Breast
    - Presents with rapidly enlarging breast associated with blue-red discoloration of skin
    - Most malignant breast tumor
  - Radiation-induced
    - Almost always high-grade and aggressive
    - Deep soft tissue
    - Tends to occur in extremities or abdominal cavity and are characterized by extensive hemorrhage and necrosis

Microscopic Pathology

- An ill-defined vascular lesion with infiltrative margins
- Appearance ranges from being so well differentiated as to appear as a benign hemangioma to so undifferentiated and solid that it appears to be a carcinoma or melanoma or other type of sarcoma
- Irregularly shaped, interanastomosing, sinusoidal-like vascular channels that dissect between cells, along collagen bundles, and tissue planes in a multifocal distribution that results in ill-defined infiltrative margins; malignant endothelial cells have variable cytologic pleomorphism, nuclear atypism, hyperchromatism, mitotic activity, and often with tufted and papillary endothelial proliferations; signet ring or primitive vascular lumina may be present in tumor cells
- Poorly differentiated areas tend to be very cellular, solid, and spindle-shaped
- Presence of necrosis is variable
- Soft-tissue lesions tend to have endothelium with an epithelioid appearance (cytoplasm granular or glassy, nuclei large and vesicular)

Special Stains

- Reticulin stain may outline vascular architecture

Immunohistochemistry

- Typically tumor cells are positive for CD31 (platelet-endothelial cell adhesion molecule—very specific) and CD34 (human hematopoietic progenitor cell antigen—less specific)
- Angiosarcomas of soft tissue often coexpress cytokeratin and EMA and are more likely to express von Willebrand factor than more conventional lesions

Electron Microscopy

- Well-differentiated cells have most of the features of normal endothelial cells (Weibel-Palade bodies, pinocytic vesicles, prominent external basal lamina along antiluminal border, and tight junctions)
- Poorly differentiated areas usually lack the features of normal endothelial cells but still have red blood cells between or in tumor cells

Molecular Alterations

- None

Differential Diagnosis

- Conventional angiosarcoma
- Benign hemangioma
- Angiomatosis
- Angiolipoma
- Angiosarcoma of soft tissue
- Poorly differentiated carcinoma and sarcoma
- Epithelioid hemangioendothelioma
- Epithelioid mesothelioma
- Epithelioid sarcoma

Treatment

- Wide excision; no benefit from lymph node dissection

Prognosis

- Cutaneous lesions have a 10% to 15% 5-year survival
- Angiosarcoma of breast has 90% mortality within 2 years of diagnosis
- Soft-tissue angiosarcomas are very aggressive; local recurrence occurs in 20%; 50% die within a year of the diagnosis

Associations

- May arise in association with longstanding lymphedema and in areas subjected to therapeutic irradiation
- Hepatic angiosarcomas associated with exposure to silver oxide-containing insecticides, vinyl chloride, intravenous thorium dioxide, and androgenic anabolic steroids

Glomus Tumor

Clinical Manifestations

- Equal sex distribution (subungual type much more common in women)
- Typically occur in the 3rd to 5th decades and present as a solitary mass in the dermis or subcutis of the extremities
- Most common site is subungual region of finger
- Reported in patella, chest wall, bone, stomach, rectum, colon, nerve, trachea, cervix, and vagina
- Usually painful and extremely sensitive to cold and touch
- May be multiple (10%); when multiple more likely to occur during childhood, less likely to be subungual, and typically asymptomatic

Gross Pathology

- Typically a small red to blue nodule in the deep dermis or subcutaneous tissue
- Most are solitary; 10% are multiple (usually in children)

Microscopic Pathology

- Variable admixture of glomus cells, vascular structures, and smooth muscle
- Variants:
  - *Classic glomus tumor*
    - Circumscribed nest of uniform, round cells with pale to pink cytoplasm arranged in solid sheets surrounding capillary-sized vessels; nuclei tend to be round and hyperchromatic; mitoses are rare
    - Tumor at least partially surrounded by a rim of collagen with small vessels and nerves; isolated nests of glomus cells may be in these small peripheral vessels
  - *Glomangioma*
    - A cavernous hemangiomalike arrangement of vaguely circumscribed groups or clusters of glomus cells in and around gaping blood vessels
    - Secondary thrombosis may be present
  - *Glomangiomyoma*
    - Least frequent variant
    - Characterized by cells in transition between glomus cells and smooth muscle cells

- *Symplastic glomus tumor*
  - Characterized by marked cytologic atypia without any other worrisome features such as large size, deep location, necrosis, or mitotic activity
- *Malignant glomus tumor (glomangiosarcoma)*
  - 2 types: spindle cell (resemble leiomyosarcoma) and round cell
  - To be considered malignant, tumor must be >2 cm, be located in a subfascial or visceral location, be mitotically active, have atypical mitotic figures, and/or show marked nuclear atypia

Special Stains

- PAS or toluidine blue will highlight a "chicken-wire" network of basal lamina material encircling individual glomus cells

Immunohistochemistry

- Neoplastic cells stain positively for vimentin and smooth muscle actin
- Type IV collagen surrounds cells
- Desmin staining quite variable

Electron Microscopy

- Tumor cells are round and have a round nucleus with a prominent nucleolus; cytoplasm contains bundles of thin actin-like filaments; cells are closely packed together, interdigitate with each other, and are surrounded by a thick basal lamina

Molecular Alterations

- When multiple may have an autosomal dominant pattern of inheritance (chromosome 1p21-22)

Differential Diagnosis

- Hemangioma
- Adnexal tumor (hidradenoma)
- Paraganglioma
- Hemangiopericytoma
- Melanoma

Treatment and Prognosis

- Simple excision
- Recurrence rate approximately 10% after surgical excision

Associations

- None

Hemangioendothelioma

Clinical Manifestations

- A vascular tumor that is intermediate in both behavior and histologic appearance between a benign hemangioma and a conventional angiosarcoma
- Variants
  - *Epithelioid hemangioendothelioma*
    - Men and women affected equally
    - Tends to occur in the distal extremities of adolescents and young adults; rare in children
    - 50% arise in the wall of a vein
    - Typically develops as a solitary slightly tender mass in either superficial or deep soft tissue; more often subfascial than subcutaneous; 10% occur in dermis; may involve bone, lung, pleura, liver, peritoneum, lymph nodes and the region of the head and neck
    - Tumors that arise in parenchymal organs (lung, liver, bone, etc.) are more common in women than men and tend to be multifocal (grow along small vessels)
  - *Retiform hemangioendothelioma*
    - Usually a red-blue plaque or nodule involving skin and subcutaneous tissue of distal extremities
  - *Spindle cell hemangioma* (formally spindle cell hemangioendothelioma)
    - Tends to present as an asymptomatic mass in distal extremities (especially the hand) of adolescents and young adults
    - More common in males than in females
    - 50% occur in patients <25 years of age
  - *Malignant endovascular papillary angioendothelioma (Dabska tumor)*
    - Typically located in skin and soft tissue of children and infants; rare in adults
    - May present as a diffuse subcutaneous indurated area or a fairly circumscribed intradermal mass that infiltrates into subcutaneous tissue and beyond

- *Kaposiform hemangioendothelioma*
    - Occurs exclusively in children and adolescents in superficial or deep soft tissue
    - Features common to both capillary hemangioma and Kaposi sarcoma
    - May arise in association with lymphangiomatosis

Gross and Microscopic Pathology

- *Epithelioid hemangioendothelioma*
    - Lesions that arise from vessels extend from the lumen circumferentially into surrounding tissue while preserving the vessel architecture; the cut surface superficially resembles an organizing thrombus with a variegated red-white color
    - Tumors that do not arise from a vessel tend to be gray-white and may not appear to be particularly vascular
    - Tumor cells usually arranged in short strands or solid nests and have an epithelial or histiocytic appearance with abundant eosinophilic cytoplasm; nucleus is typically bland, round, vesicular and occasionally indented; intracellular cytoplasmic lumina ("vacuoles") may be present and contain erythrocytes; rare mitoses, little pleomorphism and usually no necrosis; osteoclasticlike multinucleated giant cells may be present; stroma consists of a sulfated acid-rich matrix which varies from light blue (chondroidlike) to deep pink (hyaline)
- *Retiform hemangioendothelioma*
    - Diffuse involvement of dermis, frequent involvement of underlying subcutaneous tissue
    - Characterized by elongated, narrow, arborzing vascular channels quite reminiscent of the normal rete testis
    - Vessels lined by uniform, hyperchromatic endothelial cells with prominent nuclei that protrude into lumens (hobnail)
    - Pleomorphism and mitotic figures rare
    - A prominent stromal and perivascular lymphocytic infiltrate present in 50%
- *Spindle cell hemangioma* (formally spindle cell hemangioendothelioma)
    - On gross examination, tumors are small, well circumscribed, with reddish nodules that may contain phleboliths
    - Microscopically neoplasm combines features of cavernous hemangioma and Kaposi sarcoma; tumor cells have a bland spindled appearance and are arranged in a multinodular pattern with gapping vascular channels at the periphery; scattered epithelial cells have rudimentary (signet ring-like) cytoplasmic lumina and resemble the cells of epithelioid hemangioendothelioma
- *Malignant endovascular papillary angioendothelioma (Dabska tumor)*
    - Tumor consists of papillary tufts of plump endothelial cells located within dilated, well-formed vascular spaces partially filled with clear fluid (may have a glomeruloid configuration); nuclei tend to be located on luminal surface (hobnail)
    - Cytoplasmic lumina may be present and may contain intraluminal erythrocytes
    - Typically intraluminal and perivascular lymphocytes present
- *Kaposiform hemangioendothelioma*
    - Deep (soft tissue) lesions characterized by ill-defined grey to red nodules
    - Intersecting curved or flat fascicles of bland spindle cells admixed with capillaries; fascicles may be compact with few interspersed spaces or hypocellular with interspersed slit-like, sievelike, or crescent-shaped vascular lumens
    - Scattered throughout the lesion are glomeruloid nests of rounded or epithelial endothelial cells with eosinophilic cytoplasm, hemosiderin granules, hyaline globules and cytoplasmic vacuoles; red cells and microthrombi may be present between cells and in the spindled endothelium
    - Both cellular atypia and mitotic figures are rare
    - When the tumor develops in association with lymphangiomatosis, a well-defined interface between the 2 lesions is usually present

Special Stains

- Reticulin stain highlights fibrous strands surrounding individual cells and nests of cells

Immunohistochemistry

- *Epithelioid hemangioendothelioma*
    - Usually cytokeratin negative
    - Factor VIII-associated antigen present
- *Retiform hemangioendothelioma*
    - Tumor cells positive for CD31, CD34, and von Willebrand factor

- *Spindled cell hemangioma*
    - Factor VIII-associated antigen highlights cells lining vascular spaces and epithelioid endothelium; the spindled cells are usually negative
- *Malignant endovascular papillary angioendothelioma (Dabska tumor)*
    - Tumor cells positive for factor VIII-associated protein
- *Kaposiform hemangioendothelioma*
    - Most cells express CD31 and CD34, but not factor VIII-associated antigen

Electron Microscopy

- Cells have characteristics of endothelial cells with basal lamina, pinocytotic vesicles, and occasional Weibel-Palade bodies
- Spindle cells of spindle cell hemangioma appear as mesenchymal cells resembling fibroblasts

Molecular Alterations

- None

Differential Diagnosis

- *Epithelioid hemangioendothelioma:*
    - Signet-ring carcinoma, melanoma, epithelioid angiosarcoma, epithelioid sarcoma, epithelioid MPNST, and mesothelioma
- *Retiform hemangioendothelioma*
    - Dabska tumor
- *Spindle cell hemangioma*:
    - Spindle cell angiosarcoma, Kaposi sarcoma, and Kaposiform hemangioendothelioma
- *Malignant endovascular papillary angioendothelioma (Dabska tumor)*
    - Lymphangioma, epithelioid hemangioendothelioma, spindle cell hemangioma, and angiosarcoma
- *Kaposiform hemangioendothelioma*
    - Kaposi sarcoma
    - Capillary (cellular) hemangioma of infancy

Treatment

- *Epithelioid hemangioendothelioma*
    - Most are cured by simple excision
    - When liver primary site of disease, orthotopic transplantation provides a 75% 5-year survival
- *Retiform hemangioendothelioma*
    - Wide local excision
- *Spindle cell hemangioma*
    - Conservative excision for limited disease
    - Radical excision for recurrent disease
- *Malignant endovascular papillary angioendothelioma (Dabska tumor)*
    - Wide local excision
- *Kaposiform hemangioendothelioma*
    - Superficial tumors can be cured with wide local excision; deep-seated neoplasms often unresectable

Prognosis

- *Epithelioid hemangioendothelioma*
    - Recurrence rate approximately 15%
    - Metastasis in 30%, but fewer than 50% die of disease
    - Overall tumor mortality 15%
    - Mortality 65% when the primary site of disease is the lung, and 35% when primary site is the liver
- *Retiform hemangioendothelioma*
    - No reports of metastases
- *Spindle cell hemangioma*
    - Recurrence rate as high as 60%; recurrences may occur within several centimeters of the original tumor
    - Regional and distant metastasis have not been reported
- *Malignant endovascular papillary angioendothelioma (Dabska tumor)*
    - Uniformly good prognosis despite the presence of regional nodal metastasis
- *Kaposiform hemangioendothelioma*
    - No reports of distant metastasis

Associations

- *Spindle cell hemangioma*
    - Maffucci syndrome, Klippel-Trenaunay syndrome, and congenital lymphedema
- *Kaposiform hemangioendothelioma*
    - *Kasabach-Merritt syndrome*: Consumption coagulopathy and thrombocytopenia (seen with deep-seated tumors especially in the retroperitoneum)
    - Lymphangiomatosis

Hemangioma

Clinical Manifestations

- Typically regarded as a neoplasm because it produces a mass
- High percentage occur in children (may be present at birth); most common tumor of infancy and childhood
- Most occur in the area of the head and neck; fewer involve the trunk or extremities; may occur in internal organs, but most are superficial and localized
- Most are solitary (when multiple, with or without associated lesions in internal organs, the condition is known as *multifocal angiomatosis*)

Gross and Microscopic Pathology

- *Capillary hemangioma*
  - Most common variant is cellular hemangioma of infancy; other variants include pyogenic granuloma and epithelioid hemangioma
  - Seen in fewer than 1% of children and typically involves the soft tissue in the region of the parotid gland (cellular hemangioma)
  - Appears shortly after birth, enlarges rapidly, and then often regresses spontaneously
  - Microscopically, plump to flattened endothelial cells with variable number of pericytes arranged in a multilobular architectural pattern with branching, small vascular channels arising from a small arteriole ("feeder" vessel); vascular lumina may be inconspicuous; mitoses may be present; interstitial fibrosis becomes a component as the lesion ages
- *Acquired tufted angioma*
  - Slow-growing macule in dermis of upper body of adults
  - Microscopically vague nodules of capillary-sized vessels irregularly distributed in the deep dermis
- *Hobnail hemangioma (targetoid hemosiderotic hemangioma)*
  - Exophytic mass on skin of extremities of young adults
  - Microscopically, superficial portion consists of dilated vessels lined by hobnail endothelial cells; deep portion consists of think, slitlike capillaries
- *Verrucous hemangioma*
  - Occur as solitary lesion on lower extremity of child
  - Capillary or cavernous hemangioma with hyperkeratosis of overlying skin
- *Cherry angioma (senile angioma)*
  - Red papule with pale halo on trunk and extremities of adults
  - Microscopically, dilated, thin-walled capillaries with atrophy of overlying epidermis
- *Cavernous hemangioma*
  - Typically involves the upper body of children
  - Tends to be deeper, larger, and less circumscribed than a capillary hemangioma
  - Does not spontaneously regress
  - May destroy neighboring structures
  - Microscopically, medium to large caliber blood vessels with flattened endothelium arranged in a lobular or diffuse pattern; dystrophic calcifications may be present
- *Arteriovenous hemangioma*
  - Most diagnosed as intramuscular hemangioma, angiomatosis, or capillary hemangioma
  - Can be deep or superficial
  - Superficial form tends to occur as a solitary subcutaneous or submucosal nodule in an adult
  - Deep form typically occurs in the region of the head and neck or the lower extremities of children and may be characterized by local hypertrophy and significant arterial shunting
  - Microscopically, capillary and cavernous hemangiomalike areas consisting of medium to large caliber arteries and veins with intimal thickening of the veins
- *Venous hemangioma*
  - Typically a deep-seated lesion affecting adults
  - Microscopically, thick-walled blood vessels with a disorganized muscular wall; calcification and phleboliths common
- *Spindle cell hemangioma (spindle cell hemangioendothelioma)*
  - Tend to consist of multiple nodules in the same general anatomic area
  - Microscopically, thin-walled cavernous vessels lined by flat endothelium and separated from each other by spindled areas that contain epithelioid cells with cytoplasmic vacuoles or lumens
- *Epithelioid hemangioma (angiolymphoid hyperplasia with eosinophilia)*

- Typically presents in the dermis and subcutis of the head and neck region (usually near the ear) of women in the 3rd to 5th decades of life
- Usually solitary but may be multiple
- Microscopically, epithelioid endothelial cells with vacuolated, eosinophilic cytoplasm and round to oval nuclei arranged in a multilobular pattern; usually a large central vessel surrounded by smaller vessels; lymphocytes with germinal centers, eosinophils, mast cells, and plasma cells may be present

- *Pyogenic granuloma (granulation tissue-type capillary hemangioma)*
  - A polypoid growth involving the skin or mucosa of the head and neck or hands
  - Equal sex distribution and evenly distributed through all decades
  - May occur and undergo recrudescence with pregnancy (granuloma gravidarum)
  - May be intravascular (intravenous pyogenic granuloma)
  - Microscopic features include a well-circumscribed area of arborizing capillary channels arranged in a polypoid or lobular pattern; stromal edema and myxoid change are usually present; mitoses may be present; epithelial ulceration may be present (very reminiscent of granulation tissue)
- *Intramuscular hemangioma*
  - Typically occurs in young adults (<30 years); men and women affected equally
  - Thigh most common location
  - Most are of the capillary type (may be cavernous or mixed)
  - Microscopically, capillary-sized vessels with plump nuclei infiltrate between individual muscle fibers
- *Synovial hemangioma*
  - Most commonly occur in the region of the knee during childhood
  - Typically present with pain and/or effusion
  - May be localized or diffuse
  - Microscopically, a localized or diffuse cavernous hemangioma in an edematous, myxoid, or hyalinized stroma covered by a synovial membrane; hemosiderin deposition, inflammatory cells, and synovial hyperplasia may be present
- *Perineural hemangioma (hemangioma of peripheral nerve)*
  - Typically occurs in patients under age of 40 years
  - Associated with pain, numbness, and muscular atrophy
  - Microscopic appearance typical of cavernous-type hemangioma involving the epineurium of the peripheral nerve
- *Angiomatosis (diffuse hemangioma)*
  - Affects infants and children and involves a large area of the body (limb or visceral organ)
  - Affected areas are hypertrophic and frequently discolored
  - May be fatal if vital structures involved
  - Microscopically, a proliferation of irregularly shaped and sized, small to medium blood vessels that diffusely infiltrate dermis, subcutaneous tissue, skeletal muscle, bone and/or viscera; lymphoid aggregates and mature fat may be present
- *Papillary endothelial hyperplasia (intravascular hemangioendothelioma of Masson)*
  - An organizing thrombus that arises within a blood vessel and occasionally extends into adjacent soft tissue
  - Often superimposed on an underlying vascular lesion such as a benign hemangioma
  - Superficial veins of the head and neck, fingers or trunk unusually involved (first described in hemorrhoidal vessels)
  - Microscopically, a well-defined area of interanastomosing channels and papillary structures lined by benign endothelium; papillary cords may be fibrous or hyalinized; endothelial cell nuclei tend to be large and hyperchromatic; mitoses rare
  - Residual organizing thrombi frequently an associated finding

Special Stains

- Not helpful

Immunohistochemistry

- Factor VIII-associated antigen

Electron Microscopy

- Endothelial cells typically contains rod-shaped bodies (Weibel-Palade bodies) that contain parallel tubules
- Endothelium lies on thin-based lamina of collagen

Molecular Alterations

- None

Differential Diagnosis

- Capillary hemangioma
  - Cellular angiolipoma
- Kaposi sarcoma
- Hemangiopericytoma
- Angiosarcoma
- Cavernous hemangioma
  - Angiomatosis
  - Intramuscular lipoma
  - Benign mesenchymoma
  - Angiosarcoma
- Arteriovenous hemangioma
  - Intramuscular lipoma
  - Capillary/cavernous hemangioma
  - Benign mesenchymoma
  - Angiomatosis
  - Kaposi sarcoma
- Venous hemangioma
  - Same as for arteriovenous hemangioma
- Spindle cell hemangioma
  - Cavernous hemangioma
  - Angiosarcoma
  - Kaposi sarcoma
- Epithelial hemangioma
  - Bacillary angiomatosis
  - Epithelial hemangioendothelioma
  - Spindle cell hemangioendothelioma
  - Epithelioid angiosarcoma
- Pyogenic granuloma (granulation tissue-type hemangioma)
  - Well-differentiated angiosarcoma
  - Angiomatous form of Kaposi sarcoma
- Intramuscular hemangioma
  - Intramuscular lipoma
  - Benign mesenchymoma
  - Angiomatosis
  - Hemangiopericytoma
  - Angiosarcoma
  - Liposarcoma
- Synovial hemangioma
  - Synovitis
  - Vascular malformation
- Perineural hemangioma
  - Intramuscular hemangioma with perineural involvement and angiosarcoma
- Angiomatosis (diffuse hemangioma)
  - Intramuscular hemangioma
  - Arteriovenous hemangioma
- Papillary endothelial hyperplasia (hemangioendothelioma of Masson)
  - Hematoma
  - Hemangioma
  - Angiosarcoma

Treatment and Prognosis

- Capillary hemangioma
  - Surgery not indicated unless life-threatening
  - Corticosteroids or interferon-α
- Verrucous hemangioma
  - Tends to recur and develop satellite lesions if not completely excised
- Cavernous hemangioma
  - Steroids and irradiation
  - Recombinant interferon-α2a and pentoxifylline
- Spindle cell hemangioma
  - 60% recur
- Epithelioid hemangioma
  - Rarely spontaneously regress
  - 30% recur
  - Surgical excision
  - Superficial radiotherapy produces an 80% response rate
- Pyogenic granuloma
  - Surgical excision
  - Recurrence rate 15% to 20%; may recur as multiple satellite nodules

- Intramuscular hemangioma
  - Recurrence rate up to 50% and depends on adequacy of first excision
- Synovial hemangioma
  - Simple surgical excision
  - Diffuse lesions treated with low dose radiation
- Perineural hemangioma
  - Surgical excision (requires meticulous intrafascicular dissection)
- Angiomatosis
  - 90% recur (40% recur more than once)
- Papillary endothelial hyperplasia
  - Simple excision

Associations

- Capillary hemangioma occasionally associated with:
  - Kasabach-Merritt syndrome (consumption coagulopathy)
- Cavernous hemangiomas associated with:
  - Kasabach-Merritt syndrome
  - Blue rubber bleb nevus syndrome (cutaneous hemangiomas and GI (small intestine) hemangiomas)
  - Maffucci syndrome (enchondromas and multiple cavernous hemangiomas); 20% develop chondrosarcoma
- Venous hemangiomas (on feet) may be associated with Turner syndrome
- Spindle cell hemangioma associated with:
  - Maffucci syndrome
  - Klippel-Trénaunay syndrome
  - Early-onset varicosities
  - Congenital lymphedema
  - Epithelioid hemangioendothelioma (rare)
- Pyogenic granuloma may develop in response to trauma (30%)
- Angiomatosis associated with:
  - Kasabach-Merritt syndrome

Kaposi Sarcoma

Clinical Manifestations

- A multifocal disease that classically affects older men of Mediterranean or Jewish extraction
- Usually involves the skin of the distal extremities
- Has a progressive course that tends to wax and wane and may regress
- Probably a viral-associated tumor (may actually be viral induced) such as human herpesvirus 8 (HHV-8)
- Often associated with immunodeficiency

Variants

- *Classic (indolent) Kaposi sarcoma*
  - 90% in elderly men of predominantly Mediterranean/East European descent
  - Onset of disease characterized by ≥1 cutaneous lesions usually on the distal portion of the lower extremity; lesions tend to begin as blue-red nodules often accompanied by edema of the involved extremity; with time the nodules coalesce into plaques that may ulcerate
  - Spontaneous regression may occur
- *Lymphadenopathic (African) Kaposi sarcoma*
  - Occurs primarily in young African children who present with lymphopathy and adult men with progressive disease of the lower extremities
  - Children have a rapidly progressive course with tendency toward internal organ involvement
  - Adults rarely develop internal organ involvement
- *Transplantation-associated (iatrogenic immunosuppression) Kaposi sarcoma*
  - Incidence of post-transplantation Kaposi sarcoma is approximately 1%
  - Typically develops an average of 16 months after transplantation
  - Usually an indolent course and may spontaneously regress with cessation of immunotherapy
- *AIDS-related Kaposi sarcoma*
  - Kaposi sarcoma develops in 30% of patients with AIDS
  - Homosexual men have the highest incidence of AIDS-related Kaposi sarcoma
  - Lesions begin as small flat pink patches that evolve into more typical blue-red nodules

- □ Widespread skin lesions and oral mucosal involvement typical
- □ 50% have lymph node involvement
- □ 30% have GI tract involvement

Gross Pathology

- Skin lesions appear as patches, plaques, and/or nodules
- Typically small (2 to 3 cm), elevated, hemorrhagic, spongy dermal nodules

Microscopic Pathology

- Microscopic features of all the clinical forms of Kaposi sarcoma are similar
- Patch stage (earliest): Characterized by a dense aggregate of small, thin-walled, narrow vessels dissecting through dermal collagen and surrounding preexisting dermal structures and larger ectatic vessels; vessels lined by endothelial cells with plump hyperchromatic nuclei and little cytoplasm; stroma contains plasma cells, scattered spindled cells, extravasated red blood cells, and hemosiderin
- Plaque stage: Characterized by a network of irregular vessels that tend to resemble a well-differentiated angiosarcoma except that the endothelial cells are bland; spindle cell component much more prominent than in patch stage; spindle cells uniform and have eosinophilic cytoplasm; intra- and extracytoplasmic hyaline globules usually present; few lymphocytes and plasma cells aggregate around the lesion
- Well-established lesions (nodular): Characterized by a well-circumscribed, unencapsulated mass of curvilinear fascicles of bland spindle cells that architecturally resemble a fibrosarcoma and surround proliferating vascular channels; hyaline globules present inside and outside the spindle cells; slitlike vascular spaces containing red blood cells separate the spindle cells and vascular channels (when seen in cross-section the spindled cells and slitlike vascular spaces give the lesion a sievelike pattern); chronic inflammatory cells and dilated vessels are present at the periphery; mitoses, pleomorphism, and vascular invasion rare

Special Stains

- Intracellular and intracellular hyaline globules characteristic of plaque and nodular stages of disease are PAS-positive diastase resistant

Immunohistochemistry

- Spindle cells of nodular lesions strongly immunoreactive for CD34 and CD31 and weakly or focally positive for von Willebrand factor and *Ulex europaeus*; always negative for factor VIII
- Nuclei of tumor cells stain positively for HHV-8
- Nuclear immunoreactivity for FLI1 always present

Electron Microscopy

- Morphology of most spindle cells closely resembles endothelial differentiation

Molecular Alterations

- Polyclonal; no consistent chromosomal abnormality

Differential Diagnosis

- Spindle cell angiosarcoma
- Spindle cell hemangioendothelioma
- Fibrosarcoma
- Bacillary angiomatosis
- Hemorrhagic fibrohistiocytoma
- Hemorrhagic nodular fasciitis
- Arteriovenous malformation
- Nodal angiomatosis
- Castleman disease
- Hemangioma

Treatment

- Patients with cutaneous/local disease (stage I) usually treated by local irradiation
- Patients with AIDS-related Kaposi (usually stage III or IV) treated with chemotherapy (etoposide, doxorubicin, bleomycin, vinblastine sulfate, interferon-α, and zidovudine)

Prognosis

- Chronic form of disease often has an indolent course lasting of 8 to 10 years; 25% die of a second malignant tumor
- Patients with AIDS-related Kaposi have a mortality of approximately 40%

- Patients with transplantation-associated Kaposi inevitably die of disease if internal organs involved; if disease confined to skin, a 50% reduction in immunosuppression therapy will often result in a 100% response rate

Associations

- Chronic Kaposi sarcoma
  - 30% incidence of a second malignancy, 50% of which are lymphoreticular (leukemia, lymphoma and multiple myeloma)
  - Pure red cell aplasia
  - Autoimmune hemolytic anemia
  - No association with HIV-1
- Lymphadenopathic Kaposi sarcoma
  - No association with HIV-1
- Transplantation-associated Kaposi sarcoma
  - Systemic Castleman disease
  - Angioimmunoblastic lymphadenopathy

Myopericytoma

Clinical Manifestations

- Usually subcutaneous on distal extremities
- Middle-aged adults of both sexes
- Usually painless slow growing subcutaneous nodule
- Occasionally painful
- May be present for years
- Usually solitary, but may be multiple (metachronous); when multiple tend to involve 1 anatomic site

Gross Pathology

- Tends to be well-circumscribed and <2 cm

Microscopic Pathology

- Unencapsulated, but usually well circumscribed
- A multilayered concentric growth of rather monomorphic spindle-to-oval shaped cells around numerous, variably sized lesional blood vessels
- Tumor cell appear myoid with eosinophilic or amphophilic cytoplasm and may be arranged in a whorled or fasicular pattern in a myxoid stroma
- Subendothelial proliferation of lesional cells frequently present (entire lesion may be entirely in the lumen of a vein)
- Mitotic figures and foci of necrosis rare

Special Stains

- Not helpful

Immunohistochemistry

- Tumor cells usually diffusely positive for SMA, but may only be focally positive
- Focal desmin and CD34 positivity may be present
- Typically negative for S-100 and cytokeratins

Electron Microscopy

- Not helpful

Molecular Alterations

- No familial cases reported to date

Differential Diagnosis

- See comment later in this section

Treatment

- Complete excision

Prognosis

- May recur (inadequate excision or new lesion in same area)

Associations

- None

Comment

- Myopericytoma part of a spectrum of lesions that includes myofibromatosis, myofibroma, infantile hemangiopericytoma, glomangiopericytoma, and myopericytoma

References

Dabbs DJ. *Diagnostic Immunohistochemistry.* New York: Churchill Livingstone, 2002.

Fletcher CDM, Unni KK, Mertens F (eds). *World Health Organization Classification of Tumours. Pathology and Genetics of Tumours of Soft Tissue and Bone.* Lyon: IARC Press, 2002.

Kempson RL, Fletcher CDM, Evans HL, Hendrickson MR, Sibley RK. *Tumors of Soft the Tissues: Atlas of Tumor Pathology, 3rd Series, Fascicle 30.* Washington DC: Armed Forces Institute of Pathology, 2001.

Meis-Kindblom JM, Enzinger FM. *Color Atlas of Soft Tissue Tumors.* St Louis: Mosby-Wolfe, 1996.

Mills S, Carter D, Greenson JK, Oberman HA, Reuter V, Stoler MH (eds). *Sternberg's Diagnostic Surgical Pathology. 4th ed.* Philadelphia: Lippincott Williams & Wilkins, 2004.

Rosai J. *Rosai and Ackerman's Surgical Pathology. 9th ed.* St. Louis: Mosby, 2004.

Scheithauer BW, Woodruff JM, Erlandson RA. *Tumors of the Peripheral Nervous System: Atlas of Tumor Pathology, 3rd Series, Fascicle 24.* Washington DC: Armed Forces Institute of Pathology, 1999.

Weiss SW, Goldblum JR. *Enzinger and Weiss's Soft Tissue Tumors. 4th ed.* St. Louis: Mosby Inc, 2001.

Appendix

Syndromes

Syndromes

Ataxia-Telangiectasia

- Autosomal recessive
  - Characterized by cerebellar ataxia (hallmark of disease; patients unable to walk by age 10), oculocutaneous telangiectasias, progeric skin changes, immune dysfunction, and increased cancer susceptibility
  - ATM gene located on chromosome 11q22-23
  - Mutation of ATM gene which encodes a protein kinase that senses DNA double strand breaks. ATM normally phosphorylates p53 causing cell arrest in G, which leasds to apoptosis
- Individuals extremely sensitive to ionizing radiation
  - Cancers prone to develop include leukemia and lymphoma, breast, pancreatic, stomach, bladder, and ovarian cancer
  - Heterozygous carriers may have as much as a 5- to 8-fold increased risk of breast cancer over normal population

Beckwith-Wiedemann Syndrome (11p15)

- Increased risk of hepatoblastoma and rhabdomyosarcoma
- Renal pathology
  - Predisposition to develop Wilms tumor
  - Renal medullary cysts
  - Mesoblastic nephroma (case reports)
- Adrenal pathology
  - Enlarged adrenal glands with cortical cytomegaly
  - Adrenal cortical carcinoma
  - Neuroblastoma
- Pancreatic pathology
  - Pancreatic islet cell hyperplasia
  - Pancreatoblastoma
- Hemihypertrophy
- Organomegaly
- Exophthalmos and macroglossia
- Omphalocele

Carney Syndrome

- Autosomal dominant mutation of *PRKAR1A*, type 1x-regulatory subunit of a protein kinase that acts on a tumor suppressor gene on chromosome 17q22-24 in 50%
- Remainder have abnormalities at locus 2p16
- Autosomal dominant
- More frequent in whites than blacks
- ***Myxomas***
  - *Cardiac*:
    - Present in 65%
    - Most serious component of disorder
    - Causes death in 20% of patients and responsible for serious embolic sequelae in 20%
  - *Skin*:
    - Present in 30%
    - Multiple in 75%
    - Head (eyelid, ear canal, scalp and cheek) most common site followed by trunk (nipples, chest, back and flank); perineum, genitalia, buttocks, and groin; upper and lower limb
  - *Breast:*
    - Present in 25% of female patients
    - Bilateral in the majority
- ***Lentiginosis and blue nevi***
  - Location in decreasing order of frequency: face (periocular and perioral), eyelids, ears, vermilion borders of lips, trunk, neck, conjunctiva or sclera, vulva (especially labia minora), extremities, and backs of hands
- ***Endocrine tumors***
  - *Adrenal:*
    - Bilateral pigmented nodular adrenal disease with associated Cushing syndrome in 20%
    - Microscopically, nodules are composed of enlarged, globular, cortical cells with granular, eosinophilic cytoplasm that often contains lipofuscin
  - *Testis:*
    - 30% of males
    - Bilateral in 75% and multicentric in each affected testis
    - Median age 14 years (range 5-33 years)
    - Present as sexual precocity
    - Microscopically, lesions are large-cell calcifying Sertoli cell tumor and steroid-type tumor (Leydig cell tumor or adrenocortical rest tumor)
    - No reports of metastasis
  - *Pituitary:*
    - 10% have adenoma associated with the gigantism or acromegaly; plasma levels of GH always elevated

- *Schwannomas*
  - 50% of psammomatous melanotic schwannomas occur in patients with Carney syndrome
  - Most common sites are upper alimentary tract (esophagus and stomach) and paravertebral sympathetic chains
  - 10% malignant and fatal

Carney Triad

- Gastric epithelial leiomyosarcoma
- Pulmonary chondroma
- Functioning extra-adrenal paraganglioma

Coffin-Siris Syndrome

- Medulloblastoma
- Mental and growth retardation
- Joint laxity
- Brachydactyly of fifth digit with hypoplasia/aplasia of nail bed

Familial Medullary Thyroid Cancer

- A variant of MEN IIA
- A strong predisposition to medullary thyroid cancer without the other clinical manifestations of MEN IIA (or MEN IIB)
- Most cases of medullary cancer are sporadic; as many as 25% may be familial.

Gorlin Syndrome (Nevoid Basal Cell Carcinoma Syndrome)

- An autosomal dominant disorder
- Tumor suppressor gene located on chromosome 9q
- PTCH gene. People with Gorlin syndrome born with germ line mutation in one allele acquire a second mutation in the other allele
- Skeletal anomalies (including craniomegaly), lamellar calcium deposition in the falx cerebri and diaphragma sellae
- Cutaneous epidermoid cysts
- Bifid ribs and vertebral anomalies
- Pits on the palms and soles
- Odontogenic keratocysts
- Calcifying ovarian fibromas
- Multifocal basal cell carcinomas occurring at an early age
- Medulloblastoma (usually develops before age of 5 and occurs in 3% to 5% of patients with Gorlin syndrome)

Li-Fraumeni Syndrome

- Also known as *SBLA syndrome* (sarcoma, breast cancer, leukemia, and adrenocortical cancer)
- Autosomal dominant
- Affected family members carry a *p*53 mutation located on chromosome 17p13 in all somatic cells
- Patients have increased sensitivity to radiation
- Multiple primary neoplasms in children and young adults: soft tissue sarcomas, osteosarcomas, and breast cancer
- Other associated malignancies include brain tumors (70% astrocytic tumors and 17% medulloblastomas, leukemia, and adrenocortical carcinoma
- Diagnostic criteria include:
  - Occurrence of sarcoma before age 45
  - At least 1 1st degree relative with any cancer before age 45
  - A 1st (or 2nd) degree relative with cancer before age 45 or a sarcoma at any age
- Target organs:
  - Breast (25%)
  - Bone sarcoma (12%)
  - Brain tumors (12%)
  - Soft tissue sarcomas (12%)
  - GI tract tumors (7%)
  - Gynecological malignancy (5%)
  - Hematological malignancy (5%)
  - Adrenocortical carcinoma (4%); if occurring in a child, considered almost diagnostic

Mazabraud Syndrome

- Polyostotic fibrous dysplasia
- Soft tissue (usually intramuscular) myxomas

McCune-Albright Syndrome

- Occurs sporadically as a result of mutation in *GNAS1* gene located in chromosome band 20q13
- Polyostotic fibrous dysplasia
- Multiple endocrinopathies:
  - Sexual precocity

- Pituitary adenoma (acromegaly)
- Adrenocortical adenoma (Cushing)
- Hyperthyroidism
- Hyperparathyroidism

■ Other reported abnormalities:
- GI polyps; hyperplasia of spleen, thymus, and pancreatic islets
- Hepatobiliary disease; cardiac disease; failure to thrive; metabolic acidosis; abnormalities in serum electrolytes, glucose, or insulin levels; hyperphosphaturic hypophosphatemia; malignant bone tumors (osteosarcoma and conventional chondrosarcoma); benign bone tumors (aneurysmal bone cysts and unicameral bone cysts); developmental delay; microcephaly; sudden or premature death; mucoceles of head and neck; cutaneous pigmentation (cafe-au-lait with serpiginous borders); intramuscular myxoma

Multiple Endocrine Neoplastic (MEN) Syndromes

■ *MEN I (Wermer Syndrome):* encoded protein called menin that is a tumor suppressor (11q13)
- Parathyroid—5%-100% (hyperplasia); 15% have a 5th parathyroid gland
- Pancreatic—60% (dysplasia and tumor)
- Pituitary—40% (adenomas)
- Adrenocortical tumors—5%-20%
- Thyroid (benign adenomas)—20%
- Bronchi (carcinoid tumors)—5%-10%
- Thymus (male)—1%-2%
- Stomach—1%-2%
- Subcutaneous (lipomas)—2%-5%

■ *MEN IIA (Sipple or William syndrome):* Germ line mutation in *ret* protooncogene, which is a tyrosine kinase receptor that is constitutively activated, causing a gain of function (chromosome 10q11)
- C cell hyperplasia, medullary carcinoma (tend to be bilateral)—100%
- Adrenal medullary hyperplasia, pheochromocytoma (tend to be bilateral)—0%
- Parathyroid hyperplasia, adenoma—10%-20%
  - (probably not 2° to high calcitonin, but 2° to congenital abnormality causing hyperplasia)
- Chief cell hyperplasia or multiglandular adenomas
- Conservative surgery—remove only the enlarged glands (high incidence of hypoparathyroidism if more radical surgery perfomed)
- Cutaneous lichen amyloidosis (2° to repeated scratching of neurological pruritis)

■ *MEN IIB (III)*
- C cell hyperplasia—medullary carcinoma
- Adrenal medullary hyperplasia—pheochromocytoma
- GI & ocular ganglioneuromas
- Marfanoid habitus
- Characteristic facies
  - Soft tissue prognathism
  - Bumpy lips
  - Broad base of nose
  - Everted eyelids
  - Low set ears
- Bowel dysfunction—diarrhea/constipation

Neurofibromatosis I (17q11.2)

■ *NF1* tumor supressor gene elicits protein product neurofibromin, which is a GTPase-activating protein that transforms RAS from active to inactive state. Loss causes RAS to be active

■ NF-1 is diagnosed in a patient with two or more of the following:
- 6 or more cafe-au-lait macules over 5 mm in greatest diameter in a prepubertal patient, and over 15 mm in greatest diameter in a postpubertal individual
- 2 or more neurofibromas of any type or 1 plexiform neurofibroma
- Presence of freckles in the axillary or inguinal region
- Optic glioma (tumor of optic pathway)
- 2 or more Lisch nodules (benign pigmented iris hamartomas)
- An osseous lesion such as a sphenoid dysplasia or thinning of long bone cortex with or without pseudoarthrosis
- A 1st degree relative with NF-1 by the above criteria
- NF-1 associated tumors:
  - Bilateral pheochromocytoma

    - Angiomyolipoma
    - Rhabdomyosarcoma
    - Duodenal paraganglioma and carcinoid tumor
    - Somatostatinoma
    - Ganglioneuroma
    - Juvenile chronic myelogenous leukemia (JCML)
    - Juvenile xanthogranuloma
    - Non-ossifying fibroma
  - NF-1 associated central nervous system tumors:
    - Astrocytomas; to include unilateral and bilateral optic gliomas (15%), pilocytic astrocytoma, and fibrillary astrocytoma
  - NF-1 associated central nervous system lesions:
    - Neuroglial and retinal glial hamartomas
    - Macrocephaly and hydrocephaly
    - Learning disabilities and epilepsy
  - Other NF-1 associated lesions:
    - Skeletal dysplasias
    - Congenital pseudoarthroses
    - Arterial intimal hyperplasia and fibrosis with aneurysm or stenosis
    - Hypertrophic (obstructive) cardiomyopathy

Neurofibromatosis II

- Chromosome 22q12 encodes a protein Merlin, which mediates contact inhibition of growth. In NF-II, cells lacking normal Merlin protein function are insensitive to normal growth arrest signals generated by cell-cell contact
- NF-II is diagnosed in a patient who has the following:
  - Bilateral 8th cranial nerve (vestibular branch of acoustic nerve) schwannomas or a first degree relative with NF-2 plus
    - Unilateral 8th cranial nerve schwannoma and any two of the following:
      - Neurofibroma
      - Meningioma
      - Glioma
      - Schwannoma
      - Juvenile posterior subcapsular lenticular opacity/juvenile cortical cataract
- NF-II associated central nervous system lesions:
  - Multiple glial microhamartomas
  - Spinal cord cellular ependymal ectopias
  - Syringomyelia

Sturge-Weber Disease

- Sporadic not inherited
- Capillary-venous lesions on face (port-wine stain, a special type of nevus flammeus; always include portion innervated by ophthalmic division of trigeminal nerve) and leptomeninges (usually include parieto-occipital region)
- Facial and leptomeningal lesions usually on same side; may be bilateral
- Intracranial lesions may produce seizures and result in cortical atrophy and diminished intellect
- Angiomas also involve mucosal, gingival, orbital soft tissue, retina, and choroid plexus
- Spinal counterpart *(Klippel-Trenaunay-Weber disease)* associated with limb enlargement

Tuberous Sclerosis (Bourneville Disease or Epiloia)

- Autosomal dominant neurocutaneous syndrome characterized by cutaneous and neurologic manifestations (mental retardation and seizures), and tumors
- Mutations in either chromosome 9q34 (TSC1) or 16p13 (TSC2)
- Tubers (cerebral hemispheres)
- Sclerosis (characterized by areas of decreased neurons and overgrowth of fibrillary astrocytes that may differentiate into malignant astrocytomas)
- Cutaneous manifestations:
  - Adenoma sebaceum (80%)
  - Ash-leaf spots (90%)
  - Shagreen patches (35%)
  - Cafe-au-lait spots (7%-16%)
  - Fibromas (trunk, gingivae, periungual region, hairline, and eyebrows)
  - Angiomas
- Neurologic manifestations:
  - Seizures (90%)
  - Mental retardation (60%-70%)

- Tumors:
  - Retinal (50 %-80%)
    - Nodular astrocytoma of retina or optic nerve
    - Hamartomas
  - Renal (50%-80%)
    - Angiomyolipomas
  - Heart (50%)
    - Cardiac rhabdomyoma
  - Cutaneous (20%)
    - Subungual fibromas (Koenen tumors)
  - Intracranial (15%)
    - Astrocytomas (subependymal giant cell astrocytoma)
  - Oral
    - Fibromas or papillomas
- Other manifestations:
  - Respiratory
    - Cystic or fibrous lesions in lungs (lymphangioleiomyomatosis)
  - Musculoskeletal
    - Cystic changes and periosteal thickening of bones of hands and feet

von Hippel-Lindau Disease

- Autosomal dominant neurocutaneous syndrome characterized by hemangioblastomas (cerebellar and retinal), visceral cysts and tumors
- Mutations on chromosome 3p25-26 encodes pVHC protein that forms complex with tumor suppressor function
- Cerebellar hemangioblastomas (80%-85%)
- Retinal hemangioblastoma (45%)
- Visceral cysts:
  - Pancreatic (70%)
  - Renal (60%)
  - Hepatic (15%-20%)
  - Epididymis (papillary cystadenoma) (5%-10%)
- Other tumors:
  - Pheochromocytomas (15%-20%)
  - Renal cell carcinoma (50%)
  - Angiomyolipoma
  - Neurofibromas
  - Endolymphatic sac tumor (aggressive papillary middle-ear tumor)

Zollinger-Ellison Syndrome

- Gastrinoma (pancreas, duodenum, stomach, or upper jejunum)
- Massive gastric acid-hypersecretion with elevated basal serum gastrin levels (above 200 pmol/L)
- Peptic ulceration; ulcers frequently multiple and occur in unusual site)

Myelodysplastic Syndromes

Classification (WHO)

- Refractory anemia (RA)
- Refractory anemia with ring sideroblasts (RARS)
- Refractory cytopenia with multilineage dysplasia (RCMD)
- Refractory anemia with excess blasts (RAEB)
- 5q– syndrome
- Therapy-related myelodysplastic syndromes and acute myeloid leukemia
- Myelodysplastic syndrome, unclassifiable
- Chronic myelomonocytic leukemia (CMML)

Clinical Manifestations

- Myelodysplastic syndromes are irreversible diseases of bone marrow stem cells that lead to ineffective and disorderly hematopoiesis characterized by abnormal division, maturation, and production of erythrocytes, granulocytes, monocytes, and platelets
- Typically diagnosed between the ages of 60 and 75 (rare in children)
- Males affected slightly more frequently than females
- Symptoms consist primarily of fatigue, weakness and malaise (anemia)
- Occasionally patients present with infections (neutropenia) or hemorrhage (thrombocytopenia)
- Patients with chronic myelomonocytic leukemia (CMML) may present with splenomegaly
- Hepatomegaly rare

Gross and Microscopic Pathology

- *Refractory anemia (RA)*
    - Ineffective erythropoiesis in bone marrow: erythroid hyperplasia, anemia, and reticulocytopenia
    - Anemia may be normocytic or macrocystic with anisopoikilocytosis
    - Some degree of neutropenia or thrombocytopenia may be present
    - Neutrophils and platelets show little or no evidence of dysplastic change
    - Bone marrow may be hypercellular or normocellular; dyserythropoiesis may be present, but usually not severe; dysgranulopoiesis and dysmegakaryopoiesis are absent; less than 15% of the erythroblasts are ringed sideroblasts
- *Refractory anemia with ringed sideroblasts (RARS)*
    - 15% or more of the bone marrow erythroblasts are ringed sideroblasts
    - Some erythrocytes have coarse basophilic stippling (including Pappenheimer bodies)
    - Neutropenia and thrombocytopenia are usually absent
        - Bone marrow may be hypercellular or normocellular with erythroid hyperplasia and marked increased iron stores
    - Myeloblasts are rarely increased
        - Mild dyserythropoiesis may be present; no dysplastic changes in granulocytes and megakaryocytes
- *Refractory cytopenia with multilineage dysplasia (RCMD)*
    - One or more peripheral cytopenias with dysplastic changes in two or more major hematopoietic lineages
    - Blood and bone marrow myeloblasts <5%
- *Refractory anemia with excess blasts (RAEB)*
    - Characterized by pancytopenia or bicytopenia
    - Dysplastic changes usually present in erythrocytes, granulocytes and platelets
    - Myeloblasts constitute <20% of leukocytes in blood
        - Bone marrow is normocellular or hypercellular with granulocytic and/or erythroid hyperplasia; bone marrow myeloblasts are increased to at least 5% but always less than 20%
    - Dyserythropoiesis is more pronounced than in RA or RARS
    - Dysgranulopoiesis is usually prominent and dysmegakaryopoiesis may be present
    - 2 types:
        - Type 1: 5 to 9% blasts in blood or bone marrow
        - Type 2: 10 to 19% blasts in blood or bone marrow
- *5q– syndrome*
    - Macrocytic anemia, usually with thrombocytosis, erythroblastopenia, megakaryocyte hyperplasia
    - Therapy-related myelodysplastic syndromes and acute myeloid leukemia
    - Occur in patients previously treated with chemotherapy (alkylating and type II topoisomerase inhibitors) and radiotherapy
    - Onset of disease ~ 5 years after treatment with alkylating agents and ~ 3 years after treatment with type II topoisomerase inhibitors
    - Usually a severe panmyelopathy with dysplastic changes in blood and bone marrow
- *Myelodysplastic syndrome, unclassifiable*
    - Criteria for making the diagnosis of myelodysplastic syndrome, unclassifiable:
        1. Presence of Auer rods with < 5% blasts
        2. Refractory neutropenia or thrombocytopenia without anemia
        3. Hypocellular bone marrow
        4. Significant leukocytosis or thrombocytosis
        5. Myelofibrosis
- Chronic myelomonocytic leukemia (CMML)
    - Morphologic features similar to those of RA, RCMD, or RAEB with the addition of monocytosis
    - Total leukocyte count is variable and may be elevated
    - Splenomegaly in 30 to 50%; hepatomegaly in 2%
    - Myeloblast count in the bone marrow is usually less than 5%

Special Stains, Immunohistochemistry, and Electron Microscopy

- Not helpful

Syndromes>Myelodysplastic Syndromes

Molecular Alterations

- Point mutations of *ras* oncogene in 10 to 15%
- Point mutations of *p53* and *Rb* genes in 5 to 10%
- 5q– syndrome has interstitial deletion of chromosome 5
- Therapy-related myelodysplastic syndromes secondary to alkylating agents associated with cytogenetic abnormalities involving chromosomes 5 and/or 7

Differential Diagnosis

- Megaloblastosis secondary to vitamin B_{12} or folate deficiency
- Heavy metal intoxication: arsenic, lead, etc.
- Acute alcohol intoxication
- Drug effects: primarily anti-neoplastic
- Congenital dyserythropoietic anemia
- Chronic infectious disease
- Acquired immune deficiency syndrome
- Acute myeloid leukemia (M2, M4, M6)
- Any condition with unexplained cytopenias or myelodysplasia

Treatment

- Conventional antileukemic chemotherapy is usually ineffective
- Patients under the age of 50 may be candidates for bone marrow transplantation (may be curative)
- Growth factors (colony stimulating factor) may be of benefit

Prognosis

- *Refractory anemia (RA)*
  - Most have chronic course with blood transfusions as needed
  - Few evolve into a more aggressive MDS and bone marrow failure or AML
  - Refractory anemia with ringed sideroblasts (RARS)
  - More aggressive than RA
  - Refractory cytopenia with multilineage dysplasia (RCMD)
  - Clinical course similar to RAEB
- *5q– syndrome*
  - Typically a stable clinical course with blood transfusions as needed
  - Patients with therapy-related MDS usually evolve to frank AML in a relatively short period of time
- Factors associated with improved prognosis include:
  - Young age
  - Normal or moderately reduced neutrophil and platelet counts
  - Low blast counts in bone marrow and no blasts in blood
  - No Auer rods
  - Presence of ringed sideroblasts
  - Normal karyotypes without complex chromosomal abnormalities
  - In vitro bone marrow culture that reveals non-leukemic growth pattern
- Factors associated with a poor prognosis:
  - Advanced stage
  - Severe neutropenia or thrombocytopenia
  - 20%-30% blasts in the bone marrow
  - Presence of Auer rods
  - Absence of ringed sideroblasts
  - Abnormal localization of immature granulocyte precursors in sections of bone marrow
  - Abnormal karyotypes or complex chromosomal abnormalities
  - In vitro bone marrow culture that reveals leukemic growth pattern
  - Patients with RA and RARS tend to do better than patients with the other myelodysplastic syndromes

Associations

- See above

Index

B

C

F

G

H

I

L

Liver—Lung

O

P

S

Soft—Stewart-Treves

Stomach—Syndromes

V

W

X

Y

Z